ASSISTED VENTILATION *of the* NEONATE

ASSISTED VENTILATION *of the* NEONATE

FOURTH EDITION

Jay P. Goldsmith, MD

Former Chairman, Department of Pediatrics and Co-Director of Nurseries
Ochsner Clinic and Foundation Hospital
Clinical Professor
Department of Pediatrics
Tulane University School of Medicine
New Orleans, Louisiana

Edward H. Karotkin, MD

Professor of Pediatrics
Eastern Virginia Medical School
Norfolk, Virginia
Medical Director, Neonatal-Perinatal Outreach Center of Virginia and North Carolina
Community Outreach Medical Coordinator
Children's Hospital of The King's Daughters
Norfolk, Virginia

Illustrations by
Barbara L. Siede, MS
Medical Illustrator
Alton Ochsner Medical Foundaton
New Orleans, Louisiana

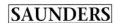

An Imprint of Elsevier Science

SAUNDERS
An Imprint of Elsevier Science

The Curtis Center
Independence Square West
Philadelphia, PA 19106

ASSISTED VENTILATION OF THE NEONATE   0-7216-9296-6
Copyright © 2003, Elsevier, Inc. All rights reserved.

NOTICE

Medical Assisting is an ever-changing field. Standard safety precautions must be followed, but as new research and clinical experience broaden our knowledge, changes in treatment and drug therapy may become necessary or appropriate. Readers are advised to check the most current product information provided by the manufacturer of each drug to be administered to verify the recommended dose, the method and duration of administration, and contraindications. It is the responsibility of the treating physician, relying on experience and knowledge of the patient, to determine dosages and the best treatment for each individual patient. Neither the Publisher nor the author assume any liability for any injury and/or damage to persons or property arising from this publication.

Previous editions copyrighted 1996, 1988, 1981

Library of Congress Cataloging-in-Publication Data

Assisted ventilation of the neonate / [edited by] Jay P. Goldsmith, Edward H. Karotkin.–
  4th ed.
    p. ; cm.
  Includes index.
  ISBN 0-7216-9296-6
   1. respiratory therapy for newborn infants. 2. Artificial respiration. I. Goldsmith, Jay P.
II. Karotkin, Edward H.
  [DNLM: 1. Infant, Newborn, Diseases—therapy. 2. Respiration,
Artificial–methods—Infant, Newborn. WS 420 A848 2003
RJ312.A87 2003
615.8'36'0832–DC21   2003041523

Acquisitions Editor: Judith Fletcher
Development Director: Lynne Gery
Production Manager: Mary Stermel

Printed in the United States of America

Last digit is the print number: 9   8   7   6   5   4   3   2   1

DEDICATION

To all babies and their heroic families who have consented to participate in randomized controlled trials of various drugs, therapies and devices, not knowing if they were assigned to the control or treatment group, and whose contributions have brought us in great measure to our present art of practice and paved the way for the care of infants in the future.

JPG

EHK

CONTRIBUTORS

STEVEN H. ABMAN, MD
Professor, Department of Pediatrics, University of Colorado
School of Medicine; Director, Pediatric Heart
and Lung Center, The Children's Hospital, Denver, Colorado
Special Ventilatory Techniques and Modalities III:
Inhaled Nitric Oxide Therapy

NAMASIVAYAM AMBALAVANAN, MD, MBBS
Assistant Professor, Department of Pediatrics, Division of
Neonatology, University of Alabama at Birmingham,
Birmingham, Alabama
Ventilatory Strategies

ROBERT MASON ARENSMAN, MD
Professor of Surgery in Pediatrics, Northwestern University;
Chief, Pediatric Surgery, Children's Memorial Hospital,
Chicago, Illinois
Extracorporeal Membrane Oxygenation
Surgical Management of the Airway

W. THOMAS BASS, MD
Associate Professor of Pediatrics, Eastern Virginia Medical
School; Neonatologist, Pediatrics Department, Children's
Hospital of The King's Daughters, Norfolk, Virginia
Central Nervous System Morbidity

MICHAEL A. BECKER , AS, RRT
Respiratory Care Clinical Specialist, Holden Neonatal
Intensive Care Unit, Critical Care Support Services
Department, C.S. Mott Children's Hospital/Holden
Hospital/University of Michigan Medical Center, Ann Arbor,
Michigan
Special Ventilatory Techniques and Modalities I:
Patient-Triggered Ventilation

ROBERT C. BECKERMAN, MD
Professor of Pediatrics and Physiology and Chief, Pediatric
Pulmonology, Tulane University School of Medicine and
Tulane University Hospital for Children, New Orleans,
Louisiana; Medical Director, Sudden Infant Death Syndrome
(SIDS) Program, State of Louisiana
Control of Ventilation and Apnea

EDWARD F. BELL, MD
Professor of Pediatrics, University of Iowa; Director of
Neonatology, Children's Hospital of Iowa, Iowa City, Iowa
Nutritional Support

VINOD K. BHUTANI, MD, FAAP
Professor, Department of Pediatrics, University of
Pennsylvania; Pediatrician, Pennsylvania Hospital,
Philadelphia, Pennsylvania
Pulmonary Function and Graphics

JUDD BOLOKER, MD
Children's Hospital at Oakland,
Oakland, California
Blood Gases: Technical Aspects and Interpretation

DAVID J. BURCHFIELD, MD
Professor of Pediatrics and Physiology, Pediatrics
Department, University of Florida, Gainesville, Florida
Pharmacologic Adjuncts I

WALLY CARLO, MD
Edward M. Dixon Professor of Pediatrics
and Director, Division of Neonatology,
Department of Pediatrics, University of Alabama
at Birmingham, Birmingham, Alabama
Ventilatory Strategies

GERALYNN M. CASSERLY, RRT
Neonatal Critical Care Respiratory Therapist,
Respiratory Therapy Department,
Evanston Hospital,
Evanston, Illinois
Pulmonary Care

STEVEN M. DONN, MD
Professor, Pediatrics and Communicable Diseases,
University of Michigan Health System; Director,
Division of Neonatal-Perinatal Medicine,
C.S. Mott Children's Hospital, Ann Arbor, Michigan
Volume-Controlled Ventilation
Special Ventilatory Techniques and Modalities I:
Patient-Triggered Ventilation

DAVID J. DURAND, MD
Division of Neonatology, Children's Hospital and Research
Center of Oakland, Oakland, California
Blood Gases: Technical Aspects and Interpretation

MOHAMMAD A. EMRAN, MD
Surgery Department, University of Illinois Metropolitan
Group Hospitals Residency in General Surgery, Chicago,
Illinois
Surgical Management of the Airway

WILLIAM W. FOX, MD
Professor of Pediatrics, Division of Neonatology,
University of Pennsylvania School of Medicine;
Children's Hospital of Philadelphia, Philadelphia,
Pennsylvania
Positive-Pressure Ventilation: Pressure-Limited
and Time-Cycled Ventilation
Special Ventilatory Techniques II: Lung Protective
Strategies and Liquid Ventilation

MARK E. GERBER, MD
Assistant Professor of Surgery, The Feinberg
School of Medicine, Northwestern University,
Chicago, Illinois
Surgical Management of the Airway

HARLEY G. GINSBERG, MD
Section Head, Section of Neonatology,
Ochsner Clinic Foundation, New Orleans, Louisiana
Cardiovascular Aspects

JAY P. GOLDSMITH, MD
Clinical Professor, Department of Pediatrics,
Tulane University School of Medicine;
Former Chairman, Department of Pediatrics,
and Co-Director of Nurseries, Ochsner Clinic
and Foundation Hospital, New Orleans,
Louisiana
Introduction to Assisted Ventilation
Resuscitation
Ventilatory Management Casebooks

JAY S. GREENSPAN, MD
Professor and Vice Chairman, Director of Neonatology,
Department of Pediatrics, Thomas Jefferson University,
A.I. duPont Hospital for Children, Wilmington, Delaware
Positive-Pressure Ventilation: Pressure-Limited
and Time-Cycled Ventilation
Special Ventilatory Techniques II: Lung Protective
Strategies and Liquid Ventilation

JOSEPH HAGEMAN, MD
Associate Professor of Pediatrics, Feinberg School
of Medicine, Northwestern University; Medical Director
of Inpatient Pediatrics, Department of Pediatrics,
Evanston Hospital, Evanston, Illinois and Children's
Memorial Hospital, Chicago, Illinois
Pulmonary Care

HARRIET HAWKINS, RN, CCRN
Resuscitation Education Coordinator,
Clinical Education Department,
Children's Memorial Hospital,
Chicago, Illinois
Pulmonary Care

M. GARY KARLOWICZ, MD
Professor of Pediatrics, Eastern Virginia Medical School;
Children's Hospital of The King's Daughters, Norfolk,
Virginia
Resuscitation

EDWARD H. KAROTKIN, MD
Professor of Pediatrics, Eastern Virginia Medical School;
Medical Director, Neonatal-Perinatal Outreach
Center of Virginia and North Carolina;
Community Outreach Medical Coordinator,
Children's Hospital of The King's Daughters,
Norfolk, Virginia
Introduction to Assisted Ventilation
Resuscitation

BRYAN S. KING, MD
Instructor in Anaesthesia, Harvard Medical School;
Assistant in Anaesthesia, Massachusetts General Hospital,
Boston, Massachusetts
Intraoperative Management

JOHN KINSELLA, MD
Professor of Pediatrics, University of Colorado School of
Medicine; Medical Director, ECMO Service and Emergency
Medical Transport Service, The Children's Hospital, Denver,
Colorado
Special Ventilatory Techniques and Modalities III:
Inhaled Nitric Oxide Therapy

ARTHUR E. KOPELMAN, MD
Professor of Pediatrics/Neonatology, Pediatrics Department,
Brody School of Medicine at East Carolina University;
Attending Neonatologist, Pediatrics Department, Pitt County
Memorial Hospital, Greenville, North Carolina
Central Nervous System Morbidity

SHELDON B. KORONES, MD
Alumni Distinguished Service Professor of Pediatrics
and Obstetrics and Gynecology, the University of Tennessee
health Science Center; Director, Newborn Center, Pediatrics
Department, Regional Medical Center at Memphis, Memphis,
Tennessee
Complications

FAWN C. LEWIS, MD
Clinical Instructor in Surgery, Department of Surgery,
Pediatric Surgery, Northwestern University Medical School;
Attending Physician, Pediatric Surgery Critical Care
Department, Children's Memorial Hospital, Chicago, Illinois
Extracorporeal Membrane Oxygenation

VICTOR W. LUCAS, JR., MD
Pediatric Cardiologist, Department of Pediatrics, Ochsner
Clinic Foundation, New Orleans, Louisiana
Cardiovascular Aspects

CAROLYN HOUSKA LUND, RN, MS, FAAN
Assistant Clinical Professor, Department of Family Health
Care Nursing, University of California, San Francisco, San
Francisco, California; Neonatal Clinical Nurse Specialist,
Intensive Care Nursery, Children's Hospital Oakland,
Oakland, California
Nursing Care

MARK C. MAMMEL, MD
Professor of Pediatrics, University of Minnesota,
Minneapolis, Minnesota; Director, Newborn Research
and Education, Neonatology Department,
Children's Hospital—St. Paul, St. Paul, Minnesota
High-Frequency Ventilation

GERALD B. MERENSTEIN, MD
Professor of Pediatrics and Senior Associate Dean,
Education, University of Colorado School of Medicine,
Aurora, Colorado
Transport of Ventilated Infants

JAY M. MILSTEIN, MD
Department of Pediatrics, University of
California-Davis, Davis, California
Pharmacologic Adjuncts I

CHERYL MARCO NAULTY, MD
Associate Professor, Department of Pediatrics,
Uniformed Services University of the Health Sciences,
Bethesda, Maryland; Medical Director, Exceptional Family
Member Program, Department of Pediatrics, Walter Reed
Army Medical Center and North Atlantic Regional Medical
Command, Washington, DC
Pulmonary Outcome and Follow-Up

JOHN J. PARIS, SJ, PhD
Walsh Professor of Bioethics, Department of Theology,
Boston College, Waltham, Massachusetts
*Ethical and Legal Issues in Assisted Ventilation
of Newborns*

GARY PETTETT, MD
Chair, Institutional Review Board and Director,
Truman Medical Center Nurseries,
Department of Neonatology,
Children's Mercy Hospital and Clinics,
Kansas City, Missouri
Transport of Ventilated Infants

BARRY PHILLIPS, MD
Medical Director, Neonatal Intensive Care Unit,
Children's Hospital at Oakland, Oakland, California
Blood Gases: Technical Aspects and Interpretation

FRANK E. REARDON, JD, MPh
Partner, Hassan & Reardon, P.C., Boston, Massachusetts
*Ethical and Legal Issues in Assisted Ventilation
of Newborns*

MARLETA REYNOLDS, MD
Professor of Surgery, Department of Pediatric Surgery,
Northwestern University Medical School;
Attending Physician, Department of Pediatric Surgery,
Children's Memorial Hospital, Chicago, Illinois
Extracorporeal Membrane Oxygenation

THERESA P. ROCA, MD
Pediatric Cardiologist, The Heart Group, Mobile, Alabama
Ventilatory Management Casebooks

ROBERT L. SCHELONKA, MD
Assistant Professor of Pediatrics, University of Alabama
at Birmingham, Birmingham, Alabama
Ventilatory Strategies

MICHAEL D. SCHREIBER, MD
Associate Professor, Department of Pediatrics,
University of Chicago, Chicago, Illinois
*Ethical and Legal Issues in Assisted Ventilation
of Newborns*

THOMAS SHAFFER, III, PhD
Professor Emeritus of Physiology and Pediatrics
and Director, Physiology Research Section,
Temple University School of Medicine;
Professor of Pediatrics, Thomas Jefferson University,
Philadelphia, Pennsylvania; Associate Director of Biomedical
Research and Director, Office of Technology Transfer,
and Director, Nemours Research Lung Center,
A. I. duPont Hospital for Children, Wilmington,
Delaware
*Special Ventilatory Techniques II: Lung Protective
Strategies and Liquid Ventilation*

NARONG SIMAKAJORNBOON, MD
Assistant Professor of Pediatrics, Tulane University School
of Medicine; Medical Director, Comprehensive Sleep
Medicine Center, Tulane University Hospital and Clinics,
New Orleans, Louisiana
Control of Ventilation and Apnea

SUNIL K. SINHA, MD, PhD, FRCP, FRCPCH
Professor, School for Health, University of Durham,
United Kingdom; Consultant Paediatrician
and Neonatologist, The James Cook University Hospital,
Middlesbrough, United Kingdom
Volume-Controlled Ventilation

EMIDIO SIVIERI, MS
Biomedical Engineer, Section on Newborn Pediatrics,
Pennsylvania Hospital, University of Pennsylvania
School of Medicine, Philadelphia, Pennsylvania

KAREN SLOTARSKI, RRT
Neonatal Critical Care Respiratory Therapist,
Respiratory Therapy Department, Evanston Hospital,
Evanston, Illinois
Pulmonary Care

ROGER F. SOLL, MD
Professor of Pediatrics, University of Vermont College
of Medicine, Burlington, Vermont
Pharmacological Adjuncts II: Exogenous Surfactants

ALAN R. SPITZER, MD
Professor of Pediatrics, State University of New York
at Stony Brook; Chief, Division of Neonatology
and NICU Director, Department of Pediatrics,
Stony Brook University Hospital, Stony Brook,
New York
*Positive-Pressure Ventilation: Pressure-Limited
and Time-Cycled Ventilation*
*Special Ventilatory Techniques II: Lung Protective
Strategies and Liquid Ventilation*

PINCHI SRINIVASAN, MD
Department of Pediatrics, Wyckoff Heights
Medical Center, Brooklyn,
New York
Continuous Positive Airway Pressure

GAUTHAM K. SURESH, MD, DM, MS
Assistant Professor, Neonatal Division,
Pediatrics Department, University of Vermont College
of Medicine, Burlington, Vermont
  Pharmacological Adjuncts II: Exogenous Surfactants

MICHAEL D. WEISS
Department of Pediatrics, University of
Florida College of Medicine,
Gainesville, Florida
  Pharmacologic Adjuncts I

THOMAS E. WISWELL, MD
Professor of Pediatrics, State University of New York
at Stony Brook; Director of Neonatal Research,
Stony Brook University Hospital, Stony Brook, New York
  Continuous Positive Airway Pressure

BRIAN R. WOOD, MD
Neonatologist, Department of Pediatrics/Neonatology,
Mission-St. Joseph's Health System, Asheville,
North Carolina
  Physiologic Principles

FOREWORD

". . . I, that am curtail'd of this fair proportion,
Cheated of feature by dissembling Nature,
Deform'd, unfinished, sent before my time
Into this breathing world, scarce half made up,
And that so lamely and unfashionable
That dogs bark at me as I halt by them"

—William Shakespeare, Richard III, I, I, 18

This passage from the opening soliloquy of Shakespeare's famous play depicts the type of patient that neonatologists deal with every day. I can remember in 1967, as an intern in the "sick nursery," staring at the long green tubing (often several feet) connecting a baby to a ventilator. Neonatology was in its infancy. Therapies were anecdotal and untested. It seemed as if there were no limits to the future of neonatal care.

This is the fourth edition of *Assisted Ventilation of the Neonate*. Many of the chapters retain the same titles but are expanded appropriately as our knowledge has increased. The expansion of cellular biology, genetics, infectious diseases, pharmacology, nutrition, and pulmonary function has enabled the "neonatal team" to save babies of lower gestational age. As new therapies have emerged, controversies have abounded. The use of sedation, the use and misuse of nitric oxide and postnatal steroids, and the employment of conventional versus nonconventional ventilatory strategies are only a few of the hot topics that have been discussed. Is ventilatory management, which is essential to the survival of premature infants and sick full-term babies, science, or art, or both?[1] In the past, neonatologists believed that "EBM" meant expressed breast milk. Today, we think of "evidence-based medicine."

We are realizing that there are certain limits to what we can do. Embryonic, fetal, and postnatal lung development have been described anatomically and physiologically. We are able to ventilate babies in the saccular phase of lung development. Can we, or should we, approach the canalicular stage with the same fervor? Better understanding of gas exchange, the potential to implant type II cells, and the development of new ventilators and ventilation strategies may lead us to focus just on the respiratory system and not the total baby. We no longer describe a "neonatal team." It is now the "multidisciplinary health provider team." The concept of family-oriented care has reduced the sterility of the neonatal intensive care unit and has stimulated family interaction. Caring intensively and intensely has softened the beeps and flashing lights of the newest technological equipment. Ethical considerations focusing on prenatal consultation and resuscitation decisions have become as important as choosing an appropriate ventilator setting. The adjunctive therapies that we use may ultimately affect morbidity as we save infants of lower gestational age.

Jay Goldsmith, Edward Karotkin, and the many contributors to this fourth edition have remained abreast of current approaches to ventilatory care of the newborn. Understanding that "just because we can does not mean that we should" has led to a more global approach to neonatal intensive care. These physicians are doing what they do best ... taking care of babies.

Gilbert I. Martin, M.D.
Medical Director, NICU
Citrus Valley Medical Center
Clinical Professor of Pediatrics
The University of California (Irvine)
Emeritus Editor, The Journal of Perinatology
PEDIATRIX Medical Group

1. Mariani GL, Carlo WA. Ventilatory management in neonates. Science or art? Clinic Perinat 1998; 25:33–48.

PREFACE

For nearly four decades we have had a tool for treating neonates with respiratory failure: ventilatory assist devices. At first, our goal was to improve survival, especially of the severely immature baby with surfactant deficiency. Over the years, smaller and more immature-gestation infants were rescued; often, however, they were doomed to lead a life of handicap and hardship. In the early 1990s, we hit the wall—the gestational age at which conventional gas exchange could not adequately occur because of the anatomic and physiologic immaturity of the premature infant's lung. Controversy exists as to where that line is: 22 to 24 weeks' gestation, 400 to 600 grams? Biologic variability allows that the line need not be drawn too sharply, so that each baby can be evaluated individually for viability and suitability for aggressive intervention. In the late 1990s the decades-long trend of improving outcomes for babies of 500 to 1500-gram birth weight also leveled off.

In recent years, emphasis has shifted from pushing back the envelope of gestational age and birth weight viability to improving functional outcomes of those babies who had the potential to be treated effectively. Despite anecdotal evidence of survival of the smallest and most immature babies without handicaps, most healthcare providers have been disturbed by the high incidence of handicap in infants who have been "saved" by our therapies. A large inter-institutional variance in the incidence of the two most recognizable sequelae of our treatment regimes—chronic lung disease and central nervous system injury—has led to an evidence-based search for the best therapies and protocols.

With particular reference to the topic of the text—assisted ventilation—we continue to search for ways to ventilate infants without causing harm. We know that the vast majority of lung injury is manmade. However, until there are social, molecular and technological solutions to prematurity and its associated diseases, we must continue to use the tools we have, despite their potentially damaging side effects. In this regard, the words of Dr. George Cassidy, writing in 1988 in the Foreword to the second edition of this text, are worth repeating: "The managements and techniques described in this text are nearly all empiric. . . . Since the methods proposed are those used by the experts, one might assume that these are the methods that work best. Not so. . . . Until we've had the opportunity to compare the 'best therapies' with each other, we'll continue to have uncertain truths to guide us. Awareness of this uncertainty makes us better doctors." Over the last fifteen years many of the "best therapies" have been evaluated and compared with other forms of treatment. Evidence evaluation, Cochrane meta-analysis reviews, and other studies in the field of neonatal pulmonary medicine have helped guide us to the treatment modalities that we use today. However, many therapies are still empiric, and the application of even "standard" therapies is so varied that inter-institutional outcomes are quite divergent.

The incidence of chronic lung disease subsequent to ventilation in the neonatal period has not decreased since the introduction of exogenous surfactant in 1990. Strategies to decrease prematurity have not worked, and basic science research has yet to identify the molecular mediators of lung injury and their potential therapies. But for the clinician at the bedside, the keys to prevention of chronic lung disease are effective ventilatory devices, strategies for ventilatory assistance, and support protocols that will decrease barovolutrauma to the immature lung. Thus this text is no longer a "how-to" manual of the mechanics for utilizing ventilatory assistance and its supportive components. Survival is no longer the goal; survival without handicap must be our new paradigm.

In 1999, L. D. Hudson wrote that "...the concept of ventilatory induced lung injury (VILI) has come of age" (JAMA). However, over 250 years earlier, Fothergill recognized the potential for VILI from mechanical assistance of lung function: "Mouth to mouth resuscitation may be better than using a mechanical bellows to inflate the lung because ... the lungs of one man may bear, without injury, as great as those of a man can exert, which by the bellows can not always be determined" (J Philos Trans Royal Society, 1745).

Thus, the theme for this Fourth Edition has shifted from the "why" and "how" of neonatal ventilation to "how best" to support the newborn's respiratory system to achieve optimal outcomes without sustaining damage from the known sequelae of ventilatory devices. Perhaps the best treatment is no treatment at all: that is, not to intervene when the infant is too immature or has no reasonable chance of intact survival. Or if intervention is chosen, to follow the "Columbia approach" of respiratory assistance and attempt to not intubate or mechanically ventilate the infant. This is accomplished by early use of nasal continuous positive airway pressure (CPAP), permissive hypercapnia, and a variety of other strategies that are discussed in the text.

If ventilatory assistance is necessary and used in neonatal intensive care units, the following principles (borrowed heavily from Evan Richards, RRT) should be followed.

These are called the LOVE principles—the Laws Of Ventilatory Efficiency.

1. Know thy ventilator and disease pathology.
2. Develop a specific strategy for the pathophysiology in each individual infant.
3. Change the ventilatory strategy as the pathophysiology changes.
4. Always strive to wean the patient off of ventilatory assistance (i.e., have an exit strategy).

This Fourth Edition of *Assisted Ventilation of the Neonate* attempts to follow these principles by offering the reader evidence-based recommendations and empiric opinions where insufficient data exists. In this edition, all previous chapters have been updated to reflect the most recent data available. New chapters on ethical considerations, nitric oxide, and ventilatory strategies expand limited sections of previous editions. Eight ventilatory management casebooks comprise the last chapter and reflect the same subjects that were presented in the second edition (1988). However, the management of these common neonatal respiratory cases (drawn from actual clinical files) has changed so dramatically in the last fifteen years as to warrant a reprise.

While pathophysiology and pulmonary mechanics are discussed as integral to the mechanics of ventilatory assistance, the reader is referred to other textbooks for detailed descriptions of the pathologic conditions and the radiographic findings of neonatal pulmonary disorders that lead to respiratory failure. As in previous editions, authors have used brand names and given representative examples of specific devices and drugs when necessary to illustrate treatment protocols and approaches. However, these representations are not endorse-

ments of these devices or drugs, and exclusion is not meant to be viewed as criticism.

Over the four editions and 22-year span of this textbook, we have seen our specialty grow and we have learned much about our capabilities and limitations. We hope each successive edition has reflected that growth and a maturation of the practitioners in this very unique field of medicine. Our failures continue to frustrate us and the temptation to adopt new and unproven therapies is great. However, we must continue to rely on evidence-based therapies and apply rigorous scientific principles to our research. Hopefully, this book will stimulate you and your colleagues to continue in that pursuit. As we wait for the solution(s) to prematurity, we should remember the wisdom of an old editorial. "The tedious argument about the virtues of respirators not invented over those readily available can be ended now that it is abundantly clear that the success of such apparatus depends on the skill with which it is used" (Lancet 2:1227,1965).

J.P.G.
E.H.K.

CONTENTS

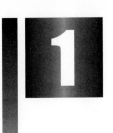

1
INTRODUCTION TO ASSISTED VENTILATION

JAY P. GOLDSMITH, MD
EDWARD H. KAROTKIN, MD

DEFINITION AND PURPOSE

Dramatic reductions in both neonatal and infant mortality have occurred over the past 50 years. A variety of medical advances have been responsible for this improvement, including better obstetric care, improved pharmacologic agents, development of respiratory support devices, micromethods for measuring a variety of parameters in the neonate, and use of surfactant. This chapter presents an introduction to neonatal assisted ventilation for medical personnel involved in this area of patient care. A brief overview of the history of neonatal medicine hopefully provides the perspective to better appreciate the contributions neonatal assisted ventilation has made to the field of newborn care.

Assisted ventilation can be defined as the movement of gas into and out of the lung by an external source connected directly to the patient. The external source may be a resuscitation bag, a continuous distending pressure device, or a mechanical ventilator. Attachment to the patient can be via a face mask, endotracheal tube, nasal prongs, or tracheostomy. Although not in general use today in modern intensive care nurseries, negative-pressure ventilation can be applied by an apparatus surrounding the infant's thorax.

In the neonate, assisted ventilation is a measure for supporting pulmonary function until the patient can breathe adequately without help. In more recent years, with the increased survival of babies born at the lower limits of gestational age, infants are requiring prolonged assisted ventilation for months and, in the case of patients with severe chronic lung disease, years. The purposes of mechanical ventilation are to facilitate alveolar ventilation and carbon dioxide removal, provide adequate tissue oxygenation, and reduce the work of breathing. This is accomplished through the use of a device that augments or replaces the bellows action of the respiratory musculature.

Mechanical ventilation of the neonate is a complex and highly invasive procedure and must not be undertaken in a casual manner. Effective ventilation of the diseased lung requires that the clinician understand the normal pulmonary physiology, as well as the pathophysiology of pulmonary diseases in the neonate. The clinician also must correlate the type of therapy to the stage of pulmonary growth and development and to the severity of the disease. In addition, he or she must understand the basic mechanical principles of the specific ventilator in use. The beneficial effects of ventilatory therapy are dependent on a strong knowledge of these subjects, skill, and experience in management, combined with constant vigilance by medical, nursing, and respiratory personnel during treatment.

HISTORY

And he went up, and lay upon the child, and put his mouth upon his mouth, and his eyes upon his eyes, and his hands upon his hands; and he stretched himself upon the child and the flesh waxed warm.

II Kings 4:34

From the earliest recorded description of mouth-to-mouth resuscitation in the Old Testament (one by Elijah, I Kings 17:17, and another quoted in the preceding passage by Elisha),[1] we have been fascinated with the idea of sustaining respiration by artificial means. The medical literature of the past several thousand years contains many references to early attempts. Hippocrates (circa 400 BC) was the first investigator to record his experience with intubation of the trachea to support pulmonary ventilation.[2] His preliminary work was ignored for almost 2000 years, until Paraclesus (1493–1541) reported the use of bellows and an oral tube in this endeavor.[2]

The 16th and 17th Centuries

The scientific renaissance in the 16th and 17th centuries rekindled interest in the physiology of respiration and in techniques for tracheostomy and intubation. By 1667, simple forms of continuous and regular ventilation had been developed.[2] With these developments, the emergence of a better understanding of the basic physiology of pulmonary ventilation can be seen.

The 19th Century

In the early 1800s, interest in resuscitation and mechanical ventilation of newborn infants flourished. In 1800, the first report describing nasotracheal intubation as an adjunct to mechanical ventilation was published by Fine in Geneva.[3] At about the same time, the principles for mechanical ventilation of adults were established; the rhythmic support of breathing was accomplished with mechanical devices, and, on occasion, ventilatory support was carried out with tubes passed into the trachea.

In 1806, Vide Chaussier, a professor of obstetrics in the French Academy of Science, described his experiments with the intubation and mouth-to-mouth resuscitation of asphyxiated and stillborn infants.[4] The work of his successors led to the development in 1879 of the aerophore pulmonaire (Fig. 1-1), the first device specifically designed for the resuscitation and

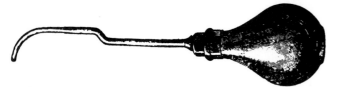

Figure 1-1. Aerophore pulmonaire of Gairal. (From DePaul. *Dictionnaire Encyclopédique*, vol. XIII, 13th series.)

short-term ventilation of newborn infants.[2] This device was a simple rubber bulb connected to a tube. The tube was inserted into the upper portion of the infant's airway, and the bulb was alternately compressed and released to produce inspiration and passive expiration. Subsequent investigators refined these early attempts by designing devices that were used to ventilate laboratory animals.

Charles-Michel Billard (1800–1832) wrote one of the finest medical texts dealing with clinical-pathologic correlations of pulmonary diseases in newborn infants. Dr. Billard's book, *Traite des Maladies des Enfants Nouveau-Nes et a la Mamelle,* was published in 1828.[5] His concern for the fetus and intrauterine injury is evident as he writes: "During intrauterine life man often suffers many affectations, the fatal consequences of which are brought with him into the world . . . children may be born healthy, sick, convalescent, or entirely recovered from former diseases."[5] His understanding of the difficulty newborns may have in establishing normal respiration at delivery is well illustrated in the following passage: ". . . the air sometimes passes freely into the lungs at the period of birth, but the sanguineous congestion which occurs immediately expels it or hinders it from penetrating in sufficient quantity to effect a complete establishment of life. There exists, as is well known, between the circulation and respiration, an intimate and reciprocal relation, which is evident during life, but more particularly so at the time of birth. . . . The symptoms of pulmonary engorgement in an infant are, in general, very obscure, and consequently difficult of observation; yet we may point out the following: the respiration is laboured; the thoracic parietes are not perfectly developed; the face is purple; the general color indicates a sanguineous plethora in all the organs; the cries are obscure, painful and short; percussion yields a dull sound."[5] It seems remarkable that these astute observations were made more than 170 years ago.

The advances made in the understanding of the pulmonary physiology of the newborn and the devices designed to support a newborn's respiration undoubtedly were stimulated by the interest shown in general newborn care that emerged in the latter part of the 19th century and continued into the first part of the 20th century.[6] In France in 1880, Dr. Eteinne Tarnier, an obstetrician and leading figure in the European Infant Welfare Movement, appreciated the importance of keeping the premature infant warm and introduced a closed water-jacketed incubator. In 1884 he introduced and popularized gavage feedings for the "debile" and "weakling."[6] A few years later, his colleague Pierre Budin developed the principles of neonatal medicine and stressed the importance of weekly physician examinations of the newborn, maternal education, and sterilized milk. In 1892 Budin opened his "consultation for nurslings." The experience he gained in the care of premature infants resulted in a book on the subject. Budin was the first to dignify the newborn with a separate hospital chart in which

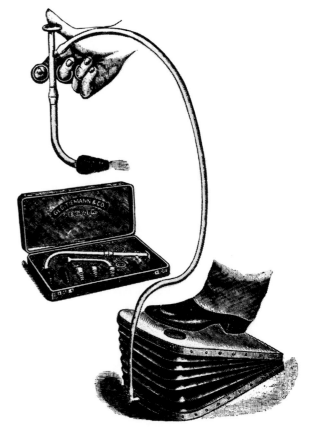

Figure 1-2. Fell-O'Dwyer apparatus for provision of intermittent positive-pressure ventilation. (From Northrup. M & S Rep Presbyterian Hospital, New York, 1896.)

weight, temperature, and breast milk intake were plotted daily. He also published survival data and established follow-up programs for his high-risk newborn patients.[6] As a result of these initiatives, he may well be regarded as the "father of neonatology." (How ironic he was an obstetrician.)

These advances were followed by the work of Dr. Ballantyne, an Edinburg obstetrician who emphasized the importance of prenatal care and recognized that syphilis, malaria, typhoid, tuberculosis, and maternal ingestion of toxins such as alcohol and opiates were detrimental to the development of the fetus.[6]

Better understanding of pulmonary physiology led to further refinements in ventilation. O'Dwyer[7] reported the first successful use of long-term positive-pressure ventilation in a large series of children when he published the results of his studies in 1887 (Fig. 1-2). Shortly thereafter, Egon Braun and Alexander Graham Bell independently developed intermittent body-enclosing devices for the negative-pressure/positive-pressure resuscitation of newborns.[8,9]

The 20th Century

In the early 20th century in the United States, three principles of public health emerged that led to further improvements in newborn survival. (1) Saving of infant lives is best achieved by protection and education of mothers before and after pregnancy. (2) Infant mortality rate is the best available index of the overall health and welfare of a community. (3) Infant mortality is related to multiple factors, and multiple interventions are necessary to lower the rate.[6]

In the 1920s, obstetrics became a full-fledged surgical discipline and pediatricians assumed the care for all children. One of Budin's students, Courney, took advantage of the public fascination with premature infants and displayed them at the Chicago Exposition in 1914. A similar display featuring warming incubators was a popular venue at the World's Fair in 1939. Shortly thereafter, Dr. Julius Hess opened the first Premature Center at the Michael Reese Hospital in Chicago and other centers soon followed. Modern neonatology was born with the recognition that premature infants required particular attention with regard to temperature control, administration of fluids and nutrition, and protection from infection. In the 1930s and 1940s premature infants were given new stature, and it was acknowledged that their death was the greatest contribution to the infant mortality rate.[6]

The early years of the second half of the 20th century were marked by soaring birth rates, the proliferation of labor and delivery services, antibiotics, positive-pressure resuscitators, miniaturization of laboratory determinations, x-ray facilities, and microtechnology that made intravenous therapy possible for neonatal patients. These advances and a host of other advances heralded the modern era of neonatal medicine.

Improvements in intermittent negative-pressure and positive-pressure ventilation devices in the early 20th century led to the development of a variety of techniques and machines for supporting ventilation in infants. In 1929, Drinker and Shaw[10] reported the development of a technique for producing constant thoracic traction to effect an increase in end-expiratory lung volume. In the early 1950s, Bloxsom[11] reported the use of a positive-pressure air lock (AL) for resuscitation of infants with respiratory distress in the delivery room.[12] This device was similar to an iron lung; it alternately created positive and negative pressure in a tightly sealed cylindrical steel chamber that was infused with warmed humidified 60% oxygen. Clear plastic versions of the AL quickly became commercially available in the United States in the early 1950s (Fig. 1-3). However, a study by Apgar and Kreiselman in 1953[12a] on apneic dogs and another study by Townsend in 150 premature infants[12b] demonstrated that the device could not adequately support the apneic newborn. The linkage of oxygen administration and retinopathy of prematurity and a randomized controlled trial of the AL versus care in an Isolette at Johns Hopkins University[12c] revealed no advantage to either study group and heralded the hasty decline in the use of Bloxsom's device.

In the late 1950s, body-tilting devices were designed that shifted the abdominal contents in order to create effective movements of the diaphragm. Phrenic nerve stimulation[13] and the use of intragastric oxygen[14] also were reported in the literature but had little clinical success. In the 1950s and early 1960s, many centers also used bag and face mask ventilation to support infants for relatively long periods of time.

The modern era of mechanical ventilation for infants can be dated back to the 1953 report of Donald and Lord,[15] who described their experience with a patient-cycled, servocontrolled respirator in the treatment of several newborn infants with respiratory distress. They claimed that three or possibly four infants were successfully treated with their apparatus.

In the decades following Donald and Lord's pioneering efforts, the field of neonatal ventilation made dramatic advances; however, the gains were accompanied by several temporary setbacks. Because of the epidemic of poliomyelitis in the 1950s, experience was gained with the use of the tank-

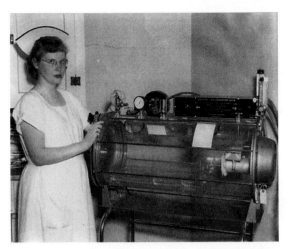

Figure 1-3. Commercial Plexiglas version of the positive-pressure oxygen air lock. Arrival of the unit at the Dansville Memorial Hospital, Dansville, New York, June 1952. (Photo courtesy of James Gross and the *Dansville Breeze,* June 26, 1952.)

type negative-pressure ventilators of the Drinker design.[16] The success of these machines with children encouraged physicians to try modifications on neonates, with some anecdotal success. However, initial efforts to apply *intermittent positive-pressure ventilation* (IPPV) to premature infants with respiratory distress syndrome (RDS) were disappointing overall. Mortality was not demonstrably decreased, and the incidence of complications—particularly that of pulmonary air leaks—seemed to increase.[17] During this period, clinicians were hampered by the types of ventilators that were available and by the techniques for their use.

In accordance with the findings of Cournand et al. in adult studies conducted in the late 1940s, standard ventilatory technique often required that inspiratory positive-pressure times be very short. Cournand et al. had demonstrated that prolongation of the inspiratory phase of the ventilator cycle in patients with normal lung compliance could result in impairment of thoracic venous return, a decrease in cardiac output, and the unacceptable depression of blood pressure. To minimize cardiovascular effects, they advocated that the inspiratory phase of a mechanical cycle be limited to one third of the entire cycle.[18] Some ventilators manufactured in this period even were designed with the inspiratory-to-expiratory ratio fixed at 1:2.

Unfortunately, the findings of Cournand et al. were not applicable to patients with significant pulmonary parenchymal disease and with reduced lung compliance, such as premature infants with RDS. Neonates with pulmonary disease, which is generally characterized by increased chest wall compliance and terminal airway and alveolar collapse, did not generally respond to IPPV techniques that had worked well in adults and older children. Thus, clinicians were initially disappointed with the outcome of neonates treated with assisted ventilation using these techniques.

The birth of a premature son to President John F. Kennedy and Jacqueline Kennedy on August 7, 1963, focused the world's attention on prematurity and the treatment of hyaline membrane disease. Patrick Bouvier Kennedy was born by cesarean section at 34 weeks' gestation. He weighed 2.1 kg. He was transported from Cape Cod, Massachusetts, to Boston, where he died at 39 hours of age (Fig. 1-4). The Kennedy baby was treated with the most advanced therapy of the time, hyperbaric

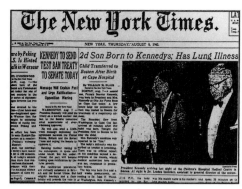

Figure 1-4. Front page of *The New York Times*, August 8, 1963. (Copyright © 1963 by *The New York Times* Co. Reprinted by permission.)

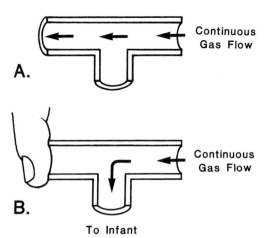

Figure 1-5. Ayre's T-piece forms the mechanical basis of most neonatal ventilators currently in use. *A,* Continuous gas flow from which an infant can breathe spontaneously. *B,* Occlusion of one end of the T-piece diverts gas flow under pressure into an infant's lungs. The mechanical ventilator incorporates a pneumatically or electronically controlled time-cycling mechanism to occlude the expiratory limb of patient circuit. Between sequential mechanical breaths, the infant can still breathe spontaneously. The combination of mechanical and spontaneous breaths is intermittent mandatory ventilation. (From Kirby RR: Mechanical ventilation of the newborn. Perinatol Neonatol 5:47, 1981.)

oxygen,[19] but he died of progressive hypoxemia. In response to his death, *The New York Times* reported: "About all that can be done for a victim of hyaline membrane disease is to monitor the infant's blood chemistry and try to keep it near normal levels." The Kennedy tragedy, followed only 3 months later by the President's assassination, stimulated further interest and research in neonatal respiratory diseases and resulted in increased federal funding in these areas.

Breakthroughs in Ventilation

A breakthrough occurred in 1971 when Gregory et al.[20] reported on clinical trials with *continuous positive airway pressure* (CPAP) for the treatment of RDS. Recognizing that the major physiologic problem in RDS was the collapse of alveoli during expiration, they applied positive pressure to the airway via an endotracheal tube during both expiration and inspiration; dramatic improvement was achieved. Although infants receiving CPAP breathed spontaneously during the initial studies, later combinations of IPPV and CPAP in infants weighing less than 1500 g were not as successful.[20] Nonetheless, the concept of CPAP was a major advance. It was later modified by Bancalari et al.[21] for use in a constant distending negative-pressure chest cuirass and by Kattwinkel et al.,[22] who developed nasal prongs for the application of CPAP without the use of an endotracheal tube.

Meanwhile, Reynolds and Taghizadeh,[23,24] working independently in Great Britain, also recognized the unique pathophysiology of neonatal pulmonary disease. Having experienced difficulties with IPPV similar to those noted by clinicians in the United States, Reynolds and Taghizadeh suggested prolongation of the inspiratory phase by delaying the opening of the exhalation valve. This "reversal" of the standard inspiratory-to-expiratory ratio, or "inflation hold," allowed sufficient time for the recruitment of atelectatic alveoli with lower inflating pressures and gas flows, which, in turn, decreased turbulence and limited the effect on venous return. The excellent results of Reynolds and Taghizadeh could not be duplicated uniformly in the United States, perhaps because their American colleagues used different ventilators.

Until the early 1970s, ventilators used in neonatal intensive care units (NICUs) were modifications of adult devices; these devices delivered intermittent gas flows, thus generating IPPV. The ventilator initiated every mechanical breath, and clinicians tried to eliminate the infants' attempts to breathe between IPPV breaths ("fighting the ventilator"), which led to

rebreathing of dead air. In 1971, a new prototype neonatal ventilator was developed by Kirby and coworkers. This ventilator used continuous gas flow and a timing device to close the exhalation valve modeled after the Ayre's T-piece used in anesthesia (Fig. 1-5).[15,23,25] Using the T-piece concept, the ventilator provided continuous gas flow and allowed the patient to breathe spontaneously. Occlusion of the distal end of the T-piece diverted gas flow under pressure to the infant. In addition, partial occlusion of the distal end generated CPAP. This combination of mechanical and spontaneous breathing under continuous gas flow was called *intermittent mandatory ventilation* (IMV).

IMV became the standard method of neonatal ventilation and has been incorporated into all infant ventilators. One of its advantages was the facilitation of weaning by progressive reduction in IMV rate, which allowed the patient to gradually increase spontaneous breathing against distending pressure. Clinicians no longer needed to paralyze or hyperventilate patients to prevent their "fighting the ventilator." Moreover, because patients continued to breathe spontaneously and lower cycling rates were used, mean intrapleural pressure was reduced and venous return was less compromised than with IPPV.[26]

From 1971 to 1995, myriad new ventilators specifically designed for neonates were manufactured and sold. The first generation of ventilators included the BABYbird I; the Bournes BP 200; and a volume ventilator, the Bournes LS 104/150. All operated on the IMV principle and were capable of incorporating CPAP into the respiratory cycle [known as *positive end-expiratory pressure* (PEEP) when used with IMV].[27]

The BABYbird I and the Bournes BP 200 used a solenoid-activated switch to occlude the exhalation limb of the gas circuit in order to deliver a breath. Pneumatic adjustments in the inspiratory-to-expiratory ratio and rate were controlled by inspiratory and expiratory times, which had to be timed with a stopwatch. A spring-loaded pressure manometer monitored peak inspiratory pressure and PEEP. These early mechanics created time delays within the ventilator, resulting in problems in obtaining short inspiratory times (<0.5 second).

In the next generation of neonatal ventilators, the incorporation of electronic controls, microprocessors, and microcircuitry allowed the addition of light-emitting diode (LED) monitors and provided clinicians with faster response times, greater sensitivity, and a wider range of ventilator parameter selection. These advances were incorporated into ventilators such as the Sechrist 100 and Bear Cub to decrease inspiratory times to as short as 0.1 second and to increase ventilatory rates to 150 breaths per minute. Monitors incorporating microprocessors measured inspiratory and expiratory times and calculated inspiratory-to-expiratory ratios and mean airway pressure. Ventilator strategies abounded, and controversy regarding the best (i.e., least harmful) method for assisting neonatal ventilation arose. High-frequency positive-pressure ventilation with the use of conventional ventilators was proposed as a beneficial treatment of RDS.[28]

Meanwhile, extracorporeal membrane oxygenation (ECMO) and true high-frequency ventilation (HFV) were being developed at a number of major medical centers.[29,30] These techniques initially were offered as rescue therapy for infants who did not respond to conventional mechanical ventilation. The favorable physiologic characteristics of HFV led some investigators to promote its use as an initial treatment of respiratory failure, especially RDS.[31]

A third generation of neonatal ventilators began to appear in the early 1990s. Advances in microcircuitry and microprocessors, developed as a result of the space program, allowed new dimensions in neonatal assisted ventilation. The use of synchronized IMV, assist/control mode ventilation, and pressure support ventilation—previously used in the ventilation of only older children and adults—became possible in neonates because of the very fast ventilatory response times. Although problems with sensing a patient's inspiratory effort sometimes limited the usefulness of these new modalities, the advances gave hope that ventilator complications could be limited and that the need for sedation or paralysis during ventilation could be decreased. Direct measurement of some pulmonary functions at the bedside became a reality and allowed the clinician to make ventilatory adjustments based on physiologic data rather than on a "hunch."

Surfactant Replacement Therapy

Perhaps the most important advance in treating RDS in the last 40 years was the development of surfactant replacement therapy. The discovery by Avery and Mead[32] in 1959 that surfactant deficiency was the critical factor in neonatal RDS was the first step in a tremendous 40-year research effort that culminated in the licensing of two exogenous surfactant preparations in the United State in the early 1990s. (In 1990, the United States Food and Drug Administration approved exogenous surfactant for general use, heralding a new era in the treatment of neonatal respiratory failure.) Surfactant replacement therapy has clearly been shown to improve lung function and mechanics in premature infants with RDS. Most studies have demonstrated decreased duration of assisted ventilation, lower fractions of inspired oxygen (FIO_2), lower peak inflating pressures, and decreases in morbidity and mortality associated with its use in infants weighing from 600 to 1500 g.[33] Although

originally developed for use in premature infants with RDS, exogenous surfactant therapy has been proposed for patients with other diseases (e.g., meconium aspiration syndrome, pneumonia) that cause neonatal respiratory failure.[34] Unresolved questions remain regarding the best formulation of surfactant, timing of administration (prophylactic vs rescue), number of doses needed, technique of administration, and quantity to be administered. Nonetheless, it was obvious that a new era of treatment of neonatal pulmonary disease had arrived. The biochemistry and physiology of surfactant and surfactant replacement therapy are discussed in detail in Chapter 20.

Assisted ventilation represents the hallmark of neonatal intensive care. Improvements in devices, the appearance of new techniques and better support systems, and the development of exogenous surfactant and other pharmacologic agents all have contributed to improving weight-specific survival rates for infants with neonatal respiratory failure. A report in the mid 1970s of all neonates ventilated from 1966 to 1969 proudly announced a survival rate of 33%.[35] A more recent study looking at the outcome of infants born in the United States in the 1990s reports survival rates of 0% to 21% for infants born at 22 weeks' gestation, 5% to 46% for infants born at 23 weeks' gestation, 40% to 59% for infants born at 24 weeks' gestation, 60% to 82% for infants born at 25 weeks' gestation, and 75% to 93% for infants born at 26 weeks' gestation.[36] It is generally recognized that survival rates for infants born at 32 weeks' gestation afforded modern neonatal intensive care are essentially the same as those of infants born at term.

Unfortunately, complications associated with infants born at the lower extremes of viability (bronchopulmonary dysplasia, blindness, and neurodevelopmental disability) remain significant. The data on the incidence of major disabilities are much more difficult to analyze, but it appears that the variation in reported disability rates varies more than survival rates for a given gestational age.[36] Approximately 75% of premature infants who survive the neonatal period will be free of disability. However, between 20% and 25% of survivors will have at least one major disability-impaired mental development, cerebral palsy, blindness, or deafness. The most common disability is impaired mental development (17%–21%), followed by cerebral palsy (12%–15%); blindness and/or deafness affect less than 8% of survivors. Studies examining surviving infants born weighing between 750 and 1000 g report that approximately another half will have one or more subtle neurodevelopmental disabilities that will become apparent later in childhood.[36] In a recent publication, Horbar et al.[37] report that the significant advances in obstetric and neonatal care that occurred during the early 1990s have been associated with decreased mortality and morbidity for very-low-birth-weight infants born during the first half of that decade. Unfortunately, this group concludes that since 1995 there have been no additional improvements in mortality or morbidity and that neonatal mortality and morbidity rates have reached a plateau. The survival rate of ventilated infants weighing between 1000 and 1249 g after surfactant therapy is greater than 90%.[38] The survival rate for similar infants weighing between 750 and 999 g is greater than 80%.[38] These statistics represent considerable improvements in survival compared with those of the presurfactant era of the late 1980s.[38] Unfortunately, increased survival rates have not resulted in a corresponding improvement in long-term neurodevelopmental outcome, which has remained stable for the past 30 years.[36]

Most morbidity and mortality occur among infants with birthweights less than 1000 g. In the infant weighing less than 750 g, surfactant may have a lesser effect because of the structural immaturity of the pulmonary system. Liquid ventilation with perfluorochemicals has been shown to improve oxygenation, promote lung expansion, and increase blood flow to the lung without systemic effects and with minimal barotrauma.[39] Although still in the experimental stage, this exciting new technique has been touted as a future potential treatment of "micropremies" who are at greatest risk for morbidity and mortality.

Certainly, the treatment of neonatal respiratory failure has improved dramatically over the last three decades, and many exciting developments are on the horizon. Better ventilators, improvement of surfactant formulation, and advances in monitoring equipment can be expected in the coming years. The goal of future care is the application of effective therapy without iatrogenic consequences.

In all probability, improvements in neonatal and infant mortality will continue to occur with improved intensive care. However, further dramatic reductions in both neonatal and infant mortality and decreases in low-birthweight-associated morbidity will not occur until many of the societal and economic disparities in our society are rectified so that the disproportionately high number of low-birthweight infants born in these disadvantaged, high-risk groups of pregnant women is lowered.

FIVE *W*'S OF ASSISTED VENTILATION

Who: Which infants are candidates for ventilation? Who is an inappropriate candidate? What are the ethical and legal considerations?

Where: Which hospital should undertake assisted ventilation of the neonate? What equipment and personnel are necessary? What is meant by regionalized perinatal care?

When: When is a patient in respiratory failure? What are the causes of inadequate ventilation?

Why: What are the neurologic and physical outcomes of babies who are ventilated? What are the financial ramifications?

What: What are the types and classifications of ventilators?

In the previous editions of *Assisted Ventilation of the Neonate,* the questions *Who* and *Why* were briefly presented as part of this section. In view of the amount of new literature and information that has been written on these two topics, the editors believe that they deserved to be covered in a separate chapter on Ethical Considerations (Chapter 5).

Therefore, the remaining three questions *Where, When,* and *What* are discussed in this chapter.

Where: Regionalization of Perinatal Care

The National Center for Health Statistics defines an NICU as a "hospital facility or unit staffed and equipped to provide continuous mechanical ventilatory support for more than 24 hours." The complex techniques involved in the treatment of respiratory failure of the newborn require an NICU staffed by specially trained nurses; a geographically accessible full-time staff of physicians composed of neonatologists, the full complement of pediatric subspecialists, and 24-hour-per-day, 7-day-per-week in-house coverage by staff physicians (i.e., neonatologists/hospitalists); pediatric house officers; and/or neonatal nurse practitioners.

Thirty years ago the vast majority of neonatal intensive care was provided in large teaching hospitals or large community hospitals. Today, sophisticated neonatal care is provided in many tertiary medical centers, as well as in many smaller hospitals that may not fulfill the expectations implied by Downes[40] in 1971. The proliferation of NICUs in hospitals with relatively small delivery services or limited ancillary services that provide care for infants with the most complex of conditions is a consequence of the "deregionalization of perinatal care." This has necessitated the development and maintenance of neonatal transport systems capable of transporting the "sickest" infants to NICUs in which the full array of pediatric subspecialists, experienced NICU nurses, respiratory therapists, and laboratory and diagnostic services is available to support these patients.

Concurrent with the tremendous advances in perinatal technology, innovation, and knowledge and the movement of neonatal services away from the larger medical centers to smaller facilities (deregionalization), there is an attempt to preserve the regionalized approach to prenatal care. A comprehensive report by the Committee on Perinatal Health[41] and the more recent publication of the March of Dimes, *Toward Improving the Outcome of Pregnancy: The 90s and Beyond,*[42] promote the concept of designating certain hospitals for the care of high-risk newborns based on each hospital's ability to provide a certain level of care. Such regionalization programs were advanced under three assumptions: that the regionalization of prenatal care (1) increased the availability of medical services; (2) decreased morbidity and mortality; and (3) decreased costs. Hospitals were traditionally designated in terms of three levels of prenatal care.[41]

Level I: Hospitals that provide services primarily for uncomplicated maternity and newborn patients.

Level II: Large urban and suburban hospitals at which the majority of deliveries occur. Because they have a highly trained staff and modern equipment, these facilities are capable of treating most perinatal complications.

Level III: Hospitals that serve a delivery population of 8,000 to 12,000 births annually and are capable of treating all types of maternal-fetal and neonatal illnesses. A level III hospital also is responsible for the education of medical providers, transport of critically ill neonates or mothers, and evaluation of the overall quality of perinatal care in its region. Typically level III centers are designated the *perinatal center* for a region.

In the past few years, some centers providing ECMO and/or heart transplantation have adopted the term *level IV centers* or *regional level III centers*. These centers have also been responsible for continuing education of their region and, in some cases, regionalized transport systems and quality assurance review.

The American Academy of Pediatrics is now considering a subdivision of level III NICUs into A, B, C, and D. The definitions proposed are as follows:

Level IIIA
Hospital or state-mandated restriction on type and/or duration of mechanical ventilation

Level IIIB
No restrictions on type or duration of mechanical ventilation
No major surgery (see below)
Level IIIC
Major surgery performed on site (e.g., omphalocele repair, tracheoesophageal fistula or esophageal atresia repair, bowel resection, myelomeningocele repair, ventriculoperitoneal shunt, myelomeningocele closure)
No surgical repair of serious congenital heart anomalies that require cardiopulmonary bypass and/or ECMO
Level IIID
Major surgery
Surgical repair of serious congenital heart anomalies that require cardiopulmonary bypass and/or ECMO for medical conditions

In some states such as Virginia, numerical designations, which may be confusing or misleading, have been replaced by more descriptive terminology:

General: Newborn service that provides care to low-risk newborns weighing at least 2000 g or who have completed 34 weeks of gestation.
Intermediate level: Newborn service that provides care for moderately ill neonates or stable-growing, low-birth-weight neonates. Intermediate nurseries have the ability to insert and maintain umbilical arterial catheters, monitor blood gases, and care for infants in environments of not more than 40% oxygen.
Specialty level: Service that provides care for high-risk neonates who may require central and/or peripheral arterial lines with constant pressure monitoring; insertion and maintenance of chest tubes; and administration of pressors, surfactant, support CPAP, and short-term ventilation.
Subspecialty level: Service that provides care for high-risk, critically ill neonates with complex neonatal illness. In-house neonatology is available constantly, with a full range of pediatric medical and surgical subspecialties available.

If these guidelines are applied, prolonged assisted ventilation should be limited to level III units B to D and subspecialty NICUs. However, for many reasons, a deregionalization of care with a proliferation in the number of NICUs,[43]—all of which want to offer a full array of neonatal services, including assisted ventilation—has been observed since the mid-1980s and has persisted into the new millennium.

Recently, certain powerful chief executive officers from the largest companies in the United States have formed an advisory group (Leapfrog Group) that, among other issues, has tried to mobilize health care purchasers to reward improvements in patient safety and consumer value in health care. The Leapfrog Evidence-Based Hospital Referral (EHR) standards were developed after review of published outcomes research and consultation with experts on neonatal intensive care. Their initial criteria would require that an infant less than 32 weeks' gestation or with an expected birthweight of less than 1500 g, or who has a prenatal diagnosis of a major congenital anomaly, be delivered at or transferred to a facility that is a *regional NICU* maintaining an average daily census of 15 or more. Although controversial, the Leapfrog Group believes such "regulation" would improve outcome, patient safety, and con-

sumer value. Using their purchasing power, the group hopes to encourage members to have half of their enrollees' hospitalizations in facilities that meet their criteria by December 31, 2004.

The tremendous growth in the number of NICUs in community hospitals has occurred for a number of reasons. The growing number of neonatologists graduating from more than 100 fellowship training programs in the United States has increased the availability of such physicians to community hospitals. Experience in some well-prepared and well-staffed community hospitals has demonstrated results with ventilated babies that are similar to those reported by university centers.[44] Neonatal care is a highly visible activity that generates good public relations; thus, community hospitals, which operate in a competitive environment, wish to demonstrate to their potential consumers that all services can be provided. Obstetricians not wishing to transfer high-risk expectant mothers to other facilities have put pressure on hospital administrators to hire neonatologists at level II and community level III centers.[45] Moreover, if indigent patients are excluded (or at least limited), NICUs can be highly profitable for individual hospitals and private practicing physicians.

Medicolegal considerations have undoubtedly caused many obstetricians to demand hospital administrators provide delivery room coverage by neonatologists for cesarean sections or unexpected high-risk deliveries. However, in response to the changing patterns of reimbursement that started in the 1990s, there may be a shift away from the concept of deregionalization because small hospitals that provide expensive neonatal care are finding it difficult to compete with larger institutions because of low census and high staffing costs.

Providers in level I hospitals argue that if they transfer all sick newborns to level II and level III centers, they will lose the skills necessary for the management of neonatal respiratory emergencies.[45] Moreover, on occasion, no beds are available at the perinatal center or conditions preclude transport. Under such circumstances, the level I hospital must ventilate infants until transport can be arranged. This dilemma does not have an easy solution, but the following basic principles may apply:

1. All hospitals with delivery services should have resources to intubate infants and maintain ventilation for up to 8 hours.
2. No infant should be more than 4 hours away from neonatal intensive care with appropriate transport.
3. Every infant should have access to optimal respiratory care, regardless of financial or geographic considerations.

The skills necessary to successfully carry out prolonged assisted ventilation cannot be learned easily, nor can they be maintained with limited numbers of ventilatory cases. All personnel (physicians, nurses, and respiratory therapists) must be extensively trained for all aspects of ventilatory assistance so that optimal outcome can be achieved.

Data collected in 1980 confirmed that hospitals ventilating fewer than 50 babies per year demonstrated twice the mortality of level III larger centers in the same area (all level III hospitals at that time ventilated more than 50 babies per year). These data have been validated by more recent studies that documented enhanced survival and fewer morbidities for infants cared for in level III perinatal centers.[46,47]

The responsibility for improved pregnancy outcome rests with obstetricians, as well as with pediatricians. Responsible prenatal health care professionals should encourage the transport of a high-risk mother and her unborn fetus to a level III center for the delivery and subsequent care of the neonate. Studies comparing very-low-birthweight infants (<1500 g) born outside level III centers with those born in level III hospitals have shown shorter hospital stays,[48] lower costs per survivor,[48] and reduced morbidity and mortality[49,50] for the inborn infants. These differences are accentuated when patients require assisted ventilation. Spitzer et al.[51] evaluated out born and inborn infants with RDS and found that inborn infants had significantly lower mean maximal F_{IO_2}, decreased duration of required O_2 administration, lower peak inspiratory pressure, and shorter duration of IPPV.

The qualifications of personnel and types of equipment necessary to maintain infants on assisted ventilation are the subjects of considerable discussion. Guidelines have been written and debated throughout the country. A modified rating system initially devised by Indyk and Cohen[52] (Table 1-1) describes some of the necessary qualifications of units that are to undertake intensive care measures such as mechanical ventilation. A unit should score 25 points or better in this system if it is to be considered adequately prepared to care for ventilated infants. Although in 2003 this rating system appears outdated, nonacademic hospitals nonetheless should review the requirements before pursuing a course to establish a high-cost, high-intensity neonatal intensive care program. The most important aspect of prolonged ventilatory care, however, is the continuous presence of skilled personnel. A person able to perform endotracheal intubation, chest tube placement, and cardiopulmonary resuscitation must be in the hospital at all times.[53] Complications such as dislodgment of the endotracheal tube or pulmonary air leaks occur suddenly, often without warning, and require immediate correction. Often, a patient cannot wait for a physician to be summoned from the office or home. Assigning the responsibility for such emergencies to untrained or uncertified staff nurses, respiratory therapists, or inexperienced emergency room physicians is not justified at the present time, when more appropriate resources are available.

Further information regarding what personnel and equipment requirements a hospital should satisfy if it is to provide a certain level of perinatal and neonatal care can be found in the most recent editions of *Toward Improving the Outcome of Pregnancy: The 90s and Beyond*[42] and *Guidelines for Perinatal Care, Fifth Edition*,[54] published by The American College of Obstetricians and Gynecologists and the American Academy of Pediatrics in 2002.

Transport systems are equipped and staffed to be capable of stabilizing infants in referring hospitals and moving them to health care centers safely. Hospital, community, and physician pride or economic considerations should not prevent the provision of optimal care to all infants.

TABLE 1-1. Modified Indyk-Cohen (INCO) Rating System for Regional Newborn Units*

Category	Two Points	One Point	No Points
Nursing ratio (patients:nurses for infants being ventilated)	1:1	2:1 or 3:1	4:1 or less
Nursing education	Full-time in-service coordinator; formal courses given routinely	Infrequent formal courses given	Apprentice system
Director of unit	Board-certified neonatologist with no other responsibilities	Physician with other responsibilities	Part-time director
Respiratory care	Respiratory therapist(s) assigned exclusively to unit	Respiratory therapist in hospital at all times	Less than full-time coverage
Working relationship between neonatologist and surgeon	24-hr availability of immediate pediatric surgical care	24-hr availability of general surgeon	Less than full-time coverage
In-house personnel responsibilities (gases, radiography, ventilation)	Physician or neonatal nurse practitioner in unit on 24-hr basis. Can run ventilators, read radiographs, interpret gases	Nurse or respiratory therapist for these functions	No formal plan
Enthusiasm and awareness of new ideas	Up-to-date, with studies ongoing	Aware, not innovative; no research	No awareness or activity
Availability of monitoring	Virtually unlimited, including capability to perform pulse oximetry	One respiration and heart rate monitor per two patients; no pulse oximetry	Fewer than one monitor per two patients
Availability of subspecialists (e.g., pediatric neurologists, cardiologists)	24-hr availability of all specialists	Some subspecialists available	No pediatric subspecialty coverage
Type of monitoring equipment	Respiration, heart, blood pressure, temperature, central venous pressure, and oxygen saturation monitoring	Lacking one type	Lacking two or more types
Data collection and analysis	Computer records, quality improvement program	Some mechanism of statistical collection	No collection and follow-up
Laboratory services (blood gases)	Available in the unit	Available within 15 min at all times	Available after 15 min
Radiography	Radiography machine in unit; radiography files easily accessible	Quickly available from central service	Slow and infrequently used
Facilities (O_2, air suction, power, air-O_2 blender at each bed)	Everything available; adequate emergency power	Lacking one utility or incomplete power coverage, or both	Use of extension cords, 3/2 adapters
Transport	Send staff member(s) with a transporter (two-way transport)	Infant brought in unaccompanied (one-way transport)	No special neonatal transport scheme

* Units performing prolonged ventilation should have a score of >25 points.
Modified from Indyk L, Cohen S: Newborn intensive care in the United States: East and West. Clin Pediatr 10:320, 1971.

When: Causes of Respiratory Failure and Indications for Ventilation

Although there are many reasons for beginning assisted ventilation in neonates, the most common is respiratory failure. In any infant, this condition may take one of two forms. The first is apnea, a condition in which mechanical ventilation is necessary because a patient does not breathe. If the lungs are normal, the cause most often is related to the control of respiration by the central nervous system. Potential causes include apnea of prematurity, asphyxia, intracranial hemorrhage, and drug overdose.

In the second form of respiratory failure, the mechanism of pulmonary gas exchange has been compromised. The cause most often is a primary lung disease or an airway disease (e.g., RDS). In these instances, physiologic alterations in gas exchange cause acidosis, hypercapnia, and hypoxemia. If organ damage or death is to be prevented, mechanical assistance is required.

The classic constellation of findings in respiratory failure consists of an acute increase in the partial pressure of arterial carbon dioxide ($Paco_2$) and a decrease in pH. The presence of hypoxemia by itself does not indicate respiratory failure, as illustrated by patients with cyanotic congenital heart disease. Respiratory failure may be caused by the failure of organ systems other than the central nervous system and the lungs (Table 1-2). When the lungs are primarily responsible, however, it is important to make a simplistic distinction between two physiologic types of lung disease: atelectatic disease and obstructive disease (Table 1-3).

An atelectatic disease is characterized by decreased lung volume and decreased functional residual capacity. Examples are RDS and pneumonia. Increased lung volumes and increased functional residual capacity, as seen in aspiration syndromes and bronchopulmonary dysplasia, characterize an obstructive disease. In many pulmonary conditions, both types of disease exist (e.g., RDS in combination with pulmonary air leaks). Even though the physiologic distinction is not absolute, it may be important for the clinician to make such a distinction before he or she addresses the criteria for the initiation of assisted ventilation, the choice of ventilator, or the parameters of ventilator control.

The physician can make a diagnosis of respiratory failure guided by both clinical manifestations and the results of blood

TABLE 1-2. Causes of Respiratory Failure

Problem Area	Possible Causes
Pulmonary	Respiratory distress syndrome
	Aspiration syndromes
	Pneumonia
	Pulmonary hemorrhage
	Pulmonary alveolar proteinosis
	Wilson-Mikity syndrome
	Bronchopulmonary dysplasia
	Pulmonary insufficiency of prematurity
	Pneumothorax
	Tumor
	Diaphragmatic hernia
	Chylothorax
	Congenital malformations (lobar emphysema, cystic adenomatoid malformation, lymphangiectasis)
Airway	Laryngomalacia
	Choanal atresia
	Pierre Robin syndrome
	Micrognathia
	Nasopharyngeal tumor
	Subglottic stenosis
Abnormalities of muscles of respiration	Phrenic nerve palsy
	Spinal cord injury
	Myasthenia gravis
	Werdnig-Hoffmann syndrome
Central problems	Apnea of prematurity
	Drugs: morphine, magnesium sulfate, mepivacaine, meperidine
	Seizures
	Birth asphyxia
	Hypoxic encephalopathy
	Intracranial hemorrhage
	Ondine's curse
	Rapid eye movement sleep
Miscellaneous	Congestive heart failure
	Persistent fetal circulation
	Postoperative anesthesia/sedation
	Tetanus neonatorum
	Extreme immaturity
	Shock
	Sepsis
	Hypoglycemia
	Electrolyte abnormalities
	Acid-base imbalance
	Infant botulism
	Hydrops fetalis

TABLE 1-3. Theoretical Classification of Neonatal Pulmonary Disorders

	Atelectatic	Obstructive
Example	Respiratory distress syndrome	Meconium aspiration syndrome
Physiology	↓ Lung volume	↑ Lung volume
	↓ Compliance	↓ Compliance
	↓ Functional residual capacity	↑ Functional residual capacity
	Normal airway resistance	↑ Airway resistance
	Normal time constant	↑ Time constant
Clinical appearance	Severe retractions; pectus excavatum	↑ Anteroposterior diameter
	Prematurity—common	Term or post term—common
Management	Early positive-pressure ventilation	Avoid positive-pressure ventilation
	Correct hypoventilation	Avoid overventilation
	Pulmonary air leaks: 10%–15%	Pulmonary air leaks: ≥30%
	Persistent pulmonary hypertension—rare	Persistent pulmonary hypertension—common

↓, decrease; ↑, increase.

SILVERMAN-ANDERSON RETRACTION SCORE

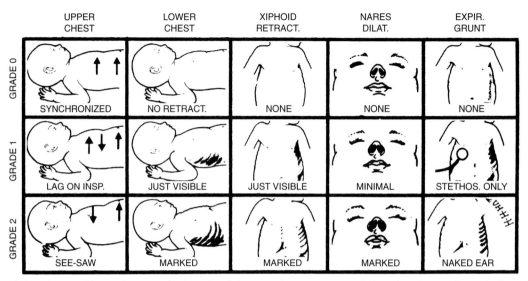

Figure 1-6. Index designed to provide continuous evaluation of an infant's respiratory status. An index of respiratory distress is determined by grading each of five arbitrary criteria: chest lag, intercostal retraction, xiphoid retraction, nares dilatation, and expiratory grunt. The "retraction score" is computed by adding the values (0, 1, or 2) assigned to each factor that best describes the infant's condition at the time of a single observation. A score of zero indicates the absence of respiratory distress; a score of 10 indicates severe respiratory distress. DILAT, dilatation; EXPIR, expiratory; INSP, inspiration; RETRACT, retraction; STETHOS, stethoscope. (Adapted from Silverman WE, Andersen DH: Controlled clinical trial of effects of water mist on obstructive respiratory signs, death rate and necroscopy findings among premature infants. Pediatrics 171:1,1956, with permission of *Pediatrics*.)

gas analysis. Clinically, the physician should look for the following signs:

1. Increase in respiratory rate
2. Decrease in respiratory rate accompanied by increasing effort or increasing retractions
3. Prolonged apnea with cyanosis, bradycardia, or both
4. Cyanosis not relieved by O_2 administration
5. Hypotension, pallor, and decrease in peripheral perfusion
6. Tachycardia (leading to bradycardia)
7. Periodic breathing with prolonged respiratory pauses
8. Gasping, and the use of accessory respiratory muscles

The Silverman-Anderson[55] retraction score has also been helpful in evaluating respiratory distress (Fig. 1-6). A score of 7 or greater indicates impending respiratory failure.

Blood gas analysis can be used to identify candidates for assisted ventilation. The selection of criteria differs from center to center. As the ability to use assisted ventilation has improved and resulted in the enhancement of outcomes and a decrease in complications, indications have become less rigid. For example, the indications of Gregory et al.[20] for CPAP administration in 1971 was PaO_2 less than 50 mm Hg in 100% O_2. Today, most centers would begin CPAP or assisted ventilation when infants cannot maintain PaO_2 greater than 50 mm Hg in 60% O_2. Although there is general consensus that PaO_2 less than 50 mm Hg is unsatisfactory, there is considerable debate on what maximal inspired O_2 should be used before CPAP or mechanical ventilation is initiated. A level of 60% FIO_2 is chosen for two reasons. First, O_2 toxicity to the lungs increases with higher inspired O_2 concentration, and "early" respiratory assistance may allow the use of lower O_2 concentrations and decrease the total duration of O_2 therapy.[56,57] Second, in most infants with respiratory failure, intrapulmonary and intracardiac right-to-left shunting are the primary causes of hypoxemia. If

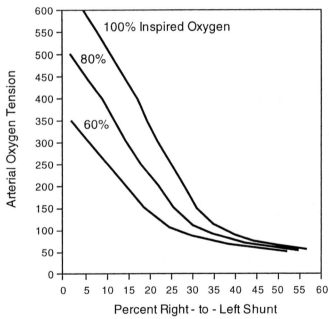

Figure 1-7. Graph for estimating the shunt at different inspired O_2 mixtures. Calculations were based on an assumed hemoglobin concentration of 16 g per 100 mL, arteriovenous difference of 4 vol %, respiratory quotient of 0.8, and $PaCO_2$ of 40 mm Hg. The graph was constructed with the aid of a Severinghaus nomogram.

the shunt is greater than 30%, an increase in FIO_2 from 60% to 100% should have very little effect on PaO_2 (Fig. 1-7).[58]

The infant's age, weight, and disease are factors that should be considered in the determination of criteria for respiratory failure. Generally, pH less than 7.25, PaO_2 less than 50 mm Hg, and $Paco_2$ greater than 60 mm Hg in 60% O_2 indicate the need for some form of respiratory assistance. However, the normal intrauterine umbilical artery pH is approximately 7.25.[59] Thus, blood gases obtained immediately after birth must be interpreted with awareness of the normal physiologic adaptation process. In infants weighing less than 1500 g, $Paco_2$ criteria for ventilatory assistance may be modified to values greater than 50 mm Hg, because respiratory acidosis may increase the incidence of intraventricular hemorrhage.[60] A contrary view is held by many neonatologists and researched by the group at Columbia University, where pH is allowed to decrease to 7.25 or lower and $Paco_2$ to increase to 55 to 60 mm Hg (permissive hypercapnia), resulting in no apparent increase in intraventricular hemorrhage or neurologic sequelae.[61] This concept is discussed more fully in Chapter 15. CPAP failure, and thus the need for mechanical ventilation, is indicated by the presence of $Paco_2$ greater than 55 to 60 mm Hg in 100% O_2 and distending pressure of 10 to 12 cm H_2O (depending on the CPAP system).

Our criteria are also modified by the pathophysiology of the disease process. In atelectatic disease with decreased lung volume (e.g., RDS), CPAP or IMV may be initiated early to increase lung volume, provide alveolar stabilization, and increase functional residual capacity. In such diseases, some physicians initiate CPAP at birth.[61,62] However, in obstructive disease (e.g., aspiration syndrome), we try to avoid positive pressure and provide ambient O_2 up to 100% before intubation is considered. The incidence of pulmonary air leaks can be extremely high when infants with obstructive lung disease are ventilated.[63] A scoring system used for the selection of infants based on the results of blood gas analysis is shown in Table 1-4. Indications for assisted ventilation are (1) a score of 3 or greater, (2) Pao_2 less than 50 mm Hg in 60% O_2, or (3) CPAP failure (i.e., CPAP ≥10 cm H_2O at 100% Fio_2).

Decisions to institute assisted ventilation should be made after the risks and benefits have been evaluated; they should not be based strictly on blood gas criteria. Even in the presence of near-normal blood gas values, certain conditions may necessitate ventilator support. A trend of deterioration may indicate the need for respiratory assistance, even though severe hypercapnia and acidosis are not yet present. In addition, repeated episodes of prolonged apnea unresponsive to other measures (i.e., theophylline administration, cutaneous stimulation) and associated with bradycardia or cyanosis should be treated with assisted ventilation. Many infants may be placed on ventilatory

assistance early in the course of progressive atelectatic disease to reduce the work of breathing and, theoretically, to conserve surfactant by alveolar stabilization before absolute criteria are met. Very-low-birthweight infants may be intubated and placed on assisted ventilation before criteria are met so that exogenous surfactant therapy can be initiated immediately after birth. Furthermore, clinical judgment and the experience of the clinician may dictate when intubation and mechanical ventilation are initiated. The criteria for the initiation of artificial surfactant therapy are discussed in detail in Chapter 20.

What: Types and Classification of Mechanical Ventilators

The classification of ventilators can be confusing because it may be based on the pressure relationship to the patient, the cycling mode, the power source, or the ventilatory rate (Table 1-5). The following approach, although somewhat simplistic, should serve as an introduction to Chapters 2 through 29.

Mechanical ventilation can be achieved through the use of intermittent negative-pressure or positive-pressure devices. Negative-pressure ventilators are mainly of historical interest and represent only a small percentage of machines currently in use in the United States. Negative-pressure respirators can provide assisted ventilation without the need for endotracheal intubation; thus, trauma to the airway is avoided and the risk of infection is reduced. They can also provide effective continuous negative pressure.[64] The only commercially available equipment for newborns, the Isolette Respirator (Airshields, Inc., Hatboro, PA, USA), is no longer manufactured. In the early 1990s, this form of ventilation experienced a minor resurgence of interest because of reported success in the ventilation of infants with persistent pulmonary hypertension who met ECMO cannulation criteria.[65] The Isolette Respirator has not been proven effective in the ventilation of very-low-birthweight infants, who represent the largest group of the NICU population. Comparison of the advantages and disadvantages of negative-pressure ventilators is presented in Table 1-6.

Positive-pressure devices are most commonly classified based on cycling mode (i.e., usually the way in which the inspiratory cycle is terminated). There are six basic types of cycling[66]:

1. *Volume cycling:* Inspiration ends when a certain volume is reached
2. *Pressure cycling:* Inspiration ends when a preset pressure is reached
3. *Time cycling:* Inspiration ends when a preset time is reached
4. *Flow cycling:* Inspiration ends when flow has reached a critical low level
5. *Mixed cycling:* Two or more independent cycling mechanisms are present in the same ventilator
6. *High-frequency ventilators:* Ventilators capable of cycling at rates greater than 150 breaths per minute

---

TABLE 1-4. Blood Gas Scoring System for Assisted Ventilation*†

	Points			
	0	**1**	**2**	**3**
Pao_2 (mm Hg)	>60	50–60	<50‡	<50‡
pH	>7.30	7.20–7.29	7.1–7.19	<7.1
$Paco_2$ (mm Hg)	<50	50–60	61–70	>70

*A score of 3 or more indicates need for CPAP or IMV.
†Ambient oxygen failure → CPAP
  CPAP failure (CPAP 10 cm H_2O and 100% Fio_2) → IMV
‡May indicate need for CPAP or IMV by itself, if cyanotic heart disease is not present.
CPAP, continuous positive airway pressure; IMV, intermittent mandatory ventilation.

TABLE 1-5. Classification of Neonatal Ventilators

By pressure relationship to patient (positive or negative)
By cycling mode (at termination of inspiration)
By power source
By rate

The vast majority of positive-pressure neonatal ventilators fall under the first three categories. Chapter 9 discusses pressure-cycled and time-cycled ventilators, and Chapter 10 addresses volume-cycled ventilators.

A surge of interest that began in the 1980s has led to the development of a new class of ventilators that cannot be classified based on conventional mechanical ventilation criteria. Because of respiratory complications, including oxygen toxicity, barotrauma, and cardiovascular compromise, HFV has been tried as an alternative to conventional mechanical ventilation when the latter has failed. HFV now is being used in many centers in the United States. Currently, there are three major types of HFV: high-frequency positive-pressure ventilation, which is produced by conventional or modified conventional mechanical ventilators operating at rapid rates; high-frequency jet ventilation, which is produced by ventilators that deliver a high-velocity jet of O_2 or gas directly into the airway; and high-frequency oscillation, which moves air back and forth at the airway opening and produces a minimum of bulk gas flow. HFV is not a specific type of ventilator but rather a pattern of ventilation that uses very high rates such that tidal volumes are less than or equal to the patient's anatomic dead space.[67] This mode of ventilation is discussed in Chapter 11.

In pressure-cycled, time-cycled, and volume-cycled ventilation, compliance varies pressure and volume as independent variables. Compliance equals that unit of volume change produced by a unit of pressure change (cm^3/cm H_2O). In volume-cycled ventilation, identical volumes delivered to two infants generate greater pressure in the infant with poorer compliance. In pressure-cycled ventilation, identical peak inspiratory pressures delivered to two infants result in greater tidal volumes in the infant with better compliance; also, the infant with poor compliance has a shorter inspiratory time. If time-cycled ventilators are not pressure limited, the volume of gas delivered to the infant is determined by inspiratory time and gas flow. Long inspiratory times and high gas flows generate increased volumes and pressures. In the case of identical inspiratory times and gas flow in two infants, the infant with the poorer compliance receives less volume and greater pressure, as shown in Figure 1-8.[68] Physiologic principles of mechanical ventilation are discussed in Chapter 2.

Devices can be added to the ventilator that prevent excessive pressure or volume as the compliance of an infant's lung changes. A pressure-limiting device regulates the maximal pressure by means of a pop-off valve. A volume-limiting device allows the ventilator to deliver less (but never more) than a specified amount. In all three types of positive-pressure ventilators, tidal volume is determined by lung compliance and, if present, a pressure-limiting device.

Ventilators also can be classified according to the manner in which they control ventilation, often termed the *ventilator mode*. To start inspiration, the machine can be triggered by the patient (assistor type), by the ventilator only (controller type), or by both the patient and the ventilator (assistor-controller type). In assistor-controller ventilators, a device allows the patient to initiate some respirations; however, it also has a pre-

---

TABLE 1-6. Negative-Pressure Ventilators

Advantages	Disadvantages
Less pulmonary O_2 toxicity (bronchopulmonary dysplasia)	High cost
	Patient inaccessible for routine procedures and resuscitation
Doubles as an incubator	Cooling of infants
Decrease in pulmonary infections	Neck abrasions
Decrease in atelectasis	Monitoring of pulmonary status based on blood gas analysis is more difficult
Decrease in pulmonary air leaks	Patient usually removed for radiography
Decrease in airway trauma	Decreased airway patency in neurologically depressed infants
May be effective in persistent pulmonary hypertension of the newborn	Compression of trunk during inspiration decreases effectiveness
	Not effective for very-low-birthweight infants (<1500 g)

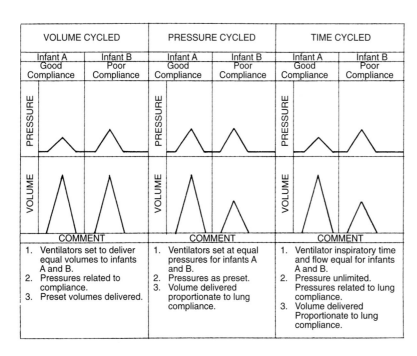

Figure 1-8. Diagrammatic pressure and volume curves generated in infants with different compliance on volume-cycled, pressure-cycled, and time-cycled ventilators. (From Gottschalk SK, King B, Schuth CR: Basic concepts in positive pressure ventilation of the newborn. Perinatol Neonatol 4:15, 1980.)

determined frequency of IMV that can be used as backup. In neonatal ventilators, the assistor device must be extremely sensitive to the slightest inspiratory effort. IMV, with or without an assistor device, has become an important aspect of neonatal ventilation, especially during weaning from respiratory support. Newer neonatal ventilators have incorporated synchronized IMV, pressure support, or both in their cycling modes. Synchronized IMV generates breaths that do not stack on top of or combine with the patient's spontaneous breaths while maintaining a preset rate as a background for periods of patient apnea. Pressure support ventilation provides a preset gas flow where each breath is completely spontaneous (i.e., it is patient triggered). These modes of ventilation are discussed in Chapter 12.

The power source for the ventilator can be either pneumatic (i.e., gas powered) or electrical. Other devices can be added to the ventilator for flow pattern and exhalation classification. The delivery of PEEP is widely used in neonatal ventilation for maintaining CPAP and improving oxygenation. With a PEEP device, the patient is allowed to exhale but the expiratory pressure never reaches zero; thus, functional residual capacity is increased, and the patient is able to retain a large amount of gas in the alveoli.

Dozens of conventional neonatal ventilators are commercially available. None of them is perfect for the complete management of every type of respiratory disease. A satisfactory neonatal ventilator should fulfill the following requirements:

1. All modes of ventilation should be possible, including IMV, CPAP, PEEP, and some form of synchronized IMV, assistor-controller ventilation, or pressure support ventilation.
2. The ventilator should be easy to operate.
3. The ventilator should be reliable (i.e., have few mechanical failures).
4. The machine should be relatively quiet, small, and "inexpensive."
5. The conventional ventilator should offer a wide range of respiratory rates up to 150 breaths per minute.
6. FIO_2 concentrations should be adjustable and accurate (from 21%–100%).
7. The ventilator should possess a low compliance system both inside and outside.
8. The conventional ventilator should accurately deliver a wide range of tidal volumes (<5–200 mL).
9. The ventilator should have a quick response time.
10. The device should have an alarm system(s) (visual and audible) to warn about mechanical failures or patient disconnects.
11. The system should offer user-variable flow rates that remain constant at a set flow.
12. The ventilator should be able to adequately humidify and heat inspired gas (60% humidity at 37°C).
13. Variable-pressure or volume-limiting devices should be available.
14. The device should offer a wide range of pressure or volume capacities.
15. The ventilator should have the capacity to digitally read out a variety of pulmonary function parameters.

Appendix 1 compares commonly used ventilators classified by pressure characteristic, cycling mode, power source, and rate and comments on principles of operation, advantages, and disadvantages.

REFERENCES

1. II Kings 4:34.
2. Daily WJR, Smith PC: Mechanical ventilation of the newborn infant: I. Curr Probl Pediatr 1:1, 1971.
3. Thatcher VS: History of Anesthesia, with Emphasis on the Nurse Specialists. Philadelphia, JB Lippincott, 1953.
4. Faulconer A Jr, Keys TE: Foundation of Anesthesiology. I. Springfield, Charles C Thomas, 1965.
5. Dunn PM: Charles-Michel Billard (1800–1832): Pioneer of neonatal medicine. Arch Dis Child 65:711, 1990.
6. Desmond MM: A review of newborn medicine in America: European past and guiding ideology. Am J Perinatol 8:308, 1991.
7. O'Dwyer J: Fifty cases of croup in private practice treated by intubation of the larynx with a description of the method and of the danger incident thereto. Med Res 32:557, 1887.
8. Doe OW: Apparatus for resuscitating asphyxiated children. Boston Med Surg J 9:122, 1889.
9. Stern L, Ramos, AD, Outerbridge EW, Beaudry PH: Negative pressure artificial respiration use in treatment of respiratory failure of the newborn. Can Med Assoc J 102:595, 1970.
10. Drinker P, Shaw LA: An apparatus of the prolonged administration of artificial respiration: 1. A design for adults and children. J Clin Invest 7:229, 1929.
11. Bloxsom A: Resuscitation of the newborn infant: Use of positive pressure oxygen-air lock. J Pediatr 37:311, 1950.
12. Kendig JW, Maples PG, Maisels MJ: The Bloxsom air lock: A historical perspective. Pediatrics 108, e116, 2001.
12a. Apgar V, Kreiselman J: Studies on resuscitation. An experimental evaluation of the Bloxsom air lock. Am J Obstet Gynecol 65:45, 1953.
12b. Townsend EH Jr: The oxygen air pressure lock I. Clinical observations on its use during the neonatal period. Obstet Gynecol 4:184, 1954.
12c. Reichelderfer TE, Nitowski HM: A controlled study of the use of the Bloxsom air lock. Pediatrics 18:918, 1956.
13. Cross K, Roberts P: Asphyxia neonatorum treated by electrical stimulation of the phrenic nerve. Br Med J 1:1043, 1951.
14. James LS, Apgar B, Burnard ED, et al: Intragastric oxygen and resuscitation of the newborn. Acta Pediatr Scand 52:245, 1963.
15. Donald I, Lord J: Augmented respiration: Studies in atelectasis neonatorum. Lancet 1:9, 1953.
16. Stahlman MT: Assisted ventilation in newborn infants. In Smith GF, Vidyasagar D (eds): Historical Reviews and Recent Advances in Neonatal and Perinatal Medicine, vol. II. Evansville, Ind., Mead Johnson Nutritional Division, 1984.
17. Kirby RR: Mechanical ventilation of the newborn. Perinatol Neonatal 5:47, 1981.
18. Cournand A, Motley HL, Werko L, et al: Physiological studies of the effects of intermittent positive pressure breathing on cardiac output in man. Am J Physiol 152:162, 1948.
19. Cochran, WD, Levison, H, Muirhead, DM, et al: A clinical trial on high oxygen pressure for the respiratory distress syndrome. N Engl J Med 212:347, 1965.
20. Gregory GA, Kitterman, JA, Phibbs RH, et al: Treatment of the idiopathic respiratory-distress syndrome with continuous positive airway pressure. N Engl J Med 284:1333, 1971.
21. Bancalari E, Garcia OL, Jesse MJ: Effects of continuous negative pressure on lung mechanics in idiopathic respiratory distress syndrome. Pediatrics 51:485, 1973.
22. Kattwinkel J, Fleming D, Cha CC, et al: A device for administration of continuous positive airway pressure by nasal route. Pediatrics 52:131, 1973.
23. Reynolds EOR: Pressure waveform and ventilator setting for mechanical ventilation in severe hyaline membrane disease. Int Clin Anesthesiol 12:269, 1974.
24. Reynolds EOR, Taghizadeh A: Improved prognosis of infants mechanically ventilated for hyaline membrane disease. Arch Dis Child 49:505, 1974.
25. Kirby R, Robison E, Schulz J, DeLemos RA: Continuous flow ventilation as an alternative to assisted or controlled ventilation in infants. Anesth Analg 51:871, 1972.
26. Kirby RR: Intermittent mandatory ventilation in the neonate. Crit Care Med 5:18, 1977.
27. Cassani VL III: We've come a long way baby! Mechanical ventilation of the newborn. Neonatal Netw 13:63, 1994.
28. Bland RD, Sedin EG: High frequency mechanical ventilation in the treatment of neonatal respiratory distress. Int Anesthesiol Clin 21:125, 1983.

29. Slutsky AS, Drazen FM, Ingram RH Jr, et al: Effective pulmonary ventilation with small-volume oscillations at high frequency. Science 209:609, 1980.

30. Pesenti A, Gottinoni L, Bombino L: Long-term extracorporeal respiratory support: 20 years of progress. Intern Ext Care Digest 12:15, 1993.

31. Frantz ID III, Werthammen J, Stark AR: High-frequency ventilation in premature infants with lung disease: Adequate gas exchange at low tracheal pressure. Pediatrics 71:483, 1983.

32. Avery ME, Mead J: Surface properties in relation to atelectasis and hyaline membrane disease. Am J Dis Child 17:517, 1959.

33. Jobe AH: Pulmonary surfactant therapy. N Engl J Med 328:861, 1993.

34. Brown DL, Pattishall EN: Other uses of surfactant. Clin Perinatol 20:761, 1993.

35. Johnson JD, Malachowski NC, Grobstein R, et al: Prognosis of children surviving with the aid of mechanical ventilation in the newborn period. J Pediatr 84:272, 1974.

36. Lorenz JM: The outcome of extreme prematurity. Semin Perinatol 25:348, 2001.

37. Horbar, JD, Badger, GJ, Carpenter JH, et al: Trends in mortality and morbidity for very low birthweight infants, 1991–1999. Pediatrics 110:143, 2002.

38. Schwartz RM, Luby AM, Scanlon JW, Kellogg RJ: Effect of surfactant on morbidity, mortality, and resource use in newborn infants weighing 500 to 1500 g. N Engl J Med 330:1476, 1994.

39. Greenspan JS: Liquid ventilation: A developing technology. Neonatal Netw 12:23, 1993.

40. Downes JJ: Mechanical ventilation of the newborn. Anesthesiology 34:116, 1971.

41. Committee on Perinatal Health, National Foundation–March of Dimes: Toward Improving the Outcome of Pregnancy. White Plains, NY, March of Dimes, 1976.

42. March of Dimes Birth Defects Foundation: Toward Improving the Outcome of Pregnancy: The 90s and Beyond. White Plains, NY, March of Dimes, 1993.

43. Goldsmith JP, Graf MA: A modest proposal [editorial]. J Perinatol 8:1, 1988.

44. Perl H: Can a community hospital NICU measure up? Contemp Pediatr, 2:38, 1985.

45. Garrett FF, Goldsmith JP: Perinatal-neonatal regionalization: A view from the outlying hospital. Respir Care 23:873, 1978.

46. Cordero L, Zuspan FP: Very low-birth weight infants: Five years experience of a regional perinatal program. Ohio Med 84:976, 1988.

47. Rosenblatt RA, Mayfield JA, Hart LG, Baldwin LM: Outcomes of regionalized perinatal care in Washington State. West J Med 149:98, 1988.

48. Levy DL, Noelke K, Goldsmith JP: Maternal and infant transport program in Louisiana. Obstet Gynecol 57:500, 1981.

49. Harris TR, Isaman J, Giles HR: Improved neonatal survival through maternal transport. Obstet Gynecol 52:294, 1978.

50. Moore TR, Resnick R: Special problems of VLBW infants. Contemp Obstet Gynecol, June 23, 1984, p. 174.

51. Spitzer AR, Fox WW, Delivoria-Papadopuolos M: Respiratory distress syndrome: The perinatal center versus infant transport in relation to severity of disease [abstract]. Pediatr Res 15:4, 1981.

52. Indyk L, Cohen S: Newborn intensive care in the United States, East and West. Comments on representative facilities and programs, and a proposed new point scoring system for evaluation. Clin Pediatr 10:320, 1971.

53. Louisiana Perinatal Commission: Maternal and neonatal guidelines for regionalization of perinatal care in the state of Louisiana. New Orleans, La., Department of Health and Human Resources, 1980, p 26.

54. Guidelines for Perinatal Care, 5th ed. Elk Grove Village, Ill., American Academy of Pediatrics and American College of Obstetrics and Gynecologists, 2002.

55. Silverman WE, Andersen DH: Controlled clinical trial of effects of water mist on obstructive respiratory signs, death rate and necropsy findings among premature infants. Pediatrics 17:1, 1956.

56. Gerard P, Fox WW, Outerbridge EH, Beaudry PH: Early versus late introduction of continuous negative pressure in the management of idiopathic respiratory distress syndrome. J Pediatr 87:591, 1975.

57. Gregory GA: Devices for applying continuous positive airway pressure. In Thibault DW, Gregory GA (eds): Neonatal Pulmonary Care. Reading, Mass., Addison-Wesley, 1979, p 187.

58. Pontoppidan H, Geffin B, Lowenstein E: Acute respiratory failure in the adult. 2. N Engl J Med 287:743, 1972.

59. Avery ME, Fletcher BD, Williams RG: The Lung and Its Disorders in the Newborn Infant, 4th ed. Philadelphia, WB Saunders, 1981, pp 40, 69.

60. Wigglesworth JS: A new look at intraventricular hemorrhage. Contemp Obstet Gynecol 98, 1985.

61. Transwell AK, Clubb RA, Smith BT, Boston RW: Individualized continuous distending pressure applied within 6 hours of delivery in infants with respiratory distress syndrome. Arch Dis Child 55:33, 1980.

62. Avery ME, Tooley WH, Keller JB, et al: Is chronic lung disease in low birthweight infants preventable? A survey of eight centers. Pediatrics 79:26, 1987.

63. Gregory GA, Gooding CA, Phibbs RH, Tooley WH: Meconium aspiration syndrome in infants: A prospective study. J Pediatr 85:848, 1974.

64. Outerbridge EW, Stern L: Negative pressure ventilators. In Goldsmith JP, Karotkin EH (eds): Assisted Ventilation of the Neonate. Philadelphia, WB Saunders, 1981, p 161.

65. Sills JH, Cvetnic WG, Pietz J: Continuous negative pressure in the treatment of pulmonary hypertension and respiratory failure. J Perinatol 9:43, 1989.

66. Williams TJ: Mechanical ventilation. In Williams TJ, Hill JW (eds): Handbook of Neonatal Respiratory Care. Riverside, Calif., Bourns, 1971, p 91.

67. O'Rourke PP, Crone RK: High-frequency ventilation: A new approach to respiratory support. JAMA 250:2845, 1983.

68. Gottschalk SK, King B, Schuth CR: Basic concepts in positive pressure ventilation of the newborn. Perinatol Neonatol 4:15, 1980.

2

PHYSIOLOGIC PRINCIPLES

BRIAN R. WOOD, MD

It is the responsibility of those who care for critically ill infants to have an understanding of respiratory physiology and the functional limitations imposed on gas exchange by anatomic and developmental constraints. The first tenet of the Hippocratic Oath states *"primum non nocere"* ("first do no harm"). The respiratory system of the premature infant is fragile. In clinical practice we are faced with the difficult task of supporting adequate gas exchange in an immature respiratory system, using powerful tools that by their very nature perturb ongoing developmental processes, often resulting in alterations in end-organ form and function.

In our efforts to provide ventilatory support, the infant's lungs and airways are subjected to forces that lead to acute and chronic tissue injury. This results in alterations in the way the lungs develop and the way they respond to subsequent noxious stimuli. Injury leads to alterations in lung development, which result in alterations in lung function as the infant's body attempts to heal and continue to develop. Superimposed on this is the fact that the ongoing development of the respiratory system is hampered by the healing process itself, which further complicates the situation.

This complexity makes caring for infants with respiratory failure both interesting and challenging. To effectively provide support for these patients, the clinician must have an understanding not only of respiratory physiology but also of respiratory system development, growth, and healing.

BASIC BIOCHEMISTRY OF RESPIRATION: OXYGEN AND ENERGY

. The energy production required for a newborn infant to sustain his or her metabolic functions is dependent upon the availability of oxygen and its subsequent metabolism. During the breakdown of carbohydrates, oxygen is consumed as carbon dioxide and water are produced. The energy derived from this process is generated as electrons are transferred from electron donors to electron acceptors. Oxygen has a high electron affinity and therefore is a good electron acceptor. The energy produced during this process is stored as high-energy phosphate bonds, primarily in the form of adenosine triphosphate (ATP). The enzyme systems within the mitochondria couple the transfer of energy to oxidation in a process known as *oxidative phosphorylation.*[1]

For energy production to occur, oxygen must be available to the mitochondria. The transfer of oxygen from the air outside the infant to the mitochondria, within the infant's cells, involves a series of steps: convection of air into the lung, diffusion of oxygen into the blood, convective flow of blood to the tissues, diffusion of oxygen into the cells, and finally diffusion into the mitochondria. The driving force for these transfer processes is an oxygen pressure gradient, which drives this cascade from the air outside the body to intracellular mitochondria (Fig. 2-1).

The lungs of the newborn infant transfer oxygen to the blood by diffusion, driven by the oxygen pressure gradient. For gas exchange to occur efficiently, the infant's lungs must remain expanded, the lungs must be both ventilated and perfused, and the ambient partial pressure of oxygen in the air must be greater than the partial pressure of oxygen of the blood. The efficiency of the newborn infant's respiratory system is determined by both structural and functional constraints; therefore, the clinician must be mindful of both aspects when caring for the infant.

The infant's cells require energy in order to function. This energy is obtained from high-energy phosphate bonds (e.g., ATP) formed during oxidative phosphorylation. Only a small amount of ATP is stored within the cells. Muscle cells contain an additional store of ATP, but in order to meet metabolic needs beyond those that can be provided for by the stored ATP, new ATP must be made by phosphorylation of adenosine diphosphate (ADP). This can be done anaerobically through glycolysis, but this is an inefficient process and leads to the formation of lactic acid. Long-term energy demands must be met aerobically through ongoing oxidative phosphorylation within the mitochondria, which is a much more efficient process and results in the formation of carbon dioxide and water.

There is a hierarchy of how energy is used by the infant. During periods of high-energy demand, muscles initially draw upon the available stores of ATP, then use glycolysis to make more ATP from ADP, and then use oxidative phosphorylation to supply the infant's ongoing energy requirements. Oxidative phosphorylation and oxygen consumption are so closely linked

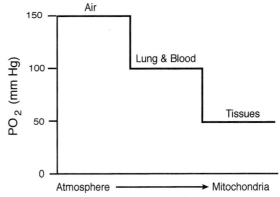

Figure 2-1. Transfer of oxygen from outside air to intracellular mitochondria via an oxygen pressure gradient.

to the newborn infant's energy requirements that total oxygen consumption is a reasonably good measure of the total energy needs of the infant. When the infant's workload is in excess of that which can be sustained by oxidative phosphorylation (aerobic metabolism), the muscle cells will revert to anaerobic glycolysis to produce ATP. This anaerobic metabolism results in the formation of lactic acid, which accumulates in the blood and causes a decrease in pH (acidosis/acidemia).

ONTOGENY RECAPITULATES PHYLOGENY: A BRIEF OVERVIEW OF DEVELOPMENTAL ANATOMY

Lung Development

The tracheobronchial airway system begins as a ventral outpouching of the primitive foregut, which leads to the formation of the embryonic lung bud. The lung bud subsequently divides and branches, penetrating the mesenchyma and progressing toward the periphery. Lung development is divided into five phases.[2]

Phases of Lung Development

- Embryonic phase (weeks 3–6)
- Pseudoglandular phase (weeks 6–16)
- Canalicular phase (weeks 16–26)
- Terminal sac phase (weeks 26–36)
- Alveolar phase (week 36–3 years)

Embryonic phase (weeks 6–6): development of proximal airways. The lung bud arises from the foregut 21 to 26 days after fertilization.

Aberrant development during the embryonic phase may result in

- Tracheal agenesis
- Tracheal stenosis
- Tracheoesophageal fistula
- Pulmonary sequestration (if an accessory lung bud develops during this period)

Pseudoglandular phase (weeks 6–16): development of lower conduction airways. During this phase the first 20 generations of conducting airways develop. The first 8 generations (the bronchi) ultimately acquire cartilaginous walls. Generations 9 to 20 comprise the nonrespiratory bronchioles. Lymph vessels and bronchial capillaries accompany the airways as they grow and develop.

Aberrant development during the pseudoglandular phase may result in

- Bronchogenic cysts
- Congenital lobar emphysema
- Congenital diaphragmatic hernia

Canalicular phase (weeks 16–26): formation of gas-exchanging acini. The formation of respiratory bronchioles (generations 21–23) occurs during the canalicular phase. The relative proportion of parenchymal connective tissue diminishes. The development of pulmonary capillaries occurs. Gas exchange is dependent upon the degree of acinus–capillary coupling.

Terminal sac phase (weeks 26–36): refinement of acini. The rudimentary primary saccules divide into subsaccules and alveoli during the terminal sac phase. The interstitium continues to dissipate. Capillary invasion leads to an increase in alveolar–blood barrier surface area. The development of the surfactant system occurs during this phase.

Birth during the terminal sac phase may result in

- Transient tachypnea of the newborn
- Respiratory distress syndrome (RDS)
- Pulmonary interstitial emphysema (PIE)

Alveolar phase (week 36–3 years): alveolar proliferation and development. Subsaccules become alveoli as a result of the thinning of the acinar walls, dissipation of interstitium, and invagination of alveoli by pulmonary capillaries during the alveolar phase. The alveoli attain a polyhedral shape.

MECHANICS

The lung has a variety of functions, but we will concern ourselves here with its primary function, that of gas exchange. The respiratory system is composed of millions of air sacs that are connected to the outside air via airways. The lung behaves like a balloon in that it is in an expanded state by the intact thorax and will deflate should the integrity of the system be compromised. The interior of the lung is partitioned so as to provide a large surface area to facilitate efficient gas diffusion. The lung is expanded by forces generated by the diaphragm and the intercostal muscles. It recoils secondary to elastic and surface tension forces. This facilitates the inflow and outflow of respiratory gases required to allow the air volume contained within the lung to be ventilated. During inspiration the diaphragm contracts. The diaphragm is a "dome-shaped" muscle at rest. As it contracts, the diaphragm flattens, and the volume of the chest cavity is enlarged. This causes the intrapleural pressure to decrease and results in gas flow into the lung.[3] During unlabored breathing the intercostal and accessory muscles serve primarily to stabilize the rib cage as the diaphragm contracts, countering the forces resulting from the decrease in intrapleural pressure during inspiration. This limits the extent to which the infant's chest wall is deformed inward during inspiration.

Although in the premature infant the chest wall is very compliant, the rib cage offers some structural support, serves as an attachment point for the respiratory muscles, and limits lung deflation on end-expiration. The elastic elements of the respiratory systems, the connective tissue, are stretched during inspiration and recoiled during exhalation. The air–liquid interface in the terminal air spaces and respiratory bronchioles generates surface tension that opposes lung expansion and supports lung deflation. The conducting airways, which connect the gas exchange units to the outside air, provide greater resistance during exhalation than during inspiration. The abdominal muscles can aid in exhalation by active contraction if required, but because expiration is generally passive, they make little contribution during unlabored breathing. The respiratory system is designed to be adaptable to a wide range of workloads; however, in the newborn infant, several structural and functional limitations make the newborn susceptible to respiratory failure.

Differences between the shape of a newborn infant's chest and that of an adult put the infant at a mechanical disadvantage. Unlike the adult's thorax, which is ellipsoid in shape, the infant's thorax is more cylindrical and the ribs are more horizontal rather than oblique. Because of these anatomic differences, the intercostal muscles in infants have a shorter course and provide less mechanical advantage for elevating the ribs and increasing intrathoracic volume during inspiration than do those of adults. Also, because the insertion of the infant's diaphragm is more horizontal than in the adult, the lower ribs tend to move inward rather than upward during inspiration. The compliant chest wall of the infant exacerbates this inward deflection with inspiration. This is particularly evident during rapid eye movement (REM) sleep, when phasic changes in intercostal muscle tone are inhibited. Therefore, instead of stabilizating the rib cage during inspiration, the intercostal muscles are relaxed. This results in inefficient respiration, which may be manifested clinically by intercostal and substernal retractions associated with abdominal breathing. The endurance capacity of the diaphragm is determined primarily by muscle mass and the oxidative capacity of muscle fibers. Infants have low muscle mass and a low percentage of type 1 (slow twitch) muscle fibers compared to adults.[4] In order to sustain the work of breathing, the diaphragm must be provided with a continuous supply of oxygen. Respiratory muscle fatigue is a common cause of respiratory failure in premature infants.

During expiration the main driving force is elastic recoil. Elastic recoil depends on the surface tension produced by the air–liquid interface, the elastic elements of tissue, and the bony development of the rib cage. Expiration is largely passive. Because the chest wall of premature infants is compliant, it offers little resistance against expansion upon inspiration and little opposition against collapse upon expiration. This collapse at end-expiration can lead to the development of atelectasis. In premature infants the largest contributor to elastic recoil is surface tension. Surfactant serves to reduce surface tension and stabilize the terminal airways. In circumstances where surfactant is deficient, the terminal air spaces have a tendency to collapse or become atelectatic. RDS is caused by a primary surfactant deficiency. Mechanical ventilation and the administration of exogenous surfactant directly into the lung is the treatment of choice for moderate-to-severe RDS. Pressure in the form of peak inspiratory pressure (PIP), positive end-expiratory pressure (PEEP), or continuous positive airway pressure (CPAP) may be applied to the infant's airway to counter the tendency toward collapse and the development of atelectasis. The application of airway distending pressure also serves to stabilize the chest wall.

Lung compliance and airway resistance are related to lung size. The smaller the lung, the lower the compliance and the greater the resistance. If, however, lung compliance is corrected to lung volume (specific compliance), the values are nearly identical for term infants and adults.[5] In term infants, immediately after delivery, specific compliance is low but normalizes as fetal lung fluid is absorbed and a normal functional residual capacity (FRC) is established. In premature infants, specific compliance remains low, due in part to persistent atelectasis and failure to achieve a normal FRC. Chest wall compliance is very high in the newborn.

The resistance within lung tissue during inflation and deflation is called *viscous resistance.* Viscous resistance is elevated in the newborn. In small lungs, there are relatively fewer terminal air spaces and relatively more stroma (cells and interstitial fluid). This is manifested by a low ratio of lung volume to lung weight. Although in absolute terms airway resistance is elevated in the newborn infant, when corrected to lung volume (specific conductance, which is the reciprocal of resistance per unit lung volume) the relative resistance is lower than in adults. It is important to remember that because of the small diameter of the airways in the lungs of the newborn infant, even a modest narrowing will result in a marked increase in resistance. That the newborn's bronchial tree is short and that inspiratory flow velocities are low are teleologic advantages for the newborn because both of these factors decrease airway resistance.

Overcoming the elastic and resistive forces during ventilation requires energy expenditure and accounts for the work of breathing. The normal work of breathing is essentially the same for newborns and adults when corrected for metabolic rates.[5] When the work of breathing increases, as it does in response to various disease states, the newborn is at a decided disadvantage. The newborn infant lacks the strength and endurance to cope with a significant increase in ventilatory workload. An increase in ventilatory workload can lead to respiratory failure.

Elastic and resistive forces of the chest, lungs, abdomen, airways, and ventilator circuit oppose the forces exerted by the respiratory muscles and/or ventilator. The terms *elastic recoil, flow resistance, viscous resistance,* and *work of breathing* are used to describe these forces. The terms *elasticity, compliance,* and *conductance* characterize the properties of the thorax, lungs, and airways. The static pressure-volume curve illustrates the relationships between these forces at different levels of lung expansion. Dynamic pressure-volume loops illustrate the pressure-volume relationship during inspiration and expiration (Figs. 2-2 to 2-4).

Elastic recoil refers to the tendency of stretched objects to return to their original shape. When the inspiratory muscles relax during exhalation, the elastic elements of the chest wall, diaphragm, and lungs, which were stretched during inspiration, recoil to their original shapes. These elastic elements behave like springs (Fig. 2-5). The surface tension forces at the air–liquid interfaces in the distal bronchioles and terminal airways decrease the surface area of the air–liquid interfaces (Fig. 2-6). At some point, the forces that tend to collapse are counterbalanced by those that resist further collapse. The point at which these opposing forces balance is called the *resting state of the respiratory system* and corresponds with FRC (Fig. 2-7; see also Fig. 2-2). Because the chest wall of the newborn infant is compliant, it offers little opposition to collapse at end-expiration; thus, the newborn, especially the premature newborn, has a relatively low FRC and thoracic gas volume, even when the newborn does not suffer from primary surfactant deficiency. This low FRC and the relative underdevelopment of the conducting airways structural support explain the tendency for early airway closure and collapse with resultant gas trapping in premature infants. The respiratory system's resting volume is very close to the closing volume of the lung. The closing volume is the volume at which dependent lung regions cease to ventilate because the airways leading to them have collapsed. In newborns, closing volume may occur even above resting volume (see Fig. 2-2).[6] Gas trapping related to airway closure has been demonstrated experimentally by showing situations in which the thoracic gas volume is greater than the FRC. For this to occur, the total gas volume measured in the chest at end-expiration is

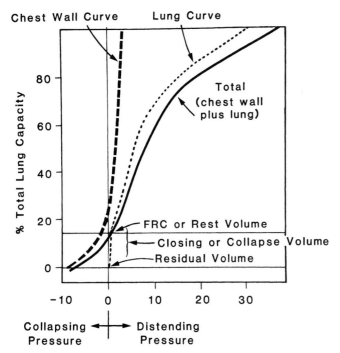

Figure 2-2. Static pressure-volume curves for the chest wall, the lung, and sum of the two for a normal newborn infant. Functional residual capacity (FRC) or rest volume (<20% of total lung capacity) is the point at which collapsing and distending pressures balance out to zero pressure. The lung would empty to residual volume if enough collapsing pressure (forced expiration) was generated to overcome chest wall elastic recoil in the opposite direction. The premature infant has an even steeper chest wall compliance curve than that shown here, whereas his or her lung compliance curve tends to be flatter and shifted to the right, depending on the degree of surfactant deficiency.

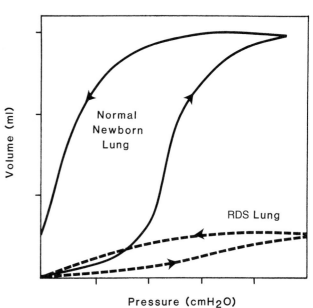

Figure 2-4. Comparison of the pressure-volume curve of a normal infant *(solid line)* with that of a newborn with respiratory distress syndrome *(dotted line)*. Note that very little hysteresis (i.e., the difference between the inspiratory and expiratory limbs) is observed in the respiratory distress syndrome curve because of the lack of surfactant for stabilization of the alveoli after inflation. The wide hysteresis of the normal infant's lung curve reflects changes (reduction) in surface tension once the alveoli are opened and stabilized. RDS, respiratory distress syndrome.

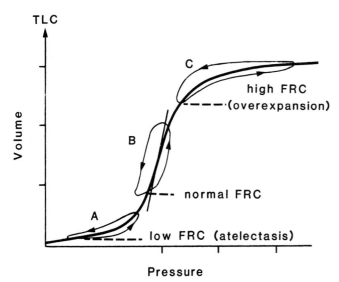

Figure 2-3. Extended compliance or lung expansion curve with "flattened" areas (*A* and *C*) at both ends. Area *A* represents the situation in disease states leading to atelectasis or lung collapse. Area *C* represents the situation in an overexpanded lung, as occurs in diseases involving significant air trapping (e.g., meconium aspiration) or in the excessive application of distending pressure during assisted ventilation. FRC, functional residual capacity.

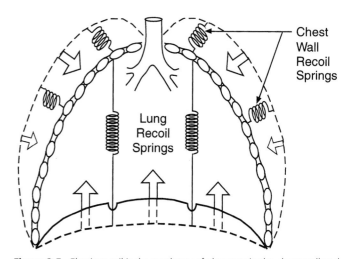

Figure 2-5. Elastic recoil is the tendency of elements in the chest wall and lungs that are stretched during inspiration to snap back or recoil *(arrows)* to their original state at the end of expiration. At this point (functional residual capacity or rest volume), the "springs" are relaxed and the structure of the rib cage allows no further collapse. Opposing forces of the chest wall and elastic recoil balance out, and intrathoracic and airway pressures become equal (this further defines functional residual capacity or rest volume; see also Fig. 2-2).

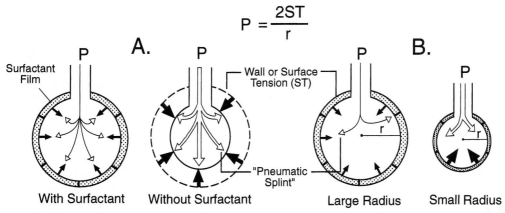

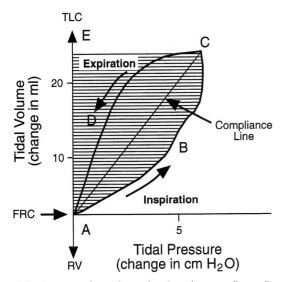

Figure 2-6. Diagrammatic illustration of the Laplace relationship and the effects of surfactant film *(A)* and alveolar radius *(B)* on wall or surface tension. The degree (reflected in the size of the *open arrows*) of airway or intra-alveolar pressure (P) needed to counteract the tendency of alveoli to collapse (represented by the *solid arrows*) is directly proportional to double the wall or surface tension (ST) and inversely proportional to the size of the radius (r). Distending airway pressure applied during assisted ventilation can be likened to a "pneumatic splint."

Figure 2-7. Pressure-volume loop showing the compliance line *(AC,* joining points of no flow); work done in overcoming elastic resistance *(ACEA),* which incorporates the frictional resistance encountered during expiration *(ACDA);* work done in overcoming frictional resistance during inspiration *(ABCA);* and total work done during the respiratory cycle *(ABCEA,* or the entire *shaded area).*

greater than the amount of gas that is in communication with the upper airway (FRC).

The main contributor to lung elastic recoil in the newborn is surface tension. The pressure required to counteract the tendency of the bronchioles and terminal air spaces to collapse is described by the Laplace relationship:

$$P = 2\,ST\,/\,r$$

Simply stated, this relationship illustrates that the pressure (P) needed to stabilize the system is directly proportional to twice the surface tension (2ST) and inversely proportional to the radius of curvature (r). (In infants, the relationship must be modified because there is an air–liquid interface on only one side of the terminal lung unit, so P = ST/r more accurately describes the situation in the infant.) The surface tension in the lung is primarily governed by the presence or absence of surfactant. Surfactant is a surface active material released by type II pneumocytes. It is composed mainly of dipalmitoyl phosphatidylcholine. Surfactant has a variety of unique properties that enable it to decrease surface tension at end-expiration and thereby prevent further lung deflation below resting volume and allow an increase in surface tension upon lung expansion that facilitates elastic recoil at end-inspiration. In addition, surfactant reduces surface tension when lung volume is decreased.[7] A reduction in the quantity of surfactant results in an increase in surface tension and necessitates the application of more distending pressure to counter the tendency of the bronchioles and terminal air spaces to collapse (Fig. 2-6A). As can be seen from the Laplace relationship, the larger the radius of curvature of the terminal bronchioles or air spaces, the less pressure is needed to hold them open or to expand them further (Fig. 2-6B). The smaller the radius of curvature (e.g., in premature infants), the more pressure is required to hold the airways open. Surfactant helps this situation throughout the respiratory cycle. As the radii of the air–liquid interfaces become smaller during exhalation, the effectiveness of surfactant in reducing surface tension increases; as the radii become larger, its effectiveness decreases.

Infants with RDS must generate high negative intrapleural pressures in order to expand and stabilize their distal airways and alveoli (see Fig. 2-4). The lung volumes achieved with the high opening pressures during inspiration are rapidly lost as the lung collapses to its original resting volume during expiration. In untreated RDS, each breath requires significant energy expenditure. If the burden imposed by this large work of breathing outstrips the infant's ability to maintain this level of output, the infant develops progressive respiratory failure. In order to expand atelectatic lungs, relatively high ventilator pressures may be required. Once the lungs are expanded, the inspiratory pressures should be quickly reduced because once the lungs are inflated, the radii of the bronchioles and terminal air spaces are larger and less pressure is required to hold them open or to expand them further. If one fails to reduce the inspiratory pressure once a normal lung volume has been established, overdistention and dilation of the conducting airways may result. This overdistention (volutrauma) is thought to be a factor in the development of the proliferate airway lesions that characterize chronic lung disease (CLD).[8] Lung overdistention also may lead to air leak conditions such as PIE and pneumothorax (see Chapter 21).

Compliance

Compliance is a measure of the change in volume resulting from a given change in pressure.

$$C_L = \Delta V / \Delta P$$

where ΔV is change in volume and ΔP is change in pressure.

Static Compliance

When measured under static conditions, compliance reflects only the elastic properties of the lung. Static compliance also is referred to as *elastance,* the pressure required to stretch the system. It is the inverse of elastic recoil. Static compliance measures are obtained by measuring the transpulmonary pressure before and after inflating the lungs with a known volume of gas. Transpulmonary pressure is the pressure difference between alveolar pressure and pleural pressure. It is approximated by measuring pressure at the mouth and in the esophagus. To generate a pressure-volume curve, pressure measurements are made at several different volumes (see Fig. 2-2, "Lung Curve"). If one measures the difference between pleural pressures (esophageal) and atmospheric pressures (transthoracic) at different levels of lung expansion, the plotted curve will be a chest wall compliance curve (see Fig. 2-2, "Chest Wall Curve"). This kind of plot shows the elastic properties of the chest wall. In the newborn, the chest wall is very compliant; thus, large volume changes are achieved with small pressure changes. Taking the lung and chest wall compliance curves together gives the total respiratory system compliance (see Fig. 2-2, "Total").

Dynamic Compliance

If one measures compliance during spontaneous breathing, the result is called *dynamic compliance.* Dynamic compliance reflects the elastic recoil of the lungs. Although this is the compliance that is generally measured during infant pulmonary function testing in the clinical setting, it should be understood that interpretation can be problematic.[9] If the patient is breathing rapidly, the instant of zero flow may not coincide with the point of lowest pressure. This is because compliance is rate dependent. Dynamic compliance may underestimate static compliance, especially in infants who are breathing rapidly and those with obstructive airway disease. Two additional factors further complicate the interpretation of compliance measurements. In premature infants, REM sleep is associated with paradoxical chest wall motion, so pressure changes recorded from the esophagus may correlate poorly with intrathoracic or pleural pressure changes. Chest wall distortion generally results in underestimation of esophageal pressure changes.[10] Also, because lung compliance is related to lung volume, measured compliance is dependent on the initial lung volume above which the compliance measure is made. Ideally comparisons should be normalized to the degree of lung expansion, for example, to FRC. Lung compliance divided by FRC is specific lung compliance.

Some clinicians use simultaneously recorded pressure and volume changes to examine the dynamic pressure-volume rela-

tionship. The pressure-volume loop allows one to quantify the work done to overcome airway resistance and to determine lung compliance (Figs. 2-4 and 2-7). Figure 2-3 shows a static lung compliance curve upon which three pressure-volume loops are superimposed. Each of the loops shows a complete respiratory cycle, but each is taken at a different lung volume. The overall compliance curve is sigmoidal. At the lower end of the curve (at low lung volume), the compliance is low, that is, there is a small change in volume for a large change in pressure (see Fig. 2-3, region A). This correlates with underinflation. Pressure is required to open up terminal airways and atelectatic terminal air spaces before gas can move into the lung. The lung volume is starting below critical opening pressure. At the center of the curve, the compliance high; there is a large change in volume for a small change in pressure. This is where normal tidal breathing should occur (see Fig. 2-3, region B). This is the position of maximum efficiency in a mechanical sense. At the upper end of the curve (at high lung volume), the compliance low; again, there is a small change in volume for a large change in pressure (see Fig. 2-3, region C). This correlates with a lung that already is overinflated. Applying additional pressure yields little in terms of additional volume but may contribute significantly to airway injury. The steeper the slope of the curve connecting the points of zero flow, the greater the compliance.

Compliance is reduced at both high and low lung volumes. Low lung volumes are seen in restrictive lung diseases such as primary surfactant deficiency (e.g., RDS), whereas high lung volumes are seen in obstructive lung diseases such as CLD. Reductions in both specific compliance and thoracic gas volume have been measured in infants with RDS.[11,12] Teleologically, premature infants with surfactant deficiency can compensate for chest wall instability to a certain extent by breathing rapidly, which results in gas trapping that tends to normalize their FRC. They also use end-expiratory grunting as a method of expiratory retardation or braking to help normalize FRC. In RDS, serial measurements of FRC and compliance have been shown to be sensitive indicators of illness severity.[13]

Dynamic lung compliance has been shown to decrease as the clinical course worsens and to improve at the recovery phase begins. When ventilation is used in infants with noncompliant lungs due to surfactant deficiency, elevated distending pressures may be required initially in order to establish a reasonable FRC. Figure 2-4 shows the pressure-volume loop of a normal infant and that of an infant with RDS. A higher pressure is required to establish an appropriate lung volume in the infant with RDS than in the normal infant. Mechanical ventilation without PEEP can lead to a reduction in lung compliance. Positive-pressure ventilation without the use of PEEP results is a decrease in surfactant production, and the repeated cycling of the terminal airways from below critical opening pressure leads to cellular injury and inflammation (atelectatrauma). This results in alveolar collapse, atelectasis, interstitial edema, and elaboration of inflammatory mediators. The resulting atelectasis leads to a further reduction in lung compliance, which necessitates higher inspiratory pressures and further compromises surfactant production. Atelectatrauma leads to an increased diffusion barrier, which necessitates increased levels of mean airway pressure (Paw) and/or increased levels of inspired oxygen (FIO_2). The increase in FIO_2 may lead to oxidative injury and further cellular dysfunction. Early establishment of an appropriate FRC, administration of surfactant, use of CPAP or PEEP to avoid the repeated collapse and reopening of small airways (atelectatrauma), avoidance of overinflation caused by using supraphysiologic tidal volumes (volutrauma), and avoidance of use of more oxygen than is required (oxidative injury) all are important to achieve the best possible outcome and long-term health of patients.[14]

The level of PEEP at which static lung compliance is maximized has been termed *best* or *optimum PEEP.* This is the level of PEEP at which O_2 transport (cardiac output $\times$ O_2 content) is greatest. If the level of PEEP is raised above the optimal level, dynamic compliance decreases rather than increasing.[15] One hypothesis for this reduction in dynamic lung compliance is that some alveoli become overexpanded due to the increase in pressure, which puts them on the "flat" part of the compliance curve (see Fig. 2-3, region C). Therefore, despite the additional pressure delivered, little additional volume is obtained, so the contribution of this "population" of alveoli may be sufficient to reduce the total lung compliance. It has been shown that dynamic lung compliance was reduced in patients with congenital diaphragmatic hernia (CDH) even though some of the infants had normal thoracic gas volumes.[11] The reduction in dynamic lung compliance in patients with CDH is attributed to overdistention of the lung remnant into the "empty" hemithorax after surgical repair of the defect. After repair of CDH, infants have a reduction in the total number of alveoli and have areas of pulmonary emphysema that persist at least into early childhood.[16] Based on available evidence, in the treatment of CDH it seems prudent to avoid rapid re-expansion and to attempt to avoid overexpansion by allowing adequate time for exhalation.

Clinicians must be alert to any sudden improvement in lung compliance in infants receiving assisted ventilation (i.e., immediately after administration of surfactant). If inspiratory pressure is not reduced as compliance improves, cardiovascular compromise may develop because proportionately more pressure is transmitted to the mediastinal structures as lung compliance improves. The distending pressure that was appropriate prior to the compliance change may become excessive and lead to alveolar overexpansion and ultimately air leak.[17] Because the chest wall is compliant in the premature infant, use of paralytic agents to reduce chest wall impedance should not be necessary. Little pressure is required to expand the chest wall of a premature infant (see Fig. 2-2, "Chest Wall Curve"). In studies investigating the use of paralytic agents in premature infants at risk for pneumothoraces, no change in lung compliance or resistance was demonstrated after 24 or 48 hours of paralysis, and many of the infants studied required more rather than less ventilator support after paralysis.[18,19] One study demonstrated a modest improvement in chest wall compliance after paralysis, but the lung compliance was 20- to 30-fold greater than chest wall compliance; therefore, paralysis would not likely contribute to reducing the need for elevated distending pressures.[20] Paralysis should be restricted to larger infants who are "fighting the ventilator" or are actively expiring against it despite the use of sedation and/or analgesia.[18] Many centers use synchronized intermittent mandatory ventilation or assist/control modes of ventilation in these situations and attempt to avoid paralysis whenever possible.

Resistance

Resistance is the result of friction. Viscous resistance is the resistance generated by tissue elements moving past one another. Airway resistance is the resistance that occurs between moving molecules in the gas stream and between these moving molecules and the wall of the respiratory system (e.g., trachea, bronchi, bronchioles). The clinician must be aware of both types of resistance, as well as the resistance to flow as gas passes through the ventilator circuit and the endotracheal tube. In infants, viscous resistance may account for as much as 40% of total pulmonary resistance.[21] The relatively high viscous resistance in the newborn is due to increases in tissue density (i.e., a low ratio of lung volume to lung weight) and the relative amount of pulmonary interstitial fluid. This increase in pulmonary interstitial fluid is especially prevalent after cesarean section delivery[22] and in conditions such as transient tachypnea of the newborn or delayed absorption of fetal lung fluid. A reduction in tissue and airway resistance has been shown after administration of furosemide.[23] Airway resistance (R) is defined as the pressure gradient (P1 – P2) required to move gas through the airways at a constant flow rate ($\dot{V}$ or volume per unit time). The standard formula is as follows:

$$R = (P1 - P2) / \dot{V}$$

Airway resistance is determined by flow rate, length of the conducting airways, viscosity and density of the gases, and inside diameter of the airways. This is true for both laminar and turbulent flow conditions.

Time Constant

The time constant of a patient's respiratory system is a measure of how quickly his or her lungs can inflate or deflate or how long it takes for alveolar and proximal airway pressures to equilibrate. Passive exhalation depends on the elastic recoil of the lungs and chest wall. Because the major force opposing exhalation is airway resistance, the expiratory time constant (Kt) of the respiratory system is directly related to both lung compliance (C_L), which is the inverse of elastic recoil, and airway resistance (R):

$$Kt = C_L \times Raw.$$

The time constants of the respiratory system are analogous to those of electrical circuits. One time constant of the respiratory system is defined as the time it takes the alveoli (capacitor) to discharge 63% of its tidal volume (V_T); (electrical charge) through the airways (resistor) to the mouth or ventilator (electrical) circuit. By the end of three time constants, 95% of the V_T is discharged. When this model is applied to a normal newborn with a compliance of 0.005 L/cm H_2O and a resistance of 30 cm H_2O/L/sec, one time constant = 0.15 second and three time constants = 0.45 second.[24] In other words, 95% of the last V_T should be emptied from the lung within 0.45 second of when exhalation begins in a spontaneously breathing infant. In a newborn infant receiving assisted ventilation, the exhalation valve of the ventilator would have to be open for at least that length of time.

The concept of time constant provides a framework for understanding the interactions between the elastic and resistive forces and how the mechanical properties of the respiratory system work together to modulate the volume and distribution of ventilation. A working knowledge of time constants aids the clinician in choosing the safest and most effective ventilator settings for an individual patient at a particular point in the course of a specific disease process that necessitates the use of assisted ventilation.

Patients are at risk for incomplete emptying of previously inspired breath when their lung condition involves an increase in airway resistance without a reduction in lung compliance.

They also are at risk when the pattern of assisted ventilation does not allow sufficient time for exhalation, that is, the lungs have an abnormally long time constant, or there is a mismatch between the time constant of the respiratory system (time constant of the patient + that of the endotracheal tube + that of the ventilator circuit) and the expiratory time setting on the ventilator. In these situations, the end result is gas trapping. This gas trapping is accompanied by an increase in lung volume and a build-up of pressure in the alveoli and distal airways. Weigl[25] termed this pressure build-up *inadvertent PEEP.*

Important clinical and radiographic signs of gas trapping and inadvertent PEEP include (1) radiographic evidence of overexpansion (e.g., increased anteroposterior diameter of the thorax, flattened diaphragms below the ninth posterior ribs, intercostal pleural bulging; (2) decreased chest wall movement during assisted ventilation; (3) hypercapnia that does not respond to an increase in ventilator rate; and (4) signs of cardiovascular compromise, such as mottled skin color, a decrease in arterial blood pressure, an increase in central venous pressure, or the development of metabolic acidosis.

The time constant should be considered whenever the lung condition for which a baby is receiving assisted ventilation involves increased compliance (with normal or abnormal airway resistance) or increased airway resistance (with or without normal compliance). For example, RDS is associated with decreased compliance but usually normal airway resistance. This means that the time constant of the respiratory system is extremely short. Equilibration or equalization of the airway and alveolar pressures occurs very quickly (i.e., early in the inspiratory cycle). Reynolds[26] estimated that the time constant in RDS may be as short as 0.05 second. This means that 95% of the pressure applied to the airway is delivered to the alveoli within 0.15 second. Ventilator adjustments that decrease the risk of gas trapping and inadvertent PEEP include (1) decreasing PIP (on a pressure-preset ventilator), (2) reducing V_T (on a volume-preset ventilator), (3) shortening the I-time (Ti), and (4) increasing PEEP. Increasing PEEP has been shown to reduce inadvertent PEEP in a lung model.[27] However, overexpansion of the lung with PEEP decreases dynamic compliance, as previously described. Decreased compliance results in a short time constant and thus fast lung emptying. Proximal airway PEEP level does not indicate the level of alveolar PEEP, nor does it demonstrate the occurrence of alveolar gas trapping. Even under conditions of zero proximal airway PEEP, alveolar PEEP levels and the degree of gas trapping may be dangerously high if the baby has compliant lungs, increased airway resistance, or both (i.e., a prolonged time constant).

Although it is useful clinically to think of the infant's respiratory system as having a single compliance and a single resistance, we know this is not really the case. The resistance and compliance values we obtain from pulmonary function measurements are essentially weighted averages for the respiratory system. There are populations of respiratory subunits with a range of discrete compliance and resistance values, whereas what we measure at the airway are averaged values for those populations of subunits.

Flow Rate

Average values for airway resistance in normal, spontaneously breathing newborn infants are between 20 and 30 cm $H_2O/L/sec$,[28] and these values can increase dramatically in disease states. Nasal airway resistance makes up approximately two thirds of total upper airway resistance; the glottis and larynx contribute less than 10%; and the trachea and first four or five generations of bronchi account for the remainder (Fig. 2-8).[29] Average peak inspiratory and expiratory flow rates in spontaneously breathing term infants are approximately 2.9 and 2.2 L/min, respectively.[28] Maximal peak inspiratory and expiratory flow rates average about 9.7 and 6.4 L/min, respectively.[30] The range of flow rates generated by spontaneously breathing newborns (including term and premature infants) is approximately 0.6 to 9.9 L/min. Turbulent flow is produced in standard infant endotracheal tubes whenever flow rates exceed approximately 3 L/min through 2.5-mm internal diameter (ID) tubes or 7.5 L/min through 3.0-mm ID tubes.[31] Flow rates that exceed these critical levels produce disproportionately large increases in airway resistance. For example, increasing the rate of flow through a 2.5-mm ID endotracheal tube from 5 to 10 L/min raises airway resistance from 32 to 84 cm $H_2O/L/sec$, more than twice its original value.[31]

Flow conditions are likely to be at least partially turbulent ("transitional") when ventilator flow rates exceed 5 L/min in infants intubated with 2.5-mm ID endotracheal tubes or when rates exceed 10 L/min in infants with 3.0-mm ID endotracheal tubes. With turbulent flow, resistance increases exponentially. Because resistance is measured as a pressure drop, when flow is turbulent the pressure delivered to the baby's alveoli is less than indicated on the pressure manometer at the airway. The volume delivered is also less than would be expected, especially if the

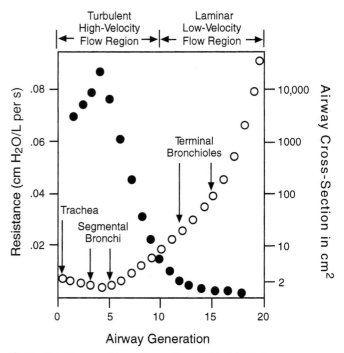

Figure 2-8. Airway resistance to gas flow *(solid circles)* is inversely proportional to the total cross-sectional area of the airways *(open circles)*. Approximately 80% of airway resistance is encountered in the first few generations of bronchi, where total cross-sectional area is the least. Pressure decreases exponentially in regions of high-velocity turbulent flow, whereas pressure decreases more linearly in regions of low-velocity laminar flow further out in the periphery. (Reprinted and adapted by permission of the publisher from *The Pathway for Oxygen: Structure and Function in the Mammalian Respiratory System* by Edward R. Weibel, pp. 285–286, 295, Cambridge, Mass.: Copyright © 1984 by the President and Fellows of Harvard College.)

ventilator rate is high or the I-time is short. The resistance produced by infant endotracheal tubes is equal to or higher than that in the upper airway of a normal newborn infant breathing spontaneously. The increased resistance due to the endotracheal tube poses little problem as long as the baby receives pressure support from the ventilator. The machine can generate the additional pressure needed to overcome the resistance due to the endotracheal tube. However, when the infant is being weaned from the ventilator or if the infant is disconnected from the ventilator with the endotracheal tube still in place, the infant may not be capable of generating sufficient effort to overcome the increase in upper airway resistance created by the endotracheal tube.[32] LeSouef et al.[33] measured a significant reduction in respiratory system expiratory resistance after extubation in premature newborn infants recovering from a variety of respiratory illnesses, including RDS, pneumonia, and transient tachypnea of the newborn.

Airway or Tube Length

The shorter the tube, the lower the resistance. Shortening a 2.5-mm ID endotracheal tube from 14.8 cm (full length) to 4.8 cm reduces the flow resistance in vitro to essentially that of a full-length tube of the next size (3.0-mm ID endotracheal tube). Shortening the length of a 3.0-mm ID endotracheal tube by 10 cm makes the tube comparable to a full-length, 3.5-mm ID endotracheal tube in terms of flow resistance. These relationships are consistent for the range of flows generated by spontaneously breathing newborns.[34]

Airway or Tube Diameter

In a single-tube system the radius of the tube is the most significant determinant of resistance. When flow is laminar, resistance can be described by Poiseuille's Law:

$$R = L / r^4.$$

Resistance is a function of the tube length divided by the radius of the tube to the fourth power. Therefore, reduction in the radius by half results in a 16-fold increase in the driving pressure required to maintain a given flow. In a multiple tube system, like the human lung, resistance is dependent on the total cross-sectional area of all of the tubes. Although the individual

bronchi decrease in diameter as they extend toward the periphery, the total cross-sectional area of the airway (see Fig. 2-8) increases dramatically.[35] Because resistance increases to the fourth power as the airway is narrowed, even mild airway constriction can cause significant increases in resistance to flow. This effect is exaggerated in newborn infants compared to adults because of the narrowness of the infant's airways. Resistance during inspiration is less than resistance during expiration because the airways dilate upon inspiration (Fig. 2-9). This is true even though gas flow during inspiration usually is greater than that during expiration. There is an inverse, nonlinear relationship between airway resistance and lung volume, because airway size increases as FRC increases. Any process that results in an increase in lung volume (other than gas trapping caused by airway obstruction) should in theory reduce resistance to airflow. Any processes that cause a reduction in lung volume, such as atelectasis or restriction of expansion, should result in increases in airway resistance. At extremely low volumes, resistance approaches infinity because the pressure drops below the critical closing pressure as residual volume is approached (see Fig. 2-2).

The preponderance of evidence suggests that application of PEEP and CPAP decreases airway resistance.[36–38] Endotracheal tube resistance is of considerable clinical importance. It has been shown that successful extubation is accomplished more often in infants coming directly off of intermittent mandatory ventilation (IMV) than after a 6-hour pre-extubation trial of endotracheal CPAP.[32] Nasal CPAP circuit design and the means by which nasal CPAP is attached to the patient are the most important determinants of CPAP success or failure.[39]

Viscosity and Density

Gas viscosity is negligible in the determination of airway resistance. However, gas density can be of clinical significance. The relationship between airway resistance and the density of the gas in turbulent flow is directly proportional and linear. Decreasing the density of the gas by two thirds, such as occurs when a heliox mixture of 80% helium and 20% O_2 is administered, reduces airway resistance to one third compared to that when room air is breathed. Heliox can be useful for reducing upper airway resistance (and work of breathing) in patients with obstructive disorders such as laryngeal edema, tracheal stenosis, and CLD.[40] Gas density is influenced by barometric

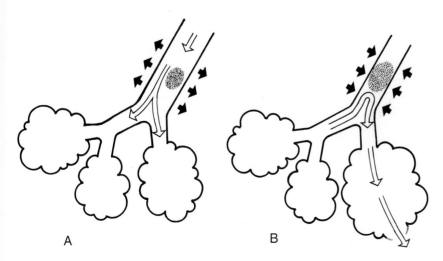

A   B

Figure 2-9. Air trapping behind particulate matter (e.g., meconium) in an airway, which leads to alveolar overexpansion and rupture. This illustrates the so-called ball-valve mechanism, in which tidal gas passes the particulate matter on inspiration, when the airways naturally dilate *(A)*, but does not exit on expiration, when the airways naturally constrict *(B)*. (From Harris TR, Herrick BR: Pneumothorax in the Newborn. Tucson, AZ, Biomedical Communications, Arizona Health Sciences Center, 1978.)

pressure, so airway resistance is slightly decreased at high altitudes.

Work of Breathing

Breathing requires the expenditure of energy. For gas to be moved into the lungs, force must be exerted in order to overcome the elastic and resistant forces of the respiratory system.

Work of breathing = Pressure (force) × Volume (displacement)

Work of breathing is the force generated to overcome the frictional resistance and static elastic forces that oppose lung expansion and gas flow into and out of the lungs during respiration. The workload depends on the elastic properties of the lung and chest wall, airway resistance, V_T, and respiratory rate. Approximately two thirds of the work of spontaneous breathing is to overcome the static elastic forces of the lungs and thorax (tissue elasticity and compliance). Approximately one third of the total work is to overcome the frictional resistance produced by the movement of gas and tissue components (air flow and viscous).[41] In healthy infants exhalation is passive. A portion of the energy generated by the inspiratory muscles is stored (as potential energy) in the lungs' elastic components; this energy is returned during exhalation. If the energy required to overcome resistance to flow during expiration exceeds the amount of elastic energy stored during the previous inspiration, work must be done not only during inspiration but also during expiration; thus, exhalation is no longer entirely passive.

In infants, energy expenditure correlates with oxygen consumption. Resting oxygen consumption is elevated in infants with RDS and CLD.[42] Mechanical ventilation reduces oxygen consumption by decreasing the infant's work of breathing.[13,43] Work of breathing is illustrated in a dynamic pressure-volume loop (see Fig. 2-7). Pressure changes during breathing can be measured with an intraesophageal catheter or balloon, and volume changes can be measured simultaneously with a pneumotachograph. During inspiration (ascending limb of the loop) and expiration (descending limb of the loop), both elastic and frictional resistance must be overcome by work. If only elastic resistance needed to be overcome, the breathing pattern would follow the compliance line; however, because airway resistance and tissue viscous resistance must also be overcome, a loop is formed (hysteresis). The areas ABCA and ACDA in Figure 2-7 represent the inspiratory work and the expiratory work, respectively, performed to overcome frictional resistance. The area ABCEA represents the total work of breathing during a single breath.

The diaphragm is responsible for the majority of the workload of respiration. The most important determinant of the diaphragm's ability to generate force is its initial position, the length of its muscle fibers at the beginning of a contraction. The longer and more curved the muscle fibers of the diaphragm, the greater the force the diaphragm can generate. In situations in which the lung is hyperinflated (overdistended), the diaphragm is flattened and thus at a mechanical disadvantage.

The application of PEEP or CPAP (continuous distending pressure, or CDP) may reduce the work of breathing for an infant whose breathing is on the initial flat part of the compliance curve secondary to atelectasis (see Fig. 2-3, region A). In this situation, CDP should reduce the work of breathing by increasing FRC and bringing breathing to a higher level on the pressure-volume curve where the compliance is lower (see Fig. 2-3, region B). Reductions in respiratory work with the application of CDP have been shown in newborns recovering from RDS[44] and in babies after surgery for congenital heart disease.[37] If the lung already is overinflated, increasing CDP will not result in a decrease in the work of breathing (see Fig. 2-3, region C). Alveolar overdistention due to excessive CDP may be accompanied by an increase in $Paco_2$ (indicating decreased alveolar ventilation) and a decrease in Pao_2, despite an increase in FRC.[36,45]

GAS TRANSPORT

Mechanisms of Gas Transport

Ventilation or gas transport involves the movement of gas by convection or bulk flow through the conducting airways and then by molecular diffusion into the alveoli and pulmonary capillaries. This makes possible gas exchange (oxygen [O_2] uptake and carbon dioxide [CO_2] elimination) that matches the minute-by-minute metabolic needs of the patient. The driving force for gas flow is the difference in pressure at the origin and destination of the gases; for diffusion, it is the difference in the concentrations between gases in contiguous spaces. Gas flows down a pressure gradient and diffuses down a concentration gradient. The predominant mechanism of gas transport by convection is bulk flow, whereas the predominant mechanism of gas transport by diffusion is Brownian motion.

Ventilation of the alveoli is an intermittent process that occurs only during inspiration, whereas gas exchange between alveoli and pulmonary capillaries occurs throughout the respiratory cycle. This is because a portion of gas remains in the lungs at the end of exhalation (FRC); the remaining gas provides a source for ongoing gas exchange and maintains approximately equal O_2 and CO_2 tensions in both the alveoli and the blood returning from the lungs.

During spontaneous breathing, inspiration is achieved through active contraction of the respiratory muscles. A negative pressure is produced in the interpleural space, a portion of which is transmitted via the parietal and visceral pleura through the pulmonary interstitial space to the lower airways and alveoli. A pressure gradient between the outside atmospheric pressure and the airway and alveoli pressures results in gas flowing down the pressure gradient into the lungs (Fig. 2-10). Interpleural pressure is more negative than alveolar pressure, which is more negative than mouth and atmospheric pressures.

When an infant receives negative-pressure ventilation, pressure is decreased around the infant's chest and abdomen to supplement the negative-pressure gradient used to move gas into the lungs. During positive-pressure ventilation the upper airway of the infant (Fig. 2-11) is connected to a device that generates a positive-pressure gradient down which gas can flow during inspiration. The pressure in the ventilator circuit and in the upper airway is greater than alveolar pressure, which is greater than interpleural pressure, which is greater than atmospheric pressure.

Expiration [except in high-frequency oscillatory ventilation (HFOV)] is a passive event. Part of the energy produced by the muscles during inspiration is stored in the respiratory system's elastic components. At end-inspiration, the respiratory muscles relax or the exhalation valve opens, and the lungs and chest

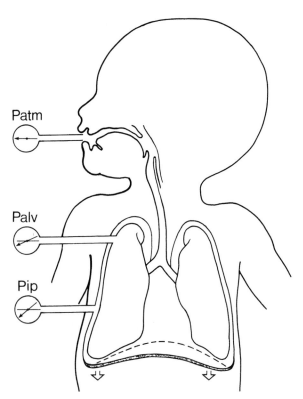

Figure 2-10. Negative-pressure gradient produced upon inspiration by the descent of the diaphragm in a spontaneously breathing infant. Pressures are measured in the interpleural space (Pip), in the alveoli (Palv), and at opening of mouth or atmosphere (Patm). Pip < Palv < Patm.

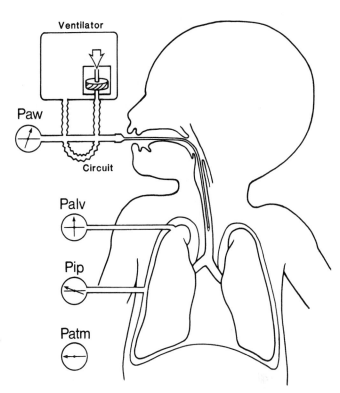

Figure 2-11. Positive-pressure gradient produced by a ventilator. Pressures are measured in the airway (Paw) and as shown in Figure 2-10. Paw > Palv > Pip > Patm. Abbreviations as in Figure 2.10.

wall return to their resting state due to elastic recoil. Exhalation is passive in that no active muscular work is performed during expiration under normal circumstances.

The amount of gas inspired in a single spontaneous breath or delivered through an endotracheal tube during a single cycle of the ventilator is called the *tidal volume* (VT). VT in milliliters (mL) multiplied by the number of breaths per minute or respirator frequency (f) is called *minute ventilation* (V_E):

$$V_E = V_T \times f.$$

The portion of the incoming VT that fails to arrive to the level of the respiratory bronchioles and alveoli but instead remains in the conducting airways occupies the space known as the *anatomic dead space*. Another portion of VT may be delivered to unperfused alveoli. Because gas exchange does not take place in these units, the volume that they constitute is called *alveolar dead space*. Together, anatomic dead space and alveolar dead space make up *total* or *physiologic dead space* (VDS). The ratio of dead space to tidal volume (VDS/VT) defines *wasted ventilation,* which reflects the proportion of tidal gas delivered that is not involved in actual gas exchange.

A number of mechanisms of gas transport other than bulk convection and molecular diffusion have been described. They include axial convection, radial diffusive mixing, coaxial flow, viscous shear, asymmetrical velocity profiles, and pendelluft effect.[46]

Henderson et al.[47] noted that during rapid shallow breathing or panting in dogs, adequate gas exchange was maintained even though the volume of gas contained in each "breath" was less

than that of the physiologic dead space. They hypothesized that low-volume inspiratory pulses of gas moved down the center of the airway as axial spikes and that these spikes dissipated at the end of each "breath" (Fig. 2-12). The faster the inspiratory pulse, the further it penetrated down the conducting airway and the more expansive the boundary of mixing between the molecules of the incoming gas (with high O_2 and low CO_2) and the outgoing gas (with high CO_2 and low O_2). During this kind of breathing, both convection and molecular diffusion are enhanced or facilitated. The provision of a greater interface or boundary area between inspiratory and expiratory gases with their different O_2 and CO_2 partial pressures is known as *radial diffusive mixing*. During high-frequency ventilation (HFV), with each inspiration gas molecules near the center of the airway flow further than those adjacent to the walls of the airway, because the gas traveling down the center of the airway is exposed to less resistance. Figure 2-13A illustrates the velocity profiles using vectors that demonstrate the intra-airway flow patterns of gas molecules in a representation of the airway during inspiration. At the end of the inspiratory phase, the contour of the leading edge of the inspired gas is cone shaped (Fig. 2-13B), having a larger diffusion interface with the preexisting gas than would be present if the leading edge was disk shaped. During exhalation, the velocity profiles are more uniform across the entire lumen rather than being cone shaped (Fig. 2-13C).[48] The pulse of gas originally occupying the lumen of the airway is displaced to the right (i.e., toward the patient's alveoli), and an equal volume gas is displaced to the left (Fig. 2-13D). This occurs even though the net displacement of the piston during a cycle of HFOV is zero. The back-and-forth currents of gas recalculating through units of lung are called *pendelluft.*[46,49] This gas flow is produced because of local differences in airway resistance and lung compliance that are accentuated under conditions of high-velocity flow. This leads to regional differences in rates of inflation and deflation. "Fast units" with short time constants inflate and deflate more rapidly, emptying out into the conducting airways to be "inhaled" by "slow units" still in the process of filling (Fig. 2-14). These recalculating currents of gas flow within the lung result in more homogeneous gas mixing and exchange.

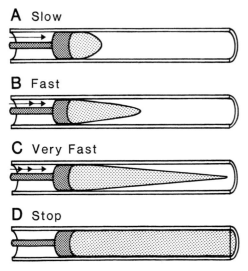

Fig. 2-12. Spike theory of panting or high-frequency ventilation. *A–C,* The quicker or more "energy dense" the puff (or inspiratory pulse), the sharper the spike and the further it extends into the airway. *D,* If the pulse is suddenly stopped at end-inspiration, mixing instantaneously occurs. (Modified from Henderson Y, Chillingworth FP, Whitney JL: The respiratory dead space. Am J Physiol 38:1, 1915.)

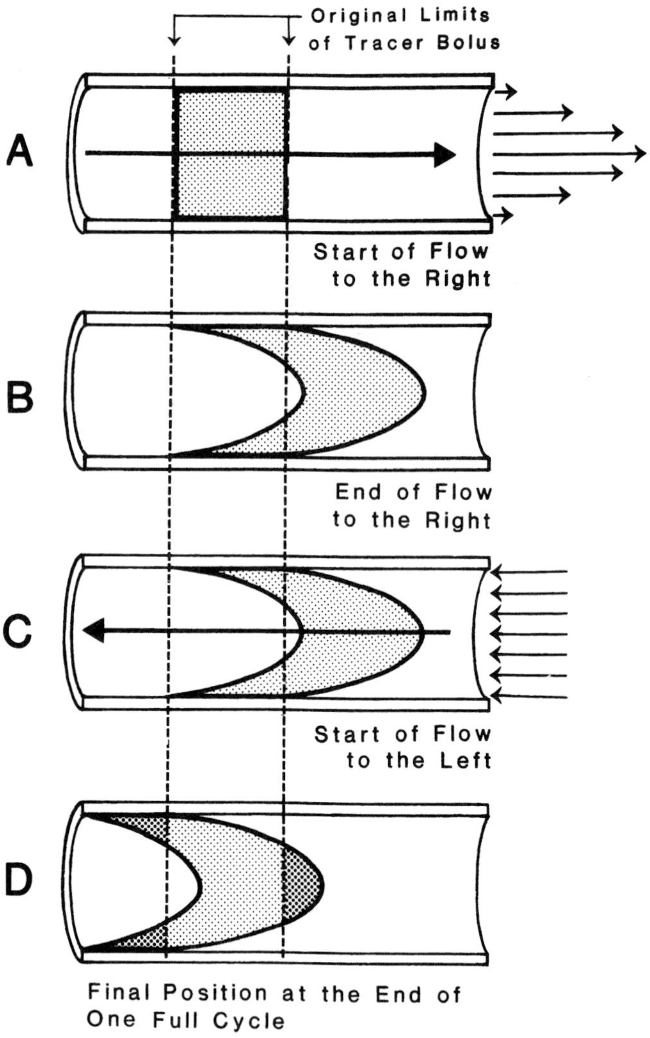

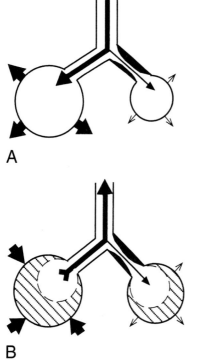

Figure 2-13. Viscous shear and inspiratory-to-expiratory velocity profiles associated with respiratory cycling. *A,* During inspiration or movement toward the right, the gas molecules of a cylindrical tracer bolus that are situated near the center of the tube travel further and faster than the gas molecules near the wall, as represented by the velocity profiles arrows at the right. *B,* At the end of the inspiratory half of the respiratory cycle, a paraboloid front has formed. *C,* During exhalation or movement toward the left, the velocity profiles are essentially uniform across the lumen. *D,* The end result after a complete respiratory cycle (with zero net directional flow) is displacement of axial gas to the right and wall gas to the left. (Modified with permission from Haselton FR, Scherer PW: Bronchial bifurcations and respiratory mass transport. Science 208:69, 1980. Copyright 1990 American Association for the Advancement of Science.)

Figure 2-14. Effects of different time constants on the uneven distribution of ventilation and the production of "pendelluft." *A,* On inspiration, the fast unit receives the majority of ventilation, whereas the slow unit fills slowly (owing to local increase in airway resistance). *B,* At the beginning of expiration, the slow unit may still be filling and actually "inspires" from the exhaling fast unit. These effects are accentuated at higher frequencies, with gas "pendeling" back and forth between neighboring units with inhomogeneity of time constants. (Modified from Otis AB, McKerrow CB, Bartlett RA, et al: Mechanical factors in distribution of pulmonary ventilation. J Appl Physiol 8:427, 1956.)

Original Limits of Tracer Bolus

A Start of Flow to the Right

B End of Flow to the Right

C Start of Flow to the Left

D Final Position at the End of One Full Cycle

OXYGENATION

Oxygen transport in the infant depends on the oxygen carrying capacity of the blood and the rate of blood flow. The concentration of oxygen in arterial blood is called *oxygen content* (CaO_2).

$$CaO_2 = (1.34 \times Hb \times SaO_2) + (0.003 \times PaO_2)$$

where Hb is hemoglobin concentration and SaO_2 is arterial oxygen saturation. The contribution of hemoglobin to oxygen content is described in the first term of the equation, which states that each gram of hemoglobin will bind 1.34 mL O_2 when fully saturated with oxygen. The second term of the equation describes the contribution of oxygen dissolved in the plasma. Oxygen is contained in the blood in two forms: (1) a small quantity dissolved in the plasma and (2) a larger quantity bound to hemoglobin. The total O_2 content of the blood is the sum of these two quantities. The dissolved portion of O_2 in blood is linearly related to PO_2, such that an increase in PO_2 is accompanied by an increase in O_2 content. Oxygen content increases 0.003 mL per 100 mL of blood with every 1 mm Hg increase in PO_2. For an infant breathing 21% O_2, the dissolved portion of the blood's O_2 content is only about 2% of the total. However, for a patient breathing 100% O_2, the dissolved portion of the blood's O_2 content is approximately 10% of the total. The hemoglobin-bound portion of O_2 content is nonlinear with respect to PO_2. This relationship is illustrated by the oxyhemoglobin dissociation curve, which is sigmoid (Fig. 2-15). The amount of O_2 that binds to hemoglobin increases quickly at low PO_2 values but begins to level off at PO_2 values greater than 40 mm Hg. After PO_2 exceeds 100 mm Hg, the curve flattens. Once the hemoglobin is saturated, further increases in PO_2 do not increase the content of bound oxygen. Oxygen binds reversibly to hemoglobin. Each hemoglobin molecule can bind up to four molecules of O_2, and each gram of hemoglobin can carry approximately 1.34 mL of O_2 when fully saturated. The total amount of O_2 carried by hemoglobin depends on the hemoglobin concentration of the blood and the bloods' oxygen saturation. Several factors affect hemoglobin's affinity for oxygen. These factors include the (1) percentages of fetal and adult hemoglobin present in the patient's blood; (2) amount of 2,3-diphosphoglycerate; (3) pH; (4) PCO_2; and (5) temperature. A greater percentage of fetal hemoglobin (as seen in premature infants), a decrease in 2,3-diphosphoglycerate content (as occurs in premature infants with RDS), alkalization of pH (e.g., after infusion of bicarbonate), a reduction in PCO_2 (secondary to hyperventilation), and a decrease of body temperature (as occurs during open heart surgery) all increase the O_2 affinity of hemoglobin (shift the oxyhemoglobin dissociation curve to the left without changing its shape). This means that the same level of hemoglobin saturation can be achieved at lower PO_2 values. In contrast, increased production of 2,3-diphosphoglycerate (as occurs in healthy newborns shortly after birth or with adaptation to high altitudes), a reduction of the percentage of fetal hemoglobin (e.g., after transfusion of adult donor blood to a newborn infant), a more acidic pH, CO_2 retention, and febrile illness each results in a reduction in O_2 affinity (shift of the oxyhemoglobin dissociation curve to the right) (Fig. 2-15).

Some shifts in the oxyhemoglobin dissociation curve promote O_2 uptake in the lungs, O_2 release at the tissue level, or

HEMOGLOBIN-OXYGEN DISSOCIATION CURVES

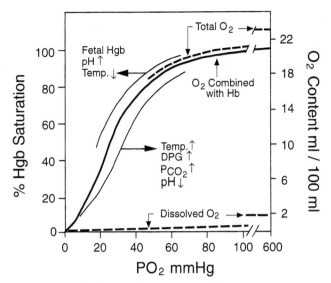

Figure 2-15. Nonlinear or S-shaped oxyhemoglobin curve and the linear or straight-line dissolved oxygen (O_2) relationships between O_2 saturation (SaO_2) and O_2 tension (PO_2). Total blood O_2 content is shown with division into a portion combined with hemoglobin and a portion physically dissolved at various levels of PO_2. Also shown are the major factors that change the O_2 affinity of hemoglobin and thus shift the oxyhemoglobin dissociation curve to either the left or the right (see also Appendix 10). (Modified from West JB: Respiratory Physiology: The Essentials, 2nd ed. Baltimore, Williams & Wilkins, 1979, pp. 71, 73.)

both. For example, when pulmonary arterial blood (which is rich in CO_2 and poor in O_2) passes through the lung's capillaries, it releases its CO_2; this raises local pH, which increases O_2 affinity. This allows more of the incoming O_2 to be bound to hemoglobin while plasma PO_2 is kept low, thus maximizing the concentration gradient down which O_2 diffuses from the alveoli into the pulmonary capillary plasma. Also, when systemic arterial blood (which is rich in O_2 and poor in CO_2) enters the tissue capillaries, it picks up CO_2 (which is in high concentration in the tissues). As a result, pH and O_2 affinity are lowered; this allows the hemoglobin to release its O_2 without significantly decreasing PO_2 and thus helps to maintain the concentration gradient down which O_2 diffuses into the tissues.[50]

SaO_2 as monitored clinically with pulse oximetry shows the percentage of hemoglobin in arterial blood that is saturated with O_2. The normal range of SaO_2 in newborn infants is different from that in adults; instead of SaO_2 levels of 95% or greater in adults, SaO_2 levels of 88% to 92% may be adequate for newborns. This is because the hemoglobin saturation curve is shifted to the left due to the high percentage of fetal hemoglobin in the infant's blood. This means that the baby has a higher PaO_2 at any given level of SaO_2. Generally the O_2 demands of most extremely premature infants can be met by maintaining PaO_2 levels just above 50 mm Hg or SaO_2 levels just above 88%.[51]

The O_2 content of the blood is only one of a number of important factors that the clinician must keep in mind. Others include (1) myocardial contractility; (2) heart rate and stroke volume (cardiac output); (3) mean systemic blood pressure and peripheral vascular resistance; and (4) venous return to the heart. These cardiovascular parameters demand the clinician's constant attention because assisted ventilation may have adverse effects on cardiac output, venous return, and pulmonary blood flow. The partial pressure of O_2 in arterial blood (PaO_2) is the amount of O_2 physically dissolved in the arterial blood plasma and is expressed in millimeters of mercury (mm Hg) or in torr. PaO_2 is measured directly as part of blood gas analysis. PaO_2 is a useful indicator of the degree of O_2 uptake through the lungs. The fraction of inspired O_2 (FIO_2) is the proportion of O_2 in the inspired gas. FIO_2 is measured directly with an O_2 analyzer and is expressed as a percentage (e.g., 60% O_2) or in decimal form (e.g., 0.60 O_2). The FIO_2 in room air is 0.21. The partial pressure of O_2 in alveolar gas (PAO_2) is the amount of O_2 present in the gas mixture delivered to the alveoli. PAO_2 relates directly to the number of O_2 molecules available for diffusion into the pulmonary capillary blood. To calculate the absolute amount of O_2 in alveolar gas, we use the alveolar gas equation:

$$PAO_2 = (\text{Barometric pressure} - \text{Partial pressure of water vapor}) \times FIO_2.$$

At sea level, the alveolar gas equation for breathing room air is as follows:

$$PAO_2 = (760 - 47) \times 0.21.$$

PAO_2 is approximately 150.

This value does not represent the exact quantity of oxygen arriving at the alveoli because the gas on its way to the alveoli mixes with CO_2 in an amount that is dependent upon the degree of alveolar ventilation. Because the sum of the partial pressures of all gases within the alveoli must remain the same (i.e., equal to barometric pressure), when PCO_2 increases, PO_2 must decrease (and vice versa). The partial pressure of CO_2 in the alveoli, or $PACO_2$, is nearly identical to the amount of CO_2 physically dissolved in the arterial blood, or $PaCO_2$. One additional correction factor must be used. This is called the *respiratory quotient,* which is the ratio of CO_2 excretion to O_2 uptake. The respiratory quotient ranges from approximately 0.8 to slightly greater than 1.0, depending on diet. A high-carbohydrate diet raises the respiratory quotient, thus decreasing CO_2 production. Generally, with a typical diet more O_2 is consumed than CO_2 is eliminated, yielding a respiratory quotient of about 0.8. The alveolar air equation allows for an accurate calculation of PAO_2 as follows:

$$PAO_2 = [(\text{Barometric pressure} - \text{Partial pressure of water vapor}) FIO_2] \times PACO_2 / R,$$

where R is the respiratory quotient.

It is important to remember that $PACO_2$ is decreased by hyperventilation and that the decrease in $PACO_2$ is matched by an equal increase in PAO_2. Barometric pressure varies with weather conditions and altitude. To demonstrate the effect of altitude on the absolute amount of oxygen available at the alveolar level, let us consider an infant with $PACO_2$ of 40 mm Hg and respiratory quotient of 0.8 who is breathing room air in Denver, Colorado, which is located 5280 feet above sea level and has an average barometric pressure of approximately 600 mm Hg. Subtracting 47 mm Hg from 600 mm Hg yields 553 mm Hg, which, when multiplied by 0.21, gives a value of around 116 mm Hg. After subtracting the dividend of 40 mm Hg/0.8, or 50 mm Hg, from 116 mm Hg, a PAO_2 value in Denver of only

66 mm Hg is obtained (instead of the approximately 100 mm Hg that would be expected at sea level). Therefore, the infant has about one third less available oxygen in the alveoli when breathing room air in Denver compared to when breathing room air at sea level. It the infant was being treated with 100% oxygen ($FIO_2 = 1.0$), the relative deficit remains. In Denver, PAO_2 while breathing 100% oxygen would be about 503 mmHg, whereas at sea level PAO_2 would be about 663 mmHg.

Some blood gas derivatives are useful as clinical indicators of disease severity. They include the following:

1. Arterial-alveolar O_2 tension ratio (PaO_2/PAO_2, or the a/A ratio)
2. Alveolar-arterial O_2 gradient or difference ($PAO_2 - PaO_2$)
3. Oxygenation index $\left(\dfrac{PAW \times FIO_2}{PaO_2}\right)$

The oxygenation index factors in the pressure cost of achieving a certain level of oxygenation. An oxygenation index greater than 15 signifies severe respiratory compromise. An oxygenation index of 40 or more on multiple occasions indicates a mortality risk approaching 80%, which justifies the need for extracorporeal membrane oxygenation in most level III neonatal centers.[52]

Effects of Altering Ventilator Settings on Oxygenation

Oxygen uptake through the lungs can be increased by (1) increasing PaO_2 (increasing the pressure gradient), or by increasing the FIO_2 (increasing the concentration gradient); (2) optimizing lung volume (increasing the surface area for gas exchange); (3) maximizing pulmonary blood flow (preventing blood from flowing left-to-right through intracardiac or ductal shunts); and (4) optimizing ventilation-to-perfusion (V/Q) matching in all parts of the lung.

There are functionally three ventilator changes available to the clinician:

1. Alter FIO_2, PaO_2, or both.
2. Alter mean airway pressure (PAW).
3. Alter the pattern of ventilation (i.e., extent and duration of the various components of applied airway pressure).

Figure 2-16 is a graphic representation of the proximal airway pressure plotted against time during a ventilation cycle with a conventional ventilator. Control variables for conventional mechanical ventilation include the following:

1. Inspiratory flow
2. PIP
3. I-time (Ti)
4. PEEP
5. Rate (f)

Control variables for high-frequency jet ventilators are similar to those for conventional ventilation.

The control variables for HFOV are as follows:

1. MAP
2. ΔP (amplitude)
3. Frequency (expressed in Hertz)
4. I-time (%)

In order to compare HFV with conventional mechanical ventilation, a composite outcome variable called the *Fujuwara ratio* is useful.[53] It is expressed as $PaO_2/FIO_2/MAP$. This ratio is

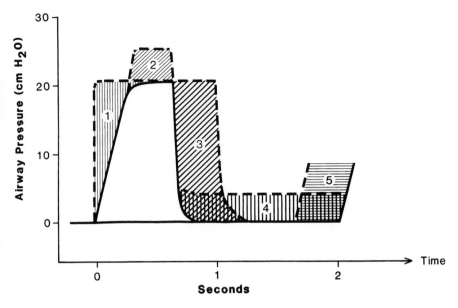

Figure 2-16. Five different ways to increase mean airway pressure: *(1)* increase inspiratory flow rate, producing a square-wave inspiratory pattern; *(2)* increase peak inspiratory pressure; *(3)* reverse the inspiratory-to-expiratory ratio or prolong the I-time without changing the rate; *(4)* increase positive end-expiratory pressure; and *(5)* increase ventilatory rate by reducing expiratory time without changing the I-time. (Modified from Reynolds EOR: Pressure waveform and ventilator settings for mechanical ventilation in severe hyaline membrane disease. Int Anesthesiol Clin 12:259, 1974.)

similar to the oxygenation index and relates oxygenation (corrected for different levels of ambient O_2 concentration) to MAP.

The clinician should formulate a hypothesis based on a physiologic rationale, make a ventilator change, and observe the response. This provides the clinician with feedback that either confirms or refutes the hypothesis. Ventilator changes may have adverse hemodynamic effects. In addition, because ventilators are powerful tools, they can cause significant damage if they are not used judiciously (Table 2-1). We must learn from experience (our own and that of others) and apply that knowledge when making ventilator setting changes during assisted ventilation of the newborn.

The effects of alterations in inspiratory flow rate on PaO_2 and right-to-left shunting (while holding frequency and V_T constant) were studied in seven newborn infants with RDS and two with meconium aspiration syndrome. The highest PaO_2 values and the lowest calculated right-to-left shunt values obtained coincided with the middle range of inspiratory flow rates (75–150 mL/sec). The investigators used a volume ventilator and maintained ventilator frequency constant; therefore they were altering the I/E ratio (calculated to range from 1:1–1:6.5) as they increased inspiratory flow rate in increments of 25 mL/sec over the machine's range of 50 to 200 mL/sec. The highest PaO_2 and the lowest calculated right-to-left shunt values coincided with I/E ratio settings in the range from 1:3 to 1:4.[54]

The effects of two different I/E ratio settings (1:2 and 2:1) on the degree of oxygenation in newborn infants receiving assisted ventilation from conventional pressure-preset ventilators for treatment of severe RDS have been studied.[55] The authors randomly assigned 69 premature infants to one or the other pattern of ventilation early in the course of their disease. Flow rates were held constant and frequency never exceeded 40 breaths per minute. All other settings, such as PIP, PEEP, and FIO_2, were adjusted to keep arterial blood gas values within specified ranges. Results showed that the study group patients (who were receiving the I/E ratio of 2:1) needed less time in O_2 concentrations greater than 60% than did the control group. They also required less time in PEEP greater than 3 cm H_2O. There were no differences in mortality or morbidity. The idea

TABLE 2-1. Cost Benefit Considerations When Applying Different Degrees of Various Components of Assisted Ventilation Therapy

Therapy	Cost	Benefit
High PIP	Barotrauma	Increase V_T Increase MAP
Low PIP	Atelectasis	Less barotrauma
High PEEP	Increase MAP Decrease V_T	Less barotrauma
Low PEEP	Atelectasis	Less barotrauma Increase V_T
High IMV rate	Increase shearing forces Increase airway resistance	Higher $\dot{V}_E$ Lower V_T
Low IMV rate	Larger airway distention	Less shearing forces Lower airway resistance
High FIO_2	Oxygen toxicity	Lower MAP
Low FIO_2	Higher MAP	Less O_2 toxicity
Long Ti	Higher MAP More pressure transmitted to terminal lung regions Inadvertent PEEP	Lower IMV Lower FIO_2
Short Ti	Lower MAP Higher IMV rates	Less pressure transmitted to terminal lung regions

FIO_2, fraction of O_2 or O_2 concentration expressed as a percentage; IMV, intermittent mandatory ventilation; MAP, mean airway pressure; PEEP, positive end-expiratory pressure; PIP, peak inspiratory pressure; Ti, inspiratory time; V_T, tidal volume.

of reverse I/E ratios as a means of improving oxygenation while lowering PIPs in newborns with severe RDS was first explored many years ago.[56] It was demonstrated that prolonging IT or reversing the I/E ratio leads to higher PaO_2 values and a reduction in calculated right-to-left shunting. It also was demonstrated that PEEP added to this method "acted synergistically" to increase PaO2 and reduce PaO_2.

Advocates for the use of short I-times argue that in situations in which the time constant is short (as in RDS), it takes very little time for pressure equilibration (or volume delivery), so a long IT will needlessly "expose" the lung to pressure, thus predisposing the airways to stretch injury and volutrauma. Remember that once the pressure reaches a plateau, no additional volume is being delivered to the lung. Using high-frequency jet ventilation (HFJV), it was shown that ventilation (CO_2 excretion) is improved by shortening It as long as Vt is kept constant. However, oxygenation varied only slightly and inconsistently with differing I/E ratios and inspiratory waveform shapes.[57,58] In newborn infants receiving HFJV for severe restrictive lung disease, it has been shown that oxygenation improves with shortening of It as long as PIP is held constant, even though MAP is thereby slightly reduced.[59,60]

The SensorMedics 3200 HFOV allows the operator to alter I/E ratios (although in practice this is rarely done). In general, most clinicians operate this high-frequency oscillator at an I/E ratio of 1:3 and do not attempt to improve oxygenation by altering this parameter. In a study in which saline lung-lavaged rabbits were treated with HFOV (SensorMedics 3200), random alteration of the I/E ratio between 2:1 and 1:2 produced no significant effect on oxygenation, ventilation, or cardiovascular function.[61] The likelihood of gas trapping is assumed to be reduced when an I/E ratio of 1:3 is used, although this claim was not directly addressed in the study by Courtney et al.[61]

Several studies have investigated the role of MAP on overcoming atelectasis and improving oxygenation.[53,62,63] It was demonstrated that MAP is the parameter that best correlates with improvement in oxygenation in premature lambs with RDS delivered by cesarean section.[63] Also, in human newborns it has been demonstrated that "the shape of the airway pressure wave per se does not appear to be particularly significant. Rather, the shape of the wave seems important only because of the changes it causes in MAP."[62] In most circumstances, MAP is the major determinant of oxygenation. This appears to hold true for conventional ventilation,[62,64,65] as well as for the various forms of HFV.[66–68] The specific alteration of pressure waveforms used to increase the MAP is a powerful means of achieving specific goals other than the improvement of oxygenation in the newborn infant receiving assisted ventilation. Table 2-2 lists the specific effects that can be achieved with alteration of the pressure waveform in various ways. Ventilator setting changes that contribute to increases in MAP during conventional ventilation produce different degrees of Pao$_2$ increase per unit increase of MAP. In an elegant study performed on 20 newborn infants treated with conventional mechanical ventilation for respiratory failure (due to RDS in 13), the changes in Pao$_2$ due to change in MAP were compared.[64] If an increase in Pao$_2$ is the primary objective and an increase in MAP is not contraindicated, then one can best achieve the goal first by increasing PEEP, then increasing PIP, and finally increasing the It. Increases in PEEP to greater than 5 or 6 cm H_2O produce decreasing effects (per unit of change) and in some cases even adverse effects on oxygenation.[69] Reports have been published about patients treated for RDS with conventional IMV or CPAP alone who had a paradoxical or reverse response to an increase in MAP.[70,71] These reports indicate that Pao$_2$ decreases instead of increasing in direct proportion to further increases in MAP. Nelson et al.[71] observed such a reverse effect of increased hypoxemia and right-to-left shunting (instead of improved oxygenation) in fewer than 3% of all newborn infants receiving CPAP for RDS or related respiratory distress. They postulated that the net effect of CPAP in these cases was overexpansion of portions of the lung leading to compression of capillaries around the alveoli, thus causing a reduction in blood flow to the

---

TABLE 2-2. Specific Effects of Different Ventilator Changes

Increasing PIP
1. Increases Vt and V̇e
2. Adds little to MAP unless combined with a reversal of I/E ratio or prolongation of Ti
3. Affects maximal dilation of alveoli already open, contributing to barotrauma
4. Opens alveoli with high critical opening pressures

Reversing the I/E Ratio (or Lengthening Ti While the Respiratory Rate Is Kept Constant)
1. Has little effect on Vt or V̇e beyond the minimum Ti needed to deliver Vt or reach desired PIP level (or both)
2. Can contribute on more than 1:1 basis to MAP, depending on original PIP and degree of reversal of I/E ratio
3. Allows expansion of atelectatic alveoli at lower PIP
4. May cause inadvertent PEEP, overinflation of alveoli, and reduction of pulmonary blood flow

Increasing Background CPAP or PEEP
1. Decreases Vt and V̇e unless significant atelectasis is overcome
2. Adds to MAP on a 1:1 basis
3. Holds open alveoli and terminal airways on end-expiration, thus raising closing volume and aiding in equal distribution of ventilation
4. Reduces likelihood of inadvertent PEEP

CPAP, continuous positive airway pressure; I/E ratio, inspiratory-to-expiratory ratio; Ti, inspiratory time; IMV, intermittent mandatory ventilation; MAP, mean airway pressure; PEEP, positive end-expiratory pressure; PIP, peak inspiratory pressure; V̇e, expiratory minute ventilation; Vt, tidal volume.

---

best-ventilated regions and shift of more blood flow to less well-ventilated areas.

A variety of modalities of HFV, applied alone or in tandem with IMV, including high-frequency positive-pressure ventilation,[72] HFOV,[73] HFJV,[74–78] and HFOV in combination with IMV,[79] have been shown to be effective in achieving comparable levels of gas exchange at lower PIPs and at the same or lower MAP in patients with intractable respiratory failure due to PIE. Significantly lower Pao$_2$/Fio$_2$/MAP values were demonstrated for the majority of patients who were switched from conventional mechanical ventilation to HFJV.[74,75,78]

A controlled study performed by Boros and Campbell[53] compared the effects on oxygenation of high-frequency, low-Vt ventilation with those of low-frequency, high-Vt ventilation using a volume-preset ventilator. The best arterial oxygenation was found to occur at the combination of settings that produced the highest MAP, once again confirming that oxygenation is predominantly related to MAP.[53] Rapid-rate IMV (otherwise known as *high-frequency positive-pressure ventilation*) has become a popular modality of ventilation for certain categories of severely ill neonatal patients. A higher rate means that less time is available for volume delivery and pressure equilibration; thus, Vt may be reduced accordingly. Also, the higher the frequency or inspiratory flow rate, the greater the proximal-to-distal airway pressure drop-off during inspiration due to the increased resistance produced by turbulent flow. Thus, the distal airways and alveoli may not be receiving the desired PIP (unless, again, It adjustments are made).[80] However, lengthening It to achieve better volume and pressure delivery to the distal airways and alveoli as the ventilator rate increases means shortening the exhalation time. When insufficient time is provided for exhalation, inadvertent PEEP may become a problem. Inadvertent PEEP and gas trapping could overexpand the lung to the point that pulmonary blood flow is compromised, thus reducing oxygenation and leading to CO_2 retention.

A study reported by Gonzalez et al.[81] demonstrates how serious inadvertent PEEP may become when rapid-rate IMV or high-frequency positive-pressure ventilation is used. Rabbits, whose lung mechanics are similar to those of human infants, were ventilated at rates of 30, 60, 90, and 120 breaths per minute, while I/E ratio and proximal distending airway pressures were kept constant at 1:2 and 17/2, respectively. In going from 30 to 60 breaths per minute under these conditions, both ventilation and oxygenation improved with only a minimal increase in tracheal pressure and lung volume (FRC). However, after the rate was increased to 120 breaths per minute, inadvertent PEEP developed, as manifest by an increase in FRC without an increase in PaO_2. Serious concern (based mainly on theoretic considerations) about the possibility of inadvertent PEEP and gas trapping has been expressed in relation to both HFOV[82] and HFJV.[24] In the case of HFOV, it is mainly the extremely high rates used (15–25 Hz, or 900–1500 cycles per minute) that have given cause for concern; in contrast, in the case of HFJV, it is the slower "passive" exhalation that worries clinicians. Kolton et al.[83] demonstrated that the mean lung volume of rabbits treated with HFOV was significantly greater than that of rabbits treated with conventional mechanical ventilation. Simon et al.[82] demonstrated that proximal MAP (as normally monitored in neonatology) is an underestimation of mean alveolar pressure. Actual measurement of inadvertent PEEP with the use of the proximal airway occlusion technique performed by Bryan and Slutsky[84] on lung-lavaged rabbits and on nine newborn infants with either RDS or persistent pulmonary hypertension (PPHN) being treated with HFOV revealed no significant trapping of air with rates of 15 to 25 Hz, which is the range usually applied to newborns.

VENTILATION

For gas exchange to occur efficiently, ventilation and perfusion must be well matched. Gas is distributed through the lung via the airways. The volume of gas moved into and out of the lung with each normal breath is the V_T. The largest volume that can be inhaled after a full exhalation is the vital capacity. The volume of gas that remains in the lung after a normal expiration is the FRC. The volume that remains in the lung after a maximal expiration is the residual volume. Residual volume and vital capacity together are the total lung capacity. The product of tidal volume and breathing frequency is the minute volume. Only a portion of our minute volume actually reaches the alveoli. The volume of the conducting airways is called the *anatomic dead space*. As respiratory rate and/or V_T are increased, minute ventilation increases. Alveolar ventilation increases even more than minute ventilation because the anatomic dead space remains constant. The dimensions of the airway system influence ventilation. With progressive dichotomous branching moving toward the lungs periphery, the overall cross-sectional area of the airways increases, so airflow velocity decreases, as does resistance.

The dimensions of the airways determine resistance to airflow; resistance falls toward the periphery of the lungs as the cross-sectional area increases. Differences in airway dimensions affect the distribution of air to the gas exchange units. The pulmonary arteries, like the airways, form a treelike structure. The pulmonary circulation is perfused by the entire cardiac output. Blood flow is determined by the pressure difference between pulmonary arteries and veins and by the vascular resistance. The pulmonary circulation is a low-pressure low-resistance system. The distribution of blood flow to the gas exchange units depends on the distribution of resistances, which are affected by contraction of the smooth muscle wall of the arteries. In hypoxia, resistance increases. There are regional differences in ventilation and perfusion. The dependent portions of the lung are better ventilated and better perfused than the upper portions. Hypoxic vasoconstriction shunts blood away from poorly ventilated acini, which helps to preserve V/Q matching. Ideally ventilation and perfusion are evenly matched, with a V/Q ratio of 1. When a lung or lung unit is relatively underventilated but normally perfused or is normally ventilated but overperfused, it is said to have a low V/Q (<1). When a lung unit is overventilated and normally perfused or is normally ventilated and underperfused, the resultant V/Q is high (>1).

With each breath, inspired gas is distributed by bulk flow to the distal airways, depending on the length of the conducting airways and the rate of flow through them. Gas flow rates are determined by local differences in driving pressure, flow resistance, tissue elasticity, and compliance. For spontaneous breathing, the driving pressure is the interpleural pressure swings generated during inspiration; during assisted ventilation, the transpulmonary pressure swings are produced by the forces exerted by the ventilator (see Figs. 2-10 and 2-11). In the healthy lung, local differences in interpleural or transpulmonary pressure are responsible for most of the regional differences in ventilation. In the sick lung, local differences in compliance and airway resistance (time constants) are the major contributors to uneven distribution of ventilation. The distribution of ventilation can be measured by having a patient breathe an inert radioactive gas such as xenon-133. Because xenon is inert and therefore is not reabsorbed, it simply fills the ventilated airways and alveoli. Scintillation counters can be used to locate and quantify the areas of ventilation. Bryan et al.[85] showed that the dependent lung regions in normal subjects have a greater regional volume expansion ratio (change in volume per unit of preinspiratory volume) than do the nondependent regions of lung. When a patient is upright, the basal regions of the lung are ventilated to a greater extent than are the apical regions. When a patient is supine, the basal and apical regions are ventilated to a similar extent, but the posterior (lowermost) regions are ventilated to a greater extent than the anterior regions (uppermost). It is important to remember, however, that at the end of a normal exhalation (at FRC) the volume in the uppermost regions of the lung is greater than that of the dependent regions (Fig. 2-17). This may appear contradictory, but these differences can be explained on the basis of regional interpleural pressure differences (Fig. 2-18). Interpleural pressure at end-expiration is more negative in the uppermost portions than in the dependent portions of the lung. Converting the interpleural pressures to transpulmonary pressures, one can plot a pressure-volume curve (lower right of Fig. 2-18). When the lungs are inflated starting from FRC, the dependent lung units will receive proportionately more of the inspired gas and the nondependent units will receive proportionally less as the height above the dependent units increases. The basilar units

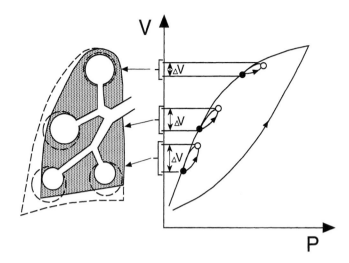

Figure 2-17. Although the upper parts of the lung are more expanded or hold a greater volume at end-expiration or the functional residual capacity level of expansion than do the lower parts, the latter show greater volume changes (i.e., ventilation changes) than do the former during tidal breathing. This occurs because the lower parts are situated on a steeper portion of the compliance or pressure-volume curve and achieve a greater ΔV per unit of ΔP. (Reprinted and adapted by permission of the publisher from *The Pathway for Oxygen: Structure and Function in the Mammalian Respiratory System* by Edward R. Weibel, pp. 285–286, 295, Cambridge, Mass.: Copyright © 1984 by the President and Fellows of Harvard College.)

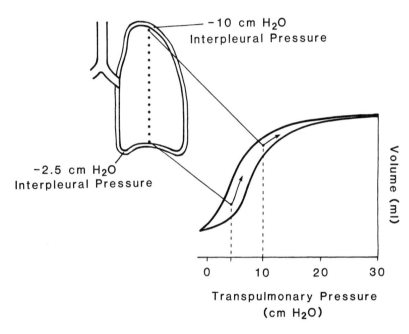

Figure 2-18. Effect of the interpleural pressure gradient up the lung upon the distribution of ventilation. The greatest negative pressure is at the top owing to the gravitational tug (weight) of the lung through its visceral pleura on the parietal pleura. Because the upper and lower areas are on different parts of the pressure-volume curve, different amounts of volume (ventilation) are achieved by the two areas given the same pressure change. The steeper compliance line for the lower area means a greater increase in volume per unit pressure change. (Modified from West JB: Respiratory Physiology: The Essentials, 2nd ed. Baltimore, Williams & Wilkins, 1979, p. 96.)

are stretched proportionately more than the higher units because they are operating on a steeper slope of the volume-pressure curve. Compliance increases progressively from the highest portion of the lung to the most dependent portion or from high starting lung volumes to lower volumes. At the beginning of a gradual inflation from FRC, the more dependent lung regions operate on a steeper part of the compliance curve than the less dependent regions, so ventilation is greater in the dependent regions.

Lung units that contain collapsed airways require large pressure changes before the airways open to permit gas transfer. These units are not ventilated as well as units in which the airways are patent from the start. Units with high resistance are ventilated poorly regardless of their position, because these units have low compliance for any given transpulmonary pressure. In newborn infants, airway closure may be present in the resting VT range, unlike older individuals in which pleural surface pressure at FRC is substantially subatmospheric throughout the lung, thus preventing airway closure while the lung is at operational volume.[86] Starting inspiration from a lung volume that is below

FRC or rest volume actually reverses the pattern of the distribution of ventilation.[87] If inspiration is started from a low level of lung volume, interpleural pressures are less negative overall (because elastic recoil is minimal at these low lung volumes) and even may be positive in the more dependent regions of the lung. When regional interpleural pressure exceeds (is more positive than) airway pressure, then airway closure occurs and no gas enters that segment for the first portion of inspiration or until regional interpleural pressure decreases to below airway pressure further along into inspiration. Thus, ventilation is reduced in dependent regions and is redirected to the upper lung regions, making them the better-ventilated areas; this is a reversal of the usual pattern. During assisted ventilation, inflation at end-inspiration is uniform, as evidenced by the observation of alveoli of equal size throughout the lung.[88] At end-expiration or FRC level, however, alveoli in the uppermost regions of the lung are found to have a volume fourfold that of alveoli at the base. Moderate levels of PEEP (<6 cm H_2O) increase FRC more in dependent regions than in upper regions of the lung because the former are less well expanded initially and are at a lower and more favorable point on their compliance curve. If significant basilar atelectasis pre-exists, the addition of PEEP or CPAP should help the most in the more dependent areas, opening them for improved regional ventilation. All forms of CDP favor uniformity of ventilation because they expand airways and thus lower resistance and because they prevent airway closure and gas trapping during forced exhalation.

Gravitational effects on the distribution of ventilation have been exploited in adult patients with or without ventilatory assistance who have unilateral lung disease[89] or who have undergone thoracotomy.[90] Improved gas exchange in these patients can be accomplished if they are positioned with their "good" side down. This technique increases ventilation to the dependent lung regions, which also receive relatively greater blood flow, resulting in better V/Q matching in the good lung. Body position affects ventilation and gas exchange in infants in the opposite way. When infants with unilateral lung disease are placed in the lateral decubitus position, the uppermost "good" lung receives a greater portion of ventilation than the dependent lung. This may be the case for infants with restrictive lung disease such as unilateral PIE. In cases of unilateral PIE, one sees ideal circumstances for the occurrence of airway closure in the "bad" lung when it is placed in the dependent position. In patients with unilateral tension PIE, interpleural pressure on the bad side already is elevated secondary to the presence of high (positive) interstitial pressure due to gas trapping outside of the terminal air spaces. Positioning patients with this side down adds the additional weight of the mediastinal structures, which causes the interpleural pressure to exceed local airway pressure and results in airway collapse. This airway closure in the dependent (bad lung) often facilitates resolution of unilateral PIE, while the infant's gas exchange needs are met by the non-dependent lung.[91,92]

The pattern of diaphragmatic motion plays a role in the distribution of ventilation in the newborn infant. When the diaphragm is paralyzed and the patient is supine, mechanical ventilation tends to produce greater motion of the superior than of the inferior portion of the diaphragm because the superior portion is less constrained by the abdominal contents and mediastinal structures. Therefore, there is preferential ventilation of the upper (anterior) segments of the lung.[93] Because perfusion still is likely to be better in the dependent regions secondary to gravitational effects, paralysis may result in V/Q mismatch with hypoxemia. The improvement in oxygenation achieved after adults with acute respiratory failure[94] or premature infants with respiratory insufficiency[95] are switched from the supine to the prone position is attributable to the enhancement of V/Q ratios (or an increase in ventilation to a level that better matches the existing degree of perfusion). In premature infants the prone position affords better distribution of ventilation throughout the lung, especially to the dependent regions that are better perfused.[95] The most common causes of uneven distribution of ventilation are conditions characterized by local differences in lung compliance, airway resistance, or both. If the patient is receiving assisted ventilation and is faced with local differences in either lung tissue elasticity or airway resistance, the distribution of gas delivered during the inspiratory phase is influenced by the mode of ventilation chosen. Local or regional (lobar) variations in compliance are determined by (1) local tissue water content; (2) presence or absence of surfactant; (3) presence of volume loss; or (4) presence of gas trapping or overexpansion. For example, pneumonia in one lung

area makes that lung less compliant than the normal lung; thus, the affected lung receives less volume per unit pressure than do the unaffected areas. Differences in distal airway resistance may be caused by local narrowing secondary to either obstruction or compression. For example, partial obstruction of a bronchus with meconium increases airway resistance and reduces alveolar ventilation in the area behind the partial obstruction (see Fig. 2-14). Many disease processes common in premature infants involve nonuniform regional compliance. During conventional mechanical ventilation, distribution of the inspired gas is largely controlled by regional variations in compliance. During HFV, the distribution of inspired gas is more dependent on the mechanical properties of the central airways and chest wall (resistance, inertance) and less so on the compliance of lung tissue. If inspiratory pressure is increased slowly (low inspiratory flow rate), the volume of gas delivered depends mainly on the compliance of the lung. If inspiratory pressure is increased quickly (high inspiratory flow rate), the distribution of gas depends mainly on local airway resistance. Consequently, the largest volumes are delivered to areas with the least resistance. This information is useful to the clinician trying to decide how best to ventilate a patient with meconium aspiration syndrome. One would like to be able to ventilate the patient's unobstructed lung regions while minimizing air trapping and overdistention in areas behind partially obstructed airways (see Fig. 2-9). One approach is to use rapid rates (high inspiratory flows) and short Its. In this fashion, only regions of the lung with short (or normal) time constants are given sufficient time for pressure equalization (volume delivery); thus, these areas are being ventilated while overdistention of lung regions with long time constants is avoided. In cases of pulmonary air leak (pneumothorax or bronchopleural fistula), a strategy incorporating short It and a high rate often is effective in decreasing the magnitude of the leak. Several reports have described the successful application of HFV in adults with airway disruption or bronchopleural fistulae[96,97] and in newborns with persistent air leaks through pneumothoraces.[98] In cases of PIE, the use of low rates and long Its might worsen the clinical situation. Because the lung regions with PIE have long time constants (due to elevated compliance and resistance), they could become further overdistended with this mode of ventilation. If ventilated with a conventional ventilator using high rates and short Its or if ventilated with an HFV, lung areas with long time constants would be less likely to become overdistended. As the PIE resolved and the compression effects on the surrounding lung tissue were alleviated, the distribution of ventilation would more homogeneous.[74,75] The clinician's choice of strategy and mode of ventilation can be important determinants of the distribution of ventilation, particularly in situations of nonhomogeneous lung disease.

During assisted ventilation, to minimize risk to the infant the minimal pressure required to achieve adequate gas flow and alveolar ventilation should be used. Enough distending pressure should be applied to prevent airway collapse and enough driving pressure should be applied so as to achieve an appropriate V_T.

Effects of Altering Ventilator Settings on Ventilation

During conventional ventilation, increasing V_T or increasing the ventilator rate are the two primary methods for increasing ventilation (enhancing CO_2 removal). The ventilator rate is controlled either directly or by altering the I/E ratio. V_T is controlled in different ways depending on the type of ventilator. With "volume ventilators," V_T can be manipulated directly. With time-cycled pressure-limited devices, adjustments that increase ΔP (difference between PIP and PEEP) generally will increase V_T. For example, if one increases PIP and leaves PEEP alone, V_T will increase. To control ventilation or CO_2 elimination during HFJV, the operator manipulates basically the same parameters in the same direction as during conventional ventilation.[57-59,99-103] Ventilation during HFOV is generally controlled by altering the amplitude, which controls the stroke length of the piston. The larger the amplitude, the greater the CO_2 removal. V_T delivered during HFOV is frequency dependent and decreases as the operating frequency increases.[104] This means that in the unusual clinical setting in which amplitude settings are maximized, frequency may need to be reduced if an improvement in ventilation is desired. At the other extreme, when V_T or amplitude settings are approaching minimum levels, operating frequency may have to be increased in order to decrease CO_2 removal.[105,106]

PERFUSION

Before delivery, only 8% to 10% of cardiac output flows to the lungs.[107] In the fetus, pulmonary vascular resistance is high and systemic vascular resistance is low. Most of the blood coming out of the fetal heart flows from right to left through the foramen ovale and ductus arteriosus, thus bypassing the lungs. Under normal circumstances after delivery, a rapid transition to the adult pattern of circulation occurs, after which virtually all right-sided heart output goes through the lungs, then the left side of the heart, and out the aorta. Key to this transition is a decrease in pulmonary vascular resistance and an increase in pulmonary blood flow preceding closure of the fetal shunts. Experiments carried out on fetal lambs[108-113] and investigations into the actions of certain mediators,[109,114-116] including nitric oxide (NO) (Table 2-3),[117,118] have demonstrated a number of factors that contribute to the decrease in pulmonary vascular resistance that occurs at birth. These include (1) expansion of

the lung with a gas,[111] (2) increase in Pao_2,[113] (3) increase in Pao_2,[112] (4) increase in pH,[110] and (5) elaboration of vasoactive substances such as bradykinin,[109] the prostaglandins [PGE_1, PGA_1, PGI_2 (prostacyclin),[114,115] and PGD_2[116]], and endothelium-derived relaxing factor,[117] which subsequently was shown to be the gas NO.[118] Blood flow through the pulmonary circuit is directly proportional to the pressure gradient across the pulmonary vessels and the total cross-sectional area of the vessels that make up the pulmonary vascular bed. Blood flow is inversely proportional to the blood's viscosity. Increased blood viscosity interferes with gas exchange by reducing pulmonary perfusion.

As the lung expands after birth, pulmonary vascular resistance decreases and pulmonary blood flow increases.[111] With inflation of the lungs, some "straightening out" of pulmonary vessels occurs. The larger vessels are pulled open by traction of the lung parenchyma that surrounds them. The perialveolar capillary lumens enlarge due to the action of surface tension produced by the newly established air–fluid interfaces. There are two types of pulmonary blood vessels: alveolar vessels, which are composed of capillaries and the slightly larger vessels in the alveolar walls (these vessels are exposed to alveolar pressure); and extra-alveolar vessels, which include the arteries and veins that run through the lung parenchyma but are surrounded by interstitial tissue rather than alveoli (Fig. 2-19).[119] The diameter of alveolar vessels is determined by the balance between the alveolar pressure and the hydrostatic pressure within the vessel. The vessel walls contain little elastic tissue and virtually no muscle fibers. Alveolar vessels collapse if alveolar pressure exceeds pulmonary venous pressure. Extra-alveolar vessels have structural support in their walls and are not significantly

TABLE 2-3. Factors Affecting Pulmonary Blood Flow

Increasing Flow	Decreasing Flow
1. Volume expansion of the lungs	1. Lung atelectasis
2. Increase in Pao_2	2. Decrease in Pao_2
3. Increase in Pao_2	3. Hypoxemia (reduction in Pao_2)
4. Alkalosis (repiratory or metabolic)	4. Acidosis (respiratory or metabolic)
5. Release of mediator substances (e.g., bradykinin, prostaglandins)	5. Mast cell degranulation with release of histamine
6. Left-to-right shunting (intracardiac or ductal)	6. Right-to-left shunting (intracardiac or ductal)
7. Endogenous production of NO or endothelium-derived releasing factor	7. Systemic hypotension (when right-to-left shunting is already present)
8. Inhalation of exogenous NO	8. Lung overexpansion

NO, nitric oxide; Pao_2; partial pressure of oxygen in arterial blood; Pao_2, partial pressure of oxygen in the alveoli.

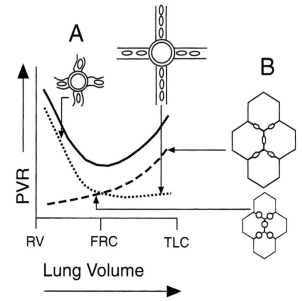

Figure 2-19. Effects of lung volume on pulmonary vascular resistance (PVR, *solid curved line*). *A,* "Extra-alveolar" vessels pose high resistance (*dotted curved line*) at low and high lung volumes, at the former because they become narrow and at the latter because they become stretched. *B,* "Alveolar" vessels pose the least resistance (*dashed curved line*) when they are open widest at the functional residual capacity (FRC) lung volume level, but they become compressed under conditions of lung overinflation. RV, residual volume; TLC, total lung capacity. (Modified from West JB: Respiratory Physiology: The Essentials, 2nd ed. Baltimore, Williams & Wilkins, 1979, p. 39.)

influenced by alveolar pressure. The vessel diameter of extra-alveolar vessels is affected by lung volume, because expanding the lung tends to pull these vessels open. If an airless lung is inflated to total lung capacity, pulmonary vascular resistance shows a U-shaped response, with high resistance at the low and high ends of inflation and low resistance in the middle (see Fig. 2-17). Resistance is high at low lung volumes because the extra-alveolar vessels are narrowed (they are not being pulled open). Resistance is high at high inflation volumes because the alveolar vessels are narrowed due to compression (they may even collapse). The lowest pulmonary vascular resistance is found when the lung is neither underinflated nor overinflated.

The rapid rise in oxygen tension in the alveoli (P_{AO_2}) and in the arterial blood (Pa_{O_2}) perfusing the pulmonary vessels plays a major role in the circulatory adaptation that occurs during transition of extrauterine life. It is the influence of P_{AO_2} on adjacent arteries that exerts the greatest effect on decreasing pulmonary vascular resistance with the initiation of breathing air.[113] With the initiation of breathing air, the lung is exposed to a P_{O_2} of approximately 100 mm Hg or greater if the infant is given supplemental O_2. Even if the O_2 tension of the mixed venous blood perfusion in the pulmonary arteries is low, the arteries themselves are rich with O_2 from the surrounding alveoli as long as P_{AO_2} is elevated. Sobel et al.[112] demonstrated that gas diffuses from the alveoli to the pulmonary arteries. Pa_{O_2} in the central circulation of the newborn infant rises from the fetal range between 25 and 30 mm Hg to greater than 60 mm Hg within the first hours following birth.

Many mediator substances have been implicated in the pulmonary vasodilation seen in the newborn infant. Bradykinin is a vasoactive peptide that produces pulmonary vasodilation in fetal lambs.[109] Bradykinin concentration increases transiently in blood that has passed through the lungs of fetal lambs ventilated with oxygen, but it does not increase if the lungs are ventilated with nitrogen. Bradykinin stimulates the local production of prostacyclin, which is also a potent pulmonary vasodilator.[114] PGA_1, PGE_1, and prostacyclin decrease pulmonary vascular resistance by dilating both pulmonary veins and arteries.[114,115,120] Prostacyclin production is stimulated by lung expansion with air and by mechanical ventilation. The decrease in pulmonary vascular resistance associated with mechanical ventilation can be attenuated by prior administration of a prostaglandin synthesis inhibitor (indomethacin).[115] PGD_2, another prostaglandin, is a semiselective pulmonary vasodilator. It promotes pulmonary vasodilation without causing the systemic vasodilatory effect produced by other prostaglandins.[116] The pulmonary vasodilatory effect of PGD_2 is present only during the first few days after birth; thereafter, it becomes a pulmonary vasoconstrictor. This observation suggests that PGD_2 plays a role in the transition from fetal to adult-type circulation after birth. PGD_2, like histamine, is released through mast cell degranulation. The number of mast cells in the lungs increases just before birth and then declines after delivery.[121] Mast cells play an important role in the pulmonary vasoconstrictive response to hypoxia.[122] Mast cells are abundant in the lung and are ideally located for modulation of vascular tone. Mast cell degranulation has been demonstrated to occur after acute alveolar hypoxia.[123] Pretreatment with cromolyn sodium (a mast cell degranulation blocking agent) prevents the pulmonary vasoconstriction normally induced by alveolar hypoxia.[124]

NO, previously known as *endothelium-derived relaxing factor,* plays an important role in regulating pulmonary vascular resistance. Its action reduces pulmonary vasoconstriction, thereby increasing pulmonary blood flow.[117,118,125–127] Endogenous NO is generated in vascular endothelial cells by enzymatic cleavage of the terminal nitrogen from L-arginine; production is accelerated at birth due to the increase in P_{O_2}. NO diffuses into the vascular smooth muscle cells and stimulates the production of cyclic guanosine monophosphate (cGMP), which causes smooth muscle relaxation.

The primary factor keeping pulmonary vascular resistance high in the fetus is relative hypoxia. Because of the preferential perfusion of the pulmonary circuit with the most desaturated blood (venous blood returning from the fetus's head), the Pa_{O_2} of blood perfusing the lungs of a fetal lamb is around 18 to 21 mm Hg.[107] Profound fetal hypoxemia causes further pulmonary vasoconstriction. A decrease in pulmonary arterial P_{O_2} to about 14 mm Hg diminishes pulmonary blood flow in the fetus to approximately 50% its base level.[128] Hypoxemic stress produces progressively greater increases in pulmonary vascular resistance as the gestational age of a fetus advances.[129] Chronic hypoxia in the fetus produces an increase in the medial smooth muscle of the pulmonary arterioles, which may lead to pulmonary hypertension and increased pulmonary vasoreactivity.[130] This may be an etiology for PPHN in the newborn infant.

A variety of mediator substances are contained in mast cells, including histamine, bradykinin, serotonin, acetylcholine, leukotrienes, and various prostaglandins (predominantly PGD_2).[121,131] Mast cells are activated by different stimuli in different ways, both in terms of increasing the synthesis of mediator substances and their release through degranulation. The same mediator substance may exert opposite effects at different times in the newborn period. Because the "net effect," such as vasoconstriction or vasodilation, is the result of many different substances acting in different directions, the regulation of pulmonary vascular tone is complicated and remains an active area of investigation.

Infants living at high altitudes have an increase in pulmonary vascular resistance that persists into childhood. They have relative pulmonary hypertension and are at increased risk for developing cor pulmonale.[132] Infants with cyanotic congenital heart disease and chronic hypoxemia are also at risk for developing pulmonary hypertension and cor pulmonale, as are oxygen-dependent infants with CLD. The vasoconstriction response to alveolar and arterial hypoxemia is potentiated by acidosis.[110]

PPHN of the newborn is associated with a variety of conditions, including RDS, pneumonia, meconium aspiration syndrome, and CHD (see Chapter 23).[133–137] It is also seen in infants with chronic fetal distress or peripartum stress. The mechanism of PPHN is right-to-left shunting at the atrial and ductal levels secondary to persistent elevation of pulmonary vascular resistance. Infants with PPHN exhibit hypoxemia secondary to extrapulmonary right-to-left shunting; near-systemic or suprasystemic pulmonary artery pressures; and lability in pulmonary artery pressure secondary to pulmonary vasoreactivity (Fig. 2-20). Hyperventilation of infants with PPHN has been shown to decrease pulmonary artery pressure.[138,139] Right-to-left shunting may occur at the foramen ovale and ductus arteriosus when pulmonary artery pressure exceeds systemic blood pressure. This results in pulmonary hypoperfusion and hypoxemia due to the contribution of the venous admixture crossing the shunts. In PPHN it is the pressure difference (ratio of pulmonary arterial-to-systemic arterial pressure) that is important, rather than any specific pressure values. A normal blood pressure in the systemic circulation may be inadequate to prevent right-to-left shunting if the pressure in the pulmonary artery is greater than that in the systemic circulation. P_{AO_2} – PaO_2 does not begin to decrease (indicating an improvement in oxygenation or a reduction in shunting) until pulmonary artery pressure drops below aortic pressure (systolic blood pressure). Dopamine is used clinically for treatment of PPHN. Dopamine causes an increase in systemic blood pressure (decreasing the magnitude of right-to-left shunting) and improves myocardial contractility.[140] The clinical usefulness of intravenous pulmonary vasodilators is limited because these medications are nonspecific; they dilate the systemic and the pulmonary vasculature.[141] Inhaled NO causes a dose-dependent decrease in pulmonary vascular resistance and an increase in pulmonary blood flow, without affecting systemic arterial pressure. It is a selective pulmonary vasodilator. When used in low concentrations (<80 ppm), it is inactivated prior to entering the systemic circulation (see Chapter 14).[126,127,137,142–148]

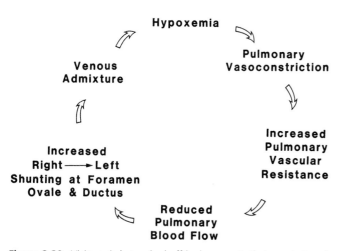

Figure 2-20. Vicious circle touched off by hypoxemia that reverts transitional circulation back to the fetal type, as seen in persistent pulmonary hypertension.

The more dependent the lung region, the greater its perfusion.[149] The vessels in dependent regions of the lung are more distended and thus present less resistance to flow because their transmural pressure is greater. Transmural pressure is the difference between the pressures inside and the pressure outside the vessel wall. Inside "hydrostatic" pressure increases the more dependent a vessel's position in the lung. Outside interstitial pressure reflects interpleural pressure (see Fig. 2-16). Interpleural pressure decreases the more dependent the lung region. Because the hydrostatic pressure increase (inside the vessel) is greater than the interpleural pressure decrease (outside the vessel), the transmural pressure increases the more dependent the lung region. In the upright adult, the lung is divided into four perfusion zones (Fig. 2-21) based on up-and-down distance and specific pressure differences.[149] Zone I is the least dependent (uppermost) region and has almost no blood flow because alveolar pressure exceeds pulmonary capillary pressure. This causes collapse of the capillaries around the alveoli. Zone II is the upper middle region and has some flow because pulmonary artery pressure exceeds alveolar pressure. Zone III is the lower middle region, where flow is determined by the difference in pressure between the pulmonary arteries and pulmonary veins. Zone IV is the most dependent region, where interstitial pressure is great enough to cause narrowing of extra-alveolar vessels and, thus, reduce blood flow due to increased pulmonary vascular resistance. In infants, under normal circumstances the entire lung is considered to have zone III characteristics from a physiologic standpoint. In some situations, as in the presence of air trapping or alveolar overdistention, a portion of the lung may behave as zone I or II, with a decrease in pulmonary blood flow. In other conditions such as interstitial edema (fluid overload; left-sided heart failure, as in congenital heart disease or significant patent ductus arteriosus; capillary leakage following hypoxic insult or asphyxia; CLD), much of the dependent portion of the lung behaves like zone IV, with increased vascular resistance and decreased pulmonary blood flow. In this clinical situation, fluid restriction, administration of a diuretic, or both may result in significant improvements in gas exchange due to an improvement in pulmonary blood flow (as well as an improvement in lung

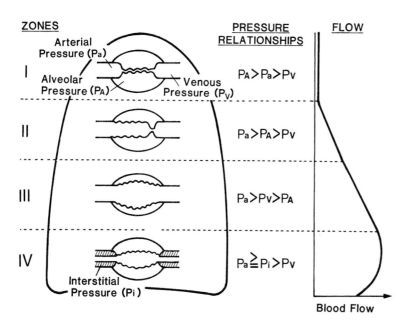

Figure 2-21. Various intraluminal and extraluminal pressure effects on the alveolar vessels of the lung in relation to blood flow in the four perfusion zones. Alveolar vessels represent "Starling resistors," which consist of collapsible tubes in pressure chambers. Note the situation in zone II, where there is a constriction in the "downstream end" of the collapsible vessel. Here, chamber (alveolar) pressure exceeds intraluminal downstream (venous) pressure and the vessel collapses; pressure inside the tube at the constriction is equal to the chamber (alveolar) pressure. Flow is thus determined by the arterial–alveolar pressure difference rather than by the usual arterial–venous pressure difference. (Modified from West JB, Dollery CT, Naimark A: Distribution of blood flow in isolated lung: relation to vascular and alveolar pressures. J Appl Physiol 19:713, 1964.)

compliance and a decrease in airway resistance). Conditions in which significant left-to-right shunting and pulmonary hyperperfusion occur tend to abolish the unevenness of blood flow in the lungs.[85]

Regional hypoventilation produces local pulmonary vasoconstriction that diverts blood flow away from underventilated areas. This is a protective mechanism that decreases the perfusion of nonventilated or poorly ventilated areas of the lung. Term newborn and premature lambs are capable of redirecting blood flow away from hypoxic regions produced by atelectasis or bronchial obstruction.[150,151] The flow directed away from atelectatic and hypoxic lung segments is directly proportional to the amount of lung volume loss.[152] Lung scans in infants have identified perfusion deficits in areas of atelectasis.[153] Alveolar overdistention secondary to air trapping may reduce area blood flow by collapsing surrounding capillaries.

When CPAP or positive-pressure ventilation is used to recruit atelectatic lung units, improvement in both local ventilation and perfusion may result in those regions. However, those areas of the lung, which already are well expanded, may be further inflated, which can increase rather than decrease pulmonary vascular resistance in those areas. The overall effect on pulmonary blood flow produced by positive-pressure ventilation depends on the initial lung volume status of the various functional lung regions and the net result of the therapy on global pulmonary blood flow.

CONTROL OF VENTILATION

In the newborn infant, neurologic and chemical control of respiration differs in several ways from that in the adult. First, the central respiratory control center is immature and therefore more easily influenced by medications, acid/base status, sleep state, temperature, hypoxia, and other variables. Second, the central and peripheral chemoreceptors that respond to changes in arterial O_2 and CO_2 tensions act both quantitatively and qualitatively different from those in adults. Third, a set of chest wall stretch proprioceptors is able to reflexively inhibit or drive respiration.[154–157] REM sleep also has a significant effect on the control of respiration in the newborn infant. During REM sleep, the normal phasic tone changes in the intercostal muscles, which are important for stabilizing the rib cage during inspiration, are inhibited. Because the intercostal muscles fail to tighten with inspiration, the infant's chest wall deforms during inspiration. Contraction of the diaphragm worsens the paradoxical movement, increases its O_2 consumption measured during REM sleep, and may lead to fatigue-induced apnea.[156] Application of CPAP or PEEP causes the infant's respiratory rate to slow and his or her respiratory efforts to become more regular. Generally one observes a reduction in periodic breathing and apneic episodes.[158,159] The distending pressure stabilizes the infant's compliant chest wall by providing a "pneumatic splint" that counters the tendency of the chest wall to collapse during inspiration. The application of continuous distending pressure shortens and intensifies inspiratory effort while prolonging expiration. Xanthines such as caffeine and aminophylline (or theophylline) increase alveolar ventilation through central stimulation.[160] They cause a shift of the CO_2 response curve to the left so that an increase in V_T occurs in response to an increase in CO_2. Increased diaphragmatic con-

tractility and resistance to fatigue are other effects of methylxanthines.[161,162] A further discussion on the control of ventilation can be found in Chapter 3.

CONCLUSION

Based on an understanding of the physiologic principles of assisted ventilation, we know that ventilator strategies must be individualized for each patient. We also know that the strategy used to provide mechanical ventilatory support is more important than the specific type of device used to deliver that support. Each time we encounter an infant in respiratory distress, we must determine what level of support is required: CPAP,[163] noninvasive ventilation, some form of HFV,[164–167] liquid ventilation,[168,169] conventional ventilation,[170–174] or perhaps some combination.[175]

We must be cognizant of how our strategies and techniques of providing assisted ventilation to infants impact their long-term outcomes. Repeated cycling of the terminal airways from below critical opening pressure leads to cellular injury and inflammation (atelectatrauma). This results in alveolar collapse, atelectasis, interstitial edema, and elaboration of inflammatory mediators. The resulting atelectasis leads to a further reduction in lung compliance that necessitates higher inspiratory pressures, which further compromises surfactant production. Atelectatrauma leads to increased diffusion barrier, which necessitates increased levels of mean airway pressure (Paw) and/or increased levels of inspired oxygen (FIO_2). The increase in FIO_2 may lead to oxidative injury and further cellular dysfunction. There are more questions than answers. We know that mechanical ventilation causes lung injury that leads to inflammatory response[176]; oxygen exposure is harmful[177,178]; lung overdistention (volutrauma) causes lung injury[179]; lung injury and inflammation exacerbate the deleterious effects of oxygen toxicity and volutrauma[180]; and atelectatrauma is a source of lung injury.[181]

Establishment of an appropriate FRC, administration of surfactant, avoidance of mechanical ventilation (if possible), use of adequate PEEP to avoid the repeated collapse and reopening of small airways, avoidance of lung overinflation caused by using supraphysiologic tidal volumes, and avoidance of use of more oxygen than is necessary all are important in order to achieve the best possible outcomes and long-term health of our patients. While caring for your patients, always remember the words of Hippocates, "first do no harm."

REFERENCES

1. Lehninger AL: Principles of Biochemistry. New York, Worth, 1982.
2. Langston C, Kida, K, Reed, M, Thurlbeck, WM: Human lung growth in late gestation and in the neonate. Am Rev Respir Dis 129:607–613, 1984.
3. Muller NL, Bryan AC: Chest wall mechanics and respiratory muscles in infants. Pediatr Clin North Am 26:503, 1979.
4. Keens TG, Bryan AC, Levison H, et al: Developmental pattern of muscle fiber types in human ventilatory muscles. J Appl Physiol 44:909, 1978.
5. Polgar G: Opposing forces to breathing in newborn infants. Biol Neonate 11:1, 1967.
6. Mansell AL, Bryan C, Levison H: Airway closure in children. J Appl Physiol 33:711, 1972.
7. Avery ME, Mead J: Surface properties in relation to atelectasis and hyaline membrane disease. Am J Dis Child 97:517, 1959.

8. Coalson JJ, Kuehl TJ, Escobedo MB, et al: A baboon model of bronchopulmonary dysplasia: II. Pathologic features. Exp Mol Pathol 37:35–63, 1982.

9. Bancalari E: Pulmonary function testing and other diagnostic laboratory procedures. In Gregory GA, Thibeault DW (eds): Neonatal Pulmonary Care, 2nd ed. Norwalk, Conn., Appleton-Century-Crofts, 1986, p. 195.

10. LeSouef PN, England SJ, Bryan AC: Influence of chest wall distortion on esophageal pressure. J Appl Physiol 55:3563, 1983.

11. Helms P, Stocks J: Lung function in infants with congenital pulmonary hypoplasia. J Pediatr 101:918–922, 1982.

12. Heaf DP, Belik J, Spitzer AR, et al: Changes in pulmonary function during the diuretic phase of respiratory distress syndrome. J Pediatr 101:918, 1982.

13. Bose C, Wood B, Bose G, et al: Pulmonary function following positive pressure ventilation initiated immediately after birth in infants with respiratory distress syndrome. Pediatr Pulmonol 9:244–250, 1990.

14. Downs JB, Klein EF Jr, Desautels D, et al: Intermittent mandatory ventilation: A new approach to weaning patients from mechanical ventilators. Chest 64:331, 1973.

15. Bancalari E, Garcia OL, Jesse MJ: Effects of continuous negative pressure on lung mechanics in idiopathic respiratory distress syndrome. Pediatrics 51:485–493, 1973.

16. Thurlbeck WM, Kida K, Langston C, et al: Postnatal lung growth after repair of diaphragmatic hernia. Thorax 34:338, 1979.

17. Hall RT, Rhodes PG: Pneumothorax and pneumomediastinum in infants with idiopathic respiratory distress syndrome receiving continuous positive airway pressure. Pediatrics 55:493, 1975.

18. Greenough A, Morley CJ, Wood S, et al: Pancuronium prevents pneumothoraces in ventilated premature babies who actively expire against positive pressure inflation. Lancet 1:1, 1984.

19. Burger RS, Fanconi S, Simma B: Paralysis of ventilated newborn babies does not influence resistance of the total respiratory system. Eur Respir J 14:357–362, 1999.

20. Boros SJ, Orgill AA: Mortality and morbidity associated with pressure and volume-limited ventilators. Am J Dis Child 132:865, 1978.

21. Polgar G, String ST: The viscous resistance of the lung tissues in newborn infants. J Pediatr 69:787, 1966.

22. Milner AD, Saunders RA, Hopkin IE: Effects of delivery by caesarean section on lung mechanics and lung volume in the human neonate. Arch Dis Child 53:545–548, 1978.

23. Kao LC, Warburton D, Sargent CW, et al: Furosemide acutely decreases airways resistance in chronic bronchopulmonary dysplasia. J Pediatr 103:624–629, 1983.

24. Bancalari E: Inadvertent positive end-expiratory pressure during mechanical ventilation. J Pediatr 108:567, 1986.

25. Weigl, J: The infant lung: A case against high respiratory rates in controlled neonatal ventilation. Respir Ther 3:57, 1973.

26. Reynolds E: Pressure waveform and ventilator settings for mechanical ventilation in severe hyaline membrane disease. Int Anesthesiol Clin 12:259, 1974.

27. Donahue LA, Thibeault DW: Alveolar gas trapping and ventilator therapy in infants. Perinatol Neonatol 3:35, 1979.

28. Swyer PR, Reiman RC, Wright JJ: Ventilation and ventilatory mechanics in the newborn. J Pediatr 56:612, 1960.

29. Ferris BG, Mead J, Opie LH: Partitioning of respiratory flow resistance in man. J Appl Physiol 19:653, 1964.

30. Long EC, Hull WE: Respiratory volume-flow in the crying newborn infant. Pediatrics 27:373, 1961.

31. Cave P, Fletcher G: Resistance of nasotracheal tubes used in infants. Anesthesiology 29:588, 1968.

32. Kim EH, Boutwell WC: Successful direct extubation of very low birth weight infants from low intermittent mandatory ventilation rate. Pediatrics 80:409, 1987.

33. LeSouef PN, England SJ, Bryan AC: Total resistance of the respiratory system in preterm infants with and without an endotracheal tube. J Pediatr 104:108, 1984.

34. Wall MA: Infant endotracheal tube resistance: Effects of changing length, diameter, and gas density. Crit Care Med 8:38, 1980.

35. Weibel ER: Morphometrics of the human lung. In Fenn WO, Rahn H (eds): Handbook of Physiology. Section 3: Respiration. Washington, DC, American Physiological Society, 1964.

36. Suter PM, Fairley HB, Isenberg MD: Optimal end-expiratory airway pressures in patients with acute pulmonary failure. N Engl J Med 292:284, 1975.

37. Cogswell JJ, Hatch DJ, Kerr AA, et al: Effects of continuous positive airway pressure on lung mechanics of babies after operation for congenital heart disease. Arch Dis Child 50:799–804, 1975.

38. Saunders RA, Milner AD, Hopkin IE: The effects of continuous positive airway pressure on lung mechanics and lung volumes in the neonate. Biol Neonate 29:178–186, 1976.

39. Harris TR, Stevens RC, Nugent M: On the use of nasal continuous positive airway pressure [letter]. Pediatrics 53:768, 1974.

40. Wolfson MR, Bhutani UK, Shaffer TH, et al: Mechanics and energetics of breathing helium in infants with bronchopulmonary dysplasia. J Pediatr 104:752–757, 1984.

41. Mortola JP, Fisher JT, Smith B, et al: Dynamics of breathing in infants. J Appl Physiol 52:1209, 1982.

42. Weinstein MR, Oh W: Oxygen consumption in infants with bronchopulmonary dysplasia. J Pediatr 99:958, 1981.

43. Grenvick A: Respiratory, circulatory and metabolic effects of respirator treatment. Acta Anaesthesiol Scand 19(Suppl):1, 1966.

44. Gregory GA, Brooks J, Wiebe H, et al: The time course changes in lung function after a change in CPAP. Clin Res 25:193A, 1977.

45. Richardson CP, Jung AL: Effects of continuous positive airway pressure on pulmonary function and blood gases in infants with respiratory distress syndrome. Pediatr Res 12:771, 1978.

46. Chang HK: Mechanisms of gas transport during ventilation by high-frequency oscillation. J Appl Physiol 55:553, 1984.

47. Henderson Y, Chillingworth FP, Whitney JL: The respiratory dead space. Am J Physiol 38:1, 1915.

48. Schroter RC, Sudlow MF: Flow patterns in models of the human bronchial airways. Respir Physiol 7:341, 1969.

49. Fredberg JJ, Keefe DH, Glass GM, et al: Alveolar pressure non-homogeneity during small-amplitude high-frequency oscillation. J Appl Physiol 57:788, 1984.

50. Weibel ER: The Pathway for Oxygen: Structure and Function in the Mammalian Respiratory System. Cambridge, Mass., Harvard University Press, 1984, p. 144.

51. Dudell G, Cornish JD, Bartlett RH: What constitutes adequate oxygenation? Pediatrics 85:39, 1990.

52. Ortega M, FamosAD, Platzker ACG, et al: Early prediction of ultimate outcome in newborn infants with severe respiratory failure. J Pediatr 113:744, 1988.

53. Boros SJ, Campbell K: A comparison of the effects of high frequency-low tidal volume and low frequency-high tidal volume mechanical ventilation. J Pediatr 97:108, 1980.

54. Owen-Thomas JB, Ulan OA, Swyer PR: The effect of varying inspiratory gas flow rate on arterial oxygenation during IPPV in the respiratory distress syndrome. Br J Anaesth 40:493, 1968.

55. Spahr RC, Klein AM, Brown DR, et al: Hyaline membrane disease: A controlled study of inspiratory to expiratory ratio in its management by ventilator. Am J Dis Child 134:373, 1980.

56. Herman S, Reynolds EOR: Methods for improving oxygenation in infants mechanically ventilated for severe hyaline membrane disease. Arch Dis Child 48:612, 1973.

57. Paloski WH, Barie PS, Mullins RJ, et al: Effects of changing inspiratory to expiratory time ratio on carbon dioxide elimination during high-frequency jet ventilation. Am Rev Respir Dis 131:109, 1985.

58. Weisberger SA, Carlo WA, Chatburn RL, et al: Effect of varying inspiratory and expiratory times during high-frequency jet ventilation. J Pediatr 108:596, 1986.

59. Harris TR, Bunnell JB: On the use of high frequency jet ventilation. Pediatr Res 17(A):1983, 1983.

60. Harris TR, Bunnell JB: On understanding the mechanism of action of high frequency jet ventilation. Clin Res 32(A):131, 1984.

61. Courtney SE, Weber KR, Spohn WA, et al: Cardiorespiratory effects of changing inspiratory to expiratory ratio during high-frequency oscillation in an animal model of respiratory failure. Pediatr Pulmonol 13:113, 1992.

62. Boros SJ: Variations in inspiratory:expiratory ratio and airway pressure wave form during mechanical ventilation: The significance of mean airway pressure. J Pediatr 94:114, 1979.

63. Boros SJ, Matalon SV, Ewald R, et al: The effect of independent variations in inspiratory-expiratory ratio and end expiratory pressure during mechanical ventilation in hyaline membrane disease: The significance of mean airway pressure. J Pediatr 91:794, 1977.

64. Stewart AR, Finer NN, Peters KL: Effects of alterations of inspiratory and expiratory pressures and inspiratory/expiratory ratios on mean airway pressure, blood gases, and intracranial pressure. Pediatrics 67:474, 1981.

65. Ciszek TA, Modanlou HD, Owings D, et al: Mean airway pressure: Significance during mechanical ventilation in neonates. J Pediatr 99:121, 1981.

66. Marchak BE, Thompson WK, Duffty P, et al: Treatment of RDS by high-frequency oscillatory ventilation: A preliminary report. J Pediatr 99:287, 1981.

67. Rouby JJ, Fusciardi J, Bourgain JL, et al: High-frequency jet ventilation in postoperative respiratory failure: Determinants of oxygenation. Anesthesiology 59:281, 1983.

68. Frantz IDI, Werthammer J, Stark AR: High-frequency ventilation in premature infants with lung disease: Adequate gas exchange at low tracheal pressure. Pediatrics 71:483, 1983.

69. Fox WW, Gewitz MH, Berman LS, et al: The PaO_2 response to changes in end expiratory pressure in the newborn respiratory distress syndrome. Crit Care Med 5:226, 1977.

70. Kanarek DJ, Shannon DC: Adverse effect of positive end-expiratory pressure on pulmonary perfusion and arterial oxygenation. Am Rev Respir Dis 112:457, 1975.

71. Nelson RM, Egan EA, Eitzman DV: Increased hypoxemia in neonates secondary to the use of continuous positive airway pressure. J Pediatr 91:87, 1977.

72. Eyal FG, Arad ID, Godder K, et al: High-frequency positive-pressure ventilation in neonates. Crit Care Med 12:793, 1984.

73. Clark RH, Gerstmann DR, Null DM, et al: Pulmonary interstitial emphysema treated by high-frequency oscillatory ventilation. Crit Care Med 14:926, 1986.

74. Harris TR, Christensen RD: High frequency jet ventilation treatment of pulmonary interstitial emphysema. Pediatr Res 19(A):141, 1984.

75. Wood BR, Eggert LD, Bolam DL, et al: High frequency ventilation in neonatal pulmonary interstitial emphysema. Nebr Med J 72:362–366, 1987.

76. Donn SM, Nicks JJ, Bandy KP, et al: Proximal high-frequency jet ventilation of the newborn. Pediatr Pulmonol 1:267, 1985.

77. Pokora T, Bing D, Mammel M, et al: Neonatal high-frequency jet ventilation. Pediatrics 72:27, 1983.

78. Boros SJ, Mammel MC, Coleman JM, et al: Neonatal high-frequency jet ventilation: Four year's experience. Pediatrics 75:657, 1985.

79. Boynton BR, Mannino FL, Davis RF, et al: Combined high-frequency oscillatory ventilation and intermittent mandatory ventilation in critically ill neonates. J Pediatr 105:297, 1984.

80. Heicher DA, Kasting DS, Harrod JR: Prospective clinical comparison of two methods for mechanical ventilation of neonates: Rapid rate and short inspiratory time versus slow rate and long inspiratory time. J Pediatr 98:957, 1981.

81. Gonzalez F, Richardson P, Carlstrom JR, et al: Rapid mechanical ventilation effects on tracheal airway pressure, lung volume, and blood gases of rabbits. Am J Perinatol 3:347, 1986.

82. Simon BA, Weinmann GG, Mitzner W: Mean airway pressure and alveolar pressure during high frequency ventilation. J Appl Physiol 57:1069, 1984.

83. Kolton M, Cattran CB, Kent G, et al: Oxygenation during high-frequency ventilation compared with conventional mechanical ventilation in two models of lung injury. Anesth Analg 61:323, 1982.

84. Bryan AC, Slutsky AS: Lung volume during high frequency oscillation. Am Rev Respir Dis 133:928, 1986.

85. Bryan AC, Bentivoglio LG, Beerel F, et al: Factors affecting regional distribution of ventilation and perfusion in the lung. J Appl Physiol 19:395, 1964.

86. Milic-Emili J: Static distribution of lung volumes. In Fishman AP, Mead J (eds): Handbook of Physiology. Section 3: The Respiratory System, volume 3. Washington, DC, American Physiological Society, 1986, p. 561.

87. Kaneko K, Milic-Emili J, Dolovich MB, et al: Regional distribution of ventilation and perfusion as a function of body position. J Appl Physiol 21:767, 1966.

88. Glacier JB, Hughes JMB, Maloney JE, et al: Vertical gradient of alveolar size in lungs of dogs frozen intact. J Appl Physiol 26:65, 1969.

89. Remolina C, Khan AU, Santiago TV, et al: Positional hypoxemia in unilateral lung disease. N Engl J Med 304:523, 1981.

90. Seaton D, Lapp NL, Morgan WKC: Effect of body position on gas exchange after thoracotomy. Thorax 34:518, 1979.

91. Cohen RS, Smith DW, Stevenson DK, et al: Lateral decubitus position as therapy for persistent focal pulmonary interstitial emphysema in neonates: A preliminary report. J Pediatr 104:441, 1984.

92. Swingle HM, Eggert LD, Bucciarelli RL: New approach to management of unilateral tension pulmonary interstitial emphysema in premature infants. Pediatrics 74:354, 1984.

93. Froese AB, Bryan AC: Effects of anesthesia and paralysis on diaphragmatic mechanics in man. Anesthesiology 41:242, 1974.

94. Douglas WW, Rehder K, Beynen FM, et al: Improved oxygenation in patients with acute respiratory failure: The prone position. Am Rev Respir Dis 115:559, 1977.

95. Martin RJ, Herrell N, Rubin D, et al: Effect of supine and prone positions on arterial oxygen tension in the preterm infant. Pediatrics 63:528, 1979.

96. Turnbull AD, Carlon GC, Howland WS, et al: High frequency jet ventilation in major airway or pulmonary disruption. Ann Thorac Surg 32:468, 1981.

97. Derderian SS, Rajagapal KR, Albrecht PH, et al: High frequency positive pressure jet ventilation in bilateral bronchopleural fistulae. Crit Care Med 10:119, 1982.

98. Gonzalez F, Harris TR, Black P, et al: Decreased gas flow through pneumothoraces of neonates receiving high frequency jet vs. conventional ventilation. J Pediatr 110:464, 1987.

99. Carlon GC, Miodawnik S, Ray C, et al: Technical aspects and clinical implications of high frequency jet ventilation with a solenoid valve. Crit Care Med 9(1):47, 1981.

100. Waterson CK, Militzer HW, Quan SF: Airway pressure as a measure of gas exchange during high-frequency jet ventilation. Crit Care Med 12:74, 1984.

101. Schlachter MD, Perry ME: Effect of continuous positive airway pressure on lung mechanics during high-frequency jet ventilation. Crit Care Med 12:755, 1984.

102. Banner MJ, Gallagher TJ, Banner TC: Frequency and percent inspiratory time for high-frequency jet ventilation. Crit Care Med 13:795, 1985.

103. Harris TR, Bunnell JB: High-frequency jet ventilation in clinical neonatology. In Pomerance JJ, Richardson CJ (eds): Neonatology for the Clinician. Norwalk, Conn., Appleton & Lange, 1993, p. 311.

104. Fredberg JJ, Glass GM, Boynton BR, et al: Factors influencing mechanical performance of neonatal high-frequency ventilators. J Appl Physiol 62:2485, 1987.

105. Clark RH, Null DM: High-frequency oscillatory ventilation. In Pomerance JJ, Richardson CJ (eds): Neonatology for the Clinician. Norwalk, Conn., Appleton & Lange, 1993, p. 289.

106. Bryan AC, Cox PN: History of high frequency oscillation. Schweiz Med Wochenschr 129:1613–1616, 1999.

107. Rudolph AM: Congenital Diseases of the Heart: Clinical-Psychological Considerations in Diagnosis & Management. Chicago, Year Book Medical Publishers, 1974, p. 29.

108. Dawes GS, Mott JC: The vascular tone of the foetal lung. J Physiol (Lond) 164:465, 1962.

109. Heymann MA, Rudolph AM, Niew AS, et al: Bradykinin production associated with oxygenation of the fetal lamb. Circ Res 25:521, 1969.

110. Rudolph AM, Yuan S: Response of the pulmonary vasculature to hypoxia and H+ ion concentration changes. J Clin Invest 45:399, 1966.

111. Einhorning G, Adams FH, Norman A: Effect of lung expansion on the fetal lamb circulation. Acta Paediatr Scand 55:441, 1966.

112. Sobel B, Boltex G, Emirgil C, et al: Gaseous diffusion from alveoli to pulmonary vessels of considerable size. Circ Res 13:71, 1963.

113. Lauer RM, Evans JA, Aoki H, et al: Factors controlling pulmonary vascular resistance in fetal lambs. J Pediatr 67:568, 1965.

114. Kadowitz PJ, Joiner PD, Hyman AL: Physiological and pharmacological roles of prostaglandins. Ann Rev Pharmacol 15:285, 1975.

115. Cassin S, Tod M, Philips J, et al: Effects of prostacyclin on the fetal pulmonary circulation. Pediatr Pharmacol 1:197, 1981.

116. Cassin S, Tod M, Philips J, et al: Effects of prostaglandin D2 in perinatal circulation. Am J Physiol 240:755, 1981.

117. Abman S, Chatfield B, Hall S, McMurtry I: Role of endothelium-derived relaxing factor during transition of pulmonary circulation at birth. Am J Physiol 250:1921, 1990.

118. Palmer R, Ferrige A, Moncada S: Nitric oxide release accounts for the biological activity of endothelium-derived relaxing factor. Nature 327:524, 1987.

119. West JB: Respiratory Physiology, 4th ed. Baltimore, Williams & Wilkins, 1990, p. 32.

120. Lee DS, Bevan MG, Olson DM: Stimulation of prostaglandin synthesis by hyperoxia in perinatal rat lung cells. Am J Physiol 259(2 Pt 1):L95–L101, 1990.

121. Schwartz LS, Osburn BI, Frick OL: An ontogenic study of histamine and mast cells in the fetal rhesus monkey. J Allergy Clin Immunol 56:381, 1974.

122. Haas F, Bergofsky EH: Role of the mast cell in the pulmonary pressor response to hypoxia. J Clin Invest 51:3154, 1972.

123. Ahmed T, Oliver W, Robinson M, et al: Hypoxic pulmonary vasoconstriction in conscious sheep: Role of mast cell degranulation. Am Rev Respir Dis 126:291, 1982.

124. Taylor BJ, Fewell JE, Dearns GL, et al: Cromolyn sodium decreases the pulmonary vascular response to alveolar hypoxia in lambs. Pediatr Res 20:834, 1986.

125. Tiktinsky MH, Moran FC III: Increasing oxygen tension dilates the fetal pulmonary circulation via endothelium-derived relaxing factor. Am J Physiol 265:376, 1993.

126. Dobyns EL, Griebel J, Kinsella JP, et al: Infant lung function after inhaled nitric oxide therapy for persistent pulmonary hypertension of the newborn. Pediatr Pulmonol 28:24–30, 1999.

127. Cuesta EG, Diaz FJ, Renedo AA, et al: Transient response to inhaled nitric oxide in meconium aspiration in newborn lambs. Pediatr Res 43:198–202, 1998.

128. Cohen HE, Sacks EJ, Heymann MA, et al: Cardiovascular response to hypoxemia and acidemia in fetal lambs. Am J Obstet Gynecol 120:817, 1974.

129. Lewis AB, Heymann MA, Rudolph AM: Gestational changes in pulmonary vascular responses in fetal lambs in utero. Circ Res 39:536, 1976.

130. Goldberg SJ, Levy RA, Siassi B, et al: The effects of maternal hypoxia and hyperoxia upon the neonatal pulmonary circulation. Pediatrics 48:528, 1971.

131. MacGlashan DW, Schleimer RP, Peters SP, et al: Generation of leukotrienes by purified human lung mast cells. J Clin Invest 70:747, 1982.

132. Sime F, Bachero N, Penaloze D, et al: Pulmonary hypertension in children born and living at high altitudes. Am J Cardiol 11:150, 1963.

133. Gersony WM, Duc GV, Sinclair JC: PFC syndrome (persistent fetal circulation). Circulation 40(Suppl):87, 1969.

134. Siassi B, Goldberg SJ, Emmanouilides GC, et al: Persistent pulmonary vascular obstruction in newborn infants. J Pediatr 78:610, 1971.

135. Peckham GJ, Fox WW: Physiologic factors affecting pulmonary artery pressure in infants with persistent pulmonary hypertension. J Pediatr 93:1005, 1978.

136. Levin DL, Heymann MA, Kitterman JA, et al: Persistent pulmonary hypertensions of the newborn infant. J Pediatr 89:626, 1976.

137. Hutchison AA: Respiratory disorders of the neonate. Curr Opin Pediatr 6:142–153, 1994.

138. Fox WW, Duara S: Persistent pulmonary hypertension in the neonate: Diagnosis and management. J Pediatr 103:505, 1983.

139. Drummond WH, Gregory GA, Heymann MA, et al: The independent effects of hyper-ventilation, tolazoline, and dopamine on infants with persistent pulmonary hypertension. J Pediatr 98:603, 1981.

140. Fiffler GI, Chatrath R, Williams GJ, et al: Dopamine infusion for the treatment of myocardial dysfunction associated with a persistent transitional circulation. Arch Dis Child 55:194, 1980.

141. Stevens DC, Schreiner RL, Bull MJ, et al: An analysis of tolazoline therapy in the critically ill neonate. J Pediatr Surg 15:964, 1980.

142. Gommers D, Hartog A, van't Veen A, et al: Improved oxygenation by nitric oxide is enhanced by prior lung reaeration with surfactant, rather than positive end-expiratory pressure, in lung-lavaged rabbits. Crit Care Med 25:1868–1873, 1997.

143. Jaillard S, Riou Y, Klosowski S, et al. Effects of inhaled nitric oxide on gas exchange and acute lung injury in premature lambs with moderate hyaline membrane disease. Eur J Cardiothorac Surg 18:334–341, 2000.

144. Storme L, Riou Y, Dubois A, et al: Combined effects of inhaled nitric oxide and hyperoxia on pulmonary vascular permeability and lung mechanics. Crit Care Med 27:1168–1174, 1999.

145. Zavek M, Cleveland D, Morin FC III: Treatment of persistent pulmonary hypertension in the newborn lamb by inhaled nitric oxide. J Pediatr 122:743, 1993.

146. Roberts JD, Polaner DM, Lang L, et al: Inhaled nitric oxide in persistent pulmonary hypertension of the newborn. Lancet 340:818, 1992.

147. Kinsella JP, Neish SR, Shaffer E, et al: Low-dose inhalational nitric oxide in persistent pulmonary hypertension of the newborn. Lancet 340:819, 1992.

148. Kinsella JP, Abman SH: Inhalational nitric oxide therapy for persistent pulmonary hypertension of the newborn. Pediatrics 91:997, 1992.

149. West JB, Dollery CT, Naimark A: Distribution of blood flow in isolated lung: Relation to vascular and alveolar pressures. Am J Physiol 19:713, 1964.

150. Hyman AL, Kadowitz PJ: Effects of alveolar and perfusion hypoxia and hypercapnia on pulmonary vascular resistance in the lamb. Am J Physiol 228:379, 1975.

151. Berry D, Jobe A, Jacobs H, et al: Distribution of pulmonary blood flow in relation to atelectasis in premature ventilated lambs. Am Rev Respir Dis 132:500, 1985.

152. Marshall BE, Marshall C, Benumof J, et al: Hypoxic pulmonary vasoconstriction in dogs: Effects of lung segment size and oxygen tension. J Appl Physiol 51:1543, 1981.

153. Leonidas JC, Moylan FMB, Kahn PC, et al: Ventilation-perfusion scans in neonatal regional pulmonary emphysema complicating ventilatory assistance. Am J Roentgenol 131:243, 1978.

154. Krauss A: The regulation of breathing. In: Scarpelli EM (ed): Newborn and Child. Pulmonary Physiology of the Fetus. Philadelphia, Lea & Febiger, 1975, p. 83.

155. Avery MA, Fletcher BD, Williams RG: The Lung and Its Disorders in the Newborn Infant, 4th ed. Philadelphia, WB Saunders, 1981, p. 48.

156. Bryan AC, Bryan MH: Control of respiration in the newborn. In Gregory GA, Thibeault DW (eds): Neonatal Pulmonary Care, 2nd ed. Norwalk, Conn., Appleton-Century-Crofts, 1986, p. 33.

157. Fisher JT, Mortola JP, Smith JB, et al: Respiration in newborns: Development of the control of breathing. Am Rev Respir Dis 125:650–657, 1982.

158. Kattwinkel J, Nearman HS, Fanoroff AA, et al: Apnea of prematurity: Comparative therapeutic effects of cutaneous stimulation and nasal CPAP. J Pediatr 86:588, 1975.

159. Martin RJ, Nearman HS, Katona PG, et al: The effect of a low continuous positive airway pressure on the reflex control of respiration in the preterm infant. J Pediatr 90:976, 1977.

160. Davi M, Sankaran K, Simons K, et al: Physiological changes induced by theophylline in the treatment of apnea in preterm infants. J Pediatr 92:91, 1978.

161. Aubier M, DeTroyer A, Sampson M, et al: Aminophylline improves diaphragmatic contractility. N Engl J Med 305:249, 1981.

162. Carnielli VP, Verlato G, Benini F, et al: Metabolic and respiratory effects of theophylline in the preterm infant. Arch Dis Child Fetal Neonatal Ed 83:F39–F43, 2000.

163. Kavvadia VA, Greenough A, Dimitriou G: Effect on lung function of continuous positive airway pressure administered either by infant flow driver or a single nasal prong. Eur J Pediatr 159:289–292, 2000.

164. Thome U, Kossel H, Lipowski G, et al: Randomized comparison of high-frequency ventilation with high-rate intermittent positive pressure ventilation in preterm infants with respiratory failure. J Pediatr 135:39–46, 1999.

165. Clark RH: Support of gas exchange in the delivery room and beyond: How do we avoid hurting the baby we seek to save? Clin Perinatol 26:669–681, vii–viii, 1999.

166. Kalenga M, Battisti O, Francois A, et al: High-frequency oscillatory ventilation in neonatal RDS: Initial volume optimization and respiratory mechanics. J Appl Physiol 84:1174–1177, 1998.

167. Hachey WE, Eyal FG, Curt-Eyal NL, et al: High-frequency oscillatory ventilation versus conventional ventilation in a piglet model of early meconium aspiration. Crit Care Med 26:556–561, 1998.

168. Cox CA, Wolfson MR, Shaffer TH: Liquid ventilation: A comprehensive overview. Neonatal Netw 15:31–43, 1996.

169. Kuo CY, Hsueh C, Wang CR: Liquid ventilation for treatment of meconium aspiration syndrome in a piglet model. J Formos Med Assoc 97:392–399, 1998.

170. Carlo WA, Ambalavanan N: Conventional mechanical ventilation: Traditional and new strategies. Pediatr Rev 20:e117–e126, 1999.

171. Mrozek JD, Bendel-Stenzel EM, Meyers PA, et al: Randomized controlled trial of volume-targeted synchronized ventilation and conventional intermittent mandatory ventilation following initial exogenous surfactant therapy. Pediatr Pulmonol 29:11–18, 2000.

172. Schulze A: Enhancement of mechanical ventilation of neonates by computer technology. Semin Perinatol 24:429–444, 2000.

173. Degraeuwe PL, Thunnisen FB, Vos GD, et al: High-frequency oscillatory ventilation, partial liquid ventilation, or conventional mechanical ventilation in newborn piglets with saline lavage-induced acute lung injury. A comparison of gas-exchange efficacy and lung histomorphology. Biol Neonate 75:118–129, 1999.

174. Mariani GL, Carlo WA: Ventilatory management in neonates. Science or art? Clin Perinatol 25:33–48, 1998.

175. Smith KM, Bing DR, Meyers PA, et al: Partial liquid ventilation: A comparison using conventional and high-frequency techniques in an animal model of acute respiratory failure. Crit Care Med 25:1179–1186, 1997.

176. Ranieri VM, Suter PM, Tortorella C, et al: Effect of mechanical ventilation on inflammatory mediators in patients with acute respiratory distress syndrome: A randomized controlled trial. JAMA 282:54–61, 1999.

177. Coalson JJ, Kuehl TJ, Prihoda TJ, deLemos RA: Diffuse alveolar damage in the evolution of bronchopulmonary dysplasia in the baboon. Pediatr Res 24:357–366, 1988.

178. Saugstad OD: Is oxygen more toxic than currently believed? Pediatrics 108:1203–1205, 2001.

179. Dreyfuss D, Saumon G: Ventilator induced lung injury: Lesions from experimental studies. Am J Respir Crit Care Med 157:294–323, 1998.

180. Jobe AH, Ikegami M: Mechanism initiating lung injury in the preterm. Early Hum Dev 53:81–94, 1999.

181. Muscedere JG, Mullen JB, Gan K, Slutsky AS: Tidal ventilation at low airway pressures can augment lung injury. Am J Respir Crit Care Med 149:1327–1334, 1994.

3 CONTROL OF VENTILATION AND APNEA

NARONG SIMAKAJORNBOON, MD
ROBERT C. BECKERMAN, MD

Assisted ventilation often is used to treat respiratory control disorders in neonates. The basic knowledge of sleep and control of breathing in infants is important for understanding the pathophysiology of apnea in these patients. Intrauterine breathing patterns have been observed in a sheep fetus as early as 5 to 14 weeks of gestation (20 weeks term).[1] The irregular breathing movements in the human fetus have been detected as early as 11 weeks of gestation, with a rate ranging from 30 to 70 movements per minute and lasting between 55% and 99% of the day.[2] The breathing pattern is altered from a periodic non–air-breathing pattern in the fetus to a continuous air-breathing pattern in infants. Sleep and breathing patterns in infants undergo a significant maturation change during the first year of life. Prematurity profoundly affects the respiratory pattern with highly irregular and frequent apnea. Understanding this developmental change in sleep and breathing patterns is important for the neonatologist and pediatrician in the diagnosis and management of apnea and respiratory dysrhythmias in neonates. Adequate establishment of functional residual capacity (FRC) in newborns is essential if their lungs are to meet the metabolic demands placed on them. Although premature infants maintain their FRC through the tonic activity of the diaphragm and intercostal muscles during expiration, babies born at term combine prolonged postinspiratory muscle activity with laryngeal control of the expiratory flow. An infant who is unable to maintain an adequate FRC may progress to respiratory insufficiency and require mechanical ventilatory support, which is associated with an obvious risk of morbidity and mortality.

In this chapter, the development of sleep and respiratory control is reviewed. The pathophysiology, diagnosis, and management of common conditions that cause abnormal control of breathing in neonates and infants are discussed (Table 3-1).

DEVELOPMENTAL ASPECT OF SLEEP AND RESPIRATORY CONTROL

Fetus

The fetal respiratory center is active in utero as evidenced by phrenic nerve activity; however, this activity is minimal and has a different pattern than that present after birth.[3,4] In the human fetus, breathing movement can be identified at the 10th to 12th week of gestation.[5,6] By 20 to 28 weeks of gestation, rhythmical breathing activity is observed in utero and is characterized by long silent periods with no respiratory movement alternating with active periods.[7] This cycle varies between 40 and 60 minutes.[8]

Preterm Infants

In the preterm infant, active sleep is prominent and accounts for 90% of total sleep time at 31 weeks of gestation. The amount of active sleep decreases to 50% at term. Irregular breathing and apnea are common and occur primarily during active sleep.[9] Premature infants have greater breath-to-breath variability in minute ventilation compared to term infants. In contrast to term infants, preterm infants respond to hypoxia with a sustained decrease in ventilation with no initial hyperpnea, which may reflect an immaturity of the central nervous system involved in breathing control.[10,11] The reduced hypercapnic response may indicate reduced CO_2 sensitivity of the central chemoreceptors, and the response increases progressively with gestational age to the adult level at term.[12] In addition, stimulation of irritant receptors in the carina in preterm infants leads to apnea; term infants respond to the same stimuli with increased respiratory efforts. This paradoxical response to respiratory stimuli may be related to immaturity of vagal myelination.[13] Chest wall instability in preterm infants may contribute to apnea secondary to intermittent airway closure and decreased FRC.[14] Increasing lung volume by continuous

---

TABLE 3-1. Anatomic Classification of Respiratory Control: Disorders in the Neonate

Brainstem
Infection
Infarction
Hemorrhage
Trauma
Apnea of prematurity
Congenital central hypoventilation syndrome

Spinal Cord
Trauma
Spinal muscular atrophy

Myoneural Junction
Congenital myasthenia gravis
Familial infantile myasthenia gravis
Muscle
Myotonic dystrophy
Chest wall, airways, and lung
Congenital scoliosis
Skeletal dysplasias
Craniofacial anomalies
Airway anomalies
Bronchopulmonary dysplasia

Miscellaneous
Gastroesophageal reflux
Inborn error of metabolism

positive airway pressure (CPAP) results in resolution of the apnea (see Chapter 8).[15]

Term Infants

The amount of quiet sleep increases with age, with a reciprocal decrease in active sleep. Most apneas occur during active sleep. Several studies have shown that most apneas in healthy term infants are central apnea; obstructive and mixed apnea are rare.[16–18] The number of apneas decreases with gestational age.

Most term infants have a normal hypercapnic ventilatory response, with an appropriate increase in minute ventilation.[19] However, the ventilatory response to hypoxia is less effective and is characterized by a biphasic pattern. In response to mild hypoxemia (F_{IO_2} 0.15), term newborns respond by an increase in minute ventilation, followed by a decrease in ventilation below baseline.[20]

Periodic Breathing

Periodic breathing (PB) is a respiratory pattern of neonates and infants seen during the first few weeks of life. It presumably is caused by immaturity of the respiratory center. PB is characterized by alternation between respiratory pauses of 3 to 10 seconds and breathing periods of 10 to 15 seconds.[21,22] PB does not represent a dramatic alternation in respiratory control but illustrates on a large scale an oscillation found in all infants. The incidence of PB in infants of gestational ages less than 37 weeks is twice that of term infants and three-fold that of infants with adequate birthweight.[21] PB cycle duration progressively shortens over the first 3 months of life, suggesting maturation of peripheral chemoreceptors over this time period.[1,23] PB can account for 2% to 6% of breathing time in healthy term infants and as much as 19% to 25% in preterm infants.[24]

The pathophysiology of PB is unknown. Possible explanations include maturation of the respiratory system and imbalance between the contributions of central and peripheral chemoreceptors.[23] Animal models suggest that the occurrence of PB is associated with suppression of central chemoreceptors with heightened metabolic responses of the peripheral chemoreceptors to hypoxia and hypercapnia. The number and duration of PB cycles can be shortened by reduction of the alveolus/chemoreceptor circulation time; decrease in the time that the chemoreceptor takes to respond to hypoxemia by sending a signal to the central integrative mechanism; or improvement in the efficiency of the respiratory pump, which causes a more rapid correction of the hypoxemia and hypercapnia associated with the apneic pause.[23] The continuous oscillation in sleep state from active to quiet sleep or vice versa may increase respiratory instability during sleep in infants. Rigatto and Brady[10] reported an increase incidence of PB when the rate of change in ventilation was maximal.

PB in infants is a situational, episodic, and developmental phenomenon. There are no universally accepted standards for quantification of PB. Acceptable (nonpathologic) values noted in the literature range from 2% to 12% in preterm infants and 2% to 6% in term infants. PB can be considered a benign and transient disturbance in the breathing pattern of term infants if it comprises less than 6% of the respiratory pattern and is not associated with clinically significant hypoxemia or bradycardia.[25] PB should be considered abnormal if it is preceded by hypoxemia or is associated with bradycardia or prolonged apnea with alveolar hypoventilation (Fig. 3-1).

APNEA OF PREMATURITY

Definition and Incidence

Apnea of prematurity is the most common disorder of breathing in neonates. The term generally applies to apneas that occur in infants of less than 37 weeks of gestation without any other identifiable cause. It is defined by cessation of air flow greater than 20 seconds or less than 20 seconds if accompanied by oxygen desaturation, bradycardia, or changes of muscle tone. The prevalence of apnea of prematurity is inversely related to gestational age and birthweight.[26] In infants weighing less than 1500 g, the incidence of apnea is approximately 25% to 50%, and it approaches 90% for those weighing less than 1000 g.[27–29] The majority of very-low-birthweight premature babies will exhibit apnea in the first week unless they receive mechanical ventilatory support.[26] Apnea often starts after the first week of life in babies who manifest uncomplicated respiratory problems, and it may coincide with the time of weaning from ventilator support.[27,30]

Pathophysiology

Three different types of apneic episodes can be identified: (1) *central apnea* is characterized by a cessation of both air flow and respiratory efforts; (2) *obstructive apnea* is defined as an absence of air flow despite continued respiratory efforts; and (3) *mixed apnea* is defined as a central apnea that either is preceded or followed by obstructive apnea. The percentage of each type of apnea varies among studies and depends on the definition of the duration of apnea. Upton et al.[31] used an apnea duration of at least 5 seconds and found that 58% were central, 35.5% were mixed, and 6.5% were obstructive. In addition, airway closure was identified in the majority of apneas, including central and mixed apnea. This finding suggests that airway obstruction is important in the pathophysiology of apnea; therefore, central and mixed apnea are not distinct entities but are part of the continuum of airway closure.[31]

Several pathophysiologic mechanisms have been proposed as the cause of apnea. The most acceptable theory proposes abnormal control of breathing caused by neuronal immaturity of the brainstem believed to be secondary to the lack of axo-dendritic synaptic connections leading to decreased afferent signal from peripheral chemoreceptors to brainstem rhythm generators.[32] Using brainstem auditory evoked response, Henderson-Smart et al.[33] demonstrated a decrease in the number and severity of apnea with maturation as evidenced by reduced brainstem conduction time. As dendritic and other synaptic interconnections multiply in the maturing brain, apnea of prematurity tends to resolve at approximately 34 to 52 weeks of postconceptional age.[27,28] Immature respiratory drive may play a role in the pathogenesis of apnea of prematurity. As mentioned previously, the hypoxic ventilatory responses in preterm infants are less vigorous than in older infants and involve a significant component of hypoxic ventilatory depression.[10,20] Ventilatory responses to hypercapnia are significantly reduced in preterm infants with apnea, especially during rapid eye movement (REM) sleep (Fig. 3-2).[34–36]

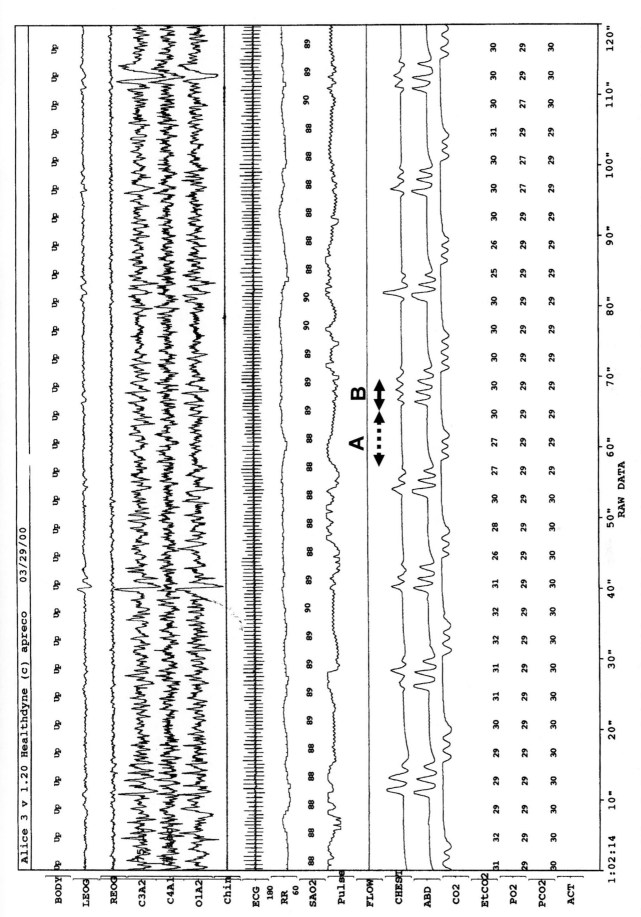

Figure 3-1. Multichannel polysomnography in 2-month-old full term infant. Recordings from top to bottom are the left and right electrooculogram, three-channel electroencephalogram, chin electromyogram, electrocardiogram, R-R interval, pulse oximetry, pulse waveform, thoracic and abdominal inductance plethysmography, end-tidal CO_2, and transcutaneous pO_2 and pCO_2. Recording reveals periodic breathing characterized by alternation between apnea of 3 to 10 seconds (A) and breathing periods (B) of 10 to 15 seconds during active sleep associated with oxygen desaturation.

43

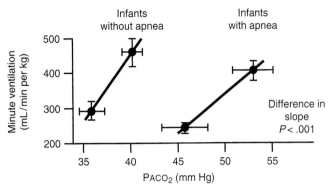

Figure 3-2. Comparison of carbon dioxide sensitivity obtained from ventilatory responses to changing alveolar P_{CO_2} (P_{ACO_2}) in preterm infants with and without apnea. Note the less steep ventilatory response in the apneic group. (From Gerhardt T, Bancalari E: Apnea of prematurity: I. Lung function and regulation of breathing. Pediatrics 74:58, 1984. Reproduced with permission of Pediatrics.)

The role of upper airway obstruction in the pathogenesis of apnea cannot be overemphasized. Intrinsic instability of the upper airway muscles may compromise upper airway patency, especially in premature infants. Cohen and Henderson-Smart[37] reported that inspiratory upper airway muscle activity did not show the usual progressive augmentation in response to nasal occlusion. Another factor that may decrease upper airway patency in premature infants is delayed chemoreceptor activation of upper airway muscles compared with that of the diaphragm.[38] This mechanism could be responsible for the common observation of obstructive breaths when inspiratory efforts resume, particularly after long central apneic episodes. Posture also may play a role in airway narrowing during neck flexion in preterm infants.[39] Upper airway reflexes (i.e., laryngeal chemoreceptor reflex) have been demonstrated in preterm infants; water induces a greater apneic response and more severe response when instilled into the hypopharynx than the nose.[40,41] Pickens et al.[42] showed that the majority of spontaneous prolonged apneic episodes in preterm infants have multiple features that are characteristic of an exaggerated airway protective response to an upper airway fluid stimulus. Endogenous upper airway secretions may be an important source of stimuli-inducing apneic episodes.[42] Finally, an exaggerated underlying oscillating breathing pattern has been proposed as a mechanism for apnea. Supplemental oxygen can decrease this oscillation by reducing breath-by-breath variability, leading to a decreased number of apneic episodes.[43]

Gastroesophageal reflux of both acid and alkaline fluids is a normal developmental phenomenon in both full-term and preterm infants. It usually is self-limited and occurs in infants between 1 month and 6 to 12 months of age. Because apnea of prematurity also occurs in that age/developmental window, it has been difficult to assign a cause-and-effect relationship among apnea, hypoxia, bradycardic events, and reflux of stomach acid. Symptoms associated with gastroesophageal reflux disease (GERD) are listed in Table 3-2. Most clinicians and investigators believe that GERD generally triggers either obstructive or mixed apnea type of events. However, acid reflux even into the distal third of the esophagus may uncommonly provoke vagal-mediated central apneas, known as *reflux apnea*. Apnea events that are presumed to be triggered by acid reflux occur more often while the infant is in the awake state and has recently been or is concurrently being fed. Because

TABLE 3-2. Clinical Symptoms Associated with Gastroesophageal Reflux

Cough
Stridor
Hiccups
Hoarseness
Bronchospasm
Failure to thrive
Aspiration pneumonia

preterm infants are fed so frequently and often by gavage, their tendency to have GERD is increased compared to full-term infants. They also have intense pharyngeal and laryngeal acid chemoreceptor responses (from 32 weeks of gestational age). The latter response usually is one of airway collapse and laryngeal spasm, thereby explaining the occurrence of obstructive events with associated hypoxia and bradycardia. Any disorder, whether congenital or acquired, that effects upper airway obstruction may result in increased GERD. These events presumably are caused by wide fluctuation in negative intrathoracic pressures during inspiration against a resistant or anatomically obstructed extrathoracic airway. Figure 3-3 shows the association between GERD and infant apnea.

The effect of apnea on cardiovascular function can be significant. The most apparent effect on cardiovascular function is abrupt bradycardia during apnea. Bradycardia may be initiated by hypoxemia or may represent a chemoreceptor-mediated vagal reflex.[44] Henderson-Smart et al.[44] reported that the incidence of bradycardia was greater in mixed and obstructive apnea than in central apnea, suggesting an important role of vagal reflex stimulation during obstructed breathing. Other cardiovascular changes during apnea involve an increase in pulse pressure and peripheral vasoconstriction; however, there is little clinical change in blood pressure.[45,46] The majority of bradycardias in these premature infants are related to apnea, and the incidence of bradycardia increases significantly with the length of apnea.[44] Bradycardia can occur at the onset of apnea if there is already substantial chemoreceptor drive, such as during disconnection of the ventilator for suction.

Diagnosis

The diagnosis of apnea of prematurity is made by excluding all other causes of neonatal apnea. The etiology of neonatal apnea includes infection, metabolic disorders, thermal instability, gastroesophageal reflux, and neurologic causes (Table 3-3). In addition, the presence of these disorders may accentuate apnea of prematurity, especially when there is a sudden appearance or increase in the frequency of apnea in a previously stable infant. The infant's history should include prenatal, perinatal, and postnatal information that may guide the clinician to a specific disease entity. Physical examination should focus on the infant's breathing pattern during awake and sleep periods, and a complete respiratory, cardiac, and neurologic examination. Clinical observation can give some clue to the diagnosis; however, studies have shown that a large percentage of apnea episodes were not detected by nursing staff.[47,48] Nursing detection not only identified significantly less true apnea and bradycardia, but it also misclassified the type of events in a significant number of infants.[49]

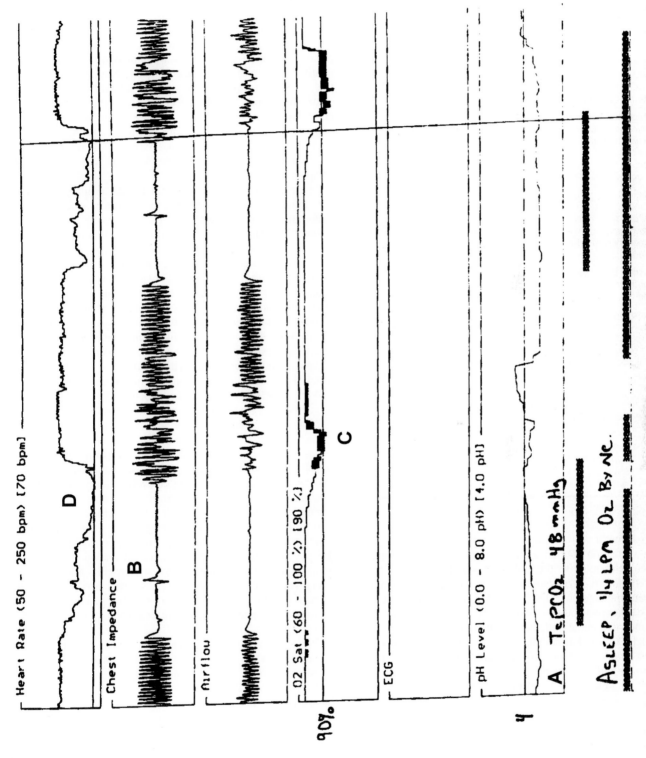

Figure 3-3. Multichannel physiologic recording in a 10-week-old male infant born at 30 weeks of gestational age shows a sequence of gastroesophageal reflux (A) (pH <4) to the lower and upper esophagus. These reflux episodes were followed by severe mixed apnea (B), hypoxia (C), and bradycardia (D), which were life threatening and resolved rapidly after a Nissen fundoplication was performed (tracing not shown).

TABLE 3-3. Apnea in Neonates: Differential Diagnosis

Infection
Meningitis
Sepsis

Metabolic Disorder
Hypoglycemia
Hyperbilirubinemia
Hyponatremia
Hypocalcemia
Hypomagnesemia
Hypochloremia
Inborn error of metabolism

Intracranial Pathology
Intracranial bleeding
Arteriovenous malformation
Tumors
Seizures
Hypoxic-ischemic encephalopathy

Impaired Oxygenation
Anemia
Cyanotic heart disease
Patent ductus arteriosus
Pulmonary hemorrhage
Pneumonia/bronchiolitis (respiratory syncytial virus)

Thermal Disturbance
Hypothermia
Hyperthermia

Anatomic Narrowing or Obstruction of the Airways
Choanal atresia
Micrognathia
Macroglossia
Vocal cord paralysis
Subglottic stenosis
Laryngomalacia
Tracheobronchomalacia

Developmental Cause
Apnea of prematurity

Miscellaneous
Gastroesophageal reflux
Hypotension
Drug depression

An overnight polysomnographic study is the most complete test for evaluation of infant apnea. The standard infant montage includes assessment of the following parameters: body position, left and right electrooculogram, central and occipital electroencephalogram (C3A1, C4A1), chin electromyogram, electrocardiogram, pulse oximetry and pulse waveform, thoracic and abdominal inductance plethysmography, air flow, end-tidal CO_2, and transcutaneous PO_2 and PCO_2. The study allows accurate assessment of the apnea and its effect on cardiovascular and pulmonary function (Fig. 3-3). It provides not only the data on the cardiorespiratory events but also information on sleep architecture, sleep organization, and the relationship between sleep states and apnea (Fig. 3-4). This complete study also offers accurate assessment of apnea and differentiation of true apnea from artifact.

Management

Treatment of apnea includes supportive care, oxygen, methylxanthine therapy, CPAP, and assisted ventilation. General supportive care may include proper positioning of the head and neck with the head in the midline and the neck in the neutral position or slightly extended to minimize airway obstruction. Tactile stimulation may be appropriate for occasional apneic events and can be done manually or by placing the infant on an oscillating waterbed. Precipitating factors, which include anemia, hypoxemia, hypothermia, and hyperthermia, should be corrected. Blood transfusion may be considered in significantly anemic infants.[50,51] If the apnea is prolonged with severe hypoxemia and bradycardia, mechanical ventilatory support should be considered. Nasal CPAP is effective, especially when there is a significant component of obstructive apnea.[52,53] The effect of nasal CPAP is believed to be secondary to improvement in upper airway patency and an increase in the stability of the lower rib cage.[52] The usual distending pressure is between 2 and 5 cm H_2O. Nasal CPAP has no effect on central apnea and may interfere with feeding (see Chapter 8).

Pharmacologic therapy is considered the primary treatment for apnea of prematurity. Methylxanthines (theophylline, caffeine) are the mainstay of pharmacologic therapy (see Chapter 19). The specific mechanisms of action on respiratory control are unknown. Several mechanisms have been proposed, including increased CO_2 sensitivity, increased respiratory center output, increased diaphragmatic contraction, increased catecholamine activity, increased metabolic rate, and decreased diaphragmatic fatigue.[54,55] Theophylline has greater efficacy as a diuretic and bronchodilator; however, it is associated with more cardiac side effects. Caffeine is more effective in central nervous system and respiratory stimulation and appears to penetrate cerebrospinal fluid better than does theophylline.[56,57] Theophylline is metabolized by methylation reaction to caffeine. It has a mean half-life in newborns of 30 hours, which is six times longer than in adults.[55,58] The half-life of caffeine varies between 86 and 277 hours; the majority of the drug is cleared by the kidneys due to inability of the neonate to metabolize caffeine through hepatic pathways.[59] The recommended dosages for methylxanthines are as follows: theophylline, a loading dose of 5 to 6 mg/kg and maintenance doses of 1 to 2 mg/kg every 8 hours; and caffeine, a loading dose of 10 mg/kg and maintenance doses of 2.5 mg/kg per day. The therapeutic serum level range for theophylline is 5 to 15 mg/mL and that for caffeine is 8 to 20 mg/mL. For a given serum level, caffeine may have fewer side effects than theophylline. Therefore, for premature infants who may require higher doses, caffeine may be the preferred drug. Another respiratory stimulant, doxapram, has been used in neonates with refractory apnea. It acts through stimulation of a peripheral chemoreceptor and has been shown to increase minute ventilation and tidal volume.[27]

Previous studies have shown that apnea of prematurity and PB resolve when oxygen concentration is increased to the threshold level.[21,43,60] Rigatto and Brady[61] reported that inhalation of 100% O_2 is associated with a decrease in PB and an increase in minute ventilation (VE).[61] Subsequent studies demonstrated that modest increases in oxygen decrease apnea and periodicity in preterm infants, not via an increase in ventilation but through a decrease in breath-to-breath variability in VE.[43] We recently studied the effect of low-flow supplemental oxygen on sleep architecture and cardiorespiratory function in premature infants. Low-flow supplemental oxygen not only significantly reduced the amount of apnea and PB, but it also altered sleep architecture by an increase in the amount of quiet

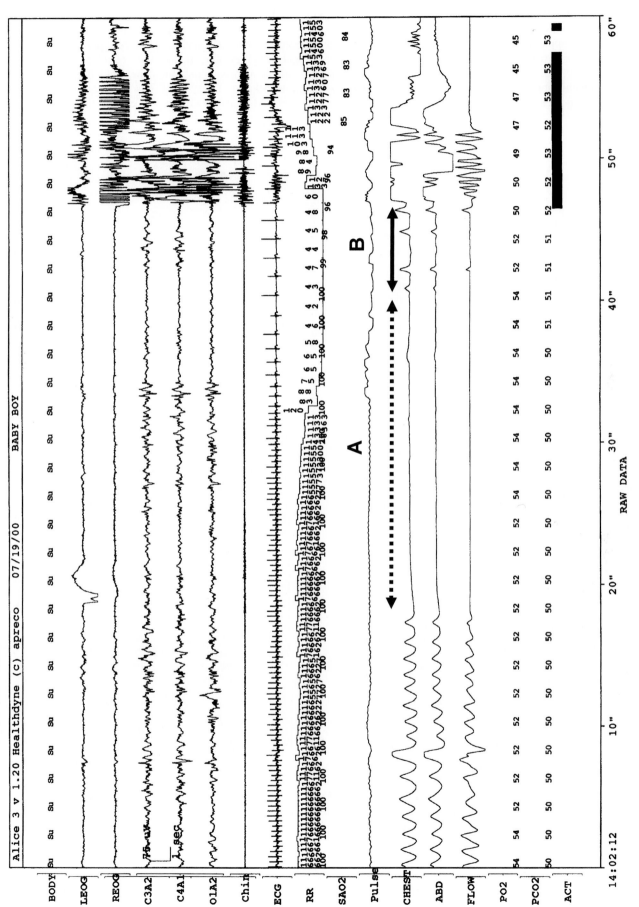

Figure 3-4. Overnight polysomnographic sleep study in a 4-week-old infant, former premature 30-week-gestation infant. Recording demonstrates prolonged mixed apnea with initial central apnea (A), followed by an obstructive component (B) at the end. This episode of apnea occurred during quiet sleep and was associated with oxygen desaturation, electroencephalographic arousal, and significant bradycardia.

47

sleep with a reciprocal decrease in the amount of active sleep.[61a] No adverse effects on alveolar ventilation were observed with the use of low-flow supplemental oxygen (Fig. 3-5).

Apnea of prematurity usually resolves by 40 to 50 weeks of postconceptional age; however, some premature infants continue to have idiopathic apnea and require both medical therapy and home monitoring after this period has elapsed. The decision to discontinue pharmacologic therapy in these infants is empirical. It is prudent to discontinue the medication when infants have been asymptomatic and have reached appropriate postconceptional age. Premature infants with or without a history of apnea are at increased risk for apnea and bradycardia after general anesthesia. Because of this increased risk, elective surgery should be deferred, if possible, until the infants' respi-

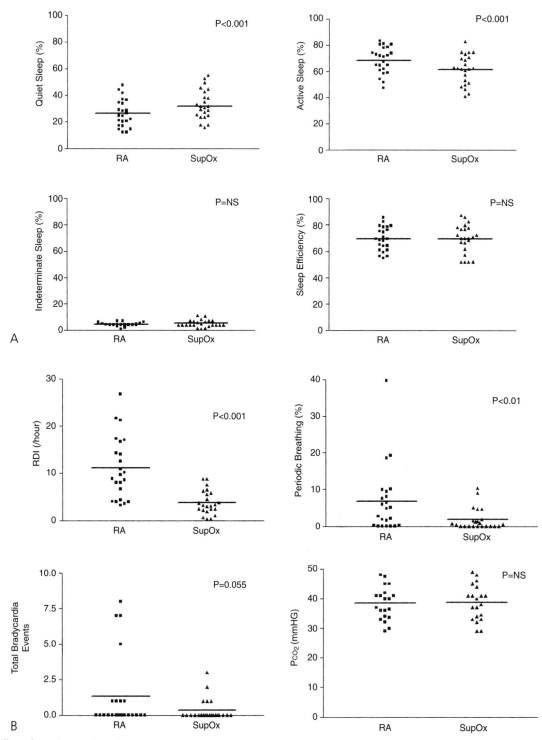

Figure 3-5. Effect of supplemental oxygen on sleep architecture and cardiorespiratory events in preterm infants. *A,* Use of supplemental oxygen is associated with an increase in percentage of quiet sleep with reciprocal decrease in time spent in active sleep. *B,* In terms of cardiorespiratory events, use of supplemental oxygen decreases the frequency of apnea, percentage of periodic breathing time, and number of bradycardias with no adverse effect on alveolar ventilation. RA, room air; RDI, respiratory disturbance index; SupOx, supplemental oxygen.

ratory control mechanism is more mature (approximately 50–60 weeks of postconceptional age). If deferral is not possible, the infants should be monitored in the hospital for apnea and bradycardia for at least 12 hours after surgery. Methylxanthine therapy may be considered postoperatively.

BRONCHOPULMONARY DYSPLASIA

Bronchopulmonary dysplasia (BPD) is a chronic lung disease of infants that results from mechanical ventilation in neonates who require supplemental oxygen at 28 days of postnatal age and/or 36 weeks of postconceptual age (see Chapter 21). This term is now often replaced by *chronic lung disease of infancy.* First described in 1967 by Northway et al.,[62] infants with BPD have abnormal respiratory control, especially during sleep, which predisposes them to episodes of respiratory failure, cor pulmonale, and sudden unexpected death.

Infants with BPD have abnormal pulmonary mechanics, predominantly an increase in airway resistance and a decrease in lung compliance.[63,64] The measurement of this resistance, however, is not a sensitive test for lower airway dysfunction. Infants with BPD also have decreased dynamic pulmonary compliance and marked elevation of FRC. These infants are at risk for developing tracheobronchomalacia that results from a lack of cartilage development and airway injury due to prolonged mechanical ventilation, barotrauma, oxygen toxicity, pulmonary infections, mucociliary abnormalities, and malnutrition.[65]

Abnormalities of sleep architectures and cardiovascular disturbances occur during sleep in infants with BPD. Harris and Sullivan[66] demonstrated that infants with BPD had significant sleep disruption and reduced REM sleep that may be secondary to increased arousal response to minimize oxygen desaturation. Sleep fragmentation was reversed with the use of supplemental oxygen. Garg et al.[67] reported that infants with BPD aroused normally to the hypoxic challenge; however, they required vigorous stimulation after the initial arousal response. These data suggest that such infants may have an abnormal response to hypoxia after arousal that may lead to prolonged apnea and bradycardia.[67] Clinically unexpected hypoxemia during sleep and feeding has been reported despite acceptable awake oxygen saturation.[68–72] In addition, the total desaturation time in these infants correlated with airway resistance, indicating the important role of airway obstruction.[68] In these infants, a decrease in the inspired fraction of oxygen increased airway restriction that was alleviated with the use of supplemental oxygen.[73,74] Sleep-related hypoxemia also has an adverse effect on cardiac function. Praud et al.[75] reported a decrease in both right and left ventricular ejection fractions in severe BPD with significant nocturnal desaturations. In addition, abnormal autonomic control of heart rate variability was observed in patients with severe BPD in relation to sleep stages and mild changes in oxygen saturation.[76] A previous study showed an association between BPD and sudden infant death syndrome (SIDS)[77]; however, a subsequent study suggested that infants with BPD were not at increased risk from SIDS if appropriate management that included supplemental oxygen and monitoring was provided.[78]

Management of BPD involves the use of long-term oxygen supplementation. As mentioned earlier, several studies have shown the benefit of supplemental oxygen. In addition, supplemental oxygen has been shown to improve central respiratory stability by decreasing central apnea and PB densities[69] and to promote growth when oxygen saturation is maintained above 92%.[79] Supplemental oxygen also may be useful for the treatment of pulmonary hypertension associated with BPD.[80,81] Awake oxygenation status does not accurately predict sleep-related hypoxemia; therefore, overnight polysomnographic evaluation is necessary to assess the need for oxygen support and to determine when to discontinue oxygen therapy.

Patients with severe BPD may require mechanical ventilatory support. Pressure-plateau ventilation allows breath-by-breath compensation of variable leaks from the delivery system. This technique of ventilation uses a volume ventilator in the assist/control mode with a set pressure limit. Large tidal volumes can be provided, and, with use of a pressure limit, the peak pressure can be sustained, thus allowing the excess volume to be discarded. This ventilation approach is especially useful in young infants and obviates the need for cuffed endotracheal tubes.[82] Infants who have undergone mechanical ventilation for long periods of time may be at risk for poor ventilatory muscular endurance because of deconditioning. In addition, hypoexcitability of the respiratory center secondary to chronic hypercapnia increases the susceptibility of these infants to respiratory arrest when small doses of sedative drugs are administered.[83] Therefore, elective surgery performed on these infants should be planned carefully so that the complications of apnea and alveolar hypoventilation secondary to poor muscular endurance can be prevented.

Several medications have been used for the treatment of BPD; however, no specific treatment guidelines have been established. Diuretics using the combination of furosemide or thiazides and spironolactone improve the dynamic compliance of infants with BPD and their specific airway conductance and airway resistance. However, use of diuretics may impair respiratory control by leading to hypochloremic and hypokalemic metabolic alkalosis with secondary retention of bicarbonate that may worsen hypercapnia.[84,85] Inhaled bronchodilators (e.g., albuterol) have been used to reduce airway obstruction in ventilator-dependent infants with BPD. Use of methylxanthines is more controversial. These drugs improve the function of ventilatory muscles and central ventilatory drive and relax bronchial smooth muscle, causing mild diuresis and stimulating ciliary motility. However, the frequent side effects of vomiting, irritability, tachycardia, and diarrhea require the monitoring of drug levels and make their use difficult.[64,83] Steroids should be used only for chronically ventilated infants with significant oxygen and ventilator requirements who have not responded to conventional therapies.[84,85] Use of steroids has been associated with an increase in adverse neurologic sequelae in premature infants, thus prompting the Committee of the Fetus and Newborn of the American Academy of Pediatrics to advise against their routine use except under investigational protocol.[85a] Further discussion of these pharmacologic therapies can be found in Chapter 19.

CONGENITAL CENTRAL HYPOVENTILATION SYNDROME

Congenital central hypoventilation syndrome (CCHS) is an uncommon respiratory control disorder characterized by failure of autonomic respiratory control. CCHS previously was named *Ondine's curse* and was first described in 1962 in three patients who became apneic after cervical spinal cord and brainstem surgery. The first case of an infant with CCHS was reported in 1970 by Mellins et al.[86] Infants with CCHS develop alveolar hypoventilation with concomitant hypercapnia and hypoxemia without primary cardiac, pulmonary, or neuromuscular disease (NMD).[87] The severity of hypoventilation is state dependent and is most severely affected during non-REM sleep, for which metabolic respiratory control is predominant. Respiratory control abnormalities are also present to a lesser degree during awake and REM sleep due to breathing drive from behavioral inputs.[13]

Several hypotheses have been proposed to explain the etiologies of CCHS. CCHS is associated with neural crest migrational abnormalities such as Hirschsprung disease[88] and ganglioneuroma.[89] Because the *re*arranged during *t*ransfection (RET) proto-oncogene is associated with Hirschsprung disease,[90] an RET mutation is speculated to be an important gene in the pathogenesis of CCHS. RET knockout mice have demonstrated reduced hypercapnic ventilatory responses[91]; however, genetic screening in patients with CCHS has not revealed an RET gene mutation.[92] Previous studies reported hypoplasia of the arcuate nucleus in one patient[93] and the presence of abnormal evoked potential responses to auditory stimuli,[94,95] suggesting structural abnormalities of the central nervous system. Subsequent study by Weese-Mayer et al.[96] revealed normal brainstem and spinal cord imaging by magnetic resonance. Patients with CCHS have absent hypoxic and hypercapnic ventilatory responses during wakefulness and sleep. An abnormality in central integration of central and peripheral chemoreceptors has been speculated.[97] In addition to loss of ventilatory control, there appears to be loss of heart rate variability, indicating a disturbance of autonomic nervous control.[98]

Clinical presentation of infants with CCHS is variable and depends on the severity of the disorder.[99] In severe cases, infants present with severe hypoventilation that requires ventilatory support at birth. This group of infants does not breathe spontaneously and will need 24-hour assisted ventilation during the first few months of life, but they may improve to a pattern of adequate ventilation during wakefulness over time.[82] In less severe cases, infants may present at a later age with cyanosis, edema, and signs of right heart failure, and they often may be incorrectly diagnosed as having cyanotic congenital heart disease.[99] Some patients may present with unexplained apnea and an apparent life-threatening event (ALTE). In late-onset CCHS, patients may present with tachycardia, diaphoresis, and cyanosis during sleep.[100] The proposed diagnostic criteria include the following: (1) shallow breathing or cyanosis and apnea that is worse during sleep than in wakefulness and has a perinatal onset; (2) hypoventilation that is worse during sleep than wakefulness; (3) absence of primary lung disease or ventilatory muscle dysfunction that can explain the hypoventilation; and (4) no evidence of primary heart disease.[101] The diagnostic approach should include careful evaluation of the infant's respiratory pattern and gas exchange abnormalities by polysomnographic study. Other investigations consist of cardiac evaluation, including chest roentgenogram, echocardiogram, diaphragm fluoroscopy to rule out diaphragmatic paralysis, extensive neurologic evaluation if significant hypotonia is present, imaging studies of the central nervous system, and metabolic studies.[82]

Medical therapy with respiratory stimulants has failed to demonstrate improvement in patients with CCHS. Doxapram, a central and peripheral respiratory stimulant, has been used primarily to counteract postanesthetic respiratory depression. Clinical trials of doxapram and almitrine bimesylate have not shown consistent improvement in spontaneous ventilatory or gas exchange parameters.[102,103] The most important aspect of management of patients with CCHS is mechanical ventilatory support through a tracheostomy tube. Negative-pressure ventilation has been used with some success in patients with CCHS[104]; however, it is cumbersome and may lead to upper airway obstruction.[105] Use of noninvasive positive-pressure ventilation through nasal mask has been reported in older patients who required nocturnal ventilatory support.[106,107] Bilateral diaphragmatic pacing with the use of a high-frequency radiotransmitter has been an effective mode of ventilation after the neonatal period, especially for infants who require daytime ventilation support. The patient who benefits most from diaphragmatic pacing is the child who is ventilator dependent 24 hours a day, has no intrinsic lung disease, does not require supplemental oxygen, and has preservation of the cervical nerve roots of the phrenic nerve (C3–C5), the phrenic nerve itself, and the diaphragm. Bilateral rather than unilateral pacing usually is necessary for adequate alveolar ventilation because of the infant's highly compliant rib cage and increased metabolic rate corrected for body weight. Tracheostomy has been necessary for prevention of upper airway obstruction due to the absence of laryngeal and pharyngeal dilator muscle activation during noncentrally (i.e., paced) inspirations. All patients who undergo diaphragm pacing should have pulse oximetric monitoring during sleep as an alarm for pacer malfunction. The arguments against diaphragmatic pacing include its high cost, development of nerve injury or diaphragm fatigue, and discomfort associated with surgical revisions due to pacer malfunction.[87,108,109]

There is no evidence that patients with CCHS outgrow their abnormal respiratory control problem. With proper management, severe medical complications such as cor pulmonale, poor growth, seizure disorder, mild cerebral palsy, and developmental delay[99] can be minimized. Early diagnosis and appropriate ventilatory support of infants with these conditions will limit the morbidity from hypoxia and improve long-term outcome.[87]

APNEA OF INFANCY

During the first 6 months of life, normal full-term infants may have isolated apnea that lasts from 5 to 15 seconds with or without PB.[110] *Apnea of infancy* is defined as apnea of more than 20 seconds or shorter if it is associated with color change or bradycardia. The term is used for infants born after 38 weeks of gestation to differentiate it from apnea of prematurity, which occurs in infants of less than 37 weeks of gestation.[111]

Apparent life-threatening events (ALTEs) refer to episodes that are frightening to the observer and usually consist of some combination of apnea, color change, decreased tone, choking, or gagging. This term replaces the term *near-miss SIDS,* which imprecisely indicated an association of these events with SIDS (Consensus Statement[111]). The etiologic factors of ALTE include infection, gastroesophageal reflux, seizure disorder, cardiac disease, and metabolic disease. Approximately 50% of ALTEs are idiopathic and sometimes are classified as apnea of infancy. Most studies report high survival rates in infants with ALTE; however, a small percentage of infants with ALTE progress to sudden and unexpected death.[112] Studies of cardiorespiratory function in infants with ALTE have revealed inconclusive results. Several studies showed an increased number of mixed apnea, obstructive apnea, and PB in patients with ALTE.[16,113,114] Other studies revealed a blunted hypoxic and arousal response in these infants.[115,116] Some investigations failed to note a difference in hypoxic and hypercapnic response between control and ALTE infants.[117,118] An abnormal cardiac rhythm (prolonged QT) interval was reported initially in these infants but was not confirmed by subsequent studies.

Management of ALTE requires identification of the specific etiology. When a specific cause of an ALTE is identified, an appropriate treatment may then be initiated. The benefit of home apnea monitoring is controversial. There is no evidence that home apnea monitoring prevents any deaths, but it may be cost effective compared with continued hospitalization and may alleviate anxiety in some families.

CRANIOFACIAL SYNDROMES

Neonates with craniofacial anomalies (CFAs) may have airway obstruction secondary to anatomic abnormalities that narrow the opening of the nasal or pharyngeal airway or displace the tongue posteriorly into the pharyngeal airway. Structural and functional airway narrowing in infants who have a variety of CFAs may lead to sleep disordered breathing (SDB) and is a major predisposing factor to infant morbidity and mortality. The inability to maintain upper airway patency during sleep in patients with CFA is the result of complex interactions between abnormal airway anatomy and alteration of the normal neuromuscular control of breathing. These structural abnormalities can predispose the infant to obstructive and mixed apnea, episodes of which tend to occur more often while the infant is sleeping in the supine position or during feeding or crying.

The most common structural anatomic abnormalities in infants and children with CFAs are nasal obstruction, malformation of the cranial base and midface, macroglossia, and hypoplasia of the lower jaw (see Chapter 22). Patients with these abnormalities often present with SDB or sleep-related disturbance. In the neonate, nasal obstruction may be due to choanal atresia. These malformations can present as an isolated entity or may be associated with facial clefting, as occurs in Treacher Collins syndrome. Nasopharyngeal hypoplasia can occur secondary to malformations of the cranial base or midface, as seen in Apert, Crouzon, and Down syndromes. The relatively small nasopharyngeal space resulting from hypoplasia is highly vulnerable to obstruction, even from normal adenotonsillar tissue. Hypoplasia of the lower jaw can compromise the upper airways, either because of retroglossia or by intrusion of retromandibular structures. In addition to the obstructive lesion, a central respiratory defect may play an important role in the morbidity of these patients.

Craniofacial dysostosis frequently is associated with hindbrain herniation, which may lead to abnormalities of respiratory control. In infants and young children, the obstructive mechanism can lead to central apnea. In obese children, central apnea can be the result of low lung volume. Upper airway obstruction can lead to chronic alveolar hypoventilation, which results in hypoxemia or hypercapnia with respiratory acidosis. These gas exchange abnormalities may cause a constrictive

TABLE 3-4. Prototypical Craniofacial Syndromes and Associated Sleep Disordered Breathing

Craniofacial Abnormalities	Disorders	Sleep Abnormalities
Craniosynostosis	Crouzon syndrome Apert syndrome	OA
Mandibular hypoplasia	Pierre Robin syndrome Treacher Collins syndrome	OA
Skeletal disorders	Achondroplasia	Hypoventilation, CA, OA
Miscellaneous	Down syndrome	Hypoventilation, OA
	Arnold-Chiari malformation	Hypoventilation, OA, CA

CA, central apnea; OA, obstructive apnea.

response of the pulmonary vascular bed, resulting in increased right ventricular work and eventual cor pulmonale and heart failure. In achondroplasia, severe obstructive sleep apnea is associated with absence of slow-wave sleep and deficiency of overnight growth hormone secretion. Correction of apnea by tracheostomy can improve growth rates postoperatively.[119] SDB abnormalities in infants with craniofacial syndromes are summarized in Table 3-4.

Infants with CFA usually present with upper airway obstruction during wakefulness and sleep that may lead to chronic respiratory failure. The symptoms of SDB are similar in infants who have obstructive sleep apnea syndrome, which is characterized by loud snoring, difficulty breathing during sleep, breathing pauses, nocturnal enuresis, nocturnal sweats, restless sleep, and frequent awakening. Infants often differ in the frequency and severity of such symptoms. In addition, morning headaches, failure to thrive, respiratory failure, and cor pulmonale more frequently accompany SDB in children with CFA. The increased energy that is required for breathing to overcome the resistance created by the upper airway obstruction is associated with sweating, poor growth, and other signs of high metabolic rate. Alveolar hypoventilation results in chronic hypercapnia that can reduce the respiratory center sensitivity to CO_2, with a decrease in respiratory drive and further hypoventilation during sleep. The hypoexcitability of the respiratory center in patients with CFAs makes them, like infants with BPD, susceptible to respiratory arrest when small doses of a sedative are administered.

Overnight polysomnography is considered the most objective physiologic study for baseline evaluation of cardiorespiratory functions in infants with CFA. Daytime nap studies in patients with Down syndrome have been shown to underestimate the presence and severity of SDB[120] and are considered unreliable. Polysomnograms will quantify the severity of the problem and determine the need for further intervention. Chest and abdominal wall movement are recorded simultaneously so that paradoxical inward movement of the chest can be documented during periods of partial airway obstruction. The study can objectively document the type of apnea present, that is, central, obstructive, or mixed, and its relationship to sleep stage and body position during sleep (Fig. 3-6). The study also can reveal if there is hypopnea, significant hypoxemia, or hypoventilation. Repeat sleep studies provide valuable information on the efficacy of treatment in the follow-up of these children.

The underlying cause of SDB must be clearly defined before treatment recommendations are made. Central apnea has been

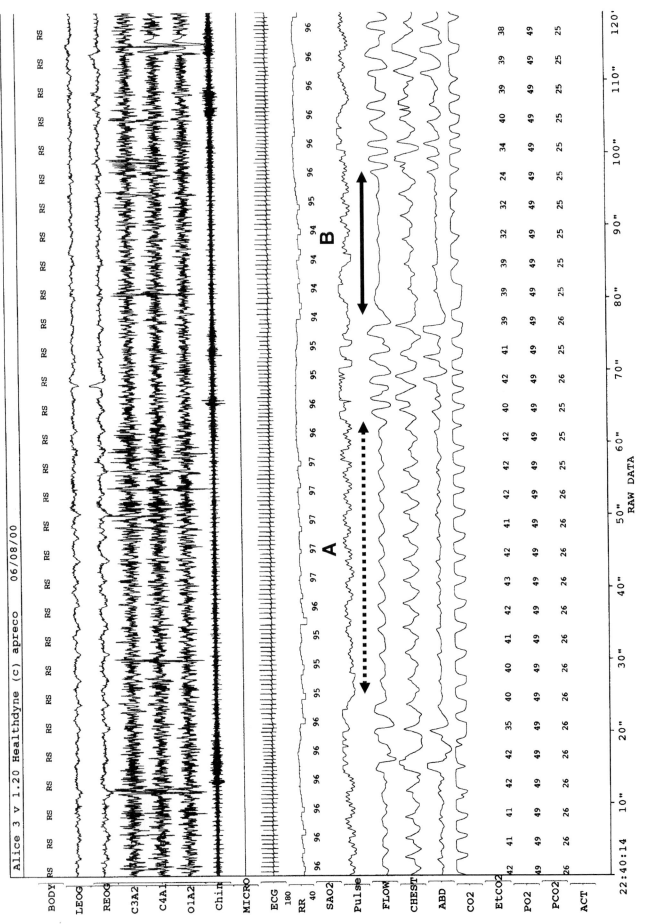

Figure 3-6. Example of polysomnographic study in an infant with Pierre Robin syndrome. Repetitive episodes of obstructive hypopnea and apnea (A) occur during rapid eye movement sleep and are associated with mild oxygen desaturation and arousal (B).

52

successfully treated with a number of medications, most commonly methylxanthines such as caffeine and theophylline. Another respiratory stimulant, acetazolamide, has been shown to improve SDB in some infants with Arnold-Chiari malformation.[121] Protriptyline has been reported to benefit some patients who have Down syndrome and SDB.[122] If the patient is obese, weight loss is important in the management of SDB.

Any indications for surgical intervention of the airway should be based upon careful evaluation of anatomic and physiologic abnormalities. Tonsillectomy and adenoidectomy (T&A) are the initial surgical procedures for relief of the signs and symptoms of SDB in infants and children. Patients with Down syndrome and SDB usually show partial benefit from T&A. However, complications of simple T&A in infants and children with Down syndrome include hypernasality and nasal regurgitation, which sometimes can result in translaryngeal aspiration. Some patients may have residual apnea after T&A and may require second-stage surgery with uvulopalatopharyngoplasty and tongue reduction.[123] Infants with CFA who have SDB, failure to thrive, chronic respiratory failure, and cor pulmonale are at significantly increased risk for prolonged intensive care stays and repeated endotracheal intubations postoperatively. Alternative management includes topical nasal decongestants, nasopharyngeal or oral airways, and nasal CPAP. The latter is technically difficult to initiate under acute conditions in the young child. If these approaches fail or if prolonged endotracheal intubation is required, permanent tracheotomy may be necessary, particularly in the infant with CFA. Tracheotomy will immediately reduce airway resistance and anatomic dead space, ameliorate respiratory failure, and ultimately reverse cor pulmonale and promote growth. Experience has shown that reconstructive surgical airway management can allow successful decannulation of the airway in the young child with CFA.[124] Reconstructive surgical approaches in children with CFA involve skeletal expansion in combination with soft tissue reduction, which can facilitate increases in the nasooropharyngeal volumes.[125] Definitive reconstructive airway surgery in the absence of a tracheotomy is less likely to be successful in the infant with CFA and is associated with a greater incidence of complications.[126] Infants who have severe upper airway obstruction secondary to CFA need to be positioned prone and upright for sleep. They also may need to be fed through a nasogastric tube. Gastrostomy tube placement and continuous nighttime feedings should be considered for the long term in an effort to provide adequate calories to promote growth.

Successful use of noninvasive positive-pressure ventilation through nasal mask has been reported in infants and children with CFA. A previous study demonstrated that CPAP is a safe and effective treatment option that may reduce the number of airway operations performed in children with craniofacial syndromes.[127] A problem with this therapy in any age group, especially when psychomotor retardation is significant, is poor acceptance of the nasal mask by the patients. Follow-up polysomnography is needed to evaluate the effectiveness of this treatment.

NEUROMUSCULAR DISEASES

Cardiorespiratory failure is the most common cause of morbidity and mortality in infants and children with neuromuscular disease (NMD). Respiratory insufficiency may present acutely or may develop insidiously as a result of progressive respiratory muscle weakness. Physiologic changes during sleep place a high demand on the respiratory muscles and may exaggerate awake abnormalities in respiratory function. Several NMDs present in early neonatal life.

Sleep-related respiratory dysfunction in infants with NMD is primarily caused by abnormalities in the respiratory muscle "pump" (chest wall and diaphragm). However, other factors predispose infants and children with NMD to manifest signs and symptoms of SDB. First, the physiologic alteration in respiratory mechanics during sleep results in decreases in tidal volume, minute ventilation, and FRC. These abnormalities are accentuated by baseline awake deficiencies in respiratory muscle and lung function. Hypotonia of the upper airway and intercostal muscles in infants with NMD is associated with increased chest wall compliance, rib cage deformability, and reduced FRC.[128] Infants with NMD may have selective bulbar involvement, resulting in additional hypotonia of the upper airway muscles and reduction in protective reflexes that can lead to aspiration of upper airway secretions during sleep. Certain NMDs [e.g., spinal muscular atrophy and Duchenne muscular dystrophy (DMD)] can involve the diaphragm and predispose the affected infant to significant hypoxemia or hypoventilation during REM sleep. In addition, patients with bilateral diaphragmatic paralysis have been reported to have profound oxygen desaturation and hypoventilation during REM sleep.[129] Infants who have a high percentage of active or REM sleep are particularly vulnerable to unsuspected respiratory failure. The reduction in FRC (~20%–30%) during sleep is accentuated in the supine position and after meals because of hydrostatic fluid pressure from abdominal contents on the weakened diaphragm. In addition, patients with progressive NMD and chronic hypercapnia may develop a secondary reduction in hypoxic and hypercapnic response.[130] It is difficult, however, to differentiate between a primary reduction in respiratory drive from a change in chest wall and lung mechanical properties caused by muscle weakness. Most published studies in NMD have failed to demonstrate true primary abnormalities in respiratory control.[131,132] To the contrary, some studies suggest that central respiratory drive is intact and may be increased to overcome abnormal respiratory mechanics.[133] Finally, most infants and children with NMD, especially those who are wheelchair bound, eventually develop progressive thoracolumbar scoliosis that further compromises lung volumes, respiratory mechanics, and pulmonary clearance.

Many NMDs can present early in the neonatal period. Infants with myasthenia gravis may have the transient or congenital form. Transient myasthenia gravis occurs in 12% of neonates born to mothers with myasthenia. The most common presenting symptom is recent-onset feeding problems. Congenital myasthenia usually is associated with significant involvement of extraocular muscles, but severe generalized muscle weakness is uncommon. Neither of these types of myasthenia in neonates is likely to be associated with recurrent apnea or respiratory failure. Familial infantile myasthenia, however, is associated with recurrent apnea and respiratory depression and may be the cause of sudden infant death. This type of neonatal myasthenia is characterized by (1) absence of myasthenia in the mother, (2) occurrence of a similar disorder among siblings, (3) respiratory depression at birth, (4) episodic weakness and apnea during the first 2 years of life, and (5) improvement with age.[134] The condition responds to anticholinesterase medication; it requires early diagnosis and intervention to prevent morbidity and mortality.[134]

Congenital myotonic dystrophy is one of the most frequent muscular diseases manifested during the neonatal period, with an incidence of approximately 1 per 3500 live births.[135] It is a dominantly inherited disorder; the affected parent is the mother, who may have a history of miscarriage, still births, and neonatal deaths. The respiratory complications of congenital myotonic dystrophy start in utero with poor fetal breathing, resulting in pulmonary and diaphragmatic hypoplasia.[135]

A short umbilical cord (<40 cm) secondary to fetal akinesia may be an early clue to diagnosis. Neonates with mild expression of the disease are hypotonic and have a poor sucking reflex, difficulty swallowing, facial diplegia, and limb contractures. Severely affected infants present with perinatal asphyxia due to respiratory muscle weakness and respiratory failure; they require positive-pressure ventilatory support if they are to survive. Difficulty in swallowing may lead to recurrent aspiration, and respiratory problems cause recurrent morbidity and mortality in the first 2 years of the affected infant's life.

Spinal muscular atrophy (Werdnig-Hoffmann disease) is transmitted as an autosomal recessive trait. The primary pathologic change is atrophy of anterior horn cells in the spinal cord and motor nuclei in the brainstem. The disease can be detected at birth in about 30% of cases. Infants with spinal muscular atrophy show weakness and hypotonia of the axial and proximal muscles.[136] Although the diaphragm is relatively normal, the weakness of intercostal muscles may cause paradoxical breathing and progressive respiratory paralysis. Infants with Werdnig-Hoffman disease have recurrent atelectasis and aspiration pneumonia, which can lead to respiratory failure and death.[137,138] Distal infantile spinal muscular atrophy differs from classic Werdnig-Hoffman disease in that it is characterized by a predominant involvement of distal limb muscles and the diaphragm. Pulmonary hypoplasia can occur in utero; therefore, diaphragmatic paralysis can be present at birth or occur soon thereafter.[136]

Skeletal dysplasias secondary to a generalized disorder of connective tissue can cause respiratory difficulties because of abnormalities of thoracic anatomy or airway mechanics. Infants with skeletal dysplasia have one or more of the following abnormalities: a barrel-shaped thorax, which accounts for decreased tidal volume; laryngomalacia, tracheomalacia, or bronchomalacia; and cervical spine instability with resultant compression of the upper cervical spinal cord or of the arterial supply to the base of the medulla, which may lead to abnormalities of respiratory control.[139] Thanatophoric dysplasia, Jeune syndrome, and spondyloepiphyseal dysplasia congenita are some examples of serious congenital thoracic dystrophies that produce severe respiratory problems during the neonatal period that may lead to respiratory failure and death.

Polysomnography is an essential tool in the evaluation of cardiorespiratory function in infants with NMD and skeletal dysplasia. Polysomnography also is important for the planning and implementation of elective nocturnal assisted ventilation; assessment of the adequacy of respiratory support; and evaluation of preoperative and postoperative status of patients with NMD.[140] A measurement of noninvasive ventilation such as end-tidal or transcutaneous CO_2 is essential in evaluation of SDB in children with NMD. In addition to apnea of any type, it is important to quantitate sleep disruption, paradoxical movement of the chest wall and diaphragm, and nocturnal alveolar hypoventilation. Nocturnal hypoventilation ($\uparrow CO_2$) may be documented in the absence of significant oxygen desaturation. REM-related oxygen desaturation correlates with diaphragm weakness and the need to initiate assisted ventilatory support (Fig. 3-7).[141] In the later stages of these diseases, hypoventilation and hypoxia will occur in all sleep stages. If polysomnography is initially normal, repeat studies should be performed on a yearly basis.

The importance of general supportive care in the management of SDB in NMD cannot be overemphasized. These measures include adequate hydration, nutritional support, and airway clearance techniques. It is important to carefully assess the caloric need of each patient, because obesity can develop insidiously in patients with significant disability caused by muscle weakness. Correction and spinal stabilization procedures for paralytic scoliosis should be performed before significant loss of lung function occurs.

A variety of modalities have been attempted to improve sleep-related respiratory disturbances in these diseases. Respiratory stimulants, such as theophylline, have been shown to be effective in infants with congenital myotonic dystrophy, although the therapeutic mechanism of theophylline is unclear. Methylxanthines may work by stimulating the infant's central respiratory drive or by directly increasing the strength of muscle contractions.[135] Nocturnal use of supplemental oxygen has been shown to alleviate the REM-related oxygen desaturation associated with respiratory muscle weakness in patients with DMD. However, the total sleep time, sleep stage distribution, and frequency and duration of arousals are not different between control and oxygen-treated groups, and supplemental oxygen may prolong the duration of apnea and hypopnea.[142] Simple elevation of the upper body while the patient is in bed can increase FRC and may prevent dependent airway closure and atelectasis. A rocking bed may have the same effect as body positioning, but it also may help drain secretions from the lower airways. Furthermore, this form of therapy may ameliorate daytime hypercapnia and subjective sleepiness with resultant improvement in sleep fragmentation by inhibiting the arousal associated with phasic accessory muscle activation.[143]

Mechanical ventilatory support remains the mainstay treatment for SDB in infants and children with severe NMD. Negative-pressure ventilation may be suitable in some patients. These devices include plexiglas lung, cuirass shell, and pulmowrap. Negative-pressure ventilation replaces the bellows function of failing respiratory muscles by artificially generating subatmospheric pressure around the chest. Use of negative-pressure ventilation in these infants and children, however, often is associated with increased frequency of SDB caused by collapse of upper airway muscles.[144,145] Although positive-pressure ventilation via tracheotomy is the most effective mode of long-term assisted ventilation, it is not easily accepted by patients and parents as first-line therapy. Nasal mask ventilation has become the preferred and effective method of nocturnal ventilation because it may obviate the need for a tracheotomy tube. Nasal mask ventilation can be provided by CPAP or by nocturnal intermittent positive-pressure ventilation through either bilevel positive airway pressure or a conventional ventilator. Long-term nasal ventilation by any of these methods has been shown to normalize gas exchange and alleviate symptoms of hypercapnia.[146,147] It also has been shown to stabilize declining lung function and prolong life expectancy of patients with DMD.[148]

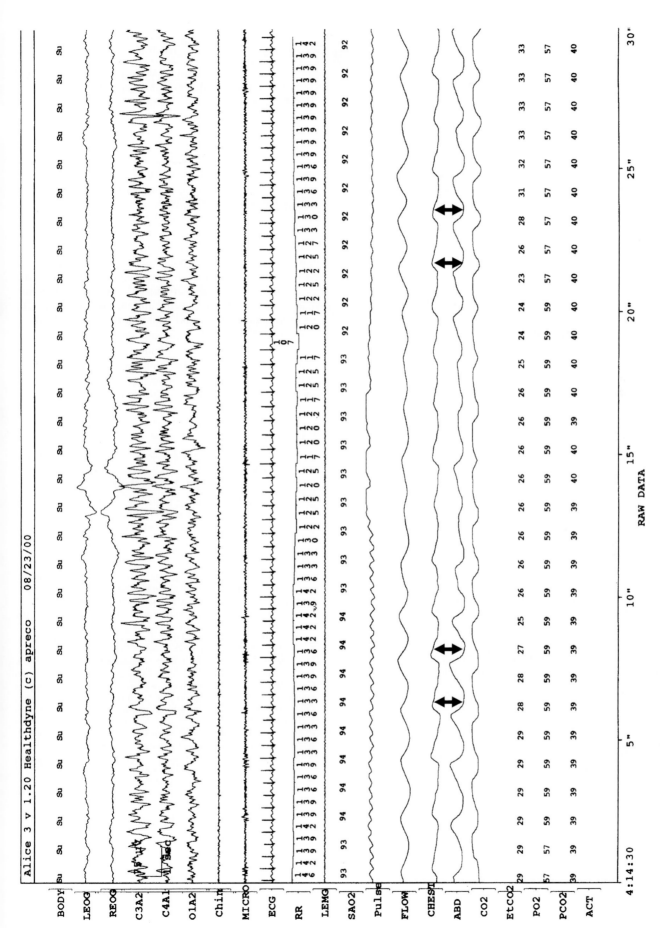

Figure 3-7. Polysomnographic segment recorded from an infant with spinal muscular dystrophy Episodes of nonapneic oxygen desaturation and paradoxical breathing between chest and abdomen (arrows) that occurred during rapid eye movement sleep indicated the need for nocturnal ventilatory support.

55

INBORN ERRORS OF METABOLISM

Inborn errors of metabolism have been associated with ALTE and SIDS. However, this association may remain undetected unless postmortem material is examined with individual metabolic disorders in mind.[149–152] Although the incidence is unknown, Arens et al.[150] found inborn errors of metabolism in 4.2% of infants referred for apnea evaluation and in about 8% of infants initially referred for ALTE. Establishing the relationship between ALTE and these metabolic errors is difficult because the infant's age at the initial episode is not helpful in making the diagnosis.

Disorders that affect energy metabolism and glucose homeostasis, including glycogen storage disorders, gluconeogenic enzyme defects, and defects of fatty acid oxidation, can present as ALTE or SIDS.[152] When the child has been fed, the principal substrate for energy metabolism is glucose. With increased duration of fasting, however, fat replaces glucose. In the neonate, this replacement can start after only 12 hours of fasting. Most reported cases of ALTE or SIDS have involved abnormalities in fatty acid oxidation. The metabolic pathway through which fatty acids provide energy is that of mitochondrial beta oxidation, and the main tissues involved are the liver, heart, and skeletal muscles.

Medium-chain acyl coenzyme A dehydrogenase deficiency is the most common inherited disorder of fatty acid oxidation associated with unexpected death. However, this deficiency is not a frequent cause of SIDS, as evidenced by a study reporting the G985 mutation was found in only three heterozygotes of P 1224 tissue samples from SIDS victims.[151] Infants with this deficiency commonly present with episodes of encephalopathy and hepatomegaly triggered by a viral infection and fasting; its clinical presentation resembles that of Reye syndrome.[153,154] Deficiency of long-chain acyl coenzyme A appears to be less common but more severe; it occurs in the neonatal period and is characterized by hypoglycemia, cardiorespiratory arrest, cardiomegaly, and hepatomegaly.[153] Other inherited disorders of fatty acid oxidation associated with SIDS are primary carnitine deficiency, ornithine transcarbamylase deficiency, glutaric aciduria type II and IIB, multiple acyl coenzyme A deficiency, 3-hydroxyl-3-methylglutaryl coenzyme A lipase deficiency, carnitine palmitoyl transferase deficiency, and deficiencies of short-chain acyl coenzyme A dehydrogenase and long-chain 3-hydroxy acyl coenzyme A dehydrogenase.[155]

ASPHYXIA, TRAUMA, AND HEMORRHAGE

Various types of perinatal injuries may affect ventilatory control on either a temporary or a permanent basis (Table 3-5).[156,157] The level of ventilatory support depends on the level of the lesion; for example, brainstem and upper cervical spinal injury may be permanent and require full support. Central alveolar hypoventilation and apnea associated with hypoxic ischemic encephalopathy, intracranial hemorrhage, brainstem hemorrhage, or hydrocephalus may be self-limiting and reversible.

TABLE 3-5. Ventilatory Control Abnormalities Secondary to Asphyxia, Trauma, or Hemorrhage

Intracranial hemorrhage or infection involving brainstem structures
Brainstem infarction secondary to perinatal asphyxia
Brainstem injury from precipitous delivery, breech presentation, both
High cervical cord injury (C1–C3) from breech presentation causing respiratory failure
Midcervical cord injury (C3–C5) causing unilateral or bilateral phrenic nerve injury with or without respiratory failure

---

SUMMARY

Sleep and respiratory control in neonates and infants undergo significant maturational changes in an orderly developmental sequence. Several factors can interfere with the normal progression of developmental changes, including immaturity, stress, neonatal insults and injuries, alterations of normal anatomic structure, and neuromuscular control. These changes can lead to disorders of sleep and respiratory control. In this chapter, the normal development of sleep and ventilatory control was discussed, with emphasis on the pathophysiology and clinical aspects of a diverse group of disorders of respiratory control in neonates and infants.

REFERENCES

1. Dawes GS, Fox HE, Leduc BM, et al: Respiratory movements and paradoxical sleep in the foetal lamb. J Physiol 210:47P–48P, 1970.
2. Boddy K, Dawes GS: Fetal breathing. Br Med Bull 31:3–7, 1975.
3. Bahoric A, Chernick V: Electrical activity of phrenic nerve and diaphragm in utero. J Appl Physiol 39:513–518, 1975.
4. Bystrzycka E, Nail BS, Purves MJ: Central and peripheral neural respiratory activity in the mature sheep foetus and newborn lamb. Respir Physiol 25:199–215, 1975.
5. de Vries JI, Visser GH, Prechtl HF: The emergence of fetal behaviour. I. Qualitative aspects. Early Hum Dev 7:301–322, 1982.
6. Hoppenbrouwers T, Ugartechea JC, Combs D, et al: Studies of maternal-fetal interaction during the last trimester of pregnancy: Ontogenesis of the basic rest-activity cycle. Exp Neurol 61:136–153, 1978.
7. Parmelee AH Jr, Wenner WH, Akiyama Y, et al: Sleep states in premature infants. Dev Med Child Neurol 9:70–77, 1967.
8. Sterman MB, Hoppenbrouwer T: The development of sleep-waking and rest-activity patterns from fetus to adult in man. In Sterman MB, McGinty DJ, Adinolfi AM (eds): Brain Development and Behavior. New York, Academic Press, 1971, pp 203–225.
9. Curzi-Dascalova L: Phase relationships between thoracic and abdominal respiratory movement during sleep in 31–38 weeks CA normal infants. Comparison with full-term (39–41 weeks) newborns. Neuropediatrics 13(Suppl):15–20, 1982.
10. Rigatto H, Brady JP: Periodic breathing and apnea in preterm infants. II. Hypoxia as a primary event. Pediatrics 50:219–228, 1972.
11. Alvaro R, Alvarez J, Kwiatkowski K, et al: Small preterm infants (less than or equal to 1500 g) have only a sustained decrease in ventilation in response to hypoxia. Pediatr Res 32:403–406, 1992.
12. Rigatto H: Ventilatory response to hypercapnia. Semin Perinatol 1:363–367, 1977.
13. Fleming PJ, Bryan AC, Bryan MH: Functional immaturity of pulmonary irritant receptors and apnea in newborn preterm infants. Pediatrics 61:515–518, 1978.
14. Heldt GP: Development of stability of the respiratory system in preterm infants. J Appl Physiol 65:441–444, 1988.
15. Kattwinkel J. Neonatal apnea: Pathogenesis and therapy. J Pediatr 90:342–347, 1977.
16. Guilleminault C, Ariagno R, Korobkin R, et al: Mixed and obstructive sleep apnea and near miss for sudden infant death syndrome: 2.

Comparison of near miss and normal control infants by age. Pediatrics 64:882–891, 1979.

17. Flores-Guevara R, Plouin P, Curzi-Dascalova L, et al: Sleep apneas in normal neonates and infants during the first 3 months of life. Neuropediatrics 13(Suppl):21–28, 1982.

18. Kahn A, Groswasser J, Sottiaux M, et al: Clinical symptoms associated with brief obstructive sleep apnea in normal infants. Sleep 16:409–413, 1993.

19. Rigatto H, Brady JP, de la Torre Verduzco R: Chemoreceptor reflexes in preterm infants: II. The effect of gestational and postnatal age on the ventilatory response to inhaled carbon dioxide. Pediatrics 55:614–620, 1975.

20. Rigatto H, Kalapesi Z, Leahy FN, et al: Ventilatory response to 100% and 15% O_2 during wakefulness and sleep in preterm infants. Early Hum Dev 7:1–10, 1982.

21. Fenner A, Schalk U, Hoenicke H, et al: Periodic breathing in premature and neonatal babies: Incidence, breathing pattern, respiratory gas tensions, response to changes in the composition of ambient air. Pediatr Res 7:174–183, 1973.

22. Waggener TB, Frantz ID III, Stark AR, et al: Oscillatory breathing patterns leading to apneic spells in infants. J Appl Physiol 52:1288–1295, 1982.

23. Barrington KJ, Finer NN, Wilkinson MH: Progressive shortening of the periodic breathing cycle duration in normal infants. Pediatr Res 21:247–251, 1987.

24. Glotzbach SF, Tansey PA, Baldwin RB, et al: Periodic breathing in preterm infants: Influence of bronchopulmonary dysplasia and theophylline. Pediatr Pulmonol 7:78–81, 1989.

25. Miller MJ, Carlo WA, DiFiore JM, et al: Airway obstruction during periodic breathing in premature infants. J Appl Physiol 64:2496–2500, 1988.

26. Henderson-Smart DJ: The effect of gestational age on the incidence and duration of recurrent apnoea in newborn babies. Aust Paediatr J 17:273–276, 1981.

27. Martin RJ, Miller MJ, Carlo WA: Pathogenesis of apnea in preterm infants. J Pediatr. 109:733–741, 1986.

28. Gerhardt T, Bancalari E: Apnea of prematurity: II. Respiratory reflexes. Pediatrics 74:63–66, 1984.

29. Alden ER, Mandelkorn T, Woodrum DE, et al: Morbidity and mortality of infants weighing less than 1,000 grams in an intensive care nursery. Pediatrics 50:40–49, 1972.

30. Daily WJ, Klaus M, Meyer HB: Apnea in premature infants: Monitoring, incidence, heart rate changes, and an effect of environmental temperature. Pediatrics 43:510–518, 1969.

31. Upton CJ, Milner AD, Stokes GM: Upper airway patency during apnoea of prematurity. Arch Dis Child 67(4 Spec No):419–424, 1992.

32. Purpura DP, Schade IP: Growth and maturation of the brain. In: Progress in Brain Research, vol 4. Amsterdam, Elsevier, 1964.

33. Henderson-Smart DJ, Pettigrew AG, Cambell DJ: Clinical apnea and brain-stem neural function in preterm infants. N Engl J Med 308:353–357, 1983.

34. Moriette G, Van Reempts P, Moore M, et al: The effect of rebreathing CO_2 on ventilation and diaphragmatic electromyography in newborn infants. Respir Physiol 62:387–397, 1985.

35. Praud JP, Egreteau L, Benlabed M, et al: Abdominal muscle activity during CO_2 rebreathing in sleeping neonates. J Appl Physiol 70:1344–1350, 1991.

36. Cohen G, Xu C, Henderson-Smart D: Ventilatory response of the sleeping newborn to CO_2 during normoxic rebreathing. J Appl Physiol 71:168–174, 1991.

37. Cohen G, Henderson-Smart DJ: Upper airway muscle activity during nasal occlusion in newborn babies. J Appl Physiol 66:1328–1335, 1989.

38. Carlo WA, Martin RJ, Difiore JM: Differences in CO_2 threshold of respiratory muscles in preterm infants. J Appl Physiol 65:2434–2439, 1988.

39. Thach BT, Stark AR: Spontaneous neck flexion and airway obstruction during apneic spells in preterm infants. J Pediatr 94:275–281, 1979.

40. Davies AM, Koenig JS, Thach BT: Upper airway chemoreflex responses to saline and water in preterm infants. J Appl Physiol 64:1412–1420, 1988.

41. Perkett EA, Vaughan RL: Evidence for a laryngeal chemoreflex in some human preterm infants. Acta Paediatr Scand 71:969–972, 1982.

42. Pickens DL, Schefft G, Thach BT: Prolonged apnea associated with upper airway protective reflexes in apnea of prematurity. Am Rev Respir Dis 137:113–118, 1988.

43. Weintraub Z, Alvaro R, Kwiatkowski K, et al: Effects of inhaled oxygen (up to 40%) on periodic breathing and apnea in preterm infants. J Appl Physiol 72:116–120, 1992.

44. Henderson-Smart DJ, Butcher-Puech MC, Edwards DA: Incidence and mechanism of bradycardia during apnoea in preterm infants. Arch Dis Child 61:227–232, 1986.

45. Storrs CN: Cardiovascular effects of apnoea in preterm infants. Arch Dis Child 52:534–540, 1977.

46. Girling DJ: Changes in heart rate, blood pressure, and pulse pressure during apnoeic attacks in newborn babies. Arch Dis Child 47:405–410, 1972.

47. Southall DP, Levitt GA, Richards JM, et al: Undetected episodes of prolonged apnea and severe bradycardia in preterm infants. Pediatrics 72:541–551, 1983.

48. Carroll JL, Marcus CL, Loughlin GM: Disordered control of breathing in infants and children. Pediatr Rev 14:51–65, 1993.

49. Razi NM, Humphreys J, Pandit PB, et al: Predischarge monitoring of preterm infants. Pediatr Pulmonol 27:113–116, 1999.

50. Sasidharan P, Heimler R: Transfusion-induced changes in the breathing pattern of healthy preterm anemic infants. Pediatr Pulmonol 12:170–173, 1992.

51. DeMaio JG, Harris MC, Deuber C, et al: Effect of blood transfusion on apnea frequency in growing premature infants. J Pediatr 114:1039–1041, 1989.

52. Miller MJ, Carlo WA, Martin RJ: Continuous positive airway pressure selectively reduces obstructive apnea in preterm infants. J Pediatr 106:91–94, 1985.

53. Ryan CA, Finer NN, Peters KL: Nasal intermittent positive-pressure ventilation offers no advantages over nasal continuous positive airway pressure in apnea of prematurity. Am J Dis Child 143:1196–1198, 1989.

54. Lopes JM, Aubier M, Jardim J, et al: Effect of caffeine on skeletal muscle function before and after fatigue. J Appl Physiol 54:1303–1305, 1983.

55. Aranda JV, Turmen T: Methylxanthines in apnea of prematurity. Clin Perinatol 6:87–108, 1979.

56. Turmen T, Louridas TA, Aranda JV: Relationship of plasma and CSF concentrations of caffeine in neonates with apnea. J Pediatr 95:644–646, 1979.

57. Kriter KE, Blanchard J: Management of apnea in infants. Clin Pharm 8:577–587, 1989.

58. Aranda JV, Louridas AT, Vitullo BB, et al: Metabolism of theophylline to caffeine in human fetal liver. Science 206:1319–1321, 1979.

59. Lee TC, Charles B, Steer P, et al: Population pharmacokinetics of intravenous caffeine in neonates with apnea of prematurity. Clin Pharmacol Ther 61:628–640, 1997.

60. Rigatto H: Apnea and periodic breathing. Semin Perinatol 1:375–381, 1977.

61. Rigatto H, Brady JP: Periodic breathing and apnea in preterm infants. I. Evidence for hypoventilation possibly due to central respiratory depression. Pediatrics 50:202–218, 1972.

61a. Simakajornboon N, Beckerman RC, Mack C, et al: Effect of supplemental oxygen on sleep architecture and cardiorespiratory events in preterm infants. Pediatrics 110:884–888, 2002.

62. Northway WH Jr, Rosan RC, Porter DY: Pulmonary disease following respirator therapy of hyaline-membrane disease. Bronchopulmonary dysplasia. N Engl J Med 276:357–368, 1967.

63. Motoyama EK, Fort MD, Klesh KW, et al: Early onset of airway reactivity in premature infants with bronchopulmonary dysplasia. Am Rev Respir Dis 136:50–57, 1987.

64. Rooklin AR, Moomjian AS, Shutack JG, et al: Theophylline therapy in bronchopulmonary dysplasia. J Pediatr 95(5 Pt 2):882–888, 1979.

65. Duncan S, Eid N: Tracheomalacia and bronchopulmonary dysplasia. Ann Otol Rhinol Laryngol 100:856–858, 1991.

66. Harris MA, Sullivan CE: Sleep pattern and supplementary oxygen requirements in infants with chronic neonatal lung disease. Lancet 345:831–832, 1995.

67. Garg M, Kurzner SI, Bautista D, et al: Hypoxic arousal responses in infants with bronchopulmonary dysplasia. Pediatrics 82:59–63, 1988.

68. Garg M, Kurzner SI, Bautista DB, et al: Clinically unsuspected hypoxia during sleep and feeding in infants with bronchopulmonary dysplasia. Pediatrics 81:635–642, 1988.

69. Sekar KC, Duke JC: Sleep apnea and hypoxemia in recently weaned premature infants with and without bronchopulmonary dysplasia. Pediatr Pulmonol 10:112–116, 1991.

70. Durand M, McEvoy C, MacDonald K: Spontaneous desaturations in intubated very low birth weight infants with acute and chronic lung disease. Pediatr Pulmonol 13:136–142, 1992.

71. Zinman R, Blanchard PW, Vachon F: Oxygen saturation during sleep in patients with bronchopulmonary dysplasia. Biol Neonate 61:69–75, 1992.

72. McEvoy C, Durand M, Hewlett V: Episodes of spontaneous desaturations in infants with chronic lung disease at two different levels of oxygenation. Pediatr Pulmonol 15:140–144, 1993.

73. Teague WG, Pian MS, Heldt GP, et al: An acute reduction in the fraction of inspired oxygen increases airway constriction in infants with chronic lung disease. Am Rev Respir Dis 137:861–865, 1988.

74. Tay-Uyboco JS, Kwiatkowski K, Cates DB, et al: Hypoxic airway constriction in infants of very low birth weight recovering from moderate to severe bronchopulmonary dysplasia. J Pediatr 115:456–459, 1989.

75. Praud JP, Cavailloles F, Boulhadour K, et al: Radionuclide evaluation of cardiac function during sleep in children with bronchopulmonary dysplasia. Chest 100:721–725, 1991.

76. Filtchev SI, Curzi-Dascalova L, Spassov L, et al: Heart rate variability during sleep in infants with bronchopulmonary dysplasia. Effects of mild decrease in oxygen saturation. Chest 106:1711–1716, 1994.

77. Werthammer J, Brown ER, Neff RK, et al: Sudden infant death syndrome in infants with bronchopulmonary dysplasia. Pediatrics 69:301–304, 1982.

78. Gray PH, Rogers Y: Are infants with bronchopulmonary dysplasia at risk for sudden infant death syndrome? Pediatrics 93:774–777, 1994.

79. Moyer-Mileur LJ, Nielson DW, Pfeffer KD, et al: Eliminating sleep-associated hypoxemia improves growth in infants with bronchopulmonary dysplasia. Pediatrics 98(4 Pt 1):779–783, 1996.

80. Abman SH, Wolfe RR, Accurso FJ, et al: Pulmonary vascular response to oxygen in infants with severe bronchopulmonary dysplasia. Pediatrics 75:80–84, 1985.

81. Halliday HL, Dumpit FM, Brady JP: Effects of inspired oxygen on echocardiographic assessment of pulmonary vascular resistance and myocardial contractility in bronchopulmonary dysplasia. Pediatrics 65:536–540, 1980.

82. Gozal D: Congenital central hypoventilation syndrome: An update. Pediatr Pulmonol 26:273–282, 1998.

83. Nickerson BG: Bronchopulmonary dysplasia. Chronic pulmonary disease following neonatal respiratory failure. Chest 87:528–535, 1985.

84. O'Brodovich HM, Mellins RB: Bronchopulmonary dysplasia. Unresolved neonatal acute lung injury. Am Rev Respir Dis 132:694–709, 1985.

85. Davis JM, Sinkin RA, Aranda JV: Drug therapy for bronchopulmonary dysplasia. Pediatr Pulmonol 8:117–125, 1990.

85a. American Academy of Pediatrics, Committee on Fetus and Newborn; and Canadian Pediatric Society, Fetus and Newborn Committee: Postnatal corticosteroids to treat or prevent chronic lung disease in preterm infants. Pediatrics 109:330–338, 2002.

86. Mellins RB, Balfour HH Jr, Turino GM, et al: Failure of automatic control of ventilation (Ondine's curse). Report of an infant born with this syndrome and review of the literature. Medicine (Baltimore) 49:487–504, 1970.

87. Weese-Mayer DE, Silvestri JM, Menzies LJ, et al: Congenital central hypoventilation syndrome: Diagnosis, management, and long-term outcome in thirty-two children. J Pediatr 120:381–387, 1992.

88. Minutillo C, Pemberton PJ, Goldblatt J: Hirschsprung's disease and Ondine's curse: Further evidence for a distinct syndrome. Clin Genet 36:200–203, 1989.

89. Swaminathan S, Gilsanz V, Atkinson J, et al: Congenital central hypoventilation syndrome associated with multiple ganglioneuromas. Chest 96:423–424, 1989.

90. Romeo G, Ronchetto P, Luo Y, et al: Point mutations affecting the tyrosine kinase domain of the RET proto-oncogene in Hirschsprung's disease. Nature 367:377–378, 1994.

91. Burton MD, Kawashima A, Brayer JA, et al: RET proto-oncogene is important for the development of respiratory CO_2 sensitivity. J Auton Nerv Syst 63:137–143, 1997.

92. Bolk S, Angrist M, Schwartz S, et al: Congenital central hypoventilation syndrome: Mutation analysis of the receptor tyrosine kinase RET. Am J Med Genet 63:603–609, 1996.

93. Folgering H, Kuyper F, Kille JF: Primary alveolar hypoventilation (Ondine's curse syndrome) in an infant without external arcuate nucleus. Case report. Bull Eur Physiopathol Respir 15:659–665, 1979.

94. Long KJ, Allen N: Abnormal brain-stem auditory evoked potentials following Ondine's curse. Arch Neurol 41:1109–1110, 1984.

95. Beckerman R, Meltzer J, Sola A, et al: Brain-stem auditory response in Ondine's syndrome. Arch Neurol 43:698–701, 1986.

96. Weese-Mayer DE, Brouillette RT, Naidich TP, et al: Magnetic resonance imaging and computerized tomography in central hypoventilation. Am Rev Respir Dis 137:393–398, 1988.

97. Paton JY, Swaminathan S, Sargent CW, et al: Hypoxic and hypercapnic ventilatory responses in awake children with congenital central hypoventilation syndrome. Am Rev Respir Dis 140:368–372, 1989.

98. Woo MS, Woo MA, Gozal D, et al: Heart rate variability in congenital central hypoventilation syndrome. Pediatr Res 31:291–296, 1992.

99. Marcus CL, Jansen MT, Poulsen MK, et al: Medical and psychosocial outcome of children with congenital central hypoventilation syndrome. J Pediatr 119:888–895, 1991.

100. Del Carmen Sanchez M, Lopez-Herce J, Carrillo A, et al: Late onset central hypoventilation syndrome. Pediatr Pulmonol 21:189–191, 1996.

101. Congenital central hypoventilation syndrome. In: Diagnostic Classification Steering Committee of the American Sleep Disorders Association. The International Classification of Sleep Disorders: Diagnostic and Coding Manual. Lawrence, Kan., Allen Press, 1990, pp. 205–209.

102. Hunt CE, Inwood RJ, Shannon DC: Respiratory and nonrespiratory effects of doxapram in congenital central hypoventilation syndrome. Am Rev Respir Dis 119:263–269, 1979.

103. Oren J, Newth CJ, Hunt CE, et al: Ventilatory effects of almitrine bismesylate in congenital central hypoventilation syndrome. Am Rev Respir Dis 134:917–919, 1986.

104. Hartmann H, Jawad MH, Noyes J, et al: Negative extrathoracic pressure ventilation in central hypoventilation syndrome. Arch Dis Child 70:418–423, 1994.

105. Olson TS, Woodson GE, Heldt GP: Upper airway function in Ondine's curse. Arch Otolaryngol Head Neck Surg 118:310–312, 1992.

106. Nielson DW, Black PG: Mask ventilation in congenital central alveolar hypoventilation syndrome. Pediatr Pulmonol 9:44–45, 1990.

107. Kerbl R, Litscher H, Grubbauer HM, et al: Congenital central hypoventilation syndrome (Ondine's curse syndrome) in two siblings: Delayed diagnosis and successful noninvasive treatment. Eur J Pediatr 155:977–980, 1996.

108. Weese-Mayer DE, Morrow AS, Brouillette RT, et al: Diaphragm pacing in infants and children. A life-table analysis of implanted components. Am Rev Respir Dis 139:974–979, 1989.

109. Fitzgerald D, Davis GM, Gottesman R, et al: Diaphragmatic pacemaker failure in congenital central hypoventilation syndrome: A tale of two twiddlers. Pediatr Pulmonol 22:319–321, 1996.

110. Richards JM, Alexander JR, Shinebourne EA, et al: Sequential 22-hour profiles of breathing patterns and heart rate in 110 full-term infants during their first 6 months of life. Pediatrics 74:763–777, 1984.

111. Consensus Statement: National Institutes of Health Consensus Development Conference on Infantile Apnea and Home Monitoring. Pediatrics 79:292, 1987.

112. Kelly DH, Shannon DC, O'Connell K: Care of infants with near-miss sudden infant death syndrome. Pediatrics 61:511–514, 1978.

113. Kelly DH, Shannon DC: Periodic breathing in infants with near-miss sudden infant death syndrome. Pediatrics 63:355–360, 1979.

114. Bazzy AR, Haddad GG, Chang SL, et al: Respiratory pauses during sleep in near-miss sudden infant death syndrome. Am Rev Respir Dis 128:973–976, 1983.

115. van der Hal AL, Rodriguez AM, Sargent CW, et al: Hypoxic and hypercapneic arousal responses and prediction of subsequent apnea in apnea of infancy. Pediatrics 75:848–854, 1985.

116. Hunt CE: Abnormal hypercarbic and hypoxic sleep arousal responses in near-miss SIDS infants. Pediatr Res 15:1462–1464, 1981.

117. Coleman JM, Mammel MC, Reardon C, et al: Hypercarbic ventilatory responses of infants at risk for SIDS. Pediatr Pulmonol 3:226–230, 1987.

118. Parks YA, Paton JY, Beardsmore CS, et al: Respiratory control in infants at increased risk for sudden infant death syndrome. Arch Dis Child 64:791–797, 1989.

119. Goldstein SJ, Wu RH, Thorpy MJ, et al: Reversibility of deficient sleep entrained growth hormone secretion in a boy with achondroplasia and obstructive sleep apnea [published erratum appears in Acta Endocrinol (Copenh) 1987 Dec;116(4):568]. Acta Endocrinol (Copenh) 116:95–101, 1987.

120. Marcus CL, Keens TG, Bautista DB, et al: Obstructive sleep apnea in children with Down syndrome. Pediatrics 88:132–139, 1991.

121. Milerad J, Lagercrantz H, Johnson P: Obstructive sleep apnea in Arnold-Chiari malformation treated with acetazolamide. Acta Paediatr 81:609–612, 1992.

122. Clark RW, Schmidt HS, Schuller DE: Sleep-induced ventilatory dysfunction in Down's syndrome. Arch Intern Med 140:45–50, 1980.

123. Donaldson JD, Redmond WM: Surgical management of obstructive sleep apnea in children with Down syndrome. J Otolaryngol 17:398–403, 1988.

124. Sculerati N, Gottlieb MD, Zimbler MS, et al: Airway management in children with major craniofacial anomalies. Laryngoscope 108:1806–1812, 1998.

125. Cohen SR, Simms C, Burstein FD: Mandibular distraction osteogenesis in the treatment of upper airway obstruction in children with craniofacial deformities. Plast Reconstr Surg 101:312–318, 1998.

126. Januszkiewicz JS, Cohen SR, Burstein FD, et al: Age-related outcomes of sleep apnea surgery in infants and children. Ann Plast Surg 38:465–477, 1997.

127. Jarund M, Dellborg C, Carlson J, et al: Treatment of sleep apnoea with continuous positive airway pressure in children with craniofacial malformations. Scand J Plast Reconstr Surg Hand Surg 33:67–71, 1999.

128. Papastamelos C, Panitch HB, Allen JL: Chest wall compliance in infants and children with neuromuscular disease. Am J Respir Crit Care Med 154(4 Pt 1):1045–1048, 1996.

129. Skatrud J, Iber C, McHugh W, et al: Determinants of hypoventilation during wakefulness and sleep in diaphragmatic paralysis. Am Rev Respir Dis 121:587–593, 1980.

130. Riley DJ, Santiago TV, Daniele RP, et al: Blunted respiratory drive in congenital myopathy. Am J Med 63:459–466, 1977.

131. Begin R, Bureau MA, Lupien L, et al: Control of breathing in Duchenne's muscular dystrophy. Am J Med 69:227–234, 1980.

132. Newsom-Davis J: The respiratory system in muscular dystrophy. Br Med Bull 36:135–138, 1980.

133. Baydur A: Respiratory muscle strength and control of ventilation in patients with neuromuscular disease. Chest 99:330–338, 1991.

134. Robertson WC, Chun RW, Kornguth SE: Familial infantile myasthenia. Arch Neurol 37:117–119, 1980.

135. Rutherford MA, Heckmatt JZ, Dubowitz V: Congenital myotonic dystrophy: Respiratory function at birth determines survival. Arch Dis Child 64:191–195, 1989.

136. Bertini E, Gadisseux JL, Palmieri G, et al: Distal infantile spinal muscular atrophy associated with paralysis of the diaphragm: A variant of infantile spinal muscular atrophy. Am J Med Genet 33:328–335, 1989.

137. Eng GD, Binder H, Koch B: Spinal muscular atrophy: Experience in diagnosis and rehabilitation management of 60 patients. Arch Phys Med Rehabil 65:549–553, 1984.

138. Kuzuhara S, Chou SM: Preservation of the phrenic motoneurons in Werdnig-Hoffmann disease. Ann Neurol 9:506–510, 1981.

139. Harding CO, Green CG, Perloff WH, et al: Respiratory complications in children with spondyloepiphyseal dysplasia congenita. Pediatr Pulmonol 9:49–54, 1990.

140. American Thoracic Society: Standards and indications for cardiopulmonary sleep studies in children. Am J Respir Crit Care Med 153:866–878, 1996.

141. White JE, Drinnan MJ, Smithson AJ, et al: Respiratory muscle activity and oxygenation during sleep in patients with muscle weakness. Eur Respir J 8:807–814, 1995.

142. Smith PE, Edwards RH, Calverley PM: Oxygen treatment of sleep hypoxaemia in Duchenne muscular dystrophy. Thorax 44:997–1001, 1989.

143. Iber C, Davies SF, Mahowald MW: Nocturnal rocking bed therapy: Improvement in sleep fragmentation in patients with respiratory muscle weakness. Sleep 12:405–412, 1989.

144. Levy RD, Bradley TD, Newman SL, et al: Negative pressure ventilation. Effects on ventilation during sleep in normal subjects. Chest 95:95–99, 1989.

145. Hill NS, Redline S, Carskadon MA, et al: Sleep-disordered breathing in patients with Duchenne muscular dystrophy using negative pressure ventilators. Chest 102:1656–1662, 1992.

146. Heckmatt JZ, Loh L, Dubowitz V: Night-time nasal ventilation in neuromuscular disease. Lancet 335:579–582, 1990.

147. Hill NS, Eveloff SE, Carlisle CC, et al: Efficacy of nocturnal nasal ventilation in patients with restrictive thoracic disease. Am Rev Respir Dis 145(2 Pt 1):365–371, 1992.

148. Vianello A, Bevilacqua M, Salvador V, et al: Long-term nasal intermittent positive pressure ventilation in advanced Duchenne's muscular dystrophy. Chest 105:445–448, 1994.

149. Emery JL, Howat AJ, Variend S, et al: Investigation of inborn errors of metabolism in unexpected infant deaths. Lancet 2:29–31, 1988.

150. Arens R, Gozal D, Williams JC, et al: Recurrent apparent life-threatening events during infancy: A manifestation of inborn errors of metabolism. J Pediatr 123:415–418, 1993.

151. Arens R, Gozal D, Jain K, et al: Prevalence of medium-chain acyl-coenzyme A dehydrogenase deficiency in the sudden infant death syndrome. J Pediatr 122(5 Pt 1):715–718, 1993.

152. Bonham JR, Downing M: Metabolic deficiencies and SIDS. J Clin Pathol 45(11 Suppl):33–38, 1992.

153. Harpey JP, Charpentier C, Paturneau-Jouas M: Sudden infant death syndrome and inherited disorders of fat metabolism. Lancet 2:1332, 1986.

154. Roe CR, Millington DS, Maltby DA, et al: Recognition of medium-chain acyl-CoA dehydrogenase deficiency in asymptomatic siblings of children dying of sudden infant death or Reye-like syndromes. J Pediatr 108:13–18, 1986.

155. Chittayat D: Sudden infant death and inherited disorders of fatty acid oxidation. In Beckerman RC, Brouillete RT, Hunt CE (eds): Respiratory Control Disorders in Infants and Children. Baltimore, Williams & Wilkins, 1992, p. 278.

156. Graham JM: Breech presentation deformation. In Gram JM (ed): Smith's Recognizable Pattern of Human Deformation, 2nd ed. Philadelphia, WB Saunders, 1988, p. 82.

157. Mengurten HH: Birth injuries. In Faranoff AA, Martin R (eds): Neonatal-Perinatal Medicine: Disease of the Fetus and Infants, 5th ed. St. Louis, Mosby-Year Book, 1992, p. 346.

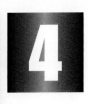

RESUSCITATION

M. GARY KARLOWICZ, MD, FAAP
EDWARD H. KAROTKIN, MD
JAY P. GOLDSMITH, MD

Resuscitation is a word derived from the Latin *resuscitare*, meaning "to arouse again." In neonatology, this term is used in two separate clinical settings. The first is the emergency situation, in which unexpected respiratory or cardiac arrest occurs in the nursery or neonatal intensive care unit (NICU) and measures to restore life are taken. Often, a new complication that is not predictable or preventable (e.g., tension pneumothorax) requires immediate intervention (e.g., thoracentesis and tube thoracostomy), as well as resuscitation. Sometimes, resuscitation is necessary because a patient has deteriorated through measurable stages of respiratory or cardiac failure because of inadequate therapy, poor judgment, or less-than-optimal observation on the part of the health care team.

In the second setting, resuscitation is used to assist the newly-born infant in making the transition from dependent fetal to independent neonatal life. Complex changes occur in the fetus during the transition from intrauterine to extrauterine life, yet the birth process usually is accomplished with relative ease. Birth asphyxia accounts for approximately 19% of five million deaths that occur annually worldwide.[1] Using these calculations, one might speculate that the outcome of one million newborns might be improved using appropriate resuscitation techniques. Approximately 10% of newly born infants require some assistance to initiate spontaneous respirations at birth.[2] More intensive resuscitation, including positive-pressure ventilation, is required by 1% of newly born infants.[3,4] In contrast to resuscitation attempts made on older children or adults, skillful resuscitation of a newborn usually is successful and gratifying experience for the health care team.

Often, one can predict which newborn infants will require assistance in the delivery room. Information regarding antepartum or intrapartum risk factors collected during gestation, labor, or delivery can be used by the clinician to prepare for resuscitation (Table 4-1). Although the mature fetus may make the crucial adjustments at birth without significant intervention, the preterm or asphyxiated infant may need immediate and skillfully performed life-preserving measures to make this transition. Of critical importance are expansion of the lungs, establishment of respirations, and conversion from fetal to adult circulation so that blood returning to the heart is directed through the lungs. Asphyxia is the major pathologic event that requires correction in both types of resuscitation.

Perinatal asphyxia usually implies a complex combination of hypoxemia, hypercapnia, and circulatory insufficiency that may be induced by a variety of perinatal events (e.g., placental insufficiency, abruption placenta, meconium aspiration, pneumothorax, blood loss). The aim of a resuscitation protocol should be the immediate reversal of hypoxemia, hypercapnia, and circulatory insufficiency in order to prevent permanent central nervous system damage or damage to other organs. If optimal outcome is to be achieved, a resuscitation protocol should be directed immediately toward (1) clearing the upper airway of secretions, meconium, or other materials so that alveolar expansion can occur; (2) providing adequate oxygenation and elimination of excessive carbon dioxide; (3) ensuring adequate cardiac output; and (4) keeping oxygen consumption to a minimum.

TABLE 4-1. Risk Factors Associated with the Need for Neonatal Resuscitation

Antepartum Factors
Maternal diabetes
Pregnancy-induced hypertension
Chronic hypertension
Rhesus factor sensitization
Previous stillbirth
Bleeding in second or third trimester
Maternal infection
Polyhydramnios
Oligohydramnios
Post-term gestation
Multiple gestation
Size-date discrepancy
Drug therapy
    Reserpine
    Lithium
    Magnesium
    Adrenergic blocking agents
Maternal drug abuse

Intrapartum Factors
Cesarean section (other than uncomplicated repeat section)
Abnormal presentation
Premature labor
Rupture of membranes earlier than 24 hours before delivery
Foul-smelling amniotic fluid
Precipitous labor
Prolonged labor
Prolonged second stage of labor
Ominous fetal heart rate patterns
General anesthesia
Uterine tetany
Narcotics given to mother within 4 hours of delivery
Meconium-stained amniotic fluid
Prolapsed cord
Abruptio placentae
Placenta previa

From Bloom RS: Delivery room resuscitation of the newborn. In Fanaroff AA, Martin RJ (eds): Neonatal-Perinatal Medicine: Diseases of the Fetus and Infant, 5th ed. Chicago, Mosby-Year Book, 1992, p. 305.

In this chapter, we briefly discuss the pathophysiology of neonatal asphyxia and the steps needed to successfully resuscitate newborn infants, either in the delivery room or in the nursery.

PHYSIOLOGIC CHANGES DURING ASPHYXIA AND RESUSCITATION

When antepartum or intrapartum factors impair fetal-placental gas exchange, asphyxia may result. Dawes[5] and Adamsons et al.[6] described the classic changes of acute and total perinatal asphyxia in a rhesus monkey experimental model, which probably approximates events in human neonates. Figure 4-1 illustrates the changes in physiologic factors during 10 minutes of total asphyxia and subsequent resuscitation. Immediately after delivery by cesarean section, the head of the monkey was covered with a saline-filled bag to prevent air entry during breathing, and the umbilical cord was ligated. Approximately 30 seconds later, the experimental animal began gasping. The gasping ceased after about 1 minute and was followed by primary apnea, which also lasted about 1 minute. During the period of primary apnea, spontaneous respirations could be induced by tactile stimulation. A decrease in heart rate from the normal range of 180 to 220 beats/min to about 100 beats/min occurred and was accompanied by a transient increase in blood pressure. After primary apnea, the monkey made deep gasping efforts for a period of 4 to

5 minutes. The gasping weakened gradually until they ceased completely; the last gasp occurred after about 8 minutes of total asphyxia. Secondary apnea began after the last gasp. Heart rate and blood pressure steadily declined. Striking changes in pH, carbon dioxide tension (P_{CO_2}), and oxygen tension (P_{O_2}) occurred during 10 minutes of total asphyxia in the rhesus monkey: pH decreased from 7.3 to 6.8, P_{CO_2} increased from 45 to 150 mm Hg, and P_{O_2} decreased from 25 mm Hg to nearly zero. Serum lactate concentration also rapidly increased. Death occurred after several minutes of secondary apnea, unless the animal was resuscitated. Tactile stimulation did not induce spontaneous respirations during secondary apnea. The longer the delay in initiating adequate resuscitation after the last gasp, the longer the time to the first gasp. For every 1-minute delay, the time to first gasp was prolonged by 2 minutes and time to onset of spontaneous respirations was delayed by approximately 4 minutes.

During the period of total anoxia, a variety of changes involving the cardiovascular system, pulmonary circulation, and other organ systems and tissues occurred in the fetus in response to asphyxia. These changes reflect the response of the fetus to asphyxia (Table 4-2). In view of these experimental observations, one could speculate that several phenomena characterize asphyxia in the human infant. First, the entire sequence of events may start in utero and continue after delivery. Second, the irregular and weak gasp of the asphyxiated infant may not generate sufficient intrathoracic pressure to expand the lungs. Third, if the effects of asphyxia are to be reversed, both ventilation and pulmonary perfusion are needed; either alone is not sufficient.

In most animal models of asphyxia, the experiment provides acute onset total asphyxia to a previously healthy animal fetus. In contrast, in human fetuses, asphyxia often is intermittent, subacute, and chronic. This makes it difficult for clinicians to apply the knowledge gained from animal models of total asphyxia to partial and subacute asphyxia in human fetuses and newborns. For example, the duration of secondary apnea probably is longer in humans than in the rhesus monkey, and the

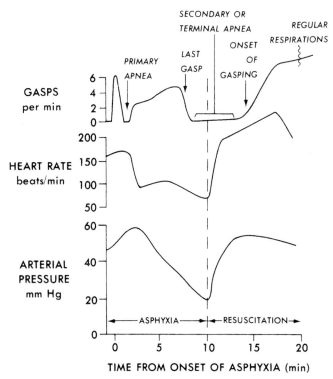

Figure 4-1. Changes in physiologic factors during asphyxia and resuscitation in newborn rhesus monkeys. (Adapted from Adamsons K Jr, Behrman R, Dawes G, et al: The treatment of acidosis with alkali and glucose during asphyxia in foetal rhesus monkeys. J Physiol 169:679, 1963, and Dawes GS: Foetal and Neonatal Physiology. Chicago, Year Book Medical Publishers, 1968. By permission of Mosby-Year Book.)

TABLE 4-2. Fetal Changes in Response to Asphyxia

Parameter	Change*
pH	↓
P_{CO_2}	↑
P_{O_2}	↓
Lactate level	↑
Plasma potassium level	↑
Free fatty acid level	↑
Glycerol level	↑
Catecholamine level	↑
Blood pressure	Transient ↑, then ↓ with prolonged asphyxia
Heart rate	Modest ↑, then ↓ with prolonged asphyxia
Umbilical blood flow	↓
Cardiac output	↓
Skin perfusion	↓
Pulmonary vascular resistance	↑
Oxygen consumption	↓
Shunting of blood through foramen ovale	↑
Glucose metabolism	Shifts from aerobic to anaerobic

* ↓, decrease; ↑, increase.

human fetus may tolerate more prolonged intermittent asphyxia before it develops permanent brain or other organ damage.

True intrapartum asphyxia cannot easily be differentiated clinically from neonatal depression from a variety of causes. Initial resuscitation responses are similar in both situations, but the diagnosis of "asphyxia" should only be made when certain clinical criteria are met. The major causes of neonatal depression at birth are listed in Table 4-3.

Moreover, in the clinical setting, primary and secondary apnea cannot be readily distinguished. Therefore, when an infant is born with apnea, it is assumed to be secondary apnea. Neonatal resuscitation, such as that taught in the American Heart Association and American Academy of Pediatrics Neonatal Resuscitation Program (AHA-AAP NRP),[1] should be initiated immediately.

TABLE 4-3. Major Causes of Neonatal Depression in the Delivery Room

Cause	Major Effect	Examples
Drugs	Respiratory depression	Anesthetics, narcotics, alcohol, magnesium sulfate, tranquilizers
Physical/mechanical	Interruption of blood supply	Prolapsed cord, head entrapment
Hemorrhage	Hypovolemia/shock	Abruptio placentae, ruptured umbilical cord, fetomaternal transfusion
Developmental anomalies	Cardiac, pulmonary insufficiency	Congenital heart disease, diaphragmatic hernia, choanal atresia, Potter syndrome
Environmental	Hypothermia	Delivery in cool environment, lack of external heat source
Postmaturity	Pneumonia, pulmonary hypertension	Meconium aspiration syndrome, persistent pulmonary hypertension of the newborn
Iatrogenic		
Excessive airway pressure generated at resuscitation	Pulmonary and cardiac embarrassment	Pulmonary air leak syndrome
Excessive suctioning	Vagal stimulation	Bradycardia, apnea
Misplacement of endotracheal tube	Hypoxia, bradycardia	Intubation of esophagus/right mainstem bronchus
Placental insufficiency	Hypoxia, acidosis	Abnormal fetal heart rate pattern, tetanic contraction
Severe immaturity (weight, <1000 g)	Pulmonary insufficiency	Respiratory distress syndrome, inadequate respiratory effort
Extrinsic or intrinsic pulmonary compression or hypoplasia	Pulmonary insufficiency	Diaphragmatic hernia, pleural effusion, pulmonary hypoplasia

METHOD: GENERAL PRINCIPLES

The four principal elements necessary for successful neonatal resuscitation are (1) anticipation of incidents that require the application of resuscitation efforts; (2) preparation of a treatment area, equipment, and drugs; (3) availability of qualified personnel; and (4) organized response to emergencies when they occur.

Anticipation

Although most cardiorespiratory arrests in the nursery are not anticipated, the delivery of a baby requiring resuscitation often can be predicted. In the past, an additional physician for the baby attended "high-risk" deliveries (especially cesarean sections) in anticipation of circumstances in which neonatal resuscitation might be needed. However, in modern surgical obstetrics, a repeat cesarean birth of a term infant usually is a benign event.

Because the need for resuscitation cannot reliably be predicted, the American Academy of Pediatrics (AAP) has recommended that at least one person who is capable of initiating resuscitation and whose primary responsibility is the neonate should attend *every* delivery. The *Guidelines for Perinatal Care* further elaborate: "Either that person or someone else who is immediately available should have the skills required to perform a complete resuscitation, including ventilation with bag and mask, endotracheal intubation, chest compressions, and the use of medication. It is not sufficient to have someone 'on call' (either at home or in a remote area of the hospital) for newborn resuscitation in the delivery room" (see Appendix 27).[7]

Many other conditions should alert the obstetrician to the need for pediatric assistance. The term *high-risk pregnancy* is not necessarily indicative or predictive of the need for resuscitation of an infant at birth. This classification is broad, and only a small percentage of high-risk pregnancies result in perinatal asphyxia. The AAP and the American College of Obstetricians and Gynecologists have published guidelines urging each institution to develop a list of maternal and fetal indications for the presence of an individual qualified in newborn resuscitation in the delivery room.[7] According to these guidelines, elective repeat cesarean delivery is not necessarily a high-risk situation. A review by Press et al.[8] on the cesarean delivery of full-term infants showed that interventions in the delivery room for *repeat* cesarean delivery are rare (tracheal intubation was required in 1 of 111 deliveries), whereas resuscitations following cesarean deliveries performed because of fetal distress were common (intubation was required in 24 of 66 deliveries). Moreover, these investigators noted that, in their hospital, the rate of tracheal intubation in the repeat cesarean group infants was lower than that for infants delivered vaginally. Levine et al.[9] reported no increased incidence of low Apgar scores in cesarean deliveries using regional anesthesia for non-fetal reasons compared to vaginal deliveries and concluded that there was no need for pediatrician attendance at such deliveries. Thus, a graded response to the so-called high-risk delivery seems appropriate, and traditional hospital policies for mandatory pediatric attendance at certain types of deliveries (e.g., cesarean deliveries using regional anesthesia for non-fetal indications) should be reviewed.

The truly high-risk pregnancy resulting in a high-risk delivery can be anticipated in most cases. Under certain circumstances, and if time allows, the mother may be transferred to a level III center (see Chapter 1), where the infant can be delivered under optimal conditions. However, advanced labor and imminent delivery preclude transfer of the mother. Often, telephone consultation or request for the neonatal transport team before delivery is worthwhile.

Pregnancies identified as high-risk require special management and intensive monitoring during gestation, labor, and delivery. Fisher and Paton[10] divide antepartum monitoring into the following four phases: (1) evaluation of the fetal placental unit during gestation; (2) estimation of fetal growth; (3) evaluation of fetal maturity, especially pulmonary maturity; and (4) acute monitoring of the fetus during labor and delivery. Problems detected during any phase of monitoring allow for prenatal identification of most infants who have difficulty in making the transition from intrauterine to extrauterine life.

Preparation

Preparation for a neonatal resuscitation is a two-stage procedure. The first stage occurs days, weeks, or months before the emergency. During this time, an area in or near the delivery room is designated as the *resuscitation area*. Provision is made for adequate space, ample heat (e.g., radiant warmer), blended O_2, and suction. Supplies and drugs are identified, obtained, and placed in a code cart or bag, or they are pegged to a wall board for easy access.[11] A resuscitation protocol should be written out, identifying procedures to be followed and personnel responsibilities during the emergency. A standardized neonatal cardiac arrest record can be developed and copies of it placed in the resuscitation area to simplify record-keeping during the procedure (see Appendix 26). In hospitals in which actual resuscitations are infrequent, periodic mock resuscitations performed to practice the procedure may be necessary.

The second stage of preparation occurs only when a resuscitation can be predicted in a high-risk patient. With adequate time, the resuscitation team can be alerted and arrangements made to have appropriate personnel present in the delivery room to assume care of a potentially depressed infant. The person in charge of the resuscitation should review the mother's chart, looking for clues in the perinatal history that signal the possibility of asphyxia in the baby. Of particular importance is the mother's medication record, especially if analgesics, which are known to depress the respiratory drive of infants in the perinatal period, have been used. This is also an excellent time for the pediatric team to talk with the parents, explaining the procedures that are to be carried out and the difficulties that can be expected. Meanwhile, everything needed for resuscitation following delivery can be prepared so that confusion is minimized: equipment can be organized; medications can be drawn up and made ready for administration; the proper operation of the laryngoscope's light can be checked; and O_2 can be turned on.

Personnel

The most important aspect of resuscitation is the availability of competent personnel who are able to respond immediately to any emergency. If a high-risk delivery is anticipated, the necessary personnel can be summoned to the hospital. If ventilation of neonates is underway in the hospital, competent personnel should be available "in house" at all times.

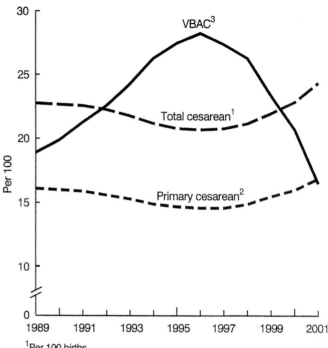

Figure 4-2. Number of total and primary cesarean sections and vaginal births after cesarians (VBAC) per 100 live births from 1989 to 2001. (From MacDorman MF, Minino AM, Strobino DM, Guyer B: Annual summary of vital statistics—2001. Pediatrics 110:1037, 2002.)

Smith[12] describes an individual properly prepared to lead a resuscitation effort as having "the diagnostic competence of a pediatrician and an internist, the technical skills of an anesthesiologist and a surgeon, and the organizational ability of a gang boss." As Smith notes, these talents are rarely found in one person (even a neonatologist!). Fortunately, not every high-risk delivery requires all of these skills. The person attending a high-risk delivery should be able to initiate resuscitation, and that person or someone "immediately available" should be able to perform ventilation and cardiopulmonary resuscitation and administer medications. It is our belief that this person does not have to be a physician (see Appendix 27).[7,13] A properly qualified neonatal nurse-clinician skilled in resuscitation may be the appropriate person to attend a moderate-risk delivery. This deviation from traditional practice has economic advantages as well, especially because approximately 20% to 25% of deliveries are now operative procedures (Fig. 4-2).[14] The true high-risk delivery requires a full-team approach. Various tasks are assigned to team members, and everyone on the team knows his or her role in the resuscitation process.

Response

The three steps in an appropriate resuscitation response are evaluation, diagnosis, and treatment.

Evaluation

The evaluation of an infant before treatment is started is essential in an emergency situation if mistakes are to be avoided. For newborn infants, the Apgar scoring system can be

TABLE 4-4. The Apgar Score

Sign	Score		
	0	1	2
Heart rate	Absent	Slow (<100 beats/min)	≥100 beats/min
Respirations	Absent	Slow, irregular	Good, crying
Muscle tone	Limp	Some flexion	Active motion
Reflex irritability (catheter in nares, tactile stimulation)	No response	Grimace	Cough, sneeze, cry
Color	Blue or pale	Pink body with blue extremities	Completely pink

helpful in assessing the infant's condition (Table 4-4)[15]; however, in most cases of neonatal asphyxia, resuscitation commences before the first Apgar score is assigned.

The Apgar scoring system was devised as a means for documenting a newborn's condition at specific intervals after birth.[15] The five signs usually are assessed at 1 and 5 minutes of age. If the score at 5 minutes is less than 7, additional scores are obtained every 5 minutes until the score is greater than 6 or until the infant is 20 minutes old. The Apgar scoring system has been used in the past for guiding resuscitative efforts. It is not used in the AHA-AAP NRP for decision-making regarding resuscitation because delays of even 1 minute could be critically important in the severely asphyxiated infant. Instead, frequent and repeated assessment of breathing, heart rate, and color are performed for evaluation of successful resuscitation.

Perinatal asphyxia is not the only factor that affects the Apgar score. Tone, color, and reflex irritability depend on the physiologic maturity of the infant. A preterm infant with no evidence of perinatal hypoxia normally has a reduced Apgar score because of immaturity.[16] Other factors depress the Apgar score, including maternal sedation and analgesia, neonatal neuromuscular disease, cerebral malformations, and congenital cardiac malformations.

Apgar scores do not correlate with the results of umbilical cord arterial blood gas analysis (i.e., low Apgar scores are not associated with severely acidotic pH values, and vice versa).[17] It is noteworthy, however, that a large, retrospective cohort analysis showed that the 5-minute Apgar score predicted neonatal death more accurately than the umbilical-artery pH value.[18] In fact, the risk of neonatal death in term infants with a 5-minute Apgar score of 3 or less was eight times that in term infants with umbilical-artery pH values of 7.0 or less. In an accompanying editorial, Lu-Ann Papile[19] concluded that until a more useful tool for assessing newborns is developed, the 5-minute Apgar score is still valid as a rapid method for evaluating the effectiveness of resuscitative efforts and risk of neonatal mortality in the 21st century.

Nelson and Ellenberg[20] have shown that the Apgar scores obtained at 1 and 5 minutes are poor predictors of neurologic disability. Therefore, low Apgar scores, by themselves, should not be considered evidence of severe asphyxia. Nevertheless, Apgar scores are useful for prognostication when combined with other clinical indicators of asphyxia. The AAP Committee on Fetus and Newborn and the American College of Obstetricians and Gynecologists Committee on Maternal and Fetal Medicine have defined criteria for identifying perinatal asphyxia that is sufficiently severe to cause neurologic damage. *All* of the following must be present: profound metabolic or mixed acidemia (pH <7.00) in an umbilical cord arterial blood sample; persistence of an Apgar score less than 4 for longer than 5 minutes; neonatal neurologic sequelae (e.g., seizures, hypotonia, coma); and multi-organ system dysfunction (e.g., cardiovascular, gastrointestinal, hematologic, pulmonary, renal).[7] Scoring systems can be used to rapidly identify infants at risk of acute multi-organ dysfunction from asphyxia and to facilitate clinical management. Carter et al.[21] have shown that a scoring system consisting of graded abnormalities in fetal heart rate monitoring, umbilical arterial base deficit, and 5-minute Apgar score was useful in rapidly identifying term and near-term infants at risk for multi-organ system morbidity after acute perinatal asphyxia.

Diagnosis

The most important requirement for a successful resuscitation is accurate diagnosis. Although treatment must be immediate, each step should be undertaken based on clinical and historical information, findings after evaluation, and accurate diagnosis. When a clinician is presented with decreased breath sounds in the left hemathorax, procedures that are life saving in one situation (needle thoracostomy in tension-generating pneumothorax) may be harmful in another clinically similar situation (diaphragmatic hernia).

Although the causes of asphyxia are numerous, several pieces of clinical and historical information should guide the clinician in his or her response. The differential diagnosis can be narrowed considerably, depending on whether the emergency takes place in the delivery room, nursery, or NICU; whether the infant is preterm or term; and whether the infant was receiving assisted ventilation before the emergency.

The response to an "arrest" of an intubated, mechanically ventilated infant in the NICU must be directed initially toward the correction of a possible mechanical problem (e.g., dislodgment or displacement of an endotracheal tube, pneumothorax, plugging of a tube, and ventilator malfunction) whenever cardiopulmonary resuscitation is started. The most important and effective action in neonatal resuscitation is to ventilate the baby's lungs with oxygen. Once cardiac compressions are initiated, the true cause of the emergency may be obscured. With adequate anticipation and preparation, the organized response to the expected diagnosis is simplified; however, adequate anticipation and preparation are not always possible. While evaluating the situation, determining the proper diagnosis, and organizing the emergency care, the clinician should bear in mind three important principles: (1) *primum non nocere* (Latin, meaning "first do no harm"); (2) avoid useless diagnostic or therapeutic procedures that waste time; and (3) do not initiate a costly procedure to prolong life when the situation is hopeless or irreversible.

The performance of cord blood gas studies may greatly assist the pediatric team in resuscitating the depressed newborn infant in the delivery room. A section of cord is clamped during the first 30 seconds of life, and a small sample of umbilical artery blood is obtained for determination of pH, Pco_2, and base deficit. The results of this examination may be available within minutes and can be helpful in determining the magnitude of the resuscitation team's response by indicating the acid-base status of the baby immediately after birth. Often, the results obtained on this test do not correlate with the Apgar score at 1 minute,[17] and performance of the test may precede by many minutes the obtaining of neonatal blood gas values for samples collected from an umbilical artery catheter or a radial artery puncture. Occasionally, venous blood is drawn from the umbilical cord and mislabeled as arterial. Although usually the arterial-venous (A-V) difference between the arterial and venous pH is 0.02 to 0.06 units, simultaneous evaluations of arterial and venous cord pH have shown a difference of 0.5 in some cases. Because arterial cord blood is desaturated, a Po_2 greater than 30 mm Hg in a sample should cause the clinician to question its origin.

A review of 30,839 births by Perlman and Risser[22] revealed that only 39 infants (0.12%) required chest compressions, epinephrine, or both, as part of delivery room resuscitation. Severe fetal acidemia (pH <7.00, or a base deficit >14 mEq/L) occurred in approximately one third of infants and portended poor outcome. In the other two thirds of neonates without fetal acidemia, malposition of the endotracheal tube combined with ineffective or improper initial ventilatory support was the presumed mechanism for the continued neonatal depression.[22] This insightful study highlights the importance of accurate diagnosis, the usefulness of cord blood gas studies, and the necessity of appropriately administered positive-pressure ventilation for successful resuscitation.

TREATMENT PROTOCOL

Resuscitation should proceed according to a predetermined protocol; the protocol that has received national acceptance is the -AHA-AAP NRP (Appendix 27).[1] The protocol for neonatal resuscitation is outlined in the algorithm.[23]

American Heart Association-American Academy of Pediatrics Neonatal Resuscitation Program

The following discussion of a neonatal resuscitation protocol is derived mostly from the 2000 AHA-AAP *Textbook of Neonatal Resuscitation* (4th ed.),[1] the *International Guidelines for Neonatal Resuscitation,*[23] and the 2002 *Guidelines for Perinatal Care* (5th ed.).[7]

Preparation for Delivery

Universal Precautions

Universal precautions should be followed because exposure to blood and other body fluids is likely in the delivery room. Gloves and other protective barriers should be worn when handling newly born infants and potentially contaminated equipment. Any technique that involves mouth suction (e.g., DeLee suction) must be avoided.

Personnel

At least one person skilled in initiating newborn resuscitation should be present at every delivery. Qualifications for this person should be determined by hospital protocol following

---

TABLE 4-5. Recommended Equipment and Supplies for Neonatal Resuscitation

Radiant warmer
Stethoscope
Cardiotachometer with electrocardiogram (oscilloscope desirable)
Suction with manometer
Bulb syringe
Meconium aspirator
Wall O_2 with flowmeter and tubing
Suction catheters (5- or 6-French, 8-French, and 10-French)
Neonatal resuscitation bag (manometer optional)
Face masks in newborn and premature infant sizes
Oral airways in newborn and premature infant sizes
Endotracheal tubes (2.5-, 3.0-, 3.5-, and 4.0-mm)
Endotracheal tube stylets
Laryngoscope(s)
Laryngoscope blades (straight no. 0 and 1)
Umbilical catheters (3.5- and 5-French)
Three-way stopcocks
Sterile umbilical vessel catheterization tray
Twenty-milliliter syringe and 8-French feeding tube for gastric suction
Needles, syringes
Medications
   Epinephrine (1:10,000 solution)
   Naloxone hydrochloride (1 mg/mL or 0.4 mg/mL solution)
   Volume expander
   Sodium bicarbonate (0.5 mEq/mL solution)

From Neonatal resuscitation. JAMA 268:2277, 1992. Coyright 1992, American Medical Association.

---

standard guidelines, including completion of the AHA-AAP NRP course. Course renewal is required every 2 years. At least two persons are required for resuscitation of a severely depressed neonate, one to ventilate and intubate, if necessary, and another to monitor heart rate and perform chest compressions, if indicated. When extensive resuscitation (including medication administration) is anticipated, a team of three to five persons with designated roles is recommended, including team leader. With multiple gestation delivery, a separate team should be present for each infant.

Equipment

A complete inventory of resuscitation equipment and medications should be present and in fully operational condition wherever deliveries occur. Table 4-5 lists the recommended equipment, supplies, and medications.

Initial Evaluation and Basic Steps of Resuscitation

Initial Evaluation

The initial assessment of the newborn infant should be performed within a few seconds of birth and should determine if routine care is indicated or if some form of resuscitation is required. The algorithm (Fig. 4-3) shows the initial steps of evaluation, decision, and action. Five signs (Fig. 4-3, top box) that need to be evaluated rapidly and simultaneously because they are indications for further evaluation and intervention are meconium in the amniotic fluid or on the skin; apnea or gasping; absence of flexor tone; central cyanosis; and preterm birth. Most newborn infants who are not meconium-stained will respond to the stimulation of the extrauterine environment

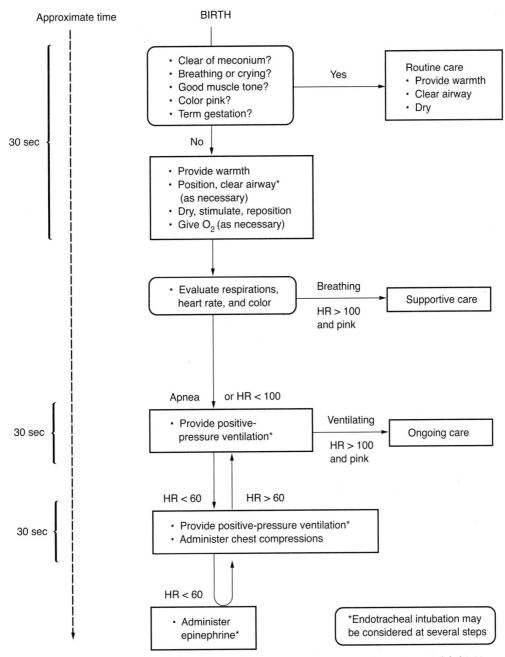

Approximate time

BIRTH

- Clear of meconium?
- Breathing or crying?
- Good muscle tone?
- Color pink?
- Term gestation?

Yes →

Routine care
- Provide warmth
- Clear airway
- Dry

30 sec

No ↓

- Provide warmth
- Position, clear airway* (as necessary)
- Dry, stimulate, reposition
- Give O_2 (as necessary)

- Evaluate respirations, heart rate, and color

Breathing

HR > 100 and pink

→ Supportive care

Apnea   or HR < 100 ↓

30 sec

- Provide positive-pressure ventilation*

Ventilating

HR > 100 and pink

→ Ongoing care

HR < 60 ↓   HR > 60 ↑

30 sec

- Provide positive-pressure ventilation*
- Administer chest compressions

HR < 60 ↓

- Administer epinephrine*

*Endotracheal intubation may be considered at several steps

Figure 4-3. Algorithm for resuscitation of the newly born infant. (From Niermeyer S, Kattwinkel J, Van Reempts P, et al. International Guidelines for Neonatal Resuscitation: An excerpt from the Guidelines 2000 for Cardiopulmonary Resuscitation and Emergency Cardiovascular Care: International Consensus on Science. Pediatrics 2000;106:E29, p. 7. Reproduced with permission.)

with a vigorous cry and movement of all extremities. If these responses are intact, color rapidly improves from cyanotic to pink, and it can be assumed that heart rate is adequate. The vigorous term infant can remain with the mother to receive routine care (providing warmth, clearing the airway, and drying).

Basic Steps of Resuscitation

Warmth. Newborn infants do not tolerate cold stress, and hypothermia delays recovery from acidosis.[24] Cold stress can increase oxygen consumption and hinder effective resuscitation.[25,26] The newborn infant should be placed under a radiant

warmer, the skin rapidly dried, and wet linen removed immediately. The baby should be left uncovered to permit full visualization and to allow effective radiant warming. Hyperthermia should be avoided because it is associated with respiratory depression in the neonate.[27,28]

Research suggests that selective hypothermia of the asphyxiated infant may protect against brain injury.[29,30] However, therapeutic hypothermia for treatment of severe asphyxia should not be used outside of randomized, controlled, multicenter trials.

Positioning and suctioning. The baby should be positioned supine or lying on its side, with the neck slightly extended in the

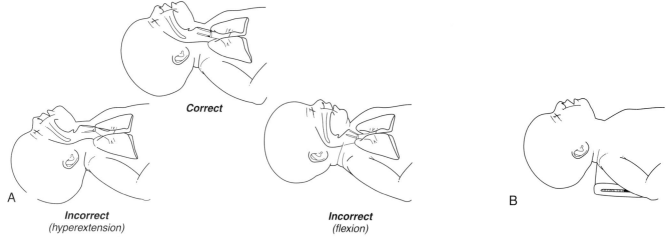

Figure 4-4. *A*, Correct and incorrect head positions for resuscitation. *B*, Optional shoulder roll for maintaining correct head position.

"sniffing" position. This position will facilitate unrestricted air entry by bringing the posterior pharynx, larynx, and trachea in line (Fig. 4-4*A*). Overextension or flexion of the neck should be avoided because these positions obstruct the airway. A rolled blanket or towel under the shoulders may help maintain the correct position, especially if the baby has a large occiput secondary to molding, edema, or prematurity (Fig. 4-4*B*).

The person assisting delivery of the baby should suction its mouth and nose with a bulb syringe after delivery of the shoulders but before delivery of the chest. Vigorous newly born infants do not need suctioning after delivery.[31,32] When fluid appears to be blocking the airway, secretions should be cleared first from the mouth and then the nose ("m" before "n") with a bulb syringe or suction catheter (8- or 10-French). The mouth is suctioned before the nose to ensure that there is nothing to aspirate if the infant should gasp when the nose is suctioned. The negative suction pressure should not exceed 100 mm Hg. If there are copious secretions, the head should be turned to the side because it allows secretions to collect in the cheek where they can be easily removed. Prolonged or deep suctioning with the catheter should be avoided because stimulation of the posterior pharynx during the first minutes after birth can produce a vagal response consisting of apnea or severe bradycardia.[33]

Tactile stimulation. Most newborn infants are stimulated to breathe with drying and suctioning. Gentle rubbing of the back or flicking the soles of the feet are two safe methods of tactile stimulation. Tactile stimulation may stimulate spontaneous respirations in newborns with primary apnea. If there is no response to one or two flicks of the soles of the feet or rubbing the back once or twice, the infant is in secondary apnea, and positive-pressure ventilation should be initiated.

Oxygen administration. Color can range from normal acrocyanosis to pallor to central cyanosis. If central cyanosis is present in the spontaneously breathing newborn, 100% free-flow O_2 should be provided. The O_2 can be delivered via a face mask and flow-inflating bag, an oxygen mask, or a hand cupped around oxygen tubing held close to the face (for maximization of O_2 concentration). Self-inflating bags will not passively deliver sufficient oxygen flow through the mask. The O_2 source should deliver at least 5 L/min. Oxygen administration is not a hazard during a brief period of resuscitation.

Clearing the airway of meconium. Meconium is present in the amniotic fluid in approximately 12% of deliveries.[34] The person assisting the delivery of the baby should thoroughly suction the mouth, posterior pharynx, and nose of the infant of meconium-stained amniotic fluid as soon as the head is delivered but before the chest is delivered (intrapartum suctioning), regardless of whether the meconium is thick or thin (Fig. 4-5).[35] A large-bore suction catheter (12- to 14-French) should be used with regulated negative-pressure suction of 100 mm Hg. Many obstetricians prefer to use a bulb syringe for intrapartum suctioning. This practice is supported in a report by Locus et al.[36] showing that there was no significant difference in the amount of meconium found below the vocal cords in a cohort study comparing catheter suction to bulb suction. Thorough suctioning of the mouth, posterior pharynx, and nose before delivery of the body decreases the risk of meconium aspiration syndrome.[35] Nevertheless, despite thorough intrapartum suctioning, 20% to 30% of meconium-stained infants will have meconium in the trachea in the absence of spontaneous respirations.[37,38] The possibility of meconium aspiration in utero suggests a need for tracheal suctioning of depressed infants after delivery.

Wiswell et al.[39] performed a large, randomized, controlled multicenter trial of delivery room intubation of the apparently *vigorous* meconium-stained neonate and found no difference in a 3% rate of meconium aspiration syndrome between prophylactically intubated and non-intubated infants. They concluded that routine tracheal suctioning of the *vigorous* newborn with meconium-stained fluid does not improve outcome and may cause complications. Therefore, as shown in Figure 4-5, the AHA-AAP NRP recommends suctioning the mouth and trachea of the meconium-stained newborn only if the child is *not* vigorous. *Vigorous* is defined as good muscle tone, strong respiratory efforts, and heart rate greater than 100 beats/min immediately after delivery.

Management of the vigorous meconium-stained infant should proceed with the remainder of the initial steps of resuscitation. The non-vigorous infant should be placed in the bed of the radiant warmer immediately after intrapartum suctioning and direct laryngoscopy should be performed in order to suction residual meconium from the hypopharynx (under direct

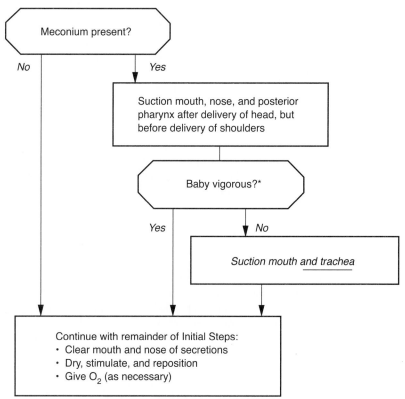

Meconium present?

No   Yes

Suction mouth, nose, and posterior
pharynx after delivery of head, but
before delivery of shoulders

Baby vigorous?*

Yes   No

Suction mouth and trachea

Continue with remainder of Initial Steps:
• Clear mouth and nose of secretions
• Dry, stimulate, and reposition
• Give O$_2$ (as necessary)

*"Vigorous" is defined as strong respiratory efforts, good muscle tone,
and a heart rate greater than 100 bpm.

Figure 4-5. Steps in clearing the airway of the newly born infant with meconium-stained amniotic fluid. (From the American Heart Association/American Academy of Pediatrics: Textbook of Neonatal Resuscitation. Dallas, American Heart Association, 2000, p. 2-7. Reproduced with permission.)

vision) and to intubate and suction the trachea. Drying and stimulation should be delayed. Tracheal suctioning should be accomplished by applying suction through a meconium aspirator device attached directly to the endotracheal tube, applying suction as the endotracheal tube is withdrawn from the airway (Fig. 4-6). Suction catheters inserted through endotracheal tubes may be too small to successfully accomplish initial removal of particulate meconium. After suctioning of particulate meconium is accomplished, use of suction catheters through the endotracheal tube may adequately remove residual meconium. Repeat intubation and suctioning until there is minimal residual meconium, but stop if the baby's heart rate is severely depressed, and begin positive-pressure ventilation. Previous AHA-AAP NRP recommendations suggested that endotracheal suctioning should depend upon whether meconium was "thick" or "thin." Although thick meconium may be more hazardous than thin, there are no clinical studies that offer suctioning guidelines based upon meconium consistency.

Gastric suctioning may be performed to prevent aspiration of swallowed meconium, but only after resuscitation is successfully completed. Large amounts of meconium-stained fluid can be present in the stomach of the newborn,[40] so the stomach should be suctioned but only after the infant is stable (generally, 5 minutes after birth).[41]

It is important to understand that if apnea or respiratory distress develops in meconium-stained infants, they should receive tracheal suctioning before positive-pressure ventilation, even if they had been initially vigorous.[23]

Subsequent Evaluation and More Advanced Resuscitation

After initial stabilization, subsequent evaluation of the newly born infant uses the triad of respiration, heart rate, and color. Apnea or gasping indicates the need for positive-pressure ventilation.[5] Heart rate is determined by auscultation of the precordium with a stethoscope or by palpating pulsations at the base of the umbilical cord. The AHA-AAP NRP recommends counting the number of heart beats for 6 seconds and multiplying by 10 to make a quick estimate of beats per minute. If the heart rate is less than 100 beats/min, positive-pressure ventilation is indicated. Persistent central cyanosis despite 100% oxygen is also an indication for positive-pressure ventilation.

Ventilation

Most neonates can be effectively ventilated with a bag and mask. Positive-pressure ventilation is indicated for any neonate with (1) apnea or gasping; (2) heart rate less than 100 beats/min; or (3) persistent central cyanosis the delivery of 100% free-flow O$_2$.

A tight seal between the face and mask is necessary for successful bag-and-mask ventilation; therefore, face masks with cushioned rims that fit preterm, term, and large newborns must be available in the delivery room. The recommended ventilation rate is 40 to 60 breaths per minute. Normal, not excessive, chest wall movement is the sign of successful positive-pressure ventilation. When starting ventilation of the newly born infant,

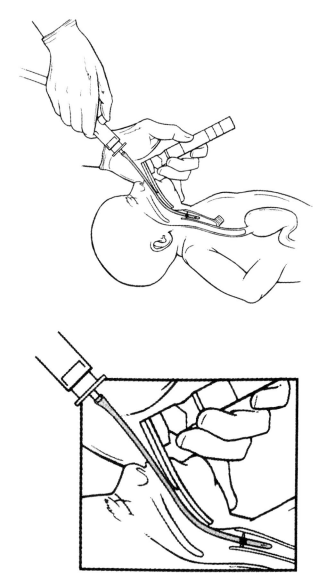

Figure 4-6. Visualizing the glottis and suctioning meconium from the trachea using a laryngoscope and endotracheal tube. (From the American Heart Association/American Academy of Pediatrics: Textbook of Neonatal Resuscitation. Dallas, American Heart Association, 2000. Reproduced with permission.)

visible chest expansion is the most reliable sign of appropriate inflation pressure, not any specific inflation pressure. Chest expansion should be the focus of attention, not the pressure manometer.[42] At first, inflation pressures may need to be 30 to 40 cm H_2O or higher. Asphyxiated neonates who are born apneic with fluid-filled lungs may need an initial prolonged inflation lasting 3 to 5 seconds for prompt establishment of a functional residual capacity.[43,44] Less pressure and shorter inspiratory times usually are adequate for subsequent ventilation. If chest wall movement is not adequate, (1) reapply the mask, ensuring that a tight seal has been obtained; (2) reposition the head; (3) repeat suctioning if secretions are present; or (4) increase the inflation pressure. If chest wall movement does

not improve, immediately intubate the infant to secure the airway. If bag-and-mask ventilation is prolonged, it may produce gastric distention; this is relieved with insertion of an 8-French orogastric tube that is aspirated with a syringe and left open to air.

One controversial aspect of the AHA-AAP NRP protocol is its reliance on bag-and-mask ventilation in the severely depressed infant (i.e., with a 1-minute Apgar score <3). Bag-and-mask ventilation initiates a gasp in approximately 85% of cases and has proved to be an acceptable and efficient way of resuscitating the mildly or moderately asphyxiated or depressed infant. However, in a comparison of face-mask ventilation with the intubation and ventilation of a small group of asphyxiated term newborns, Milner et al.[45] concluded that the face-mask system was relatively inefficient because tidal volume exchange is less than one third of that seen after intubation and because it may not be sufficient to produce adequate alveolar ventilation. Despite this, all babies resuscitated with bag-and-mask ventilation responded satisfactorily and were breathing within 4 minutes of birth. The authors concluded that successful resuscitation depended on stimulation of a baby to make his or her own respiratory efforts (Head's paradoxical reflex). Therefore, when severe depression is present at birth (e.g., heart rate is zero) and it is unlikely that the infant will be able to initiate and sustain ventilation on his or her own, intubation is suggested. Moreover, when prolonged ventilation is necessary during any resuscitation, insertion of an endotracheal tube is preferable because it affords greater airway stability than other ventilatory measures. On the other hand, proper tracheal intubation is of paramount importance in successful resuscitation. In a study on the use of capnography in the delivery room of a major university level III hospital to evaluate placement of the endotracheal tube, 41% (11/27) of intubations were incorrectly placed on the initial attempt.[46] Thus, the experience of the person managing the airway must be taken into account when deciding between bag-mask ventilation and intubation.

After positive-pressure ventilation has achieved good chest wall movement for 30 seconds, heart rate should be re-evaluated. If the heart rate is greater than 100 beats/min and if spontaneous breathing is present, positive-pressure ventilation can be gradually discontinued. Tactile stimulation can be provided while the infant is closely monitored to ensure that effective spontaneous respirations continue. Assisted ventilation must continue if spontaneous respirations are absent or ineffective, or if heart rate is less than 100 beats/min. If heart rate is less than 60 beats/min, continue positive-pressure ventilation, begin chest compressions, and consider endotracheal intubation.

Establishing adequate ventilation is the key to successful neonatal resuscitation. Satisfactory inflation of fluid-filled lungs with air or oxygen expedites reversal of bradycardia, hypoxia, and acidosis.[47] For rapid reversal of hypoxia during resuscitation, 100% oxygen has been traditionally used, but biochemical evidence and preliminary clinical studies suggest that resuscitation with 21% oxygen may be equally effective with less oxidative stress.[48–50] In a small randomized, controlled trial, Vento et al.[50] found no apparent clinical disadvantages in using room air instead of 100% oxygen for ventilation of asphyxiated neonates. Neonates resuscitated with room air - demonstrated quicker recovery as determined by time to first cry and time to sustained respirations. Furthermore, Vento et al.[50] showed that in contrast to neonates resuscitated with room air, infants resuscitated with 100% oxygen showed biochemical evidence of prolonged oxidative stress 4 weeks after birth. Nevertheless, the 2000 AHA-AAP NRP recommends delivery of 100% oxygen by positive-pressure ventilation if assisted ventilation is required. If supplemental oxygen is not available, resuscitate the neonate with positive-pressure ventilation and room air via a self-inflating bag because it does not require an oxygen source to function.[23]

Ventilation Bags

Newly born babies have small tidal volumes (5–8 mL/kg). Resuscitation bags for neonates should be no larger than 750 mL because it is difficult to deliver small tidal volumes with bigger bags. There are two types of ventilation bags (Fig. 4-7): self-inflating bags and flow-inflating bags.

The self-inflating bag is more commonly found in the delivery room and resuscitation cart because it is somewhat easier to use. The recoil of the bag enables the self-inflating bag to refill even with no compressed gas source. Self-inflating bags have an air inlet at one end that permits rapid re-inflation but which will pull in room air and dilute oxygen flowing into the bag and deliver only 40% oxygen to the patient. An oxygen reservoir must be attached to the air inlet (Fig. 4-8) to enable the self-inflating bag to deliver 90% to 100% oxygen to the patient. Most self-inflating bags have a pressure-release valve to prevent excessive pressure build-up and should release at approximately 30 to 35 cm H_2O pressure. The pressure-release valve should have an override feature that permits delivery of higher pressures if necessary to achieve good chest expansion. Some self-inflating bags have a pressure manometer attachment site that can be attached to an in-line manometer. Self-inflating bags cannot be used to deliver 100% free-flow O_2 through the mask because the flow of oxygen is unreliable unless the bag is being squeezed.

The flow-inflating (anesthesia) bag will only inflate when compressed gas is flowing into it and the patient outlet is occluded. Proper use of the flow-inflating bag requires successful coordination of three tasks: (1) adjusting the flow of gas into the bag and (2) adjusting the flow of gas out of the bag through the flow-control valve while (3) maintaining a tight seal between the mask and the face of the infant. More training and practice are required to effectively and safely use a flow-inflating bag in contrast to the self-inflating bag.[51] A manometer must be connected to the flow-inflating bag to monitor peak and end-expiratory pressures because the flow-inflating bag can deliver very high pressures. Advantages of the flow-inflating bag include the common belief that the stiffness of the baby's lungs can be "felt" when squeezing the bag, in contrast to a self-inflating bag, and that 100% free-flow O_2 can be delivered through the mask with a flow-inflating bag.

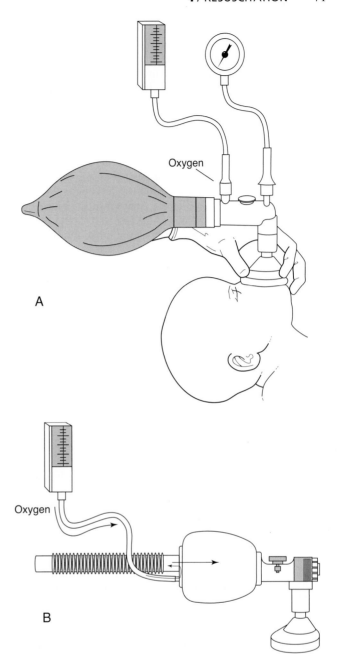

A

Oxygen

Oxygen

B

Figure 4-7. Types of ventilation bags. *A,* Flow-inflating bag inflates only with compressed gas source and with mask sealed on face; otherwise, the bag remains deflated. *B,* Self-inflating bag remains inflated without gas flow and without mask sealed on face. However, it is shown with oxygen line attached because oxygen is recommended for resuscitation. (From the American Heart Association/American Academy of Pediatrics: Textbook of Neonatal Resuscitation. Dallas, American Heart Association, 2000, pp. 3-4, 3-5. Reproduced with permission.)

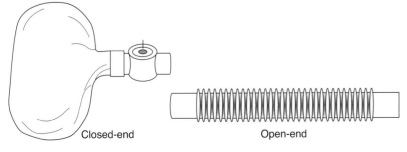

Closed-end   Open-end

Figure 4-8. Types of oxygen reservoirs. (From the American Heart Association/American Academy of Pediatrics: Textbook of Neonatal Resuscitation. Dallas, American Heart Association, 2000, p. 3-15. Reproduced with permission.)

Face Masks

Face masks should be cushioned and of the correct size so that the rim covers the tip of the chin, mouth, and nose, but not the eyes. It is important to have three sizes of masks in order to fit full-term infants, premature infants, and extremely-low-birthweight infants. Masks that are too large may cause damage to the infant's eyes and will not provide a good seal. Masks that are too small will not cover the mouth and nose and may occlude the nose. Cushioned masks conform more easily to the shape of the newborn's face, thus creating an effective seal; require less pressure to make a seal; and are less likely to damage eyes if the masks are positioned incorrectly. Masks can be round or anatomically shaped. Anatomically shaped masks are designed to fit the contours of the face and should be placed on the face with the pointed part of the mask fitting over the nose.

The laryngeal mask airway (Fig. 4-9), a mask designed to fit over the laryngeal inlet, may be an effective alternative for establishing an airway during resuscitation of the newborn infant,[52,53] but it cannot be recommended for routine use at this time because of insufficient clinical evidence of its efficacy and ease of use.

Endotracheal Intubation

Timing of endotracheal intubation depends upon the experience and skill of the resuscitator. Endotracheal intubation may be considered at several steps during neonatal resuscitation (indicated by an asterisk in the NRP algorithm in Fig. 4-3):

1. When tracheal suctioning for meconium is required
2. When bag-mask ventilation is ineffective or prolonged
3. When chest compressions are performed
4. When tracheal administration of medications is planned, or
5. With special resuscitation circumstances, including diaphragmatic hernia and extremely-low-birthweight infants

The technique of tracheal intubation is discussed fully in Chapter 6. Supplies and equipment for endotracheal intubation need to be readily available. Endotracheal tubes should have uniform diameter, a natural curve, a radiopaque indicator line, and markings to indicate depth of insertion. Use of a stylet is optional; if used, the stylet must never protrude beyond the tip of the tube. Table 4-6 shows recommended tracheal tube size and depth according to weight and gestational age. Figure 4-10 illustrates proper placement of the laryngoscope and the landmarks that should be seen on intubation. The clinician can avoid inserting the endotracheal tube too deeply by using a length of tubing measuring no more than 6 cm (from tip of the tube to the lip of the infant) plus the infant's weight in kilograms. For example, a 2-kg infant should have a "tip-to-lip" distance of $6 + 2 = 8$ cm.[54] This rule may not apply in infants with hypoplastic mandibles (e.g., Pierre-Robin syndrome) or with short necks (e.g., Turner syndrome). Babies weighing less than 750 g may require only 6 cm or less of tracheal tube insertion.

The clinician needs to confirm successful endotracheal intubation by the following:

1. Observing symmetrical chest-wall movement,
2. Listening for equal breath sounds, especially in the axilla, and for absent breath sounds over the stomach,
3. Confirming absence of gastric inflation,

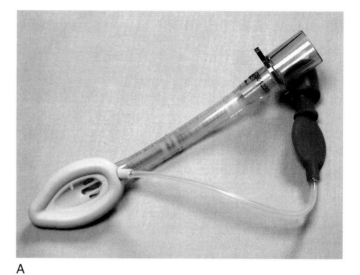

A

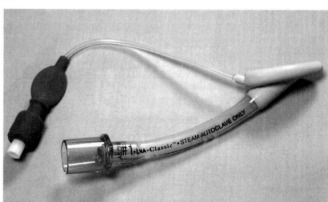

B

Figure 4-9. Laryngeal mask airway, number 1, for use in neonates weighing less than 5 kg. *A,* Frontal view. *B,* Side view.

TABLE 4-6. Guidelines for Endotracheal Tube Size

Tube Size (mm, Inside Diameter)	Infant Weight (g)
2.5	<1000
3.0	1000–2000
3.5	2000–3000
3.5–4.0	>3000

From the American Heart Association/American Academy of Pediatrics: Textbook of Neonatal Resuscitation. Dallas, American Heart Association, 1994, p. 5–10. Reproduced by permission. © Textbook of Neonatal Resuscitation, 1987, 1990, 1994. Copyright American Heart Association.

4. Observing condensation in the tube during exhalation, and
5. Noting improvement in heart rate, color, and spontaneous respirations.

CO_2 levels usually are much higher in the trachea than the esophagus because the lungs are the primary organ for removal of CO_2 from the body. Monitoring of exhaled CO_2 may be useful in secondary confirmation of tracheal intubation in the newly born infant.[55,56] There are two types of CO_2 detec-

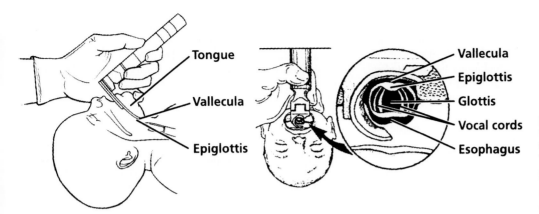

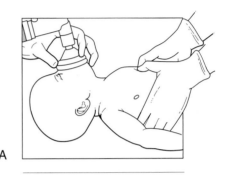

Figure 4-10. Identification of landmarks before placing endotracheal tube through glottis. (From the American Heart Association/ American Academy of Pediatrics: Textbook of Neonatal Resuscitation. Dallas, American Heart Association, 2000. Reproduced with permission.)

tors: colorimetric devices, which change color in the presence of CO_2, and capnographs, which display a specific CO_2 level and should read greater than 2% CO_2 if the tube is in the trachea.[57] In some patients, CO_2 monitoring can be misleading because extremely-low-birthweight infants and infants with very poor cardiac output may not exhale enough CO_2 to be reliably detected, despite proper position of the endotracheal tube. In one study, however, capnography identified all infants who had esophageal intubations and improved the median times to recognition of improper intubation by 21 seconds ($P \leq 001$).[46] There is limited clinical evidence on sensitivity and specificity of exhaled CO_2 detectors and successful endotracheal tube placement in newly born infants, so routine use in neonatal resuscitation cannot be recommended at this time.

If there is any doubt that the tracheal tube was passed through the glottis, repeat visualization of the larynx with a laryngoscope must be performed for verification. If the infant is to remain intubated, a chest radiograph should be obtained for confirmation of proper tube position.

Chest Compressions

Chest compressions should be started after 30 seconds of positive-pressure ventilation with 100% oxygen if heart rate is less than 60 beats/min. The 2000 AHA-AAP NRP no longer recommends chest compressions for heart rate that is between 60 and 80 beats/min and not increasing because cardiac output probably is adequate when heart rate is 60 beats/min or greater. Ventilation should be the priority in neonatal resuscitation, and chest compressions may compete with provision of effective ventilation. Figure 4-11*A* and *B* shows the two different techniques for performing chest compressions. The two-thumb technique is the preferred method for performing chest compressions.[58–61] Both thumbs are placed on the lower third of the sternum,[62,63] superimposed or adjacent to each other according to the size of the chest, and the fingers encircle the chest to support the back. The thumbs should be placed on the sternum just below an imaginary line passing between the nipples (Fig. 4-11*C*). Abdominal organs can be damaged with direct compressions of the xiphoid or lower end of the sternum. If the resuscitator's hands are too small to encircle the chest, then two-finger compressions should be performed with the other hand supporting the back (Fig. 4-11). The thumbs or fingers

A

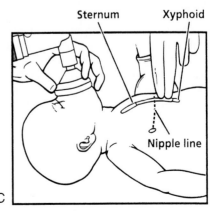

B

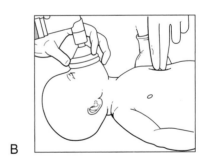

C

Figure 4-11. Two methods of applying chest compression. *A,* Thumb method. *B,* Two-finger method. *C,* Correct finger position on the sternum. (From the American Heart Association/American Academy of Pediatrics: Textbook of Neonatal Resuscitation. Dallas, American Heart Association, 2000, pp. 4-5, 4-7. Reproduced with permission.)

must remain in contact with the sternum in all phases of compression. The sternum should be compressed approximately one third of the diameter of the chest in a smooth fashion. Compression phase duration slightly shorter than relaxation phase is recommended because this technique has resulted in improved blood flow in neonatal animal experiments.[64]

Simultaneous chest compressions and ventilations that have been under investigation in older children and adults must not be used in babies,[65] because effective ventilation should be the priority in neonatal resuscitation. Chest compressions should be interposed with ventilation in a 3:1 ratio. This means that the combined rate of chest compressions and ventilations is approximately 120 events per minute, that is, 90 compressions and 30 breaths. It is recommended that the compressor count aloud so that the ventilator knows when to perform the ventilation. The cadence should be "one-and-two-and-three-and breathe-and … ." Heart rate should be checked every 30 seconds. Chest compressions should be discontinued when the heart rate is 60 beats/min or greater.[23]

Medications

Medications are rarely indicated in resuscitation of the neonate.[22] Bradycardia in the newly born infant usually occurs because of inadequate lung expansion and hypoxia. Effective positive-pressure ventilation is the most important step in correcting bradycardia. Medications should be administered if heart rate remains less than 60 beats/min after 30 seconds of chest compressions and adequate ventilation.

Epinephrine

Epinephrine is indicated when heart rate is less than 60 beats/min, and especially when asystole is present, despite a minimum of 30 seconds of chest compressions and adequate ventilation with 100% oxygen. Although epinephrine has both α- and β-adrenergic–stimulating properties, α-adrenergic–mediated vasoconstriction probably is the more important action during cardiac arrest.[66] Vasoconstriction enhances delivery of oxygen to the heart and brain by elevating perfusion pressure during chest compression.[67] Epinephrine also increases heart rate, stimulates spontaneous contractions, and strengthens the contractile state of the heart.

The recommended dose of endotracheal or intravenous epinephrine is 0.1 to 0.3 mL/kg of a 1:10,000 solution (0.01 to 0.03 mg/kg), repeated every 3 to 5 minutes. Endotracheal epinephrine is effective because trans-pulmonary absorption of epinephrine is not decreased during times of hypoxia-induced low pulmonary blood flow in neonatal animal experiments.[61] The endotracheal route is associated with somewhat lower blood levels of epinephrine, so the higher end of the dosage range (0.3 mL/kg) should be considered. When giving epinephrine by endotracheal tube, be sure to give it directly into the tube and follow the drug by several positive-pressure breaths to distribute it throughout the lungs to maximize absorption. Higher doses (>0.3 mL/kg of 1:10,000 solution) of epinephrine have been associated with extreme hypertension and low cardiac output in animal experiments.[68,69] When hypotension is followed by hypertension, the risk of intracranial hemorrhage is increased, especially in preterm infants.[70] Therefore, routine use of higher doses (>0.3 mL/kg of 1:10,000 solution) of epinephrine is not recommended.

Volume Expanders

Volume expanders should be considered whenever an infant appears to be in shock (pale, poor perfusion, weak pulse) or when the infant has not responded to chest compressions, effective ventilation, and epinephrine administration. The initial dose of volume expander is 10 mL/kg given over 5 to 10 minutes by slow intravenous push. Although higher-bolus volumes of volume expander have been recommended for resuscitation of older infants, intracranial hemorrhage or volume overload may result from inappropriate intravascular volume expansion in asphyxiated newborn infants and especially preterm infants.[71] Normal saline is the fluid of choice. Ringer's lactate is an alternative volume expander but may not be as readily available as normal saline. Administration of O-negative packed red blood cells should be considered for replacement of large volume blood loss. Administration of albumin-containing solutions is no longer recommended for initial volume expansion because of an association with increased mortality,[72] as well as limited availability and risk of transmission of infectious diseases.

Bicarbonate

Routine use of sodium bicarbonate is not recommended in neonatal resuscitation because of insufficient data supporting the practice. In addition, sodium bicarbonate may be harmful to myocardial and cerebral function because of its hyperosmolarity and CO_2-generating properties.[73–75] Use of sodium bicarbonate should be discouraged during brief resuscitation. If bicarbonate is used during prolonged cardiopulmonary arrests unresponsive to other therapy, it should be given only after adequate ventilation and circulation are established.[76] After an infant has been successfully resuscitated, use of bicarbonate for treatment of persistent severe metabolic acidosis or hyperkalemia should be directed by blood gas levels or serum chemistries. The recommended dose of sodium bicarbonate is 2 mEq/kg of a 0.5 mEq/mL solution given by slow intravenous push over at least 2 minutes after adequate ventilation and perfusion have been established. Bicarbonate should never be given faster than 1 mEq/kg/min.

Concern about the CO_2-generating properties of bicarbonate led to development of 0.3 N tromethamine, or THAM, which is a carbon dioxide-consuming alkalinizing agent. Unfortunately, THAM has not been shown to be safer than bicarbonate during resuscitation. THAM has been reported to cause hepatic necrosis in neonates, as well as hyperkalemia, hypoglycemia, and ventilatory depression[77]; therefore, THAM is not recommended for routine use in neonatal resuscitation and should not be substituted for bicarbonate.

Naloxone

Use of the narcotic antagonist naloxone hydrochloride is indicated for the neonate with severe respiratory depression attributable to narcotics given to the mother within 4 hours of delivery. Naloxone should be given only if severe respiratory depression persists *after* positive-pressure ventilation with 100% oxygen has restored a normal heart rate and color.[1] The dose is 0.1 mg/kg.[78] An endotracheal or intravenous route of administration is preferred, but intramuscular or subcutaneous routes are acceptable with adequate perfusion. The initial dose can be repeated once in 3 to 5 minutes if there are still no spontaneous respirations. The duration of action of narcotics can exceed that of naloxone. Continuous monitoring is required for at least 6 hours in an infant who requires naloxone for reversal of respiratory depression. Use of naloxone is contraindicated in a neonate whose mother is suspected of being narcotic-dependent because sudden narcotic withdrawal can induce severe seizures.[79] In this setting, the neonate should receive mechanical ventilation until narcotic-induced respiratory depression resolves. Monitoring for signs of fetal abstinence syndrome should be initiated in infants of narcotic-dependent mothers.

Despite standard recommendations by AHA-AAP NRP, variability in use of naloxone among hospitals is considerable,[80] which cannot be explained by differences in maternal exposure to opiates. Herschel et al.[81] evaluated use of naloxone at a university hospital and a community hospital and reported that in neither hospital was naloxone given as recommended by AHA-AAP NRP. They found that naloxone was given even when mothers did not receive opiates within 4 hours of delivery; it was given to infants who did not have severe respiratory depression; and it was given without first supporting ventilation. Naloxone may be given by some practitioners because of a belief that endogenous opiates might play a role in the pathogenesis of perinatal asphyxia. Chernick et al.[82] performed a blinded clinical trial of naloxone in newly born infants with low 1-minute Apgar scores who were born to women who had not received opiates within 4 hours of delivery and who had not received general anesthesia. Naloxone had no significant effect on heart rate or restoration of spontaneous respirations in these infants. The investigators concluded that naloxone showed no benefit in resuscitation of the asphyxiated newborn infant; therefore, naloxone should be used only when there is a history of maternal narcotic administration within the past 4 hours and only *after* positive-pressure ventilation has restored normal heart rate and color. Other drugs given to the mother can depress respirations in the newly born infant, such as magnesium sulfate or general anesthetic, but will not respond to naloxone.

Routes of Medication Administration

The endotracheal route is the most rapidly accessible route for drug administration during resuscitation in the delivery room. Although the tracheal route can be used for administration of epinephrine or naloxone, it must not be used to administer caustic substances such as sodium bicarbonate.

If an infant fails to respond to intratracheal epinephrine, intravenous access needs to be established. The umbilical vein is the recommended site for intravenous administration of drugs in the delivery room because it can be identified and catheterized fairly rapidly. A 3.5- or 5-French radiopaque catheter with a single end hole should be inserted only far enough (approximately 2 to 4 cm below the skin, less in preterm infants) to yield a free flow of blood return. If the catheter is inserted too deeply, there is risk of damaging infusion of hypertonic and vasoactive drugs directly into the liver. During cardiac arrest in neonates, it usually is impossible to administer drugs through a peripheral vein because venous collapse makes cannulation difficult and drug delivery to the central circulation may be impaired. Resuscitation drugs should not be administered through the umbilical artery because it is not rapidly accessible and there is a high risk of complications if vasoactive or hypertonic drugs are given by this route.

Intraosseous lines are not often placed in newly born infants. It is believed that the umbilical vein is more readily accessible; the intraosseous space is small in the premature infant; and neonatal bones are fragile. Nevertheless, Ellemunter et al.[83] reported a series of 27 term and preterm infants who were successfully resuscitated within 5 hours of birth via rapid intravascular access with intraosseous lines. They used an intraosseous infusion needle with an 18-gauge internal diameter (Cook Critical Care, Bloomington, IN, USA). Nine of the patients had birthweight less than 1000 g, including a 515-g infant. There were no failed attempts, and the entire procedure took less than 2 minutes. Previously reported complications with use of intraosseous needles in infants include osteomyelitis, skin infection, skin necrosis, subcutaneous abscess, fractures, and compartment syndrome.[84] In the case series reported by Ellemunter et al.,[83] three patients had dislocation and malfunction of the bone marrow needle requiring placement of a new intraosseous needle. The only other complications included one case each of subcutaneous necrosis and hematoma. No adverse effects on limb growth as a result of intraosseous needle use occurred during follow-up in the 15 long-term survivors. Intraosseous access is considered an acceptable, safe, and useful alternative route for medications/volume expanders if umbilical venous access is not readily available.[23] This route may be especially important in the emergency room and other resuscitations of babies up to several weeks of age when intravenous access is difficult. Abe et al.[85] reported that intraosseous line placement was significantly faster and easier than umbilical venous catheterization in newborn emergency vascular access models in their study of 42 medical students without prior experience in intraosseous or umbilical venous catheterization. Skill with placement of intraosseous lines is easily mastered even with limited opportunity for practice.[84] The recommended method of emergency vascular access in the newly born infant may needs to be reconsidered pending further study. In the meantime, intraosseous infusion needles (18 gauge) should be available on neonatal code carts and clinicians should be experienced in their use (Fig. 4-12).

Special Considerations
Preterm Neonates

Whenever a preterm birth is anticipated, it is important that specially trained personnel receive sufficient notification so that they can prepare the necessary equipment and environment. Asphyxia and the need for resuscitation are much more common in the preterm than the term neonate.[86] Preterm infants are at increased risk for heat loss, intraventricular hemorrhage, and respiratory distress. Susceptibility to heat loss increases with decreasing gestational age because extremely premature infants have an increased ratio of surface area to body mass and decreased thickness of the epidermis. Minimizing heat loss in preterm infants improves survival.[87] The preterm infant's brain has a fragile subependymal germinal matrix that is prone to intraventricular hemorrhage; therefore, the volume and rate of infusion of volume expanders should be monitored closely so that sudden changes in vascular pressure can be prevented.[88]

Preterm infants have an increased need for assisted ventilation because they have decreased lung compliance, respiratory musculature, and respiratory drive. Early elective intubation of extremely-low-birthweight (<1000 g) neonates at birth has

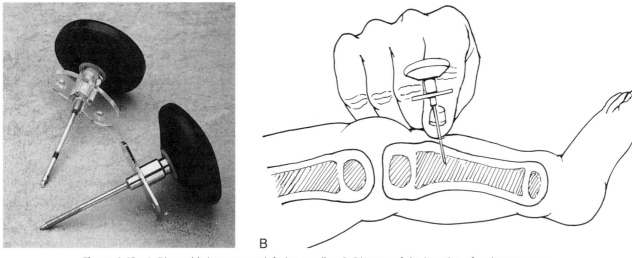

Figure 4-12. *A,* Disposable intraosseous infusion needles. *B,* Diagram of the insertion of an intraosseous needle into the femur of a neonate.

become common practice in many medical centers.[89] Other centers practice early initiation of nasal continuous positive airway pressure (CPAP) instead of intubation to establish an air-fluid interface in extremely preterm infants[90] (see Chapter 8). Many infants less than 31 weeks of gestation will require intubation for surfactant administration after successful resuscitation in the delivery room[91] (see Chapter 20).

Progressive Distress After Birth

Occasionally, an infant deteriorates rapidly in the delivery room without evidence of perinatal asphyxia. Diagnostic evaluation must be systematic if treatment is to be prompt. An infant with diaphragmatic hernia develops asymmetrical breath sounds with a scaphoid abdomen and shift in the cardiac apex. Avoidance of bag-and-mask ventilation with the application of early intubation and nasogastric suctioning can decrease the amount of air in the intrathoracic gastrointestinal tract that is compressing the lungs. Unilateral pneumothorax also manifests as a decrease in breath sounds on the affected side, with a shift in the cardiac apex to the opposite side. Emergency chest radiography definitively demonstrates both diaphragmatic hernia and pneumothorax. Needle aspiration or chest tube insertion may be needed for treatment of pneumothorax.

Bilateral choanal atresia with obstruction of both posterior nares can cause progressive respiratory distress immediately after birth. Insertion of an oral airway provides an unobstructed pathway for air through the mouth. Severe micrognathia and a posterior displacement of the tongue in Pierre Robin syndrome can block the airway and cause rapid respiratory deterioration. Prone positioning and insertion of a nasopharyngeal airway displace the tongue and permit the movement of air through the mouth. A nasopharyngeal airway can be life saving for an infant with Pierre Robin syndrome because even experienced neonatologists may have difficulty intubating the trachea.

Hydrops Fetalis

The survival rate can be as high as 50% in infants with non-immune hydrops fetalis without chromosomal abnormalities or major malformations.[92] Close collaboration between perinatologists and neonatologists is essential for successful management of infants with prenatal diagnosis of hydrops fetalis. The perinatologist may need to remove excess fluid from either the fetal abdomen or thoracic cavity before delivery. The neonatologist and perinatologist need to collectively decide on the appropriate timing and route of delivery. Queenan[93] recommends cesarean section for neonates with hydrops fetalis because vaginal delivery frequently leads to severe asphyxia and postpartum hemorrhage. Table 4-7 lists the additional equipment and supplies recommended for the resuscitation of the infant with hydrops fetalis. Immediate and vigorous resuscitation usually is required, with multiple procedures necessary for effective ventilation of the infant.[94] Personnel experienced in performing paracentesis and thoracentesis should be present, in addition to staff members who can ventilate, perform cardiac compressions, insert umbilical vessel catheters, and administer medications. If any difficulty with effective ventilation occurs after intubation, paracentesis should be performed immediately. If ventilation is still ineffective, thoracentesis should be performed. Infants with hydrops fetalis often have extremely stiff lungs and may require high ventilatory pressures and high end-expiratory pressures for initial stabilization. They often are premature with an increased risk for respiratory distress syndrome, and they may benefit from surfactant therapy. In 1980, Giacoia[95] recommended avoiding the use of salt-poor albumin as a volume expander because the albumin quickly moves into the extravascular space, worsening hydrops fetalis and increasing the risk of pulmonary edema. Albumin is no longer recommended as a volume expander in the AHA-AAP NRP because a systematic review of the use of albumin-containing solutions was associated with increased mortality in critically ill patients.[72] Intravenous furosemide 2 mg/kg may be given in the delivery room to help mobilize edema fluid. Both umbilical vein and artery catheters should be inserted in hydropic infants because peripheral venous access can be difficult. If severe anemia is present, partial exchange transfusion with O-negative packed red blood cells cross-matched against the mother can be performed immediately upon admission to the NICU. Transferring the infant from the delivery suite to the intensive

TABLE 4-7. Suggested Additional Equipment and Supplies for Delivery Room Resuscitation of Newborns with Hydrops Fetalis

1. Four thoracentesis/paracentesis kits (one for each side of the chest, and one for each side of the abdomen)
2. Normal saline for infusion (avoid 5% albumin)
3. If severe anemia is suspected, O-negative blood cross-matched with the mother
4. Three doses of epinephrine already prepared for estimated fetal weight
5. Furosemide 10 mg (1 mL); recommended dose for severe hydrops fetalis is 2 mg/kg IV
6. Heparinized blood gas syringe
7. Cardiac arrest orders/record (Appendix 26)

care unit for the partial exchange transfusion facilitates continuous monitoring of O_2 saturation and vital signs and ensures radiologic confirmation of proper position of the umbilical vein and artery catheters.

Ethics

Noninitiation of Resuscitation

Current evidence indicates that resuscitation of certain types of newly born infants is unlikely to result in survival or survival without severe disability. Therefore, the 2000 AHA-AAP NRP considers noninitiation of resuscitation in the delivery room appropriate for infants with confirmed gestation less than 23 weeks or birthweight less than 400 g,[4,96] anencephaly, or confirmed trisomy 13 or 18.[23]

Often, antenatal information is unreliable and incomplete. In the delivery room, resuscitation should be initiated when prognosis and gestational age are uncertain. Initiation of resuscitation in the delivery room does not mandate continued aggressive intervention. Delayed withdrawal of support and noninitiation of resuscitation are considered ethically equivalent. Later withdrawal of support allows clinicians time to collect more complete clinical information and to provide counseling to the family. There should be ongoing evaluation of the infant's clinical condition and discussion between the parents and the health care team to guide continuation versus withdrawal of support. In the case of extremely-low-birthweight infants, there is no advantage to delayed or partial resuscitation in the delivery room. If the infant survives, outcome may be worse because of such an approach.[23] Ethical considerations are reviewed in Chapter 5.

Unsuccessful Resuscitation

It is reasonable to want to avoid prolonged resuscitation that results in only delayed death or in the survival of a severely disabled infant. Jain et al.[97] reviewed the outcome of 93 infants who received resuscitation despite their having no detectable heartbeat at birth because signs of life were observed shortly before birth ("apparently stillborn infants"). Developmental assessment of 23 long-term survivors available for follow-up showed normal outcome in 14 (62%). Similar results have been reported by other investigators.[98,99] Therefore, aggressive resuscitation should be initiated in previously undiagnosed fresh stillborn infants. However, Jain et al.[97] also reported that

58 of the 93 infants had no heartbeat at 10 minutes of life. All but one of these infants died, and the one survivor had cerebral palsy. These findings led to the suggestion by Jain et al. that resuscitation be performed for up to 10 minutes after birth if a heartbeat remains undetectable. Ballard[100] recommended discontinuing resuscitation at 15 minutes in an infant with no heartbeat who does not respond to ventilation, cardiac compression, and resuscitative medications. The 2000 AHA-AAP NRP concluded that discontinuation of resuscitative efforts may be appropriate if resuscitation of an infant with cardiorespiratory arrest does not result in spontaneous circulation in 15 minutes.[23]

Postresuscitation Care

After an infant has been stabilized, a thorough re-evaluation should be made. The infant should undergo a complete physical examination to determine whether any congenital anomalies that might have contributed to the asphyxia are present. Persistent cyanosis with adequate ventilation and normal pH may alert the physician to consider primary structural heart defects or persistent pulmonary hypertension of the newborn (see Chapter 23). An orogastric tube should be passed into the stomach as a diagnostic and therapeutic device. By removing air and gastric secretions, the stomach can be decompressed, which allows better movement of the diaphragm and prevents regurgitation and possible aspiration. Failure to pass the tube may indicate esophageal atresia. Finding less than 20 mL of gastric contents may indicate a high bowel atresia or stenosis. This is also a good time for abdominal palpation for assessment of kidney size because air in the bowel makes this procedure more difficult. Absent or abnormal kidneys may be a diagnostic clue to pulmonary hypoplasia.

If an infant has required vigorous resuscitation or if the extended Apgar scores are low, he or she should be admitted to a special or intensive care unit for close observation and monitoring for at least 24 hours. Seizures may develop, indicating the need for treatment. Initial tests should include determination of serum electrolyte, glucose, and calcium levels; arterial blood gas analysis; and chest radiography.

All tubes and monitoring devices should be securely fastened in place while preparations are made for transfer of the patient to the NICU. A transport incubator with a portable electrocardiographic monitor facilitates movement of the infant from the delivery room to the NICU without loss of heat or interruption of intensive care. All specimens collected during the resuscitation (e.g., samples for culture and blood samples) should be delivered promptly to the laboratory. All notes (e.g., those on the cardiac arrest record; see Appendix 26) made during the procedure should become part of the patient's permanent record. Before the transfer begins, the NICU should be alerted so that preparations for the accommodation of the infant can be made.

REFERENCES

1. Kattwinkel J, Bloom RS: Textbook of Neonatal Resuscitation, 4th ed. Dallas, American Heart Association, and Elk Grove Village, Ill., American Academy of Pediatrics, 2000.
2. Saugstad OD: Practical aspects of resuscitating asphyxiated newborn infants. Eur J Pediatr 157(Suppl 1):S11–S15, 1998.
3. Palme-Kilander C: Methods of resuscitation in low-Apgar-score newborn infants: A national survey. Acta Paediatr 81:739–744, 1992.

4. Tyson JE, Younes N, Verter J, et al: Viability, morbidity, and resource use among newborns of 501- to 800-g birth weight. National Institute of Child Health and Human Development Neonatal Research Network. JAMA 276:1645–1651, 1996.

5. Dawes GF: Foetal and Neonatal Physiology: A Comparative Study of the Changes at Birth. Chicago, Ill., Year Book Medical Publishers, 1968, pp. 149–151.

6. Adamsons K Jr, Behrman R, Dawes G, et al: The treatment of acidosis with alkali and glucose during asphyxia in foetal rhesus monkeys. J Physiol 169:679, 1963.

7. American Academy of Pediatrics and American College of Obstetricians: Guidelines for Perinatal Care (fifth edition). Elk Grove Village, Ill., American Academy of Pediatrics, 2002.

8. Press S, Tellechea C, Pregen S: Caesarean delivery of full-term infants: Identification of those at high risk for requiring resuscitation. J Pediatr 106:477–479, 1985.

9. Levine EM, Ghai V, Barton JJ, et al: Pediatrician attendance at cesarean delivery: Necessary or not? Obstet Gynecol 93:338–340, 1999.

10. Fisher DE, Paton JB: Resuscitation of the newborn infant. In Klaus MH, Fanaroff AA (eds): Care of the High-Risk Neonate, 2nd ed. Philadelphia, WB Saunders, 1978, p. 28.

11. Clark JM, Brown ZA, Jung AL: Resuscitation equipment board for nurseries and delivery rooms. JAMA 236:2427–2428, 1976.

12. Smith R: The critically ill child: Respiratory arrest and its sequelae. Pediatrics 46:108–116, 1970.

13. American Academy of Pediatrics, Committee on Fetus and Newborn: Care of the newborn in the delivery room. Pediatrics 64:970, 1979.

14. MacDorman MF, Minino AM, Strobino DM, et al: Annual summary of vital statistics—2001. Pediatrics 110:1037, 2002.

15. Apgar V: A proposed new method of evaluation of the newborn infant. Curr Res Anesth Analg 32:260, 1953.

16. Catlin EA, Carpenter MW, Brann BS IV, et al: The Apgar score revisited: Influence of gestational age. J Pediatr 109:865–868, 1986.

17. Hermansen MC: Intrapartum asphyxia and cerebral palsy. Pediatrics 83(4 Pt 2):653–654, 1989.

18. Casey BM, McIntire DD, Leveno KJ: The continuing value of the Apgar score for the assessment of newborn infants. N Engl J Med 344:467–471, 2001.

19. Papile LA: The Apgar score in the 21st century. N Engl J Med 344:519–520, 2001.

20. Nelson KB, Ellenberg JH: Apgar scores as predictors of chronic neurologic disability. Pediatrics 68:36–44, 1981.

21. Carter BS, McNabb F, Merenstein GB: Prospective validation of a scoring system for predicting neonatal morbidity after acute perinatal asphyxia. J Pediatr 132:619–623, 1998.

22. Perlman JM, Risser R: Cardiopulmonary resuscitation in the delivery room. Associated clinical events. Arch Pediatr Adolesc Med 149:20–25, 1995.

23. Niermeyer S, Kattwinkel J, Van Reempts P, et al: International Guidelines for Neonatal Resuscitation: An excerpt from the Guidelines 2000 for Cardiopulmonary Resuscitation and Emergency Cardiovascular Care: International Consensus on Science. Contributors and Reviewers for the Neonatal Resuscitation Guidelines. Pediatrics 106:E29, 2000.

24. Adamsons K Jr, Gandy GM, James LS: The influence of thermal factors upon oxygen consumption of the newborn human infant. J Pediatr 66:495, 1965.

25. Dahm LS, James LS: Newborn temperature and calculated heat loss in the delivery room. Pediatrics 49:504–513, 1972.

26. Gandy GM, Adamsons K Jr, Cunningham N, et al: Thermal environment and acid-base homeostasis in human infants during the first few hours of life. J Clin Invest 43:751–758, 1964.

27. Lieberman E, Lang J, Richardson DK, et al: Intrapartum maternal fever and neonatal outcome. Pediatrics 105(1 Pt 1):8–13, 2000.

28. Perlman JM: Maternal fever and neonatal depression: Preliminary observations. Clin Pediatr 38:287–291, 1999.

29. Battin MR, Dezoete JA, Gunn TR, et al: Neurodevelopmental outcome of infants treated with head cooling and mild hypothermia after perinatal asphyxia. Pediatrics 107:480–484, 2001.

30. Edwards AD, Wyatt JS, Thoresen M: Treatment of hypoxic-ischaemic brain damage by moderate hypothermia. Arch Dis Child Fetal Neonatal Ed 78:F85–F88, 1998.

31. Carrasco M, Martell M, Estol PC: Oronasopharyngeal suction at birth: Effects on arterial oxygen saturation. J Pediatr 130:832–834, 1997.

32. Estol PC, Piriz H, Basalo S, et al: Oro-naso-pharyngeal suction at birth: Effects on respiratory adaptation of normal term vaginally born infants. J Perinatal Med 20:297–305, 1992.

33. Cordero LJ, Hon EH: Neonatal bradycardia following nasopharyngeal stimulation. J Pediatr 78:441–447, 1971.

34. Wiswell TE, Tuggle JM, Turner BS: Meconium aspiration syndrome: Have we made a difference? Pediatrics 85:715–721, 1990.

35. Carson BS, Losey RW, Bowes WAJ, et al: Combined obstetric and pediatric approach to prevent meconium aspiration syndrome. Am J Obstet Gynecol 126:712–715, 1976.

36. Locus P, Yeomans E, Crosby U: Efficacy of bulb versus DeLee suction at deliveries complicated by meconium stained amniotic fluid. Am J Perinatol 7:87–91, 1990.

37. Falciglia HS: Failure to prevent meconium aspiration syndrome. Obstet Gynecol 71:349–353, 1988.

38. Rossi EM, Philipson EH, Williams TG, et al: Meconium aspiration syndrome: Intrapartum and neonatal attributes. Am J Obstet Gynecol 161:1106–1110, 1989.

39. Wiswell TE, Gannon CM, Jacob J, et al: Delivery room management of the apparently vigorous meconium-stained neonate: Results of the multicenter international collaborative trial. Pediatrics 105:1–7, 2000.

40. Gregory GA, Gooding CA, Phibbs RH, et al: Meconium aspiration in infants: A prospective study. J Pediatr 85:848–852, 1974.

41. Karlowicz MG: More on meconium aspiration. Pediatrics 86:1007–1008, 1990.

42. Milner AD: Resuscitation of the newborn. Arch Dis Child 66:66–69, 1991.

43. Vyas H, Field D, Milner AD, et al: Determinants of the first inspiratory volume and functional residual capacity at birth. Pediatr Pulmonol 2:189–193, 1986.

44. Vyas H, Milner AD, Hopkin IE, et al: Physiologic responses to prolonged and slow-rise inflation in the resuscitation of the asphyxiated newborn infant. J Pediatr 99:635–639, 1981.

45. Milner AD, Vyas H, Hopkin IE: Efficacy of facemask resuscitation at birth. Br Med J (Clin Res Ed) 289:1563–1565, 1984.

46. Repetto JE, Donohue PA-C PK, Baker SF, et al: Use of capnography in the delivery room for assessment of endotracheal tube placement. J Perinatol 21:284–287, 2001.

47. de Burgh Daly M: Interactions between respiration and circulation. In Cherniack NS, Widdicombe JG (eds). Handbook of Physiology, Section 3, The Respiratory System. Bethesda, Md., American Physiological Society, 1986, pp. 529–595.

48. Rootwelt T, Odden J, Hall C, et al: Cerebral blood flow and evoked potentials during reoxygenation with 21 or 100% O_2 in newborn pigs. J Appl Physiol 75:2054–2060, 1993.

49. Saugstad OD, Rootwelt T, Aalen O: Resuscitation of asphyxiated newborn infants with room air or oxygen: An international controlled trial: The Resair 2 Study. Pediatrics 102:e1, 1998.

50. Vento M, Asensi M, Sastre J, et al: Resuscitation with room air instead of 100% oxygen prevents oxidative stress in moderately asphyxiated term neonates. Pediatrics 107:642–647, 2001.

51. Kanter RK: Evaluation of mask-bag ventilation in resuscitation of infants. Am J Dis Child 141:761–763, 1987.

52. Gandini D, Brimacombe JR: Neonatal resuscitation with the laryngeal mask airway in normal and low birth weight infants. Anesth Analg 89:642–643, 1999.

53. Paterson SJ, Byrne PJ, Molesky MG, et al: Neonatal resuscitation using the laryngeal mask airway. Anesthesiology 80:1248–1253, discussion 27A, 1994.

54. Tochen ML: Orotracheal intubation in the newborn infant: A method for determining depth of tube insertion. J Pediatr 95:1050–1051, 1979.

55. Aziz HF, Martin JB, Moore JJ: The pediatric disposable end-tidal carbon dioxide detector role in endotracheal intubation in newborns. J Perinatol 19:110–113, 1999.

56. Bhende MS, Thompson AE, Orr RA: Utility of an end-tidal carbon dioxide detector during stabilization and transport of critically ill children. Pediatrics 89:1042–1044, 1992.

57. Rozycki HJ, Sysyn GD, Marshall MK, et al: Mainstream end-tidal carbon dioxide monitoring in the neonatal intensive care unit. Pediatrics 101(4 Pt 1):648–653, 1998.

58. David R: Closed chest massage in the newborn infant. Pediatrics 81:552–554, 1988.

59. Houri PK, Frank LR, Menegazzi JJ, et al: A randomized, controlled trial of two-thumb vs two-finger chest compression in a swine infant model of cardiac arrest. Prehosp Emerg Care 1:65–67, 1997.

60. Menegazzi JJ, Auble TE, Micklas KA: Two-thumb versus two-finger chest compression during CPR in a swine infant model of cardiac arrest. Ann Emerg Med 22:240–243, 1993.

61. Whitelaw CC, Goldsmith LJ: Comparison of two techniques for determining the presence of a pulse in an infant. Acad Emerg Med 4:153–154, 1997.

62. Orlowski JP: Optimum position for external cardiac compression in infants and young children. Ann Emerg Med 15:667–673, 1986.

63. Phillips GW, Zideman DA: Relation of infant heart to sternum: Its significance in cardiopulmonary resuscitation. Lancet 1:1024–1025, 1986.

64. Dean JM, Koehler RC, Schleien CL, et al: Age-related effects of compression rate and duration in cardiopulmonary resuscitation. J Appl Physiol 68:554–560, 1990.

65. Berkowitz ID, Chantarojanasiri T, Koehler RC, et al: Blood flow during cardiopulmonary resuscitation with simultaneous compression and ventilation in infant pigs. Pediatr Res 26:558–564, 1989.

66. Zaritsky A, Chernow B: Use of catecholamines in pediatrics. J Pediatr 105:341–350, 1984.

67. Berkowitz ID, Gervais H, Schleien CL, et al: Epinephrine dosage effects on cerebral and myocardial blood flow in an infant swine model of cardiopulmonary resuscitation. Anesthesiology 75:1041–1050, 1991.

68. Berg RA, Otto CW, Kern KB, et al: A randomized, blinded trial of high-dose epinephrine versus standard-dose epinephrine in a swine model of pediatric asphyxial cardiac arrest. Crit Care Med 24:1695–1700, 1996.

69. Burchfield DJ, Preziosi MP, Lucas VW, et al: Effect of graded doses of epinephrine during asphyxia-induced bradycardia in newborn lambs. Resuscitation 25:235–244, 1993.

70. Pasternak JF, Groothuis DR, Fischer JM, et al: Regional cerebral blood flow in the beagle puppy model of neonatal intraventricular hemorrhage: Studies during systemic hypertension. Neurology 33:559–566, 1983.

71. Funato M, Tamai H, Noma K, et al: Clinical events in association with timing of intraventricular hemorrhage in preterm infants. J Pediatr 121:614–619, 1992.

72. Cochrane Injuries Group Albumin Reviewers: Human albumin administration in critically ill patients: Systematic review of randomised controlled trials. BMJ 317:235–240, 1998.

73. Kette F, Weil MH, Gazmuri RJ: Buffer solutions may compromise cardiac resuscitation by reducing coronary perfusion pressure [published erratum appears in JAMA 266:3286, 1991]. JAMA 266:2121–2126, 1991.

74. Papile L, Burstein R, Koffler H, et al: Relationship of intravenous sodium bicarbonate infusions and cerebral intraventricular hemorrhage. J Pediatr 93:834–836, 1978.

75. Simmons MA, Adcock EW III, Bard H, et al: Hypernatremia and intracranial hemorrhage in neonates. N Engl J Med 291:6–10, 1974.

76. Hein HA: The use of sodium bicarbonate in neonatal resuscitation: Help or harm? Pediatrics 91:496–497, 1993.

77. Adrogue HJ, Madias NE: Management of life-threatening acid-base disorders. First of two parts. N Engl J Med 338:26–34, 1998.

78. American Academy of Pediatrics: Emergency drug doses for infants and children and naloxone use in newborns: Clarification. Pediatrics 83:803, 1989.

79. Gibbs J, Newson T, Williams J, et al: Naloxone hazard in infant of opioid abuser. Lancet 2:159–160, 1989.

80. Fagerli I, Hansen TWR: Use of naloxone at Norwegian maternity centers. Tidsskr Nor Laegeforen 114:305–307, 1994.

81. Herschel M, Khoshnood B, Lass NA: Role of naloxone in newborn resuscitation. Pediatrics 106:831–834, 2000.

82. Chernick V, Manfreda J, De Booy V, et al: Clinical trial of naloxone in birth asphyxia. J Pediatr 113:519–525, 1988.

83. Ellemunter H, Simma B, Trawoger R, et al: Intraosseus lines in preterm and full term neonates. Arch Dis Child Fetal Neonatal Ed 80:F74–F75, 1999.

84. Fiser DH: Intraosseus infusion. N Engl J Med 322:1579–1581, 1990.

85. Abe KK, Blum GT, Yamamoto LG: Intraosseous is faster and easier than umbilical venous catheterization in newborn emergency vascular access models. Am J Emerg Med 18:126–129, 2000.

86. Low J, Wood SL, Killen HL, et al: Intrapartum asphyxia in the preterm fetus <2,000 grams. Am J Obstet Gynecol 162:378–382, 1990.

87. Silverman WA, Fertig JW, Berger AP: The influence of the thermal environment upon the survival of newly born premature infants. Pediatrics 22:876, 1958.

88. Finberg L: The relationship of intravenous infusions and intracranial hemorrhage: A commentary. J Pediatr 91:777–778, 1977.

89. Poets CF, Sens B: Changes in intubation rates and outcome of very low birth weight infants: A population-based study. Pediatrics 98:24–27, 1996.

90. Avery ME, Tooley WH, Keller JB, et al: Is chronic lung disease in low birth weight infants preventable? A survey of eight centers. Pediatrics 79:26–30, 1987.

91. Kattwinkel J: Surfactant. Evolving issues. Clin Perinatol 25:17–32, 1998.

92. Etches PC, Lemons JA: Nonimmune hydrops fetalis: Report of 22 cases including three siblings. Pediatrics 64:326–332, 1979.

93. Queenan JT: Polyhydramnios, oligohydramnios, and hydrops fetalis. In Fanaroff AA, Martin RJ (eds): Neonatal-Perinatal Medicine—Diseases of the Fetus and Infant. St. Louis, Mosby-Year Book, 1992, p. 249.

94. Goldsmith JP, Chen C: Ventilatory management casebook. Resuscitation in hydrops fetalis. J Perinatol 11:285–289, 1991.

95. Giacoia GP: Hydrops fetalis (fetal edema). A survey. Clin Pediatr 19:334–339, 1980.

96. Finer NN, Horbar JD, Carpenter JH: Cardiopulmonary resuscitation in the very low birth weight infant: The Vermont Oxford Network experience. Pediatrics 104(3 Pt 1):428–434, 1999.

97. Jain L, Ferre C, Vidyasagar D, et al: Cardiopulmonary resuscitation of apparently stillborn infants: Survival and long-term outcome. J Pediatr 118:778–782, 1991.

98. Casalaz DM, Marlow, N, Speidel BD: Outcome of resuscitation following unexpected apparent stillbirth. Arch Dis Child Fetal Neonatal Ed 78:F112–F115, 1998.

99. Yeo CL, Tudehope DI: Outcome of resuscitated apparently stillborn infants: A ten year review. J Paediatr Child Health 30:129–133, 1994.

100. Ballard RA: Resuscitation in the delivery room. In Taeusch HW, Ballard RA, Avery ME (eds): Schaffer and Avery's Diseases of the Newborn. Philadelphia, WB Saunders, 1991, p. 204.

5

ETHICAL AND LEGAL ISSUES

JOHN J. PARIS, SJ, PHD
MICHAEL D. SCHREIBER, MD
FRANK E. REARDON, JD

In the nearly 2 decades since the now infamous "Baby Doe" Regulations[1] attempted to provide federally mandated rules on treatment of neonates, the norms on who is to make treatment decisions for newborns and on what standard have been significantly altered and revised. There is now a strong consensus in the medical, legal, and ethical literature that it is the best interests of the infant—not the desires of the parents or the determination of the physician—that must prevail in the care of newborns.[2] That standard, unlike *substituted judgment*, does not rest on autonomy or self-determination but solely on the protection of the patient's welfare. That protection is particularly important with regard to infants and children because with it they are now seen not merely as the property of parents but as patients in their own right.[3] The implication is that although parents may continue to be involved in decision making for their children, they do not have an absolute right to refuse or require medical treatment for their infant. It is the child's best interests, and those alone, that are to be the focus and goal of medical treatment decisions.

Translated into practice, this standard means that if the burden on the infant is overwhelming or the prospects are extremely bleak, as is true in the presence of a lethal abnormality, there is no obligation to subject the infant to further procedures.[4] In such cases, the parents' decision to omit further treatment is to be respected. Alternatively, if out of ignorance, fear, misguided pessimism, or simple refusal to accept a compromised infant the parents were to decline relatively low-level, high-benefit interventions that would save the life of a child, even if the child were to evidence some permanent handicap, there is no question today that the physicians should treat.[5]

Before applying these standards to the use of assisted ventilation in newborns, it would be helpful to place them in the context of some nearly 40 years of shifting practice patterns. That is best done by reviewing some of the landmark medicolegal cases of the last 4 decades, cases that have not only shaped our present posture but at times have warped and distorted our prospective on how best to care for seriously compromised infants.

FROM THE JOHN HOPKINS BABY TO BABY MILLER

The first of these issues to come to public attention is the now infamous 1963 Johns Hopkins[6] case in which a child born with Down syndrome and duodenal atresia was left untreated and allowed to starve to death over a 15-day period. The parents, a nurse and a lawyer, determined to forgo the relatively easy corrective surgery because the child would be "a financial and emotional burden on the rest of the family." The doctors at Hopkins concurred in that decision. In the words of the treating physician, "In a situation in which the child has a known, serious abnormality ... I think it unlikely that a court would sustain an order to operate on the child against the parents' wishes." In fact, as the studies by Shaw et al.[7] and Todres et al.[8] demonstrate, an overwhelming majority of pediatricians and pediatric surgeons in the United States surveyed in 1977 agreed that in a case similar to that in the Johns Hopkins Hospital they would abide by a parental decision to omit surgery and let the child die.

One of the first significant court involvements to challenge that approach was *Maine Medical Center v Houle*,[9] a 1974 case that involved a profoundly compromised newborn suffering from multiple maladies whose family and physician decided to forgo medical treatment. Other physicians in the hospital objected and the case was brought to court. Maine Superior Court Judge David Roberts began his analysis this way: "Though recent decisions may have cast doubt upon the legal rights of an unborn child, at the moment of live birth there does exist a human being entitled to the fullest protection of the law." Then, in words that presage his order, Judge Roberts states, "The most basic right enjoyed by every human being is the right to life itself." In his view, the issue before the court was not the prospective quality of the life to be preserved but the medical feasibility of the proposed treatment compared with the almost certain risk of death should the treatment (surgical correction of the tracheoesophageal fistula) be withheld. With that premise, the judge then asked whether there is a medical need and a medically feasible response. If these two questions could be answered affirmatively, then, Judge Roberts argued, regardless of the quality of life, the surgery must be performed. In this case the surgery was performed, but the child nonetheless died.

That stark "life-at-all-cost" stance occasioned a scathing criticism in a now oft cited 1974 *JAMA* article by Richard

McCormick[10] entitled "To Save or Let Die: The Dilemma of Modern Medicine." McCormick, the most renowned Jesuit moral theologian of his era, noted that there was no moral obligation to impose treatment on a patient who was dying or who was totally dependent on intensive measures to sustain life, nor was there an obligation to do so for a patient whose potential for relationships is nonexistent. That article, which was the first to attempt to establish practical norms or guidelines for seriously compromised newborns, has been quoted with approval by nearly every group that has subsequently tried to design standards for such decisions.

An even more frequently cited essay published by Duff and Campbell[11] a year earlier in *The New England Journal of Medicine* was the first to bring the topic of ethical dilemmas in the newborn nursery to the public's attention. In their essay the authors revealed that decisions were regularly being made in major neonatal intensive care units to forgo treatment and let infants die. They reported that of 299 deaths in the special care nursery of the Yale-New Haven Hospital between 1970 and 1972, 43 (14%) were associated with discontinuance of treatment. In cases of children with multiple abnormalities, trisomy, cardiopulmonary crippling, and central nervous system disorders, the parents and physicians in a group decision concluded that if prognosis for "meaningful life" was extremely poor or hopeless, no further treatment was warranted. The children were left untreated and allowed to die. In Duff and Campbell's view the decision to withhold or withdraw treatment belonged to those who bore the responsibility for the consequences of treatment—the families.

In a subsequent essay Paris and McCormick[12] had occasion to critique the Duff and Campbell position as "normless." They had provided no guidelines, no standards, or any norms on which to base the decision. Under this schema the treatment decision could equally be made on concern for siblings or "family convenience" as on the best interests of the infant. What the approach failed to realize is that even good and caring parents acting out of fear, ignorance, or misreading of the clinical situation can make decisions antithetical to the best interests of the child.

As illustrated in the well-known *Stinson* case, chronicled in Robert and Peggy Stinson's *The Long Dying of Baby Andrew,*[13] physicians can also err in their judgments on the value of medical intervention for a hopelessly compromised newborn. The Stinsons's son Andrew was delivered 4 months prematurely as a "marginally viable" 800-g newborn. In the early 1980s, infants in his category had a survival rate of less than 5%. Recognizing this fact, his parents told the pediatrician not to attempt any "heroics." The doctors at Community Hospital promised that they would follow the parents' wishes.

Stinson and his wife each kept a journal of the experiences of their son's life. Those journal entries reflected their initial joy at the baby's successful delivery and their fear that he might be maintained "by science-fiction means in a state of pain or hopeless deterioration." That fear was realized when Andrew developed problems in fluid adjustment and was transferred to a well-known but unidentified pediatric hospital center (now publicly acknowledged to be the Children's Hospital of Philadelphia). There the commitment to care provided at Community Hospital was transformed into a "no stops, no exit, no appeal" stance. The family was informed that "[a] baby must be saved at all costs: anything less is illegal and immoral."

When the parents asked the doctors not to use a respirator, they were castigated for violating the sacredness of life and seeking a "return to the law of the jungle." Brain death was the only criterion the doctors would recognize as a legitimate basis for stopping treatment. With such a standard, the parents helplessly stood by as the doctors treated Andrew for brain hemorrhage, respiratory failure, necrosis of the right leg, gangrene, rickets, multiple bone fractures, retrolental fibroplasia, blindness, and finally pulmonary hypertension—a terminal disease occasioned by the ventilator. Through all of this, there was no hint of a willingness to accede to the parents' repeated requests to allow Andrew to die a natural death. Only when Andrew accidentally pulled out his endotracheal tube and began breathing on his own did doctors allow "nontreatment," that is, an inadequate oxygen supply, to bring Andrew's life to a close.

"Babe Doe" Regulations

The attitude of the physicians in the *Stinson* case briefly became the standard in the United States in what is now known as the "*Baby Doe" Regulations*. Those federal regulations rose from the Reagan administration's disapproval of the nontreatment in the *Bloomington Baby Doe* case.[14] There an infant with Down syndrome and a tracheoesophageal fistula was allowed to die untreated when the attending obstetrician recommended, and the family agreed, to no surgical intervention. Although three courts, including the Indiana Supreme Court, upheld the parental decision, the subsequent public outcry led to federal involvement. Under the original regulations issued by the US Department of Health and Human Services, physicians were required to provide life-sustaining medical interventions to every infant. As a highly critical editorial in *The New England Journal of Medicine* stated, "The Regulations are based on the premise that *all* life, no matter how miserable, should be maintained if technically possible."[15]

Those regulations were struck down on procedural grounds by a federal court. Their legacy, however, continues in the 1984 amendments to the Child Abuse Protection Act,[16] the so-called "Baby Doe Regs," which mandate that state child protective agencies, as a condition for receiving federal funding, must have procedures in place for oversight of medical neglect. Despite the fact, as Alan Fleischman[17] correctly observes, that "[t]hese regulations . . . do not mandate unnecessary or inappropriate treatments," more than one third of the neonatologists in a 1988 national survey stated that because of the Baby Doe regulations they provided medical interventions for seriously compromised infants that in their judgment were not medically indicated. In fact, the regulations do not allow but direct physicians to make treatment recommendations to the parents based on "reasonable medical judgment."

Linares and Messenger

The test of those standards was found in the *Linares*[18] and *Messenger*[19] cases, each a highly dramatic case in which a father was charged with homicide for turning off a ventilator used to treat his infant son.

Linares

In the first case, Sammy Linares, a 1-year-old child who suffered massive anoxic damage when he ingested a balloon at a birthday party, was diagnosed as being in a persistent vegetative condition. In the words of the director of the pediatric intensive care unit at Chicago's Rush-Presbyterian-St. Luke's Medical Center, recovery "was not possible." Both the father and the treating physician agreed that given the child's physical status, it would be medically and morally appropriate to remove the respiratory support. The hospital attorney, however, informed the physician that "while Illinois law permits hospitals to withdraw life-support mechanisms from patients who have no brain activity, there is no precedent governing those who have minimal brain activity even if they have virtually no prospect of regaining consciousness." The attorney told the parents to seek a court order for the removal of the ventilator. In the meantime the attending physician, understandably, declined to remove the life-sustaining machinery.

The father, rather than petitioning for a court injunction to terminate the treatment, entered the pediatric intensive care unit with a magnum .357, held it to the child's head, and threatened to kill his son if anyone approached. He himself then removed the infant from the ventilator and waited a half hour to be sure the child was dead before dropping his weapon. The district attorney sought homicide charges. One of us (JJP) wrote an "op-ed" piece for the *Chicago Tribune* on the case entitled "A Desperate Act But Not Murder," which argued that a patient in a well-diagnosed persistent vegetative state has no obligation to undergo life-sustaining interventions.[20] The father's act, reprehensible though it might be as a way of proceeding in a medical case, was not murder; rather, it was the freeing of his son from an unwanted medical intervention that the son had no obligation to undergo and the physician no duty to impose. The grand jury in this case agreed. It refused to return a homicide indictment against the father.

Messenger

Homicide charges were likewise brought in a dramatic 1996 case against Dr. Gregory Messenger, a dermatologist from Lansing, Michigan, for removing his extremely premature infant son from a ventilator in Sparrow Hospital's neonatal intensive care unit. The newborn infant had been placed on mechanical life support despite the explicit instruction of the parents that they did not want aggressive or resuscitative measures used on their 780-g, 25-week gestational-age son.

In week 25 of the pregnancy, the mother, who suffered from hypertension, went into pulmonary edema that precipitated premature labor. Concern about maternal complications led to delivery by cesarean section. Prior to delivery the parents had been told by the neonatologist that the child had a 30% to 50% possibility of survival and that if he did survive there was a 20% to 40% chance of severe intraventricular hemorrhage. The parents informed the neonatologist they did not want any extraordinary efforts undertaken, nor did they want any attempts at resuscitation. The neonatologist preferred a "wait and see" approach. She instructed her physician's assistant (PA) that if the child were "vigorous" at birth and needed ventilatory support, she was to intubate. At birth the infant was hypotonic and hypoxic, purple-blue in color, "floppy," and "appearing lifeless." He did, however, have an umbilical cord pulse of 80 to 90 beats/min. The PA immediately intubated the infant.

The father informed the PA that he and the boy's mother did not want resuscitation. The PA told him that she was not author-

ized to withdraw treatment. The neonatologist returned to the hospital, saw the infant was pink and stable, and indicated she wanted to try surfactant to see how the child would respond before coming to any decision to remove the ventilator support.

Gregory Messenger asked to be left alone with his son and then he turned off the ventilator. Some 10 minutes later the father opened the door and indicated that his newborn son had died. The pathologist found the infant's condition was not terminal. He ruled the cause of death was respiratory failure due to the removal of ventilatory support. The district attorney claimed that the father had failed to provide proper medical treatment for his son and charged him with manslaughter.

One of us (JJP) testified at the trial that the focus in this case, as in all treatment decisions, must be centered on the patient. It is the patient's condition and the patient's desires—not the wishes of the parents or the goals of the physician—that ought to govern these treatment decisions. The issue here was how to discern what the infant patient would want. Although some, such as the Massachusetts Supreme Judicial Court, believe that through a process of "substituted judgment"[21] we can discern the mind of the never competent, including newborn infants,[22] most commentators believe this admitted "legal fiction"[23] is so farfetched as to be judicial fantasy.[24]

As noted, the consensus now in the literature seems to be that for the "never competent" the "best interests" standard is the one that should be used. There is no question that if the Messengers had requested aggressive treatment for their 25-week gestational-age son, it would have been provided. The question is: Did the information given to the parents warrant a predelivery decision to withhold resuscitation and other aggressive medical interventions? Or, as the neonatologist wanted, must the parents authorize resuscitation and the use of aggressive life-sustaining measures until it becomes clear, if not certain, that the child will not survive or that if he does, he will be in such a devastated state as to justify removal of life-sustaining measures?[25]

Under any schema a 50% to 70% risk of mortality puts a newborn into that broad area of gray in which the degree of burden and the prospects of benefit are so suffused in ambiguity and uncertainty that a decision as to whether to continue treatment properly belongs to those who bear the responsibility for the infant, in this case the parents.[26] That stand, as the Hastings Center Project on "Imperiled Newborns" reports, is contrary to the medical practice in the United States where we respond to uncertain outcome in neonatal medicine by giving "a chance" to every infant who is even potentially viable. Active treatment is then continued until it is nearly certain that the particular baby will either die or be so severely impaired that, under any substantive standard, parents would legitimately opt for termination of treatment. Then, and only then, do we present a choice of withdrawal of treatment to the parents.

The "wait and see" approach is appropriate when we face complete uncertainty, that is, when decision makers have no knowledge at all about the probabilities of various outcomes. But, as the Hastings Center group put it, "It is not particularly well-suited to moral situations in which there are data on which to base predictions." The Messengers had such data. The prospect of a 50% to 70% death rate, a 20% to 40% risk of a severe brain bleed, and the probability of respiratory distress syndrome was more than sufficient evidence of the disproportionate burden that awaited this child to justify a decision to withhold resuscitation.

The jury in the *Messenger* case believed the parental decision not to initiate ventilatory support and, once it had been initiated over the parents' objection, the decision to terminate it was a morally acceptable choice. With minimal debate the jury unanimously found Gregory Messenger's actions neither grossly negligent nor a breach of his legal duty to provide proper medical treatment for his son.

HCA v Miller

A recent 2-1 ruling of the Texas Court of Appeals, *HCA v Miller*,[27] puts the emphasis on parental authority in decision making for newborns into question. Early on August 17, 1990 Karla Miller was admitted to the Woman's Hospital of Texas in premature labor. Ultrasound revealed a 629-g fetus of 23 weeks of gestational age. The mother was believed to have a life-endangering infection. The obstetrician and neonatologist informed the parents that if the baby survived, she would most likely suffer severe impairments. The Millers requested that no heroic measures be performed. That request was placed in the medical record, and the obstetrician informed the nursing staff that no neonatologist would be needed at delivery.

After subsequent consultation with hospital administrators the obstetrician concluded that if the baby were born alive and weighed more than 500 g, then the staff was obliged by law and hospital policy to administer life-sustaining procedures even if the parents did not consent. Sidney, the Miller's daughter, was born alive weighing 629 g. The neonatologist determined the baby was viable and so instituted resuscitative measures. Sidney survived, but she suffers severe physical and mental impairments that harbinger a lifelong dependence on others for her care.

The parents sued and a jury awarded the family $29,400,000 for past and future medical expenses. In addition the jury awarded $13,500,000 in punitive damages against the hospital for having violated the parental instructions. (An additional $17,503,066 in accrued interest was added to the award.) The $13 million in punitive damages reflected the jury's outrage at the physicians' and hospital's action in overriding the parents' request. That very substantial sum was designed to punish the facility for imposing its values on the patient rather than following the parents' care directives. It also was intended to serve as a deterrent to other institutions that might be inclined to act in a similar manner.

On December 28, 2000 the Texas Court of Appeals reversed the trial court's decision on the grounds that although Texas law allows the withholding of life-sustaining medical treatment for those who are "certified in writing by a physician to be terminal," there is no similar provision to withhold treatment from "children with non-terminal impairments, deformities, or disabilities, regardless of their severity." Consequently, it ruled that until a determination of a terminal condition has been established, the physician does not violate tort duties by instituting resuscitative measures on a newborn, even if the parents object.

The Texas Court of Appeals took the position that "a parents' right to refuse urgently-needed life-sustaining medical treatment for their child exists only under provisions of the Texas Health and Safety Act, i.e., only where the child's condition is certifiably terminal." It follows then, as the court itself ruled, that unless and until that child has been certified as terminally ill "a health care provider is under no duty to follow a parent's instruction to withhold urgently-needed life-sustaining medical treatment for their child."

That ruling, even if correct, ought not be read too broadly. Read within the context of a lawsuit seeking multimillion dollar damages for violation of a tort duty, the *Miller* opinion is not a directive mandating medical treatment of all potentially "viable" newborns; rather, it is a ruling that absolves from legal liability physicians who act to preserve the life of a newborn until an adequate diagnosis of the neonate's medical status could be ascertained. That ruling had the secondary effect of freeing the hospital and physicians from the $60 million judgment.

An insight into the limited nature of the court's ruling on neonatal treatment decisions is its concession that good public policy might carve out an exception that would allow the withholding or withdrawing of medical interventions on infants born markedly premature even prior to a determination of a terminal condition. Further, there is no indication in the *Miller* opinion (as there was, for example, in the ruling in *Maine Medical Center v Houle*) that in a life-threatening situation, if there is a medical need and there exists a medically feasible response, the physician *must* treat the infant even if both the parents and doctor agree that withholding medical interventions is the best course for the infant. Further evidence that the Texas court did not share the *Houle* court's belief that there was an obligation to attempt to save every newborn's life indifferent to the degree of devastation is its observation that when a difficult birth can be anticipated, "the circumstances might allow the parents to remove the child from the health provider's care."

The Texas Court of Appeals reinforced its rather odd stance of encouraging mothers to leave the hospital in order to avoid unwanted medical treatment for their newborns with the comment that "under existing legal principles, the treatment cannot lawfully be provided without consent before the need for it becomes acute." Here the court is saying that because prior to the birth there is no "emergency" situation with regard to the baby, there is, prior to delivery, no justification for the doctor to impose unconsented treatment. The court here seems to imply that pregnant women who do not want aggressive medical treatment for their marginally viable newborns should not wait until the delivery results in an "emergency" situation; rather, they should flee the designs of the medical personnel while they are still free to do so.

The holding of the majority in *HCA v Miller* ought not lead physicians to believe that by refraining from certifying a very early gestational age newborn as "terminally ill" they can override the parents' explicit treatment requests limiting aggressive treatments. The specific ruling in this case, based on the Texas Court of Appeals' statutory interpretation of that state's Advance Directive Act, is not final. It is still subject to further appellate review. Further, its precedental force is confined to the limited jurisdiction of that court. Elsewhere, the widespread consensus on the standard of care with regard to resuscitation of neonates at the very margins of viability remains what it has been for the past 2 decades: the "best interests" of the infant.[28]

IMPLICATION OF BEST INTERESTS STANDARD

That focus forces us to consider the future of infants being saved by current technology, including assisted ventilation in neonatal intensive care units. A study by Wood et al.[29] of children born at 25 or fewer weeks of gestation revealed about half of all survivors had major psychomotor development impairments at 30 months of age. One fourth of the children met the criteria for severe disability.[29] In a startlingly frank critique of such outcomes, Battle[30] questions whether we have adequately assessed the consequences of our technologic successes in neonatology. The advances accomplished through technology, not only of keeping some babies alive but also of restoring some of these tiny infants from near certain death, is a marvel. However, as Battle notes, the health care professionals who achieve these miracles disappear from the life of the child and the family within days, weeks, or months. For the remaining months or years, the child and family are left to wonder about the appropriateness of those miracles as they struggle to live with or to support one of those "successes." Battle's challenge demonstrates the need to consider outcome data and long-term commitments, as well as the technical ability to save infants at the margins of viability, in evaluating progress in neonatology.

FUTILITY DEBATE

One troubling area of dispute in the progress in extending life is the intense and ongoing debate noted by Helft and colleagues[31] on the limits, if any, to parents' claims to requested medical treatment.[31] Before 1990 there was scant mention of the issue of physician reluctance to comply with patient or family requests for treatment. The pressing ethical concern had been to gain recognition of patients' rights to refuse unwarranted treatments. However, with the US Supreme Court's *Cruzan*[32] opinion and the Patient Self-Determination Act of 1990,[33] the issue that first arose with the 1976 *Quinlan*[34] case—the right of a patient, competent or incompetent, to decline unwanted medical interventions—had been definitely resolved. Patients have that right.

The focus then shifted to a little noted but increasingly difficult problem: what to do with requests for treatment believed by the physician to be futile, ineffective, or inappropriate. Until the article in *The New England Journal of Medicine* in 1990 about the by now-famous "Baby L" case,[35] in which the physicians at Boston Children's Hospital who had cared for a profoundly compromised baby for some 23 months refused a mother's request to put her child on a ventilator, the issue had been confined to simple questions such as whether to comply with patient requests for antibiotics for viral infections or computed tomographic scans for routine headaches.

Although theoretically agreeing that such treatments ought not to be given, many physicians found it easier to go along with patient requests than to try to persuade them otherwise. The placebo effect frequently would convince patients that they felt better, and the insurance company would pay for the treatment. That approach, however, fed the consumer-dominated mindset of both patient and physician. It also contributed to the erosion of physician authority and, more important, of professional responsibility. The physician was transformed from the one with the knowledge and expertise to diagnose and prescribe into an entity whose role was to respond to whatever the patient desired.

So long as that interaction involved rather innocuous medications or relatively simple and inexpensive technologies, there was no concern on the part of medicine. However, as the consumer model began to dominate, the requests escalated into demands for increasingly more exotic and inappropriate treat-

ment. With that shift, the belief began to grow that informed consent and patient autonomy not only implied that patients had the right to accept or reject proposed therapies, but they had the right to propose the therapy itself.

Autonomy, or the right of self-determination, was seen not only as a significant moral principle but became in the minds of some bioethicists, such as Veatch and Spicer,[36] the overriding moral principle. They believe that families have a right to demand, and physicians an obligation to provide, whatever life-prolonging treatments the family requests. Veatch goes so far as to insist that if no other physician can be found who is willing to provide the requested treatment, the attending physician is obliged to do so. This holds true, he argues, even if a surrogate's request "deviates intolerably" from established standards or is, from the physician's perspective, "grossly inappropriate." Veatch's position places the physician in a terrible dilemma. It would require the physician to relentlessly impose aggressive procedures on devastated infants if requested to do so by the parents, even in the face of overwhelming evidence that the interventions cannot reverse or ameliorate the child's condition.

That dilemma was raised in dramatic form by Hackler and Hiller[37] in an essay in which they described their experience with a 6-year-old child who had undergone multiple abdominal surgeries and repeated resuscitation over a 10-month period.[38] The physicians did not believe there was any hope of survival, but hospital policy required approval by the next of kin for "do not resuscitate" (DNR) status. In this case the mother refused to consider any limitation of treatment. As the authors report, "During her final resuscitation, [the patient] was asystolic for 30–45 minutes. Her mother was called during the course of resuscitation but would not allow it to be stopped." The physicians, subsequent to the mother's urging, succeeded in reestablishing a heartbeat in what was now a neurologically devastated child.

Such a situation has led physicians to ask if they are, in fact, obliged to do what they believe to be futile or ineffective. The so-called futility debate centers primarily on cardiopulmonary resuscitation (CPR) and the requirement of patient or family consent for DNR orders.[39] It is now well documented that in certain clearly defined categories of patients there is nearly 100% mortality.[40] In light of these data, Blackhall[41] argues that in such circumstances, even if the family requests CPR, the physician should refuse. In such instances she states, "[T]he issue of patient autonomy is irrelevant." It is irrelevant because in such cases the requested intervention will not work.

Although the medical literature continues to bombard us with articles on "medical futility,"[42] as Helft and colleagues[31] observe there is no agreement on what the term means or what implications it conveys. Younger[43] has queried: Does it signify absolute impossibility? Is it purely physiologic? Does it include the ability to revive heartbeat but not to achieve discharge from the hospital? How much quality of life and social value does the term embrace?

Lantos et al.[44] noted that even among physicians there is no consensus on the meaning of the term. Physicians disagree on both the chances of success and the goals of therapy. Some invoke futility only if the success rate is 0%, whereas others declare a treatment futile with a success rate as high as 18%. Furthermore, social and psychologic factors may cloud a physician's estimate of success.[45] For example, some consider liver transplantation for an alcoholic patient futile because of the likelihood of recidivism. Others consider a treatment futile if all it can provide is a chance for a couple of days or weeks in an intensive care unit. However, as Lantos et al. note, "Such a goal can be of supreme value to a dying patient or the patient's family."

This lack of agreement on the meaning of the term and its already abundant misuse as a shorthand way for physicians to truncate discussions on treatment decisions make it ever more apparent that its usefulness in the medical lexicon has been short-lived. Perhaps as Truog et al.[46] suggest, its rapid intrusion into bioethics should be met by its equally swift demise. Jettisoning this new buzzword would be no loss. The debate on futility not only distracts, it distorts the real issue. It is not the meaning of a word but the moral basis of the participant's actions that ought to be the focus of our attention.

APPROACH TO RESUSCITATION OF NEWBORNS AT THE MARGIN OF VIABILITY

At the end of their article on repeated resuscitation of a devastated child, Hackler and Hiller[37] pleaded for a better approach to the care of the hopelessly dying child. The same might be asked of the newborn at the margins of viability. It is not unrelenting aggressive interventions but the appropriate response to the physical status and continuing interests of the newborn that commands and should direct our care.

To arrive at that response, the first question ought not be what should we do but "what is going on?"[47] In medicine, that necessitates beginning with facts. Our first task is to identify the physical findings and the data on those findings reported in the literature to come to a determination of the patient's medical condition. Once the diagnosis is made the physician is to draw on training and experience to formulate a prognosis and recommendation. The patient or, in the case of neonates, the parents evaluate that recommendation in light of their personal psychosocial values. They can then accept or reject the recommendation, seek an alternative treatment, or decide to forgo medical interventions altogether.

Society's role is to assure that the patient is not undertreated by omission of beneficial therapies or overtreated with unwanted or unwarranted interventions. In that delicate balancing, as noted by the President's Commission report on *Deciding to Forego Life-Sustaining Treatment,* great discretion is to be afforded to parents whenever the outcome is uncertain or ambiguous.[48]

How does this apply to resuscitation and assisted ventilation for extremely-low-birthweight, early gestational age newborns? In an article on neonatal practice, Partridge et al.[49] remind us that even as we enter the 21st century, "It is not clear which infants born at the margins of viability should be resuscitated and provided neonatal intensive care." From their study these authors conclude that at extremely low birthweight or gestational ages, "There are no standards for appropriate levels of intervention or few factors which should be considered relevant to discussions about resuscitation at birth."

Although it is true that prognostic uncertainty for survival or long-term morbidity make antenatal counseling for parents expecting a very premature infant difficult, the failure of physicians to provide parents with the known mortality and morbidity data or an inadequate discussion of that information hinders or even precludes informed decision making.

What do the current studies tell us about mortality and morbidity in extremely-low-birthweight, early gestational age infants? More importantly, what do they indicate is the practice among neonatologists regarding this class of patients? The reported outcomes from several large neonatal centers are consistent. Although there is now some survival of preterm infants at the lower levels of weight (<500 g) and age (<23 weeks of gestation), the prospects for survival and, more importantly, intact survival are exceedingly small.[50–54] For example, a 1993 study by Allen et al.[51] reveals that for infants born at 22 to 25 weeks of gestation at Johns Hopkins during the period 1988 to 1991, none of 29 infants born at 22 weeks of gestation survived, 15% survived at 23 weeks of gestation, and 56% survived at 24 weeks of gestation. Of those born at 23 weeks of gestation, only 2% survived without severe abnormalities noted on cranial ultrasound.

When weight rather than gestational age is used as the determinant of the lower margins of viability, similar bleak outcomes are found. Hack et al.[54] report that in their study of outcomes of extremely-low-birthweight infants at Cleveland's Rainbow Babies Hospital during the two periods from 1982 to 1988 and from 1990 to 1992, "only 8 of 159 infants of <500 gm birth weight received active delivery room treatment during the whole 9-year period, of whom 2 survived." In a 12-year historical cohort study of 1193 infants weighing less than 500 g born between 1983 and 1994 in Alberta, Canada, Sauve et al.[55] report that of the 382 infants born alive, neonatal care was provided in 113 cases (29.6%). Of those, 95 (84.1%) died and 18 (15.9%) were discharged alive, 5 of whom subsequently died of respiratory complications. Of the 13 (11%) survivors, 4 had no serious disabilities. The remaining 9 had one or more major disabilities, including cerebral palsy, profound mental retardation, blindness, and deafness.

As the study by Allen et al.[56] demonstrates, the introduction of antenatal steroids and post delivery use of surfactant in the early 1990s significantly improved the prospects of these early gestational age infants. However, there is and will always be a level below which survival is both increasingly small and highly precarious. That reality is challenged by reports of "miracle babies," such as the intact survival of a 360-g girl born at 26 weeks 1 day of gestation, or the even more startling news of a 280-g twin girl born at 26 weeks 6 days of gestation who at 2 years of age is developing normally.[57] Such cases have led to the expectation that medicine can rescue almost every neonate beyond 22 weeks of gestation. Confirmation of this belief is found in a 1998 essay by Sanders et al.,[58] who note that 82% of neonatologists surveyed would ventilate an infant born at 23 weeks of gestation. That number increases to 95% for infants delivered at 24 weeks of gestation. For the respondents in the survey by Sanders et al., any prediction of less than 100% mortality justifies an attempt at resuscitation. These data on the willingness of physicians to attempt resuscitation on infants at the very margins of viability are confirmed in other multiple studies done over the past decade, such as that reported by Hack and Faranoff.[59]

WITHHOLDING AND WITHDRAWAL OF TREATMENT

Even in cases of extremely-low-birthweight infants the possibility of intact survival makes resuscitation, with subsequent reassessment and willingness to terminate treatment in the face of declining status, an acceptable approach. The same justification that applies to the withholding of a treatment governs its withdrawal. In fact, there is an even greater warrant for instituting a therapy to determine if it might work and then withdrawing it if it fails than in never instituting it. The patient has the benefit of a trial course of the therapy, and we have assurance that the therapy did not work.

Still, as Weir[60] observes, the feeling still mistakenly persists among some caregivers that the withdrawal of life-sustaining treatment is morally more significant and certainly more legally serious than the withholding of treatment. Several reasons contribute to this misunderstanding. It is psychologically easier not to start than to stop. Further, withdrawing a treatment once it is instituted gives a sense that the physician's action, rather than the underlying illness, "caused" the death of the patient. There is also belief that the physician is duty bound to do everything possible to sustain life, and there is the lingering belief by some that the law prohibits the removal of life-sustaining technology. From *Quinlan* to *Cruzan,* the US Supreme Court and every state supreme court that has addressed the issue have unambiguously stated that there is no moral, ethical, or legal difference between withholding or withdrawing medical interventions. Further, as the US Supreme Court made clear in its 1990 *Cruzan* opinion, it is legitimate with patient or family permission to withdraw life-sustaining assisted ventilation in the face of imminent death or irreversible loss of consciousness.

The moral issue now facing critical care physicians involved in the withdrawal of medical interventions is to assure the patient and family that the withdrawal will not produce suffering for the patient.[61] This, as Civetta[62] notes, is of particular concern when ventilatory support is withdrawn. If the withdrawal is done too rapidly or without close attention, air hunger or dyspnea may result in gagging, gasping, and struggle in the patient. Neither the patient nor the family or caregivers should be subjected to such insensitive circumstances. To prevent that situation, physicians should take care to premedicate patients with a sedative, usually morphine, to alleviate dyspnea and pain and a benzodiazepine for anxiety. Because the goal of these medications is symptom relief, not death, they should be titrated to the intended effect.

Although it might appear beneficial to paralyze the patient before extubation or weaning, most commentators agree that it is unethical to use neuromuscular blocking agents at the time ventilatory support is withdrawn.[63] In addition to blurring the threshold between allowing to die and actively causing the patient's death, these agents mask potential patient pain and anxiety. They are not necessary to assure absence of pain and ought not be used for that purpose.

LIMITING THE USE OF ASSISTED VENTILATION

Physician unwillingness to limit or omit interventions when the outcome is anything less than 100% certain, coupled with the dominant role parents have in the contemporary American setting, virtually assures that if the parents request it, resuscitation will be attempted on nearly every infant, even those at the outer margins of viability. The ethical concern today is what happens when the prognosis of infants at the margin of viability shifts from uncertain to dim to dismal. In the present medicolegal environment, the tendency is still to do whatever the parents demand.

Given that situation, what should be done? Does the treating physician mindlessly continue providing "everything possible" to satisfy parental hopes, fears, or denial? For a physician to do so, as Ingelfinger[64] pointedly reminds us in an essay on the patient-physician relationship, is to be "guilty of shirking [one's] duty, if not malpractice." Ingelfinger's position on the positive role of the physician to intervene in order to protect the interests of the patient, even over the objections of the family, is supported by the American College of Obstetricians and Gynecologists (ACOG) and the American Academy of Pediatrics (AAP) statement that in such situations the role of parents is not absolute.[65] Although their informed decision must be given great weight, the parents' decision is not dispositive. The focal point for the neonatologist, as of every physician, is the best interests of the patient. That standard, as the AAP's guidelines on foregoing life-sustaining medical treatment reminds us, must weigh the benefits and burdens of treatment from the infant's—not the parents'—perspective. Such an assessment requires calculating the chance the therapy will succeed and the degree to which it will extend life if successful; the risks, pain, and discomfort involved with the treatment or nontreatment; and the anticipated quality of life with or without the treatment.[66]

Tyson et al.,[67] whose research on viability and morbidity among infants of birthweight 501 to 800 g provides the most complete US data on these issues, hold that ventilation is not necessarily justified simply because it affords a modest chance of survival. They argue that although most immature infants will die without such an intervention, mechanical ventilation can make for worse outcomes—death after days or months of distress or morbidity so severe it might be considered worse than death.[68] To prevent that outcome they propose that medical interventions on extremely premature infants be judged for individual infants as mandatory, optional, investigational, or unreasonable. The classification allows for a more nuanced analysis of what is being done. It also broadens the decision-making process beyond merely asking the parents, "What do you want?"

The categories are explained as follows.

Mandatory

If, as we observed in an earlier article, the parents ask the physician to withhold or withdraw a ventilatory support that has a very high likelihood of significantly benefiting a child, the treating physician's independent obligation to foster the best interests of the patient prohibits following the parents' request. The physician is morally obliged to provide such treatment even over the family's protests. (The legal questions on the need for court involvement, protective custody, or guardianship are beyond the scope of the moral analysis we address here.)

Optional

When the risks are very high and the benefits are at best uncertain or extremely low, the parents have the option of accepting or rejecting the proposed resuscitation. In this "gray zone" the parents' decision to either accept or reject ventilatory support should be followed.

Investigational

As Lantos et al.[69] commented in their 1988 insightful analysis of resuscitation in babies of very low birthweight, the outcome data available for some procedures are such that at best we can tell parents that "this intervention is so new or its effect on this class of patients so unproven that it is an 'innovative' or 'experimental' procedure." What both the physician and parents have to understand at this point is that they are embarking into the realm of the unknown. We proceed in such situations on a hypothesis and a hope. The latter may be dashed and the former discarded as we test the hypothesis and assess the results. This joint venture into the investigational requires a willingness on the part of both physician and parents to assess and reassess at every step. If the hoped for effect is not achieved or if the evolving data indicate there is no evidence that it can be attained, there is no basis for continuing the "investigation."

At the point at which the ventilation fails to check or reverse the patient's progressive deterioration, the justification for the initial intervention has ceased and, unless there is another overriding rationale for carrying on, there is no warrant to continue the procedure. A "time limited trial" is the hallmark of this investigational process. The endpoint of such a trial is two-fold: the withdrawal of consent *or* the "failure" of the investigational intervention to reverse or affect the disease process.

Unreasonable

Once a procedure, drug, or process under investigation has failed to attain the desired goal, there is no justification to continue it.[70] That point was forcefully stated by the California Court of Appeal in *Barber v Superior Court* when it noted, "Although there may be a duty to provide life-sustaining machinery in the *immediate* aftermath of a cardio-respiratory arrest, there is no duty to continue its use once it has become futile in the opinion of qualified medical personnel.[71] Here the court was giving legal recognition to the position eloquently articulated by Francis Moore[72] that "[t]here must be a rationale on which the desperately ill patient may be offered not merely pain, suffering, and cost, but also a true hope of prolonged survival [without devastating sequelae]."

CURRENT PRACTICE OF NEONATOLOGISTS IN THE FACE OF FAILED THERAPIES

What is the practice of neonatologists when they are confronted with a deteriorating patient receiving life-sustaining treatment? A study by Wall and Partridge[73] reveals that in the face of imminent death, most neonatologists recommend the withdrawal or withholding of treatment. Some centers such as the University of North Carolina at Chapel Hill report that "[I]n most cases death occurred after life-sustaining treatment was withdrawn."[74]

A different perspective is taken by Meadow,[75] who reports that at the University of Chicago Children's Hospital, "The overwhelming majority of these patients are not withdrawn from the ventilator simply because the ethical consensus in our nursery is that if the patients are going to die anyway, and die soon, it is an unnecessary burden to ask parents to participate in a decision to withdraw care from their infant." "This practice," he notes, "reflects the fairly consistent beliefs of the

parents in our patient population." The postulate of Meadow's position is data from his study that 80% of low-gestational-age, low-birthweight deaths occurred in the first 3 days of life. From this he argues not only to "the reasonableness of physicians offering NICU care to extremely low birthweight (ELBW) infants with unlikely prospects for survival, but to the continuation of that support lest the physician 'unnecessarily burden the parents' by asking them to participate in a decision to withdraw ventilatory support from their infant."

In contrast to Meadow's position, Hack and Fanaroff[59] found that although aggressive treatment of infants with birthweights less than 750 g did not affect mortality, it did increase the mean age of death form 72 to 880 hours. Allen[56] reports a similar frequency of late deaths in her study at Johns Hopkins. This led her to conclude that "although an argument can be made in favor of keeping an infant alive long enough for the parents to say goodbye, deliberately prolonging death beyond a few hours is difficult to justify." For Allen, prolonging death is not relieving the parents of a burden, it is "prolonging suffering, not only for the infant, but also for the family and members of the staff."

Although imposing heroic suffering on one's self in the hope of a therapeutic benefit or even the altruistic advancement of science is acceptable,[76] the same does not hold for imposing that suffering on others. The lesson from the Willowbrook experiments, in which severely retarded children were subjected to hepatitis infection in the search for a cure, is that there are limits to which children may be subjected in clinical investigation.[77] The requirements for proceeding in such investigational situations are substantially higher than having parental consent.[78]

The issue in research ethics is how to protect vulnerable populations, such as children who cannot protect themselves, from the injury that can occur as a result of investigational procedures. To guard their interests we need to recast the issue in cases such as resuscitation of infants at the very margins of viability from "autonomy"—which it is not—to the rules governing research subjects. In such cases, as Lantos noted, "[T]he effectiveness of therapy replaces patient preference as the primary factor governing decisions to use or discontinue therapy."

The importance of the distinction between requirements governing therapeutic and research interventions is reiterated in two recent *The New England Journal of Medicine* articles on ethical aspects of randomized trials. In a study of the harm that can be done to patients in randomized trials, Alexander Capron[79] reminds us that "the lessons of the past half-century is that suffering, death, and violation of human rights can arise not only when dictators give inhumane scientists free reign to treat human beings as guinea pigs, but also when well-meaning physicians conduct research in a free and enlightened society." That reality leads Truog et al.[80] to insist that, unlike conventional therapy, investigational procedures require more than informed consent; they demand heightened protection of the subject by the investigator.

Although the consent of the subject or proxy is a necessary prerequisite to begin an investigational procedure, it is not a sufficient basis to continue. The scientist-investigator, as the Nuremberg Code makes clear, must exercise independent judgment on the safety and efficiency of the intervention under investigation.[81] In particular, the scientist is charged with protecting the subject from "all unnecessary physical and mental suffering and injury."

This obligation continues to be the duty of neonatologists who use innovative or unproven methods to sustain the life of infants at the margins of viability. That neonatologists honor the obligation is seen in reports such as those of Allen and colleagues at Johns Hopkins that if there is no positive response in the delivery room to bag and mask ventilation in infants with poor respiratory effort and low heart rate, no prolonged resuscitation is attempted.[56] These physicians know from the literature and their extensive experience that additional efforts in such cases would at best only delay the inevitable outcome and would be accompanied by painful and potentially harmful interventions. They do not engage in such action.

As the cases of *MacDonald v Milleville*[82] and *Hall v DeSoto Memorial Hospital*[83] show, parental permission to stop the attempted resuscitation in such circumstances is not legally required. The same holds true for those infants who, despite an initial positive response to assisted ventilation, develop a physical condition as incompatible with survival as that evidenced in newborns whose heart rate cannot be increased beyond 40 to 50 beats/min. The problem in these cases is not one of science. Every neonatologist knows that a 410-g, 23-week gestational-age neonate with progressively deteriorating pulmonary function cannot survive. The problem lies in the practice developed over the past 2 decades of giving parents the cruel option between continuing the now failed attempts at restoring health or letting their child die. For many parents the latter choice is too difficult even to contemplate. Overwhelmed by anguish, they are in no position to make a reasoned choice, let alone one that will dash forever their hopes for a healthy child.

When there is no realistic choice to be made or when one of the choices fails and thereby ceases to be an option, *no choice should be offered*. The words we use when undertaking an investigational procedure, "[W]e will initiate the process and see how the child declares himself," should be followed. If, as sometimes happens, a newborn receiving assisted ventilation evidences pulmonary insufficiency incompatible with survival, the parents should be informed that although "everything possible" has been tried, all the efforts have failed. The most we can do now for such infants is to keep them comfortable.

As Gordon Avery[84] commented in a 1987 editorial in *The New England Journal of Medicine* on care of extremely small infants, "Do not continue with intensive care in the face of accumulating evidence of hopelessness." In blunt words he exhorted his colleagues to "[T]ake a stand." Had neonatologists heeded that challenge, we would not be entering the 21st century still pondering our obligations to infants for whom medicine's exquisite interventions have failed. It still is not too late to respond to that call.

REFERENCES

1. Kopelman LM, Irons TG, Kopelman AE: Neonatologists judge the "Baby Doe" regulations. N Engl J Med 318:677–683, 1988.
2. Caplan A, Cohen CB (eds): Imperiled newborns. Hastings Cent Rep 17:5–32, 1987.
3. Bartholomew WG: The child-patient: Do parents have the right to decide? In Spicker S, Englehardt T, Healty J, et al. (eds): The Law-Medicine Relation: A Philosophical Explanation. Dordrecht, The Netherlands, Reidel, 1981, pp. 126–132.
4. Paris JJ, Weiss AH, Soifer S: Ethical issues in the use of life-prolonging interventions for an infant with trisomy 18. Ethical Issues Perinatol 12:366–368, 1992.
5. Paris JJ, Bell AJ: Guarantee my child will be "normal" or stop all treatment. J Perinatol 13:469–472, 1993.

6. Gustafson JM: Mongolism, parental desires, and the right to life. Perspect Biol Med 16:524, 529–533, 1973.
7. Shaw A, Randolph J, Manard B: Ethical issues in pediatric surgery: A national survey of pediatricians and pediatric surgeons. Pediatrics 60:588–589, 1977.
8. Todres ID, Krane D, Howell MC, et al: Pediatrician's attitudes affecting decision-making in defective newborns. Pediatrics 60:197–201, 1977.
9. *Maine Medical Center v Houle*, No. 74-145 (Super Ct, Cumberland Cty., ME, February 14, 1974).
10. McCormick RA: To save or let die: The dilemma of modern medicine. JAMA 229:172–176, 1974.
11. Duff RS, Campbell AGM: Moral and ethical dilemmas in the special care nursery. N Engl J Med 289:890–894, 1973.
12. Paris JJ, McCormick RA: Saving defective infants: Options for life or death. America 313–317, April 23, 1983.
13. Stinson R, Stinson P: The Long Dying of Baby Andrew. Boston, Little Brown and Company, 1983.
14. Pless JE: The story of Baby Doe. N Engl J Med 309:664, 1983.
15. Angell MA: Handicapped children: Baby Doe and Uncle Sam. N Engl J Med 309:659–661, 1983.
16. Child Abuse and Prevention Act of 1984. Federal Register 50:14878–14901, April 15, 1985.
17. Fleischman AR: Ethical issues in neonatology: A U.S. perspective. Ann N Y Acad Sci 530:83–91, 1988.
18. Blau R: Father killed son "because I love him." Chicago Tribune, April 27, 1989:S1, at 1.
19. Paris JJ: Manslaughter or a legitimate parental decision? The Messenger case. J Perinatol 16:60–64, 1996.
20. Paris JJ. A desperate act, but not murder. Chicago Tribune, May 15, 1989:S1, at 15.
21. *Superintendent of Belchertown State School v Saikewicz*, 373 Mass 728, 370 NE 2d 417 (1977).
22. *Custody of a Minor (No. 1)*, 385 Mass 697, 434 NE 2d 601 (1982).
23. *Guardianship of Jane Doe*, 411 Mass 512, 583 NE2d 1263 (1992).
24. Capron AM: Substituting our judgment. Hastings Cent Rep 22:58–59, 1992.
25. Rhoden NK: Treating Baby Doe: The ethics of uncertainty. Hastings Cent Rep 34:42–48, 1986.
26. Paris JJ, Newman V: Ethical issues in quadruple amputation in a child with meningococcal septic shock. J Perinatol 13:56–58, 1993.
27. 2000 WL 1867775 (Tex App, Hous.) December 28, 2000.
28. Spense K: The best interest principle as a standard for decision making in the care of neonates. J Adv Nursing 31:1286–1292, 2000.
29. Wood NS, Marlow N, Costeloe K et al: Neurologic and developmental disability after extremely premature birth. N Engl J Med 343:378–430, 2000.
30. Battle CUL: Beyond the nursery door: The obligation to survivors of technology. Clin Perinatol 14:417–427, 1987.
31. Helft PR, Siegler M Lantos J: The rise and fall of the futility movement. N Engl J Med 343:293–296, 2000.
32. *Cruzan v Director, Missouri Department of Health*, 110 Super Ct 2841 (1990).
33. Paris JJ, O'Connell K: The patient self-determination act of 1990. Clin Ethics Rep 5:1–10, 1991.
34. *In re Quinlan*, 70 NJ 10, 355 A2d 647 (1976).
35. Paris JJ, Crone R, Reardon FE: Physician refusal of requested treatment: The case of Baby L. N Engl J Med 322:1012–1014, 1990.
36. Veatch RM, Spicer CM: Medically futile care: The role of the physician in setting limits. Am J Law Med 18:15–36, 1992.
37. Hackler JC, Hiller MD: Family consent to orders not to resuscitate. JAMA 264:1281–1283, 1990.
38. *Byran v University of Virginia*, 95 F3d 349 (1996).
39. Weil MH, Weil CJ: How to respond to family demands for futile life support and cardiopulmonary resuscitation. Crit Care Med 28:3339–3340, 2000.
40. Bedell SE, Pelle D, Maher PL, et al: Do-not-resuscitate orders for critically ill patients in the hospital: How are they used and what is their impact? JAMA 256:233–237, 1986.
41. Blackhall L: Must we always use CPR? N Engl J Med 317:1281–1285, 1987.
42. Paris JJ, Schreiber MD: Physicians refusal to provide life-prolonging medical interventions. Clin Perinatol 23:563–571, 1996.
43. Younger SJ: Who defines futility? JAMA 260:2094–2095, 1990.
44. Lantos JD, Singer PA, Walker RM, et al: The illusion of futility in clinical practice. Am J Med 87:81–84, 1989.
45. Pinkerton J, Finnerty JJ, Lombardo PA, et al: Parental rights at the birth of a near-viable infant: Conflicting perspectives. Am J Obstet 177:283–288, 1997.

46. Truog RD, Brett AS, Frader: The problem with futility. N Engl J Med 326:1560–1564, 1992.
47. Niebuhr HR: The Responsible Self: An Essay in Christian Moral Philosophy. New York, Harper & Row, 1963.
48. President's Commission for the Study of Ethical Problems in Medicine and Biomedical and Behavioral Research: Deciding to Forego Life-Sustaining Treatment. Washington, DC, US Government Printing Office, March 1983, p. 220.
49. Partridge JF, Freeman H, Weiss I, et al: Delivery room resuscitation decisions for extremely low birthweight infants in California. J Perinatol 21:27–33, 2001.
50. Fanaroff AA, Wright LL, Stevenson DK, et al: Very low birthweight outcomes of the National Institute of Child Health and Human Development Neonatal Research Network, May 1991 through December 1992. Am J Obstet Gynecol 173:1423–1431, 1995.
51. Muraskas JK, Weiss MG, Myers TF: Neonatal viability in the 1990's: Held hostage by technology. Pediatr Res 39:234, 1996.
52. Sauve R, Robertson C, Etches P, et al: Initiation of intensive care and outcome in infants who weighed 500 grams or less at birth: A geographically-based study. Pediatr Res 39:1657, 1996.
53. Davis DJ: How aggressive should delivery room cardiopulmonary resuscitation be for extremely low birth weight neonates? Pediatrics 92:447–450, 1993.
54. Hack M, Friedman H, Fanaroff AA: Outcomes of extremely low birth weight infants. Pediatrics 98:931–937, 1996.
55. Sauve RS, Robertson C, Etches P, et al: Before viability: A geographically based outcome study of infants weighing 500 grams or less at birth. Pediatrics 101:438–445, 1998.
56. Allen MC, Donohue PK, Dusman AE: The limit of viability: Neonatal outcome of infants born at 22 to 25 weeks' gestation. N Engl J Med 329:1597–1601, 1993.
57. Muraskas J, Bhola M, Tomich P, et al: Neonatal viability: Pushing the envelope. Pediatrics 101:1095–1096, 1998.
58. Sanders MR, Donohue PK, Oberdorf MA, et al: Impact of the perception of viability on resource allocation in the neonatal intensive care unit. J Perinatol 18:347–351, 1998.
59. Hack M, Fanaroff A: Outcomes of extremely low birth-weight infants between 1982 and 1988. N Engl J Med 321:1642–1647, 1989.
60. Weir R: Withholding and withdrawing therapy and actively hastening death. In Goldworth A, Silverman W, Stevenson DK, et al. (eds): Ethics and Perinatology. New York, Oxford University Press, 1995, pp. 173–183.
61. Brody H, Campbell ML, Faber-Langedoen K, et al: Withdrawing intensive life-sustaining treatment: Recommendations for compassionate clinical management. N Engl J Med 336:652–657, 1997.
62. Civetta JM: Futile care or caregivers frustration? A practical approach. Crit Care Med 24:346–351, 1996.
63. Daly BJ, Newlon B, Montenegrott D, et al: Withdrawal of mechanical ventilation: Ethical principles and guidelines for terminal weaning. Am J Crit Care 2:217–223, 1993.
64. Ingelfinger FJ: Arrogance. N Engl J Med 303:107–1511, 1980.
65. American Academy of Pediatrics Committee on Fetus and Newborn; American College of Obstetricians and Gynecologists Committee on Obstetric Practice: Perinatal care at the threshold of viability. Pediatrics 96:974–976, 1995.
66. American Academy of Pediatrics Committee on Bioethics: Guidelines on foregoing life-sustaining medical treatment. Pediatrics 93:532–536, 1994.
67. Tyson JE, Younes N, Verter J, et al: Viability, morbidity, and resource use among newborns of 501- to 800-g birth weight. JAMA 276:1645–1651, 1996.
68. Mitchell C: When living is a fate worse than death. Newsweek, August 20, 2000, p. 12.
69. Lantos J, Miles SH, Silverstein MD, et al: Survival after cardiopulmonary resuscitation in babies of very low birth weight. N Engl J Med 318:91–95, 1988.
70. Paris JJ, Schreiber M, Statter M, et al: Beyond autonomy: Physicians' refusal to use life-prolonging extracorporeal membrane oxygenation. N Engl J Med 329:354–357. 1993.
71. *Barber v Superior Court*, 147 Cal App 3rd 1006 (1983).
72. Moore FD: The desperate case: CARE (costs, applicability, research, ethics). JAMA 261:1483–1484, 1989.
73. Wall SN, Partridge JC: Death in the intensive care nursery: Physician practice of withdrawing and withholding life support. Pediatrics 99:64–70, 1997.
74. Doron MW, Veness-Meehan KA, Margolis LH, et al: Delivery room resuscitation decisions for extremely premature infants. Pediatrics 102:574–582, 1998.
75. Meadow W, Reimshisel T, Lantos J: Birth weight-specific mortality for extremely low birth weigh infants vanishes by four days of life: Epidemiology and ethics in the neonatal intensive care unit. Pediatrics 97:636–643, 1996.
76. Jonas H: Philosophical reflections or experimenting with human subject. In Jonas H (ed): Philosophical Essays. Chicago, University of Chicago Press, 1980, pp. 105–131.
77. Krugman S, Giles JP: Viral hepatitis: New light on an old disease. JAMA 212:1019–1021, 1970.
78. McCormick RA: Proxy consent in the experimental situation. Perspect Biol Med 18:2–20, 1974.
79. Capron AM: Ethical and human-rights issues in research and mental disorders that may affect decision-making capacity. N Engl J Med 340:1430–1434, 1999.
80. Truog RD, Robinson W, Randolph A, et al: Is informed consent always necessary for randomized, controlled trials? N Engl J Med 340:804–807, 1999.
81. Shuster E: Fifty years later: The significance of the Nuremberg Code. N Engl J Med 337:1436–1440, 1997.
82. Paris JJ, Goldsmith JP, Cimperman M: Resuscitation of a micropremie: The case of MacDonald v. Milleville. J Perinatol 18:302–305, 1998.
83. *Hall v DeSoto Memorial Hospital*, 774 So2d 41 (Fla App 2 Dist, 2000).
84. Avery GD: Comments on Hack M, Fanaroff AA. Changes in the delivery room care of extremely small infant (<750 g): Effects on morbidity and outcome. N Engl J Med 314:640, 1986.

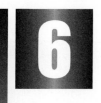

PULMONARY CARE

JOSEPH R. HAGEMAN, MD, FCCM
KAREN SLOTARSKI, RRT
GERALYNN CASSERLY, RRT
HARRIET HAWKINS, RN, CCRN

In addition to establishing and maintaining the artificial airway, the clinician must demonstrate a working knowledge of the multiple supportive pulmonary care skills that are essential for optimal care of the intubated ventilated neonate. This chapter presents the principles and guidelines required for the safe intubation and successful pulmonary care of these critically ill infants. Some of the guidelines addressed will reflect significant changes in cardiopulmonary resuscitation (CPR) of the newborn presented in the revised Neonatal Resuscitation Program (NRP)[1] (see Chapter 4). With the "explosion" of new information available in the care of the neonate who requires assisted ventilation, we attempt to focus the discussion on pulmonary care. The reader will be referred to other chapters of the book for a more in-depth presentation of specific topics.

All caretakers involved in the management of these babies need to be aware of the safety issues with regard to the transmission of pathogenic organisms by bodily fluids and closely follow the Occupational Safety and Health Administration (OSHA) standards outlined in Appendix 30.

INDICATIONS FOR INTUBATION

Resuscitation at Delivery

Despite the well-known limitations of the Apgar score, it is still the most widespread method of recording the caretaker's assessment of the neonate after delivery.[2,3] The original intent was to assess the newly born infant's need for CPR at 1 minute of age and the progress of resuscitation at 5 minutes of age. In the new NRP course, the emphasis is no longer on the Apgar score; it is now on a "global assessment" of the baby's status immediately after delivery.[1] The assessment includes any additional information gathered during the pregnancy and the peripartum period that is made available to the perinatal team (see Chapter 4 for more detailed information). The assessment is ongoing and is done at intervals of seconds, as interventions can be performed based upon these frequent reassessments. The Apgar score is still assigned at 1 and 5 minutes of age and every 5 minutes for the first 20 minutes or until the score is 7.[1,2] The appropriate time for endotracheal intubation should be based on the ongoing global assessment of the baby.

If meconium is seen in the amniotic fluid, preparations should be made for the possible need for endotracheal intubation and suctioning of the airway using a meconium aspirator (Fig. 6-1) inserted into the adapter, which is attached to the endotracheal tube. Another technique involves using the meconium suction device (Fig. 6-2) devised by Kurtis.[4] Studies by Wiswell et al.[5] have resulted in a simpler assessment to make the decision to intubate. If there is meconium in the amniotic fluid and the baby is lethargic and/or hypotonic, the intubation should be performed.[1,5,6] If the infant is vigorous, endotracheal intubation and suctioning of the airway may not be warranted.[1,7]

The DeLee trap, which utilized oral suction, is no longer being used; one reason is the possible acquisition of infection from the secretions being suctioned using the DeLee trap.[1,6] Some obstetricians attach a modified trap to wall suction; if this is done, the pressure should not exceed 100 mm Hg or last for more than 5 seconds.

Positive-Pressure Ventilation

Tracheal intubation is well established as a requirement for infants receiving positive-pressure ventilation. "Noninvasive ventilation" has been receiving more attention in the literature.[8] Noninvasive ventilation using a face mask had been used to ventilate infants for several days;[9] however, the problems and complications reported include increased cerebellar hemorrhage, added dead space, gastrointestinal insufflation, rupture of an abdominal viscus, pressure necrosis of the nose and scalp, and inability to obtain a good seal. At this time, face masks are not recommended for long-term assisted ventilation of neonates.[9]

When gastrointestinal distention must be avoided, as in congenital diaphragmatic hernia or esophageal atresia with tracheoesophageal fistula, mask ventilation may be detrimental and serious consideration should be given to careful intubation of the airway and placement of a nasogastric tube for diagnostic and therapeutic purposes.[1,10]

Obstructive Lesions of the Airway

Certain lesions may cause obstruction at the level of the nasopharynx, larynx, and upper trachea and may necessitate careful and timely endotracheal intubation of affected neonates.[10] Beginning at the nasal level, these lesions include bilateral or severe unilateral choanal atresia or stenosis; pharyngeal hypotonia; and micrognathia, such as may be seen in the Robin sequence (which may include cleft palate and glossoptosis).[11] At the level of the larynx, obstructive problems may include laryngomalacia (or laryngotracheomalacia), laryngeal

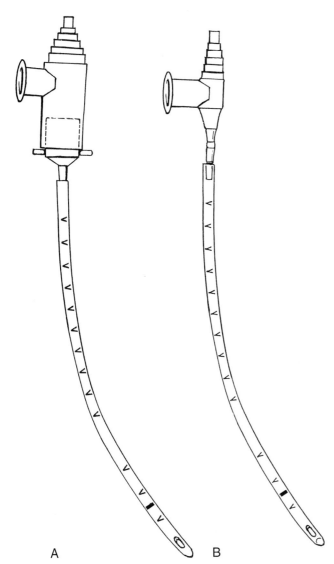

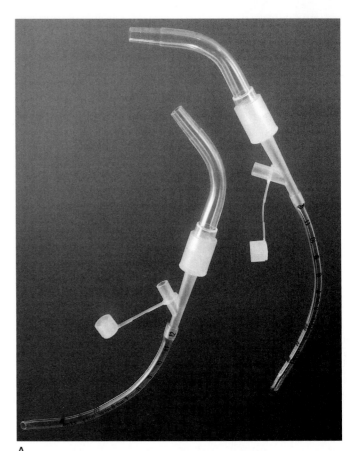

A

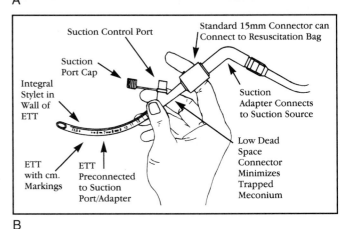

B

Figure 6-1. *A*, Custom suction adapter fitted to the 15-mm tracheal tube adapter for suctioning of meconium. *B*, "Home-made" equivalent. The catheter was cut from the thumb control and attached directly to the tracheal tube.

Figure 6-2. *A*, Kurtis meconium suction device (MSD). *B*, Illustration and labeling of the components of the Kurtis MSD. Sizes include 3.0 and 3.5 mm, both with and without an internal suction device.

web, bilateral vocal cord paralysis, and congenital or acquired subglottic obstruction.[12,13] In addition, critical airway obstruction may be secondary to other lesions that may compress the airway and impair normal respiration. These may include cystic hygroma, goiter, or hemangioma.[14] For additional examples and discussion, see Chapters 22 and 26.

ROUTES OF INTUBATION

Intubation can be performed orally or nasally. The choice of route depends on the circumstances and the preference of the clinician. Both oral and nasal endotracheal intubation have their unique complications and share a few as well.[13,15] Oral intubation is easier, faster, and less traumatic to perform, and it may be preferable in an emergency. Available data have failed to demonstrate statistically significant differences between oral and nasal intubation with respect to tracheal injury, frequency

of tube retaping, or tube replacement.[16] However, a higher incidence of postextubation atelectasis has been noted in nasally intubated patients, especially in preterm infants with birthweight less than 1500 g; atelectasis was associated with a marked reduction in nasal airflow through the previously intubated nares and stenosis of the nasal vestibule.[17,18] Midface hypoplasia has been reported to be associated with long-term intubation for bronchopulmonary dysplasia.[19]

On the other hand, proponents of nasal intubation believe that fixation of the tube to the infant's face is easier and more stable because it minimizes the chance for accidental dislodg-

TABLE 6-1. Problems in Newborn Infants with Oral and Nasal Endotracheal Tubes

Common Problems
Postextubation atelectasis—more common with nasal endotracheal tubes
Pneumonia/sepsis
Accidental extubation
Intubation of mainstem bronchus
Occlusion of tube from thickened secretions
Tracheal erosion
Pharyngeal, esophageal, tracheal perforation
Subglottic stenosis

Problems Unique to Nasal Endotracheal Tubes
Nasal septal erosion
Stricture of the nasal vestibule

Problems Unique to Oral Endotracheal Tubes
Palatal grooving
Interference with subsequent primary dentition

From Spitzer AR, Fox WW: The use of oral versus nasal endotracheal tubes in newborn infants. J Cal Perinatol Assoc 4:32, 1984.

TABLE 6-2. Equipment Needed for Intubation

Laryngoscope with premature (Miller no. 0) and infant blades (Miller no. 1)
Endotracheal tubes, sizes 2.5, 3.0, 3.5, and 4.0 mm 1D
Suction apparatus (wall)
Suction catheters 5.0, 6.5, 8.0, 10.0
Non–self-inflating bag (0.5 L), manometer, and tubing
Newborn and premature mask
Source of compressed air/O_2 with capability for blending
Humidification and warming apparatus for air/O_2
Tape: ½-inch pink (Hytape)
Magill neonatal forceps
Elastoplast (elastic bandages)
Cardiorespiratory monitor
Pulse oximeter (Spo_2)

TABLE 6-3. Selecting the Appropriate-Sized Endotracheal Tube

Tube Size (inside diameter in mm)	Weight (g)	Gestational Age (wk)
2.5	<1000	<26
3.0	1000–2000	28–34
3.5	2000–3000	34–38
3.5–4.0	>3000	>38

Used with the permission of the American Academy of Pediatrics, Neonatal Resuscitation Textbook, 3rd ed. American Academy of Pediatrics and the American Heart Association, 2000.

TABLE 6-4. Selecting the Appropriate-Sized Suction Catheter

Endotracheal Tube Size (mm)	Catheter Size (French)
2.5	5 or 6
3.0	6 or 8
3.5	8
4.0	8 or 10

Used with the permission of the American Academy of Pediatrics, Neonatal Resuscitation Textbook, 3rd ed. American Academy of Pediatrics and the American Heart Association, 2000.

ment and decreases tube movement, which can result in subglottic stenosis. Prolonged oral intubation can result in palatal grooving[20] and defective dentition.[21] Furthermore, there is evidence that acquired subglottic stenosis is increased in patients who were orally intubated and whose birthweight was less than 1500 g. The same study and one other offer evidence that the nasotracheal tube is easier to stabilize than an oral tube and that extubation occurs less frequently than in oral intubation.[15,22]

Acquired subglottic stenosis secondary to oral intubation may be a sequela of tracheal mucosal damage from the endotracheal tube itself or from repeated intubations. Most significantly, severe damage can occur from the up-and-down movement of the endotracheal tube.[16] Even with perfect fixation of the tube, up-and-down movement of 7 to 14 mm has been reported owing to the varying degrees of flexion of the neck. The caretaker team can minimize palatal grooving and defective dentition by rotating the fixation site from side to side during periodic retaping. Continuing attention to the quality of fixation, together with stabilization of the infant's head position, minimizes tube shifting and accidental extubation with the oral approach. However, both the oral and nasal techniques will continue to have a place in the care of the ventilated neonate. Problems associated with oral and nasal endotracheal tube use are summarized in Table 6-1.

EQUIPMENT

The equipment needed for intubation is listed in Table 6-2,[1] and the guidelines for choosing the correct tube size and suction catheters are listed in Tables 6-3 and 6-4.[1]

The use of tubes of appropriate size minimizes trauma, airway resistance, and excessive leak around the tube. A standard kit containing all of the equipment, as listed in Table 6-2, can be prepared and stocked, but it must be checked regularly to ensure that all of the necessities are present. The infant should be placed under a radiant warmer for endotracheal intubation. A laryngoscope with a Miller no. 0 and 1 blade should be used to visualize the vallecula, epiglottis, and glottis. The

no. 0 blade is used for almost all newborns. The no. 1 blade is used for infants who are several months old or newborns whose birthweight is greater than 4 to 5 kg.[1,23] A Miller "00" blade has been touted for use in extremely-low-birthweight infants because its smaller blade is more easily accommodated in the mouths of micropremies. However, because the light source is set back farther from the blade tip, some clinicians believe the visualization is not as good as with the "0" blade. In cases where the baby requires bag-and-mask ventilation prior to intubation, a non–self-inflating bag with a manometer and the appropriate-sized mask should be used. The mask should be clear and have a soft, form-fitting cushion that extends around the circumference. The alternative is the rigid but anatomically shaped Rendell-Baker/Soucek mask, which may have less dead space but has been demonstrated to be more difficult to use; this often results in ineffective ventilation.[24]

Two different types of resuscitation bags or manual resuscitators are available to provide assisted ventilation via mask

TABLE 6-5. Neonatal Manual Resuscitators

	Self-Inflating Bag	Non–Self-Inflating Bag
Types	Laerdal, Hope II, PMR II, and a host of disposable equivalents	"Anesthesia bag" with spring-loaded or variable-orifice bleed port
Operator	Requires education on bag characteristics	Requires both experience and knowledge of bag characteristics for adjustment of flow and bleed
Oxygen-air source positive F_{IO_2} delivery	Operates with room air	Requires compressed gas
	Efficacy of O_2 delivery dependent on correct use of closed reservoir system and closure of pop-off valve (use of open reservoir or pop-off valve reduces F_{IO_2})	Delivers F_{IO_2} of gas source unambiguously
	Many brands deliver room air on spontaneous breaths (in-house verification of brand performance is recommended)	Oxygen delivery same on spontaneous breaths as it is on mandatory breaths
Pressure delivery	Having excessive trust in pop-off feature is unwise; occlusion of pop-off valve and use of manometer allow performance equal to that of non–self-inflating bags	With manometer attached, any pressure can be easily given
Comments	Relatively complex mechanism with possibility of failure, particularly when reusable units are reassembled	Simple, reliable mechanism dependent on gas supply
	If pop-off pressure is adequate, allows removal of bulky manometer for transport	Manometer is bulky

or endotracheal tube: the self-inflating bag and the non–self-inflating or "anesthesia" bag.[1] The non–self-inflating bag is also commonly referred to as a *flow-inflating bag*.[1] Both come in a wide variety of configurations, but all configurations share some basic attributes, including an oxygen inlet, patient outlet, flow-control valve, and pressure manometer attachment site. The self-inflating bag, as the name implies, reinflates after squeezing and does not require the flow of oxygen to reinflate. However, this bag with an oxygen source can deliver only about 40% oxygen because as the bag reinflates, room air is drawn into the bag and mixes with 100% oxygen from the oxygen source. A reservoir will not allow room air to come into the bag; therefore, the self-inflating bag attached to an oxygen source with a reservoir is able to deliver 90% to 100% oxygen to the baby. Two other important characteristics of most self-inflating bags are a "popoff valve," which is "set" at 30 to 40 mm Hg, and a non-rebreathing valve, which is built into the bag and prevents the reliable delivery of free-flow oxygen.[25] In order to deliver free-flow oxygen, the operator needs to disconnect the oxygen tubing from the bag and hold the oxygen tubing close to the nose of the baby. In contrast, the non–self-inflating bag is an excellent source of free-flow oxygen, especially with the use of the appropriate-sized mask attached to the bag. Finally, both of these bags require a pressure manometer in order to provide safe and effective ventilation to the newborn.[25] Table 6-5 compares the two ventilation bags (or manual resuscitators).

TYPES OF TUBES

The endotracheal tube should be made of a nontoxic, thermolabile, nonkinking material that molds to the airway. The tube should meet the standards of the American Society for Testing and Materials F1242-89 and be radiopaque or have a radiopaque line.[25] Cuffed endotracheal tubes are not routinely used in neonates because the bulk of the cuff may prevent the

practitioner from inserting as large a diameter tube as would otherwise be possible. There is always a serious concern that the inflated cuff may damage the very sensitive airway mucosa of the small bag. If sealing the space around the tube becomes a priority, cuffed tubes are available (Sheridan, Inc., Argyle, NY, USA).

The type of endotracheal tube used most commonly is the Murphy endotracheal tube (Fig. 6-3). The Murphy tube is preferred for long-term ventilation. Most frequently, Murphy tubes have centimeter markers to show the overall depth of the tube, as well as vocal cord guide markers near the tip. These markers, under laryngoscopic visualization, show the clinician the depth within the trachea. Standard default markers should be used with caution because of the range of anatomic variation. In one review of the length of the black area at the tip of endotracheal tubes produced by four major manufacturers, the marker length varied by 10 mm in 2.5-mm internal-diameter tubes.[25a]

A Murphy tube has a tip bevel that allows smooth passage through the nares and a side hole whose purpose is to allow ventilation even if the tip is partially obstructed or is placed in the right mainstem bronchus. Some clinicians avoid using side-hole ("Murphy eye") tubes for prolonged ventilation because of anecdotal evidence that these tubes can abrade the trachea and cause scarring. Exclusive use of these endotracheal tubes in one institution was associated with an increased incidence of subglottic stenosis that ended when use of the tubes was discontinued. It can be adequately maintained in the correct position if the lip marker is placed on the tube at the lip level and it is fixed to the face. After proper placement is determined, the marker can be used as a reference to ensure that the tube's position remains constant. The Murphy tube is pliable (and becomes even less firm when it is allowed to remain under a radiant warmer while preparations are made for resuscitation). Many clinicians prefer to use an obturator or stylet to facilitate insertion. The stylet should not extend beyond the distal tip of the tube if tracheal damage is to be prevented.

The vicious cycle of asphyxia is frequently in progress in the critically ill neonate who requires emergent tracheal intu-

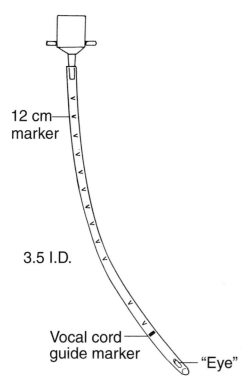

12 cm — marker

3.5 I.D.

Vocal cord — guide marker   "Eye"

Figure 6-3. Murphy-type endotracheal tube. The Murphy type is straight and relatively soft, with markings to show depth of insertion in the airway and in the trachea. An "eye" is present at the tip.

bation. The process of intubation in such an infant can exacerbate the difficulties that he or she is already experiencing. Intubation is associated with severe bradycardia, hypoxia, and elevation of arterial blood pressure and intracranial pressure.[26]

TECHNIQUES

There are a number of methods for performing endotracheal intubation in newborns, but the technique outlined in the NRP textbook should be considered the technique of choice[1] and "a common sense approach."[27] The steps are as follows, with other acceptable techniques included in parentheses:

• Stabilize the baby's head in the "sniffing position." A shoulder roll placed under the shoulders can help to maintain the baby's head in the correct position.
• Deliver free-flow oxygen during the procedure and suction the mouth and pharynx before sliding the blade into the mouth.
• Slide the laryngoscope over the right side of the tongue, pushing the tongue to the left side of the mouth, and advance the blade until the tip lies just beyond the base of the tongue.
• Lift the blade up slightly; raise the entire blade, not just the tip. The blade should be placed in the vallecula and, as the blade is raised, the epiglottis and the glottis with the vocal cords should be visualized. (Some clinicians slide the blade and raise the epiglottis to visualize the vocal cords.)
• Look for anatomic landmarks; suction as necessary for visualization.
• If the vocal cords are closed, wait for them to open. Insert the tip of the tube until the vocal cord guide is at the level of the vocal cords.

• Hold the tube firmly against the baby's hard palate while removing the laryngoscope once the tube has been placed. Hold the tube while removing the stylet as well.

The procedure should be completed in 20 seconds. This does not include setting up all of the equipment and getting the team together to help with the resuscitation.[1] Heart rate and pulse oximetry should be monitored during the intubation procedure and the infant ventilated with bag and mask. Recovery should be allowed between intubation attempts. The practitioner can improve O_2 tension during intubation by taping a suction catheter connected to a low-flow O_2 source along the laryngoscope blade.[28] Other investigators have maintained a flow of O_2 (3 to 5 L/min) through the endotracheal tube during intubation in an attempt to prevent drastic changes in oxygenation. At least two laryngoscopes have been designed with an O_2 port alongside the blade[29].

There is no apparent consensus on the use of medications such as atropine, succinylcholine, or pancuronium bromide before intubation. In some respects, atropine could be helpful in decreasing the volume of secretions and blocking a bradycardia secondary to a vagal response, and a muscle relaxant might be helpful in decreasing movement of the baby.

Nasotracheal Intubation

Nasotracheal intubation may be more time consuming and technically more difficult than orotracheal intubation for the less experienced practitioner. A nasotracheal tube is inserted into one of the nares and guided into the posterior pharynx along the floor of the nose. A laryngoscope is placed into the mouth and the glottis is visualized. A Magill forceps is held in the right hand and introduced into the mouth along the right side of the laryngoscope blade. The nasotracheal tube is grasped a short distance from its tip with the forceps. The tip of the tube is elevated until it is at the level of the glottis and is advanced between the vocal cords and into the trachea. An assistant may be needed to grasp the exterior (or distal) end of the endotracheal tube and assist with its advancement. Care should be exercised in using the Magill forceps so that the soft tissues of the oropharynx are not damaged. Experienced operators may successfully accomplish nasotracheal intubation without the Magill forceps. In addition, cooling a Murphy tube with a predetermined bend prior to intubation may facilitate the procedure.

Depth of Tube Insertion

In addition to direct visualization of the tube as it passes through the glottis, there are a number of different suggested "rules of thumb" for initial estimation of proper depth of tracheal tube placement. These rules use the centimeter markings on the side of a standard Murphy tube to gauge the depth of placement. The most common rule uses birthweight and a simple formula, *the rule of 7-8-9*. An endotracheal tube is advanced 7 cm to the lip for a 1-kg infant, 8 cm for a 2-kg infant, and 9 cm for a 3-kg infant. The rule of 7-8-9 is not appropriate for infants with hypoplastic mandibles (e.g., those with Pierre Robin syndrome) or short necks (e.g., those with Turner syndrome).[30] Similarly, nasotracheal tube insertion can be governed by adding 1 cm to the 7-8-9 rule.

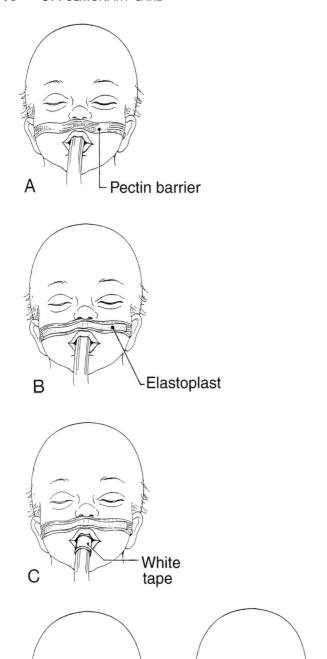

Figure 6-4. Technique for securing an endotracheal tube. *A,* Pectin barrier is applied to the infant's face from ear to ear and over the upper lip. *B,* A ¼-inch width of an elastic bandage (Elastoplast) is applied over the pectin barrier. *C,* A short strip of cloth tape or elastic bandage is wrapped around the tracheal tube to mark its point of passage at the mouth. The centimeter marking under the tape should be charted. *D,* Pink tape cut in the shape of an H is applied over the elastic bandage, with its ends extending beyond the bandage. The lower arms of the H are then wrapped around the tube. *E,* Single, ¼-inch strips of pink tape are secured over the lower part of the elastic bandage and wrapped around the tube. As an alternative to using an H-shaped piece of tape, the entire taping procedure can be done with a series of single strips of tape.

Determination of Placement

Determination of placement of the endotracheal tube after intubation is determined first clinically and then by chest radiograph. Clinical determination includes the following:

- Improvement or maintenance of heart rate in the normal range
- Good color, pulses, and perfusion after the intubation
- Good bilateral chest wall movement with each breath
- Equal breath sounds heard over both lung fields
- Breath sounds heard much louder over the lung fields than are heard over the stomach
- No gastric distention with ventilation
- Presence of vapor in the tube during exhalation
- Direct visualization by laryngoscope of the tube passing between the vocal cords
- Presence of exhaled CO_2 as determined by a CO_2 detector and/or an end-tidal CO_2 monitor or capnography[31]
- Tip to lip measurement: Add 6 to the newborn's weight in kilograms (rule of "7-8-9")

The chest radiograph can demonstrate that the tube is in the mid trachea. The position can be confirmed by following both of the mainstem bronchi back to the carina and cephalad to the tip of the tube.[1] Occasionally a lateral radiograph is necessary to confirm placement in the trachea.

Tube Fixation

Secure fixation of the endotracheal tube is important, not only to prevent accidental extubation but also to minimize tube movement during ventilation and other interventions such as suctioning or chest physiotherapy (CPT). Accidental extubation and repeated intubations have been demonstrated to be associated with the development of subglottic stenosis, as well as increased mortality.[12,13] The likelihood of accidental extubation also has been found to be associated with younger gestational age, higher level of consciousness, higher volume of secretions, and slippage of the tube.[32] It also is clear that there is no consensus as to which tube fixation method is most effective. The technique shown in Figure 6-4 represents a modification of the method described by Gregory[33] and is similar to what is used at the authors' institutions. The exception is that tincture of benzoin is no longer used, especially in "micropremies." Also, some of these techniques can be used to secure nasotracheal tubes (Fig. 6-5) without the use of tincture of benzoin. Several devices for fixation of neonatal endotracheal tubes are available from various manufacturers.

Alternative to Endotracheal Intubation: Use of the Laryngeal Mask Airway

The laryngeal mask airway (LMA) has been available for a number of years as an alternative to endotracheal intubation in babies, infants, children, and adults.[7] It is mentioned but not recommended for routine use in the new NRP textbook,[1] and a variety of papers discuss its use in various clinical scenarios, including the following:

- In neonatal resuscitation of term and preterm infants (size 1 LMA) (see Fig. 4-9)
- In the difficult airway, such as in the Robin sequence, and other situations when micrognathia is profound

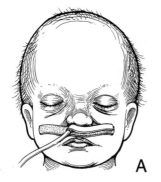

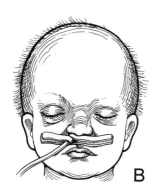

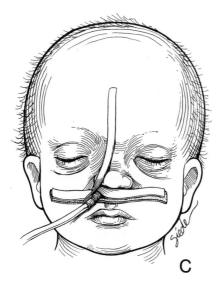

Figure 6-5. Technique for securing a nasotracheal tube. *A,* A ¼-inch strip of elastic bandage is applied over the upper lip, and a ¼-inch strip of Hytape (pink) is applied from the right side of the face and around the tube. *B,* A second piece of tape is applied from the left side of the face and around the tube. *C,* A third piece of tape is applied down the bridge of the nose and around the tube.

- As an aid to endotracheal intubation
- As an aid in flexible endoscopy
- In surgical cases in place of endotracheal intubation[34–37]

The success rate of insertion of the LMA has been reported to be greater than 90% in a number of descriptive studies of small series of infants and children[38] (see Chapter 23 for further discussion of LMA use).

MONITORING DURING VENTILATION AND HIGH-FREQUENCY OSCILLATION

Electrocardiography, respiratory impedance tracings, and serial arterial and/or capillary blood gases have been the traditional mainstays of bedside monitoring of the newborn, and they still have an important role. In general, the emphasis on noninvasive monitoring has resulted in the development and availability of new technologies that allow close monitoring without invasive procedures. The following is a list of those instruments:

- Transcutaneous monitoring of Po_2 and Pco_2
- Pulse oximetry to provide continuous measurement of hemoglobin saturation with O_2
- End-tidal CO_2 monitoring

See Chapters 7 and 17 for a more in-depth discussion of these noninvasive monitoring techniques.

For infants on high-frequency oscillation, pulmonary care involves new technology and keen observation.[39,40] These critically ill babies require a definite team approach, including an experienced respiratory therapist and nurse, and the traditional tools, including cardiorespiratory monitoring, intermittent arterial blood gases (from an arterial line), and "wiggle" assessment. A sample of a protocol used in the Infant Special Care Unit at our institution includes the following:

Assessments every 1 hour:
- Vital signs from monitors, including heart rate, arterial blood pressure, (what about respiratory rate?), body temperature (not hourly, then how frequently?)
- Vibration (or wiggle) assessment (scale +1 to +3)
- Capillary refill
- Comfort level

Assessments every 4 hours—"Hands on assessment":
- Auscultation of breath sounds on oscillator
- Palpation of pulses
- Nasogastric tube placement can be assessed without having to take the baby off of the oscillator

Assessments every 8 hours—Oscillator is turned off but the patient remains on the circuit:
- Heart rate, position of point of maximum intensity (PMI), presence or absence of a heart murmur
- Bowel sounds

Other assessments:
- Arterial blood gases after initiation of oscillation: hourly for 6 hours, every 2 hours for 6 hours, every 4 hours and as needed thereafter
- Chest radiograph schedule: just prior to being placed on the oscillator, within 1 hour after initiation of oscillation, every 12 hours twice, then daily and as needed
- Continuous monitoring of oxygen saturation using the pulse oximeter

Airway Management After Artificial Airway Placement

The keys to optimal management of the airway after placement of an endotracheal tube include knowledge of the potential problems, close monitoring of clinical parameters, thoughtful use of the technology listed previously, and intervention if problems arise. This level of care is the responsibility of all members of the team caring for each baby.

HUMIDIFICATION AND WARMING

The endotracheal tube bypasses the normal humidifying, filtering, and warming systems of the upper airway; therefore, heat and humidity must be provided to prevent hypothermia, inspissation of airway secretions, and necrosis of airway mucosa. Filtration of dry gases before humidification also is needed because of the contamination sometimes found in medical gas lines. A heater water humidifier is necessary to ensure that inspired gases are delivered at or near body temperature (37°C) and that they achieve near-total saturation with water vapor. A minimum dead space hygroscopic condenser (Hudson/RCI, Temecula, CA, USA) should be considered for use during transport or short-term ventilation. In the past, nebulizers were used in some applications, particularly in oxygen administration by head hood after extubation. Use of this system has been discarded because of impairment in oxygenation and the possibility of water intoxication due to excess delivery of particulate water and the presence of excessive noise. Sterile distilled water rather than saline is used in continuous therapy. It should be noted that water packaged "for irrigation" exceeds standards established for water packaged "for respiratory therapy" and costs less.

A modern servocontrolled heated humidifier, with its high and low temperature alarms and heated wires that prevent accumulation of condensation, should provide adequate humidification with proper operation. O'Hagan et al.[41,42] observed wide variation in the delivery of relative humidity, even when the temperature was maintained above 34.7°C; this variation resulted in failure to meet the American National Standards Institute guidelines for humidifier performance.[43] This may account for the findings of O'Hagan et al.,[42] who observed a significant increase in morbidity when temperatures below 36.5°C were maintained at the airway. These studies have led to the recommendation that relative humidity, as well as temperature, be monitored continuously. Miyao et al.[44] suggest that even maintenance of the Institute's standards (70% humidity at 37°C) may be inadequate, particularly if heated wire circuits are used. Use of circuits with heated wires was adopted primarily because of the frequency with which condensation needed to be drained and because of infection control considerations. The heated wire circuits were intended to enable the clinician to heat the gas inside the circuit to a temperature above that at which it left the humidifier, ensuring adequate absolute humidity without condensation in the circuit. This feature, which results in delivery of a hot gas with a lower relative humidity, may have caused the problems noted earlier.[44]

The increased temperature of a gas shifts the isothermal boundary (the point at which the gas completes equilibrium to body temperature and humidity levels) to a point closer to the airway opening. At first glance, this seems beneficial because less mucosa is exposed to the humidity deficit of the gas. However, because the effect of a given humidity deficit is concentrated on a smaller area of the mucosa, there is the potential for a greater degree of damage. Moreover, use of higher airway temperatures means that, even with lower humidity, there is rel-

atively less opportunity for humidified air from within the lung to recondense some of its humidity upon exhalation. The result is an increase in the humidity deficit (the difference in total water content of inspired gas and the water content it achieves within the lung). The potential for adverse effects with use of the heated wire circuit is exacerbated by inadequate monitoring of humidity levels. If the wire is so hot that the circuit is dry, it is not known whether the relative humidity is 70% (the nominally acceptable American National Standards Institute value) or less.[42]

Traditionally, probes for monitoring inspired gas have been placed as close as possible to the patient connection so that the effect of the trip down the inspiratory line on the inspired gas can be monitored. Unfortunately, in some neonatal circumstances, the probe is continuously in the presence of a heated field and may register the effect of this heat by radiation and/or convection, totally apart from the effect of the inspired gas. If this temperature is sensed by a servocontroller, the humidifier and the heated wires may automatically heat less because the temperature is actually being controlled by another heat source (Fig. 6-6). An extension adapter, which is provided by most manufacturers, allows the probe to be placed outside of the heating field, thus remedying this problem. This extension does not need to incorporate heated wires because the gas temperature is maintained by the heated field on entry.

An additional set of problems associated with heated wire circuits has been reported by the Emergency Care Research Institute (ECRI)[43] and the US Food and Drug Administration (FDA; see Appendix 31). Generic circuits that are not always compatible with the humidifier and its power source have been manufactured, leading to melting or charring of circuit components. Use of such circuits must be preceded by careful compatibility testing. In addition, the ECRI emphasizes that the circuits must never be covered by bed linens or drapes and that they must never be activated in the absence of flow through the system; otherwise, melting or charring may result. If a non-heated wire system is used, the temperature must be monitored by a thermometer placed inline to ensure proper temperature ranges. Use of inline water traps is recommended for decreasing the resistance to flow caused by condensate and for ensuring stability of oxygen concentrations. Despite all of the hazards and limitations of the current generation of heated wire circuits, their use has become widespread in most neonatal intensive care units. The clinician should adopt the following precautions specified by the ECRI and the FDA (in addition to the previously mentioned standards):

1. Temperature monitoring must take place before gas enters the heated field.
2. Temperature must be maintained at 36° to 37°C.
3. At least some visible condensation must be present on the inspiratory limb, despite previous beliefs to the contrary.

BRONCHOPULMONARY HYGIENE

The clinician must keep the chest clear of secretions in the conducting airways, and he or she must keep the artificial airway patent by ensuring proper humidification and suctioning of the endotracheal tube. These procedures may be done as needed but normally are performed immediately, followed by

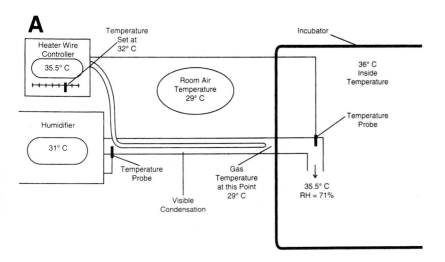

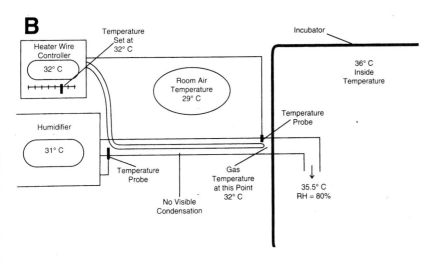

Figure 6-6. *A,* Temperature probe located inside a heated field tends to indicate a heat representative of the heated field rather than of the inspiratory gas before entry into the field. The humidifier does not provide the heat that is being detected by the wire controller. The heat source is particularly difficult to assess because most heated wire circuits operate with humidifiers that do not provide a display of the temperature of the gas immediately after it leaves the humidifier. *B,* Proper placement of the probe. If the probe is only slightly outside a radiant warmer field, it may need to be shielded, particularly if phototherapy is in use. (From Chatburn RL: Principles and practice of neonatal and pediatric mechanical ventilation. Respir Care 36:560, 1991.)

administration of aerosolized medications.[45] The frequency of suctioning should depend on the patient's need, because this and other methods of bronchopulmonary hygiene may have detrimental side effects.

CPT involving postural drainage in concert with percussion or vibration has been shown to be beneficial in removing secretions and preventing atelectasis in recently extubated neonates.[46] It also has been shown to result in removal of more secretions from intubated neonates.[47] Furthermore, oxygenation has been shown to be enhanced after completion of CPT.[46] The benefit of this procedure may lie in the periodic redistribution of the gravity-dependent regions of the lung, rather than in the physical removal of secretions. On the other hand, CPT has not gained universal acceptance. Its use should be individualized in each baby because as noted earlier, use of these techniques has been associated with a variety of negative effects, especially in infants born weighing less than 1000 g. If anything, this group of extremely-low-birthweight infants frequently is on a minimal stimulation plan of care for the first 3 to 5 days of extrauterine life.[48] The paucity of airway secretions in this group of infants during this time has led some clinicians to suction only on an "as needed" basis or not at all.

Positioning of the Patient

Postural drainage involves the use of various positions in which the different mainstem bronchi are positioned vertically so that drainage from the smaller bronchi moves into the larger bronchi (Figs. 6-7 to 6-14). The two forces at work during this procedure are gravity and air flow. Any area of the bronchial tree that is to be drained (with the exception of medial basal segment) must be uppermost.[49] These positions may not be practical for implementation in critically ill babies who have chest tubes or endotracheal tubes, who have undergone surgery, or who are at great risk for intraventricular hemorrhage. Optimally, the infant should be monitored during CPT; potential monitors include transcutaneous O_2 or CO_2, or pulse oximeter. Significant oxygen desaturation during the procedure should cause the caretaker to pause and initiate measures necessary to correct hypoxemia.

Percussion and Vibration

Two types of hand pressure can be applied to the neonatal chest to expedite adequate drainage: percussion and vibration. Percussion in the neonate can be performed with small plastic

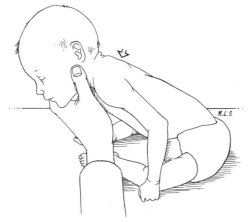

Figure 6-7. Drainage of the posterior segments of the upper lobe. The infant is leaned over at a 30° angle from the sitting position. The clinician claps and vibrates over the upper back on both sides.

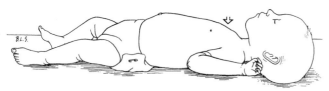

Figure 6-8. Drainage of the anterior segments of the upper lobe. While the infant is lying flat on his or her back, the clinician claps and vibrates between the nipples and the clavicle on both sides.

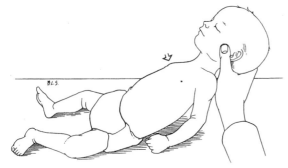

Figure 6-9. Drainage of the apical segment of the upper lobe. The infant is leaned backward about 30° from the sitting position, and the clinician claps or vibrates above the clavicle on both sides.

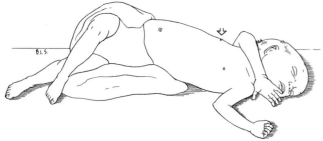

Figure 6-10. For drainage of the right middle lobe, the caregiver elevates the hips to about 5 inches above the head. He or she rolls the infant backward one-quarter turn and then claps and vibrates over the right nipple. For drainage of the lingular segments of the left upper lobe, the caregiver places the infant in the same position but with the left side lifted upward; he or she then claps and vibrates over the left nipple.

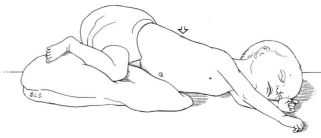

Figure 6-11. Drainage of the lateral basal segments of the lower lobes. The caregiver places the infant on the left side with the hips elevated to a level about 8 inches above that of the head. The caregiver rolls the infant forward one-quarter turn and then claps or vibrates over the lower ribs. Note that the position shown is for draining the right side. For draining the left side, the same procedure is followed, except that the infant is placed on his or her right side.

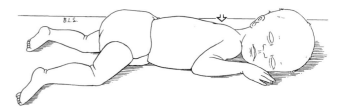

Figure 6-12. Drainage of the superior segments of the lower lobe. The clinician places the infant flat on the stomach and then claps or vibrates at top of the scapula on the back side of the spine.

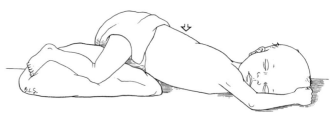

Figure 6-13. Drainage of the posterior basal segments of the lower lobe. The clinician places the infant on the stomach with the hips at a level 8 inches above that of the head. He or she then claps and vibrates over the lower ribs close to the spine on both sides.

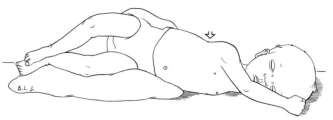

Figure 6-14. Drainage of the anterior basal segment of the lower lobes. The caregiver places the infant on the left side with the hips at a level about 8 inches above that of the head. He or she then claps and vibrates just beneath the axilla. Note that for drainage of the opposite anterior basal segment, the infant is turned on the right side.

cups with padded rims or with soft circular masks with their adapters plugged so that the air pockets are maintained. The chest is percussed over the area to be drained for 1 to 2 minutes. Percussion may be reserved for infants who weigh more than 1500 g and are older than 2 weeks of age because of the potential risk for intraventricular hemorrhage.

The traditional view of vibration is that it is effective only during exhalation because it causes secretions to move from the periphery of the lungs with the outflow of air. This technique requires careful observation of chest movements. For vibration, the wrist is extended and the arm muscles are contracted in a manner similar to that used for isometric exercises. The result can be described as a controlled quiver. The placement of fingers flat against chest walls of infants suffices. A light touch with rapidly vibrating fingers has been considered effective in mobilizing secretions in neonates.[50] Because few practitioners feel comfortable with this technique, vibrations can be done with a padded electric toothbrush, a small hand vibrator, or a commercially available pulmonary vibrator.

Vibration is tolerated by a greater number of patients than is percussion. The duration of vibration therapy is subject to the infant's tolerance and can be monitored on the basis of the parameters discussed previously.[50]

Optimization of Drug Delivery

The common practice of administering aerosolized medications before bronchopulmonary hygiene and suctioning is based on custom more than scientifically verified practice. The pharmacology of drug action is discussed in Chapter 19.

Although delivery of aerosolized medication has a number of advantages over systemic dosing, recent information has helped in the design of a few reliable aerosol delivery systems (Tables 6-6 to 6-8).[45] The basic fundamental characteristics of factors that influence neonatal aerosol delivery and deposition are listed in Table 6-6. These factors can be divided into

two groups: host-related factors and aerosol system-related factors.[51] Table 6-7 lists the characteristics of "the ideal aerosol delivery system." Table 6-8 compares the advantages and disadvantages of the three most frequently used aerosol delivery systems: the pressurized metered dose inhaler, and

---

TABLE 6-6. Overview of Factors That Influence Neonatal Aerosol Delivery and Deposition

Host-Related Factors
- Anatomic (nasal breathing, size of oropharynx, airways, lung development)
- Physiologic (breathing pattern, inspiratory flow rate, tidal volume, pulmonary mechanics)
- Pathophysiologic (inflammation, mucus, atelectasis, fibrosis)

Aerosol-System Related Factors
- Characteristics of the medication (particle size, shape, density, output)
- Generator [pressurized meter dose inhaler (pMDI) or nebulizer]
- Delivery devices–patient interfaces (face mask or endotracheal tube)
- Conditions (ventilatory, environmental)
- Provider technique (optimum use of pMDI with spacer)

Data from Cole C: The use of aerosolized medicines in neonates. Neonat Respir Dis 10:4, 2000.

TABLE 6-7. The Ideal Aerosol Delivery System

- High efficiency in aerosol delivery
- Predictable and reproducible (in same patient and different patients)
- Easy to use and maintain
- Efficient to administer
- Convenient
- Cost-effective
- Environmentally safe

Data from Cole C: The use of aerosolized medicines in neonates. Neonat Respir Dis 10:4, 2000.

TABLE 6-8. Advantages and Disadvantages of Aerosol Generators in Neonates

Aerosol Generator	Advantages	Disadvantages
Pressurized metered dose inhaler (pMDI)	• More consistent aerosol particle size and output • Less time-consuming • Less preparation time • Less contamination • Less expensive than single-use nebulizers • Some HFA formulations have more optimal aerosol particle size	• Technique problems • Lack of pure medications • Not all medications available in pMDI • New hydrofluoroalkane (HFA) formulations need clinical studies
Jet nebulizer	• Tidal breathing • Passive cooperation • Can be used for long periods to deliver high doses • Wide range of medications	• Expensive and inconvenient • Inefficient and highly variable aerosol output • Numerous environmental factors affect aerosol particle size and output • Poor aerosolization of suspensions and viscous solutions • Preparation time • Time-consuming to administer • Contamination potential • Requires compressed gas
Ultrasonic nebulizer	• Potentially more efficient than jet nebulizer and pMDI • Tidal breathing • Passive cooperation • Can be used for long periods to deliver high doses	• Expensive and inconvenient • Requires power source • Contamination potential • Limited medications available for use • Preparation time • Time-consuming to administer

Data from Cole C: The use of aerosolized medicines in neonates. Neonat Respir Dis 10:4, 2000.

the jet and ultrasonic nebulizers.[45] However, even with the progress being made in the design of aerosolized medication delivery systems, the clinician may need to test a variety of delivery devices and decide which system is most efficacious for each individual patient. The same may have to be done with the type and dose of aerosol medication[52,53] in order to establish a bronchodilator dose, that is, measuring a patient's response to a specific drug and dose using bedside pulmonary function methods detailed in Chapter 19 rather than using predetermined dose tables. In addition, it is important to understand the variables unique to the aerosol route that can affect the drug delivery device. The small internal diameter and high resistance of the neonatal endotracheal tube impair aerosol delivery in the intubated patient compared with the nonintubated patient. In studies with animals, humans, and bench models, from 0.19% to 2.14% of the total drug amount in the nebulizer cup was administered to the lung or lung model when conventional jet nebulizers were used[52,53] compared with 10% of the total dose that was shown to be deposited in the lungs of nonintubated patients.[54]

With currently available methods, the placement and operation of a nebulizer are important for maximizing drug delivery to the lung. The nebulizer should be placed at least 5 inches upstream from the patient connection (not directly on the ventilator Y), and the humidifier should be bypassed for the duration of medication delivery.[45] If the nebulizer itself can provide the necessary flow for operation of a time-cycled pressure-limited ventilator, source flow other than the nebulizer should be eliminated if dilution of medication is to be prevented; however, the nebulizer flow should not be permitted to back up into the ventilator.[55] On the other hand, for more sophisticated ventilators with which this technique would trigger an alarm, nebulizers that prime the inspiratory tubing while running only in the expiratory phase are under development.[56]

Suctioning

Standards for suctioning protocols vary among institutions and usually are not based on physiologic principles or the results of current research.[57] The role of endotracheal suctioning is important, but the potential risks are many.[58] Use of a closed "inline" suctioning system has been promoted to decrease respiratory contamination and pulmonary infections. Disadvantages of these systems include increased expense and potential increase in air leaks. Suctioning should be performed by experienced personnel because complications from the trauma of this procedure may lead to hypoxemia,[57–59] cardiovascular embarrassment, barotrauma, and intraventricular hemorrhage. However, with care, patience, and appropriate anticipation, suctioning is a highly effective method of clearing the airway. The interval should be individualized and documented at the bedside; an example is illustrated in Figure 6-15. Following are a few suggestions on how to optimize benefits and prevent complications (see Table 6-9 and Fig. 6-15 and 6-16 for additional information):

- Anticipate when setting up for suctioning by having the proper equipment available
- Be aware of ventilatory parameters and F_{IO_2}
- Perform noninvasive monitoring of oxygenation before, during, and after suctioning
- Have two people available (two-person job)

FRONT

ET TUBE PLACEMENT AND SUCTIONING RECORD
Baby's Name ——————— Weight (gm) ———
Date Tube Inserted —————————
Tube Position ——— cm Above Carina
ET Tube Size ——— Catheter Depth ——— cm

BACK

INTERTECH / OHIO		
TUBE SIZE	CUT (cm)	CATHETER DEPTH (cm)
2.5	11	14.5
3.0	13	17.0
3.5	13	17.0
4.0	14	18.0

Figure 6-15. Bedside "suction card" with values to be re-verified after every chest radiograph has been obtained. Values are based on tube position relative to the carina. Suction depth must be reduced if the tip is not 2 cm above the carina. The table on the back of the card allows compensation for the extra length of the endotracheal tube's 15-mm adapter.

- Have the proper suction catheter size (see Tables 6-3 and 6-4 and/or Figs. 6-15 and 6-16)
- Individualize suctioning interval, catheter size, and depth of instillation of suction catheter as outlined in Tables 6-3 and 6-4
- Prepare settings for vacuum pressure, from 60 to 100 mm Hg
- Ensure the suction catheter is not more than two thirds the internal diameter of the endotracheal tube
- Use normal saline for irrigation, 0.1 to 0.5 mL/kg depending on patient's tolerance

Remember, suctioning technique looks easy when it is performed by neonatal intensive care unit nurses and respiratory therapists. Close attention to the changes in the baby and adherence to suction technique are necessary to be of benefit to the sick infant.

SURFACTANT ADMINISTRATION

The following section addresses the technical aspects of instillation of surfactant. More details on the choice of surfactant and the physiology, usefulness, and efficacy of surfactants are addressed in Chapter 20. At the time of publication of the third edition of this text, only two surfactant preparations were commercially available in the United States: Survanta (beractant) and Exosurf (colfosceril). Since then, a number of preparations have become available and include the following, as listed in Table 6-10 by Dekowski and Holtzman.[51] The two most commonly used methods of administration of surfactant

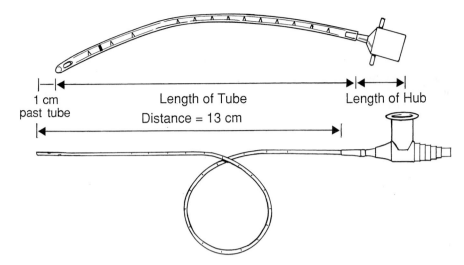

Figure 6-16. Method for determining the length of catheter advancement in an endotracheal tube. Knowledge of the placement of the tube and of the length of the tube can be applied to the use of a calibrated suction catheter for providing consistent catheter advancement to a level 1 cm above the carina.

TABLE 6-9. Endotracheal Suctioning in Newborn Infants

	Hodge	Hagedorn et al.	Fletcher and MacDonald
Irrigation solutions	Saline, but not routinely	Saline	Saline
Amount for irrigation	0.1–0.2 mL/kg	0.25–0.5 mL	Not specified
Catheter size	0.5–0.66 of tube diameter	Not specified	0.5 of tube diameter
Depth of insertion	Length of tube only	Length of tube only	1 cm beyond tip of tube
Hyperinflation	PIP 10–20% above baseline	Match PIP	PIP or PIP plus up to 10 cm H_2O
Hyperventilation	Equal total respiratory rate	Equal to ventilatory rate	Rate 40–60 breath min with long inspiratory time
Oxygen enhancement	10%–20% above baseline	If clinically indicated	10% above baseline
Suction pressure	50–80 cm H_2O	80–100 mm Hg	"Lowest possible"
Duration	Not specified	5–10 s	15–20 sec disconnect time
Intermittent vs continuous	Not addressed	Continuous on withdrawal	Not addressed
Head turn	No	No	Turn head for selective bronchial suction

PIP, peak inspiratory pressure.
Data from Hodge D: Endotracheal suctioning and the infant: A nursing care protocol to decrease complications. Neonat Network 9:7, 1991; Hagedorn MI, Gardner SL, Abman SH: Respiratory diseases. In Merenstein GB, Gardner SL (eds): Handbook of Neonatal Intensive Care. St. Louis, CV Mosby, 1989, p. 381; Fletcher MA, MacDonald MG: Atlas of Procedures in Neonatology, 2nd ed. Philadelphia, JB Lippincott, 1993, p. 292.

into the airway of the newborn were reflected by the first two products that became available. Survanta was administered using a feeding tube of a length that put the tip just below the end hole of the Murphy tube. It was injected at a steady rate so as not to cause any obstruction of the airway 1 cm above the carina. Exosurf was administered using a special tube adapter with a side hole so that the baby remained on the ventilator during administration. It was instilled at a steady rate within 30 minutes of birth.[51] Each surfactant has a procedure for optimal instillation provided in the package insert. The objective is to achieve maximal distribution of the drug to all parts of the lung. This usually requires placing the infant in different positions during instillation.

EXTUBATION

The optimal time for extubation is determined by a variety of parameters, including mean airway pressure, oxygen requirement, ventilatory requirements (see Chapters 9 and 10

TABLE 6-10. Surfactant Preparations

Surfactant Type	Material	Proteins
Bovine	Modified minced lung extracts [surfactant TA (Surfactant)]	SP-B, SP-C
Bovine	Modified minced lung extracts [beractant (Surfactant)]	SP-B, SP-C
Bovine	Calf lung lavage extracts (CLSE, Infasurf)	SP-B, SP-C
Bovine	Cow lung lavage extracts [SF-RI 1 (Alveofact)]	SP-B, SP-C
Porcine	Minced lung extracts (Curosurf)	SP-B, SP-C
Human	Human amniotic fluid extract	SP-A, SP-B, SP-C
Synthetic	DPPC-PG (artificial lung-expanding compound)	None
Synthetic	DPPC, CPHT (Exosurf Neonatal)	None

CPHT, colfosceril palmitate, hexadecanol, and tyloxapol; DPPC-PG, dipalmitoylphosphatidylcholine-phosphatidylglycerol; SP-A, surfactant apoprotein A; SP-B, surfactant apoprotein B; SP-C, surfactant apoprotein C. From Dekowski S, Holtzman RB: Surfactant replacement therapy: An update on applications. Pediatr Clin North Am 45:549–572, 1998.

on modes of ventilation), estimation of negative inspiratory force, static compliance, and, most importantly, the appearance of the baby. The clinician may use intermittent bagging of the infant to get a sense of the compliance of the lung. The baby's primary problem and the clinical course and duration of assisted ventilation can provide helpful information regarding safe time for extubation. Some experts believe that a transition period from assist mode, pressure support, and/or extubation to nasal prong or nasopharyngeal continuous positive airway pressure (CPAP) is an excellent way to facilitate extubation. Sometimes a methylxanthine is used during the weaning process because its effects include "reminding the newborn to breathe" and increasing the efficiency of the diaphragm, especially in very-low-birthweight infants.[60,61] If the infant has been on assisted ventilation for several days and there is concern about edema and inflammation in the upper airway, one or two doses of dexamethasone, given 24 to 48 hours prior to extubation, may be helpful.

Extubation Technique

Many authors advise extubation with positive pressure in order to avoid atelectasis.[33] Some clinicians, however, use negative pressure to suction the airway during the extubation process. To the best of our knowledge, no controlled clinical study has yet established the advantage of extubating with positive or negative pressure.

POSTEXTUBATION CARE

The extubated infant requires frequent clinical assessment during the postextubation period. Frequent observation of breathing patterns, auscultation of the chest, and monitoring of vital signs, pulse oximetry (continuous), transcutaneous CO_2

levels, and/or blood gases are all of value. Other interventions, including bronchopulmonary hygiene,[62] can be started in an attempt to prevent or reverse atelectasis, most frequently seen in the right middle and upper lobes. Racemic epinephrine may help to open up the airways by decreasing edema of the airway. After extubation, if there is a clinical concern, a chest radiograph can be obtained. If the baby continues to deteriorate, other techniques to consider include initiation of CPAP using the nasopharyngeal technique (NPCPAP), intermittent manual bagging using the correct-sized mask and non–self-inflating bag, racemic epinephrine, and/or corticosteroids (enterally or parenterally) if signs of upper airway obstruction are noted. If the baby is unable to maintain adequate ventilation despite interventions, then reintubation and suctioning should be accomplished. There are multiple reasons for extubation failure; Table 6-11 provides a comprehensive list. Extubation failure should prompt a search for a cause that can be corrected before the next extubation attempt.

TABLE 6-11. Major Causes of Extubation Failure

I. Pulmonary
  A. Primary disease not resolved
  B. Postextubation atelectasis
  C. Pulmonary insufficiency of prematurity
  D. Bronchopulmonary dysplasia
  E. Eventration or paralysis of diaphragm
II. Upper Airway
  A. Edema and/or excess tracheal secretions
  B. Subglottic stenosis
  C. Laryngotracheomalacia
  D. Congenital vascular ring
  E. ? Necrotizing tracheobronchitis
III. Cardiovascular
  A. Patent ductus arteriosus
  B. Fluid overload
  C. Congenital heart disease with increased pulmonary flow
IV. Central Nervous System
  A. Apnea (extreme immaturity)
  B. Intraventricular hemorrhage
  C. Hypoxic ischemic brain damage/seizures
  D. Drugs (phenobarbital)
V. Miscellaneous
  A. Unrecognized diagnosis (e.g., nerve palsy, myasthenia gravis)
  B. Sepsis
  C. Metabolic abnormality

REFERENCES

1. Kattwinkel J (ed): Textbook of Neonatal Resuscitation, 4th ed. Dallas, American Heart Association, and Elk Grove Village, Ill., American Academy of Pediatrics, 2000.
2. Apgar V: A proposal for a new method of evaluation of the newborn infant. Anesth Analg (Paris) 32:260, 1953.
3. Casey VL: Hypoxia secondary to suctioning of the neonate. Neonatal Network 3:8, 1984.
4. Kurtis PS: Letter to the editor. Meconium aspiration. Pediatrics 106:867–868, 2000.
5. Wiswell T, Gannon CM, Jacob J: Delivery room management of the apparently vigorous meconium-stained neonate: Results of the multicenter, international, collaborative trial. Pediatrics 105:1–7, 2000.
6. Hageman JR: New developments: Meconium staining of the amniotic fluid. The need for reassessment by obstetricians and pediatricians. Curr Prob Pediatr 20:396–401, 1993.
7. Linder N, Aranda J, Tsur M, et al: Need for endotracheal intubation and suction in meconium stained neonates. J Pediatr 112:613–615, 1988.
8. Venkataraman S: Noninvasive mechanical ventilation and respiratory care. New Horizons 7:353–358, 1999.
9. Pape K, Armstrong DL, Fitzhardinge P: Intracerebellar hemorrhage as a possible complication of mask applied mechanical ventilation in the low birthweight infant. Pediatr Res 9:383, 1975.
10. Avery ME, Fletcher BP, Williams R: The Lung and Its Disorders in the Newborn Infant, 4th ed. Philadelphia, WB Saunders, 1981, pp. 182–202, 305, 661–681.
11. Jones KL: Smith's Recognizable Patterns of Human Malformation. Philadelphia, WB Saunders, 1997, pp. 234–235.
12. Ratner I, Whitfield J: Acquired subglottic stenosis in the very low birthweight infant. Am J Dis Child 137:40, 1983.
13. Sherman JM, Lowitt S, Stephenson C, et al: Factors influencing acquired subglottic stenosis in infants. J Pediatr 109:322, 1986.
14. Jona J: Advances in neonatal surgery. Pediatr Clin North Am 45:605–617, 1998.
15. Spitzer A, Fox WW: The use of oral versus nasal endotracheal tubes in newborn infants in newborn infants. J Cal Perinatal Assoc 4:32, 1984.
16. Todres ID, deBros F, Kramer SS, et al: Endotracheal tube displacement in the newborn infant. J Pediatr 88:126, 1976.
17. Gowdar K, Bull MJ, Schreiner RL: Nasal deformities in neonates: Their occurrence in those treated with nasal continuous positive airway pressure and nasal endotracheal tubes. Am J Dis Child 134:954, 1980.
18. Jung AI, Thomas GK: Stricture of the nasal vestibule: A complication of nasotracheal intubation of newborn infants. J Pediatr 85:412, 1978.
19. Rotschild A, Dison A, Chitaya D, et al: Midface hypoplasia associated with long term intubation for bronchopulmonary dysplasia. Am J Dis Child 144:1302, 1990.
20. Erenberg A, Nowak AJ: Palatal groove formation in neonates and infants with orotracheal tubes. Am J Dis Child 128:974, 1985.
21. Moylan FMB, Seldin E, Shannon D, et al: Defective dentition in survivors of neonatal mechanical ventilation. J Pediatr 96:106, 1980.

22. Molho M, Lieberman P: Safe fixation of oro- and naso-tracheal tubes for prolonged ventilation in neonates, infants and children. Crit Care Med 3:81, 1975.
23. Finer NN, Muzyka D: Flexible endoscope intubation of the neonate. Pediatr Pulmonol 12:48, 1992.
24. Palme C, Nystrom B, Tunell R: An evaluation of the efficiency of face masks in the resuscitation of newborn infants. Lancet 1:207, 1985.
25. Goldstein B, Nystronam B, Twell R: The role of on-line manometers in minimizing peak and mean airway pressures during the hand-regulated ventilation of newborn infants. Respir Care 34:23,1989.
25a. Molendijk H: Use of the black area on the tube tip for rapid estimation of insertion depth of endotracheal tubes in neonates: A potential hazard. Arch Dis Child Fetal Neonatal Ed 85:F77, 2001.
26. Kelly M, Finer N: Nasotracheal intubation in the neonate: Physiologic response to effects of atropine and pancuronium. J Pediatr 105:303, 1984.
27. Hageman JR: Editor's notes: Ninth in a series. Illinois Pediatrician Newsletter, Spring/Summer:10, 2001.
28. Wung JT, Stark R, Indyk L, et al: Oxygen supplementation during endotracheal intubation of the infant. Pediatrics 59:1046, 1977.
29. Todres ID, Crone RK: Experience with a modified laryngoscope in sick infants. Crit Care Med 9:544, 1981.
30. Tochen ML: Orotracheal intubation in the newborn infant: A method for determining depth of tube insertion. J Pediatr 95:1050, 1979.
31. Repetto J, Donohue PK, Baker SF, et al: Use of capnography in the delivery room for assessment of endotracheal tube placement. J Perinatol 21:281–287, 2001.
32. Sherman JM, Lowitt S, Stephenson C: Factors influencing acquired subglottic stenosis in infants. J Pediatr 109:322, 1986.
33. Gregory G: Respiratory care of newborn infants. Pediatr Clin North Am 19:311,1972.
34. Ellis DS, Potluri PK, O'Flaherty JE: Difficult airway management in the neonate: A simple method of intubating through a laryngeal mask airway. Pediatr Anaesth 9:460–462, 1999.
35. Osses H, Poblete M, Asenjo F: Laryngeal mask airway for difficult intubation in children. Pediatr Anesth 10:399–401, 1999.
36. Paterson SJ, Byrne PJ, Molesky MG, et al: Neonatal resuscitation using the laryngeal mask airway. Anesthesiology 80:1248–1253, 1994.
37. Paterson SJ, Byrne PJ: Time required to insert the laryngeal mask airway in neonates requiring resuscitation. Anesthesiology 80:1248, 1995.
38. Gandini D, Brimacombe JR: Neonatal resuscitation with the laryngeal mask airway in normal and low birthweight infants. Anesth Analg 89:642–643, 1999.
39. Avila K, Mazza L, Morgan-Trukillo L: High-frequency oscillatory ventilation: A nursing approach to bedside care. Neonatal Network 13:23–29, 1994.
40. Truog W: High-frequency oscillatory ventilation. In Spitzer A (ed): Intensive Care of the Fetus and the Neonate. St. Louis, Mosby-Yearbook, 1996, pp. 584–593.
41. Mishoe SC, Brooks CW, Valeri KL, et al: Sound levels of humidifiers and nebulizers supplying oxygen hoods. Respir Care 37:1288,1992.
42. O'Hagan M, Reid E, Tarnow-Murdi W: Is neonatal inspired gas humidity accurately controlled by humidifier temperature? Crit Care Med 19:1370, 1991.
43. Health Devices Report: Emergency Care Research Institute (ECRI). 22:300, 1993.
44. Miyao H, Hirokawa T, Miyasaka K, et al: Relative humidity, not absolute humidity, is of great importance when using a humidifier with a heating wire. Crit Care Med 29:674, 1992.
45. Cole C: The use of aerosolized medicines in neonates. Neonatal Respir Dis 10:1–12, 2000.
46. Finer NN, Moriartery R, Boyd J, et al: Post extubation atelectasis: A retrospective review and a prospective controlled study. J Pediatr 94:110, 1979.
47. Etches A, Scott B: Chest physiotherapy in the newborn: Effect on secretions removed. Pediatrics 62:713,1978.
48. Bregman J, Kimberlin L: The Small Baby Protocol. Evanston Infant Special Care Unit, revised edition, April 2001.
49. Dunn DT, Lewis AT: Some important aspects of neonatal nursing related to pulmonary disease and family involvement. Pediatr Clin North Am 20:81, 1973.
50. King M, Phillips DM, Gross D, et al: Enhanced tracheal mucus clearance with high frequency chest wall compression. Am Rev Respir Dis 128:511, 1983.
51. Dekowksi S, Holtzman RB: Surfactant replacement therapy: An update on applications. Pediatr Clin North Am 45:549–572, 1998.
52. Rau JL, Harwood RJ: Comparison of nebulizer delivery methods through an endotracheal tube: A bench study. Respir Care 37:1233, 1991.
53. Rau JL: Delivery of aerosolized drugs to pediatric and neonatal patients. Respir Care 36:514,1991.
54. MacIntyre NR, Silver R, Miller CW: Aerosol delivery in intubated mechanically ventilated patients. Crit Care Med 13:81, 1985.
55. Cameron D, Daly M, Silverman M: Evaluation of nebulizers for use in neonatal ventilatory circuits. Crit Care Med 18:866, 1990.
56. Dahlback M, Wollmer P, Drefeldt D, et al: Controlled aerosol delivery during mechanical ventilation. J Aerosol Med 2:339, 1989.
57. Turner BS: Nursing interventions: Current concepts in endotracheal suctioning. J Cal Perinatal Assoc 3:104, 1983.
58. Cassani VL: Hypoxia secondary to suctioning of the neonate. Neonatal Network 2:8, 1984.
59. Dawford AD, Miske S, Headley J, et al: Effects of routine care procedures on transcutaneous oxygen in neonates: A quantitative approach. Arch Dis Child 58:20, 1983.
60. Harris MC, Baumgart S, Rooklin AR, et al: Successful extubation of infants with respiratory distress syndrome using aminophylline. Pediatrics 103:303, 1983.
61. Barrington K, Finer NN: A randomized controlled trial of aminophylline in ventilatory weaning of premature infants. Crit Care Med 21:846–850, 1993.
62. Bloomfield F, Teele R, Voss M: The role of neonatal chest physiotherapy in preventing postextubation atelectasis. J Pediatr 133:269–271, 1998.

NURSING CARE

CAROLYN HOUSKA LUND, RN, MS, FAAN

Newborns receiving assisted ventilation and neonatal intensive care require a multidisciplinary group of care providers. Professional nurses, physicians, respiratory therapists, social workers, developmental specialists, occupational and physical therapists, pharmacists, and clinical dietitians comprise the team who works in the neonatal intensive care unit (NICU). In this chapter, nursing care for the newborn requiring assisted ventilation is explored. After describing daily nursing assessment, the following areas are addressed in detail: thermoregulation, skin care, developmental care, comfort and pain management, and care of families. Specific nursing issues with regard to airway management and care during advanced technologies, such as high-frequency ventilation and extracorporeal membrane oxygenation (ECMO), are discussed. More extensive discussion of standard intensive care nursing and procedures can be found in the standard nursing texts.

NURSING ASSESSMENT

Neonatal nurses provide hour-by-hour care of each patient in the NICU. The experienced NICU nurse serves as the infant's link to the environment, often serving as "interpreter" for the infant through the careful assessment of physiologic data and infant behavioral responses to determine each individual infant's response to treatment. Because each nurse will generally be responsible for only two to three patients at any given time, the nurse remains in constant proximity to patients, often making observations and assessments that are reported to the health care team. Observations by nurses may stimulate further evaluation by the medical team and may result in laboratory testing and other diagnostic evaluations.

Nurses assess patients during their admission to the NICU and at regular intervals each day. This assessment includes evaluation of physical characteristics such as color, neuromuscular tone, skin integrity, vascular perfusion, and edema. Evaluation of the cardiovascular, respiratory, gastrointestinal, genitourinary, neurologic, musculoskeletal, and integumentary systems are made and documented in the medical record at least once every shift. Monitoring for disease processes such as necrotizing enterocolitis or gastrointestinal perforation includes measuring abdominal girth and observing for discoloration of the abdomen, gastric residuals, and frank or occult blood in stools. Sepsis monitoring involves assessment of hypothermia or hyperthermia, hypoglycemia, increased apnea and bradycardia, lethargy, hypotonia, and poor feeding. Other assessment activities include measuring and recording daily weights, intake, and output; temperature of the infant and

environment; heart rate; electrocardiogram; respiratory rate and quality of breathing; blood pressure and perfusion; and oxygen saturation monitoring. Neurobehavioral and developmental status includes the assessment of pain and discomfort in relation to the treatments being received, as well as the effect of other environmental stimuli.

Another aspect of assessment involves evaluating the technology used to support the infant. This includes checking the patency and functioning of all intravascular devices; evaluating the patency and security of endotracheal tubes (ETTs) and continuous positive airway pressure (CPAP) and cannula prongs; and assessing the placement and security of all other invasive tubes, such as chest tubes and nasogastric tubes. The presence and appropriate functioning of all respiratory equipment, monitoring devices, intravenous (IV) pumps, thermoregulatory devices, and emergency equipment such as bag, mask, and suctioning equipment should be confirmed with appropriate documentation.

Assessment of the family is an important responsibility shared with social workers and physicians. Nurses assist families as they come into contact with their infants, helping them understand the infant's medical problems, the type of equipment that is being used, and the infant's unique responses to the environment. Nurses often can identify behaviors in families that are commonly seen during this vulnerable period versus behaviors with significant concern for later attachment disorders or needing immediate crisis intervention. They also integrate parents and other caregivers into the daily care of the infant from the first days of hospitalization and assess how well the family is able to assume physical and emotional caregiving for their infant. This should be accomplished well before discharge to home.

Nursing the newborn requiring assisted ventilation and intensive care is complex and challenging. Nurses provide a vital link between the patient and the rest of the multidisciplinary team because of their knowledge, proximity to the patient, and skill at interpretation of physiologic, behavioral, and technical information.

THERMOREGULATION

Newborns are at risk for hypothermia and increased oxygen consumption due to their large surface area in relation to body weight. Premature infants are even more prone to hypothermia due to the absence of brown fat for thermogenesis and lack of subcutaneous fat for insulation. In addition, premature infants less than 30 weeks postconceptional age have immature skin, which results in increased evaporative heat loss. Newborns who require assisted ventilation often must be unclothed for appropriate assessment and monitoring, and they rely on thermoregulation devices such as incubators and radiant warmers to maintain their body temperature.

There are four mechanisms of heat transfer in newborns: conduction, convection, radiation, and evaporation. Although commonly seen as modes of heat loss, these mechanisms also can be used to provide heat sources for newborns. Conductive heat loss can occur with physical contact between the infant and a cooler surface (e.g., a cold bedside scale or x-ray plate). Conductive heat can be provided by warm blankets and heated mattresses and other surfaces. Convective heat loss results when infants are exposed to cool air or drafts. The primary convective heat source is the incubator with circulating warm air. Radiant heat loss is seen when the infant is placed next to cool surfaces, without direct contact, such as the wall of the incubator or a window; radiant heat emitted from the infant is transferred to the cooler surface in an effort to heat the surrounding surface. Techniques to reduce radiant heat loss include using heat shields inside incubators, double-walled incubators, and moving cribs away from windows. Radiant heat sources include radiant warming tables and heating lamps. Evaporative heat loss occurs when a surface is wet, such as an infant is covered with wet towels in the delivery room. Heat loss via evaporation also occurs when large surface areas are not covered with skin, such as in infants with abdominal wall defects. Techniques for reducing evaporative heat loss include keeping the skin surfaces dry and covering large abdominal wall defects with plastic wrap or bags. In addition, the premature infant less than 30 weeks of gestation has large evaporative heat losses due to immature skin. Reducing evaporative heat loss and excessive transepidermal water loss (TEWL) in small premature infants requires special techniques that are described in detail later in this section.

The goal of thermoregulation for newborns in the NICU is to maintain a neutral thermal environment. This is a stable environment in which the infant's temperature is maintained at 36° to 37°C while reducing oxygen consumption due to metabolic processes involved in heat loss and heat production. Neutral thermal environment temperatures (see Appendix 12) are guidelines for selecting temperature ranges that will achieve thermoregulation goals.

Radiant warmers are commonly used to provide thermal support in the delivery room and initial stabilization period. Many term newborns and large premature infants will be cared for on radiant warmers as long as assisted ventilation is required because of better accessibility during care procedures and visibility without clothing. Minimal oxygen consumption has been shown to occur when the radiant warmer is skin servocontrolled with the abdominal skin temperature maintained between 36.2° and 36.5°C.[1] Infants cared for on radiant warmers can experience both convective and evaporative heat loss. Use of plastic wrap over the sides of the radiant warmer will prevent convective heat losses and reduce radiant heat output.[2] Placing the infant on heated water-filled mattresses has also been shown to reduce heater output.[3] However, use of radiant warmers for very small prematures (<800 g) is debatable because the immature skin of these very small infants may cause massive fluid and heat losses under radiant warmers.

Incubators provide convective heat that circulates within a plexiglass enclosure. Double-walled incubators are most com-

monly used to prevent radiant heat loss by maintaining a warm inner incubator wall even in a cooler temperature room. Temperatures that achieve the neutral thermal environment can be selected using Appendix 12. Another technique is skin servocontrol, which uses a temperature probe that automatically adjusts the environment to maintain the skin temperature at 36.5°C. If the infant is clothed, swaddled, or "nested," use of skin servocontrol may prevent overheating.

For prematures less than 30 weeks of gestation, additional measures that prevent evaporative heat loss are necessary because the primary source of heat loss for these infants in the first weeks of life is evaporation due to fewer layers of stratum corneum, the uppermost layer of the skin.[4] Immediately after delivery, infants less than 28 weeks of gestation wrapped with occlusive polyethylene bags covering their torso and extremities had significantly better temperatures compared to infants who received drying and radiant heat in the delivery room due to significantly reduced evaporative heat and water loss; the wrapping was removed upon admission to the NICU. There was also a significant decrease in mortality in the infants who were wrapped.[5]

Several techniques that have been shown to reduce evaporative heat and TEWL in very-low-birthweight infants cared for in the NICU. Transparent adhesive dressings, such as Tegaderm, OpSite, and Bioocclusive, applied to large areas of skin surfaces reduce TEWL.[6–9] High humidity (>70%) added to the incubator has been shown to effectively reduce evaporative heat loss and TEWL.[10,11] Using incubators that actively heat and evaporate water separately from circulating heat prevents contamination with microorganisms (Fig. 7-1).[12,13] Application of petrolatum-based emollients, such as Aquaphor ointment (Beirsdorf), every 6 to 12 hours also reduces TEWL and can be used on infants on radiant warmers or under phototherapy without temperature increases or burns.[14] Although each of these techniques has been shown to be effective, none has been compared to another, so it is not clear which is most effective with the fewest side effects. However, addressing the important area of reducing excessive heat loss and TEWL is necessary in the care of the small premature infant with lung disease in order to maintain adequate hydration without excessive fluid intake. The goal of maintaining hydration and normal serum sodium levels on an intake of less than 150 cc/kg/day is optimal and achievable using one of these preventive strategies (see Chapter 24).

SKIN CARE

The skin of term and premature infants is a barrier against infection, toxicity from topically applied agents, and fluid and heat losses. It also is the source of tactile sensation. It is a challenge to maintain the integrity of this delicate organ when providing care to newborns requiring assisted ventilation. Trauma to skin can occur when life support or monitoring devices are removed or replaced, or when procedures such as blood sampling and chest tube insertion penetrate the skin's barrier. Significant morbidity and even mortality can be attributed to practices that cause trauma or alterations in normal skin function. Thus, understanding the developmental variations and selecting skin care practices that promote skin integrity are important aspects of nursing care in the NICU.

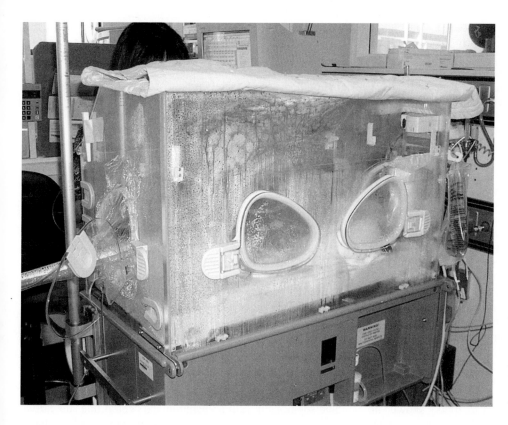

Figure 7-1. Incubator at 85% relative humidity, using specially designed heating process that prevents bacterial contamination. Moisture ("rainout") is seen when the temperature of the air inside the incubator is higher than the temperature of the incubator walls.

The term infant has a well-developed epidermis. The top layer of the epidermis, the *stratum corneum,* is structured similar to that of the adult stratum corneum with 10 to 20 layers. The premature infant has fewer layers of stratum corneum; it has been described histologically as thinner, with the cells of all strata being more compressed.[15] The result of this immature stratum corneum is increased permeability, increased risk of toxicity from substances applied to the skin, and increased evaporative heat and TEWL.

Fibrils that connect the top two layers of the skin, the epidermis and the dermis, are fewer and more widely spaced in the premature infant compared to the term infant.[15] Thus, premature infants are more vulnerable to blistering and have a tendency toward stripping of the epidermis when adhesives are removed because the adhesives may be more firmly attached to the epidermis than the epidermis is to the dermis.

The dermis is made of collagen and elastin fibers in a gel matrix; it provides mechanical strength, protection, and elasticity to the skin. The dermis of the term newborn is less developed than adult dermis.[15] Premature infants have a tendency to become edematous because they have even less collagen and fewer elastin fibers.[15] Both term and premature infants may be prone to necrotic injury from excessive edema because of alteration in blood flow to the epidermis. Edematous infants need protection from pressure and ischemic injury, including routine turning and use of surfaces that minimize pressure points, such as water beds and gelled mattresses or pads.

In the term newborn, skin surface pH immediately after birth is alkaline (mean pH 6.34) and declines to 4.95 within 4 days.[16] pH in premature infants is greater than 6 on the first day of life, decreases to 5.5 over the first week, and gradually declines to 5 by the fourth week.[17] An acid skin surface is credited with bacteriocidal qualities against some pathogens and serves in the defense against infection. A shift in skin surface pH from acidic to neutral can result in an increase in total numbers of bacteria, a shift in the species present, and a rise in TEWL.[18]

Bathing

The primary purpose of bathing in newborns is to remove waste materials. Antimicrobial cleansers are used in many newborn nurseries for the first bath but are effective in reducing colonization for only a 4-hour period after bathing; they are not indicated for daily care. Neither the Centers for Disease Control and Prevention nor the American Academy of Pediatrics recommends the initial or daily use of antimicrobial cleansers in newborns.[19,20]

The first bath should be given only when the infant's temperature has stabilized for 1 to 4 hours to prevent hypothermia, increased oxygen consumption, and respiratory distress.[21,22] Cleansers used for routine bathing include "baby" soaps, neutral pH synthetic detergents, and superfatted and even deodorant cleansers that contain antimicrobial properties. It is known that all cleansers are at least mild irritants to the skin, and frequent soaping increases the irritant effect.[23–25] A comparison of bathing with alkaline soap, compact bar, liquid synthetic detergent cleansers with a neutral pH, or water alone revealed alterations in skin surface pH, hydration of stratum corneum, and fat content of the skin with all cleansing agents in infants 1 to 16 months of age, but these effects were seen most markedly with alkaline soap.[26]

The effects of bathing on skin properties of small premature infants has not been studied to date. To reduce alterations in skin pH and to prevent dryness and irritation, the current recommendation is to limit bathing with mild cleansers to 2 to

3 times per week and to cleanse with warm water baths at other times until the skin becomes more mature. It has been shown that skin colonization with bacteria does not increase with bathing as infrequently as every 4 days.[27] Less frequent bathing may offer other advantages for premature infants, who have demonstrated physiologic and behavioral disruptions during sponge baths.[28] Immersion bathing, even of ventilated stable infants, may be soothing and less stressful (Fig. 7-2).

Moisturizers

The degree of hydration in the stratum corneum is related to the capacity of this layer to absorb and retain water. Moisturizers improve skin function by restoring intercellular lipids in dry or injured stratum corneum layers. These include products such as emollient creams, lanolin, mineral oil, and lotions. Many moisturizers have petrolatum as an ingredient because of its excellent hydrating and healing qualities.[29,30]

Beneficial effects of routine emollient use in premature infants less than 33 weeks of gestation were reported from a randomized controlled trial of 60 infants. Improved barrier function and reduced TEWL were seen in infants treated with a petrolatum-based, water-miscible emollient, and there was no increase in bacterial or fungal colonization and no evidence of altered skin temperature or burns when used under a radiant heater or concurrently with phototherapy.[14] However, a randomized trial of 1191 infants with birthweights of 501 to 1000 g showed an increase in coagulase-negative staphylococcus blood infections in infants weighing less than 750 g with routine application of petrolatum-based ointment for the first 2 weeks of life.[31] The benefits of emollient use for prevention of dermatitis and skin breakdown should be carefully weighed against the risk of infection. Emollients were used in the control group in this study to treat dryness, and there was no increase in infection when they were used on an "as needed" basis, rather than the twice daily regime.

Emollients can be safely used to treat excessive drying, skin cracking, or fissures. It is prudent to select products that are free of perfumes or dyes that can be absorbed and may result in later sensitization or toxicity.[32]

Skin Disinfectants

Decontamination of the skin before intensive procedures such as blood sampling or placement of vascular access devices is common practice in the NICU. Harmful effects from disinfectant solutions include skin necrosis, blistering, burns, and both alcohol and iodine toxicity.[33–35] Prospective studies of povidone-iodine use in nurseries document iodine absorption from the skin of premature infants with toxicity in the form of altered thyroid function.[36–39] No systemic toxicity from chlorhexidine gluconate, another skin disinfectant solution used in the NICU, has yet been reported.

Efficacy of skin decontamination is another important consideration. Povidone-iodine proved better than 70% isopropyl alcohol in reducing skin colonization in a study of pediatric patients.[40] A prospective randomized study comparing isopropyl alcohol, povidone-iodine, and 2% aqueous chlorhexidine solutions in skin preparation and central line site care in 668 adults showed that chlorhexidine significantly reduced catheter-related infections.[41] A sequential study of 254 premature and term infants in the NICU found that IV catheter colonization was reduced when 0.5% chlorhexidine in alcohol solution was used, compared to 10% povidone-iodine.[42]

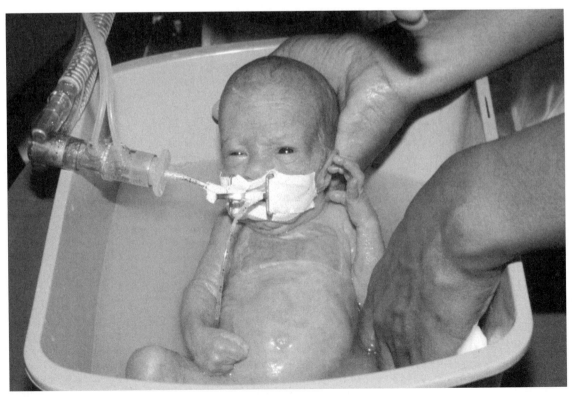

Figure 7-2. Ventilated infant during immersion bathing.

When any skin disinfectant solution is used, it is necessary to remove the preparation completely from skin surfaces when the procedure is finished. Water or saline is preferred for removing disinfectants to reduce the risk of further skin injury and toxicity from these caustic preparations.

Adhesive Application and Removal

The types of damage that result from adhesive removal include epidermal stripping, tearing, maceration, tension blisters, chemical irritation, sensitization, and folliculitis.[43] The traumatic effects of adhesive removal on premature infants have been documented and include reduced barrier function, increased TEWL, increased permeability, erythema, and skin stripping[44,45] (Fig. 7-3). Skin barrier function also is altered in adults with tape removal but requires repeated strippings.[46]

Solvents used to remove tape and adhesives contain hydrocarbon derivatives or petroleum distillates that have potential toxicity when they are absorbed. The risk of toxicity from absorption is greater in premature infants due to their immature stratum corneum and in newborns in general due to their larger surface area to body weight.[47] In addition, skin irritation and injury have been reported due to the use of solvents.[48]

Bonding agents such as tincture of benzoin or Mastisol that increase the adherence of adhesives may result in skin stripping and damage because they cause the adhesive to adhere more tenaciously to the epidermis than the fragile bond between epidermis and dermis, especially in the premature infant.[15] Such agents have previously been used to help hold ETTs in place but can no longer be recommended. Pectin-based skin barriers such as Hollihesive and DuoDERM are used between skin and adhesive, and mold well to curved surfaces while maintaining adherence in moist areas. Although studies initially described less visible trauma to skin with pectin barriers,[49–51] a study using direct measurements of skin barrier function found that pectin barriers caused a similar degree of trauma to commonly used plastic tape.[45] Despite this finding, pectin barriers continue to be used in the NICU because they mold well to curved surfaces and adhere even with moisture. Cavilon (3M), an alcohol-free plastic polymer skin protectant, has been shown to reduce measurable damage from adhesives in adults[52] and to reduce visible disruption in newborns,[53] and it is approved for use in term infants older than 30 days of age.[54] The effects of these barriers films with repeated applications or in moist environments have not been studied.

Preventing trauma from adhesives can be accomplished by minimizing use of tape when possible, dabbing cotton on tape to reduce adherence, and using hydrogel adhesives for electrodes. Delaying tape removal may be helpful because many adhesives attach less well to skin when they have been in place for more than 24 hours. Remove adhesives slowly and carefully, using water-soaked cotton balls, and pull the adhesive horizontal to the skin surface, folding the adhesive onto itself. Removal can be facilitated by using emollients or mineral oil if reapplication of adhesives at the site is not necessary.

Transparent adhesive dressings made from a polyurethane are impermeable to water and bacteria but allow the free flow of air, thus enabling the skin to "breathe" when in place. Uses for transparent dressings include securing IV catheters, percutaneous catheters and central venous lines, nasogastric tubes, chest tubes, and nasal cannulas. They also can be used to prevent skin breakdown over areas that have the potential for friction burns or pressure sores, such as the knees, elbows, or sacrum, or as a dressing over surface injuries.

Prevention and Treatment of Skin Breakdown due to Ischemic Injury

Infants at risk for ischemic injury due to pressure ulcers include those on high-frequency ventilation and ECMO because they are more difficult to turn or move. Hypotension leading to peripheral tissue hypoperfusion is another risk factor, as well as edema in critically ill patients who have leaking capillaries or require excessive fluid or blood products to maintain blood pressure. Paralyzing medications such as pancuronium, vecuronium, or high levels of sedation create poor tone and decreased movement,[55] increasing risk of skin breakdown. Therapies such as nasal CPAP require attaching devices such as nasal prongs or masks to maintain an airleak-proof "seal," which places infants at risk for necrotic injury due to the combined effects of pressure and reduced blood flow to the skin.

Sites for pressure ulcers in newborns on assisted ventilation include the occiput of the head and the ears, due to the heavy weight of the infant's head compared to the body. In addition, the circuit connected to the ETTs often is secured to avoid displacing the tube; thus, the infant cannot turn or move his or her head without assistance. With nasal CPAP, necrotic injury often occurs on the philtrum of the lip, the nares, or nasal septum.

Prevention of pressure ulcers to the head and ears involves using surfaces that alleviate pressure points. These include water mattresses or pillows, air mattresses, and gelled mattresses, pillows, wedges, or "doughnuts." Spenco gelled pads, ½-inch thick, are helpful supports for the head or under ears. Turning the infant a minimum of every 4 hours is necessary, with careful inspection of skin surfaces. Even when turning side to side is not feasible, lifting the head, shoulders, and hips and supporting these areas with pressure-reducing surfaces is helpful.

Treatment of breakdown and ischemic injury includes identifying the cause of the injury and determining if the wound is clean or infected. Skin cultures of purulent areas can be useful if the patient later becomes infected systemically, as these areas may have been the original portal of entry. Cleaning

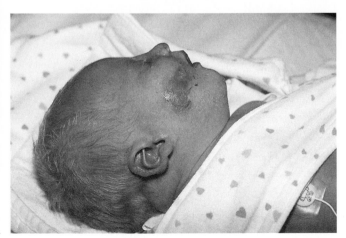

Figure 7-3. Damage caused by adhesive removal from endotracheal tube taping.

the excoriation with saline can gently debride the wound. Using a 20- to 30-mL syringe and 18-gauge Teflon catheter flushes out exudate without injuring tissue. Skin cleansers, soaps, or antiseptic solutions should not be used routinely on wounds because of cytotoxic effects that can delay the healing process.[56] This prohibition includes povidone-iodine, iodophor, hydrogen peroxide, acetic acid, Dakin's solution, or any alcohol-containing antiseptic.

Emollients or ointments are used to coat the skin breakdown or wound in order to facilitate the healing process. Petrolatum and petrolatum-based ointments such as Aquaphor ointment provide an occlusive layer that improves the migration of epithelial cells across the wound bed or skin surface, becoming part of the stratum corneum during healing.[29] Antibacterial ointments such as Polysporin, Bacitracin, and Neosporin can reduce colonization with gram-positive bacteria but may actually promote growth of gram-negative organisms.[57] Their use is not recommended because of the potential for infection and the potential sensitivity from these ointments.[58] If a culture indicates colonization with *Staphylococcus aureus,* Bactroban can be used; if a fungal organism such as *Candida albicans* is cultured, an antifungal ointment or cream is indicated.

Other dressings that provide moist healing processes include wet gauze, transparent adhesive dressings, hydrogel dressings, and hydrocolloid dressings. Indications for use of each are based on recommendations by wound experts[59] and on the particular location and other characteristics of the breakdown or wound.

With nasal CPAP, careful inspection for skin and tissue injury by removing the nasal prongs or mask is necessary every 3 to 4 hours. Despite meticulous care practices, tissue injury can occur on the philtrum of the lip or on the nasal septum (Fig. 7-4). Pectin dressings such as DuoDERM, which has a soft cushioned side, or a thin foam dressing such as Lyofoam, can be placed at strategic points around the upper lip and nose to reduce pressure and avoid injury. Some nurseries alternate between mask and prong systems to reduce pressure at any one point. Although some units apply steroid creams to the nasal prongs, the antiinflammatory effect of this practice has not been proven to be beneficial in reducing pressure necrosis.

DEVELOPMENTAL CARE

A significant aspect of providing nursing care to infants requiring assisted ventilation is to create an environment that reduces noxious stimuli, promotes positive development, and minimizes the negative effects of illness, early delivery, and separation from parents. Neonatal nurseries have become increasingly concerned about the negative effects of the NICU environment. Preventive strategies are focused on protecting the delicate, immature central nervous system of premature and ill newborns; the term *developmental care* is used to describe this process. Improved neurodevelopmental and medical outcomes have been reported in premature infants cared for in a developmentally supportive environment with caregivers specially educated in assessing premature infant behavior and modifying care practices to reduce negative or stressful responses.[60–64]

The NICU of today appears quite different than its predecessor 30 years ago: dimmed lights, crib covers, swaddling and

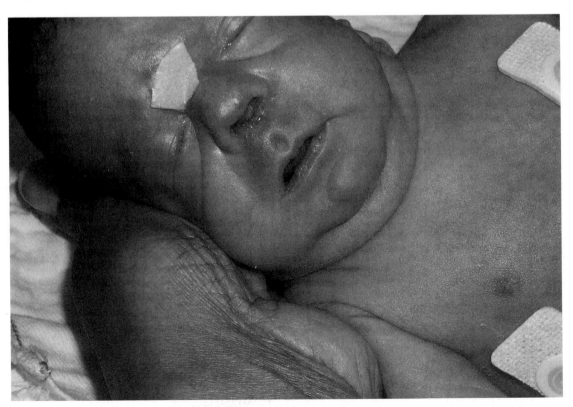

Figure 7-4. Tissue damage to the nares from nasal continuous positive airway pressure prongs.

supported positioning, decibel meters, and other techniques are familiar sights. Future research to better understand the effects and contribution of each individual intervention will shed more light on this area of neonatal nursing care.

Noise in the Neonatal Intensive Care Unit

Much of the technology used in the NICU generates a significant amount of noise and activity. Excessive noise can disturb and overstimulate the premature or ill term newborn, leading to agitation, crying, and "fighting" the ventilator. Decreased oxygenation, increased intracranial pressure, and elevated heart and respiratory rates have been reported to result from exposure to loud noise.[65–67] Noise also disrupts the sleep/wake cycle and may delay recovery and the ability to have positive interactions with parents and caregivers due to fatigue and overwhelming overstimulation.[68]

Noise levels in the NICU have been reported to range from 50 to 80 decibels. Inside the incubator, measurements from 55 to 88 decibels, with peak levels of 117, have been reported.[69] Damage to delicate auditory structures has been associated with prolonged exposure to over 90 decibels in adults; in neonates, decibel levels and length of exposure that result in hearing damage have not been identified. The possibility that immature auditory structures may be compromised because of the combination of noise and ototoxic medications makes the reduction of noise levels an important consideration.

Incubator motors generate an average of 55 to 60 decibels. Equipment and activity inside or around the incubator can add an additional 10 to 40 decibels.[69] Routine care activities, such as placing glass formula bottles on the bedside table, closing storage drawers, and opening packaged supplies, have been recorded at sound levels from 58 to 76 decibels; alarms from IV pumps and cardiorespiratory monitors also have measured 57 to 66 decibels.[70] Noise from staff talking, radios, and monitors can add to this cacophony.[71] Use of ear muffs and other similar devices have been studied,[67] but long-term studies are needed before routine use of ear coverings is recommended.

The American Academy of Pediatrics Committee on Environmental Health has concluded that exposure to environmental noise in the NICU may result in cochlear damage and may disrupt normal growth and development. Their recommendations include monitoring decibel readings and providing interventions to keep levels less than 45 decibels.[72]

Light in the Neonatal Intensive Care Unit

The effect of continuous light exposure on premature and term newborns in the NICU is another developmental consideration. Although constant light exposure in adult ICUs results in patient disorientation, effects on the newborn's behavioral state modulation are not well understood. Additional concerns about continuous light exposure include effects on eye structures such as the retina and the visual cortex.

Attempts to provide more normal lighting conditions have resulted in several studies on the effects of cycling light by alternating bright light periods with dimmed periods. Results of cycled lighting include more time spent in sleep states, increased weight gain,[73] lower motor activity levels, and lower heart rates.[74] The cycling of light periods for infants in the NICU may help in beginning the regulation of sleep/wake periods.

Concerns about the effects of light on infants in the NICU have also focused on the possible damaging effects on the developing optic structures already at risk for retinopathy of prematurity (ROP). Glass et al.[75] found a reduced incidence of ROP in infants weighing less than 2000 g when their incubators were covered with a plastic gel that reduced light intensity from 60 to 25 footcandles. Another study failed to see a change in the incidence of ROP when incubators were covered with blankets even when light levels were similarly reduced.[76] A large randomized controlled trial of 409 premature infants weighing less than 1251 g found no difference in the incidence of ROP when goggles that reduced visible light exposure by 97% and ultraviolet light by 100% were applied to each infant.[77]

Safe levels of light in NICU have not yet been established, and further research is needed to define the optimal approaches for lighting the immediate environment for the NICU patient. However, shielding the infants from light in incubators or on warming tablets reduces the unrelenting and noxious continuous exposure to light. This relatively easy intervention may prove beneficial in promoting rest, behavioral stability, and recovery.

Positioning

Body alignment and positioning has both physiologic and neurobehavioral effects. Proper positioning can prevent postural deformities such as hip abduction and external rotation, ankle eversion, retracted and abducted shoulders, increased neck hyperextension and shoulder elevation, cranial molding, or dolichocephaly, and it can improve neuromuscular development.[78–80] Learning supportive positioning techniques using rolls, nesting linens, and wedges is necessary to prevent postural abnormalities in the infant requiring assisted ventilation for either brief or longer periods of time.

Positioning can alter respiratory physiology. Placing an infant in the prone position increases oxygenation, tidal volume, and lung compliance and reduces energy expenditure compared to the supine position.[81–84] Prone positioning has become an important therapeutic intervention for adults or children with acute respiratory distress syndrome (ARDS), allowing ventilation of formerly dependent areas of the lung.[85–88] Similar effects may improve ventilation of the neonatal lung. Side-lying positions seem to have no significant effect on either oxygenation or carbon dioxide exchange.[89]

Body position affects gastric emptying and skin integrity, as well as neurobehavioral development. Activities such as hand-to-mouth ability, midline orientation, flexion, and self-soothing and self-regulatory abilities can be enhanced through facilitating body positions. Selecting positions that maintain unobstructed venous return from the head, such as keeping the infant's head in midline or side lying, may help in the prevention of intracranial hemorrhage or extension of existing head bleeds.

Gestational age, degree of illness, and use of neuromuscular blocking medications all influence positioning decisions. Critically ill premature and term infants cannot expend significant energy to move; they require assistance to attain any body position. Infants receiving neuromuscular blocking agents, such as pancuronium, must receive positioning assistance to maintain physiologic stability and comfortable appropriate postures. Thus, selecting an appropriate body position and assisting patients into it are important considerations for the nurse caring for infants receiving assisted ventilation (Table 7-1).

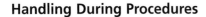

TABLE 7-1. Interventions to Position Neonates

1. Change positions every 2–3 hours for extremely ill or immature infants.
2. Promote hand-to-mouth behavior by allowing the hands to be free when caregiver is present; side-lying positioning assists in this goal.
3. "Nest" the infant by using blanket rolls or other positioning aids.
4. Place rolls under the hips when infant is prone to prevent hip abduction.
5. Roll shoulders gently forward with soft rolls when infant is both prone and supine to prevent shoulder extension.
6. Use water- or air-filled pillows under the head to minimize cranial molding; frequent position changes (every 2–3 hours) from side to side and midline facilitate this goal.
7. Support soles of feet with rolls to prevent ankle extension.
8. Swaddle with blankets or buntings when infant is stable to promote flexion and self-regulatory behavior.
9. Consider gentle massage to promote skin blood flow in infants with neuromuscular blocking agents; reposition every 2 hours to prevent pressure sores.
10. Position with right side down or prone to promote gastric emptying; prone position is best to minimize effects of gastroesophageal reflux.
11. Elevate head of bed after feedings to reduce pressure of full stomach against the diaphragm and improve respiratory capacity.
12. Hold stable infants, even when infant is on the ventilator; holding is soothing and provides vestibular stimulation similar to fetal experience.

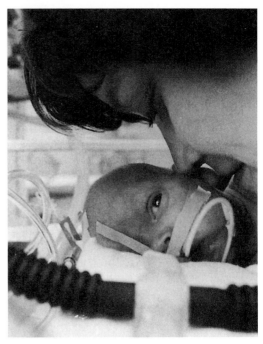

Figure 7-5. Intubated infant responding to mother's touch and whispering.

Handling During Procedures

Premature and seriously ill neonates on assisted ventilation are continually bombarded by procedures aimed at improving their physiologic status or monitoring their condition. With continuous monitoring using pulse oximetry, the effects of routine procedures on oxygenation, including heelstick blood sampling, intubation, suctioning the ETT, chest physical therapy, weighing, bathing, changing diapers, and even social interaction, were revealed; procedures often resulted in significant and prolonged reductions in oxygenation.[90–93] The extent of hypoxemia and overall distress can be dramatically reduced when personnel modify their caregiving according to the infant's responses.

Careful observations of oxygenation and behavioral reactions in ventilated infants with appropriate individualized interventions can reduce the amount of stress experienced by the infant. Supporting the infant's body position can reduce the stressful effects of procedures and other interventions. Swaddling, rolls, and use of other containment techniques have been shown to improve physiologic and behavioral organization during weighing,[94] suctioning, and heelsticks[95,96] and to provide comfort from pain.[97] The positive effects of infant massage techniques in the NICU include improved weight gain and longer rest periods,[98] but they should be used with careful observation of individual infant's reactions to this form of stimulation and should not be used in infants with physiologic instability.

Infants requiring assisted ventilation must undergo daily invasive procedures, which include heelsticks, endotracheal suctioning, IV placement, venipunctures, and adhesive removal. A descriptive study showed that infants younger than 31 weeks averaged a mean of 142 painful procedures during their NICU

stay[99]; we encourage neonatal units to question the need for each and every potentially harmful invasive procedure.

Interventions such as containment and offering a pacifier have been shown to reduce overall crying time and improve behavioral response to pain and discomfort.[96,100,101] Oral sucrose has been shown to reduce crying when it is offered to newborns during painful procedures such as heelstick blood sampling.[102] Dipping a pacifier in sucrose or sterile water has also been shown to significantly reduce pain responses in premature infants[101]; however, the use of oral sucrose for premature infants undergoing repeated painful procedures has not been studied.

Regular administration of opiates and sedatives for ventilated infants remains controversial. Use of opiates for ventilated infants during routine caregiving procedures, such as weighing, bathing, and suctioning, has been shown to reduce hypoxemia and associated distress.[103] However, the calming effects of medications, while reducing patient movement and promoting sleep, may interfere with the infant's own respiratory effort and prolong weaning from assisted ventilation. Medications are best used judiciously, taking into account the stage of illness, therapeutic goals, and individual infant characteristics. Other causes of agitation should be considered, including inadequate ventilation. In many cases, patient comfort is often the best indicator of the appropriateness of selected ventilatory support parameters, perhaps more useful than blood gas analyses. Caregivers should encourage parents to touch, talk, and interact with their baby as a calming measure to increase patient comfort and decrease stress (Fig. 7-5).

CARE OF PARENTS

During the initial phase of hospitalization, parents of critically ill infants experience significant loss of emotional equilibrium. The expected outcome for their pregnancy has been changed from a healthy, full-term newborn to a newborn who is premature or has significant medical or surgical problems. If problems are detected during prenatal evaluation or if the mother is treated for premature labor for any length of time, families may begin to form some idea of the situation they are facing. However, many families have not faced a crisis of such importance and may need help in developing coping skills, understanding complicated medical information, and learning how to be a parent and an advocate for their infant. Nurses utilize therapeutic communication, crisis intervention, and supportive techniques to assist families during this time.[104]

Because many families may have additional social risk factors, including language or cultural differences, poverty, chronic illness, or substance abuse, health professionals need knowledge about the impact of these factors on coping with crises and parenting. The importance of early intervention cannot be emphasized strongly enough, and interventions by neonatal nurses, along with NICU social workers and neonatologists, can have considerable positive effects on high-risk families during this time of disruption.

Family-centered care is both a philosophy and an approach that can enhance the potential of families to cope with the crisis and experience a positive outcome. In the NICU that embraces this philosophy, parents are partners; they become an integral part of the caregiving team from the beginning. They are not "visitors"; they have full rights to stay with their infant at all times. Siblings can visit, along with family members and friends that have been identified by the parents; some units restrict sibling visits and other family members to specific times to reduce crowding and noise levels. Parents, as partners in care, are given information specific to their baby and are requested to participate in all decisions about their baby. While advocating this enhanced involvement of parents with their own babies, it is important to recognize that most NICUs are open units and the privacy of other patients must be maintained.

Family-Centered Care

Principles for family-centered neonatal care include open and honest communication in terms of medical and ethical considerations, in-depth medical information that is provided in terms that are meaningful and understandable, and access to other parents who have had infants in similar circumstances. Whenever possible, information is provided to families during pregnancy if prenatal diagnosis about a neonatal problem is found. Parents are given the right to make decisions for their infants about aggressive treatments once they are fully informed. Additional areas addressed in family-centered care are alleviation of pain, ensuring an appropriate environment, providing safe and effective treatments, and policies and programs that promote parenting skills and maximum involvement of families with their infant in the NICU.[105–108] Key elements of family-centered care are outlined in Table 7-2.

Parent and family education is provided throughout the infant's hospitalization in the NICU. Initially, parents need information about their infant's medical condition, what it means in terms of day-to-day care and prognosis, and an orientation to the NICU in terms of the personnel they will encounter ("who does what"). Pamphlets and booklets about premature infants or specific disease conditions are helpful. There are several books written by both parents and NICU professionals that contain detailed information, illustrations, and

TABLE 7-2. Key Elements of Family-Centered Care

- Incorporating into policy and practice the recognition that the family is the constant in a child's life while the service systems and support personnel within those systems fluctuate
- Facilitating family/professional collaboration at all levels of hospital, home, and community care:
  - Care of an individual child
  - Program development, implementation, evaluation, and evolution
  - Policy formation
- Exchanging complete and unbiased information between families and professionals in a supportive manner at all times
- Incorporating into policy and practice the recognition and honoring of cultural diversity, strengths, and individuality within and across all families, including ethnic, racial, spiritual, social, economic, educational, and geographic diversity
- Recognizing and respecting different methods of coping and implementing comprehensive policies and programs that provide developmental, educational, emotional, environmental, and financial support to meet the diverse needs of families
- Encouraging and facilitating family-to-family support and networking
- Ensuring that hospital, home, and community service and support systems for children needing specialized health and developmental care and their families are flexible, accessible, and comprehensive in responding to diverse family-identified needs
- Appreciating families and children as children, recognizing that they possess a wide range of strengths, concerns, emotions, and aspirations beyond their need for specialized health and developmental services and support

Reprinted with permission from Shelton TL, Stepanek JS: Family-Centered Care for Children Needing Specialized Health and Development Services. Bethesda, Md., Association for the Care of Children's Health, 1994.

accounts of parents' reactions to the NICU experience.[109,110] The Internet is another source of information for parents. Each unit should wisely evaluate what resources on the Internet contain the most up-to-date, factual, nonbiased information about specific conditions and post these resources for parents to access if they wish. Written information is valuable, but it is not a substitute for verbal interchange with parents. Family conferences should not only focus on the specific medical problems of the baby but also on parental concerns, as well as their feelings and reactions to what is happening to them and to their infant.

An explanation about the environment surrounding the infant is important, including the type of monitors, special beds, and other equipment being used in the care of their infant. Nurses facilitate parental participation in the physical care of their infant by assisting them to learn caregiving activities such as comfort measures, bathing, skin or mouth care, changing the diaper, taking the temperature, providing breast milk, and holding the infant as soon as he or she is stable on the ventilator or in oxygen (Fig. 7-6).

Holding the infant is an important step in the process of attachment for both parents, as it helps counteract the loss of physical contact with their infant. In recent years, holding infants who require assisted ventilation has become more common in many NICUs, as staff become cognizant of the importance of holding for the parents and develop the necessary skills and comfort level themselves in assessing and handling the ventilated infant. Some nurseries have even found techniques to have parents hold infants who are on high-frequency oscillatory ventilators.[111] A special type of holding,

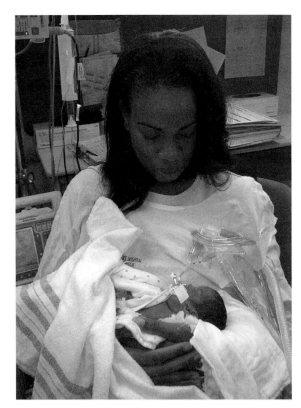

Figure 7-6. Parent holding infant receiving conventional ventilation.

skin-to-skin or "kangaroo holding," is now practiced in many nurseries, even for ventilated infants.[112]

Skin-to-Skin Holding

During skin-to-skin holding, the mother or father holds the infant clothed only in a diaper, against the skin of his or her chest. The infant then is covered with a blanket or the parent's clothing (Fig. 7-7). Practical issues during skin-to-skin holding include transfer techniques from bed/incubator to parent, selecting chairs that support parent and infant comfortably, and monitoring during holding, Transfer techniques include carefully moving the baby to the seated parent or having the mother or father stand while the infant is placed on her or his chest, then carefully lowering herself or himself with the infant to the chair. Other nurseries have invested in special lounge or reclining chairs that can be raised to the level of the infant's incubator; these chairs provide a comfortable way for the parent to relax during holding for prolonged periods. Continuous monitoring of heart rate, oxygenation, and skin temperature is necessary to determine each individual infant's tolerance during holding.

Benefits of early skin-to-skin holding on the psychological state of the parent, improved lactation, and parent-infant bonding have been proven and recognized.[113,114] A number of studies have evaluated the effects of skin-to-skin holding on the infant with sometimes conflicting results seen in temperature stability[115,116] and other physiologic parameters.[115–118] A prospective study of 53 premature infants with mean weight of 1253 g (range 631 to 1700 g) at study, including five ventilated infants, found that the infants remained clinically stable and had more efficient gas exchange, with no risk of hypothermia

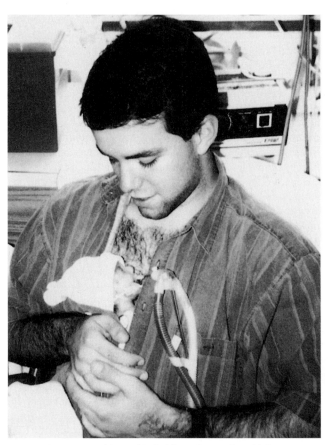

Figure 7-7. Skin-to-skin holding of a ventilated infant.

even for infants weighing less than 1000 g.[119] Adverse effects of skin-to-skin holding were reported by another study, including a significant increase in the frequency of bradycardia and hypoxemia, which may be due to an increase in temperature.[120] Careful monitoring of all physiologic parameters is necessary during skin-to-skin holding to assess each infant's response to this valuable experience and to determine when intervention is needed.

RESPIRATORY CARE

Monitoring and observing ventilation equipment, oxygen delivery systems, and patient oxygenation are ongoing activities and essential components of nursing care for infants receiving assisted ventilation; many of these activities are responsibilities shared with respiratory therapists in the NICU (see Chapter 6). Special concerns while caring for infants requiring assisted ventilation includes securing ETTs, nasal CPAP, and oxygen cannulas, and maintaining a patent airway via suctioning.

Airway Security

Accidental dislodgment of the ETT can result in serious complications, including acute hypoxia, bradycardia, and potential damage to the trachea or larynx. Preventing accidental extubations is an important responsibility of bedside care-

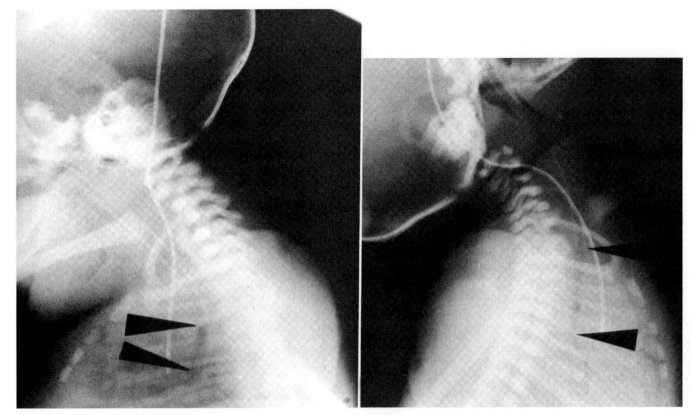

Figure 7-8. X-ray films showing movement of the endotracheal tube with head position changes. The film on the left shows the tip moving down toward the carina when the neck is flexed *(second arrow)*; the film on the right shows the tip moving up in the neck *(first arrow)* when the neck is extended. (From Todres ID, deBros F, Kramer SS, et al: Endotracheal tube displacement in the newborn infant. J Pediatr 89:126–127.)

givers. Factors associated with accidental extubations include the length of time intubated, agitation, ETT suctioning, weighing, turning patient's head, chest physiotherapy, loose tape, short ETTs, and retaping of the ETT.[121] The incidence of accidental extubations reported in the literature is variable.[122–124]

Many different techniques have been described to secure ETTs, ranging from adhesives with bonding agents[125,126] or pectin barriers,[50,51] suturing the tube to tape, and using metal or plastic bows to prevent slipping of the ETT.[127] In addition, there are now commercially available products for securing ETTs in newborns. Skin integrity should be a consideration regardless of the method used; many NICUs firmly established with adhesive bonding agents such as tincture of Benzoin or Mastisol should consider replacing these agents with pectin barriers or protective barrier films to prevent injury to the epidermis when the ETT is removed or retaped. Taping techniques are demonstrated in Figures 6-4 and 6-5.

Products that prevent palatal groove formation, acquired cleft palate, and defective dentition have been described,[128–130] but they are not in widespread use at the current time. Placing the ETT at the side of the mouth, rather than at the center, and alternating from one side to the other with retaping can minimize the pressure of the ETT on the infant's palate.

No research has identified the "best practice" for ETT taping. It is imperative that each NICU develop a standard practice that is consistently used to avoid confusion during intubations and ETT retaping and that all members of the multidisciplinary team agree on the method selected. A card specifying the depth to which the ETT is inserted should be posted at each bedside, with the centimeter marking that is at the patient's lip displayed (see Fig. 6-15). Adhesion of the ETT taping should be inspected often, and the ETT should be retaped whenever necessary to prevent accidental dislodgment. Regular monitoring of unplanned extubations can be incorporated into quality improvement audits, and practices that can reduce the number of untoward events should be implemented.

Problems with ETT movement and malposition occur. Position of the ETT may be altered with inadequate fixation of the tube, changes in patient position, and flexion and extension of the head. Because the trachea of a newborn is quite short (mean 57 mm) and even shorter in premature infants, movement of the ETT can result in displacement, causing the tube to move into the right mainstem bronchus with flexion or into the neck with extension[131,132] (Fig. 7-8). In addition to potentially altering ventilation and blood gas parameters and causing tracheal damage, ETT movement can result in misinterpretation of the ETT position on x-ray films. The infant's head should be carefully positioned in a "neutral" position to avoid extension or flexion when obtaining x-ray films. Some authors have even devised plastic forms to keep the infant's head in place when x-ray films are being obtained[133] to avoid the unrewarding activity of pushing the ETT in further, only to have to withdraw it when obtaining the next x-ray film. The ETT should also be positioned with the bevel in an anterior placement to avoid having the bevel abut against the tracheal wall with head movement or position changes[134] (Fig. 7-9).

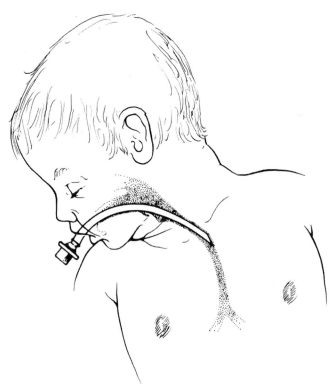

Figure 7-9. Illustration of endotracheal tube bevel abutting against the wall of the trachea. (From Brasch RC, Heldt GP, Hecht ST: Endotracheal tube orifice abutting the tracheal wall: a cause of infant airway obstruction. Radiology 141:387–391, 1981.)

Suctioning

The presence of an ETT causes irritation to tissue and increased secretions. It is necessary to clear this artificial airway on a regular basis to maintain ventilation for the infant. ETT suctioning has been associated with a number of complications in infants, including hypoxemia,[135,136] bradycardia,[135,137] atelectasis,[138] mucosal trauma, and pneumothorax.[139–141] Systemic adverse effects are also of concern, including increased blood pressure,[142,143] changes in cerebral blood volume,[142–145] and reduced oxygenation in cerebral blood flow.[142,144] Infection is a concern, in terms of both nosocomially acquired pneumonia and introduction of microorganisms into the bloodstream through injured mucosa.

Important considerations in ETT suctioning for NICU patients include frequency of suctioning, depth of suctioning, use of instillates such as normal saline, and use of closed suction devices. Because there are hazards associated with suctioning, many NICUs suction intubated patients only when assessment indicates it is needed, that is, when breath sounds are moist or congested, when secretions are visible, or when the infant is either hypoxic or agitated with no known cause.[146] During high-frequency oscillatory or jet ventilation (HFV), it is not always obvious when suctioning is needed, and some nurseries implement routine suctioning every 4 hours for patients on HFV.

Suctioning to the end of the ETT, to a premeasured depth that includes the ETT and adapter, is a common practice performed out of concern about trauma to the tracheal mucosa or introduction of microorganisms through injured mucosa[147] or bronchial[148] and esophageal perforation.[149–151] Regular use of normal saline to lubricate the ETT with volumes of 0.25 to 0.5 mL is routine in most nurseries.[152]

Closed suctioning systems that are placed inline with the ETT and ventilator circuit have become popular in many nurseries. Small studies support the reduction in transient hypoxemia and bradycardia with closed suctioning versus open suctioning methods.[153,154] Other potential advantages to closed suctioning include ease of use, with need for only one person, and reduced contamination with microorganisms. Although maintenance of lung volumes during suctioning has been mentioned as an advantage during closed suctioning because positive pressure is maintained from the ventilator, this was not seen in bench test evaluation of these systems.[155] The closed suction system (Fig. 7-10) is replaced once a day. Disadvantages include its cost and the potential for tracheal and/or bronchial injury if suctioning is done past the tip of the ETT.

Sudden Deterioration

A sudden deterioration can occur due to a multitude of factors in the ventilated neonatal patient. NICU nurses are often the first to detect the change of condition and should be prepared to respond to each situation. Among the causes of acute decompensation are malfunction of the ventilator, malpositioning or plugging of the ETT, and pulmonary air leaks.

The cause of acute deterioration is not always apparent. Often the assessment and problem solving of these events occur during resuscitation. Hand ventilation with a resuscitation bag connected to a manometer is initiated immediately and FIO_2 increased to 100%. Breath sounds are immediately auscultated; if breath sounds are equal bilaterally, the tube is likely in proper position and free from thick secretions. If the breath sounds are distant, if air entry is detected in the gastric area and is accompanied by distention, or if an audible cry is heard, the ETT may have slipped into the esophagus. An end-tidal CO_2 monitor or detection device will show an absence of CO_2 during expiration. The ETT should be removed immediately and bag-and-mask ventilation provided until the infant is reintubated. Once replaced, the ETT should be securely taped at the same place as the previous tube and an x-ray film obtained to confirm appropriate ETT position.

If the breath sounds are louder on the right side, the ETT may have slipped into the right mainstem bronchus. A quick check using the "7-8-9 rule" (weight in kilograms + 6) may alert the clinician that the tube is positioned too far in. A chest x-ray film can confirm this diagnosis and will help differentiate between a right mainstem bronchus ETT and an air leak in the left lung. If the ETT extends down into the right bronchus, the left lung may appear atelectatic on x-ray film. The appropriate adjustment to ETT position is determined by x-ray film, and the tube is repositioned and retaped securely.

If the ETT is plugged with secretions, breath sounds may be diminished bilaterally, with decreased rise of the chest wall during hand ventilation. Initially, the ETT should be suctioned with normal saline lavage in an attempt to remove the secretions. If this measure is unsuccessful, the ETT is removed and bag-and-mask ventilation initiated until the ETT is replaced.

An extremely serious and potentially life-threatening cause of sudden deterioration is tension pneumothorax. The immediate clinical presentations are cyanosis, bradycardia, decreased blood pressure, and narrowing pulse pressure, as well as a shift in the point of maximal impulse of the heart with breath sounds

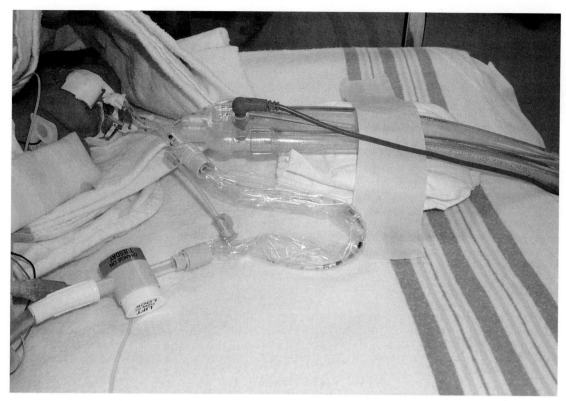

Figure 7-10. Closed suction system used for endotracheal tube suctioning.

diminished or absent on the affected side. Once the decompensation is detected, the patient is hand ventilated with 100% oxygen. The diagnosis may be confirmed by transillumination of the chest with a high-density fiberoptic light source or with a chest x-ray film. The situation may be so severe that the air in the pleural space is emergently evacuated with needle aspiration before the diagnosis is confirmed by x-ray film. Once the air is evacuated and the patient is somewhat stabilized, a chest tube is inserted and placed to water seal drainage, and vacuum is applied at 10 to 20 cm H_2O pressure. An algorithm that describes interventions for acute deterioration for infants on assisted ventilation is shown in Figure 8-9.

High-Frequency Ventilation

Assessment of the infant while he or she is receiving high-frequency ventilation is frequent and extensive, and it differs from routine nursery assessment of infants on conventional ventilation due to the absence of tidal breathing (see Chapter 11). It is not possible to auscultate the chest for either breath sounds or apical pulse while on high-frequency ventilation, and skill in observing for chest "wiggle" and other parameters of ventilation adequacy is used. In many cases, the infant's condition while he or she is undergoing high-frequency ventilation can change rapidly because of both the infant's underlying pulmonary pathology and the device in use. It is possible to interrupt or pause the ventilator briefly during the assessment process in order to auscultate breath sounds and listen for heart murmurs; however, this can destabilize the infant. Coordination among multidisciplinary team members is recommended for these assessment periods so that the time the patient is removed from high-frequency ventilation is kept to a minimum.

This concern about minimizing periods when the infant is not connected to the ventilator circuit is primarily because the mean airway pressure will fall, allowing the alveoli to collapse.[111] Closed suctioning, utilizing inline devices described in the previous section, is used to prevent disconnecting from ventilation during suctioning. Many NICUs use in-bed scales, weigh infants infrequently, or simply do not weigh patients receiving high-frequency ventilation to prevent destabilizing the respiratory system. Depending on the high-frequency ventilator in use, positioning and turning infants on high-frequency ventilation may require two persons, one to rotate the infant while a partner briefly disconnects the ventilator circuit while the ventilator itself remains in a fixed location. Some units have devised ways for parents to hold infants while they are on high-frequency ventilation,[111] although many still do not allow holding for these infants. Table 7-3 lists assessment and care practices specific to high-frequency ventilation.

Inhaled Nitric Oxide

The use of inhaled nitric oxide (iNO) is rapidly expanding in newborns receiving assisted ventilation (see Chapter 14). Following approval by the U.S. Food and Drug Administration (FDA) for treatment of pulmonary hypertension in term newborns in 1998, use of this selective pulmonary vasodilator has become mainstreamed in many NICUs for this indication.

Care of the infant receiving iNO requires comprehensive knowledge of physiology, pathology, and treatment regimes. Nursing care of the newborn receiving iNO includes careful monitoring of the gas administration and preventing any interruption of iNO administration during hand ventilation, turning, moving, or suctioning[156]; closed suctioning systems are recommended. Regular monitoring of methemoglobin levels is necessary, and gradual weaning of iNO is necessary, even in patients who are "nonresponders," due to the down-regulation of the patient's endogenous NO production during treatment with iNO and the potential for destabilizing patients with marginal oxygenation and reserves.

Extracorporeal Membrane Oxygenation

ECMO is the use of prolonged cardiopulmonary bypass to support oxygenation and ventilation (see Chapter 16). ECMO is used as a rescue technique in approximately 100 specially equipped NICUs in the United States. Patients considered for ECMO are generally term or near-term infants with life-threatening yet reversible cardiopulmonary conditions, including meconium aspiration syndrome, idiopathic pulmonary hypertension, septic shock, and diaphragmatic hernia with pulmonary hypoplasia, which have failed to respond to conventional intensive treatment.

The care team is larger than that for infants requiring mechanical ventilation alone, as described in Chapter 16. The specialized nursing care is described in Tables 7-4 and 7-5.

SUMMARY

The daily care of newborns who require assisted ventilation involves knowledge that extends beyond pulmonary anatomy and physiology, and technology. The nursing care for these infants demands advanced knowledge of multiple organ systems, precision in caregiving, and creative problem-solving. Also critical to successful outcomes are attention to developmental care and family-centered care during this vulnerable period for infants and their families.

TABLE 7-3. Nursing Interventions in Infants Receiving High-Frequency Jet and High-Frequency Oscillatory Ventilation

Intervention	HFJV	HFOV
ETT suctioning	Suction catheter inserted into ETT, continuous suction applied. Avoid manual bagging. Adjust HFJV or CMV setting to facilitate recovery.	Performed on HFOV. Suction with closed, inline suction system; reconnect to HFOV. Hand bagging is avoided. MAP increased if needed to facilitate recovery.
Positioning	Patient can be placed in all positions. Limited by short, but flexible, length of "jet" tubing to patient box. Patient box sits next to head. Can move patient while connected to HFJV.	Positioning on HFOV limited by rigid tubing that delivers bias flow. Turning "head to toe" by moving the baby 180° while the circuit remains fixed is the most common technique. Infants must always remain elevated above the rigid circuit tubing to prevent aspiration of condensed humidity.

CMV, conventional mechanical ventilation; ETT, endotracheal tube; HFJV, high-frequency jet ventilation; HFOV, high-frequency oscillatory ventilation; MAP, mean airway pressure.
Adapted from Karp T: High frequency ventilation: Life in the fast lane? Presented at Neonatal Nurses National Conference, Nottingham, England, September 25, 1993, and adapted from Inwood S: High frequency oscillation and Karp T: High frequency jet ventilation. In Nugent J (ed): Acute Respiratory Care of the Newborn (Monograph), Petaluma, Calif., Neonatal Network, 1991; Avila K, Mazza LV, Morgan-Trujillo L: High-frequency oscillatory ventilation: A nursing approach to bedside care. Neonatal Network 13:23, 1994.

TABLE 7-4. Nursing Responsibilities and Interventions for ECMO

Responsibility	Intervention
Obtain and document baseline physiologic data	Record weight, length, head circumference Draw blood samples for CBC, electrolytes, calcium, glucose, BUN, creatinine, PT/PTT, platelets, arterial blood gases Record vital signs: heart rate; respiratory rate; systolic, diastolic, and mean blood pressures; temperature
Ensure adequate supply of blood products for replacement	Draw type and cross-match samples for two units of red cells, fresh-frozen plasma Keep one unit of packed cells and fresh-frozen plasma always available in the blood bank
Maintain prescribed pulmonary support	Maintain ventilator parameters Administer muscle relaxants if indicated
Assemble and prepare equipment	Prepare infusion pumps to maintain arterial lines and infusion of parenteral fluids and medications into the ECMO circuit Place the infant on a radiant warmer with the head positioned at the foot of the bed to provide thermoregulation and access for cannulation Attach infant to physiologic monitoring devices for heart rate, intra-arterial blood pressure, transcutaneous oxygen, etc. Insert urinary catheter and nasogastric tube; place to gravity drainage Prepare loading dose of heparin (100 U/kg) Prepare heparin solution for continuous infusion (100 U/mL/D5W or 25 U/kg/mL/D5W) Prepare paralyzing drug (pancuronium bromide 0.1 mg/kg); prepare analgesic (fentanyl 15 µg/kg) Assist in insertion of arterial line (umbilical or peripheral)

TABLE 7-4. Nursing Responsibilities and Interventions for ECMO—cont'd

Responsibility	Intervention
Monitor cardiopulmonary status	Monitor heart rate, intra-arterial blood pressure, and CVP continuously Obtain blood gases after paralysis and during cannulation as indicated by the infant's response to the procedure
Be prepared to administer cardiopulmonary support	Have available medications and blood products to correct hypovolemia, bradycardia, acidosis, cardiac arrest
Administer medications	Give paralyzing and analgesic drugs systemically just prior to cannulation of internal jugular vein; give loading dose of heparin systemically when vessels are dissected free and are ready to be cannulated
Reduce ventilator parameters to minimal settings	Once adequate bypass is achieved, reduce ventilatory support to "rest settings": peak inspiratory pressure to 16–20 cm H_2O, positive end-expiratory pressure to 5–10 cm H_2O, ventilator rate to 10–20 breaths/min, and FiO_2 to 21%
Monitor and document physiologic parameters	Record hourly: heart rate, blood pressure (systolic, diastolic, mean), CVP, respirations, temperature, transcutaneous Po_2, CO_2, oxygen saturation, ACT, ECMO flow Measure hourly and accurately intake and output of all body fluids (urine, gastric contents, blood); measure every 8 hours urine pH, protein, glucose, blood, specific gravity; Hematest all stools Regularly assess color, breath sounds, heart tones, murmurs, cardiac rhythm, arterial pressure waveform, peripheral perfusion, oxygen saturation Perform ongoing neurologic check, including fontanelle tension; pupil size and reaction; level of consciousness; reflexes, tone, and movement of extremities Record ventilator parameters hourly Draw arterial blood gases from umbilical or peripheral line every 4–8 hours All other blood specimens are drawn from the ECMO circuit: electrolytes, calcium, platelets, Chemstrip, hematocrit every 4–8 hours, CBC, PT/PTT, BUN, creatinine, total and direct bilirubin, plasma hemoglobin, fibrinogen, fibrin split products, blood culture as indicated
Administer medications	Remove air bubbles and double-check dosages before infusion Administer no medications intramuscularly or by venipuncture Place all medications and fluids into the venous side of the ECMO circuit Prepare and administer the arterial line (umbilical or peripheral) infusion Administer parenteral alimentation
Provide pulmonary support	Perform endotracheal suctioning based on individual assessment and need Maintain patent airway; be alert to extubation or plugging Obtain daily chest films and tracheal aspirant culture as indicated Maintain ventilator parameters
Prevent bleeding	Avoid rectal probes, injections, venipunctures, heelsticks, cuff blood pressures, chest tube stripping, restraints; chest percussion can be done gently with vibrator Avoid invasive procedures; do not change nasogastric tube, urinary catheters, or endotracheal tube unless absolutely necessary; use premeasured endotracheal tube suction technique Observe for blood in the urine, stools, endotracheal or nasogastric tubes
Maintain excellent infection control	Change all fluids and tubing daily Change dressings daily and prn Clean urinary catheter site daily Maintain strict aseptic and hand-washing technique Use universal barrier precautions
Provide physical care	Keep skin dry and clean Pressure points on head (temporal or occiput area) should be protected with sheepskin, or water-, air-, or gel-filled pillows Give mouth care prn Provide range of motion as indicated Turn child side to side every 1–2 hours
Provide pain management, sedation, stress reduction	Minimize noise level Cluster patient care to maximize sleep periods Administer analgesia: fentanyl 9–18 microgram/kg/hr (increased dosage required due to fentanyl binding to membrane oxygenator) Manage iatrogenic physical dependency by following a dose reduction regimen (reduce dose 10% every 4 hours)

ACT, activated clotting time; BUN, blood urea nitrogen; CBC, complete blood count; CVP, central venous pressure; ECMO, extracorporeal membrane oxygenation; prn, as needed; PT/PTT, prothrombin time/partial thromboplastin time.
Reprinted and modified by permission of Neonatal Network, Acute Respiratory Care of the Neonate, 1991.

TABLE 7-5. ECMO Specialist Responsibilities and Interventions

Responsibility	Intervention
Maintain and monitor ECMO circuit	Check circuit carefully for air, clots, tightness of connectors, stopcocks Check bladder box alarm function or venous/arterial monitoring systems Monitor pump arterial and venous blood gases each shift to assess oxygenator function; pump arterial Po_2 0 mm Hg, CO_2 retention, or leaking membrane indicates oxygenator failure
Assess infant	Check cannula placement and stability; measure distance from insertion site Assess breath sounds and neurologic status Observe volume of fluid and blood drainage Monitor vital signs and laboratory values
Maintain prescribed parameters: pH 7.35–7.45; Pao_2 60–80 mm Hg; $Paco_2$ 35–45 mm Hg	Maintain infant's systemic arterial blood gases by adjusting sweep gas and pump flow
MAP 45–55 mm Hg; Hct 45%–55%; platelets 70,000–100,000; Svo_2 >70%; Sao_2 >90%	Maintain MAP, Hct, and platelets by infusion of appropriate blood products
ACT 180–250 seconds	Assess ACT hourly or as needed; titrate heparin infusion to maintain parameters
Assist nurse in care	Draw all blood samples from circuit except systemic arterial blood gases Coordinate recording of intake and output with nurse Assist in all position changes Administer and monitor all medications, blood products, and fluids placed into the pump circuit

ACT, activated clotting time; ECMO, extracorporeal membrane oxygenation; Hct, hematocrit; MAP, mean arterial blood pressure.
Reprinted and modified by permission of Neonatal Network, Acute Respiratory Care of the Neonate, 1991.

REFERENCES

1. Klaus M, Fanaroff A: The physical environment. In Klaus M, Fanaroff A (eds): Care of the High Risk Neonate, 5th ed. Philadelphia, WB Saunders, 2001 (Chapter 5, pp 130–146).
2. Baumgart S: Reduction of oxygen consumption, insensible water loss, and radiant heat demand with use of plastic blanket for low-birth-weight infants under radiant warmers. Pediatrics 74:1022–1028, 1984.
3. Topper W, Stewart T: Thermal support for the very-low-birth-weight infant: Role of supplemental conductive heat. J Pediatr 105:810–814, 1984.
4. Sedin G, Hammarlund K, Nilsson G, et al: Measurements of transepidermal water loss in newborn infants. Clin Perinatol 12:79–99,1985.
5. Vohra S, Frent G, Campbell V, et al: Effect of polyethylene occlusive skin wrapping on heat loss in very low birth weight infants at delivery: A randomized trial. J Pediatr 134:547–551, 1999.
6. Bustamante S, Steslow J: Use of a transparent adhesive dressing in very low birthweight infants. J Perinatol 9:165, 1989.
7. Knauth A, Gordin M, McNelis W, et al: Semipermeable polyurethane membrane as an artificial skin for the premature neonate. Pediatrics 83:945, 1989.
8. Mancini A, Sookdeo-Drost S, Madison K, et al: Semipermeable dressings improve epidermal barrier function in premature infants. Pediatr Res 36:306, 1994.
9. Vernon H, Lane A, Wischerath L, et al: Semipermeable dressing and transepidermal water loss in premature infants. Pediatrics 86:357–362, 1990.
10. Harpin V, Rutter N: Humidification of incubators. Arch Dis Child 60:219–224, 1985.
11. Hammarlund K, Sedon G: Transepidermal water loss in newborn infants. III. Relation to gestational age. Acta Pediatr Scand 68:795–801, 1979.
12. Drucker D, Marshall N: Humidification without risk of infection in the Drager incubator 8000. Neonatal Intens Care July/August:44–46, 1995.
13. Marshall A: Humidifying the environment for the premature neonate: Maintenance of a thermoneutral environment. J Neonatal Nurs January:32–36, 1997.
14. Nopper AJ, Horii KA, Drost SS, et al: Topical ointment therapy benefits premature infants. J Pediatr 128:660–669, 1996.
15. Holbrook KA: A histological comparison of infant and adult skin. In Maibach HI, Boisits EK (eds): Neonatal Skin: Structure and Function. New York, Marcel Dekker, 1982 (Chapter 1, pp 3–31).

16. Behrendt H, Green M: Patterns of Skin pH from Birth through Adolescence. Springfield, Ill., Charles C. Thomas, 1971.
17. Fox C, Nelson D, Wareham J: The timing of skin acidification in very low birth weight infants. J Perinatol 18:272–275, 1998.
18. Wilhelm K, Maibach H: Factors predisposing to cutaneous irritation. Dermatol Clin 8:17, 1990.
19. American Academy of Pediatrics: Standards and Recommendations for Hospital Care of Newborn Infants. Evanston, Ill., American Academy of Pediatrics, 1997.
20. Centers for Disease Control: Leads from the MMWR. Update: Universal precautions for prevention of transmission of human immunodeficiency virus, hepatitis B virus, and other bloodborne pathogens in health care settings. JAMA 260:462–465, 1988.
21. Penny-MacGillivray T: A newborn's first bath. When? J Obstet Gynecol Neonatal Nurs 25:481–487, 1996.
22. Varda KE, Behnke RS: The effect of timing of initial bath on newborn's temperature. J Obstet Gynecol Neonatal Nurs 29:27–32, 2000.
23. Frosch PJ, Kligman AM: The soap chamber test. J Am Acad Dermatol 1:35, 1979.
24. Tupker RA, Pinnagoda J, Nater JP: The transient and cumulative effect of sodium lauryl sulphate on the epidermal barrier assessed by transepidermal water loss: Inter-individual variation. Acta Derm Venereol 70:1, 1990.
25. Tupker RA, Pinnagoda J, Coenraads PJ, et al: Evaluation of detergent-induced irritant skin reactions by visual scoring and transepidermal water loss measurement. Dermatol Clin 8:33, 1990.
26. Gfatter R, Hackl P, Braun F: Effects of soap and detergents on skin surface pH, stratum corneum hydration, and fat content in infants. Dermatology 195:258–262, 1997.
27. Franck L, Quinn D, Zahr L: Effects of less frequent bathing of preterm infants on skin flora and pathogen colonization. J Obstet Gynecol Neonatal Nurs 29:584–589, 2000.
28. Peters KL: Bathing premature infants: Physiological and behavioral consequences. Am J Crit Care 7:90–100, 1998.
29. Ghadially RL, Halkier-Sorensen L, Elias P: Effects of petrolatum on stratum corneum structure and function. J Am Acad Dermatol 26:387–396, 1992.
30. Hoath S, Narendran V: Adhesives and emollients in the preterm infant. Semin Neonatol 5:112–119, 2000.
31. Edwards W, Conner J, Gerdes J, et al: The effect of Aquaphor ointment on nosocomial sepsis rates and skin integrity in infants of birthweights

501–1000g. Paper presented at the Hot Topics Neonatology Conference, Washington, DC, December 2000.

32. Cetta F, Lambert G, Ros S: Newborn chemical exposure from over-the-counter skin care products. Clin Pediatr 30:286, 1991.

33. Harpin V, Rutter N: Percutaneous alcohol absorption and skin necrosis in a preterm infant. Arch Dis Child 57:825, 1982.

34. Jackson H, Sutherland R: Effect of povidone-iodine on neonatal thyroid function. Lancet 2:992, 1981.

35. Schick JB, Milstein JM: Burn hazard of isopropyl alcohol in the neonate. Pediatrics 68:587, 1981.

36. Linder N, Davidovitch N, Reichman B, et al: Topical iodine-containing antiseptics and subclinical hypothyroidism in preterm infants. J Pediatr 131:434–439, 1997.

37. Mitchell I, Pollock C, Jamieson MP, et al: Transcutaneous iodine absorption in infants undergoing cardiac operation. Ann Thorac Surg 52:1138, 1991.

38. Parravicini E, Fontana C, Paterlini GL, et al: Iodine, thyroid function, and very low birth weight infants. Pediatrics 98:730, 1996.

39. Smerdely P, Lim A, Boyages SC, et al: Topical iodine-containing antiseptics and neonatal hypothyroidism in very-low-birthweight infants. Lancet 16:661, 1989.

40. Choudhuri J, McQueen R, Inoue S, et al: Efficacy of skin sterilization for a venipuncture with the use of commercially available alcohol or iodine pads. Am J Infect Contr 18:82–85, 1990.

41. Maki D, Ringer M, Alvarado C: Prospective randomized trial povidone-iodine, alcohol, and chlorhexidine for prevention of infection associated with central venous and arterial catheters. Lancet 338:339, 1991.

42. Garland J, Buck RK, Maloney P, et al: Local reactions to a chlorhexidine gluconate impregnated antimicrobial dressing in very-low birthweight infants. Pediatr Infect Dis J 15:912–914, 1995.

43. Hoath S, Narendran V: Adhesives and emollients in the preterm infant. Semin Neonatol 5:112–119, 2000.

44. Harpin V, Rutter N: Barrier properties of the newborn infant's skin. J Pediatr 102:419, 1983.

45. Lund C, Nonato L, Kuller J, et al: Disruption of barrier function in neonatal skin associated with adhesive removal. J Pediatr 131:367–372, 1997.

46. Lo J, Oriba H, Maibach H, et al: Transepidermal potassium ion, chloride ion, and water flux across delipidized and cellophane tape-stripped skin. Dermatologica 180:66, 1990.

47. Rutter N: Drug absorption through the skin: A mixed blessing. Arch Dis Child 57:220–221, 1987.

48. Ittman P, Bozynski M: Toxic epidermal necrolysis in a newborn infant after exposure to adhesive remover. J Perinatol 13:476–477, 1993.

49. Dollison E, Beckstrand J: Adhesive tape vs. pectin-based barrier use in preterm infants. Neonatal Network 14:35, 1995.

50. Lund C, Kuller J, Tobin C, et al: Evaluation of a pectin-based barrier under tape to protect neonatal skin. J Obstet Gynecol Neonatal Nurs 15:39, 1986.

51. McLean S, Kirchhoff KT, Kriynovich J, et al: Three methods of securing endotracheal tubes in neonates: A comparison. Neonatal Network 11:17, 1992.

52. Grove GL, Leyden JJ: Comparison of the Skin Protectant Properties of Various Film-Forming Products. Broomall, Pa., Skin Study Center, KLG, Inc., 1993.

53. Irving V: Reducing the risk of epidermal stripping in the neonatal population: An evaluation of an alcohol free barrier film. J Neonatal Nurs 7:5–8, 1999.

54. 3M Cavilon No Sting Barrier Film Brochure. 3M Health Care, St. Paul, Minnesota, 2000.

55. Lund C: Prevention and management of infant skin breakdown. Nurs Clin North Am 34:907–920, 1999.

56. Rodeaver G: Controversies in topical wound management. Wounds 1:19–27, 1989.

57. Smack DP, Harrington AC, Dunn C, et al: Infection and allergy incidence in ambulatory surgery patients using white petrolatum vs. bacitracin ointment. A randomized controlled trial. JAMA 276:972–977, 1996.

58. Marks J, Belsito D, DeLeo V, et al: North America Contact Dermatitis Group standard tray patch test results. Am J Contact Dermat 6:160–165, 1995.

59. Krasner D, Kennedy KL, Rolstad BS, et al: The ABCs of wound care dressings. Ostomy/Wound Management 39:68–72, 1993.

60. Als H, Lawhon G, Duffy FH, et al: Individualized behavioral and environmental care for the very low birth weight preterm infants at high risk for bronchopulmonary dysplasia: Neonatal intensive care unit and developmental outcome. Pediatrics 78:1123, 1986.

61. Als H, Lawhon G, Duffy FH, et al: Individualized developmental care for the very low birth weight preterm infant: Medical and neurofunctional effects. JAMA 272:853, 1994.

62. Becker P, Grunwald P, Moorman J, et al: Outcomes of developmentally supportive nursing care for very low birth weight infants. Nurs Res 40:150, 1991.

63. Buehler D, Als H, Duffy F, et al: Effectiveness of individualized developmental care for low-risk preterm infants: Behavioral and electrophysiologic evidence. Pediatrics 96:923, 1995.

64. Fleisher B, VandenBerg K, Constantinou J, et al: Individualized developmental care for very low birth weight premature infants. Clin Pediatr 34:523, 1995.

65. Long J, Lucey J, Philip A: Noise and hypoxemia in the intensive care nursery. Pediatrics 65:143, 1980.

66. Zahr L, Balian S: Responses of premature infant to routine nursing interventions and noise in the NICU. Nurs Res 44:179, 1995.

67. Zahr L, de Traversay J: Premature infant responses to noise reduction by earmuffs: Effects on behavioral and physiologic measures. J Perinatol 15:448, 1995.

68. Philbin M: Some implication of early auditory development for the environment of hospitalized preterm infants. Neonatal Network 15:71, 1996.

69. Thomas K: How the NICU environment sounds to a preterm infant. MCN Am J Matern Child Nurs 14:249, 1989.

70. DePaul D, Chambers S: Environmental noise in the neonatal intensive care unit: Implications for nursing practice. J Perinatal Neonatal Nurs 8:71, 1995.

71. Long J, Lucey J, Philip A: Noise and hypoxemia in the intensive care nursery. Pediatrics 65:143, 1980.

72. American Academy of Pediatrics, Committee on Environmental Health: Noise: A hazard for the fetus and newborn. Pediatrics 100:724, 1997.

73. Mann N, Haddow R, Stokes L, et al: Effect of day and night on preterm infants in the newborn nursery: Randomized trial. Br Med J 293:1265, 1986.

74. Blackburn S, Patteson D: Effects of cycled light on activity state and cardiorespiratory function in preterm infants. J Perinatal Neonatal Nurs 4:47, 1991.

75. Glass P, Avery G, Kolinjavada N, et al: Effect of bright light in the hospital nurseries on the incidence of retinopathy of prematurity. N Engl J Med 313:401, 1985.

76. Ackerman B, Sherwonit E, Williams J: Reduced incidental light exposure: Effect on the development of retinopathy of prematurity in low birth weight infants. Pediatrics 83:958, 1985.

77. Reynolds J, Hardy R, Kennedy K, et al: Lack of efficacy of light reduction in preventing retinopathy of prematurity. N Engl J Med 338:1572, 1998.

78. Cartlidge P, Rutter N: Reduction of head flattening in preterm infants. Arch Dis Child 63:755, 1988.

79. Long T, Soderstrom E: A critical appraisal of positioning infants in the neonatal intensive care unit. Phys Occup Ther Pediatr 15:17, 1995.

80. Updike C, Schmidt R, Macke C, et al: Positional support for premature infants. Am J Occup Ther 40:712, 1986.

81. McEnvoy C, Mendoza ME, Bowling S, et al: Prone positioning decreases episodes of hypoxemia in extremely low birth weight infants (1000 grams or less) with chronic lung disease. J Pediatr 130:305–309, 1997.

82. Bjornson K, Deitz J, Blackburn S, et al: The effect of body position on the oxygen saturation of ventilated preterm infants. Pediatr Phys Ther 4:109, 1992.

83. Lioy J, Manginello F: A comparison of prone and supine positioning in the immediate post extubation period of neonates. J Pediatr 112:982, 1988.

84. Masterson J, Zucker C, Schulze K: Prone and supine positioning effects on energy expenditure and behavior of low birth weight infants. Pediatrics 5:689, 1988.

85. Marion B: A turn for the better: Prone positioning of patients with ARDS. Am J Nurs 101:26–34, 2001.

86. Curley MA, Thompson JE, Arnold JH, et al: The effects of early and repeated prone positioning in pediatric patients with acute lung injury. Chest 118:156–163, 2000.

87. Mure M, Martling CR, Lindahl SG, et al: Dramatic effect on oxygenation in patients with severe acute lung insufficiency treated in the prone position. Crit Care Med 25:1539–1544, 1997.

88. Balas MC: Prone positioning of patients with acute respiratory distress syndrome: applying research to practice. Crit Care Nurse 20:24–36, 2000.

89. Bozynski ME, Naglie R., Nicks J, et al: Lateral positioning of the stable ventilated very-low-birth-weight infant: Effect on transcutaneous oxygen and carbon dioxide. Am J Dis Child 142:200, 1988.

90. Peters K: Bathing the premature infant: Physiologic and behavioral consequences. Am J Crit Care 7:90, 1998.

91. Peters K: Does routine nursing care complicate the physiologic status of the premature neonate with respiratory distress syndrome? J Perinatal Neonatal Nurs 6:67, 1992.

92. White-Traut R, Nelson M, Silvestri J, et al: Responses of preterm infants to unimodal and multimodal sensory intervention. Pediatr Nurs 23:169, 1997.

93. Zahr L, Balian S: Responses of premature infant to routine nursing interventions and noise in the NICU. Nurs Res 44:179, 1995.

94. Neu M, Browne J: Infant physiologic and behavioral organization during swaddled versus unswaddled weighing. J Perinatol 17:193, 1997.

95. DePaul D, Chambers S: Environmental noise in the neonatal intensive care unit: Implications for nursing practice. J Perinatal Neonatal Nurs 8:71, 1995.

96. Taquino L, Blackburn S: The effects of containment during suctioning and heelsticks on physiological and behavioral responses of preterm infants. Neonatal Network 13:55, 1994.

97. Corff K, Seideman R, Venkataraman P, et al: Facilitated tucking: A non-pharmacologic comfort measure for pain in preterm infants. J Obstet Gynecol Neonatal Nurs 24:143, 1995.

98. Field T, Sehanberg SM, Scafidi F, et al: Tactile/kinesthetic stimulation effects on preterm neonates. Pediatrics 77:654, 1986.

99. Barker DP, Rutte N: Exposure to invasive procedures in neonatal intensive care unit admissions. Arch Dis Child Fetal Neonatal Ed 72:F47–F48, 1995.

100. Corff K, Seideman R, Venkataraman P, et al: Facilitated tucking: A non-pharmacologic comfort measure for pain in preterm infants. J Obstet Gynecol Neonatal Nurs 24:143, 1995.

101. Stevens B, Johnston C, Franck L, et al: The efficacy of developmentally sensitive interventions and sucrose for relieving procedural pain in very low birth weight neonates. Nurs Res 48:35, 1998.

102. Blass EM, Hoffmeyer LB: Sucrose as an analgesic for newborn infants. Pediatrics 87:215, 1991.

103. Pokela ML: Pain relief can reduce hypoxemia in distressed neonates during routine treatment procedures. Pediatrics 93:379–383, 1994.

104. Kenner C: Caring for the NICU parent. J Perinatal Neonatal Nurs 4:78–87, 1990.

105. Institute for Family Centered-Care: Advances in Family-Centered Care (newsletter). Bethesda, Md., Institute for Family-Centered Care, Volume 7, 2001.

106. Harrison H: The principles for family-centered neonatal care. Pediatrics 82:643, 1993.

107. Johnson BH, Jeppson ES, Redburn L: Caring for Children and Families: Guidelines for Hospitals. Bethesda, Md., Association for the Care of Children's Health, 1992.

108. Stepanek JS: Moving Beyond the Medical/Technical: Analysis and Discussion of Psychosocial Practices in Pediatric Hospitals. Bethesda, Md., Association for the Care of Children's Health, 1992.

109. Linden DW, Paroli ET, Doron MW: Preemies: The Essential Guide for Parents of Prematures. New York, Pocket Books, 2000.

110. Zaichkin J: Newborn Intensive Care: What Every Parent Needs to Know, 2nd ed. Petaluma, Calif., NICU INK Book Publishers, 2001 (available in English and Spanish).

111. Avila K, Mazza LV, Morgan-Trujillo L: High-frequency oscillatory ventilation: A nursing approach to bedside care. Neonatal Network 13:23, 1994.

112. Gale G, Franck L, Lund C: Skin-to-skin (kangaroo) holding of the premature infant. Neonatal Network 12:49, 1993.

113. Anderson GC: Skin-to-skin (kangaroo) care for preterm infants: Review of the literature. J Perinatol 11:216, 1991.

114. Sloan NL, Camacho LWL, Rojas EP, et al: Kangaroo mother method: Randomised controlled trial of an alternative method of care for stabilised low-birthweight infants. Lancet 344:782–785, 1994.

115. Bosque E, Brady J, Affonso D, et al: Physiologic measures of kangaroo versus incubator care in a tertiary-level nursery. J Obstet Gynecol Neonatal Nurs 2:219–226,1995.

116. Ludington-Hoe S, Hadeed A, Cranston Anderson G: Physiologic responses to skin-to-skin contact in hospitalized premature infants. J Perinatol 11:19–24, 1991.

117. DeLeeuw R, Colin E, Dunnebier E, et al: Physiological effects of kangaroo care in very small preterm infants. Biol Neonate 59:139–155, 1991.

118. Acolet D, Sleath K, Whitelaw A: Oxygenation, heart rate, and temperature in very low birth weight infants during skin-to-skin contact with their mother. Acta Pediatr Scand 78:189, 1989.

119. Fohe K, Kropf S, Avenarius S: Skin-to-skin contact improves gas exchange in premature infants. J Perinatol 5:311–315, 2000.

120. Bohnhorst B, Heyne T, Peter CS, et al: Skin-to-skin (kangaroo) care, respiratory control, and thermoregulation. J Pediatr 138:193–197, 2000.

121. Brown MS: Prevention of accidental extubation in newborns. Am J Dis Child 143:880–881, 1989.

122. Braun D, Bosque E, Juster RP: Unexpected extubation and ETT taping factors in neonates. Pediatr Res 21(Pt 2):355A, 1987.

123. Hummel PA, Kleiber C: Spontaneous endotracheal tube extubation in the neonate. Pediatr Nurs 15:347–351, 1989.

124. Franck L, Vaughan B, Wallace J: Extubation and reintubation in the NICU: Identifying opportunities to improve care. Pediatr Nurs 18:267–270, 1992.

125. Nieves J: Avoiding spontaneous extubation of nasotracheal or oral tracheal tubes. Pediatr Nurs 12:215–218, 1986.

126. Robson LK, Tompkins J: Maintaining placement and skin integrity with endotracheal tubes in a pediatric ICU. Crit Care Nurs May/June:29–32, 1984.

127. Budd RA: The "Logan Bow" method for securing endotracheal tubes in neonates. Crit Care Nurs May/June:27–28, 1982.

128. Erenberg A, Nowak AJ: Appliance for stabilizing orogastric and orotracheal tubes in infants. Crit Care Med 12:669–671, 1984.

129. Ash SP, Orth D, Moss JP, et al: An investigation of the features of the pre-term infant palate and the effect of prolonged orotracheal intubation with and without protective appliances. Br J Orthodont 14:253–261, 1987.

130. Ginoza G, Cortez S, Modanlou H: Prevention of palatal groove formation in premature neonates requiring intubation. J Pediatr 115:133–135, 1989.

131. Todres ID, deBros F, Kramer SS, et al: Endotracheal tube displacement in the newborn infant. J Pediatr 89:126–127, 1979.

132. Donn SM, Kuhns LR: Mechanism of endotracheal tube movement with change of head position in the neonate. Pediatr Radiol 9:37–40, 1980.

133. Etches PC, Finer NN: Endotracheal tube position in neonates (letter). Am J Dis Child 146:1013, 1992.

134. Brasch RC, Heldt GP, Hecht ST: Endotracheal tube orifice abutting the tracheal wall: A cause of infant airway obstruction. Radiology 141:387–391, 1981.

135. Simbruner G, Coradello H, Fodor M, et al: Effects of tracheal suction on oxygenation, circulation and lung mechanics in newborn infants. Arch Dis Child 56:326–330, 1981.

136. Danford DA, Miske S, Headley J, et al: Effects of routine care procedures on transcutaneous oxygen in neonates: A quantitative approach. Arch Dis Child 58:20–23, 1983.

137. Cabal L, Devaskar S, Siassi B: New endotracheal tube adapter reducing cardiopulmonary effects of suctioning. Crit Care Med 7:552–555, 1979.

138. Fox WW, Schwartz JG, Shaffer TH: Pulmonary physiotherapy in neonates: Physiologic changes and respiratory management. J Pediatr 92:977–981, 1978.

139. Anderson KD, Chandra R: Pneumothorax secondary to perforation of sequential bronchi by suction catheters. J Pediatr Surg 11:687–693, 1976.

140. Vaughan RS, Menke JA, Giacoia GP: Pneumothorax: A complication of endotracheal suctioning. J Pediatr 92:633–634, 1978.

141. Alpin G, Glik, B, Peleg O, et al: Pneumothorax due to endotracheal tube suction. Am J Perinatol 1:345–348, 1984.

142. Perlman JM, Volpe JJ: Suctioning in the preterm infant: Effects on cerebral blood flow velocity, intracranial pressure and arterial blood pressure. Pediatrics 72:329–334, 1983.

143. Shah AR, Kurth CD, Gwiazdowski S, et al: Fluctuations in cerebral oxygenation and blood volume during endotracheal suctioning in premature infants. J Pediatr 120:769–774, 1992.

144. Skov L, Ryding I, Pryds O, et al: Changes in cerebral oxygenation and cerebral blood volume during endotracheal suctioning in ventilated infants. Acta Pediatr 81:389–393, 1992.

145. Bucher HU, Blum-Gisler M, Duc G: Changes in cerebral blood volume during endotracheal suctioning. J Pediatr 122:324, 1993.

146. Turner BS: Maintaining the artifical airway: Current concepts. Pediatr Nurs 16:487–493.

147. Turner BS, Loan LA: Tracheobronchial trauma associated with airway management in neonates. AACN Clin Issues 11:283–299, 2000.

148. Thakur A, Brickmiller T, Atkinson J: Bronchial perforation after closed-tube endotracheal suction. J Pediatr Surg 35:1353–1355, 2000.

149. Clarke TA, Coen RW, Feldman B, et al: Esophageal perforations in premature infants and comments of the diagnosis. J Thorac Cardiovasc Surg 139:367–368, 1980.

150. Johnson DE, Foker J, Munson D, et al: Management of esophageal and pharyngeal perforation in the newborn infant. Pediatrics 70:592–595, 1982.

151. Talbert JL, Rodgers BM, Felan AH, et al: Traumatic perforation of the hypopharynx in infants. J Thorac Cardiovasc Surg 74:152–156, 1977.
152. Turner BS: Current concepts in endotracheal suctioning. J California Perinatol Assoc 3:104–106, 1983.
153. Gunderson LP, McPhee AJ, Donovan EF: Partially ventilated endotracheal suction: Use in newborns with respiratory distress syndrome. Am J Dis Child 140:462–465, 1986.
154. Mosca F, Colnaghi M, Lattanzio M, et al: Closed versus open endotracheal suctioning in preterm infants: Effects on cerebral oxygenation and blood volume. Biol Neonate 72:9–14, 1997.
155. Monaco FJ, Meredith KS: A bench test evaluation of a neonatal closed tracheal suction system. Pediatr Pulmonol 13:121–123, 1992.
156. Craig J, Mullins D: Nitric oxide inhalation in infants and children: Physiologic and clinical implications. Am J Crit Care 4:443–450, 1995.

8 CONTINUOUS POSITIVE AIRWAY PRESSURE

THOMAS E. WISWELL, MD
PINCHI SRINIVASAN, MD

Continuous positive airway pressure (CPAP) is a form of non-invasive ventilation that is becoming increasingly more popular as a method of respiratory support in sick newborn infants. The acronym CPAP reflects a positive pressure applied to the airways of a spontaneously breathing baby throughout the respiratory cycle. *Positive end-expiratory pressure (PEEP)* refers to the positive pressure applied to a mechanically ventilated neonate during the expiratory phase of respiration. *Continuous negative-expiratory pressure (CNEP)* can be applied transthoracically to similarly distend distal airways; however, it is a technique rarely used in infants during the past 4 decades. *Continuous distending pressure (CDP)* is a general term defined as the maintenance of increased transpulmonary pressure during the expiratory phase of respiration. CPAP, PEEP, and CNEP are types of CDP. The basic goal when one treats with any form of CDP is to provide low-pressure distention of the lungs and prevent collapse of the alveoli and terminal airways during expiration.

As part of this rapidly developing field, the terminology has evolved. This has resulted in a conundrum: variations in the terminology and acronyms that are used to described methods of ventilation, CPAP, and associated parameters. Unfortunately, such variations result in confusion among readers of the neonatology literature. A compilation of the diverse acronyms we have encountered concerning this topic is given in Table 8-1. A list of the acronyms we prefer to use in this chapter is given in Table 8-2. The latter reflects what we believe to be the most commonly applied terms.

CPAP and PEEP are used to treat neonates of both preterm and term gestation with respiratory distress. The major disorder for which CPAP and PEEP are primarily used is respiratory distress syndrome (RDS) in premature infants. Additional common uses of CPAP are to provide an adjunct to weaning infants off mechanical ventilation after they have been extubate and to manage apnea of prematurity (AOP). Moreover, PEEP and CPAP are used for a variety of other respiratory conditions associated with (1) decreased functional residual capacity; (2) atelectasis; (3) right-to-left cardiac or intrapulmonary shunting; (4) ventilation-perfusion mismatch; (5) alveolar edema; (6) aspiration of noxious substances; (7) increased airway resistance; (8) chest wall and airway instability; and (9) obstructive apnea.

In this chapter, we present a broad overview of the current status of the use of CDP, particularly CPAP, in neonates. As part of this review, we refer to relevant Cochrane Collaboration Reviews. For readers unfamiliar with the Cochrane Collaboration, it is an organization in which members perform systematic reviews of randomized controlled trials (RCTs) in order to produce unbiased and precise estimates of the effect of a treatment on outcomes of clinical importance. A number of such reviews concerning CPAP have been completed. Readers interested in the various reviews concerning neonates can peruse the topics at the following web site: *http://www. nichd.nih.gov/cochrane/cochrane.htm.* This web site is provided free of charge by the National Institute of Child Health and Human Development, a division of the National Institutes of Health (NIH).

TABLE 8-1. Confusing Status of Acronyms on Continuous Distending Pressure Used in the Medical Literature

Acronym	Definition
BiPAP	Bilevel positive airway pressure
CDP	Continuous distending pressure
CNEP	Continuous negative expiratory pressure
CPAP	Continuous positive airway pressure
DPAP	Directional positive airway pressure
ETCPAP	Endotracheal tube continuous positive airway pressure
HFNC	High-flow nasal cannulae
IFD	Infant flow driver
NC	Nasal cannulae
NCPAP	Nasal continuous positive airway pressure
nCPAP	Nasal continuous positive airway pressure
N-CPAP	Nasal continuous positive airway pressure
n-CPAP	Nasal continuous positive airway pressure
NEEP	Negative end-expiratory pressure
NHFV	Nasal high-frequency ventilation
NIPPV	Nasal intermittent positive-pressure ventilation
NPCPAP	Nasopharyngeal continuous positive airway pressure
NP-CPAP	Nasopharyngeal continuous positive airway pressure
NP-CPAP	Nasal prong continuous positive airway pressure
NPPV	Noninvasive positive-pressure ventilation
NPSIMV	Nasopharyngeal synchronized intermittent mandatory ventilation
NP-SIMV	Nasal prong synchronized intermittent mandatory ventilation
NP-SIMV	Nasopharyngeal synchronized intermittent mandatory ventilation
NSIMV	Nasal synchronized intermittent mandatory ventilation
NSIPPV	Nasal synchronized intermittent positive-pressure ventilation
NV	Nasal ventilation
PDP	Positive distending pressure
PEEP	Positive end-expiratory pressure
SiPAP	Synchronized intermittent positive airway pressure
SNIPPV	Synchronized nasal intermittent positive-pressure ventilation

Note that different acronyms are used to mean the same thing and that the same acronym is used to mean different things.

TABLE 8-2. Preferred Acronyms on Continuous Distending Pressure Used in This Chapter

Acronym	Definition
CDP	Continuous distending pressure
CNEP	Continuous negative expiratory pressure
CPAP	Continuous positive airway pressure
ETCPAP	Endotracheal tube continuous positive airway pressure
IFD	Infant flow driver
NC	Nasal cannulae
NCPAP	Nasal continuous positive airway pressure
NHFV	Nasal high-frequency ventilation
NIPPV	Nasal intermittent positive-pressure ventilation
NPCPAP	Nasopharyngeal continuous positive airway pressure
NPSIMV	Nasopharyngeal synchronized intermittent mandatory ventilation
NSIMV	Nasal synchronized intermittent mandatory ventilation
NV	Nasal ventilation
PEEP	Positive end-expiratory pressure

BACKGROUND AND HISTORICAL ASPECTS

The application of positive airway pressure in the clinical management of adult patients with lung disorders dates back to the 1930s. Poulton and Oxon,[1] Bullowa,[2] and Barach et al.[3] described use of positive pressure via face masks for acute respiratory insufficiency, pneumonia, and pulmonary edema, respectively. During the 1940s, positive pressure was introduced for high-altitude flying. Because of the recognition of potential complications of CDP due to its effects on major blood vessels,[4] during the ensuing 2 decades it was used only sporadically in clinical practice. In 1967 PEEP was added to mechanical ventilation in conjunction with peak inspiratory pressure to treat hypoxemia in adults with acute respiratory distress syndrome (ARDS).[5] In neonates who were mechanically ventilated during the 1960s, it was a common practice to allow the positive pressure at end-expiration to fall to 0 cm H_2O. A classic clinical finding in premature infants with RDS is an expiratory grunt. Widespread alveolar collapse is the prominent pathophysiology of this disorder. Harrison et al.[6] recognized that the grunt was produced by infants who closed their glottises during expiration in an attempt to increase pressure in the airways and maintain dilation of their alveoli. Limited air escaping through the partially closed glottis produced the audible grunt. In a landmark report in 1971, Gregory et al.[7] described the initial clinical use of CPAP (via either an endotracheal tube or a head box) in premature infants with RDS.

Use of CPAP in neonates during the 1970s was welcomed with enthusiasm as the "missing link" between supplemental oxygen and mechanical ventilation to treat RDS.[8] During this decade, a simple approach to providing CPAP was widely used, application via binasal prongs, known as *nasal CPAP (NCPAP)*.[9,10] Alternative methods of providing CPAP were occasionally described (see subsequent section on delivery of CPAP). During the 1970s, it was commonly believed that air leaks (such as pneumothoraces) were more common with CPAP than with mechanical ventilation. Gastric distention during CPAP was frequently observed. The hard nasal prongs were often not tolerated by neonates. For these and perhaps other reasons, the use of CPAP fell out of favor during the

1980s and early 1990s. Intermittent mandatory ventilation (IMV), first described in the early 1970s, has been the standard for mechanically ventilating sick newborn infants for 3 decades. Exogenous surfactant therapy has clearly decreased the mortality rate of very-low-birthweight (VLBW) neonates weighing less than 1500 g. Other chapters in this book describe multiple other ways of ventilating infants that were developed during the 1980s and 1990s (e.g., high-frequency ventilation, patient-triggered ventilation) in an attempt to further improve pulmonary outcomes; however, none of these techniques has definitively improved either morbidity [e.g., air leaks and chronic lung disease (CLD)] or mortality. Over the past decade, there has been a resurgence of interest in CPAP. The desired effect is that CPAP will be a gentle way of maintaining patency of alveoli and allowing sufficient gas exchange.

Atelectotrauma is both a cause and consequence of lung injury.[11] It is a process of individual lung units collapsing and requiring higher pressures in order to reopen. Unfortunately, some areas of the lungs may remain collapsed while others are overventilated. The collapse of lung units, as well as over-expansion of others, may injure lung parenchymal elements, as well as the alveoli themselves. The process of closing and reopening, particularly when there is excess alveolar distention, may lead to inflammation and the release of cytokines. This process has been termed *biotrauma. Volutrauma* is regional overdistention of the lungs due to large tidal volume breathing. Such breaths may damage the pulmonary capillary endothelium and the basement membranes. As a consequence, fluid, protein, and blood may leak into the airways and alveoli. This process also promotes lung inflammation. It does not take much to initiate the cascade of lung injury. In preterm animals, as few as six manual tidal ventilations of 35 to 40 mL/kg administered to preterm lambs before surfactant treatment resulted in lung injury and decreased response to exogenous surfactant.[12] The term *barotrauma* refers to purported injury from the pressure used to inflate the lungs. Although the latter was once thought to be a major factor in producing lung injury, atelectotrauma, volutrauma, and biotrauma currently are believed to be the key elements.

Optimal lung inflation is defined as the lung volume at which the recruitable lung is open but not overinflated.[11] The art of medicine in the neonatal intensive care unit (NICU) is to achieve optimal lung volume in neonates with respiratory disorders. CPAP is one method many clinicians believe best achieves optimal lung inflation with resultant good oxygenation and ventilation and, hopefully, less CLD. Using CPAP, care must be taken not to decrease the distending pressure below the closing pressure of the majority of the alveoli. The trick is to achieve the lowest possible pressure to maintain open alveoli without overdistention.

Any review of NCPAP over the past 15 years will refer to the 1987 publication of Avery et al.,[13] who surveyed eight NICUs to assess the incidence of CLD. The frequency of CLD in that report was lowest at Babies and Children's Hospital, Columbia University, New York, New York. That center reportedly used NCPAP considerably more often than the other seven NICUs. Many clinicians have been influenced by the Columbia approach in which "bubble CPAP" is used early in the course of respiratory distress of both premature and term-gestation infants. As part of this strategy, clinicians often accept hypercapnia with $Paco_2$ levels up to 65 mm Hg (8.7 kPa) or higher, Pao_2 levels as low or lower than 50 mm Hg (6.7 kPa), and pH values as low as

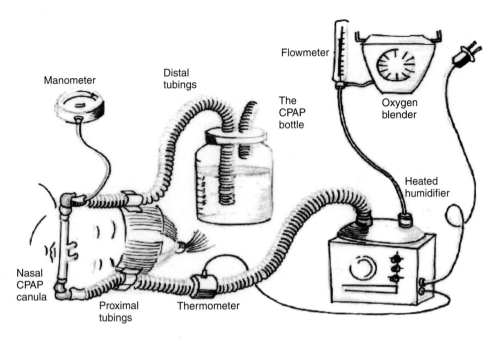

Figure 8-1. Nasal prong continuous positive airway pressure (CPAP) delivery system. Schematic diagram of the "bubble CPAP" setup. A source of blended gas is administered to the child, in this case via Hudson prongs. The distal tubing is immersed in fluid to a depth of the desired level of CPAP. (From Aly HZ: Nasal prongs continuous positive airway pressure: A simple yet powerful tool. Pediatrics 2001, 108:759–761, reproduced by permission of Pediatrics.)

7.20. This general approach has been used in that institution for more than 25 years.[14] Despite the promulgation and widespread acceptance of this approach, to date there have been no RCTs to validate its superiority over any other management strategy or technology. Additionally, there are no long-term outcome studies comparing neurologic, pulmonary, and other findings among infants treated in this manner with others managed differently. Van Marter et al.[15] assessed the differences in outcomes between the Columbia NICU and two NICUs in Boston. This was an epidemiologic survey in which outcomes of infants born between 1991 and 1993 with birthweights between 500 and 1500 g were examined. Mortality was similar between centers. Initial respiratory management in Boston was more likely to include mechanical ventilation (75% vs 29%) and surfactant treatment (45% vs 10%). The prevalence rate of CLD (defined as supplemental oxygen required at 36 weeks postmenstrual age) was 4% at Columbia and 22% in Boston. The initiation of mechanical ventilation was the biggest risk factor for CLD. The latter review has been criticized because of differences in patient populations, indications for mechanical ventilation and other treatment strategies, and the definition of CLD. Much of the apparent success of the Columbia approach has been attributed to the diligent management of sick neonates by a single senior clinician. Nevertheless, knowledge of the Columbia experience has contributed to the flurry of research concerning CPAP over the past decade.

METHODS OF GENERATING CONTINUOUS DISTENDING PRESSURE

Following the initial publication by Gregory et al.[7] demonstrating success using CPAP in premature infants, efforts were made to simplify the manner in which CDP was generated, as well as the mode of delivery. Kattwinkel et al.[9] and Caliumi-Pellegrini et al.[10] described devices in which binasal prongs were used for delivery. These methods were standard for a number of years. In the subsequent section, we describe various methods of CPAP delivery (prongs, mask). The gas mixture delivered via CPAP is derived from either continuous flow or variable flow. From the 1970s through the 1980s, only continuous flow was used. Continuous-flow CPAP consisted of gas flow generated at a source and directed against the resistance of the expiratory limb of a circuit. In ventilator-derived CPAP, a variable resistance in a valve is adjusted to provide this resistance to flow. A second method of continuous-flow CPAP is the so-called *bubble* or *waterseal* CPAP (Fig. 8-1), the method advocated at the Columbia University NICU.[14,16] With bubble CPAP, blended gas flows to the infant after the gas is heated and humidified. Typically, nasal prong cannulae are secured in the infant's nares, such as the Hudson (Hudson Respiratory Care, Inc., Temecula, CA, USA) (Fig. 8-2) or Inca (Ackrad Laboratories, Inc., Cranford, NJ, USA) prongs. The distal end of the expiratory tubing is immersed under either 0.25% acetic acid or sterile water to a specific depth to provide the desired level of CPAP (e.g., the tubing is immersed to a depth of 6 cm in order to provide 6 cm H_2O of CPAP). Lee et al.[17] observed vibrations of infants' chests during bubble CPAP at frequencies similar to those used with high-frequency ventilation. In their study, bubble CPAP was delivered via an endotracheal tube, not nasal prongs. Lee's group found that, compared to ventilator-derived CPAP, bubble CPAP resulted in decreased minute ventilation and respiratory rate. These authors speculated that the observed vibrations enhanced gas exchange. Five years previously, Nekvasil et al.[18] described oscillations produced via this bubbling phenomenon. Nevertheless, the gas-exchange mechanisms of the bubble CPAP setup have yet to be explored further to elucidate whether there is a to-and-fro oscillatory waveform that truly augments ventilation.

The Benveniste gas-jet valve (Dameca, Copenhagen, Denmark) has been used extensively in Scandinavia.[8,19–21] The device consists of two coaxially positioned tubes connected by a ring (Fig. 8-3A). The device works via the Venturi principle to generate pressure and is a continuous-flow CPAP system. The Benveniste gas-jet valve typically is connected to a blended gas source and then to the patient via either a single nasal prong or binasal prongs (Figs. 8-3A, 8-4, and 8-5).

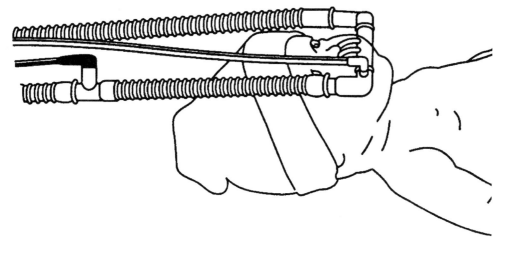

Figure 8-2. Representation of the positioning and appearance of Hudson nasal prongs, which are commonly used for nasal continuous positive airway pressure. (From Davis P, Davies M, Faber B: A randomised controlled trial of two methods of delivering nasal continuous positive airway pressure after extubation to infants weighing less than 1000 g: Binasal (Hudson) versus single nasal prongs. Arch Dis Child Fetal Neonatal Ed 2001 Sep;85:F82–F85, with permission from the BMJ.)

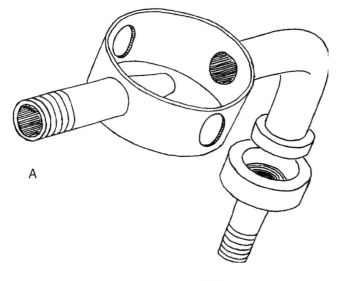

A

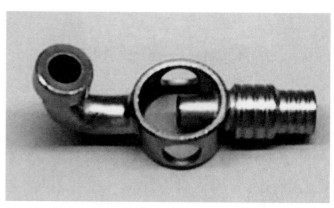

Figure 8-4. Photograph of an actual Benveniste gas-jet valve. (Photograph courtesy of Dr. Jens Kamper.)

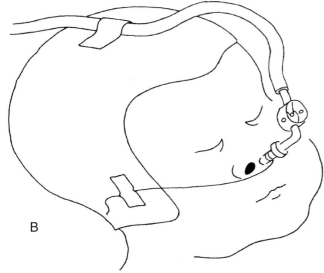

B

Figure 8-3. *A,* Schematic diagram of the Benveniste gas-jet valve. The device consists of two coaxially positioned tubes connected by a ring. *B,* Depiction of an infant being managed with nasopharyngeal continuous positive airway pressure via a nasal prong. The Benveniste gas-jet valve is connected between the blended gas and the nasal prong. No expiratory tubing is necessary, as the exhaled gas leaves the system through the jet valve. (Drawings courtesy of Dr. Gorm Greisen. Figures reproduced from Prenatal Neonatal Medicine, 1996;1:80–91, with permission.)

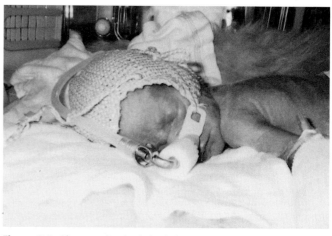

Figure 8-5. Photograph of a baby being managed with the Benveniste gas-jet valve. The infants shown is 28 weeks of gestation, birthweight 1080 g, and is being managed for respiratory distress syndrome. No expiratory tubing is necessary, as the exhaled gas leaves the system through the jet valve. (Photograph courtesy of Dr. Jens Kamper.)

Over the past decade, variable-flow CPAP has come into widespread use. The technique, which was developed by Moa et al.,[22] reduces the patient's work of breathing. Variable-flow NCPAP generates CPAP at the airway proximal to the infant's nares. Variable-flow devices use the Bernoulli effect via dual injector jets directed toward each nasal prong in order to maintain a constant pressure (Figs. 8-6 to 8-10). If the infant requires more inspiratory flow, the Venturi action of the injector jets entrains additional flow. With the variable-flow system, when the infant makes a spontaneous expiratory breathing effort, there is a "fluidic flip" that causes the flow to flip around and to leave the generator chamber via the expiratory limb (Fig. 8-11). The latter phenomenon is due to the Coanda effect. Basically, the Coanda effect is related to the phenomenon of wall attachment, which is the tendency of a fluid or gas to follow the curved surface of a wall. A stream of air (or other fluid) emerging from a nozzle will follow a nearby curved surface. In the case of variable-flow CPAP, once a child starts to exhale, the jet of gas flow easily changes direction from toward the nasal prongs to the expiratory channel (Fig. 8-11). Upon the start of passive exhalation, there is a decrease in the forward velocity of the air flow. This decrease in velocity allows for the "flip" (or reversal) of the gas flow out via the exhalation port. A residual gas pressure is provided by the constant gas flow, which enables stable CPAP delivery at a particular pressure during the entire respiratory cycle. More extensive description of the physiology of variable-flow CPAP can be found elsewhere.[22–24] The major advantage of variable-flow CPAP is reducing the work of breathing of an infant. Typically, in order to exhale while on continuous-flow CPAP, an infant must exhale against the flow of incoming air. The "fluidic flip" of the variable-flow devices assists exhalation by the infant. Klausner et al.[24] used a simulated breathing apparatus and found the work of breathing via nasal prongs to be one fourth that of continuous-flow CPAP. Pandit et al.[25] assessed work of breathing in premature infants treated with either continuous-flow or variable-flow NCPAP.

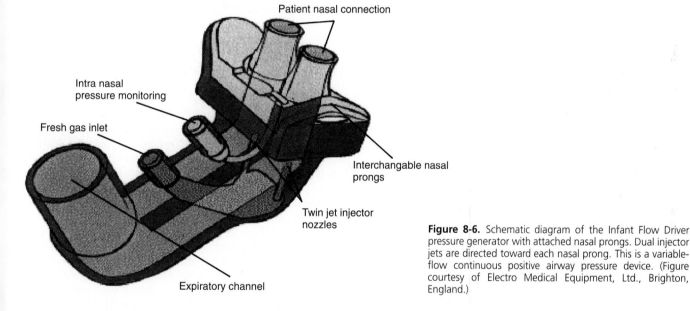

Figure 8-6. Schematic diagram of the Infant Flow Driver pressure generator with attached nasal prongs. Dual injector jets are directed toward each nasal prong. This is a variable-flow continuous positive airway pressure device. (Figure courtesy of Electro Medical Equipment, Ltd., Brighton, England.)

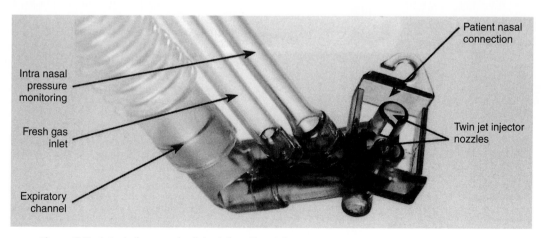

Figure 8-7. Actual photograph of the Infant Flow Driver pressure generator without the nasal prongs attached. (Figure courtesy of Electro Medical Equipment, Ltd., Brighton, England.)

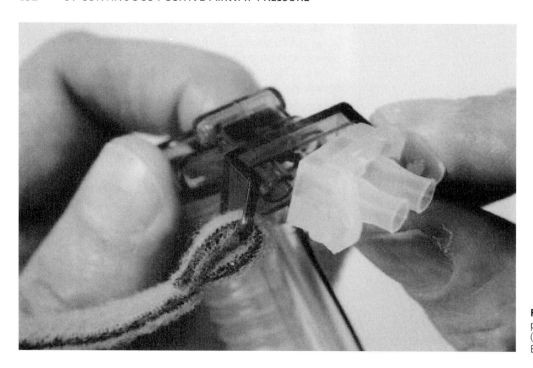

Figure 8-8. Attachment of nasal prongs to the Infant Flow Driver. (Figure courtesy of Electro Medical Equipment, Ltd., Brighton, England.)

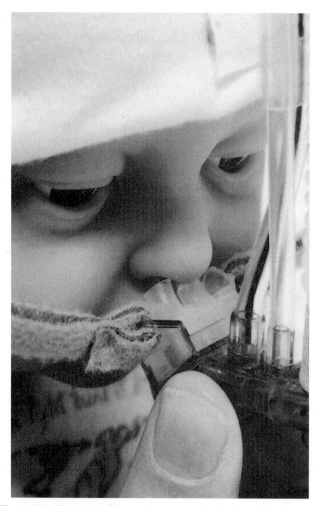

Figure 8-9. Placement of the nasal prongs and Infant Flow Driver pressure generator in the nares of a mannequin. (Figure courtesy of Electro Medical Equipment, Ltd., Brighton, England.)

They found the work of breathing to be significantly less with variable-flow NCPAP. Additionally, the variable-flow devices appear to be able to maintain a more uniform pressure level compared to continuous-flow CPAP (Fig. 8-12).[22,24]

Three variable-flow CPAP systems currently are commercially available. The Infant Flow System (Electro Medical Equipment, Ltd., Brighton, England) has been the most extensively evaluated. This system is commonly known as the *Infant Flow Driver (IFD)*. In the United States, the IFD was known as the Aladdin system. The Arabella system (Hamilton Medical, Reno, NV, USA) has a flow-generating chamber that varies from the IFD (Figs. 8-13 and 8-14), although the same principles (Venturi, Bernoulli, and Coanda) apply. The Arabella system was briefly known as the Aladdin II, although it differed from the original IFD. The name Aladdin II no longer applies to the Arabella system, and there are currently no commercially available CPAP devices known as either the Aladdin or Aladdin II. The final commercially available variable-flow CPAP system is the SensorMedics CPAP generator (Viasys, Bilthoven, The Netherlands). This system appears to function in a fashion similar to that of the IFD and Arabella systems. Although numerous published studies (in vitro and in neonates) have assessed the IFD, we are not aware of any peer-reviewed publications describing either the Arabella system or the SensorMedics CPAP generator.

DEVICES THROUGH WHICH CONTINUOUS POSITIVE AIRWAY PRESSURE IS PROVIDED

Multiple nasal devices are available through which continuous-flow CPAP can be delivered. The devices can be either short (6 to 15 mm) or long (40 to 90 mm). It probably is more accurate to refer to the former as nasal prongs and to the latter as nasopharyngeal prongs. The acronym for nasal CPAP

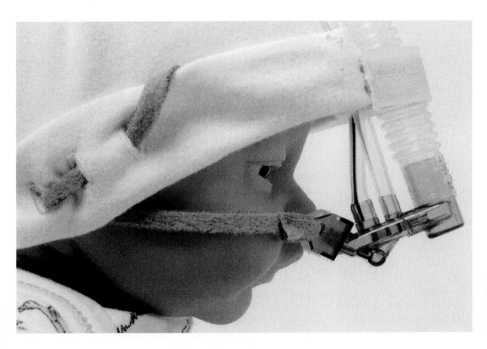

Figure 8-10. Lateral view of a mannequin on which the Infant Flow Driver is attached. Note the proper fixation of the device. (Figure courtesy of Electro Medical Equipment, Ltd., Brighton, England.)

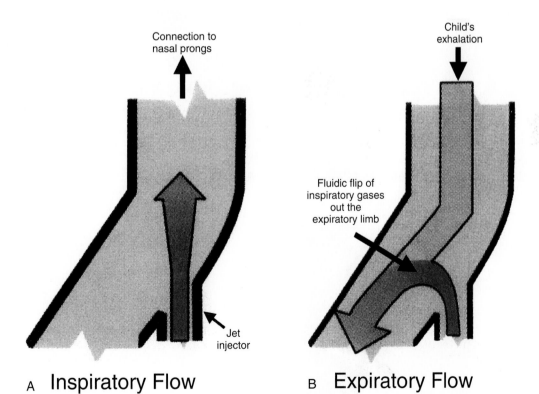

Connection to nasal prongs

Child's exhalation

Fluidic flip of inspiratory gases out the expiratory limb

Jet injector

A Inspiratory Flow

B Expiratory Flow

Figure 8-11. *A,* Schematic representation of the "fluid flip" of the variable-flow continuous positive airway pressure (CPAP) device, the Infant Flow Driver. In this figure, during the child's inspiration, the Bernoulli effect directs gas flow toward each nostril in order to maintain a constant pressure. *B,* Schematic representation of the "fluid flip" of the variable-flow CPAP device, the Infant Flow Driver. In this figure, during the child's exhalation, the Coanda effect causes inspiratory flow to "flip" and leave the generator chamber via the expiratory limb. As such, the child does not have to exhale against high inspiratory flow and work of breathing is decreased compared to continuous-flow CPAP. The residual gas pressure enables stable levels of CPAP to be delivered to the child. (Figures courtesy of Electro Medical Equipment, Ltd., Brighton, England.)

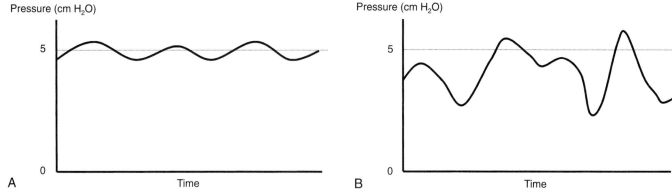

A   Pressure (cm H₂O)   Time

B   Pressure (cm H₂O)   Time

Figure 8-12. *A,* Depiction of the levels of pressure generated via a variable-flow continuous positive airway pressure (CPAP) device. The mechanics of the device allow for stable levels of CPAP during variable-flow CPAP generated via the Infant Flow Driver. *B,* Depiction of the levels of pressure generated via a continuous-flow CPAP device. The levels of pressure greatly vary over time for several reasons, such as increased work of breathing against inspiratory flow and loss of pressure through an open mouth. (Figures modeled after the work of Moa G, Nilsson K, Zetterstrom H, et al: A new device for administration of nasal continuous positive airways pressure in the newborn: An experimental study. Crit Care Med 1988, 16:1238–1242; and Klausner JF, Lee AY, Hutchinson AA: Decreased imposed work with a new nasal continuous positive airway pressure device. Pediatr Pulmonol 1996, 22:188–194.)

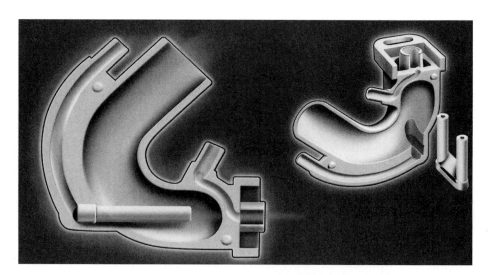

Figure 8-13. Schematic diagram of the Arabella variable-flow continuous positive airway pressure (CPAP) system. Dual injector jets are directed toward each nasal prong. This is a variable-flow CPAP device. (Figure courtesy of Hamilton Medical, Reno, NV, USA.)

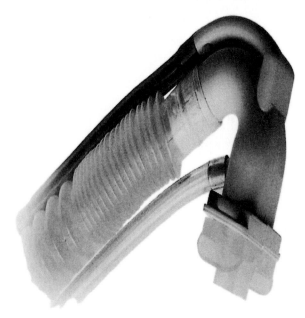

Figure 8-14. Photograph of the Arabella variable-flow continuous positive airway pressure system connected to nasal prongs. (Figure courtesy of Hamilton Medical, Reno, NV, USA.)

(NCPAP) often is used to represent both short-prong nasal CPAP and nasopharyngeal CPAP (NPCPAP). Single nasopharyngeal prongs are used to transmit CPAP and typically consist of an endotracheal tube that has been shortened considerably and is inserted through one of the nares. There are multiple manufacturers of binasal prongs. A typical example is shown in Figures 8-15 and 8-16. Hudson prongs are shown in Figure 8-17. The IFD nasal prongs are shown in Figures 8-8 and 8-9. The Arabella prongs are shown in Figures 8-14 and 8-18.

Unfortunately, there are little comparative data available to guide clinicians in determining the effectiveness of one type of prong over another. The devices may vary with regard to the type of material, length, configuration, and inner and outer diameters. These aspects will affect the resistance to flow in a particular device; as a result, the pressure entering the device may differ considerably from that entering the child's nares or nasopharynx. DePaoli et al.[26] compared the pressure drop for five different CPAP devices at various rates of gas flow and

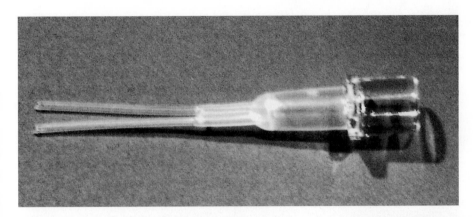

Figure 8-15. Example of nasopharyngeal prongs used for continuous positive airway pressure. (This particular device is produced by NeoTech, Inc., Chatsworth, CA, USA.)

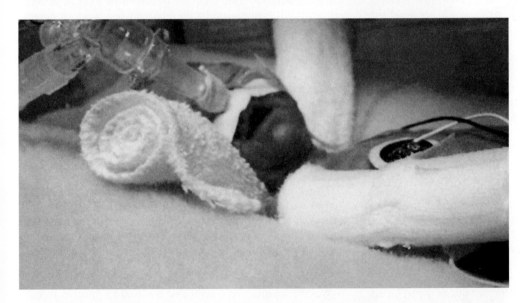

Figure 8-16. Photograph of a baby being managed with nasopharyngeal continuous positive airway pressure that is continuous flow generated by a ventilator.

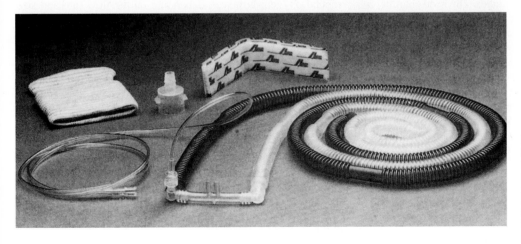

Figure 8-17. Hudson nasal continuous positive airway pressure equipment. Note the wide-bore short prongs. Depictions of children being managed with this device are shown in Figures 8-1 and 8-2. (Photograph courtesy of Hudson RCI, Temecula, CA, USA.)

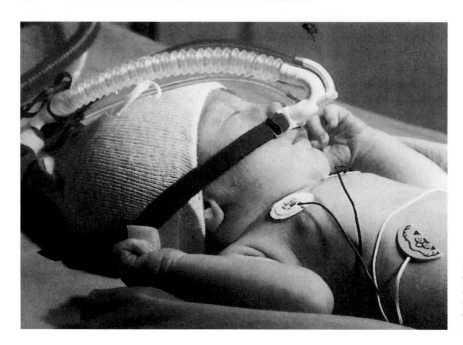

Figure 8-18. Photograph of a baby being managed with the Arabella variable-flow continuous positive airway pressure system. This device must be affixed properly to optimize function and prevent injury. (Figure courtesy of Hamilton Medical, Reno, NV, USA.)

found great variation in the pressure drop among devices. The least amount of dropoff was with the Infant Flow System. These authors cautioned that their findings do not establish clinical superiority of one mode of NCPAP or NPCPAP over any other.

Multiple other methods of delivering CPAP to neonates have been described over the past 3 decades. The initial studies describing CPAP for treatment of premature infants with RDS most often used the endotracheal tube to deliver CDP.[7] This is one of the most effective methods and has many advanatages[27]: (1) ease of use; (2) minimal to no leakage in the system; (3) ability to achieve high pressure with low flow; (4) ease of switching back and forth to mechanical ventilation; and (5) ease of fixation of the tube. Unfortunately, the resistance of endotracheal or nasotracheal tubes makes it difficult for babies to breathe through them for prolonged periods of time. The length of the tube contributes to the dead space of the respiratory system. Moreover, intubation is invasive, and there can be associated complications (trauma from the tube, vagal response).

The head chamber (head box) and face chamber, although noninvasive, never gained wide acceptance due to the technical difficulties and mechanical disadvantages. The head chamber is a closed system that permits use of low flows. It seals around the infant's neck, thus limiting access to the child's face. It is difficult to administer in infants weighing less than 1500 g. The devices are very noisy and have been associated with complications such as hydrocephalus, nerve palsies, and local neck ulceration resulting from mechanical compression by the neck seal.[7,28,29] The face chamber, originally described by Alhstrom et al.,[30] consists of the application of CPAP via a mask covering the entire face. The mask is held in place by negative pressure. This system is simple and effective, and there are no reported patient complications or mechanical problems such as loss of pressure during administration. There is reported success in using the face chamber for treating RDS[30,31] and in weaning infants.[32] The major limitations are access to the infant's face and the cumbersome method of administration.

The face mask is another simple, effective easy-to-place mode for administering CDP for treatment of RDS in preterm infants.[33,34] It is associated with relatively less work of breathing compared to nasal prong CPAP.[35] The mask must cover both the nose and mouth and be securely placed with a good seal in order to prevent loss of pressure. Severe gastric distention can be produced. An orogastric tube could relieve this distention, but there would likely be loss of pressure because of the tube's placement under the edge of the face mask. Other reported pressure-induced effects include trauma to the facial skin and the eyes, intracerebellar hemorrhage, and gastric rupture.[33,34,36] Hypercapnia due to excessive CO_2 retention from increased dead space of the mask may result if the infant cannot compensate by increasing ventilation.

Nasal masks are a relatively recent innovation available with two of the variable-flow systems (IFD and SensorMedics). A small soft mask is attached to the pressure generator (Figs. 8-19 and 8-20). Such masks are markedly smaller than face masks; hence, there is little additional dead space; however, a good seal is necessary to prevent pressure loss. There are no published data on the safety and efficacy of nasal masks.

Nasal cannulae (NC) typically are used to provide supplemental oxygen; however, depending on the flow rate and size of the nasal cannulae, these devices may also provide distending pressure.[37] Many neonatologists use relatively high-flow nasal cannulae to treat AOP (Fig. 8-21). Sreenan et al.[38] compared nasal cannula CPAP (at high flows) with nasal prong CPAP for the management of AOP and concluded that the pressure-distention effects of these methods were similar. A major drawback is that the cannulae become dislodged easily. It is not unusual to pass by a child being treated with nasal cannulae and to note that the cannulae are not in the nares but in the cheek, mouth, or elsewhere.

Nasal and nasopharyngeal prongs remain the most common method of administering CPAP in neonates. Because infants are generally obligate nose breathers, CPAP may be facilitated when delivered directly into the nose. The most common complications with these devices are obstruction by secretions

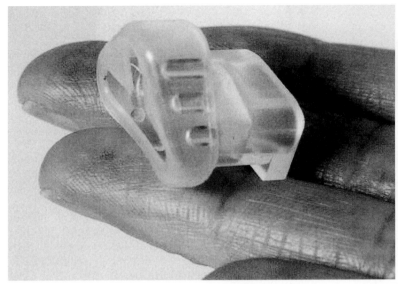
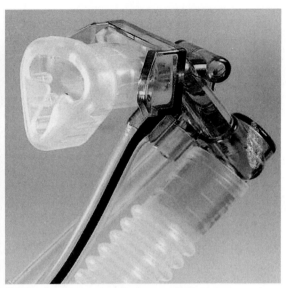

A   B

Figure 8-19. *A,* Size of a nasal mask that can be used with the Infant Flow Driver continuous-flow nasal continuous positive airway pressure (NCPAP) system. *B,* Nasal mask used with the Infant Flow Driver continuous-flow NCPAP system. The mask is attached to the pressure chamber in the same location as nasal prongs. (Figures courtesy of Electro Medical Equipment, Ltd., Brighton, England.)

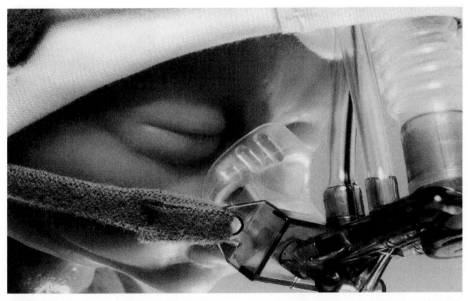

Figure 8-20. Depiction of nasal mask nasal continuous positive airway pressure (NCPAP) used via the Infant Flow Driver continuous-flow NCPAP system. (Figure courtesy of Electro Medical Equipment, Ltd., Brighton, England.)

and kinking of nasopharyngeal prongs in the pharynx. Infants may lose pressure through their open mouths while they're undergoing NCPAP or NPCPAP. Thus, some clinicians actively try to prevent pressure loss by either placing a pacifier in the child's mouth or using a strap under the infant's chin to close the mouth. When NCPAP and NPCPAP are applied, however, there often is enough downward pressure on the palate that it is frequently contiguous to the tongue, providing a natural seal so that there is minimal to no pressure loss through the mouth.

CLINICAL USE OF CONTINUOUS POSITIVE AIRWAY PRESSURE: ANECDOTAL EXPERIENCES

Most of the literature describing the use of CPAP in neonates consists of anecdotal experiences: case reports, case series, and cohort-comparison studies (concurrent or historical). It does not consist of RCTs. The former carry considerably less strength than RCTs in validating the safety and effectiveness of

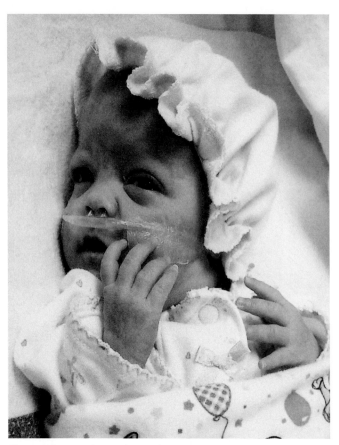

Figure 8-21. Nasal cannulae in place in a growing, premature, 4-week-old infant of 27 weeks' gestation and birthweight 960 g. The nasal cannulae were being used to generate nasal continuous positive airway pressure as therapy for apnea of prematurity.

a therapy. Nevertheless, in order to present a comprehensive review of CPAP, we report anecdotal experiences that we have not yet discussed in this section.

Use of the Benveniste gas-jet valve in neonates was first described in 1976.[19] Jacobsen et al.[39] described the "minitouch" approach in which VLBW infants (neonates weighing <1500 g) were managed with minimal handling and early use of NCPAP via the Benveniste valve. They compared this experience over 1 year with that of a previous 2-year period in which most VLBW infants with respiratory failure were intubated and treated with mechanical ventilation. Jacobsen's group found a significantly decreased use of mechanical ventilation and decreased frequency of intracranial hemorrhages with the mini-touch approach; however, there were no differences in other major outcomes (pneumothoraces, CLD, mortality).

Gittermann et al.[40] compared outcomes of VLBW infants during two periods, 1990 and 1993. In 1990, most infants were not treated with NCPAP; in 1993, generalized use of NCPAP was implemented. These authors used Hudson prongs. It is unknown whether pressure was ventilator-generated or bubble CPAP. Gittermann et al. found that during the second epoch, fewer infants required mechanical ventilation. There were no differences in CLD or mortality.

Lindner et al.[41] similarly addressed management of extremely low birthweight (ELBW) infants (birthweight <1000 g) during two different epochs. In 1994, ELBW infants were generally intubated and ventilated immediately after

delivery once initial resuscitation was accomplished with a mask and bag. In 1996, management changed; a nasopharyngeal tube was placed in the delivery room and initial continuous pressure of 20 to 25 cm H_2O was applied for 15 to 20 seconds. The infants then were managed with NPCPAP at 4 to 6 cm H_2O. The latter group occasionally received ventilator breaths via the nasopharyngeal tube until sufficient respiratory effort was achieved by the child. The authors reported that during the latter period (1996), the percentage of babies who never needed intubation and mechanical ventilation was 25%, compared with 7% during 1994. Moreover, the infants born in 1996 had lower frequencies of CLD and intracranial hemorrhages and shorter hospital stays. There were no differences in mortality.

De Klerk and De Klerk[42] performed a historical comparison of two groups of infants (birthweight 1000–1499 g) over a 5-year period. During the first part of that 5-year period, early intubation and ventilation were performed frequently; during the latter part of the period, infants were routinely placed on NCPAP when they demonstrated respiratory distress. De Klerk and De Klerk used bubble CPAP delivered via Hudson nasal prongs. These authors reported that during the second epoch, fewer infants required mechanical ventilation or exogenous surfactant; however, they did not find differences in mortality or CLD.

The "INSURE" approach to VLBW infants has been described in abbreviated form.[43–45] Basically, this consists of *in*tubation, *su*rfactant administration, and *r*apid *ex*tubation to NCPAP. Essentially, all reports are descriptive in nature, without controls.

Kavvadia et al.[46] assessed a group of 36 infants managed after extubation with (1) NCPAP via the IFD; (2) NCPAP via a single nasal prong; or (3) no CPAP. There were no differences in lung function after 24 hours. The nasal prong group had a significant reduction in supplementary oxygen concentration after 24 hours.

Kurz[47] assessed the effect of NPCPAP on breathing pattern and incidence of apneas in preterm infants. Thirteen preterm infants who were weaning from single-prong NPCPAP were evaluated for 2 hours on NCPAP and for 2 hours off any CPAP. During NPCPAP, the respiratory rate was significantly lower. Additionally, there were fewer obstructive apnea periods, less severe apnea-associated desaturation episodes, and more central apnea events. During NPCPAP, infants spent significantly more time in a state of quiet breathing.

As previously discussed, nasal cannulae are mainly used to deliver supplemental oxygen. Locke et al.[37] demonstrated that nasal cannulae could deliver CDP to infants and alter breathing patterns; however, they advised against its use. Subsequently, Sreenan et al.[38] compared the use of high-flow nasal cannulae with NCPAP generated by a ventilator using Argyle prongs (Argyle-Sherwood Medical Company, St. Louis, MO, USA) in premature infants already being treated with NCPAP for AOP. They used nasal cannulae flow rates up to 2.5 L/min. This was a crossover design study in which all infants initially started on NCPAP. After 6 hours, the infants were changed to nasal cannulae for another 6-hour period. The authors assessed delivered airway pressure by measuring esophageal pressures. Sreenan's group found that comparable CDP could be generated by the nasal cannulae. The amount of flow required to generate comparable pressures depended upon the infant's weight. There were no differences between the two systems in the frequency and duration of apnea, bradycardia, or desaturation episodes.

CLINICAL USE OF CONTINUOUS POSITIVE AIRWAY PRESSURE: RANDOMIZED CONTROLLED TRIALS

Multiple disorders in which CPAP is used have been studied in RCTs as (1) treatment for AOP, (2) postextubation management following mechanical ventilation, and (3) early management of RDS. The trials consist of comparisons of either CPAP with a standard therapy or different types of CPAP.

AOP is a common disorder in premature infants born before 34 weeks of gestation (see Chapter 3). These infants exhibit various combinations of apnea, bradycardia, and oxygen desaturation. Apnea can be classified as obstructive, central, or mixed. Methylxanthines are effective in treating AOP. The sole trial comparing CPAP with methylxanthine therapy was performed more than 20 years ago.[48] In that trial, face mask CPAP at levels of 2 to 3 cm H_2O was compared with theophylline in 32 infants of 25 to 32 weeks of gestation. The investigation found theophylline was more effective than face mask CPAP in reducing (1) prolonged apnea episodes; (2) need for intubation and ventilation because of worsening AOP; and (3) number of bradycardia spells. The Cochrane Review regarding CPAP use for AOP concludes that this area needs additional evaluation.[49] We are aware there is widespread use of NCPAP and NPCPAP for management of AOP despite the dearth of supportive evidence.

Premature infants being extubated following a period of mechanical ventilation via an endotracheal tube are at risk for developing respiratory failure, which may manifest as increased frequency or severity of apnea, CO_2 retention, diffuse atelectasis, increased work of breathing, increased oxygen requirement, or need for reintubation and mechanical ventilation. All of these findings typically are included in "treatment failure" criteria in the various trials that have assessed whether CPAP may be a good therapy for infants with AOP. Davis and Henderson-Smart[50] reviewed the literature to assess whether direct extubation of mechanically ventilated preterm infants would be as successful as extubation following a short period of endotracheal tube CPAP (ETCPAP). These authors identified three appropriate clinical trials in their review. Davis and Henderson-Smart concluded that a trial of ETCPAP prior to extubation did not provide any advantages. In fact, there was a trend toward an increased number of apnea episodes in ETCPAP-treated infants.

Engleke et al.[51] randomized 18 premature neonates recovering from RDS to either oxygen delivered via an oxyhood or NCPAP. During the 24 hours of the study, the NCPAP group of infants had lower respiratory rates, better oxygenation, lower $Paco_2$ values, higher pHs, and less radiographic atelectasis. Higgins et al.[52] similarly randomized 58 infants of birthweight less than 1000 g to either NCPAP or oxyhood at the time of extubation. They found 22 (89%) of 29 NCPAP babies remained successfully extubated compared to 6 (21%) of 29 oxyhood babies ($P < 0.0001$). Chan and Greenough[53] performed a trial in which ventilated infants with both relatively acute (<14 days of age) and chronic (≥14 days of age) respiratory distress were randomized to either NCPAP at 3 cm H_2O or head box oxygen. These authors did not find any differences in extubation failure rates in either group (NCPAP vs head box oxygen) or in acute versus chronic respiratory distress. One should note, however, that 3 cm H_2O is a relatively low amount of distending pressure. Annibale et al.[54] randomized 124 preterm infants

meeting extubation criteria to (1) a long course of NPCPAP (until lung disease was resolved); (2) a 6-hour course of NPCPAP; or (3) oxyhood. These investigators found no differences in the extubation success rate between groups. So et al.[55] randomized 50 VLBW infants in an extubation protocol to either NCPAP or oxyhood. Successful extubation was achieved in 21 (84%) of 25 NCPAP subjects compared to 12 (48%) of 25 in the oxyhood group ($P = 0.01$). Tapia et al.[56] assigned 87 preterm neonates to oxygen alone, endotracheal tube CPAP for 12 to 24 hours with subsequent extubation, or NPCPAP. They found no differences in extubation failure rates among groups.

Davis et al.[57] randomized 92 ventilated preterm infants to either NCPAP or head box oxygen when they were ready for extubation. Thirty-one (66%) of 47 were successfully extubated in the NCPAP group compared to 18 (40%) of 45 in the head box oxygen group ($P = 0.013$). Robertson et al.[58] performed a variation of the preceding trials. They randomized 58 preterm infants after extubation to either immediate NCPAP for 72 hours or head box oxygen with "rescue" NCPAP as an option if necessary. These authors found no differences between groups in successful extubation up to 2 weeks after enrollment. Dmitriou et al.[59] performed an RCT in premature infants (24 to 34 weeks of gestation) who were believed to be ready for extubation. The infants were randomized to either head box oxygen or NCPAP via either single or binasal prongs. There were no differences between groups with regard to extubation failure. Because there could have been outcome differences between the two types of NCPAP (unfortunately no subgroup analysis was presented), we do not believe that the study by Dimitriou et al. carries as much weight as other trials in which only one type of CPAP was evaluated. The Cochrane Collaboration analysis[60] of NCPAP use immediately following extubation concludes that it is an effective therapy for preventing failure of extubation. Nevertheless, the latter evaluation stresses the need for further studies to determine the gestational age and birthweight groups that would benefit most. The evaluation also stresses the need for further trials to determine optimal levels of NCPAP and optimal methods of administering NCPAP.

Several investigators have compared different types of NCPAP to determine if one method was effective following extubation of mechanically ventilated preterm infants. Davis et al.[61] compared ventilator-generated CPAP via either single or binasal prongs. Their population consisted of 87 premature infants of birthweight less than 1000 g. Single-prong NPCPAP was delivered via a shortened endotracheal tube inserted 2.5 cm into one nostril; binasal NCPAP was given through Hudson prongs. Significantly more infants [26/46 (57%)] randomized to the single-prong NPCPAP met failure criteria compared to 10 (24%) of 41 managed with binasal NCPAP ($P = 0.005$). Sun and Tien[62] compared the IFD to "conventional" binasal NCPAP that was ventilator generated. Their population consisted of 73 ventilated premature infants 30 weeks or more of gestation and birthweight at least 1250 g who met extubation criteria. Sun and Tien found 19 (54%) of 35 infants in the "conventional" group met failure criteria compared to 6 (16%) of 38 IFD-managed neonates ($P < 0.001$). Similarly, Roukema et al.[63] randomized 93 VLBW infants to either IFD or NPCPAP. The NPCPAP group [27/45 (60%)] was significantly more likely to fail extubation compared with the IFD group [18/48 (38%); $P = 0.0006$]. Murphy et al.[64] enrolled 162 ELBW infants into a RCT after extubation. The neonates were managed with either the IFD or binasal NCPAP. In contrast, these authors were unable to demonstrate any differences in extubation success rates between groups.

A number of investigators have assessed the value of nasal or nasopharyngeal CPAP as primary therapy for premature infants with RDS. Verder et al.[20] randomized premature infants with moderate-to-severe RDS to either NCPAP alone (n = 33) or NCPAP plus surfactant (n = 35). They used the Benveniste gas-jet valve to provide NCPAP in both groups. In the surfactant group, infants were transiently intubated and given Curosurf (Chiesi Farmaceutici, Parma, Italy) followed by several minutes of mechanical ventilation. These infants then were extubated and placed on NCPAP. The NCPAP plus surfactant group was significantly less likely to subsequently require mechanical ventilation [15/35 (43%)] compared to the NCPAP-only group [28/33 (85%); P = 0.003]. There were no differences in the following outcomes at 28 days of life: (1) mortality; (2) grade 3 or 4 intracranial hemorrhage or periventricular leukomalacia; or (3) need for oxygen. Verder's group[21] subsequently performed a second small trial to assess whether "early" administration of Curosurf (median age 5.2 hours) was better than "late" administration of this surfactant when infants' respiratory status had worsened (median age 9.9 hours). This was not a prophylaxis versus rescue surfactant trial. The Benveniste gas-jet valve was the method of NCPAP. The neonates who received surfactant earlier were significantly less likely to require mechanical ventilation prior to discharge [8/33 (24%) vs 17/27 (63%), P = 0.005]. In a group of 36 premature infants with RDS, Mazzella et al.[65] randomized subjects to either the IFD or bubble NPCPAP delivered via a single nasal prong. Although IFD-managed infants had more rapid declines in oxygen requirement and respiratory rate, there were no differences between groups with regard to the need for mechanical ventilation or the total duration of respiratory support.

Sandri et al.[66] randomized 230 premature infants (gestational age 28 to 31 weeks) to either prophylactic use of NCPAP (administration within 30 minutes of birth) or "rescue" NCPAP once the infants required an F_{IO_2} greater than 0.40 to maintain oxygen saturation levels greater than 93%. NCPAP was administered using the IFD in all infants. There were no significant differences between groups with regard to the need for exogenous surfactant (21.8% vs 20.8%) or mechanical ventilation (10.2% vs 9.1%). Thompson et al.[67] randomized 237 neonates (27 to 29 weeks of gestation) to one of four groups: (1) early NCPAP with prophylactic surfactant; (2) early NCPAP with rescue surfactant if needed; (3) early mechanical ventilation with prophylactic surfactant; or (4) early mechanical ventilation with rescue surfactant if needed. NCPAP was given via the IFD; Curosurf was the surfactant used in this trial. There were significantly less need for mechanical ventilation in the two NCPAP groups during the first 5 days of life. There were no significant differences among groups with regard to either mortality or oxygen dependency (at either 28 days of life or at 36 weeks of postmenstrual age).

Finally, Goldstein et al.[68] randomized seven mature infants (gestation ≥35 weeks) to either ventilator-generated NCPAP (n = 3) or negative end-expiratory pressure (NEEP; n = 4) via the Emerson negative pressure chamber (J.H. Emerson Co., Cambridge, MA, USA). The NCPAP infants were placed at 4 cm H_2O; the initial pressure in the NEEP group was −4 cm H_2O. Infants in the NEEP group were weaned to room air significantly faster than the NCPAP infants (P < 0.05).

Cochrane Collaborative Reports have addressed diverse CPAP RCTs. To date the following conclusions have been made: (1) there is insufficient evidence to assess the benefits and risks of prophylactic NCPAP in the preterm infant[69]; (2) early use of CPAP may reduce the need for mechanical ventilation[70]; and (3) early therapy with surfactant and NCPAP may be of benefit.[71] Concerning these areas, no definitive conclusions were drawn in the Cochrane evaluations and all reports stressed the need for larger prospective RCTs.

NASAL VENTILATION

Nasal ventilation (NV) is an intriguing concept that has gained popularity without substantial medical evidence. The concept is attractive: provision of positive pressure breaths non-invasively. Potentially, NV would avoid potential complications of prolonged ventilatory support via an endotracheal tube (volutrauma, subglottic stenosis, infections). Moreover, NV may have advantages over NCPAP or NPCPAP in stabilizing borderline functional residual capacity, reducing dead space, preventing atelectasis, and improving lung mechanics.[72,73] The practice was performed in the United States during the mid-1970s (Steven M. Donn, personal communication) and in Canada during the mid-1980s, with more than half of the level III NICUs in that country using the technique.[74,75] In general, NV has been studied to determine its potential usefulness (1) in preventing extubation failures[75–77]; (2) in treating AOP[74,78]; and (3) as a primary mode of treating respiratory disorders.

Friedlich et al.[76] randomized 41 premature infants to either NPCPAP or nasopharyngeal synchronized intermittent mandatory ventilation (NPSIMV) to be used after extubation. The authors used the Infant Star ventilator (Infrasonics, Inc., San Diego, CA, USA) with the "StarSync" abdominal capsule-triggering device (Infrasonics) for synchronization. Binasal nasopharyngeal prongs were used in both groups. Treatment failure was defined as one of multiple parameters: (1) pH ≤7.25; (2) increased $Paco_2$; (3) increased F_{IO_2} requirement; (4) need for NPSIMV rate greater than 20/min; (5) need for peak inspiratory pressure (PIP) on NPSIMV ≥20 cm H_2O; (6) need for PEEP on NPSIMV ≥8 cm H_2O; or (7) severe apnea. Friedlich's group reported significantly fewer extubation "failures" with NPSIMV [1/22 (5%)] compared to NPCPAP [7/19 (37%); P = 0.016]. Barrington et al.[75] randomized 54 VLBW infants to NCPAP or nasal synchronized intermittent mandatory ventilation (NSIMV) after extubation. They used binasal Hudson prongs with the Infant Star ventilator as the generating source for both groups, as well as the StarSync triggering device. Extubation failure criteria were similar to those used by Friedlich et al. Barrington et al. found that the NSIMV group had a lower incidence of failed extubation [4/27 (15%)] compared with the NCPAP group [12/27 (44%); P < 0.05]. Khalaf et al.[77] randomized 64 premature infants to either NSIMV or NCPAP applied after extubation using either the Bear Cub Model BP 2001 (Bear Medical Systems, Inc., Riverside, CA, USA) or the Infant Star ventilator, the StarSync triggering device, and Argyle nasal prongs. Failure criteria were similar to the two previous trials. Treatment failure occurred in 2 (6%) of 34 NSIMV infants compared to 12 (40%) of 30 NCPAP infants (P < 0.01).

Management of AOP using NV has been evaluated in RCTs.[74,78] Ryan et al.[74] used nasal intermittent positive-pressure ventilation (NIPPV) in a crossover study in which 20 premature infants less than 32 weeks of gestation were being treated for apnea with NCPAP and aminophylline. Infants were randomized to either continue on this regimen or be treated with NIPPV using either binasal prongs or nasopharyngeal tubes for 6 hours. The subjects then crossed over to the alternative therapy for an additional 6 hours. There were no differences in the rate of apnea between groups. Lin et al.[78] subsequently performed an RCT in which 34 premature infants (gestational age 25 to 32 weeks) were treated with aminophylline and enrolled for treatment with either NCPAP or NIPPV. Hudson nasal prongs were used in both groups. In the study by Lin et al., all infants had previously been treated with aminophylline but were not on any type of positive-pressure support (e.g., NCPAP or other support) at the time of enrollment. The infants were treated for a 4-hour period. Those treated with NIPPV had significantly fewer apnea spells ($P = 0.02$) and a trend toward fewer bradycardia spells ($P = 0.09$) compared to neonates managed with NCPAP.

Although we have heard about anecdotal experience in which clinicians used NV for primary management of respiratory disorders, we are aware of no studies (descriptive or RCTs) that have actually described such therapy. van der Hoeven et al.[79] reported using nasal high-frequency ventilation (NHFV) in which high-frequency breaths were delivered via a single nasopharyngeal tube in 21 neonates of both preterm and term-gestation. NHFV was provided by the Infant Star high-frequency flow interrupter. Six of the 21 neonates had previously received mechanical ventilation; in the other 15 infants, NHFV was used early in the course of their respiratory disease. The authors reported a decline in $Paco_2$ levels following initiation of NHFV.

In 1985 Garland et al.[80] reported an increased risk of gastrointestinal perforation among infants ventilated noninvasively with either nasal prongs or a face mask. Of note, in none of the five aforementioned RCTs did any infant develop such a perforation. As with standard NCPAP, we believe an orogastric tube should be placed in all infants undergoing NV in order to vent the stomach of swallowed air.

The conclusion of the Cochrane Collaboration Review[81] is that NV may be useful in augmenting NCPAP in preterm infants with apnea that is frequent or severe. Additional safety and efficacy data are required before recommending NV as standard therapy for apnea. The Cochrane Collaboration Review[82] assessing NV after extubation concluded that NV may augment the beneficial effects of NCPAP in preterm infants. The impact of synchronization on safety and efficacy of NV should be established in future trials.

OTHER APPLICATIONS OF CONTINUOUS POSITIVE AIRWAY PRESSURE IN NEONATES

We have mainly concentrated on describing the three primary uses of CPAP, particularly NCPAP, in newborn infants: (1) postextubation management; (2) treatment of AOP; and (3) primary therapy for RDS. CPAP has been applied in a variety of other conditions (Table 8-3),[83] but there are few data supporting CPAP use in these other conditions. Postoperatively

TABLE 8-3. Conditions For Which Continuous Distending Pressure Has Been Applied

Respiratory distress syndrome (RDS) in premature newborn infants
Apnea of prematurity
Postextubation management of premature infants
Postoperative respiratory management:
    Congenital hart disease
    Abdominal wall defects (gastroschisis, omphalocele)
    Other abdominal or thoracic surgical conditions
Differentiating congenital cyanotic heart disease from pulmonary disorders
Meconium aspiration syndrome (MAS)
Other aspiration syndromes (e.g., blood or gastric aspiration)
Transient tachypnea of the newborn ("wet lungs")
Pulmonary edema
Congestive heart failure
Patent ductus arteriosus (PDA)
Pneumonia
Laryngomalacia, bronchomalacia, and/or tracheomalacia
Resuscitation of infants in the delivery room
Increased work of breathing
"Other" disorders with radiographic findings of atelectasis, poor lung expansion, or pulmonary infiltrates
Persistent pulmonary hypertension of the newborn (PPHN)
Pulmonary hemorrhage
Provision of high positive end-expiratory pressure (PEEP) during extracorporeal membrane oxygenation (ECMO)

among infants with congenital heart disease, CPAP improved pulmonary mechanics and oxygenation.[84–86] CPAP may assist in the differentiation of congenital cyanotic heart disease from cyanotic pulmonary disorders.[87] Simplistically, the application of CPAP in infants with pulmonary disease should increase Pao_2 by more than 20 mm Hg (3 kPa). Furthermore, after surgical repair of abdominal wall defects (gastroschisis and omphalocele), increased abdominal pressure may adversely affect pulmonary function. CPAP was found to improve oxygenation in these disorders.[88] Fox et al.[89] described improved oxygenation with the application of CPAP [at 4 to 7 mm Hg (0.6 to 1 kPa)] among infants with meconium aspiration syndrome.

CPAP often is used for management of laryngomalacia, bronchomalacia, and/or tracheomalacia.[90,91] The positive pressure distends these large airways and mitigates their tendency to collapse, particularly during expiration. Conceptually, CPAP should help neonatal pulmonary disorders in which there is excessive lung fluid, such as transient tachypnea of the newborn, patent ductus arteriosus, pulmonary edema, congestive heart failure, and hydrops fetalis; however, data are lacking. Keszler et al.[92] assessed the use of different levels of background PEEP applied during extracorporeal membrane oxygenation. These investigators randomized 74 neonates requiring extracorporeal membrane oxygenation to either low PEEP (3 to 5 cm H_2O) or high PEEP (12 to 14 cm H_2O). Infants in the high PEEP group had significantly higher lung compliance and the duration of ECMO therapy was significantly shorter.

According to a recent survey, the majority of clinicians use CPAP in the delivery room during resuscitation of both preterm and term-gestation neonates (N.N. Finer, personal communication). Conceivably, CPAP could provide early noninvasive respiratory support and ameliorate or mitigate lung disease; however, the data supporting CPAP use in the delivery room are virtually nonexistent. There are commercially available devices, such as the Neopuff (Fisher & Paykel Healthcare, Auckland, New Zealand), a type of face mask CPAP, that are specifically made to provide CPAP and controlled positive pressure in the delivery room. Unquestionably, in the delivery room when infants do not respond to the initial steps of providing warmth, stimulating, drying, positioning, and administering blow-by oxygen, the key to resuscitation is positive-pressure ventilation. The vast majority of neonates will respond to the latter therapy; chest compressions, medications, and volume infusions are rarely needed. What populations should be studied in the delivery room? The preterm infant is more likely to sustain lung injury and develop CLD; hence, this population would be one in which noninvasive pulmonary therapy could be of benefit. Clearly, however, nasal CPAP can only be provided to infants who are making respiratory efforts. CPAP delivered via face mask devices can be augmented by intermittent sustained inflations or other higher volume breaths, as needed. Is there a population of term-gestation infants likely to benefit from CPAP in the delivery room? We are aware of two ongoing large RCTs that are assessing CPAP use in the delivery room:, one with the Neopuff and the other providing early nasal CPAP for extremely premature infants (25 to 28 weeks of gestation). Hopefully these trials will help determine the role of CPAP in the delivery room shortly after birth.

HAZARDS, ADVERSE EFFECTS, AND COMPLICATIONS OF CONTINUOUS POSITIVE AIRWAY PRESSURE

A major difficulty with the use of nasal cannulae or nasal prongs is keeping them in proper position. One can walk through most NICUs at any given time and note infants with malpositioned or displaced cannulae and prongs. We want to emphasize that with the variable-flow CPAP systems (IFD, Arabella, and SensorMedics devices), meticulous attention must be paid to assure proper fixation of the nasal prongs. Airway obstruction by secretions, particularly mucus, is a common finding in babies managed with CPAP. Optimal gas humidification, as well as frequent irrigation with saline followed by suctioning, should mitigate airway obstruction. Although nasopharyngeal prongs (single or binasal) are likely to be displaced, they are more easily blocked by secretions, they can kink, and they may not be as effective as the shorter prongs. Local irritation to the nares and oral cavity may occur with CPAP. Some clinicians use steroid and antibiotic ointments on the outer surfaces of CPAP devices to minimize the effects of irritation. Good oral hygiene (e.g., with lemon glycerine swabs or saline) should be considered to prevent drying and cracking.

A number of adverse side effects and complications of CPAP, PEEP, and NV have been described. The development of inadvertent PEEP may occur in ventilated babies, primarily those ventilated via endotracheal tubes. Conceivably, inadvertent PEEP could occur with NV. The mechanism is related to fast ventilatory rates and inadequate (too short) expiratory times. Inadvertent PEEP may occur in babies with minimal to no lung disease (e.g., postoperative patients) or in those with sick lungs. Healthy lungs have longer time constants; hence, passive exhalation requires a greater amount of time. Inadvertent PEEP results in air trapping that clinically may appear as hyperexpanded lungs on chest roentgenograms. Air

trapping may manifest clinically as hypoxemia and hypercapnia. Health care providers should be suspicious of this entity when oxygenation deteriorates as inspiratory pressure is increased. Air trapping contributes to the development of air leaks. Additionally, air leaks (pneumothorax, pneumomediastinum, pulmonary interstitial emphysema) may be a direct complication of CPAP/PEEP.[93–95] The mechanism may be related to overdistention of the more compliant areas of the lung. Most evidence linking CPAP/PEEP to air leaks comes from publications at least 20 years old (see Chapter 21). As a generalization, those references indicate pneumothoraces were a problem with babies in whom CPAP was the primary ventilatory therapy for RDS. We are unaware of any reported increased risk for air leaks when CPAP is used for postextubation respiratory management or as therapy for AOP. Moreover, there is no apparent increased risk among infants who are nasally ventilated. Unfortunately, no incidence rates of air leaks were provided in the large review of Van Marter et al.[15] comparing the Columbia experience with that of the Boston group. In the IFDAS trial,[67] in which two NCPAP groups are compared with two mechanically ventilated groups, there were no differences in the frequency of air leaks between the early-NCPAP and early-ventilated groups. In any future trials in which CPAP is compared to mechanical ventilation or to other therapies, air leaks remain an important outcome parameter that should be followed and reported.

Retention of carbon dioxide (CO_2) has been noted with higher levels of CPAP, particularly at levels above 8 cm H_2O. Alveolar overdistention, as well as inadequate expiratory times, may lead to reduced tidal volumes and cause CO_2 retention. Other manifestations of lung overdistention[96] include increased work of breathing, impaired systemic venous return, decreased cardiac output, and increased pulmonary vascular resistance. In addition, mechanical ventilation with PEEP may produce a decrease in glomerular filtration rate and a decrease in urine output.[97] Renal effects of CPAP in preterm infants are notable at higher levels of pressure.[98] These effects on the kidney may be due to decreased cardiac output and decreased perfusing pressure to the organs. In addition, CPAP and PEEP are known to increase intracranial pressure.[83] Nevertheless, with the widespread use of screening ultrasonography over the past 2 decades, we are unaware of any direct links between CPAP/PEEP and brain injury in premature or term-gestation neonates.

Gastrointestinal blood flow may decrease with the application of CPAP.[99] Additionally, marked bowel distention ("CPAP belly") is frequently recognized in infants treated with this therapy.[100] With nonendotracheal tube CPAP, administered gas can easily pass into the esophagus. Infants may swallow a considerable volume of gas and present with bulging flanks, increased abdominal girth, and visibly dilated intestinal loops. Upward pressure may be placed on the diaphragm and compromise the child's respiratory status. Unquestionably, routine placement of an orogastric tube should take place whenever CPAP is used. The orogastric tube should prevent or alleviate "CPAP belly." No direct link between CPAP and the overwhelming gastrointestinal disorder necrotizing enterocolitis has been demonstrated; however, it may be difficult to distinguish early nonspecific gastrointestinal distention of necrotizing enterocolitis from "CPAP belly." Garland et al.[80] reported an increased risk of gastric perforation in nasally ventilated neonates; however, virtually all recent investigations of NV do not confirm this association. Moreover, CPAP alone has not been reported to cause gastric perforation.

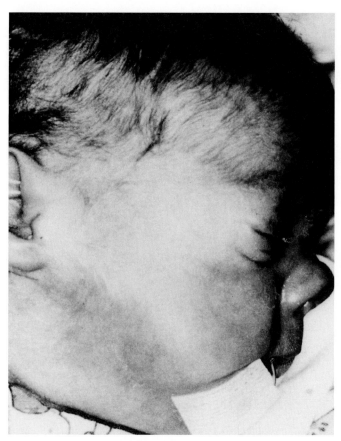

Figure 8-22. Severe nasal "snubbing" noted after prolonged nasal continuous positive airway pressure use in a 3-month-old, ex-24-week-gestational-age premature infant. (Figure courtesy of Dr. Nicola Robertson and reproduced from Robertson NJ, McCarthy LS, Hamilton PA, et al: Nasal deformities resulting from flow driver continuous positive airway pressure. Arch Dis Child Fetal Neonatal Ed 1996;75:F209–F212, with permission.)

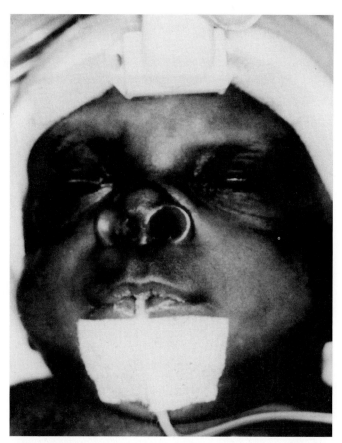

Figure 8-23. Three-month-old infant with a circumferential distortion noted after prolonged (6 weeks) nasal continuous positive airway pressure therapy. (Figure courtesy of Dr. Nicola Robertson and reproduced from Robertson NJ, McCarthy LS, Hamilton PA, et al: Nasal deformities resulting from flow driver continuous positive airway pressure. Arch Dis Child Fetal Neonatal Ed 1996;75:F209–F212, with permission.)

Nasal prongs may cause trauma to the nose that can be mild (e.g., edema or erythema) or severe. Robertson et al.[101] reported a series of cases of severe trauma, including nasal snubbing (Fig. 8-22), flaring of the nostrils (Fig. 8-23), and columella necrosis (Fig. 8-24). Nasal deformities may occur with different types of nasal prongs and NCPAP devices.[101,102] Other rare complications have been described in single case reports. Peck et al.[103] described the dislodgment of a single nasal prong that slipped into the child's stomach and ultimately needed endoscopic retrieval. Additionally, a preterm infant developed a pneumatocele approximately 24 hours after CPAP was instituted.[104] Wong et al.[105] described an infant being managed on NCPAP who developed bilateral tension pneumothoraces and extensive vascular air embolism.

CONTRAINDICATIONS TO CONTINUOUS POSITIVE AIRWAY PRESSURE

There are several contraindications to CPAP,[96,106] including the following:

- Infants who have progressive respiratory failure and are unable to maintain oxygenation, $Paco_2$ levels less than 60 mm Hg (8 kPa), and/or pH levels ≥7.25

- Certain congenital malformations (congenital diaphragmatic hernia, tracheoesophageal fistula, choanal atresia, cleft palate)
- Infants with severe cardiovascular instability (hypotension, poor ventricular function)
- Neonates with poor or unstable respiratory drive (frequent apnea, bradycardia, and/or oxygen desaturation) that is not improved by CPAP

DETERMINING OPTIMAL LEVELS OF CONTINUOUS POSITIVE AIRWAY PRESSURE AND POSITIVE END-EXPIRATORY PRESSURE

What is the best level of CPAP or PEEP? We believe it is the level at which oxygenation and ventilation occur in acceptable ranges and there are no adverse side effects. Unfortunately, there are no simple and reliable methods to determine the most advantageous pressure.[83,96,106] Clearly, each baby's respiratory problems and support needs at any given moment are those of that individual and cannot be extrapolated to all neonates with similar problems. Some investigators have used esophageal pressures or changes in the inspiratory limbs of

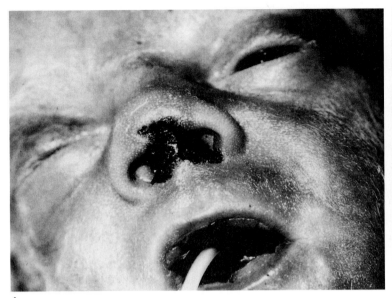

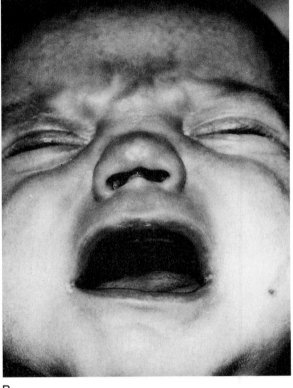

Figure 8-24. *A,* Columella necrosis noted after 3 days of nasal continuous positive airway pressure. *B,* Progression of columella necrosis to absent columella in the same infant at 4 months of age. (Figures courtesy of Dr. Nicola Robertson and reproduced from Robertson NJ, McCarthy LS, Hamilton PA, et al: Nasal deformities resulting from flow driver continuous positive airway pressure. Arch Dis Child Fetal Neonatal Ed 1996;75:F209–F212, with permission.)

pressure-volume curves to guide their efforts in finding the elusive pressure level; however, these techniques are not generally available at the bedside of most clinicians. In general, to determine whether a particular level of pressure is appropriate, clinicians should assess the chest radiograph. The appearance should be assessed for the type of disorder the baby has and the degree of lung expansion. Diseases with atelectasis (volume loss) and increased fluid (e.g., pulmonary edema) should be treated with increasing pressures. In general, we start with pressure levels of 5 to 6 cm H_2O and increase as necessary to improve oxygenation. We have used levels as high as 8 to 10 cm H_2O. Occasionally babies with particularly poor compliance have needed even higher levels. Serial chest radiographs will help one assess the degree of lung expansion. If the lungs are overinflated, air trapping may occur and the CPAP/ PEEP levels should generally be decreased. Following the child's oxygenation and carbon dioxide levels with arterial or capillary blood gases, as well as oxygen saturation monitoring, will further assist the assessment of appropriate CPAP level. As a general rule, we perform blood gas analysis within 30 to 60 minutes following any changes in pressure. If oxygenation worsens following increases in pressure, the lungs may be overdistended. Because CO_2 levels generally increase with increasing pressures, the clinician must weigh the potential advantages of improved oxygenation versus hypercapnia. If these levels are in a range acceptable to the clinician, mild CO_2 retention may be allowed. Many of the current mechanical ventilators have graphic monitors on which pulmonary mechanics are displayed. If one uses ventilator-generated CPAP or PEEP via an endotracheal tube with such a device, the monitor may be useful in determining the optimal pressures that should be used.

WEANING FROM CONTINUOUS POSITIVE AIRWAY PRESSURE

Once a child is being treated with CPAP, there are no magic guidelines as to when the infant can be weaned off. As the pressures are decreased, we assess the baby's oxygen saturation levels, occurrence of apnea and/or bradycardia, and work of breathing. Hopefully, we have been able to lower the FIO_2 to a relatively low amount. In general, infants who require an FIO_2 greater than 0.40 or are clinically unstable are unlikely to be successfully weaned off CPAP. Generally, we like to decrease pressures down to a relatively low level (~5 cm H_2O). Once we are at this level without increasing work of breathing and do not have substantial apnea, bradycardia, or oxygen desaturation levels, we attempt to discontinue CPAP. The baby's subsequent clinical findings and oxygen requirement will guide the clinician as to whether CPAP must be reinstituted.

SUMMARY

Use of continuous positive airway pressure in neonates is not a new concept. Apparent benefits were first noted more than 3 decades ago. For a 15- to 20-year period, however, treatment with CPAP and research on the technology waned. Renewed interest in the technique came about in the mid-1990s. With advances in obstetric and neonatal care, survival of increasingly smaller and less mature neonates has become possible. CPAP represents a noninvasive method of respiratory support that may lessen iatrogenic injury to newborn infants, particularly those of very low birthweight. The history of neonatology is replete with widespread enthusiastic acceptance of diverse therapies with a modicum of supportive evidence. Unfortunately, we see that CPAP is currently being similarly embraced.

The major areas in which CPAP is being used are for post-extubation management, treatment of AOP, and primary treatment of RDS. There is some evidence supporting NCPAP use after extubation; however, CPAP use for AOP currently is unfounded. There is a little evidence that early NCPAP use, particularly with early exogenous surfactant therapy, reduces the need for mechanical ventilation in premature babies with RDS. There is no evidence that early NCPAP prevents air leaks, CLD, or mortality. There is even less basis for CPAP use for conditions other than the aforementioned ones, much less in the delivery room. A similar lack of evidence does not permit us to definitively define a role for NV in infants. Simple questions have yet to be answered:

- Does CPAP use increase caloric expenditure?
- What are the long-term pulmonary and neurodevelopmental outcomes among infants who are primarily managed with CPAP?
- What are acceptable ranges of pH, Pa_{O_2}, and Pa_{CO_2} among infants receiving CPAP?
- Does early use of NCPAP delay timely administration of exogenous surfactant?

Many additional simple and complex questions concerning this therapy have not been answered. Although we believe CPAP may play a major role in our management of neonates with respiratory distress, that role has yet to be clearly defined by evidence-based medicine.

REFERENCES

1. Poulton EP, Oxon DM: Left sided heart failure with pulmonary edema: Its treatment with the "pulmonary plus pressure machine." Lancet 1936;231:981–983.
2. Bullowa JGH: The Management of the Pneumonias. New York, Oxford University Press, 1937.
3. Barach AL, Martin J, Eckman M: Positive pressure respiration and its application to the treatment of acute pulmonary edema and respiratory obstruction. Proc Soc Clin Invest 1937;16:664.
4. Armstrong HG (ed): Aerospace Medicine. Baltimore, Williams & Wilkins, 1946.
5. Ashbaugh DG, Bigelow DB, Petty TL, et al: Acute respiratory distress in adults. Lancet 1967;2:319.
6. Harrison VC, Heese H de V, Klein M: The significance of grunting in hyaline membrane disease. Pediatrics 1968;41:549–559.
7. Gregory GA, Kitterman JA, Phibbs RH, et al: Treatment of the idiopathic respiratory distress syndrome with continuous positive airway pressure. N Engl J Med 1971;284:1333–1340.
8. Kamper J: Early nasal continuous positive airway pressure and minimal handling in the treatment of very-low-birth weight infants. Biol Neonate 1999;76(Suppl):22–28.
9. Kattwinkel J, Nearmam HS, Fanaroff AA, et al: Apnea of prematurity: Comparative therapeutic effects of cutaneous stimulation and nasal CPAP. J Pediatr 1975;86:588.
10. Caliumi-Pellegrini G, Agostino R, Orzalesi M, et al: Twin nasal cannulae for administration of continuous positive airway pressure to newborn infants. Arch Dis Child 1974;49:228–229.
11. Clark RH, Gerstmann DR, Jobe AH, et al: Lung injury in neonates: Causes, strategies for prevention, and long-term consequences. J Pediatr 2001;139:478–486.
12. Björklund LJ, Ingimarsson J, Curstedt T, et al: Manual ventilation with a few large breaths at birth compromises the therapeutic effect of sub-

13. sequent surfactant replacement in immature lambs. Pediatr Res 1997;42:348–355.
13. Avery ME, Tooley WH, Keller JB, et al: Is chronic lung disease in low-birth-weight infants preventable? A survey of eight centers. Pediatrics 1987;79:26–30.
14. Wung JT, Koons AH, Driscoll JM Jr, et al: Changing incidence of bronchopulmonary dysplasia. J Pediatr 1979;95(5 Pt 2):845–847.
15. Van Marter LJ, Allred EN, Pagano M, et al: Do clinical markers of barotrauma and oxygen toxicity explain interhospital variation in rates of chronic lung disease? Pediatrics 2000;105:1194–1201.
16. Aly HZ: Nasal prongs continuous positive airway pressure: A simple yet powerful tool. Pediatrics 2001;108:759–761.
17. Lee KS, Dunn MS, Fenwick M, et al: A comparison of underwater bubble continuous positive airway pressure with ventilator-derived continuous positive airway pressure in premature neonates ready for extubation. Biol Neonate 1998;73:69–75.
18. Nekvasil R, Kratky J, Penkova Z, et al: High frequency "bubble" oscillation ventilation in the neonatal period. Cesk Pediatr 1992;47:465–470.
19. Benveniste D, Pedersen JEP: A valve substitute with no moving parts for artificial ventilation in newborn and small infants. Br J Anaesth 1968;40:464–470.
20. Verder H, Robertson B, Greisen G, et al: Surfactant therapy and nasal continuous positive airway pressure for newborns with respiratory distress syndrome. N Engl J Med 1994;331:1051–1055.
21. Verder H, Albertsen P, Ebbesen F, et al: Nasal continuous positive airway pressure and early surfactant therapy for respiratory distress syndrome in newborns of less than 30 weeks' gestation. Pediatrics 1999;103:e24.
22. Moa G, Nilsson K, Zetterstrom H, et al: A new device for administration of nasal continuous positive airways pressure in the newborn: An experimental study. Crit Care Med 1988;16:1238–1242.
23. Bachman TE: Nasal CPAP for the preterm infant: Recent technical advances Neonatal Intens Care 2002;15:19–21.
24. Klausner JF, Lee AY, Hutchinson AA: Decreased imposed work with a new nasal continuous positive airway pressure device. Pediatr Pulmonol 1996;22:188–194.
25. Pandit PB, Courtney SE, Pyon KH, et al: Work of breathing during constant- and variable-flow nasal continuous positive airway pressure in preterm neonates. Pediatrics 2001;108:682–685.
26. De Paoli AG, Morley CJ, Davis PG, et al: In vitro comparison of nasal continuous positive airway pressure devices for neonates. Arch Dis Child Fetal Neonatal Ed 2002;87:F42–F45.
27. Kornhauser MS, Needelman HW, Leahey M: Efficacy of short vs long term CPAP prior to extubation. Pediatric Res 1986;20:433A.
28. Krauss DR, Marshall RE: Severe neck ulceration from CPAP head box. J Pediatr 1975;86:286–287.
29. Vert P, Andre M, Sibout M: CPAP and hydrocephalus. Lancet 1973;2:319.
30. Ahlstrom H, Jonson B, Svenningsen NW: Continuous positive airway pressure with a face chamber in early treatment of idiopathic respiratory distress syndrome. Acta Paediatr Scand 1973;62:433–436.
31. Svenningsen NW, Jonson B, Lindroth M, et al: Consecutive study of early CPAP-application in hyaline membrane disease. Eur J Pediatr 1979 25;131:9–19.
32. Andreasson B, Lindroth M, Svenningsen NW, et al: Effects on respiration of CPAP immediately after extubation in the very preterm infant. Pediatr Pulmonol 1988;4:213–218.
33. Allen L, Blake A, Durbin G, et al: CPAP and mechanical ventilation by face mask in newborn infants. Br Med J 1975;4:137–139.
34. Rhodes PG, Hall RT: Continuous positive airway pressure delivered by face mask in infants with the idiopathic respiratory distress syndrome: A controlled study. Pediatrics 1973;52:1–5.
35. Goldman SL, Brady JP, Dumpit F: Increased work of breathing associated with nasal prongs. Pediatrics 1979;64:160–164.
36. Pape K, Armstrong D, Fitzhardinge EP: Central nervous system pathology associated with mask ventilation in the very low birth weight infant: A new etiology for intracerebellar hemorrhage. Pediatrics 1976;58:473–483.
37. Locke RG, Wolfson MR, Shaffer TH, et al: Inadvertent administration of positive end-distending pressure during nasal cannula flow. Pediatrics 1993;91:135–138.
38. Sreenan C, Lemke RP, Hudson-Mason A, et al: High-flow nasal cannulae in the management of apnea of prematurity: A comparison with conventional nasal continuous positive airway pressure. Pediatrics 2001;107:1081–1083.
39. Jacobsen T, Grønvall J, Petersen S, et al: "Minitouch" treatment of very-low-birth-weight infants. Acta Paediatr 1993;82:934–938.

40. Gittermann MK, Fusch C, Gittermann AR, et al: Early nasal continuous positive airway pressure treatment reduces the need for intubation in very low birth weight infants. Eur J Pediatr 1997;156:384–388.

41. Lindner W, Vossbeck S, Hummler H, et al: Delivery room management of extremely low birth weight infants: Spontaneous breathing or intubation? Pediatrics 1999;103:961–967.

42. De Klerk AM, De Klerk RK: Nasal continuous positive airway pressure and outcomes of preterm infants. J Paediatr Child Health 2001;37:161–167.

43. Blennow M, Jonsson B, Dahlstrom A, et al: Lung function in premature infants can be improved. Surfactant therapy and CPAP reduce the need of respiratory support. Lakartidningen 1999;31;96:1571–1576.

44. Ancora G, Sandri F, Lanzoni A, et al: Efficacy of INSURE approach (intubation-surfactant-extubation) followed by nasal continuous positive airway pressure (nCPAP) in preterm infants with respiratory distress syndrome (RDS) [abstract 2248]. Pediatr Res 2001;49:392A.

45. Blennow M, Jonsson B, Bohlin K, et al: Early surfactant administration with brief ventilation and extubation to nCPAP [abstract 2017]. Pediatr Res 2002;51;347A.

46. Kavvadia V, Greenough A, Dimitriou G: Effect on lung function of continuous positive airway pressure administered either by infant flow driver or a single nasal prong. Eur J Pediatr 2000;159:289–292.

47. Kurz H: Influence of nasopharyngeal CPAP on breathing pattern and incidence of apnoeas in preterm infants. Biol Neonate 1999;76:129–133.

48. Jones RAK: Apnoea of prematurity. 1. A controlled trial of theophylline and face mask continuous positive airways pressure. Arch Dis Child 1982;57:761–765.

49. Henderson-Smart DJ, Subramaniam P, Davis PG: Continuous positive airway pressure versus theophylline for apnea in preterm infants. Cochrane Database Syst Rev 2001;4:CD001072.

50. Davis PG, Henderson-Smart DJ: Extubation from low-rate intermittent positive airways pressure versus extubation after a trial of endotracheal continuous positive airways pressure in intubated preterm infants. Cochrane Database Syst Rev 2001;4:CD001078.

51. Engelke SC, Roloff DW, Kuhns LR: Postextubation nasal continuous positive airway pressure. Am J Dis Child 1982;136:359–361.

52. Higgins RD, Richter SE, Davis JM: Nasal continuous positive airway pressure facilitates extubation of very low birth weight neonates. Pediatrics 1991;88:999–1003.

53. Chan V, Greenough A: Randomised trial of methods of extubation in acute and chronic respiratory distress. Arch Dis Child 1993;68:570–572.

54. Annibale DJ, Hulsey TC, Engsstrom PC, et al: Randomized, controlled trial of nasopharyngeal continuous positive airway pressure in the extubation of very low birthweight infants. J Pediatr 1994;124:455.

55. So B-H, Tamura M, Mishina J, et al: Application of nasal continuous positive airway pressure to early extubation in very low birthweight infants. Arch Dis Child Fetal Neonatal Ed 1995;72:F191–F193.

56. Tapia JL, Bancalari A, Gonzalez A, et al: Does continuous positive airway pressure (CPAP) during weaning from intermittent mandatory ventilation in very low birth weight infants have risks or benefits? A controlled trial. Pediatr Pulmonol 1995;19:269–274.

57. Davis P, Jankov R, Doyle L, et al: Randomised controlled trial of nasal continuous positive airway pressure in the extubation of infants weighing 600 to 1250 g. Arch Dis Child Fetal Neonatal Ed 1998;78:F54–F57.

58. Robertson NJ, Hamilton PA: Randomised trial of elective continuous positive airway pressure (CPAP) compared with rescue CPAP after extubation. Arch Dis Child Fetal Neonatal Ed 1998;79:F58–F60.

59. Dimitriou G, Greenough A, Kavvadia V, et al: Elective use of nasal continuous positive airways pressure following extubation of preterm infants. Eur J Pediatr 2000;159:434–439.

60. Davis PG, Henderson-Smart DJ: Nasal continuous positive airways pressure immediately after extubation for preventing morbidity in preterm infants. Cochrane Database Syst Rev 2000;3:CD000143.

61. Davis P, Davies M, Faber B: A randomised controlled trial of two methods of delivering nasal continuous positive airway pressure after extubation to infants weighing less than 1000 g: Binasal (Hudson) versus single nasal prongs. Arch Dis Child Fetal Neonatal Ed 2001;85:F82–F85.

62. SunSC, Tien HC: Randomized controlled trial of two methods of nasal CPAP (NCPAP): Flow driver vs. conventional NCPAP [abstract 1898]. Pediatr Res 1999;45:322A.

63. Roukema H, O'Brien K, Nesbitt K, et al: A randomized, controlled trial of Infant Flow continuous positive airway pressure (CPAP) versus nasopharyngeal CPAP in the extubation of babies ≤1250 grams [abstract 1874]. Pediatr Res 1999;45:318A.

64. Murphy WP, Hansell BJ, Fuloria M, et al: A randomized comparison of two CPAP systems for the successful extubation of extremely low birth weight (ELBW) infants [abstract 1646]. Pediatr Res 2001;49:288A.

65. Mazzella M, Bellini C, Calevo MG, et al: A randomised control study comparing the infant flow driver with nasal continuous positive airway pressure in preterm infants. Arch Dis Child Fetal Neonatal Ed 2001;85:F86–F90.

66. Sandri F, Ancora G, Mosca F, et al: Prophylactic vs. rescue nasal continuous positive airway pressure (nCPAP) in preterm infants: Preliminary results of a multicenter randomized controlled trial [abstract 1558]. Pediatr Res 2001;49:273A.

67. Thomson MA, IFDAS Study Group: Early nasal continuous positive airways pressure (nCPAP) with prophylactic surfactant for neonates at risk of RDS. The IFDAS Multi-Centre Randomized Trial [abstract 2204]. Pediatr Res 2002;51:379A.

68. Goldstein MR, Furman GI, Sindel BD, et al: Negative pressure ventilation: An alternative to management of neonatal respiratory distress with nasal continuous positive airway pressure (NCPAP) [abstract 2297]. Pediatr Res 2001;49:400A.

69. Subramaniam P, Henderson-Smart DJ, Davis PG: Prophylactic nasal continuous positive airways pressure for preventing morbidity and mortality in very preterm infants. Cochrane Database Syst Rev 2000;2:CD001243.

70. Ho JJ, Henderson-Smart DJ, Davis PG: Early versus delayed initiation of continuous distending pressure for respiratory distress syndrome in preterm infants. Cochrane Database Syst Rev 2002;2:CD002975.

71. Stevens TP, Blennow M, Soll RF: Early surfactant administration with brief ventilation vs selective surfactant and continued mechanical ventilation for preterm infants with or at risk for RDS. Cochrane Database Syst Rev 2002;2:CD003063.

72. Kiciman NM, Andreasson B, Bernstein G: Thoracoabdominal motion in newborns during ventilation delivered by endotracheal tube or nasal prongs. Pediatr Pulmonol 1998; 25:175–181.

73. Moretti C, Gizzi C, Papoff P: Comparing the effects of nasal synchronized intermittent positive pressure ventilation (nSIPPV) and nasal continuous positive airway pressure (nCPAP) after extubation in very low birth weight infants. Early Hum Dev 1999;56:167–177.

74. Ryan CA, Finer NN, Peters KL: Nasal intermittent positive-pressure ventilation offers no advantages over nasal continuous positive airway pressure in apnea of prematurity. Am J Dis Child 1989;143:1196–1198.

75. Barrington KJ, Bull D, Finer NN: Randomized trial of nasal synchronized intermittent mandatory ventilation compared with continuous positive airway pressure after extubation of very low birth weight infants. Pediatrics 2001;107:638–641.

76. Friedlich P, Lecart C, Posen R, et al: A randomized trial of nasopharyngeal-synchronized intermittent mandatory ventilation versus nasopharyngeal continuous positive airway pressure in very low birth weight infants after extubation. J Perinatol 1999;19:413–418.

77. Khalaf MN, Brodsky N, Hurley J, et al: A prospective randomized, controlled trial comparing synchronized nasal intermittent positive pressure ventilation versus nasal continuous positive airway pressure as modes of extubation. Pediatrics 2001;108:13–17.

78. Lin C-H, Tsai W-H, Lin Y-J, et al: Efficacy of nasal intermittent positive pressure ventilation in treating apnea of prematurity. Pediatr Pulmonol 1998;26:349–353.

79. van der Hoeven M, Brouwer E, Blanco CE: Nasal high frequency ventilation in neonates with moderate respiratory insufficiency. Arch Dis Child Fetal Neonatal Ed 1998;79:F61–F63.

80. Garland JS, Nelson DB, Rice T, et al: Increased risk of gastrointestinal perforations in neonates mechanically ventilated with either face mask or nasal prongs. Pediatrics 1985;76:406–410.

81. Lemyre B, Davis PG, de Paoli AG: Nasal intermittent positive pressure ventilation (NIPPV) versus nasal continuous positive airway pressure (NCPAP) for apnea of prematurity. Cochrane Database Syst Rev 2002;1:CD002272.

82. Davis PG, Lemyre B, de Paoli AG: Nasal intermittent positive pressure ventilation (NIPPV) versus nasal continuous positive airway pressure (NCPAP) for preterm neonates after extubation. Cochrane Database Syst Rev 2001;3:CD003212.

83. Ahumada CA, Goldsmith JP: Continuous distending pressure. In Goldsmith JP, Karotkin EH (eds): Assisted Ventilation of the Newborn, 3rd ed. Philadelphia, WB Saunders, 1996, pp. 151–165.

84. Gregory GA, Edmunds LH Jr, Kitterman JA, et al: Continuous positive airway pressure and pulmonary and circulatory function after cardiac surgery in infants less than three months of age. Anesthesiology 1975;43:426–431.

85. Cogswell JJ, Hatch DJ, Kerr AA, et al: Effects of continuous positive airway pressure on lung mechanics of babies after operation for congenital heart disease. Arch Dis Child 1975;50:799–804.

86. Hatch DJ, Taylor BW, Glover WJ, et al: Continuous positive-airway pressure after open-heart operations in infancy. Lancet 1973;2:469–470.

87. Rao PJ, Marino BL, Robertson AF III: Usefulness of continuous positive airway pressure in differential diagnosis of cardiac from pulmonary cyanosis in newborn infants. Arch Dis Child 1978;53:456–460.

88. Buyukpamukcu N, Hicsonmez A: The effect of CPAP upon pulmonary reserve and cardiac output under increased abdominal pressure. J Pediatr Surg 1977;12:49–53.

89. Fox WW, Berman LS, Downes JJ Jr, et al: The therapeutic application of end-expiratory pressure in the meconium aspiration syndrome. Pediatrics 1975;56:214–217.

90. Miller RW, Pollack MM, Murphy TM, et al: Effectiveness of continuous positive airway pressure in the treatment of bronchomalacia in infants: A bronchoscopic documentation. Crit Care Med 1986;14:125–127.

91. Davis S, Jones M, Kisling J, et al: Effect of continuous positive airway pressure on forced expiratory flows in infants with tracheomalacia. Am J Respir Crit Care Med 1998;158:148–152.

92. Keszler M, Ryckman FC, McDonald JV Jr, et al: A prospective, multicenter, randomized study of high versus low positive end-expiratory pressure during extracorporeal membrane oxygenation. J Pediatr 1992;120:107–113.

93. Hall RT, Rhodes PG: pneumothorax and pneumomediastinum in infants with idiopathic respiratory distress syndrome receiving CPAP. Pediatrics 1975;55:493–496.

94. Ogata ES, Gregory GA, Kitterman JA, et al: Pneumothorax in the respiratory distress syndrome: Incidence and effect on vital signs, blood gases, and pH. Pediatrics 1976;58:177–183.

95. Theilade D: Nasal CPAP treatment of RDS: A prospective investigation in 10 newborn infants. Intens Care Med 1978;4:149–153.

96. Morley C: Continuous distending pressure. Arch Dis Child Fetal Neonatal Ed 1999;81:F152–F156.

97. Jarnberg PD, de Villota ED, Eklund J, et al: Effects of PEEP on renal function. Acta Anaesthesiol Scand 1978;22:508–514.

98. Tulassay T, Machay T, Kiszel J, et al: Effects of continuous positive airway pressure on renal function in prematures. Biol Neonate 1983;43:152–157.

99. Furzan JA, Gabriele G, Wheeler JM, et al: Regional blood flow in newborn lambs during endotracheal continuous negative pressure breathing. Pediatr Res 1981;15:874–878.

100. Jaile JC, Levin T, Wung JT, et al: Benign gaseous distension of the bowel in premature infants treated with nasal continuous airway pressure: A study of contributing factors. AJR Am J Roentgenol 1992;158:125–127.

101. Robertson NJ, McCarthy LS, Hamilton PA, et al: Nasal deformities resulting from flow driver continuous positive airway pressure. Arch Dis Child Fetal Neonatal Ed 1996;75:F209–F212.

102. Ridout RE, Townsent SF, Kelley P, et al: Nasal septal necrosis resulting from nasal synchronized intermittent mandatory ventilation in VLBW infants [abstract 2025]. Pediatr Res 2002;51:348A.

103. Peck DJ, Tulloh RM, Madden N, et al: A wandering nasal prong-a thing of risks and problems. Paediatr Anaesth 1999;9:77–79.

104. de Bie HM, van Toledo-Eppinga L, Verbeke JI, et al: Neonatal pneumatocele as a complication of nasal continuous positive airway pressure. Arch Dis Child Fetal Neonatal Ed 2002;86:F202–F203.

105. Wong W, Fok TF, Ng PC, et al: Vascular air embolism: A rare complication of nasal CPAP. J Paediatr Child Health 1997;33:444–445.

106. Morley CJ: Continuous positive airway pressure. In Sinha SK, Donn SM (eds): Manual of Neonatal Respiratory Care. Armonk, NY, Futura Publishing Company, 2000, pp. 134–140.

9

POSITIVE-PRESSURE VENTILATION
Pressure-Limited and Time-Cycled Ventilation

ALAN R. SPITZER, MD
JAY S. GREENSPAN, MD
WILLIAM W. FOX, MD

Positive-pressure mechanical ventilation with the use of pressure-limited ventilators remains the most common approach for treatment of respiratory failure in neonatal intensive care units (NICUs) in the United States. Since the last edition of this text, mechanical ventilators have changed significantly, although the fundamental physiology of positive-pressure ventilation remains intact. The most dramatic changes have involved the introduction of a variety of novel variations for the delivery of positive-pressure ventilation. Most of these new approaches are designed to reduce either volutrauma or barotrauma to the lung, theoretically diminishing the risk of bronchopulmonary dysplasia (BPD). Although many of these therapies appear promising, none has clearly been shown to either eliminate BPD or reduce hospital length of stay, especially for the extremely-low-birthweight neonate (birthweight ≤1000 g). These infants, in particular, have emerged as a primary focus of attention in the NICU. Although these babies comprise only a small part of NICU admissions (5% to 8%), they remain hospitalized for long periods of time and consume a disproportionate number of hospital days. In addition, they often have the greatest mortality and morbidity, both acute and long-term. Because of these issues, positive-pressure ventilation remains a critical focal point of care, not only from a pulmonary perspective but also from a neurodevelopmental viewpoint. At the beginning of a new millennium, it no longer is sufficient to ensure pulmonary recovery alone. Intact neurologic outcome also must be considered a priority with any approach to care of the neonate with lung disease.

For the larger infant with pulmonary problems, positive-pressure ventilation is also an essential aspect of care. For these neonates, the use of more advanced forms of ventilatory support, such as synchronized intermittent mandatory ventilation (SIMV),[1] assist/control ventilation,[2] high-frequency jet ventilation (HFJV),[3,4] high-frequency oscillatory ventilation,[5] inhalational nitric oxide therapy,[6] or extracorporeal membrane oxygenation (ECMO),[7] has not altered the central role of positive-pressure conventional mechanical ventilation. The purpose of this chapter is to review the uses of pressure-limited, time-cycled, positive-pressure ventilation in the management of neonatal respiratory failure in both the premature and term neonate.

DESIGN PRINCIPLES

Classification

Positive-pressure mechanical ventilators are referred to by most clinicians as either volume or pressure types. *Volume-controlled ventilators* deliver the same tidal volume of gas with each breath, regardless of the pressure that is needed. *Pressure-preset ventilators,* in contrast, are designed to deliver a volume of gas until a preset limiting pressure designated by the physician is reached. The remainder of volume in the unit is then released into the atmosphere. As a result, the tidal volume that is delivered to the patient by pressure-preset ventilators with each breath may be variable, but the peak pressure delivered to the airway remains constant. The flow generation necessary to drive pressure-preset ventilators may occur in the following ways: constant-flow generator (high-pressure gas source or compressor), nonconstant-flow generator (cam-operated piston), or constant-pressure generator (weighted bellows).

Ventilators have been introduced that have the capability of serving as either volume-controlled or pressure-controlled, time-cycled ventilators, depending on the operator's preference (i.e., Bird V.I.P., Bird Products Co., Palm Springs, CA, USA). These units have significant advantages for some patients and represent an important advance in ventilator technology. In addition, new modifications of ventilator circuits allow a variety of pressure assist modes designed to reduce the effort required (especially in the extremely-low-birthweight infant) to generate, sustain, and terminate a ventilator breath.[8] Termination of inspiration now is recognized to be an important component of ventilator control, because prolongation of inspiration may lead to air trapping, air leak, and chronic lung injury. Furthermore, the use of microprocessors allows modification of ventilators to perform very small, but theoretically beneficial, changes to pressure, flow, and volume throughout the ventilatory cycle. Through these mechanisms, approaches such as proportional assist ventilation and respiratory muscle unloading can be achieved during the ventilatory cycle, a feat that would have been impossible just a few years ago.[9] With these techniques, pressure at the airway is increased during inspiration proportionate to the inspired tidal volume (with restrictive lung disease) or to flow (with resistive or obstructive airway disease) to diminish the elastic work of breathing. Many of these approaches are described in greater detail elsewhere in this chapter and in other sections of the book.

Volume Versus Pressure Ventilators

For many years, there has been an ongoing debate in neonatal respiratory care as to the relative merits of volume-controlled versus pressure-controlled mechanical ventilation for the neonate (see Chapter 10).[10] This debate has been mirrored in recent years by the debate on whether it is barotrauma (pressure injury) or volutrauma (volume injury) that primarily damages the lung during mechanical ventilation in the treatment of neonatal respiratory disease.[11,12] As a result, many neonatologists base their decision to use a ventilator on their familiarity with individual units (most commonly, the ventilator used in the nursery in which they trained!), personal bias, or anecdotal information. It is apparent that each type of ventilator can provide appropriate support if the clinician understands the basic principles of physiology that support mechanical ventilation. Distinguishing features of pressure-controlled versus volume-controlled ventilators are listed in Table 10-1.

As mentioned previously, volume-controlled ventilators deliver the same tidal volume with each breath. Areas of the lung that are atelectatic due to collapsed or obstructed airways require a higher opening pressure, which often can be achieved with a volume-preset ventilator. Most of this volume, however, is preferentially delivered into segments of the lung that remain partially inflated and more compliant. Consequently, although the volume-preset ventilator delivers a more consistent tidal volume, it may overdistend the "healthier" areas of the lung and promote air leaks. Furthermore, although these ventilators deliver the preset volume, they may lose some of that volume around the endotracheal (ET) tube because the neonatal ET tube is uncuffed. Ventilator monitors can now measure the amount of this volume loss by comparing inspiratory flow and expiratory return through the ET tube adapter. Recent modifications allow some ventilators to adjust for this volume loss. In diseases in which shifting or migratory atelectasis is commonplace (e.g., BPD) with frequent compliance changes, the delivery of a consistent tidal volume may prevent the frequent episodes of oxygen (O_2) desaturation that often occur.

With pressure-controlled ventilation, the volume of gas delivered to the terminal air spaces depends on the compliance of the lungs and, to a lesser degree, that of the airway and the thoracic wall. With a decrease in compliance (increased lung stiffness), the preset pressure is reached more rapidly during gas compression and delivery, and residual volume is released to the atmosphere. As a result, tidal volume decreases. If ventilation is inadequate, the physician must compensate for this loss of volume by increasing the peak inspiratory pressure (PIP) or inspiratory time. Nevertheless, because of the types of pulmonary diseases most often encountered in the neonate, pressure-controlled ventilators often offer advantages in management of the critically ill neonate.

Theoretical Advantages of Pressure-Preset Ventilators

1. Pressure-preset ventilators can use simple flow meters or pressure meters to monitor ventilator gas delivery. These ventilators have greater simplicity of design (fewer working parts), compact design, operation by means of a pressure source alone in some models (no electricity needed), and lower cost. Volume-controlled ventilators, in comparison, require a piston or volume meter to regulate breath size, in addition to the pressure meter. Volume-controlled ventilators have more working parts, more complex metering requirements, and, in general, greater cost. In the more modern ventilator units with SIMV, assist/control capability, pressure assist modes, or both pressure and volume capability, the devices increase in complexity, and the cost typically exceeds that of the volume-controlled ventilator alone. The disadvantages in cost and complexity of such units, however, are compensated for by their enhanced flexibility in clinical use.

2. Pressure-preset ventilators are, in general, relatively simple to operate. As a result, fellows, house staff, nurse practitioners, and other personnel can be taught the basic principles of therapy more easily. The pressure delivered to the infant can be immediately read from the meter, and adjustments to therapy can be made once appropriate monitoring has been performed or an arterial blood gas level is obtained. With volume-preset ventilators, either compliance of the ventilator and tubing must be known and calculated to assess volume, or a rough guess must be made as to the volume required and delivered to the infant. The calculations often are complex and difficult for physicians in training to grasp readily. The differences between pressure-preset and volume-controlled monitors have decreased in recent years with the addition of the various other modalities used in mechanical ventilation. In general, fewer preliminary calculations must be made when using pressure-preset ventilators.

3. PIP is thought to be directly related to the likelihood of development of air leaks and chronic lung disease in the newborn infant.[13] Judicious use of PIP, with constant monitoring of that factor, may aid in reducing these complications. Again, the theoretical considerations of pressure injury, as opposed to volume injury, enter into the discussion. If one is a firm believer that volume injury is the primary reason for the development of either air leaks or chronic lung disease in neonates, cautious monitoring of volume delivery to the lung may be preferential. In actual practice, however, it is so difficult to divorce pressure-related and volume-related injury that this controversy may be far more theoretical than practical.

4. Because the same pressure is provided to the infant with each ventilator breath, one does not have to constantly review pressure delivery and the risk it poses, even as compliance, waveform, and respiratory rate change during the illness. With volume ventilation, as compliance improves [e.g., during recovery from respiratory distress syndrome (RDS)], volume delivery may become rapidly excessive and injury may occur. With pressure ventilation, excessive volume is always dumped from the ventilator circuit once the preset pressure is reached. Overdistention of the lung is less likely, although air leaks and BPD can occur with any form of mechanical ventilation.

5. The distinction between pressure-controlled and volume-controlled ventilation has continued to blur even further with the introduction of volume guarantee ventilation (Drager Babylog 8000 Ventilator), perhaps achieving simultaneously the best of both approaches to neonatal ventilation. With volume guarantee, a targeted mean tidal volume or minute ventilation for an infant can be assured while still maintaining operator control of PIP. A predetermined tidal volume is thereby assured even in the face of an elevated PIP, which nor-

mally would result in tidal volume loss to the atmosphere. A modest reduction in PIP for very-low-birthweight infants has been achieved with this form of mechanical ventilation, while gas exchange has been well maintained.[14] Further evaluation of this form of ventilation will no doubt occur in the near future.

Basic Ventilator Design

Commonly used infant pressure-preset ventilators operate on similar principles, as illustrated in Figure 9-1. Some newer technologic advances, such as the dual microprocessor units that open and close a series of solenoid valves in the Infant Star ventilator (Infrasonics, Inc., San Diego, CA, USA), modify this approach to some extent. The underlying concept, however, is the same in that a preset pressure allows a certain volume of gas to be delivered to the patient until the desired pressure is reached. In addition, the provision of additional ventilator capabilities, such as assist/control and SIMV ventilation, requires sophisticated microprocessor assistance during mechanical ventilation. The microprocessor must be able to assess ventilator cycle timing; the changeover from inspiration to expiration and expiration to inspiration; and the relative pressure, flow rate, and tidal volume levels during ventilatory cycling. Without this capability, many of the newer ventilatory modalities would not be possible. To assist in this regard, especially if one is also using ventilator graphics monitoring, flow sensor capability is needed. Many ventilators have a low-volume pressure transducer within, or added to, the ventilator circuit (usually at the proximal airway) to measure gas flow into and out of the patient. In their basic design, however, ventilators basically remain pistons that deliver a volume of gas under pressure to the lung.

In the system illustrated in Figure 9-1, a pressure source of either compressed air, O_2, or both from a wall source is introduced into chamber A. The wall pressure is approximately 50 to 150 cm H_2O. This pressure is never applied directly to the infant but acts as a driving force for the ventilator. Mixing of compressed air and O_2 occurs in a blender before the gases reach the chamber so that a known concentration of O_2 is delivered to the infant. A second chamber, chamber B, is added, and a flow meter or resistor is inserted between the two to regulate the amount of air flow delivered into chamber B, which is smaller in the diagram and operates at a much lower pressure.

From the diagram, one can see that if the flow rate between the two chambers is high, the smaller chamber (B) eventually could reach driving pressure levels if the system were closed. Because chamber B interfaces with the infant, a maximum of 70 cm H_2O should rarely, if ever, be exceeded. For this reason, a pressure gauge and a "pop-off" regulating valve are added to the system to prevent excessive pressures from developing in chamber B (and in the infant's airway).

In addition, an exhalation valve is incorporated into the system. When open, a continuous flow occurs through the system, which prevents accumulation of excessive CO_2 in the tubing. Upon closure of this valve, pressure increases in chamber B, the ventilator tubing, and the infant's airway until the preset pressure level is reached. The ventilator is cycled by the opening and closing of the expiratory valve or by the solenoid system in the Infant Star. In the Infant Star and the Bird V.I.P. ventilators, there is an additional "demand flow" modification in which the negative pressure created in the circuit during a patient's spontaneous breath is augmented by an additional fast response demand valve that increases flow through the circuit, easing work of breathing. In the Newport Wave ventilator (Newport Medical Instruments Inc., Newport Beach, CA, USA), there is a separation of the spontaneous flow system from the mechanical breath system called the Duoflow System. This system acts as a separate-standing continuous positive airway pressure (CPAP) unit during spontaneous respiration in the exhalation phase of respiration.

Finally, the design of the system is such that the "upstroke" of the ventilator during inhalation can be modified by flow rate between chambers A and B. If flow is high, inspiratory pressure is reached quickly, and the respiratory waveform is "squared" (Fig. 9-2). If flow is reduced, the rate of rise of the inspiratory pressure is lessened, and the waveform appears more sinusoidal. Because sudden distention of the airways is thought by some neonatologists to contribute to tracheobronchomalacia and BPD, most current ventilators produce a more sinusoidal waveform at standard flow rates.[15] Ventilator design during the past decade has moved toward more sinusoidal gas delivery, even though evidence for the effect of waveform on development of chronic respiratory complications is not substantial.

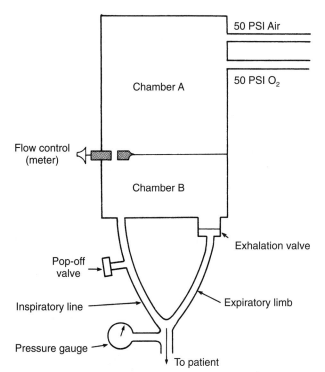

Figure 9-1. Diagram of the basic system used in infant positive-pressure ventilators. The pressure source is compressed air, O_2, or both, from a wall source to chamber A. A flow meter between chambers A and B regulates air flow to chamber B, which operates at a much lower pressure. The pressure gauge and pop-off valve prevent the pressure from exceeding 50 to 70 cm H_2O. The ventilator is cycled by the opening and closing of the expiratory valve, which prevents CO_2 accumulation in the tubing. PSI, pounds per square inch.

Cycling

In conventional positive-pressure ventilators, the cycling process determines the method by which the inspiratory phase is initiated and terminated. Volume-preset ventilators are cycled when a preset volume is attained. Most standard pressure-preset

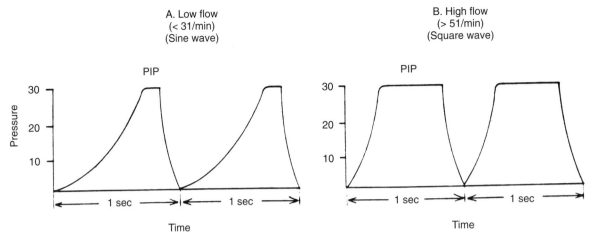

Figure 9-2. Comparison of ventilator wave forms. *A,* Relative sine wave. *B,* Relative square wave. PIP, peak inspiratory pressure.

ventilators are regulated by either an electrical timer (time-cycled) or a pneumatic timer (pressure-cycled). The pneumatic-cycled ventilators have a small chamber in which pressure increases to a preset level and subsequently closes the inspiratory valve.

Although these ventilators are called *pressure-preset ventilators* by clinicians who set the machines according to desired inspiratory pressure, they are technically known as *flow generators* because the power source produces such high pressure that even if the infant's lung compliance or airway resistance changes, the inspiratory flow rate is not affected. Examples of the most common time-cycled and pressure-cycled ventilators in current use are listed in Table 9-1. Some ventilators have two or more cycling modes and are called *mixed-cycle ventilators.* These are generally volume-cycled ventilators with an additional time-cycle control. The control capabilities of each ventilator, and the differences between the methods in which pressures and volumes are delivered, sustained, and terminated, are important to understand but beyond the scope of this discussion. Clinicians are strongly urged to carefully review the operator's manual for each specific ventilator in order to prevent any error in management.

If one operates pressure-preset ventilators at a high respiratory rate, the flow rate must be sufficiently high if one wishes to deliver a full tidal breath or reach the desired pressure in a brief period of time. In addition, if inspiratory time is short, a higher flow rate may be necessary to deliver the required volume and pressure in the limited time period.[16] Consequently, one should avoid excessive ventilator rates (>70 breaths/min) in most neonatal lung diseases. Given the reduced compliance that often is present in these restrictive lung diseases, the combination of short inspiration and reduced compliance may result in little more than dead space ventilation and gas trapping.

A recent addition to many neonatal ventilators is the concept of *termination sensitivity.* Termination sensitivity is a ventilator control that the clinician can set to terminate a ventilator breath at a specific percentage of peak flow during expiration (see Fig. 12-6). Termination sensitivity is an effective way to limit prolongation of the inspiratory phase of the ventilatory cycle. By setting a termination sensitivity of 5% to 10%, inspiration will cease when inspiratory flow decreases to 5% to 10% of peak flow. A termination sensitivity of 5% to 10% usually

---

TABLE 9-1.   Commonly Used Neonatal Positive-Pressure Ventilators

Bird V.I.P. Infant/Pediatric Ventilator
Bird V.I.P. Gold Infant/Pediatric Ventilator
Bear Cub 750 PSV Infant Ventilator (see Figure 9-3)
Infant Star Ventilator
Sechrist IV-200 SAVI Ventilator
Newport Wave Ventilator
Draeger Babylog 8000 Plus Infant Care Ventilator
Siemens Servo 300 Ventilator

---

limits inspiration to 0.2 to 0.3 seconds during neonatal mechanical ventilation. In practice, however, we have often found it preferable to simply set the inspiratory time that is desired directly on the ventilator and turn off the termination sensitivity control.

PROCEDURE FOR INITIATING MECHANICAL VENTILATION

Mechanical ventilation of the newborn, especially in the extremely-low-birthweight infant (<1000 g), is associated with numerous complications. Before using this therapy, all clinical personnel must be thoroughly familiar with the operation of ventilators and the physiologic principles that govern their use. We believe that mechanical ventilation is 5% device related and 95% physiologic principles in delivering optimal patient care. Unfortunately, too many clinicians become overly concerned with the "hardware" of mechanical ventilation and forget that the "software," or the decisions governing use of the devices, is far more important. With the increasing complexity of modern neonatal mechanical ventilators, it is becoming more difficult to avoid becoming enmeshed in hardware issues, even when it is unclear to what extent the newer modifications provide any substantial clinical benefit. It is essential to have a comprehensive understanding of both the equipment being used and the controls offered by that equipment in treating the critically ill neonate. The methods offered throughout the remainder of this chapter focus primarily on the physiologic principles of neonatal respiratory care rather than the innumerable technologic manipulations that one can achieve with modern neonatal ventilators. Additional information about the many different approaches to neonatal mechanical ventilation is discussed in Chapters 12 and 13 (Special Ventilatory Techniques I and II) and Chapter 15 (Ventilatory Strategies).

First Steps

Although the procedures discussed in this section may appear routine and simple, they are crucial because errors made at this point may be life threatening (e.g., if one does not correctly connect the gas sources to the ventilator). In addition, although this discussion focuses primarily on the pulmonary physiology and ventilator management of the infant, one should never overlook many of the important peripheral issues for successful respiratory care, such as infection surveillance and control; nutritional support; fluid and electrolyte management; comfort and pain relief of the infant; and emotional support for the family. These issues are discussed in other sections of the book. We have frequently observed throughout our careers that a discussion with the family early in the child's hospitalization about the benefits and perils of ventilatory assistance can be extremely important in reducing the understandable concern of the family.

The ventilator should be carefully cleaned when it is not in use, the circuits should be sterilized, and the unit should be stored in a clean dry area. A plastic cover should be placed over the ventilator. Periodic infection control surveillance and culturing of ventilator equipment is a valuable practice. When the ventilator is removed from storage, the following steps should be taken:

1. The electrical connections should be checked. Only grounded sources (three-pronged) should be used. Any unit that undertakes the care of neonates on ventilatory support must have access to back-up generators in case of power failure in the nursery.

2. O_2 and room air gas sources should be connected to the wall, and the required pressure must be adequate to drive most conventional ventilators (approximately 50 psi). Wall gauges should monitor this pressure.

3. All connections must fit securely, and the correct ventilator tubing and circuitry should be placed for the specific ventilator. The ET tube must fit tightly into the ventilator connector; otherwise, air leaks may result. Circuits should never be "jury-rigged" if appropriate connectors are unavailable. These kinds of modifications can be lethal to an infant if a circuit comes apart at a critical point in care.

4. Humidification systems must be properly filled and checked. Newer units that use hydrophobic humidification techniques, especially those with heated filaments in the tubing, may not show droplet formation, which indicates saturation of the gas (see Chapter 6). Alternative methods of periodically checking the humidifiers for adequate humidification are essential. Inadequately humidified gas can injure the airway and has been associated with necrotizing tracheobronchitis.[17]

5. Temperature devices should be examined periodically to ensure appropriate and accurate temperature of the gas entering the lungs. Inspired gas should be approximately at body temperature 35° to 36°C ($\pm$2°C). Inadequately warmed gas can produce bronchospasm, especially in the chronically ventilated infant; excessively heated gas can inflame the immature airway.[18]

Ventilator Controls

The ventilator controls that are found on most pressure-controlled ventilators include the following (as shown in Fig. 9-3):

1. Fraction of inspired oxygen (F_{IO_2})
2. PIP
3. Positive end-expiratory pressure (PEEP)
4. Rate
5. Ventilator flow rate
6. Inspiratory time (T_I) [Some ventilators may also have expiratory time (T_E) or inspiratory-to-expiratory (I/E) ratio]
7. Assist sensitivity
8. Termination sensitivity
9. Selection of SIMV/CPAP mode or assist/control mode for either volume or pressure ventilation
10. Graphics monitoring
11. Ventilator alarm settings

From these controls, waveform and mean airway pressure (MAP) can be indirectly selected. Newer ventilators also digitally display controls. The external waveform monitor on the Bird V.I.P. has unusually extensive capabilities, including demonstration of flow-volume and pressure-volume loops. In addition, ventilators may have the following control capabilities:

1. Demand flow (Infrasonics, Bird V.I.P.)
2. Exhalation assist
3. Manual breath
4. Pressure support modes
5. High-frequency modes (Infant Star)

Although sales representatives often stress the utility of these additional capabilities, the scientific evidence underscoring the value of these modifications is limited, although increasing numbers of investigations are emerging that appear to show some benefit from these modifications. The use of SIMV and assist/control has become widespread and appears to offer demonstrable advantages in neonatal respiratory care (see Chapter 12).[19,20]

High-frequency ventilators (see Chapter 11) have additional controls, such as peak-to-peak pressure, jet valve on-time, amplitude, and high frequency and duration. The reader is referred to Chapter 11 for more detailed discussion of these ventilators.

Fraction of Inspired Oxygen

Oxygen is probably the most commonly used drug in neonatal intensive care, yet it is rarely thought of as such by physicians. Appropriate use of O_2 is highly therapeutic in most cases of neonatal cardiopulmonary disease. In addition to relieving hypoxemia, its action as a pulmonary vasodilator in cases of persistent pulmonary hypertension of the neonate may be invaluable.[21] Inadequate O_2 administration with resultant hypoxemia, however, may result in severe neurologic injury. Excessive variation in O_2 administration has been implicated as one of the provocative factors in retinopathy of prematurity[22] (not purely a high level of supplemental oxygen as previously thought[23]), with subsequent retinal scarring and loss of vision,

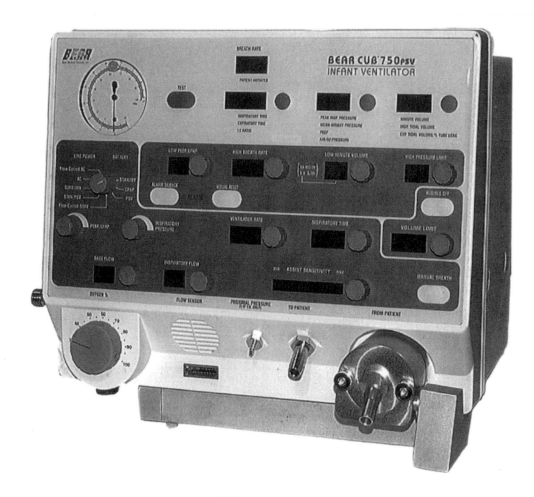

Figure 9-3. Front panel of Bear Cub 750 PSV Infant Ventilator (A), with controls identified (B).

as well as in BPD,[24] leading to further O_2 or ventilator dependency. Accurate measurement of O_2 administration and arterial O_2 tension (PaO_2) or oxygen saturation is mandatory in any neonate requiring O_2 therapy.

Regulation of ambient O_2 concentration during mechanical ventilation is performed by blenders. Commercial blenders precisely mix O_2 and compressed air into desired concentrations of O_2 as determined by the patient's O_2 requirements. Many ventilators have blenders incorporated into their design, particularly the newer units. Older ventilators have separate blenders that can be attached to the O_2 inflow source on the ventilator. Blenders usually are easy to operate and work by simply dialing in the desired O_2 concentration. Although blenders are generally very accurate, the clinician must use an additional device periodically to check that the blender is delivering the desired O_2 concentration to the patient. Portable O_2 analyzers or continuous inline sensing devices can be used to check the inspired O_2 concentration at the connection of the patient to the ventilator.

Administration of poorly humidified oxygen may result in bronchospasm and airway injury in neonates. It is important that oxygen be warmed to 35° to 36°C to reduce the risk of airway problems. When warming and humidifying any gases administered to patients, excessive humidification may enter into the circuit and produce "rainout," or the formation of droplets that can drip into the airway. A heating wire within the ventilator circuitry can reduce the severity of this problem.

Peak Inspiratory Pressure

With pressure-limited ventilators, PIP is the primary factor used to deliver tidal volume (Table 9-3). The difference in pressures between PIP and end distending pressure (i.e., the compression pressure) is the primary determinant of tidal volume in these machines. In most modern ventilators, PIP can be directly selected by the physician, but the operator should be aware that PIP may change if either flow rate or the I/E ratio is changed. In some older, pressure-cycled ventilators (BABYbird), PIP is regulated by a combination of flow rate, respiratory rate, and I/E ratio.

When starting levels of PIP are selected, several physiologic factors must be considered: the infant's weight, gestational age, and postnatal age; type and severity of the disease process; lung compliance; airway resistance; and time constant of the lung (see Chapter 2). A time constant, which is the product of compliance and resistance, refers to the unit of time necessary for the alveolar pressure to reach 63% of the total change in airway pressure during positive-pressure ventilation. Time constants can be measured during inspiration and expiration. For example, if inspiration lasts for a period of time equal to one time constant, then 63% of the difference in pressure between airway opening and alveoli equilibrates, and a proportional volume of gas enters the airways of the lung. With additional time during inspiration for further pressure equilibration, an additional 63% of the remaining pressure equilibrates [total = 86% now (or 63% + 63% × the remaining 37%)], and an additional equivalent volume of gas follows. After three to five time constants, little additional pressure change occurs, so gas volume delivery is essentially complete (Fig. 9-4).

With reduced compliance, as seen in RDS, the time constant decreases so that pressure equilibration occurs during a shortened inspiration and expiration. Inspiration and expiration,

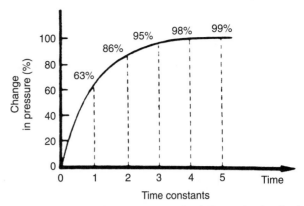

Figure 9-4. Percentage change in pressure in relation to the time (in time constants) allowed for equilibration. Because a longer time is allowed for equilibration, a higher percentage change in pressure occurs. The same rule governs the equilibration for step changes in volume. (From Carlo WA, Martin RJ: Principles of assisted ventilation. Pediatr Clin North Am 33:221, 1986.)

with volume movement of gas in and out of the lungs, occur in a shorter time period than is seen in normal lungs. When the time constant of the lung becomes so short during either inspiration or expiration that pressure equilibration cannot occur, then either inadequate delivery of volume during inspiration may result, or air trapping and incremental overdistention of the lung during expiration may ensue. This latter phenomenon appears to be important in the development of air leak syndromes during neonatal ventilation.[25]

Before any patient is connected to the ventilator, inspiratory pressure should be carefully checked to be certain that the pressure is neither excessive nor inadequate. The adapter that connects to the ET tube should be occluded and the pressure gauge on the ventilator should be checked, with adjustments made as necessary. Once the patient is attached to the ventilator, PIP should be rechecked to be certain it has not changed significantly from what was observed when the adapter occluded. If PIP has changed more than 2 to 3 cm H_2O, one must consider the possibility of air leak or an obstructed ET tube.

Considerable controversy exists regarding the level of PIP that should be used for infants with respiratory disease. This issue is considered in greater detail later in this chapter in the section on ventilator management, as well as in Chapter 13 on ventilatory techniques and lung-protective strategies. As a basic principle, it appears that the lowest PIP that adequately ventilates the patient is usually the most appropriate. Another important consideration in this regard is the overall approach to mechanical ventilation that is used. In general, the use of assist/control ventilation will result in a need for lower PIP than may be seen with either conventional mechanical ventilation (with pressure that is entirely operator selected) or SIMV. With assist/control, infants usually tend to increase their ventilatory rate somewhat to compensate for the lower PIP selected by the clinician. This strategy usually is effective unless one selects a PIP that is inadequate to provide adequate gas exchange and only dead space ventilation occurs. Simply increasing the PIP slightly may be sufficient to achieve success if PaCO_2 remains excessively elevated (>55 mm Hg). In some clinical circumstances, such as acute RDS, this style of ventilatory support may be beneficial and may reduce exposure to higher PIP. It appears that the incidence of pulmonary complications (air leaks and BPD) also may be reduced with this technique.[26]

In contrast, some neonatologists, fearful of barotrauma at all costs, may persist and use an inadequate PIP for excessively long periods. Based on the infant's size, some physicians arbitrarily set a certain PIP level above which they will not venture, even when ventilation remains grossly insufficient as seen in arterial blood gases. In contrast to the excellent and well-conceived "gentle ventilation" approach developed by Jen-Tien Wung at the Children's Hospital of New York (formerly Babies Hospital), protracted hypercapnia and respiratory acidosis can result in serious systemic and neurologic injury. A study by Vannucci et al.[27] indicates that in an animal model, extreme hypercapnia (PaCO$_2$ >100 mm Hg) may result in cardiac depression and reduced cerebral blood flow, with subsequent hypoxic-ischemic brain injury. The necessity of adequate gas exchange under all circumstances cannot be overemphasized. It does no good to avoid barotrauma while the patient dies or suffers significant injury from insufficient gas exchange that results in long-term morbidity. Appropriate PIP usually can be judged on clinical examination (chest movement and breath sounds) and on the basis of blood gas analysis.

Table 9-2 summarizes the advantages and side effects of different pressure ranges. Barotrauma can be reduced with lower PIP, and the incidence of air leaks and chronic lung disease may be decreased. There are, however, little data suggesting a definite value to extreme pressure reduction with permissive hypercapnia.[28,29] Normal lung development may be enhanced by lower PIP, although recent evidence suggests that even distribution of gas throughout the lung may be more important than low pressure. High-frequency ventilation appears to decrease barotrauma to some extent by providing such gas distribution. Again, one must provide adequate PIP to deliver an appropriate tidal volume (VT) to the patient. Low VT from low PIP may reduce minute ventilation (VE = rate × VT), resulting in elevated arterial carbon dioxide tension (PaCO$_2$) and hypoxemia. Long-term follow-up on children treated with this approach has not been extensive to date; thus, the degree of morbidity is not known.

High PIP usually should be avoided because of the risk of air leaks, such as pneumothorax, interstitial emphysema, and pneumomediastinum. Furthermore, high intrathoracic pressure, when transmitted to the myocardium, may impede venous return to the heart and decrease cardiac output. There appears to be a neutral range of PaCO$_2$. Although a high or low PaCO$_2$ by itself may not be harmful, it may be related to alterations in cardiac output that can produce injury to the central nervous system. Certain clinical conditions, however, may warrant the use of high PIP. In patients with markedly decreased compliance or in those with decreased lung volume from atelectasis, a high PIP may be needed to maintain adequate gas exchange or to reexpand collapsed sections of the lung. Some physicians treat pulmonary hypertension with high PIP to hyperventilate patients intentionally to a lower PaCO$_2$ in an effort to decrease pulmonary artery pressure.[21] As a general rule, however, hyperventilation has been shown to induce a variety of neurologic injuries in infants and is no longer a recommended therapy in persistent pulmonary hypertension of the neonate (see Chapter 23).[30]

Positive End-Expiratory Pressure

Although CPAP has been used since Gregory's original work in 1970–1971, CPAP has reemerged as a highly effective method to initiate ventilatory assistance in the lowest birth-weight babies, with the least risk of airway and neurologic injury.[31,32] Extubation to CPAP following mechanical ventilation appears to decrease the likelihood of reintubation and reduce the frequency of apnea.[33,34] In our nursery, nearly all infants receive a trial of CPAP prior to initiation on mechanical ventilation. Some information suggests that there are outcome differences in the methods by which CPAP is delivered.[35] In addition, some groups suggest that "bubble" or underwater CPAP may be more effective than ventilator-delivered CPAP. It is difficult to reconcile how relatively small pressure differences can be reflected in an infant's outcome given the normal attenuation of pressures down the airway. Further studies should be undertaken in this regard (see Chapter 8).

Use of PEEP or continuous distending pressure while the infant is on the ventilator has become a standard technique for ventilatory treatment of the neonate. The approach to treatment is similar to that recommended for CPAP in the spontaneously breathing patient. Selection of the appropriate PEEP depends on the size of the patient, the pathophysiology of the disease process, and the goals of treatment. In most clinical situations, there appears to be an "optimal PEEP" below which lung volumes are not well maintained and above which the lung becomes overdistended.[36] On most ventilators, PEEP is selected simply by setting the desired pressure. One must be aware, however, that the chosen PEEP may be altered by other

TABLE 9-2. Peak Inspiratory Pressure (PIP)

Low (≤20 cm H$_2$O)		High (≥20 cm H$_2$O)	
Advantages	**Adverse Effects**	**Advantages**	**Adverse Effects**
1. Fewer side effects, especially BPD, PAL	1. Insufficient ventilation; may not control PaCO$_2$	1. May help reexpand atelectasis	1. Associated with ↑ PAL, BPD
2. Normal lung development may proceed more rapidly	2. ↓ PaO$_2$, if too low	2. ↓ PaCO$_2$	2. May impede venous return
	3. Generalized atelectasis may occur (may be desirable in some cases of air leaks)	3. ↑ PaO$_2$	3. May decrease cardiac output
		4. Decrease pulmonary vascular resistance	

BPD, bronchopulmonary dysplasia; PAL, pulmonary air leaks.

ventilator variables. For example, if expiratory time is too short or if airway resistance is increased, a degree of inadvertent PEEP may be generated that is additive to the selected level.[37,38] In such situations, this inadvertent PEEP may contribute to gas trapping and increase the potential for air leaks (Fig. 9-5).

The major benefits of PEEP are similar to those seen with CPAP in the spontaneously breathing infant. PEEP stabilizes and recruits lung volume, improves compliance (to a certain point, after which compliance may actually decrease), and improves ventilation-perfusion matching in the lung.

Table 9-3 summarizes the effects of PEEP at various levels. PEEP less than 2 cm H_2O is not recommended, except in rare

instances, because the presence of an ET tube bypasses the normal airway mechanics that typically provide a low level of end-distending pressure during spontaneous breathing.[39] Furthermore, the resistance of the ET tube requires a certain PEEP level if the atelectasis that is produced by an inspiratory load in the face of inadequate PEEP is to be prevented.

Low PEEP levels (2 to 3 cm H_2O) usually are used during weaning phases of ventilatory management, and some extremely low birthweight babies on assist/control support may be adequately treated at these levels. When such levels are provided early in the course of disease in larger infants, however, atelectasis may result with CO_2 retention. In most clinical circumstances, medium levels of PEEP (4 to 7 cm H_2O) are

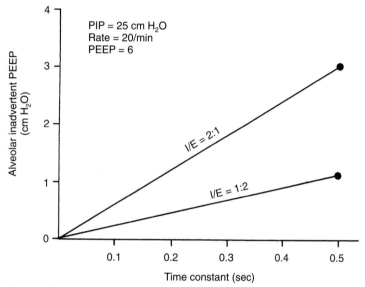

Figure 9-5. Relationship of inadvertent positive end-expiratory pressure (PEEP) to increasing time constants and reversal of the inspiratory-to-expiratory (I/E) ratio (1:2 to 2:1) in an infant recovering from respiratory distress syndrome complicated by a patent ductus arteriosus. PIP, peak inspiratory pressure. (Modified from Donahue LA, Thibeault DW: Alveolar gas trapping and ventilatory therapy in infants. Perinatol Neonatol 3:35, 1979.)

TABLE 9-3. Continuous Positive Airway Pressure or Positive End-Expiratory Pressure (CPAP or PEEP)

Low (2–3 cm H_2O)		Medium (4–7 cm H_2O)		High (>8 cm H_2O)	
Advantages	**Adverse Effects**	**Advantages**	**Adverse Effects**	**Advantages**	**Adverse Effects**
1. Used during late phases of weaning	1. May be too low to maintain adequate lung volume	1. Recruit lung volume with surfactant deficiency states (e.g., RDS)	1. May overdistend lungs with normal compliance	1. Prevents alveolar collapse in surfactant deficiency states with severely decreased C_L	1. PAL
2. Maintenance of lung volume in very premature infants with low FRC	2. CO_2 retention from V/Q mismatch, as alveolar volume is inadequate	2. Stabilizes lung volume once recruited		2. Improves distribution of ventilation	2. Decreases compliance if lung overdistends
3. Useful in some extremely LBW infants on A/C ventilation		3. Improve V/Q matching			3. May impede venous return to the heart
					4. May increase PVR
					5. CO_2 retention

A/C, assist/control; C_L, lung compliance; FRC, functional residual capacity; LBW, low birthweight; PAL, pulmonary air leaks; PVR, pulmonary vascular resistance; RDS, respiratory distress syndrome; V/Q, ventilation-perfusion.

appropriate. Such levels allow appropriate maintenance of lung volumes yet minimize the potential side effects associated with higher PEEP and pulmonary overdistention. PEEP levels above 8 cm H_2O are rarely used in conventional mechanical ventilation because of the risk of pulmonary air leaks and reduction of cardiac output. With HFJV, however, higher PEEP may be needed to ensure adequacy and maintenance of lung volume.[3] Severe respiratory failure in the larger infant may require high PEEP levels (8 to 10 cm H_2O and above) for a period, until an alternative therapy (HFJV or ECMO) can be initiated. Extreme vigilance for pneumothoraces, pneumomediastinum, increased pulmonary vascular resistance, and inadequate cardiac output is essential at any level of CPAP or PEEP, but it should always be considered at the higher levels of support.

Rate or Frequency of Ventilation

Respiratory rate is one of the primary determinants of minute ventilation in mechanical ventilation (minute ventilation = respiratory rate × V_T) (Table 9-4). No conclusive studies have demonstrated the optimal ventilatory rate for treatment of neonatal respiratory disease. Some studies have indicated improved oxygenation at higher rates (≥60 breaths/min).[40] Other studies have historically suggested more success with slower rates (≤40 breaths/min).[41] As with other previously mentioned ventilator controls, the best rate in a given situation depends on several variables, including size of the infant, type and stage of the disease, presence of complications, and clinical response. Furthermore, the successful introduction of high-frequency ventilators suggests that frequency may be important only in reference to other controls being used at that time. For example, very high rates can be successfully used if PIP (and consequently V_T) and T_I can be reduced simultaneously. Without such a reduction, high frequencies may result in severe complications. In conventional ventilation, especially during assist/control, high frequencies may be generated spontaneously by an infant with PIP kept at a minimum level. Many babies will subsequently "autowean" their rate as lung compliance improves. This circumstance is much different than the case of a patient intentionally treated with hyperventilation to deliberately lower Pa_{CO_2}.

In most instances, whether the clinician selects a high or low respiratory rate, the goal of therapy is to reduce barotrauma with an associated decrease in air leaks and chronic lung disease. Again, neurologic effects from whatever ventilatory technique is used must always be taken into consideration. Both high and low ventilatory rates can achieve these objectives if the physician has an overall strategy for ventilator management such as that outlined later in this chapter. Most complications involving ventilator rates occur because the clinician fails to recognize the impact of rate change on other aspects of ventilatory care. For example, if higher rates are selected, a prolonged T_I and an inadequate T_E may result in decreased compliance and air trapping, if the time constant of the lung does not adequately allow for gas exit. Thus, ventilatory changes cannot be entertained without evaluating the overall effects of that decision.

In addition to the considerations already noted, it is essential that the capabilities of the ventilator in use be examined to be certain that the parameters selected for the patient are actually delivered by the machine. Boros[42] and Simbruner and Gregory[43] showed that there is significant variability among ventilators in delivering pressures and V_T, especially at higher frequencies. Some ventilators have exhalation assist modes to help alleviate gas trapping in the tubing at higher rates, but this provision does not ensure consistent V_T delivery.

Physicians who prefer slower-rate ventilation often cite the work of Haman and Reynolds[41] and Boros,[42] who demonstrated that lower rates, when delivered with higher MAPs, produced better oxygenation. Again, lower rates can be used successfully, with a minimum of complications, if one is aware of the potential sources of problems for the infants being treated. Slower-rate ventilation could not have been developed without modification of ventilator circuitry to provide continuous gas flow rather than intermittent flow. This modification, introduced by Kirby et al.[44] more than 3 decades ago, has now been extended in some ventilators to include a separate circuit entirely for spontaneous breathing. Before the introduction of

---

TABLE 9-4.   Neonatal Mechanical Ventilatory Rates (f)

Slow (≤40 breaths/min)		Medium (40–60 breaths/min)		Rapid (≥60 breaths/min)	
Advantages	**Adverse Effects**	**Advantages**	**Adverse Effects**	**Advantages**	**Adverse Effects**
1. ↑ Pa_{O_2} with increased MAP	1. Must ↑ PIP to maintain minute ventilation	1. Mimics normal ventilatory rate	1. May not provide adequate ventilation in some cases	1. Higher Pa_{O_2} (may be the result of air trapping)	1. May exceed time constant and produce air trapping
2. Useful in weaning	2. ↑ PIP may cause barotrauma	2. Will effectively treat most neonatal lung diseases	2. ↑ PIP may still be needed to maintain minute ventilation	2. May allow ↓ PIP and V_T	2. May cause inadvertent PEEP
3. Used with square wave ventilation	3. Patient may require paralysis	3. Usually does not exceed time constant of lung, so air trapping is unlikely		3. Hyperventilation may be useful in PPHN	3. May result in change in compliance (frequency dependence of compliance)
4. Needed when I/E ratio is inverted				4. May reduce atelectasis (? air trapping)	4. Inadequate V_T and minute ventilation if only dead space is ventilated

I/E, inspiratory to expiratory; MAP, mean airway pressure; PEEP, positive end-expiratory pressure; PIP, peak inspiratory pressure; PPHN, persistent pulmonary hypertension of the neonate; V_T, tidal volume.

continuous flow, an infant who attempted to breathe against a closed valve would rebreathe exhaled gas, with a potential increase in $Paco_2$. With constant flow in a time-cycled device, the physician now can choose to provide a predetermined amount of mechanical ventilation in combination with spontaneous breathing. This technique is referred to as *intermittent mandatory ventilation (IMV),* and it has been a useful adjunct to ventilator weaning. With the current ability to synchronize the ventilator to the infant breath (SIMV), the technique has become increasingly important as a weaning approach. As the pulmonary disease improves, the infant receives fewer machine breaths and spontaneous breathing is allowed to increase.

Ventilator rate usually is controlled by directly selecting the rate in time-cycled machines, which comprise the majority of neonatal ventilators in use today. In some older pressure-cycled machines (BABYbird), the rate is changed by altering T_I, T_E, or the I/E ratio.

Inspiratory-to-Expiratory Ratio

Possible variations in I/E ratios are summarized in Table 9-5. The ability to select an I/E ratio varies among ventilators. In some pressure-cycled units, both T_I and T_E can be selected directly to produce the desired I/E ratio. On most units, however, the T_I is selected, and, in combination with the desired frequency, the I/E ratio is automatically set. In patient-triggered ventilation, with the termination sensitivity set at 5% to 10%, the I/E ratio may become variable as the flow characteristics of the inspiratory phase of ventilation alter the duration of inspiration from breath to breath. If a specific I/E ratio is desired, the termination sensitivity must be shut off.

I/E ratio has been considered an important variable in ventilator management strategies, beginning with the work of Reynolds and Tagizadeh[45] that emphasized its role in controlling oxygenation. In their studies, the I/E ratio was reversed (>1:1), with inspiration longer than expiration. More recently, however, the I/E ratio has been regarded as less important and

more complicated than controlling simply the T_I. There is still a great deal of debate among neonatologists regarding the optimal T_I for neonatal mechanical ventilation. Increasingly, emphasis has been placed on shorter inspiratory times, with the belief that airway and lung injury will be reduced. It is evident, however, that if T_I is reduced too much, opening pressure within the lung will not be reached and only dead space ventilation will occur. As a result, we have tried to achieve a balance between shorter inspiratory times and adequate gas entry into the lung. In general, we now use a starting T_I of 0.3 to 0.4 seconds for most neonatal ventilation, which is shorter than previously described in earlier editions of this book.

Selecting any two of the four variables (T_I, T_E, I/E ratio, and rate) automatically determines the other two. Choosing a T_I of 0.5 seconds with an I/E ratio of 1:1 automatically provides a T_E of 0.5 seconds and a rate of 60 breaths/min. If rate is decreased to 30 breaths/min and the I/E ratio is left at 1:1, then T_I increases to 1 second, possibly increasing the risk of airway overdistention and air leak. Consequently, many physicians prefer to set a T_I that they believe is adequate; they are not as concerned about the I/E ratio directly. It is our preference, in general, to select a T_I of 0.3 to 0.4 seconds during the acute phases of most neonatal lung diseases to prevent air trapping. Further recommendations about appropriate I/E ratios depend on the type, severity, and stage of the disease being treated. It is evident, however, that the I/E ratio decreases as ventilatory rates are slowed, assuming T_I remains constant. This approach provides a higher MAP and better oxygenation during the early phases of disease. As the infant's status improves, the slowing of the ventilator rate with constant T_I extends expiration and automatically decreases the I/E ratio and MAP, when it is often appropriate to do so.

An additional caution about prolonged I/E ratios involves cardiac output considerations. Increasing the duration of inspiration will enhance the amount of intrathoracic pressure that is transmitted to the heart. Venous return may be compromised, and cardiac output may be decreased. If an air leak develops, it

TABLE 9-5. Inspiratory:Expiratory (I/E) Ratio Control in Neonatal Mechanical Ventilation

| Inverse (>1:1) | | Normal (1:1 to 1:3) | | Prolonged Expiratory (<1:3) | |
Advantages	Adverse Effects	Advantages	Adverse Effects	Advantages	Adverse Effects
1. ↑ MAP	1. May have insufficient emptying time and air trapping may result	1. Mimics natural breathing pattern	1. Insufficient emptying at highest rates	1. Useful during weaning, when oxygenation is less of a problem	1. Low T_I may decrease tidal volume
2. ↑ Pao_2 in RDS	2. May impede venous return to the heart	2. May give best ratio at higher rates		2. May be more useful in diseases such as MAS, when air trapping is a part of the disease process	2. May have to use higher flow rates, which may not be optimal for distribution of ventilation
3. May enhance alveolar recruitment when atelectasis is present	3. ↑ Pulmonary vascular resistance and worsen diseases such as PPHN and CHD				3. May ventilate more dead space
	4. Worsen PAL				

CHD, congenital heart disease; I/E, inspiratory to expiratory; MAP, mean airway pressure; MAS, meconium aspiration syndrome; PAL, pulmonary air leaks; PPHN, persistent pulmonary hypertension of the neonate; RDS, respiratory distress syndrome; T_I, inspiratory time.

may further impair venous return. As a result, prolonged I/E ratio has been associated with an increased risk of intraventricular hemorrhage. We use reversed I/E ratio only as a last resort to try to improve oxygenation, most often in cases where a more effective method to increase oxygenation cannot be found. Since the introduction and widespread use of high-frequency ventilators, inhalational nitric oxide therapy, and ECMO, prolonged I/E ratio has not been used in our nurseries.

Flow Rate

Flow rates used for neonatal mechanical ventilation are summarized in Table 9-6. Flow rate is an important determinant of the ability of the ventilator to deliver desired levels of PIP, waveform, I/E ratios, and, in some cases, respiratory rate. A minimum flow at least two times an infant's minute ventilation usually is required (neonatal minute ventilation typically ranges from approximately 0.2 to 1 L/min), but the usual operating range during mechanical ventilation 4 to 10 L/min.

When low flow rates are used, it takes longer to reach PIP, and the pressure curve has a lower plateau and appears similar to a sine waveform (see Fig. 9-2). Normal neonatal spontaneous breaths are shaped like a sine waveform. Because maldistribution of ventilation occurs in many neonatal respiratory diseases, theoretically there may be a reduction of barotrauma with this pattern of waveform. With sine wave ventilation, if the flow rate is too low relative to minute ventilation, dead space ventilation may increase because effective opening pressure for the airways is not reached within an appropriate time. Hypercapnia may result. In addition, if higher ventilator rates

are used on sine wave ventilators, inadequate flows may result in dead space ventilation because the ventilator does not reach PIP in the allocated time. Opening pressure of the lung is not reached and gas exchange is reduced.

Higher flow rates are needed if square wave ventilation (see Fig. 9-2) is desired on standard ventilators. At higher rates, a high flow may be necessary to attain a high or adequate PIP (and adequate V_T) because inspiratory time (T_I) is short. Carbon dioxide rebreathing is also prevented in the ventilator tubing at higher flow rates. The most common complication of high flow rates is an increased incidence of air leaks because maldistribution of ventilation results in a rapid pressure increase in nonobstructed or nonatelectatic airways and alveoli. Very high flow rates may result in decreased V_T secondary to increased turbulence in high-resistance, small-diameter ET tubes.

Waveforms

The waveforms commonly used in neonatal ventilation are described and summarized in Table 9-7. Waveforms typically are not selected by the physician in prescribing mechanical ventilation but often are the result of other factors, including ventilator design. Many of the considerations regarding waveform were discussed in the section on flow rate. Sine wave breathing approximates normal spontaneous respiration more closely than does a square waveform. The smoother increase in inspiratory pressure may be advantageous for infants with maldistribution of ventilation, which is commonly seen in many neonatal lung diseases.

TABLE 9-6.   Flow Rate Adjustment in Neonatal Ventilation

Low Rate (0.5–3 L/min)		High (4–10 L/min or more)	
Advantages	**Adverse Effects**	**Advantages**	**Adverse Effects**
1. Slower inspiratory time, more sine wave	1. Hypercapnia, if flow rate is not adequate to remove CO_2 from the system	1. Produces more square wave ventilatory pattern	1. Increased barotrauma
2. Less barotrauma to airways	2. At high ventilator rate, low flow may not enable the machine to reach PIP	2. ↑ Po_2	2. In moderate-to-severe RDS, may produce more airway injury
	3. ↓ Pao_2 in some cases	3. Needed to deliver high PIP with rapid ventilator rates	3. ↑ Turbulence, ↓ V_T in small ET tubes
		4. Prevents CO_2 retention	

ET, endotracheal; PIP, peak inspiratory pressure; RDS, respiratory distress syndrome; V_T, tidal volume.

TABLE 9-7.   Wave Forms in Neonatal Mechanical Ventilation

Sine Wave		Square Wave	
Advantages	**Adverse Effects**	**Advantages**	**Adverse Effects**
1. Smoother increase of pressure	1. Lower mean airway pressure	1. Higher MAP for equivalent PIP	1. With high flow, the ventilation may be applying higher pressure to normal airways and alveoli
2. More like normal respiratory pattern		2. Longer time at PIP may open atelectatic areas of lung and improve distribution of ventilation	2. Impede venous return if longer T_I is used or I/E ratio is reversed

I/E, inspiratory to expiratory; MAP, mean airway pressure; PIP, peak inspiratory pressure; T_I, inspiratory time.

Square waveforms improve oxygenation when used with slower rates and longer TI. Square waves, in general, provide a higher MAP than do sine waveforms if identical PIP is used because the PIP is reached more rapidly with square waves.[42] The longer time at PIP with square waves may assist in opening atelectatic areas of the lung in some instances, although overdistention of inflated areas and air leaks may occur. With square waves and reversed I/E ratios, venous return to the heart and cardiac output may decrease.

The use of graphics monitoring is helpful when examining pressure-limited and volume-limited breaths to obtain a better understanding of how they differ. Figure 9-6 shows the differences between the waveforms in these approaches to positive-pressure ventilation.

Mean Airway Pressure

Although no conventional mechanical ventilator presently allows the operator to select MAP (the SensorMedics high-frequency oscillator is an exception), this ventilator variable is considered to be important because of its relationship to oxygenation.[46] The clinician typically measures MAP by determining the mean of instantaneous readings of pressure within the airway during a single respiratory cycle. In waveform terminology, the MAP is equal to the area under the pressure curve for a single respiratory cycle divided by the duration of the cycle, or the integral of the pressure during a respiratory cycle (see Fig. 2-20). MAP is higher in square wave ventilation than in sine wave ventilatory patterns when PIP and duration of PIP are equal. No studies to date have specifically implicated MAP as the primary determinant of air leaks or chronic lung disease. Increases in oxygenation, however, are directly related to increases in MAP. It is evident that some changes in MAP, particularly with a short TI, may not be reflected in increased oxygenation. The ventilator control variables that influence MAP are (1) PIP, (2) PEEP, (3) I/E ratio, (4) flow, and (5) waveform.

Because pulmonary barotrauma may be correlated with high PIP that is unevenly distributed throughout the lung,[47] efforts have been made to ventilate patients with lower PIP and slower ventilatory frequency, while MAP is maintained. To accomplish this pattern of ventilator support, TI must be increased, which also changes the I/E ratio. As MAP increases, alveolar recruitment occurs, which reduces the alveolar-arterial DO_2 gradient and increases arterial oxygenation. Techniques to recruit alveolar volume using sustained inflation and higher MAP during high-frequency oscillatory ventilation appear to be effective, although less so during conventional positive-pressure ventilation.[48] The use of high MAP may be required during acute phases of neonatal lung disease, especially RDS, when compliance is low. In less severely affected infants and during recovery, high MAP may interfere with venous return as seen with elevated PEEP. One must be particularly cautious after surfactant administration in the low-birthweight baby because compliance and functional residual capacity changes may occur very rapidly.[49] If efforts to reduce PIP and MAP are not made quickly, lung overdistention with the potential risk for air leaks may occur. It is also thought that sudden changes in compliance may predispose some infants to pulmonary edema and pulmonary hemorrhage.[50]

An alternative approach to ventilation, first developed by Wung et al.[51] at Babies Hospital in New York, downplays the importance of close management of higher PIP and MAP. In that approach, lower PIP and MAP are commonly selected even during acute phases of illness, and arterial blood gas measurements of pH and PCO_2 that may be outside the normal range are accepted (*permissive hypercapnia*). Wung et al. have been very successful with what often has been described as *gentle ventilation*, but the clinician should *always* attempt to ventilate infants as "gently" as possible. The goal of any strategy of ventilatory management is to provide adequate gas exchange with the lowest settings possible. Wung's approach to ventilation is discussed further in the section on ventilatory management of infants, as are a number of other management approaches, in Chapter 13 (Special Ventilatory Techniques II).

MANAGEMENT OF RESPIRATORY FAILURE WITH POSITIVE-PRESSURE VENTILATORS

Definition of Respiratory Failure

There presently is no universally accepted definition for respiratory failure in the neonatal period. Because of the complexity of interplay between clinical and laboratory relationships in determining respiratory failure, management of this problem during the neonatal period is rarely simple and straightforward. Respiratory failure usually includes two or more criteria from the following clinical and laboratory categories:

1. Clinical Criteria
   a. Retractions (intercostal, supraclavicular, suprasternal)
   b. Grunting
   c. Respiratory rate greater than 60 breaths/min
   d. Central cyanosis
   e. Intractable apnea
   f. Decreased activity and movement
2. Laboratory Criteria
   a. $PaCO_2$ >60 mm Hg
   b. PaO_2 <50 mm Hg or O_2 saturation <80%, with an FIO_2 of 1.0
   c. pH <7.25

The clinical severity of presentation of respiratory failure can be extremely variable in the neonatal period. Some infants exhibit severe distress immediately; others may have marked abnormalities in arterial blood gas levels and yet appear to be

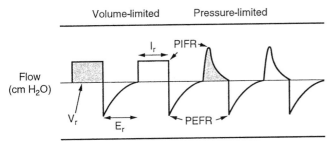

Figure 9-6. Flow waveforms for both volume-limited and pressure-limited breath types. Inspiratory flow is above baseline; expiratory flow is below baseline. Peak inspiratory flow rate (PIFR) and peak expiratory flow rate (PEFR) are shown. (From Nicks JJ: Graphics Monitoring. In Sinha SK, Donn SM (eds): Manual of Neonatal Respiratory Care. Armonk, NY, Futura Publishing Company, 2000, p. 65.)

far less compromised. Close observation of infants is critical in this setting. Retractions typically indicate a significant loss of lung volume. The infant then attempts to recruit alveolar volume by increasing respiratory effort, but the excessively compliant neonatal chest wall makes this effort somewhat futile in most cases. Rather than acting as a rigid strut, the neonatal thorax collapses, and the negative intrapleural pressure that is generated fails to reopen alveoli that are atelectatic. Grunting often accompanies retractions, particularly in the neonate with RDS. Grunting is an expiratory effort against a partially closed glottis that elevates the end-expiratory pressure in an attempt to increase residual lung volume and oxygenation. It usually is indicative of volume loss in the lung. Retractions and grunting should be considered ominous signs of impending respiratory failure during the neonatal period, particularly in the infant who weighs less than 1500 g. Both retractions and grunting occasionally may be seen in the neonate with cold stress, in which case these signs should last for no longer than 2 to 4 hours once the child has been warmed appropriately. The clinician should always maintain appropriate thermal stability for any infant, otherwise the medical care may become far more complex than is necessary. Grunting may also be an early sign of sepsis.

If significant grunting and retractions are observed in an infant, early ventilatory assistance should be offered. We very quickly place infants on nasal CPAP in an attempt to halt progressive volume loss in the lung. Nasal CPAP often is initiated in the delivery room, especially in the very smallest infants, as the need for surfactant administration is determined. We occasionally intubate an infant briefly to give surfactant, then return the baby to CPAP. If such measures are ineffective, intubation and mechanical ventilation may be required because metabolic derangement in these infants may proceed rapidly once the child can no longer support gas exchange. Late institution of mechanical support often is less effective and the complications and associated morbidity far greater than those seen with early intervention. Although the larger, more mature infant may have greater reserve and tolerate respiratory insufficiency for a longer period than the premature infant, one should keep in mind that recovery from respiratory failure rarely occurs in any infant during the neonatal period without some form of respiratory assistance. We believe that an aggressive (but gentle) early approach often is preferable in neonates, regardless of their disease.

Connecting the Patient to the Ventilator

The ventilator should be selected based on the size of the child, the disease to be treated, and the severity of the disease. It is important to try to visualize the potential changes in the disease that may await an infant in the days ahead and select a ventilator that has the capability of meeting the requirements for therapy in that child. Few events are more frustrating than having to change a ventilator in the middle of treatment because the ventilator in use does not have the needed capability. Fortunately, most neonatal ventilators introduced during the past decade have exceptional capabilities compared to earlier models that were far more limited.

Before treating a child with a ventilator, the following considerations should be kept in mind:

1. The ET tube should be well secured and appropriately positioned. The tip of the ET tube should be located about 1 to 2 cm above the carina. Breath sounds should be equal after insertion, and a chest radiograph should be obtained before mechanical ventilation is initiated to ensure correct placement of the tube and to permit the physician to follow changes in the disease with treatment.

2. Once the patient is connected to the ventilator, the clinical observations and mechanical factors listed in Table 9-8 should be followed. Vascular access is an important part of management and should occur shortly after initiation of ventilatory support, if not prior to that time. Our nursing staff is extremely adept at intravenous catheter placement and often has a catheter placed peripherally as rapidly as intubation can occur.

Ventilator Management

Since the last edition of this book, a number of ventilator variables have been added to some units that increase their capabilities. SIMV and assist/control mode ventilation have become standard approaches, but newer modalities such as proportional assist ventilation and tidal volume guarantee ventilation are more recent modifications. The benefits of these newer strategies of treatment are still somewhat uncertain, and their usefulness and effects upon long-term outcomes remain to be determined. Because many of these strategies are discussed extensively elsewhere in this book (see Chapter 13, Special Ventilatory Techniques II), this section concentrates on the basics of ventilator management that are common to most pressure-cycled and time-cycled machines. It is difficult to describe the use of positive-pressure ventilation without describing an overall management strategy for the particular circumstance of ventilator use. When appropriate, some brief discussion about the various new ventilator capabilities is provided, as well as how these capabilities might affect the patient's management.

Arterial blood gas analysis remains the "gold standard" for assessment of effective gas exchange (see Chapter 17). It is essential for the clinician to understand which ventilator controls are most likely to correct or change specific blood gas abnormalities. Table 9-9 summarizes these adjustments. In general, it is sound practice to adjust only one ventilator control at a time. Multiple changes made simultaneously are difficult to interpret, and the clinical care of the patient may be made more difficult to assess. One cannot overemphasize the importance of an overall scheme of management for ventilatory care of a neonate. Regardless of the approach to ventilation that is used, one should not simply respond randomly to blood gas measurements but rather have a specific set of goals in mind that

---

TABLE 9-8. Preliminary Review for Initiating Ventilatory Support

Clinical Observations	Mechanical Factors
Color	Oxygen supply
Respiratory rate	Endotracheal tube placement
Breathing pattern	Ventilator circuit humidification
Retractions and grunting	Humidifier and heater function
Chest and abdominal synchrony	Chest radiograph
Synchrony with the ventilator	Intravascular access
(consider assist/control or SIMV)	

SIMV, synchronized intermittent mandatory ventilation.

should be progressively approached throughout care. It is critical that the physician of record articulate this approach to everyone involved in the care of the infant. There is nothing more frustrating than coming to a child's bedside only to find that the changes made (especially during the night) on the ventilator, although not incorrect on a blood gas by blood gas basis, have resulted in a child making little overall progress because the specific goals of treatment were not clear.

The initiation of mechanical ventilation often is unnecessarily complicated. A scheme for the initiation of ventilation is shown in Figure 9-7. If one has a clear understanding of the goals of ventilatory support, steady progress toward those goals should be readily attainable. Once the clinician has decided that intervention is needed, the steps outlined in Table 9-10 should be followed. Adjustment of ventilation after stabilization of the infant is detailed in Figure 9-8. Some additional comments are appropriate relative to this approach to management.

The use of surfactant has become a standard adjunct to ventilatory management of the neonate. A more detailed discussion of surfactant therapy is presented in Chapter 20. Although optimal surfactant treatment is not established at the present time, the practice at most level III NICUs has been to use

TABLE 9-9. Mechanical Ventilator Settings Used to Adjust Arterial Blood Gases

$Paco_2$	Pao_2	Respiratory Acidosis (low pH)	Metabolic Acidosis (low pH)
1. Rate and PIP (determine minute ventilation; ↑ rate or ↑ PIP will ↓ CO_2)	1. Fio_2 (↑ O_2 will ↑ Pao_2)	1. Same controls as $Paco_2$	1. Volume expansion or sodium bicarbonate
2. I/E ratio (determines duration of inspiration and expiration; longer expiration will ↓ $Paco_2$)	2. PEEP (↑ PEEP will ↑ Pao_2)		2. May correct with improved oxygenation and ventilation, as perfusion improves
3. PEEP (if too high or too low, may ↑ $Paco_2$)	3. Ti or I/E ratio (↑ Ti will ↑ Pao_2; ↓ Ti will ↓ Pao_2 in general)		3. Caution: High PEEP may result in metabolic acidosis due to impaired venous return
	4. PIP (↑ PIP will usually ↑ Pao_2; effect is less than others listed above)		

Fio_2, fraction of inspired oxygen; I/E ratio, inspiratory-to-expiratory; PEEP, positive end-expiratory pressure; PIP, peak inspiratory pressure; Ti, inspiratory time.

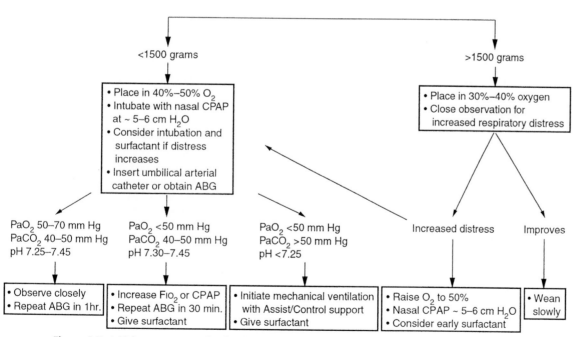

Figure 9-7. Initial management plan for the neonate with pulmonary disease. ABG, arterial blood gas analysis; CBC, complete blood count; CPAP, continuous positive airway pressure; CXR, chest x-ray; Fio_2, fraction of inspired oxygen.

TABLE 9-10. Initiation of Mechanical Ventilation in Neonatal Lung Disease

1. Intubate infant; secure endotracheal tube adequately
2. Place pressure manometer in gas flow line and begin manual ventilation to determine appropriate pressures for ventilation
3. Begin manual inflation with
   - $FIO_2 \geq 0.5$
   - Rate at 40–50 breaths/min
   - Initial PIP at 12–15 cm H_2O
   - Initial PEEP at 4–5 cm H_2O
   - I/E ratio at 1:1 to 1:2
4. Observe infant for
   - Cyanosis
   - Chest wall excursion
   - Capillary perfusion
   - Breath sounds
5. If ventilation is inadequate, increase PIP by 1 cm H_2O every few breaths until air entry seems adequate
6. If oxygenation is poor, and cyanosis remains, increase FIO_2 by 5% every minute until cyanosis is abolished
7. Draw ABG
8. Adjust ventilation as indicated by ABG results (see Fig. 9-8)

ABG, arterial blood gas; FIO_2, fraction of inspired oxygen; I/E, inspiratory to expiratory; PEEP, positive end-expiratory pressure; PIP, peak inspiratory pressure.

surfactant liberally and early in the infant diagnosed with RDS (surfactant deficiency disease). There are data suggesting that early use of surfactant, as soon as the diagnosis of RDS is made, has better results than later rescue use after the disease is well established.[52] Other neonatal lung diseases may respond to surfactant administration, given that inactivation of surfactant is commonly seen with acidosis or with the presence of meconium in the airway and lungs,[53] but the evidence in these diseases is less extensive than what has been reported for treatment of RDS. Furthermore, it appears that some differences with respect to surfactant replacement in meconium aspiration syndrome need to be considered when using exogenous surfactants. Peptide-containing surfactants (KL-4) appear to be more resistant than the modified natural surfactants currently in use.[54] Several surfactants are now approved by the US Food and Drug Administration (FDA) for use in the United States. Beractant (Survanta, Ross Laboratories, Columbus, OH, USA), colfosceril palmitate (Exosurf, Burroughs-Wellcome, Inc., Chapel Hill, NC, USA), calfactant (Infasurf, Forest Laboratories, Inc., New York, NY, USA), and poractant (Curosurf, Dey L.P., Napa, CA, USA) are available and have their various advocates among neonatologists.

Depending on the specific surfactant used and the infant's response, one to four doses of the drug are given. It is important that the clinician observe the baby closely during the surfactant administration process. Although most infants tolerate the procedure well, some babies experience oxygen desaturation. Other infants may improve rapidly, and overventilation can occur with the possibility of air leaks. Pulmonary hemorrhage appears to be slightly more common in some infants.[50] Excessively low $PaCO_2$ during the first days of life has been associated with an increased risk of cerebral palsy in some children.[55]

The use of pulmonary function testing may guide ventilator management. In recent years, use of pulmonary graphics monitoring, either as an intrinsic part of the ventilator or as an adjunct, has become increasingly widespread. Although not as precise as pulmonary functions performed independently of the ventilator, these units are extremely helpful in guiding ventilator management. Tidal volumes, minute ventilation, ventilator leak, chest wall distortion, flow-volume loops, pressure-volume loops, and several other functions can be readily evaluated. Overall lung volumes cannot be determined, however, except through measurements of functional residual capacity by either nitrogen washout or helium dilution. Recently, some interpolation methods have been studied that are less difficult to perform but somewhat less precise.[56] Improved functional residual capacity is probably the most important effect of surfactant administration in many disease conditions. Our practice traditionally has been to perform pulmonary mechanics several times per week to guide ventilator management and weaning. With newer graphics monitors, however, much of the necessary information can be evaluated several times daily during management of neonates on ventilatory support. Pulmonary function testing is described in greater detail in Chapter 18.

The management strategy outlined in Figure 9-8 is applicable to nearly all types of neonatal lung disease. The basic principles that guide this approach are as follows:

1. It is generally accepted that the most damaging aspects of neonatal ventilation, or the leading causes of lung injury, are FIO_2 and PIP. Although it is not always possible to limit the use of FIO_2 and PIP during the most critical phases of illness, one should try to reduce the levels of these controllable variables as soon as the infant shows signs of improvement. This algorithm for ventilator management is designed to reduce FIO_2 and PIP as primary initiatives while later decreasing rate and PEEP. In recent years, our practice has been to initiate positive-pressure ventilation in the assist/control mode, especially in the very-low-birthweight baby. Because of its design, assist/control weaning will occur primarily by decreasing FIO_2 and PIP, not the rate or PEEP. We have found that the basic principles outlined in the previous editions of this book not only remain applicable but actually are facilitated by using assist/control ventilation.

2. It is preferable to make frequent small changes in ventilator support rather than infrequent larger changes in degree of support. Commonly, ventilator management is approached with no overall plan in mind. In many nurseries, an arterial blood gas level is obtained at a random time, and the neonatologist makes a change based on that single blood gas analysis. Often the changes may be reasonable, yet they can be inappropriate because they do not take place within a defined strategy for weaning. The child ultimately receives a level of support that appears odd, yet ventilator changes were not necessarily incorrect on a blood gas by blood gas basis. The clinician simply did not have a coherent plan for ventilator management. For example, a child ultimately may receive a PIP of 25 cm H_2O and a rate of 5 to 10 breaths/min as weaning progresses because of low $PaCO_2$ levels. Each decision might have been correct, but the overall "balance" of ventilatory support is not optimal (although occasionally, as in a child with chronic BPD, such support levels may be necessary). It is important to develop a feel for overall balance of ventilator support, such as that listed in Table 9-11. If the ventilator settings vary much from the overall patterns across any row in this table, the physician should consider a ventilator strategy that brings the patient's support back into a more appropriate combination of settings. Table 9-11 assumes an approximate I/E ratio of 1:1 to 1:3 and an initial back-up ventilator rate of 40 to

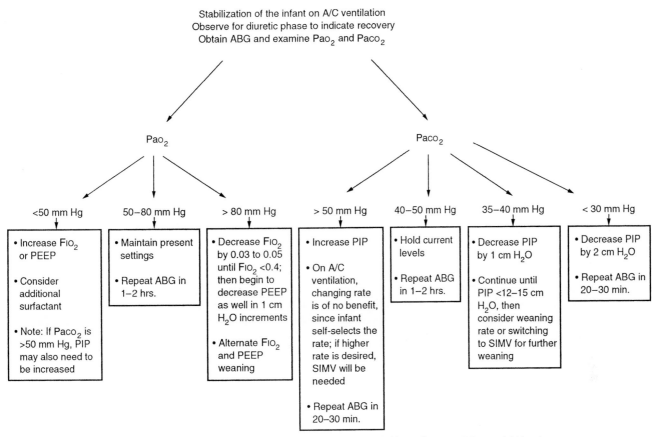

Figure 9-8. Approach to ventilator management during neonatal lung disease. ABG, arterial blood gas analysis; A/C, assist/control; PEEP, positive end-expiratory pressure; PIP, peak inspiratory pressure; SIMV, synchronized intermittent mandatory ventilation.

60 breaths/min. Normal arterial blood gas values for this table are as follows:

Pao_2 = 60 to 80 mm Hg
$Paco_2$ = 40 to 55 mm Hg
pH = 7.25 to 7.45

VENTILATOR WEANING

As previously indicated, our suggested approach to ventilator weaning is shown in Figure 9-8. Once an infant has remained stable for at least 24 hours, we gradually decrease the two factors that appear to have the greatest toxicity for the lung, namely, O_2 and PIP, while leaving the infant initially on assist/control ventilation. The weaning approach is very gradual, and frequent small changes are preferred to infrequent larger decreases in support. The goal is to allow the infant to assume gradual progressive responsibility for gas exchange while ventilator support is decreased. As Fio_2 and PIP are decreased, we usually switch an infant back to SIMV when the Fio_2 is below 0.4 and the PIP is less than 12 cm H_2O. The factor that made this approach possible was the introduction of IMV, now synchronized to the infant's own breathing as SIMV.

The general approach to SIMV weaning is to decrease the number of ventilator breaths progressively while the infant steadily increases spontaneous respiratory effort. No prospective controlled studies have clearly demonstrated the benefit of

this approach in the sick neonate, but theoretically this system affords several advantages:

1. It allows a gradual transition from mechanical ventilation to spontaneous breathing.
2. It eliminates the need for special bedside equipment to provide PEEP during weaning. (Some individuals believe that there is a difference between ventilator-delivered and underwater-delivered or "bubble" CPAP. This issue still needs to be studied. There appear to be differences among CPAP devices in some cases.[35])
3. It does not require expensive and complicated sigh mechanisms seen in some ventilators.
4. It has been shown to increase lung volume in infants.
5. There is a decreased need to use muscle relaxants or sedation to prevent patients from fighting the ventilator during weaning.
6. It may assist in coordinating respiratory muscular efforts during weaning.

In practice, simply weaning the ventilator rate, especially in the low-birthweight infant, does not work well, and it may expose the infant to excessive PIP during weaning. As a result, our approach, as shown in Figure 9-8, advocates decreasing pressure first to a low level (<15 cm H_2O) before SIMV weaning. In this way, the risks of barotrauma and late air leak development are reduced.

Weaning usually should be initiated as soon as possible after the infant has demonstrated stability for at least 4 to 8 hours and

TABLE 9-11.   Guidelines for Ventilator Care

| Inspired O_2 (%) | PEEP (cm H_2O) | PIP (cm H_2O) | | Rate (breaths/min) |
		<1500 g	>1500 g	
100%	6–8	25–30	25–30	40–60
90%	5–7	25–30	25–30	40–60
80%				
70%	5	20–25	22–30	35–50
60%				
50%	4	20–25	22–30	30–45
40%	3–4	15–20	18–25	20–35
30%	2–3	10–18	15–22	<30 (wean)

Note: These values are only guidelines that may not be appropriate in all clinical situations. In general, they should be viewed as the maximum necessary levels of support. At the highest support levels, standard positive-pressure ventilation may no longer be appropriate and alternatives (high-frequency ventilation, inhalational nitric oxide, extracorporeal membrane oxygenation) should be considered on an individual basis. The reader also should note that we have lowered the acceptable levels of PIP from prior iterations of this chart because we no longer believe infants should receive peak pressures >30 cm H_2O, except in unique cases.
PEEP, positive end-expiratory pressure; PIP, peak inspiratory pressure.

when arterial blood gas values suggest that ventilatory needs are decreasing. Before initiation of weaning, a chest radiograph should be obtained as a baseline against which subsequent radiographs can be compared if problems arise during the weaning process. Pulmonary function testing or examination of graphics monitoring is helpful in gauging the capacity for weaning. Increases in compliance and functional residual capacity typically herald recovery from pulmonary disease in the neonate. Our practice has been to follow pulmonary graphics on a daily basis in critically ill neonates to help define weaning possibilities. Improvement in compliance slope on the graphics and increasing flow rates often herald weaning and extubation potential. It has been demonstrated that, in infants with RDS, a diuretic phase occurs immediately before the improvement in pulmonary mechanics. Thus, an increase in urine output (>3 mL/kg per hour) may be a helpful observation during treatment.[57]

Studies have suggested that even the smallest infants can be weaned effectively from positive-pressure ventilation to nasal CPAP.[58] We have adopted nasal CPAP as a useful adjunct to therapy in very-low-birthweight infants (<1500 g). Without nasal CPAP, progressive atelectasis often occurs because the very compliant chest wall does not maintain lung volume well in these infants. Nasal CPAP often helps avoid the need for reintubation (see Chapter 8). Recent work has suggested that nasal SIMV may be even more advantageous, but studies thus far are limited.[53] Once extubation is planned, we usually place a baby on nasal CPAP for a minimum of 2 to 3 days, or longer in some cases. This therapy usually is well tolerated, but one must be attentive to stomach distention and nasal erosion.

During weaning, it is important to follow the infant's complete blood count, electrolytes, calcium, glucose, blood urea nitrogen levels, fluid balance, and urine specific gravity. Metabolic disturbances that manifest as abnormalities in these studies may affect weaning rate and prolong duration of support and length of stay. Appropriate caloric balance also is essential for successful weaning. The infant who is nutritionally depleted does not wean or extubate as well as the child who is in positive caloric balance. Nutrition may be given enterally or parenterally. We have not found intubation to be a contraindication to feeding in low-birthweight babies. Feeding should always be stopped at least 4 hours before an extubation attempt, or a nasogastric tube should be inserted and the stomach emptied. Following extubation, feeding should be held for a minimum of 4 to 6 hours or

until the infant can make an audible cry, which indicates the ability to oppose the vocal cords and protect the airway. Further discussion of nutritional support is found in Chapter 24.

Extubation

Some clinicians have difficulty managing the patient at the time of extubation. We have observed that even though ventilator care often is meticulous and thoughtful, extubation seems to be chaotic and haphazard. The child who is to be extubated should be prepared for the procedure, as with any medical intervention. Extubation is reasonable when the child is receiving less than 40% O_2 and when ventilator support has decreased to a rate of 10 breaths/min and PIP of 10 to 12 cm H_2O. For the past several years, we have rarely allowed a child to wean to ET tube CPAP alone and prefer to extubate from a rate of 5 to 10 breaths/min. In our experience, the child who is intubated but only on CPAP of 2 to 4 cm H_2O expends increased effort in work of breathing that wastes calories and energy unnecessarily. Our success rate has improved with extubation from low-level ventilatory support.

The decision to extubate should be made well in advance of the procedure. A chest radiograph should be obtained before extubation to be certain that a baseline study is available should problems arise after extubation. Repeat radiographs are obtained 2 and 24 hours after extubation to evaluate atelectasis. Respiratory therapists are notified, and the equipment that is desired after extubation should be immediately available. For very-low-birthweight infants, we usually extubate to a nasal CPAP of 5 to 6 cm H_2O. The child who weighs more than 1500 g is placed in a humidified oxygen hood or provided nasal cannula O_2 at the desired concentration. The child typically is treated initially with an O_2 concentration that is 5% above that given while he or she was still mechanically ventilated.

All facial tape should be carefully removed from the child who is to be extubated so that skin injury to the face can be avoided. The ET tube is connected to a Mapleson bag, and the child is given a prolonged sigh of 15 to 20 cm H_2O while the ET tube is extracted. This sigh prevents negative pressure from developing in the airway, which occurs upon tube removal and may cause atelectasis. The baby then is placed in the desired environment (often with nasal CPAP in the case of the very-low-birthweight baby) and watched closely for several minutes. Use of pulse oximetry at this time is invaluable. Oxygen saturation should be kept at a minimum of 92% to 96%. Upon extubation, there should be no significant respiratory distress, or it should last only momentarily. Signs of respiratory difficulty include tachypnea, retractions, pallor, cyanosis, agitation, and lethargy. If distress is significant, it is prudent to replace the ET tube and repeat the trial in 2 days. If a child fails two attempts at extubation, we perform flexible fiberoptic bronchoscopy on the baby to be certain there are no obstructive lesions in the airway. If the result of this study is negative, we initiate dexamethasone treatment (0.5 mg/kg per day in two divided doses beginning 48 hours before extubation, continuing for 24 hours after extubation, if successful) to reduce any airway edema. In addition, methylxanthines, such as caffeine citrate or theophylline, may decrease resistance and increase respiratory drive, enhancing the likelihood of successful extubation. There are no controlled studies demonstrating the effectiveness of this approach, but it anecdotally appears to benefit some children.

If a child cannot be extubated upon several repeated attempts, the diagnosis of laryngotracheomalacia must be considered. Some infants may not be extubated successfully, and tracheostomy must be considered. We do *not* perform a tracheostomy until we are certain a child cannot be extubated and that this fact has been demonstrated at least four times over several weeks. Such cases are exceedingly rare in the nurseries at our institutions.

Accidental extubation occasionally occurs in all nurseries for a variety of reasons. The tape around the ET may loosen, or the movement of the child may free the tube and dislodge it. If extubation occurs, we carefully assess the infant to determine his or her readiness for extubation at the time of the event. If extubation was thought to be days away and the child appears to be exerting excessive effort, the ET tube is immediately replaced. *Allowing the child to become unnecessarily distressed at this point further delays ultimate extubation and should be avoided.* If, however, the child appears comfortable, we follow pulse oximetry to be sure the infant remains well oxygenated and obtain a chest radiograph and arterial blood gas levels. If these results are acceptable, the child can remain extubated with very careful observation.

COMPLICATIONS OF MECHANICAL VENTILATION

The potential complications of neonatal mechanical ventilation are substantial, and a partial list is given in Table 9-12. Many of these complications can be prevented or minimized with the approaches to care outlined in this chapter. The most commonly seen clinical circumstance that produces immediate concern involves sudden deterioration of an infant on ventilatory support. In such circumstances, the child may appear well one moment but rapidly become cyanotic, with pallor, bradycardia, hypotension, and hypercapnia next. An approach to this situation is shown in Figure 9-9. An extensive discussion of

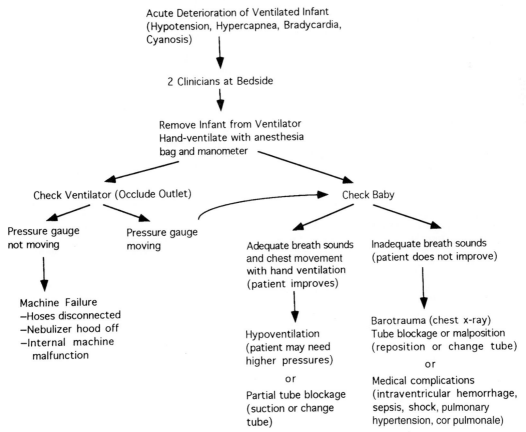

Figure 9-9. Algorithm demonstrating approach to the ventilated infant with sudden acute deterioration. (Modified from Gottschalk SK, King B, Schuth CR: Basic concepts in positive pressure ventilation of the newborn. Perinatol Neonatol 4:15, 1980.)

TABLE 9-12. Complications of Mechanical Ventilation

Airway Injury	Air Leaks
Tracheal inflammation	Pulmonary interstitial
Tracheobronchomalacia	emphysema (PIE)
Subglottic stenosis	Pneumothorax
Granuloma formation	Pneumomediastinum
Palatal grooving	Pneumopericardium
Nasal septal injury	Pneumoperitoneum
Necrotizing tracheobronchitis	Air embolism syndrome
Endotracheal Tube Complications	Cardiovascular
Dislodgment	Decreased cardiac output
Obstruction	Patent ductus arteriosus
Accidental extubation	(PDA)
Airway erosion	
	Miscellaneous
Chronic Lung Injury	Retinopathy of prematurity
Bronchopulmonary dysplasia	Apnea
(BPD)	Infection
Acquired lobar emphysema	Feeding intolerance
	Developmental delay
	Hyperinflation
	Intraventricular hemorrhage
	(IVH)

pulmonary air leaks, BPD, and retinopathy of prematurity can be found in Chapter 21.

If the physician determines that progression of lung disease is the cause of deterioration, then a more advanced form of therapy, such as high-frequency ventilation or ECMO, must be considered. These treatments appear to be effective for some infants who require rescue therapy for severe cardiopulmonary disease. These therapies are discussed in Chapters 11 and 16.

REFERENCES

1. Greenough A, Milner AD, Dimitriou G: Synchronized mechanical ventilation for respiratory support in newborn infants (Cochrane Review). Cochrane Database Syst Rev 1:CD000456, 2001.
2. Abubakar KM, Keszler M: Patient-ventilator interactions in new modes of patient-triggered ventilation. Pediatr Pulmonol 32:71, 2001.
3. Spitzer AR, Butler S, Fox WW: Ventilatory response of combined high frequency jet ventilation and conventional mechanical ventilation for the rescue treatment of severe neonatal lung disease. Pediatr Pulmonol 7:244, 1989.
4. Baumgart S, Hirschl RB, Butler SZ, et al: Diagnosis-related criteria in the consideration of extracorporeal membrane oxygenation in neonates previously treated with high frequency jet ventilation. Pediatrics 89:491, 1992.
5. Bhuta T, Clark RH, Henderson-Smart DJ: Rescue high frequency oscillatory ventilation vs conventional ventilation for infants with severe pulmonary dysfunction born at or near term (Cochrane Review). Cochrane Database Syst Rev 1:CD002974, 2001.
6. Finer NN, Barrington KJ: Nitric oxide for respiratory failure in infants born at or near term (Cochrane Review). Cochrane Database Syst Rev 2:CD000399, 2001.
7. Hintz SR, Suttner DM, Sheehan AM, et al: Decreased use of neonatal extracorporeal membrane oxygenation (ECMO): How new treatment modalities have affected ECMO utilization. Pediatrics 106:1339, 2000.
8. Donn SM, Sinha SK: Newer modes of mechanical ventilation for the neonate. Curr Opin Pediatr 13:99, 2001.
9. Schulze A, Gerhardt T, Musante G, et al: Proportional assist ventilation in low birth weight infants with acute respiratory disease: A comparison to assist/control and conventional mechanical ventilation. J Pediatr 135:339, 1999.
10. Sinha SK, Donn SM, Gavey J, et al: Randomised trial of volume controlled versus time cycled, pressure limited ventilation in preterm infants with respiratory distress syndrome. Arch Dis Child Fetal Neonatal Ed 77:F202, 1997.
11. Dreyfuss D, Saumon G: Barotrauma is volutrauma, but which volume is the one responsible? Intensive Care Med 18:139, 1992.
12. Gannon CM, Wiswell TE, Spitzer AR: Volutrauma, $PaCO_2$ levels, and neurodevelopmental sequelae following assisted ventilation. Clin Perinatol 25:159–175, 1998.
13. Ratner I, Hernandez J, Accurso F: Low peak inspiratory pressures for ventilation of infants with hyaline membrane disease. J Pediatr 100:801, 1982.
14. Cheema IU, Ahluwahia JS: Feasibility of tidal volume-guided ventilation in newborn infants: A randomized, crossover trial using the volume guarantee modality. Pediatrics 107:1323, 2001.
15. Truog WE, Jackson LC: Alternative modes of ventilation in the prevention and treatment of bronchopulmonary dysplasia. Clin Perinatol 19:621, 1992.
16. Boros SJ, Bing BR, Mammel MC, et al: Using conventional ventilators at unconventional rates. Pediatrics 74:487, 1984.
17. Hanson JB, Waldstein G, Hernandez JA, et al: Necrotizing tracheobronchitis: An ischemic lesion. Am J Dis Child 142:1094, 1988.
18. Greenspan JS, DeGuilio PA, Bhutani VK, et al: Airway reactivity as determined by a cold air challenge in infants with bronchopulmonary dysplasia. J Pediatr 114:452, 1988.
19. Schulze A: Enhancement of mechanical ventilation of neonates by computer technology. Semin Perinatol 24:429, 2000.
20. Kapasi M, Fujino Y, Kirmse M, et al: Effort and work of breathing in neonates during assisted patient-triggered ventilation. Pediatr Crit Care Med 2:9, 2001.
21. Peckham GJ, Fox WW: Physiologic factors affecting pulmonary artery pressure in infants with persistent pulmonary hypertension. J Pediatr 93:1005, 1978.
22. Cunningham S, McColm JR, Wade J, et al: A novel model of retinopathy of prematurity simulating preterm oxygen variability in the rat. Invest Ophthalmol Vis Sci 41:4275–4280, 2000.
23. STOP-ROP Study Group: Supplemental Therapeutic Oxygen for Prethreshold Retinopathy Of Prematurity (STOP-ROP), a randomized, controlled trial. I: Primary outcomes. Pediatrics 105:295, 2000.
24. Jobe AH, Ikegami M: Prevention of bronchopulmonary dysplasia. Curr Opin Pediatr 13:124–129, 2001.
25. Keszler M, Donn SM, Bucciarelli RL, et al: Multicenter controlled trial comparing high-frequency jet ventilation and conventional mechanical ventilation in newborn infants with pulmonary interstitial emphysema. J Pediatr 119:85–93, 1991.
26. Mrozek JD, Bendel-Stenzel EM, Meyers PA, et al: Randomized controlled trial of volume-targeted synchronized ventilation and conventional intermittent mandatory ventilation following initial exogenous surfactant therapy. Pediatr Pulmonol 29:11, 2000.
27. Vannucci RC, Towfighi J, Brucklacher RM, et al: Effect of extreme hypercapnia on hypoxic-ischemic brain damage in the immature rat. Pediatr Res 49:799, 2001.
28. Mariani G, Cifuentes J, Carlo WA: Randomized trial of permissive hypercapnia in preterm infants. Pediatrics 104:1082, 1999.
29. Woodgate PG, Davies MW: Permissive hypercapnia for the prevention of morbidity and mortality in mechanically ventilated newborn infants (Cochrane Review). Cochrane Database Syst Rev 2:CD002061, 2001.
30. Graziani LJ, Desai S, Baumgart S, et al: Clinical antecedents of neurologic and audiologic abnormalities in survivors of neonatal ECMO—A group comparison study. J Child Neurol 12:415, 1997.
31. Gregory GA, Kitterman JA, Phibbs RH, et al: Treatment of the idiopathic respiratory-distress syndrome with continuous positive airway pressure. N Engl J Med 284:1333, 1971.
32. De Klerk A, De Klerk R: Nasal continuous positive airway pressure and outcomes of preterm infants. J Paediatr Child Health 37:161, 2001.
33. Lemyre B, Davis PG, De Paoli AG: Nasal intermittent positive pressure ventilation (NIPPV) versus nasal continuous positive airway pressure (NCPAP) for apnea of prematurity (Cochrane Review). Cochrane Database Syst Rev 3:CD002272, 2000.
34. Davis PG, Henderson-Smart DJ: Nasal continuous positive airways pressure immediately after extubation for preventing morbidity in preterm infants [update of 20257405]. Cochrane Database Syst Rev 3:CD000143, 2000.
35. Courtney SE, Pyon KH, Saslow JG, et al: Lung recruitment and breathing pattern during variable versus continuous flow nasal continuous positive airway pressure in premature infants: An evaluation of three devices. Pediatrics 107:304, 2001.
36. Bonta BW, Vavy R, Warshaw JB, et al: Determination of optimal continuous airway pressure for the treatment of RDS by measurement of esophageal pressure. J Pediatr 91:449, 1977.

37. Stenson BJ, Glover RM, Wilkie RA, et al: Life-threatening inadvertent positive end-expiratory pressure. Am J Perinatol 12:336, 1995.

38. da Silva WJ, Abbasi S, Pereira G, et al: Role of positive end-expiratory pressure changes on functional residual capacity in surfactant treated preterm infants. Pediatr Pulmonol 18:89–92, 1994.

39. Fox WW, Berman LS, Dinwiddie R, et al: Tracheal extubation of the neonate at 2–3 cm H_2O continuous positive airway pressure. Pediatrics 59:257, 1977.

40. Bland RD, Kim MH, Light MJ, et al: High frequency mechanical ventilation in severe hyaline membrane disease. An alternative treatment? Crit Care Med 8:275, 1980.

41. Haman S, Reynolds EOR: Methods of improving oxygenation in infants mechanically ventilated for severe hyaline membrane disease. Arch Dis Child 48:617, 1973.

42. Boros SJ: Variations in inspiratory-expiratory ratio and air pressure wave form during mechanical ventilation: The significance of mean airway pressure. J Pediatr 94:114, 1979.

43. Simbruner G, Gregory GA: Performance of neonatal ventilators: The effects of changes in resistance and compliance. Crit Care Med 9:509, 1981.

44. Kirby R, Robinson EJ, Schulz J, et al: Continuous flow ventilation as an alternative to assisted or controlled ventilation in infants. Anesth Analg 51:871, 1971.

45. Reynolds EOR, Tagizadeh A: Improved prognosis of infants mechanically ventilated for hyaline membrane disease. Arch Dis Child 49:505, 1974.

46. Boros SJ, Mabaln SV, Ewald R, et al: The effect of independent variations in inspiratory-expiratory ratio and end expiratory pressure during mechanical ventilation in hyaline membrane disease: The significance of mean airway pressure. J Pediatr 91:794, 1977.

47. Meredith KS, deLemos RA, Coalson JJ, et al: Role of lung injury in the pathogenesis of hyaline membrane disease in premature baboons. J Appl Physiol 66:2150, 1989.

48. Bond DM, McAloon J, Froese AB: Sustained inflations improve respiratory compliance during high-frequency oscillatory ventilation but not during large tidal volume positive-pressure ventilation in rabbits. Crit Care Med 22:1269, 1994.

49. Goldsmith LS, Greenspan JS, Rubinstein SD, et al: Immediate improvement in lung volume after exogenous surfactant: Alveolar recruitment versus increased distension. J Pediatr 119:424, 1991.

50. Soll RF: Prophylactic synthetic surfactant for preventing morbidity and mortality in preterm infants. Cochrane Database Syst Rev 2:CD001079, 2000.

51. Wung JT, James LS, Kilchevsky E, et al: Management of infants with severe respiratory failure and persistence of the fetal circulation, without hyperventilation. Pediatrics 76:488, 1985.

52. Yost CC, Soll RF: Early versus delayed selective surfactant treatment for neonatal respiratory distress syndrome. Cochrane Database Syst Rev 2:CD001456, 2000.

53. Wiswell TE: Advances in the treatment of the meconium aspiration syndrome. Acta Paediatr Suppl 90:28, 2001.

54. Herting E, Rauprich P, Stichtenoth G, et al: Resistance of different surfactant preparations to inactivation by meconium. Pediatr Res 50:44, 2001.

55. Graziani LJ, Spitzer AR, Mitchell DG, et al: Mechanical ventilation in preterm infants: Neurosonographic and developmental studies. Pediatrics 90:515, 1992.

56. Riou Y, Storme L, Leclerc F, et al: Comparison of four methods for measuring elevation of FRC in mechanically ventilated infants. Intensive Care Med 25:1118, 1999.

57. Spitzer AR, Fox WW, Delivoria-Papadopoulos M: Maximal diuresis—A factor in predicting recovery from RDS and the development of bronchopulmonary dysplasia. J Pediatr 98:476, 1981.

58. Higgins RD, Richter SE, Davis JM: Nasal continuous positive airway pressure facilitates extubation of very low birth weight neonates. Pediatrics 88:999, 1991.

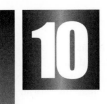

VOLUME-CONTROLLED VENTILATION

SUNIL K. SINHA, MD, PhD, FRCP, FRCPCH
STEVEN M. DONN, MD

Despite the introduction of newer strategies such as extracorporeal membrane oxygenation, inhaled nitric oxide, high-frequency ventilation, and partial liquid ventilation, conventional mechanical ventilation remains the primary treatment for respiratory failure in newborns. Until recently, this has been accomplished by using traditional time-cycled, pressure-limited ventilation, in which peak inspiratory pressure (PIP) is set by the clinician and is not exceeded by the ventilator (see Chapter 9). Because PIP is thought to be directly related to the likelihood of development of air leaks and chronic lung disease in newborn infants, it has been assumed that pressure-limited ventilation decreases barotrauma because of its ability to control PIP. This, however, is an oversimplification not supported by adequate scientific evidence. Moreover, there are indications that the injury to the neonatal lung may be more related to volutrauma than to barotrauma, and it is the amount of gas delivered to the lungs that may be more critical to the effectiveness and safety of a particular ventilatory mode.[1,2] When tidal volume is appropriate and the lung is adequately inflated, the use of high airway pressure does not seem to produce lung injury. This observation becomes more clear if one understands the concept of lung volume-pressure hysteresis (see Fig. 2-4).

Over the last decade, there has been a tremendous improvement in ventilator designs using microprocessor-based respiratory technology, and this has facilitated the introduction of a variety of newer modes of ventilation that had not been available to neonatal populations.[3] One of these newer modes is volume-controlled ventilation. Incidentally, one of the first ventilators designed specifically for use in infants was a volume-cycled ventilator, the Bourns LS 104-150, which was modified from an adult ventilator and featured in the first edition of this text (1981). Because of problems with trigger sensitivity, long response times, and lack of continuous flow during spontaneous breathing, volume-controlled ventilation fell out of favor in the 1980s. Technologic advances in the 1990s enabled reintroduction of this type of ventilation in neonatal and pediatric intensive care units, and the difference between volume ventilators of the 1970s and the present day is remarkable. These new ventilators not only incorporate sophisticated devices to trigger and deliver the smallest amount of tidal volume required by an infant weighing as little as 500 to 600 g, but they also manipulate gas delivery in order to match the patient's demand. In many respects, the mechanically delivered breaths resemble the patient's own spontaneous breaths, giving this mode of ventilation obvious physiologic advantages. Most of the modern ventilators now are also capable of providing both pressure-limited and volume-controlled ventilation with a variety of secondary options. This novel flexibility often leads to confusion, and it is crucial that clinicians familiarize themselves with the new nomenclature and differences among these newer ventilatory modes (see Chapter 12).

The key differentiating feature of volume ventilation from pressure-limited, time-cycled ventilation is that it targets a specific volume of gas to be delivered either from the ventilator or to the patient, and inspiration is terminated (cycled into expiration) when this preset volume of gas has been delivered. This initially gave rise to the name *volume-cycled ventilation.* However, because cuffed endotracheal tubes are not used in newborns, there almost always is some degree of gas leak around the endotracheal tube. Thus, true volume cycling is probably a misnomer in neonatal practice. Terms such as *volume-controlled, volume-limited,* and *volume-targeted* better describe what happens during this type of ventilation. It is important to realize that the volume of gas that leaves the ventilator is not the same volume that reaches the proximal airway. Depending on a number of factors, including circuit tubing compliance, humidification, and pulmonary compliance, there will be a loss of compressible volume. Of the devices presently available, most ventilators for neonatal use measure volume delivery at the proximal airway (wye piece). This provides a much closer estimate of what will be delivered to the lungs compared to those devices that measure volume at the ventilator and provide algorithms to determine what the patient will actually receive. Tidal volume is the volume of each breath as measured during inspiration, expiration, or averaged for both respiratory cycles. Normal values in healthy newborn infants range from 5 to 8 mL/kg body weight, but in practice it seems safer to use a range from 4 to 7 mL/kg. Volumes greater than 8 mL/kg suggest volume overdistention. When measured over a 1-minute duration, the volume data provide a reference to minute ventilation; normal values in newborns range from 240 to 480 mL/kg per minute. Minute ventilation is a surrogate measure of carbon dioxide elimination, although it is alveolar ventilation (minute ventilation minus dead space ventilation) that has a direct inverse relationship to alveolar P_{CO_2} or arterial carbon dioxide tension.

The major distinguishing features of volume-controlled and pressure-limited ventilation are summarized in Table 10-1. Major features of volume ventilation include a relatively square flow waveform and the occurrence of peak volume delivery at end-inspiration. Inspiratory time is determined by flow rate and is inversely proportional to it (Fig. 10-1). This is different from pressure-limited ventilation, where the opening pressure is reached much more quickly (spike flow waveform); this allows more time for the alveoli to fill, so alveolar ventilation and

TABLE 10-1.   Distinguishing Features of Volume-Controlled and Pressure-Limited Ventilation

Features	Volume-Controlled	Pressure-Limited
Control (fixed) variable	Volume	Pressure
Phase (changeable) variable		
Inspiratory trigger	Patient or machine	Patient or machine
Inspiratory limit	Flow	Pressure
Inspiratory cycle	Volume or flow	Time or flow
Delivered tidal volume	Constant	Variable
Recorded peak pressure	Variable	Constant
Inspiratory flow waveform	Square	Ramp-descending
Available modes	IMV, SIMV, A/C, PSV	IMV, SIMV, A/C, PSV

A/C, assist/control; IMV, intermittent mandatory ventilation; PSV, pressure-support ventilation; SIMV, synchronized intermittent mandatory ventilation.

perhaps oxygenation are greater. This may or may not be advantageous, because injury to the immature lungs depends not only upon the amount of volume or pressure but also upon the duration of lung inflation. Some of the newer machines offer the option of decelerating inspiratory flow and an inspiratory "hold" or "pause" with volume ventilation. The intention is to improve oxygenation, as described later in this chapter. The inspiratory pause must be long enough to allow the pressure to plateau or reach a stable pause pressure. The plateau pressure is more representative of alveolar pressure than is the PIP.

Detractors of volume-controlled ventilation have argued that unlike the fixed PIP used in pressure-limited ventilation, volume-controlled ventilation utilizes a high inflation pressure to deliver the preset volume in cases of decreased compliance or increased resistance. This previously had been a source of anxiety to clinicians because of perceived risks of barotrauma and its consequences. However, it must be realized that the excessive peak pressure associated with fixed-flow delivery in volume-controlled ventilation is a reflection of proximal airway pressure rather than peak lung (alveolar) pressure. When the compliance of the patient's lungs improves

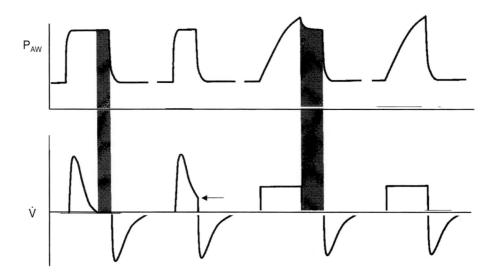

Figure 10-1. Cycles 1 and 2 represent pressure-targeted (pressure-limited) ventilation.

- Set, limited, constant inspiratory pressure level
- Nonlimited, decelerating inspiratory flow
- Control (nondependent) variable: pressure
- Dependent variable: tidal volume
- Cycling mechanisms:
  - Time: pressure control, time-cycled pressure-limited ventilation (TCPLV) (cycle 1)
  - Flow: pressure-support, flow-synchronized vent (cycle 2)
  - Arrow head: termination flow criterion (usually as percentage of peak flow)

Cycles 3 and 4 represent volume-targeted (volume-control volume-cycled) ventilation.

- Set, limited, constant inspiratory flow rate
- Gradually increasing, "shark fin" inspiratory pressure
- Control (nondependent) variable: flow
- Dependent variable: peak inspiratory pressure
- Cycling mechanisms:
  - Time: volume ventilation with set inspiratory pause time (cycle 3)
  - Volume: volume-control ventilation (cycle 4) (volume may be represented as the area under the flow curve)

Note that the inspiratory plateau period *(gray-filled area)* may exist during time-cycled modes (cycle 1 in pressure and cycle 3 in volume ventilation). (Acknowledgment to Dr. Akos Kovacs, Clinical Specialist, Viasys Health Care System, Hungary, for help in preparing this figure.)

(increases), the ventilator actually generates less pressure to deliver the same tidal volume, thus leading to automatic reduction ("autoweaning") of the PIP. Although peak airway pressure is greater for the constant flow pattern seen in volume-controlled ventilation, mean airway pressure (Paw) is less, and it is the latter that should correlate better with the mean lung pressure (assuming that resistance and compliance remain constant throughout the ventilatory cycle). For a single-compartment lung model, if tidal volume is held constant, the risk of barotrauma is the same for pressure-controlled or volume-controlled ventilation and peak alveolar pressure will be the same. For a two-compartment model with unequal time constants [as in neonatal respiratory distress syndrome (RDS)], it can be shown mathematically that volume-controlled ventilation results in a more even distribution of volume and a potentially lower risk of barotrauma.[4,5] Because of these considerations, limiting the peak pressure in volume-controlled devices (in an effort to vent excessive gas volumes) may be a misconception, as it offsets the major advantage of volume-controlled ventilation in maintaining a constant flow pattern.

There is a commonly held belief that pressure-limited ventilation of infants is superior to volume-controlled ventilation because it can maintain a constant airway pressure in the presence of leaks around uncuffed endotracheal tubes. The reasoning seems to be that constant pressure implies that the delivered volume remains constant; however, this is a misunderstanding. In addition to the effects of changing lung compliance on tidal volume delivery during pressure-limited ventilation, leaks at the tracheal level can drop the pressure in the trachea and thus affect ventilation just the same as during volume-controlled ventilation. The effect may be masked during pressure-limited ventilation. Some devices that provide volume-controlled ventilation actually supply a means to compensate for leaks by adding additional flow to the circuit to automatically maintain a stable baseline pressure.

Although it remains to be seen whether volume-controlled ventilation is a superior technique in this population, there has been a resurgence of interest in its use as a primary strategy during assisted ventilation of newborns. This may be accomplished by using volume-controlled ventilation as a primary mode or by using tidal volume delivery as a reference to adjust the level of PIP during pressure-limited ventilation. To facilitate this, most of the newer neonatal ventilators provide breath-to-breath displays of pulmonary mechanics as either real-time graphic or digital displays. Alternatively, some machines use a software algorithm to adjust tidal volume delivery according to airway resistance, lung compliance, and the strength and duration of patient inspiratory effort. Salient features of commercially available ventilators that are being used in the neonatal population are described later, but it is always advisable to review their detailed product information or share the experience of those who regularly use a particular device before incorporating it into clinical practice.

MODES UTILIZING VOLUME-CONTROLLED VENTILATION

Like pressure-limited ventilation, volume-controlled ventilation can be accomplished in a number of ways. Detailed description of each of these modes is given elsewhere in the book (see Chapter 12), but the key features of commonly used methods are discussed here.

Intermittent Mandatory Ventilation

As the name *intermittent mandatory ventilation (IMV)* implies, in this mode the clinician adjusts the ventilator to determine the minimum breaths per minute with which the patient will be ventilated. The patient is still able to breathe independently from the bias flow in the circuit between the mechanically delivered breaths. Such systems do not permit synchronization of the patient's breath with the mechanical breath, but it is possible to superimpose a generated tidal volume on the patient during inspiration or expiration. Asynchrony may result in widely variable tidal volume delivery, alveolar overdistention, and air leaks, and it has been associated with intraventricular hemorrhage (IVH) in preterm infants. To prevent these complications, patients often require sedation and occasionally neuromuscular paralysis.

Synchronized Intermittent Mandatory Ventilation

Synchronized intermittent mandatory ventilation (SIMV) is an improvement over IMV in achieving inspiratory synchrony in that the ventilator allows the patient to receive mandatory breaths whose onset is timed to the patient's inspiratory effort. The assisted breaths occur only during windows of time established by the manufacturer and set by the clinician. The time available within each window for patient triggering varies, but it is usually a function of the set respiratory rate. If a patient's inspiratory effort is detected while the window is open, a synchronized breath is delivered. If no patient effort is detected at the time the window closes, the ventilator delivers a mandatory breath. Spontaneous breaths taken by the patient between the SIMV breaths are supported by positive end-expiratory pressure (PEEP) or alternatively by pressure-support ventilation (PSV), in which spontaneous breaths are fully or partially supported (described later). The flexibility of SIMV in offering a range of ventilatory support makes it useful as both an acute and weaning form of mechanical ventilation. However, a low "unsupported" SIMV rate is undesirable when the patient's ventilatory demand is high because this may result in patient fatigue and alveolar hypoventilation. Similarly, reduction of the SIMV rate to a low level (e.g., less than 20 breaths/min) without some other means of breath support, such as PSV, may be theoretically unwise when discontinuation of mechanical support is imminent. This may impose a significant work of breathing for an intubated infant and contribute to weaning failure.

Assist/Control

In *assist/control (A/C)* mode, each spontaneous breath that exceeds the trigger threshold results in the delivery of a completely supported mechanical breath (assist) (Fig. 10-2). If the patient fails to breathe or if the spontaneous breath fails to exceed the trigger threshold, a mechanical (control) breath is provided at a rate set by the clinician to ensure adequate ventilation. A/C ventilation appears to be the preferred choice as an initial mode of ventilation in many institutions. It probably is the best mode to use in the premature infant in the acute phase of respiratory failure because it requires the least amount of patient effort. It also has the safety of a guaranteed "back-up" rate to assure adequate minute ventilation in the event of apnea or insufficient patient effort. Weaning during A/C is different than it is for IMV or SIMV because many of the parameters previously set by the clinician are now controlled by the patient.[6] During A/C, as long as the patient is breathing above the control rate, reduction in the mechanical rate brings about no change in ventilator cycling. Unlike pressure-limited A/C, where reduction in PIP is the primary weaning parameter, reduction in tidal volume delivery to a level of 3 to 4 mL/kg or the use of slower-rate SIMV with PSV is the preferred method of weaning in volume-controlled modes.

Pressure-Support Ventilation

Pressure-support ventilation is a pressure-limited, flow-cycled spontaneous mode of ventilation in which inspiratory flow is variable according to patient effort. It is intended to give the patient an inspiratory pressure "boost" during spontaneous breathing in order to overcome the imposed work of breathing created by the narrow-lumen, high-resistance, endotracheal tube; the ventilator circuit; and the demand valve system. Although PSV can be used as a singular mode (provided the patient has sufficient ventilatory drive), it most commonly is used in combination with volume-controlled SIMV.[7] The level of support can be selected by the clinician and may vary from full support (referred to as *PSMAX*) to partial support as used during weaning stages in conjunction with other modes such as SIMV (Fig. 10-3). The major function of PSV is to assist respiratory muscle activity and thus reduce the workload. Depending on the level of pressure support used, PSV can either totally or partially unload ventilatory muscles during spontaneous breathing. Partial unloading is of value, particularly in babies requiring prolonged ventilatory support, such as those with bronchopulmonary dysplasia or difficulty in weaning due to other causes. Being pressure limited, the tidal volume delivery in PSV depends on the respiratory mechanics and may be variable. To overcome this variability, some devices have combined pressure support with a guaranteed minimum tidal volume delivery as described later.

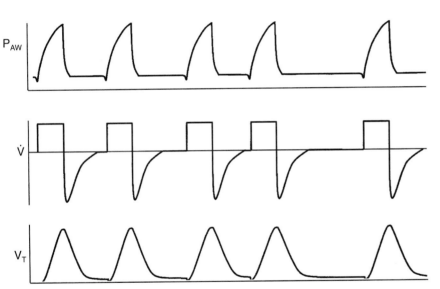

Figure 10-2. Volume ventilation modes: assist/control ventilation. Airway pressure, flow, and volume waveforms are shown. All cycles are similar mandatory; the ventilator responds to all detected spontaneous inspiratory effort. Note that the delivered volume is equal during every cycle, and the total rate is controlled by patient effort (plus the minimum set rate delivered if no spontaneous inspiration has been detected.) Measured exhaled tidal volume is always a bit less than inspiratory, representing the leak around the uncuffed endotracheal tube. (Acknowledgment to Dr. Akos Kovacs, Clinical Specialist, Viasys Health Care System, Hungary, for help in preparing this figure.)

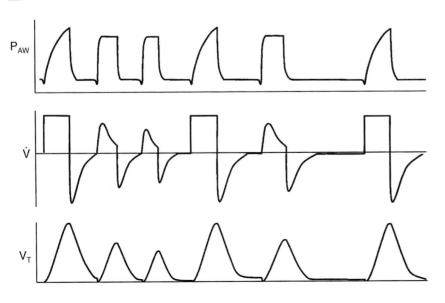

Figure 10-3. Volume ventilation modes: synchronized intermittent mandatory ventilation (SIMV) plus pressure support (PS). Airway pressure, flow, and volume waveforms are shown. Two different waveforms exist. Set number of mandatory (SIMV) cycles plus PS cycles with set inspiratory pressure and non-limited flow rate. Note that tidal volume during PS is enhanced (compared to continuous positive airway pressure) but is varying and not guaranteed. PS cycles are terminated when inspiratory flow drops to the set level. Inspiratory time and breath rate may vary during PS. For the mandatory cycles, rate and volume are guaranteed, flow is fixed, and peak pressure is patient dependent. The total rate is a sum of the set mandatory plus the spontaneous (PS) cycles. (Acknowledgment to Dr. Akos Kovacs, Clinical Specialist, Viasys Health Care System, Hungary, for help in preparing this figure.)

COMBINED FORMS OF VENTILATION (PRESSURE-LIMITED WITH VOLUME-TARGETED)

Both volume-controlled and pressure-limited modes are perceived to have certain advantages and disadvantages (Table 10-2). To obviate disadvantages, manufacturers of newer ventilators have attempted to combine the desirable features of both pressure-controlled and volume-controlled breaths in one mode. These hybrid forms, which include volume-assured pressure-support (VAPS) and pressure-regulated volume-control (PRVC) ventilation, are primarily pressure-limited modes but guarantee a desired tidal volume chosen by the clinician. Their features and the commonly available ventilators that incorporate them are summarized in Tables 10-3 and 10-4.

Volume-Assured Pressure-Support Ventilation

This modality combines the advantages of pressure and volume ventilation on a breath-to-breath basis and can be used with both A/C and SIMV or by itself in babies with reliable respiratory drive. It can be described as *variable-flow volume ventilation.* This is a blended mode with decelerating, non-limited, variable flow with guaranteed tidal volume delivery. The breath is triggered by the patient. Spontaneous breaths

TABLE 10-2.   Perceived Advantages and Disadvantages of Volume-Targeted versus Pressure-Limited Ventilation

	Volume-Targeted	Pressure-Limited
Advantages	Linear increase in minute volume delivery as V$_T$ is increased	Improves gas distribution by exposing the lungs to set PIP throughout inspiratory cycle
	Autoweaning of proximal airway pressure as lung compliance improves	Reduces work of breathing by providing high initial flow (pressure control)
	Constant V$_T$ delivery regardless of pulmonary compliance in the presence of a substantial leak around the uncuffed endotracheal tube (as used in newborns); inspired tidal volumes may overestimate the actual tidal volume delivered to the lungs	Limits excessive airway pressure and thus reduces "risk" of barotrauma
Disadvantages	Excessive airway pressure could increase risk of barotrauma	Variable V$_T$ delivery; thus, risk of excessive volume delivery as compliance improves or inadequate volume delivery if compliance worsens (if no adjustment is made)
	Patient-ventilator asynchrony from fixed inspiratory flow, which may cause difference between set flow and patient flow demand leading to "flow starvation" and increased work of breathing	Inconsistent change in V$_T$ with change in PIP and PEEP

PEEP, positive end-expiratory pressure; PIP, peak inspiratory pressure.

TABLE 10-3.   Features of Various Forms of Volume-Targeted Ventilatory Modes

Volume-control (VC; V.I.P. BIRD Gold, Siemens Servo 300)	10–1200 mL tidal volume range Flow or pressure triggered Square or decelerating flow waveform Inspiratory pause Volume delivery set on inspired or expired tidal volume as reference
Volume-assured pressure-support (VAPS; V.I.P. BIRD Gold)	Variable flow decelerating wave form Adjustable rise time Target pressure with volume guarantee on breath-to-breath basis Transition to constant flow waveform to deliver volume Flow or volume cycled Inspiratory pause May be used during weaning either in A/C or SIMV with PSV
Pressure-regulated volume-control (PRVC; Siemens Servo 300A)	Pressure-limited, time-cycled mode Closed-loop feedback system Pressure adjusted based on previous four-breath average Must be switched to volume-support mode for weaning
Volume-guaranteed (VG), pressure-limited (Draeger Babylog 8000 Plus)	Pressure-limited mode Targeted mean tidal volume delivery Volume guarantee based on the previous 8- to 10-breath average Targets expired tidal volume as reference Automated leak compensation

Note: Although often referred to as special types of volume ventilation, PRVC and VG theoretically are time-cycled, pressure-limited modes where the peak inspiratory pressure setting is not solely user determined but adjusted according to a built-in software algorithm.
A/C, assist/control; PSV, pressure-support ventilation; SIMV, synchronized intermittent mandatory ventilation.

TABLE 10-4.   Commonly Available Neonatal Ventilators That Provide Volume-Targeted Modes of Ventilation

Ventilator	Available Modes	Features
V.I.P. BIRD Gold	Volume control Combination modes VAPS	Flow cycling Variable orifice sensor Proximal airway sensor Flow triggering
Bear Cub 750 PSV	Volume-limited, pressure-controlled breaths	Requires properly installed flow sensor
Siemens Servo 300	Volume control Combination modes PRVC Volume support	Flow cycling in all modes Sensor located in machine Closed-loop feedback technology "Automode"
Draeger Babylog 8000	Combination mode Volume-guaranteed, pressure-limited	Flow cycling in PSV only with a fixed 15% termination criteria Heated wire sensor

PRVC, pressure-regulated volume-control; PSV, pressure-support ventilation; VAPS, volume-assured pressure-support.

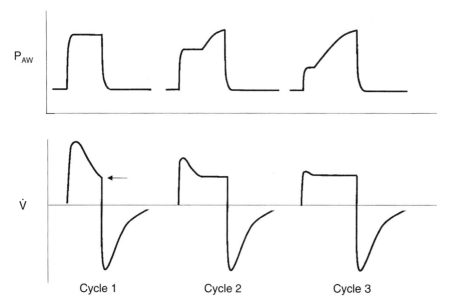

Figure 10-4. Volume-assured pressure-support ventilation. Airway pressure and flow waveforms of three typical settings are shown. Cycle 1: Set tidal volume is lower than the delivered volume (as inspiratory pressure has augmented to a relatively high level). Breath is terminated when flow decelerates to the set flow rate (arrow). Breath behaves similar to pressure support. Cycle 2: At a lower level of pressure augmentation, the set volume is not completely delivered until the decelerating flow reaches the set flow level (transition point). The flow is maintained as long as the set volume is completed. See the typical notch in the middle of the breath. Cycle 3: At a minimal pressure augmentation level, the peak flow hardly exceeds the set flow and breath behaves like volume ventilation, except for the nonlimited flow at the very beginning of the breath. (Acknowledgment to Dr. Akos Kovacs, Clinical Specialist, Viasys Health Care System, Hungary, for help in preparing this figure.)

begin as pressure-support breaths. The ventilator measures delivered volume when inspiratory flow has decelerated to the minimal set value. As long as the delivered volume exceeds the desired level (set by the clinician), the breath behaves like a pressure-support breath and is flow cycled. If the preset tidal volume has not been achieved, the breath will transition to a volume-controlled breath; the set flow will persist and the inspiratory time will be prolonged until the desired volume has been reached (Fig. 10-4). VAPS can be used both in the acute phase of respiratory illness, where the patient requires a substantial level of ventilatory support, and when a patient is being weaned from the ventilator, even in the face of unstable ventilatory drive. In this case, it is designed to supply a back-up tidal volume as a "safety net" in case the patient's effort and/or lung mechanics change.[8] In summary, VAPS is a hybrid mode of ventilation that optimizes two types of inspiratory flow patterns (VAPS = PSV + volume-controlled ventilation). There is also an adjustable rise time (flow acceleration) that controls the rate of rise of airway pressure and is set by the clinician. The optimal flow acceleration varies with patient dynamics, patient demand, and patient circuit characteristics. Pulmonary graphics are an essential tool for making the appropriate adjustment to flow acceleration. Thus, VAPS is equally suitable for both acute respiratory illness and as a facilitatory mode during weaning because of its advantage in reducing the patient's work of breathing and improving synchrony between patient and ventilator.

Pressure-Regulated Volume-Control Ventilation

This mode is a form of closed-loop ventilation that has attempted to combine the features of volume control and pressure control.[9] Essentially, the clinician sets a target tidal volume and a maximum pressure level. The ventilator logic attempts to achieve the volume target using a pressure-control gas delivery format at the lowest possible airway pressure. When activated, the first delivered breath is a test breath at 5 cm H_2O pressure, which is used to calculate the patient's compliance. The next three breaths are delivered at a pressure 75% of the calculated pressure needed to deliver the target tidal volume. After this, the pressure limit is increased by 3 cm H_2O each breath until the target volume is delivered (Fig. 10-5). If the target volume is exceeded, the pressure limit is decreased

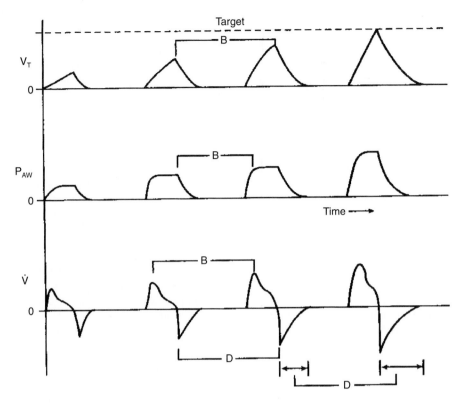

Figure 10-5. Volume, pressure, and flow waveforms[17] for four sequential breaths showing the functioning of pressure-regulated volume-control ventilation. Note the progressively increasing PIP, peak inspiratory flow, and inspiratory tidal volume (B), and the progressively increasing peak expiratory flow rate (D), as well as the duration of expiratory flow. (From Hagus CK, Donn SM: Pulmonary graphics: Basics of clinical application. In Donn SM (ed): Neonatal and Pediatric Pulmonary Graphics. Principles and Clinical Applications. Armonk, NY, Futura Publishing Company, 1998, pp. 81–127, with permission.)

by 3 cm H_2O. The inspiratory pressure is automatically regulated between PEEP and 5 cm H_2O below the set upper pressure limit. This mode is intended for use in patients in need of high peak airway pressures who supposedly are at risk for barotrauma, patients with large endotracheal tube leaks, and patients with airway obstruction. The clinician-set parameters include tidal volume, inspiratory time, ventilatory rate, PEEP, FIO_2, high and low minute ventilation alarms, high-pressure alarm, and trigger sensitivity level. This mode of ventilation provides the guarantee of volume delivery with advantages of pressure-limited ventilation in the sense that peak pressure and inspiratory flow delivery are variable. The earlier models allowed use of this mode only with mandatory breaths. Recently introduced ventilators incorporate an interactive form of ventilation called "*automode,*" which is an adaptive technology that enables the patient to breathe spontaneously while guaranteeing volume or pressure support and providing control ventilation in the event of apnea. Although microprocessor technology and a "closed-loop feedback system" (whereby pressure is decreased in response to measured tidal volume) sound sophisticated, there may be several problems, including the fact that tidal volumes are measured not at the patient wye but at the machine. This may lead to inaccurate measurements, resulting in a less than ideal feedback system. Moreover, in this mode, pressure is adjusted according to the average of the previous four breaths. It is a time-cycled mode, not a flow-cycled mode, which possibly can lead to expiratory asynchrony. The machine must be switched to volume support (which provides guaranteed tidal volume) to wean patients. Compared to other ventilators, this device has no leak compensation system and uses pressure triggering.

Because PRVC is intended for patients without sufficient breathing capability, this breath type is available in A/C mode only. The flow, pressure, and volume graphic presentations for a PRVC breath are similar to those of the pressure-controlled breath type, but the functioning of PRVC can only be assessed by evaluating sequential graphic presentations over time.

Volume-Support Ventilation

Volume-support ventilation is a hybrid mode similar to both PSV and PRVC. The volume-supported breath is patient triggered, pressure limited, and flow cycled in the same way as PSV, and it is intended for patients who are breathing spontaneously with sufficient respiratory drive. Similar to PRVC, breath rate and tidal/minute volume are preset by the clinician; however, inspiratory time is determined by the patient. Like PRVC, the ventilator algorithm adjusts the PIP limit up or down by no more than 3 cm H_2O at a time. Adjustments are made in sequential breaths until the target tidal volume is achieved. The flow, pressure, and volume graphics for a volume-supported breath are similar to those of pressure-supported breaths; however, evidence for efficacy of volume support can only be assessed by evaluating sequential graphic presentations over time, as in PRVC. The tidal volume graphic will increase in a stepwise fashion until the target volume is reached.

Pressure Augmentation

This is also a hybrid mode, similar to PRVC, which offers the benefit of matching the patient's flow demand while guaranteeing a minimal tidal volume. Pressure augmentation differs from PRVC in the following ways: (1) preset tidal volume is only a minimum and the patient can breathe a greater tidal volume than the preset minimum; (2) the minimal tidal volume is guaranteed by adjustment in flow rather than PIP, which is fixed at preset level; and (3) adjustment to flow is made within each breath rather than several sequential breaths. Pressure augmentation is interactive with the patient and is dependent on the patient's flow demand and dynamics. Pressure augmentation can be utilized in the A/C or SIMV mode, where volume-controlled breaths are selected (Fig. 10-6).

Volume-Guaranteed, Pressure-Limited Ventilation

Volume guarantee (VG) is a feature that primarily ventilates with a time-cycled, pressure-limited breath type but allows the pressure to be increased to a user-adjustable maximum pressure setting to guarantee tidal volume delivery.[10] Pressure may also be lowered with improving compliance. This is an auto-feedback feature that guarantees tidal volume, but it is based on an 8- to 10-breath average and is referenced to exhaled tidal volume. The use of exhaled tidal volume as the basis for determining delivered tidal volume is an important distinction compared to most volume-controlled ventilators. In the presence of a substantial leak around the endotracheal tube, there are concerns that this system will falsely underestimate the actual tidal volume delivered to the lung and overcompensate the subsequent breaths with excessive tidal volumes. This also may explain the difficulties encountered in avoiding hypocapnia in early clinical applications. VG can only be used in conjunction with patient-triggered modes, that is, A/C, SIMV, and pressure support. The addition of VG to one of the triggered modes allows the clinician to set a mean tidal volume to be delivered, as well as the standard ventilator settings of PIP, PEEP, inspiratory time, and respiratory rate. The inspiratory pressure is set at the upper desired pressure limit. If this pressure is reached and the set tidal volume is not, an alarm will sound. Automatic pressure changes are made in increments (theoretically) to avoid overcompensation. No more than 130% of the target tidal volume is supposed to be delivered. The usual starting target is a tidal volume of 4 to 5 mL/kg. The PIP limit is set approximately 15% to 20% above the peak pressure needed to constantly deliver the target tidal volume. If the flow sensor is removed or damaged, the ventilator will default to the set pressure limit. Because in this mode the adjustment of PIP is in response to exhaled tidal volume and adjustments are made in limited increments to prevent overcompensation, the PIP cannot be adjusted instantaneously to compensate for large breath-to-breath fluctuations in respiratory effort. One reason for this lack of variability may be attributable to the fact that VG uses historical exhaled tidal volume data to determine PIP rather than real-time data. This may be an important limiting factor in its clinical applicability. Consequently, although the delivered tidal volume certainly is more constant than in the absence of VG, it does fluctuate around the target value. The VG mode automatically compensates for changes in compliance, resistance, and spontaneous respiratory effort. VG is useful in infants with periodic breathing and apnea who are on low-maintenance respiratory support. When used appropriately, the alarm function should alert staff to worsening lung compliance, which may require immediate attention. The PIP is weaned automatically and in real time as lung compliance improves. Theoretically this should lead to faster weaning from mechanical ventilation. Most infants can be extubated when they consistently maintain tidal volume at or above the target value with delivered PIP less than 10 to 12 cm H_2O and FIO_2 less than 0.35 and show good sustained respiratory effort.

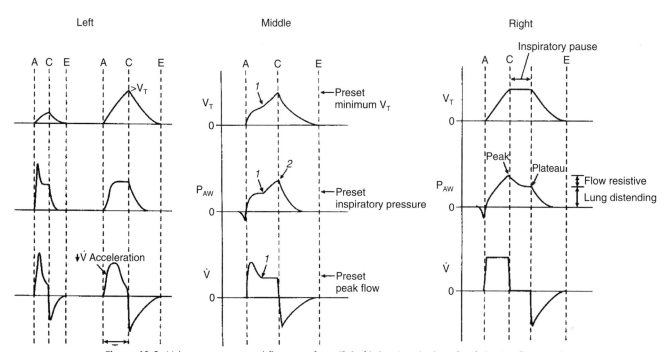

Figure 10-6. Volume, pressure, and flow waveforms[17] *(Left)* showing the benefit of slowing flow acceleration when compliance is low and airway resistance is high; *(Middle)* for a volume-assured, pressure-supported breath type; and *(Right)* for a volume-controlled breath type with an inspiratory pause. A, inspiration begins; C, inspiration ends and expiration begins; E, expiration ends. (Modified from Hagus CK, Donn SM: Pulmonary graphics: Basics of clinical application. In Donn SM (ed): Neonatal and Pediatric Pulmonary Graphics. Principles and Clinical Applications. Armonk, NY, Futura Publishing Company, 1998, pp. 81–127, with permission.)

SUGGESTED VENTILATORY MANAGEMENT GUIDELINES

Although a number of units have now started using volume-controlled or volume-targeted modes of ventilation in newborn populations, there are no published guidelines that have been truly tested in a controlled manner on a large population of newborns, especially premature infants. However, the following guidelines can be recommended because they appear to be safe and effective and have been tested in a randomized controlled trial.[5] It is imperative that the operator be well versed with these techniques and any specifications that may be unique to different ventilators before using them on a real patient population. One safety measure is to set up a sequence of parameters required for individual modes of ventilation on a test lung prior to connecting the infant to the ventilator. Although the new generation of mechanical ventilators provides adaptive software to compensate for any malfunctioning (e.g., leak-induced autotriggering), it is imperative that the operator set the alarm signals, such as "low-high limits" for pressure, volume, or rate, and understand the means to deal with any trouble shooting. It should be realized that the pathophysiology of underlying lung conditions that give rise to respiratory failure in newborns is characterized by changing pulmonary mechanics, either on its own or in response to treatment or because of secondary complications, and the initial ventilatory settings may need to be adjusted. We strongly recommend that the operator closely monitor the indices of gas exchange, hemodynamics, minute ventilation, and arterial blood gases to gauge the safety and efficacy of the ventilatory mode being applied. Online breath-to-breath pulmonary waveforms and mechanics displays may provide useful information about the trends in pulmonary function and allow the operator to make adjustments in the ventilatory settings. A brief summary of the clinical management protocol for volume-controlled ventilation and volume-guaranteed ventilation is given in Tables 10-5 and 10-6.

In volume-controlled ventilation using the V.I.P. Gold (Table 10-5), we generally initiate ventilation in the A/C mode using an inspiratory tidal volume of 4 to 6 mL/kg measured at the proximal endotracheal tube as the reference range to achieve the target blood gases. Because of the use of A/C mode, we seldom administer neuromuscular paralyzing agents. For weaning, we use the SIMV mode combined with PSV to augment spontaneous breaths and prevent increased work of breathing. We do not recommend use of SIMV at a rate lower than 15 to 20 breaths/minute. If a baby satisfies all the criteria of extubation based on clinical evaluation and information obtained from pulmonary graphics and blood gases, he or she can be extubated directly to room air, supplemental oxygen, or nasal prong continuous positive airway pressure (CPAP), depending on the clinical circumstances.

In VG using the Babylog 8000 Plus, the initial ventilation is started in synchronized intermittent positive pressure ventilation (SIPPV) mode with a trigger sensitivity set at 1, which is the most sensitive setting (Table 10-6). This may need subsequent adjustment to reduce the effect of leak-induced autotriggering. The starting tidal volume reference range is between 4 and 6 mL/kg, which can be adjusted by using – and + buttons until the appropriate value appears against V_{TSET}. This again will need adjustment during the course of ventilation based

on the results of blood gas analysis. In contrast to volume-controlled ventilation using the V.I.P. Gold machine (in which the "inspired" tidal volume usually is used as a reference breath), VG uses "expired" tidal volume as the reference breath. It takes the Babylog between six and eight breaths to reach target V_T, the exact time depending on the respiratory rate. If the PIP being used to deliver desired V_T is several centimeters of water (or mbar) below P_{INSP} (where P_{INSP} is maximum allowed pressure), then the set P_{INSP} may be left as is. This extra available peak pressure can be used by the ventilator if lung compliance decreases (or resistance increases, endotracheal tube leak increases, or respiratory effort decreases). If the PIP used by the Babylog 8000 Plus is close to or equal to set P_{INSP}, then set P_{INSP} should be increased by at

TABLE 10-5.   Methods for Using Volume-Controlled Ventilation (V.I.P. Gold)

Initial Mode	Start in A/C mode
	Adjust volume to deliver 4–6 mL/kg (measured at proximal endotracheal tube)
Time limit (A/C)	Use flow to adjust inspiratory time to 0.25–0.4 sec
Target ABG	pH: 7.25–7.4
	P_{CO_2}: 45–60
	P_{O_2}: 50–80
Weaning	Wean by reducing volume as tolerated but continue in A/C with control rate to assure normocapnia and tidal volume delivery at 4–6 mL/kg
	Switch to SIMV/PS when control rate is <30
Weaning to extubation	Decrease rate to 20
	Decrease pressure support to have similar V_T to previous settings until 10 is reached
Trial of extubation	If infant is tolerating the minimal settings and MAP <8.0 cm H_2O for at least 12 hours/or earlier self-extubation
	Load and start methylxanthine

ABG, arterial blood gas; A/C, assist/control; MAP, mean airway pressure; PS, pressure-support; SIMV, synchronized intermittent mandatory ventilation.

TABLE 10-6.   Methods for Using Volume-Guaranteed Mode of Ventilation (Draeger Babylog 8000 Plus)[18]

1. Press "vent mode" and select triggered mode of ventilation (SIMV, SIPPV = A/C, PSV)
2. Set trigger sensitivity at most sensitive
3. Set T_I, T_E (therefore back-up rate for apnea), F_{IO_2}, P_{INSP}, PEEP, flow rate
4. Press <VG>; preset V_T set by – and + buttons (start value 4–6 mL/kg[7,8])
5. Connect Babylog to the infant
6. Select <Meas 1> or <VG> screen
7. Check to see delivered V_T and PIP used by Babylog to delivery target V_T
8. Adapt P_{INSP} to actual PIP

A/C, assist/control; PEEP, positive end-expiratory pressure; P_{INSP}, maximum allowed pressure; PIP, peak inspiratory pressure; PSV, pressure-support ventilation; SIMV, synchronized intermittent mandatory ventilation; SIPPV, synchronized intermittent positive pressure ventilation; VG, volume guarantee.

least 4 to 5 mbar. This will allow the ventilator some leeway to deliver desired V_T even if compliance decreases. Once appropriate levels of V_T have been established, weaning should be an automatic process, with the amount of pressure deployed by the ventilator to provide the set V_T decreasing as the infant recovers. When this peak airway pressure used is very low, below 10 to 12 cm of H_2O, the infant may be ready for extubation. Despite considered judgment, the trial of extubation may fail and the baby may require reintubation or other support such as nasal prong CPAP. It is recommended that the operator consult the manual provided by the manufacturer (Draeger).

CLINICAL CONSIDERATIONS

Because volume-targeted modes of ventilation only recently have become available for use in neonatal practice, clinical trials are few. In one of the first neonatal trials, 50 preterm babies weighing at least 1200 g with clinical and radiographic evidence of RDS were randomly allocated to receive either volume-controlled ventilation or time-cycled, pressure-limited ventilation.[11] Tidal volume delivery in each group was deliberately controlled at 5 to 8 mL/kg so that the only difference between the two groups was the manner in which tidal volume was delivered. Success outcome criteria for this trial were determined *a priori* and consisted of either $AaDo_2$ less than 100 torr (<13 kPa) or mean airway pressure less than 8.0 cm H_2O maintained for at least 12 hours. The period of mechanical ventilation from the time of entry into the study until achievement of success criteria and the total duration of mechanical ventilation were calculated for each baby. Secondary outcome measures were noted and included complications frequently associated with mechanical ventilation, such as IVH, periventricular leukomalacia, patent ductus arteriosus, and chronic lung disease (defined as oxygen dependency beyond the 36th postconceptual week with compatible radiographic changes). Infants randomized to the volume-controlled group achieved success criteria faster than those randomized to the pressure-limited group (mean time 65.6 vs 125.6 hours; $P < 0.001$). The total duration of mechanical ventilation was significantly shorter in the volume-controlled group (mean time 122.4 vs 161.9 hours, $P < 0.001$). Among the secondary outcome measures, the frequency of major neuroimaging abnormalities (large IVH, ventriculomegaly, intraparenchymal echodensities) and chronic lung disease was lower in the volume-controlled mode. There were no significant differences in the incidence of air leaks or patent ductus arteriosus requiring intervention. Because tidal volume delivery was carefully controlled in both groups, it appears that the infants assigned to volume-controlled ventilation may have benefited from better alveolar recruitment and ventilation-perfusion matching. In this study, the inclusion criteria were such that only bigger babies could be enrolled because of technologic limitations of the ventilator (V.I.P. Bird, Bird Products Corp., Palm Springs, CA, USA), which could not deliver the tidal volumes suitable for smaller babies. Since then, a newer version of this ventilator (V.I.P. Gold) has become available. It has a superior design in terms of flow triggering, smaller minimal tidal volume delivery (as little as 10 mL), and lower minimal flow rates (3.0 L/min), theoretically allowing its use in virtually all babies. A number of neonatal units have already acquired experience in this technique and currently are involved in a randomized clinical trial of volume-controlled versus pressure-limited ventilation in this population.

It will be interesting to see if stabilization of volume delivery by volume-controlled ventilation in neonatal RDS has beneficial effects in reducing the frequency and severity of chronic lung disease. The credence to this notion comes from animal studies designed to compare the efficacy of volume-cycled or pressure-limited ventilation on pulmonary vascular resistance, cardiac index, and dynamic compliance in uninjured and injured lungs (surfactant deficiency induced by saline lavage). After a stable 30-minute baseline, animals were randomly assigned to volume-cycled ventilation or pressure-limited ventilation. Although there was no significant difference in healthy lungs, in the setting of lung injury, dynamic compliance was 1.44 ± 0.15 after 180 minutes in the volume-cycled group and 0.91 ± 0.10 in the pressure-limited group. Similarly, pulmonary vascular resistance was 100 ± 6 in the volume-cycled group and 145 ± 12 in the pressure-limited group after 180 minutes of lung injury. Cardiac index declined significantly in all groups irrespective of ventilatory mode. Although there was no difference between ventilatory modes in healthy lungs, pressure-limited ventilation, when combined with partial liquid ventilation in injured lungs (as designed in this study), had adverse effects on lung compliance and pulmonary vascular resistance. The authors concluded that volume-cycled ventilation was effective in optimizing the ability of perfluorocarbon to recruit collapsed or atelectatic lung regions.[12]

In another clinical study designed to compare the effects of PRVC with pressure-preset IMV, 60 newborns with RDS or congenital pneumonia who weighed less than 2500 g and required mechanical ventilation were prospectively recruited in a randomized manner. In babies assigned to PRVC, the tidal volume was preset and pressure-controlled breaths were delivered with PIP values adapted to achieve the preset tidal volume. The main outcome measures in this study were duration of ventilation and incidence of chronic lung disease. Pulmonary air leaks and IVH were considered major adverse effects. Demographic data, ventilation parameters, and arterial-to-alveolar oxygen tension ratio were similar at randomization. Duration of ventilation and incidence of chronic lung disease were not decreased by use of PRVC. Air leaks occurred in three infants in the PRVC group and in seven infants treated with IMV. The incidence of IVH grade greater than 2 was lower in babies treated with PRVC ($P < 0.05$). In a subgroup of newborns weighing less than 1000 g, however, the duration of ventilation and incidence of hypotension were reduced in the PRVC group ($P < 0.05$). The authors concluded that PRVC can be used safely and may contribute to a lower incidence of complications.[13]

Volume-guaranteed (or volume-targeted), pressure-limited ventilation has shown beneficial effects, although the number of infants studied has been very small. In a randomized crossover study of VG versus SIMV in very-low-birthweight infants recovering from respiratory failure, eight clinically stable infants (birth weight 853 ± 161 g, gestational age 26.7 ± 1.9 weeks, age 5 ± 2.3 days) were assigned to consecutive 60-minute epochs of VG, "clinical" SIMV (ventilator settings chosen by the care team), and "matched" SIMV (PIP adjusted to obtain same tidal volume as in VG) in random order. In comparing VG and clinical SIMV, the investigators found that total minute ventilation was the same; however, mechanical minute ventilation was lower with VG compared to clinical SIMV. Conversely, spontaneous minute ventilation was higher during VG. Mean airway pressure and mean driving pressure ($\Delta P \times$ breath duration) also were significantly lower during VG. There were no differences in oxygen saturation, transcutaneous P_{O_2}, and transcutaneous P_{CO_2}. There were no statistically significant differences between VG and matched SIMV modes.[14] These results indicate that very-low-birthweight infants frequently require less ventilatory support than that provided in the clinical situation because they are able to increase their own inspiratory effort. VG allows them to achieve this while guaranteeing a physiologic tidal volume, in contrast to SIMV, which delivers a constant PIP regardless of tidal volume delivered.

In another study, 10 infants were randomized to receive A/C ventilation or A/C with VG using the Draeger Babylog infant ventilator.[15] In this study, the authors hypothesized that the volume-targeted mode would maintain tidal volume and P_{aCO_2} within a target range from 4 to 6 mL/kg and 35 to 45 torr, respectively, more consistently than conventional modes. Arterial blood gases were obtained every 2 to 4 hours as clinically indicated. To analyze the data, the authors chose the number of breaths and P_{aCO_2} values outside the target range for comparison between the two groups. They found that VG, as used in the study, kept tidal volume within the target range more consistently than A/C alone but did not reliably prevent hypocarbia. It is unlikely that the 5 mL/kg target tidal volume used in this study was too high. There are at least two possible explanations for observed hypocarbia: (1) it may have resulted from spontaneous hyperventilation given that these infants were not sedated; or (2) overcorrection occurred due to endotracheal tube leaks because this ventilator references exhaled rather than inhaled tidal volume.

In a larger, randomized, crossover trial that used VG to assess the feasibility of tidal volume-guided ventilation in newborn infants, 40 babies (mean birthweight 1064 g, gestational age 27.9 weeks) were studied.[16] These babies were placed in two groups: those receiving A/C ventilation in the early phase of RDS (group 1, $n = 20$) and those who were being weaned during the recovery phase using SIMV (group 2, $n = 20$). Both groups of babies were studied over a 4-hour period. Data on ventilation parameters and transcutaneous carbon dioxide and oxygen were collected continuously. No adverse events were observed during the study. Analyzing the fractional inspired oxygen, transcutaneous carbon dioxide pressure, and transcutaneous partial pressure of oxygen, the study found no differences between babies receiving SIMV and A/C alone or when VG was added to these modes. The investigators found, however, that mean airway pressure recorded in SIMV and A/C plus VG was lower compared to SIMV and A/C alone. Based on these observations, they concluded that VG may be a stable and feasible method of ventilation in newborns and can achieve equivalent gas exchange using statistically significantly lower peak airway pressure during both the early and recovery stages of RDS.

FUTURE DIRECTIONS

The development of microprocessor-based respiratory technology and sophisticated yet miniature transducers has resulted in new modes of volume-targeted ventilation for treatment of neonatal respiratory failure. This further expands the therapeutic range and enables customization of ventilator management based on specific pathophysiology and patient responses.

However, many questions remain unanswered and further studies are required to confirm the safety and efficacy of volume-controlled and volume-targeted modes with respect to both short-term and long-term outcome measures, such as their impact on chronic lung disease.

The volume-controlled modes are new and represent a departure from the time-honored pressure-limited modes. The wide range of choices now available should not intimidate the clinician but should represent a challenge to determine the best clinical indications, as well as the limitations of each. Clinical information on newborns is limited, and the opportunity to design and implement randomized, controlled clinical trials may never be better. Before embarking on such studies, it is imperative that clinicians familiarize themselves with individual ventilator specifications, as well as differences among the many available commercial devices. Gone are the days when all neonatal lung diseases are treated alike.

ACKNOWLEDGMENT

We thank Dr. Jag Ahluwallia, Consultant Neonatologist Cambridge, United Kingdom, for guidance in preparing the ventilatory management guideline on volume-targeted ventilation on the Babylog 2000 Plus.

REFERENCES

1. Dreyfuss D, Saumon G: Baro-trauma is volu-trauma but which volume is the one responsible? Intensive Care Med 18:139–141, 1992.
2. Dreyfuss D, Saumon G: Role of tidal volume, FRC, and end-inspiratory volume in the development of pulmonary oedema following mechanical ventilation. Am Rev Respir Dis 148:1194–1197, 1993.
3. Donn SM, Sinha SK: Newer modes of mechanical ventilation for the neonate. Curr Opin Pediatr 13:99–103, 2001.
4. Martin RJ, Carlo WA, Chatburn RL: Mechanical ventilation in the neonatal and paediatric setting. In Tobin MJ (ed): Principles and Practice of Mechanical Ventilation. New York, McGraw-Hill, 1994, pp. 514–519.
5. Marini JJ, Crooke PS III, Truwit JD: Determinants and limits of pressure-preset ventilation: A mathematical model of pressure control. J Appl Physiol 67:1081–1092, 1989.
6. Sinha SK, Donn SM: Weaning from mechanical ventilation: Art or science? Arch Dis Child Fetal Neonatal Ed 83:F64–F70, 2000.
7. Sinha SK, Donn SM: Pressure support ventilation. In Sinha SK, Donn SM (eds): Manual of Neonatal Respiratory Care. Armonk, NY, Futura Publishing Company, 2000, pp. 157–160.
8. MacIntyre NR, Gropper C, Westfall T: Continuing pressure-limiting and volume-cycling features in a patient-interactive mechanical breath. Crit Care Med 22:253–257, 1994.
9. Product Literature, Siemens Servo 300 Ventilator reference manual, ventilation modes no. 60-26-608-E313E. Siemens, Solna, Sweden, 1992.
10. Product literature, Draeger Babylog 8000 Plus infant care ventilator operating instructions, software 5n, 1st edition, February 1997.
11. Sinha SK, Donn SM, Gavey J, et al: Randomised trial of volume controlled versus time cycled, pressure limited ventilation in preterm infants with respiratory distress syndrome. Arch Dis Child 77:F202–F205, 1999.
12. Weiswasser J, Lueders M, Stolar CJ: Pressure- versus volume-cycled ventilation in liquid-ventilated neonatal piglet lungs. J Pediatr Surg 33:1158–1162, 1998.
13. Piotrowski A, Sobala W, Kawczynski P: Patient-initiated, pressure-regulated volume-controlled ventilation compared with intermittent mandatory ventilation in neonates: A prospective, randomised study. Intensive Care Med 23:975–981, 1997.
14. Herrera CM, Gerhardt T, Everett R, et al: Randomized, crossover study of volume guaranteed (VG) versus synchronised intermittent mandatory ventilation (SIMV) in very low birth weight (VLBW) infants recovering from respiratory failure. Pediatr Res 45:304A, 1999.
15. Keszler M, Abubaker KM: Volume targeted mechanical ventilation of newborn maintains more stable tidal volume but does not prevent hypocarbia in first 24 hours of life. Pediatr Res 45:307A, 1999.

16. Cheema IU, Ahluwalia JS: Feasibility of tidal volume-guided ventilation in newborn infants: A randomised, crossover trial using the volume guarantee modality. Pediatrics 107:1323–1328, 2001.

17. Hagus CK, Donn SM: Pulmonary graphics: Basics of clinical application. In Donn SM (ed): Neonatal and Pediatric Pulmonary Graphics. Principles and Clinical Application. Armonk, NY, Futura Publishing Company, 1998, pp. 81–128.

18. Ahluwalia J, Morley C, Wahle HG: Volume guarantee, new approaches in volume controlled ventilation for neonates. Product Information Literature, Dräger Medizintechnik, GmbH, Germany.

such effects have been accounted for. A special triple-lumen (Hi-Lo jet) endotracheal tube has been designed specifically for use during HFJV. In addition to the standard endotracheal tube lumen, this tube has a pressure monitoring port located at its distal tip and a jet injector port located within the tube wall approximately 7 cm upstream from the pressure monitoring port (Fig. 11-3). In addition, a triple-lumen endotracheal tube adapter is available that allows jet ventilation without using the Hi-Lo tube. This adapter, shown schematically in Figure 11-4, houses the jet injector port and the pressure monitoring port. Jet

ventilators have been tested extensively in laboratory animals and have been used clinically in adults and neonates.[31–43]

The Bunnell Life Pulse jet ventilator (Bunnell Inc., Salt Lake City, UT, USA) was designed specifically for infants (Fig. 11.5). Using the triple-lumen endotracheal tube or the triple-lumen adapter, this device delivers its jet pulse into the endotracheal tube through the tube's injector port, then servo-controls the background pressure, or driving pressure, of the jet pulse to maintain a constant predetermined pressure at the endotracheal tube tip. This device is approved for clinical use in neonates and infants. It appears to be most effective in disorders where CO_2 elimination is the major problem, such as air block syndrome [i.e., pulmonary interstitial emphysema (PIE)]. With HFJV, CO_2 removal is achieved at lower peak and mean airway pressures than with either HFPPV or HFO.[34,35,44,45] Although effective in RDS, only one randomized multicenter trial of HFJV has been performed.[35,36,38,43] In this study, HFJV resulted in a lower incidence of chronic lung disease (CLD), defined as persistent oxygen requirement at 36 weeks adjusted age, without other adverse side effects.[43] A review of HFJV versus CMV from the Cochrane Database found a benefit in pulmonary outcomes in patients with RDS electively ventilated with HFJV. Because of concerns about the appropriate strategy and the lack of long-term pulmonary and neurodevelopmental outcome studies, this form of therapy is not been recommended at this time as a primary treatment modality.[42,46]

High-Frequency Oscillators

HFOs are essentially airway vibrators, usually piston pumps or vibrating diaphragms, that operate at frequencies ranging from 400 to 2400 breaths/min.[6,47] During HFO, inspiration and expiration are both active (proximal airway pressures are negative during expiration). Oscillators produce little bulk gas delivery. A continuous flow of fresh gas rushes past the source, generating or *powering* the oscillations. This *bias* gas flow is the system's only source of fresh gas. A controlled leak or *low-pass filter* allows gas to exit the system (Fig. 11-6).[47] Pressure oscillations within the airway produce tiny tidal volumes around a constant mean airway pressure, maintaining lung volume. Tidal volumes are determined by the amplitude of the airway pressure oscillations, which, in turn, are determined by the stroke of the device producing the oscillations.

As with HFJV, pressure monitoring is a problem. During HFO, airway pressures usually are measured either at the proximal end of the endotracheal tube or within the ventilator itself. Many practitioners question the clinical relevance of such measurements; the relationship of pressures measured during HFO to those measured during CMV is difficult to assess accurately. Depending upon the size and resonant frequency of the lung, alveolar pressures can be the same, lower, or even higher than those measured in the trachea.[47–50]

HFOs have been tested extensively in animals and humans.[43–65] Today the most commonly used neonatal HFO is the SensorMedics 3100A oscillator (SensorMedics Corp., Yorba Linda, CA, USA). This ventilator has been approved for clinical use in neonates. This device produces its oscillations via an electronically controlled piston and diaphragm. Frequency (3 to 15 Hz), percent inspiratory time, and volume displacement can be adjusted, as well as resistance at the end of the bias flow circuit (Fig. 11-7). Variations in bias flow rate and the patient circuit outflow resistor control mean airway pressures.

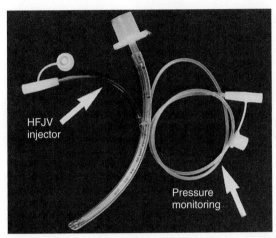

Figure 11-3. Triple-lumen endotracheal tube for use with high-frequency jet ventilation (HFJV; Hi-Lo jet tube, National Catheter Corporation, Division of Mallinckrodt, Inc.). The HFJV injector and pressure monitoring ports are labeled. The pressure monitoring port measures pressure at the distal end of the endotracheal tube; the HFJV injector enters the lumen of the tube approximately 7 cm above the monitoring port.

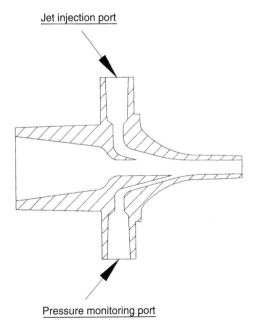

Figure 11-4. Schematic representation of the triple-lumen endotracheal tube adapter designed for use with the Bunnell Life Pulse jet ventilator. This adapter incorporates a standard lumen for connection to a conventional ventilator circuit, a jet injection port, and a pressure monitoring port. This adapter eliminates the need for reintubation prior to initiation of jet ventilation.

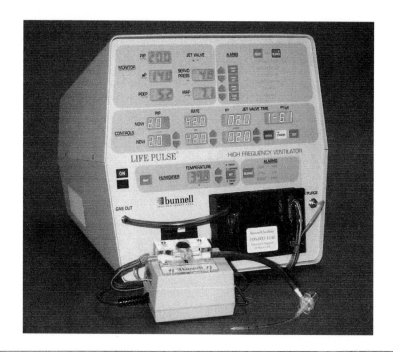

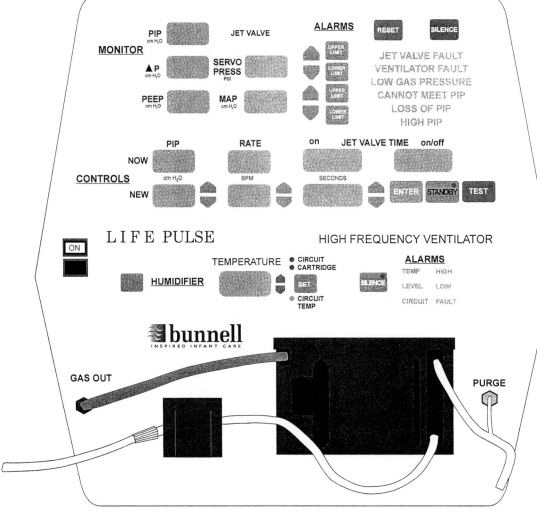

Figure 11-5. The Bunnell Life Pulse jet ventilator. This microprocessor-controlled, pressure-limited, time-cycled ventilator servocontrols delivered airway pressure as measured at the endotracheal tube tip. Frequency range is from 240 to 660 breaths/min. Pressure range is from 8 to 50 cm H_2O. Inspiratory time is adjustable from 0.02 to 0.034 seconds.

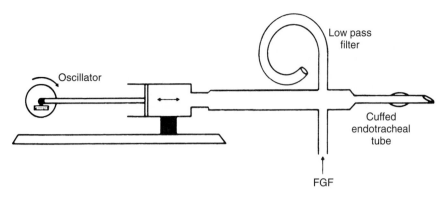

Figure 11-6. High-frequency oscillator. Fresh gases enter the system proximal to the endotracheal tube (FGF). Excess gas and mixed expired gases exit via a low-pass filter. (From Thompson WK, Marachak BE, Froese AB, et al: High frequency oscillation compared with standard ventilation in pulmonary injury model. J Appl Physiol 52:543, 1982.)

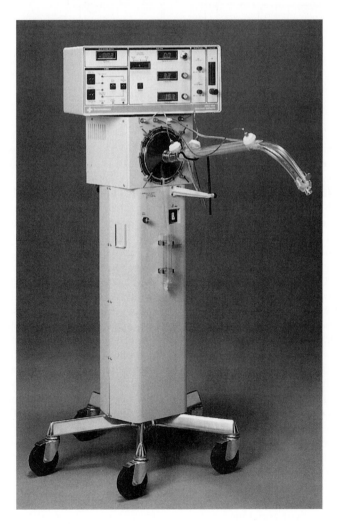

Figure 11-7. The SensorMedics 3100A high-frequency oscillator. This electronically controlled and powered ventilator uses a sealed piston with adjustable volume displacement to generate oscillations into the airway. Frequency is adjustable from 180 to 900 breaths/min (3 to 15 Hz). Mean airway pressure can be set between 3 and 45 cm H_2O; oscillatory pressure is adjustable to greater than 90 cm H_2O. Inspiratory time can be set from 30% to 50% of the total cycle.

Figure continued on following page

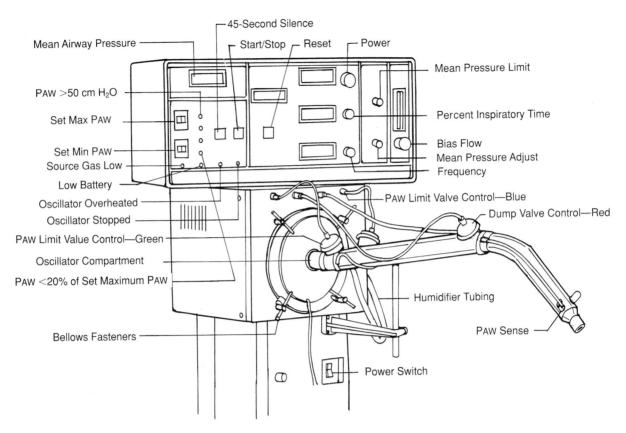

Figure 11-7. *Continued.*

The Hummingbird BMO 20N and Hummingbird II (Senko, Tokyo, Japan) are two other fairly well-known HFOs. Both are mechanical piston-driven devices. The BMO 20N was the primary ventilator used in the National Institutes of Health (NIH)-sponsored multicenter HFO-RDS (HIFI) trial. This ventilator also was studied in a similar controlled trial in Japan.[66] Unlike the results in the United States, the much smaller Japanese trial (92 infants) found no increase in complications in HFO-treated patients. Neither study showed any clear advantage to the routine use of HFO in the treatment of neonatal RDS. Even though this ventilator was used in a large nationwide clinical trial and currently is used extensively in Japan, it is not approved for clinical use in the United States.

A newer HFO device is the Dräger Babylog 8000 (Dräger Medical, Lübeck, Germany). This ventilator is based on "membrane oscillation," in which a continuous flow from 10 to 30 L/min is modulated by high-frequency oscillation of the exhalation valve membrane (Fig. 11-8). Frequency (5 to 20 Hz) and pressure amplitude are adjustable. Mean airway pressure is adjusted by automatic modulation of the active expiration, the continuous flow rate, and alteration of the I/E ratio. This ventilator is unique in its ability to measure and monitor airway pressures and tidal volumes at the airway opening during ventilation. A bench comparison of this device to the SensorMedics 3100A suggests that the Dräger ventilator in its current form is best suited for use in patients weighing less than 1500 to 2000 g due to its inability to generate large enough tidal volumes and variation in I/E ratios with frequency changes.[67]

Only the SensorMedics 3100A is approved for use in the United States and Canada. The Dräger Babylog 8000 is approved for use in Canada.

CLINICAL APPLICATIONS

The full potential of HFV has yet to be realized despite more than 20 years of intensive study. Initial animal studies suggested that HFV works at lower proximal airway pressures than CMV, reduces ventilator related lung injuries, improves gas exchange in the face of air leaks, and decreases oxygen requirements.[44,50–53,56,60,61,68–72] In human trials, however, only some of these projections have been proven true. In air leak syndromes, including PIE and bronchopleural fistula, all types of HFV improve patient outcomes.[33,34,40,73] In preoperative and postoperative congenital diaphragmatic hernias (CDHs), meconium aspiration syndromes, and some forms of pulmonary hypoplasia, HFV can provide good gas exchange, but no clear improvement in outcome has been demonstrated. HFV can be useful in seemingly intractable respiratory failure as a bridge, or alternative, to extracorporeal membrane oxygenation (ECMO). Clearly, some patients can avoid ECMO if HFV is used first.[74–76]

Neonatal RDS is the most common lung disease treated in newborn intensive care units. It is the one condition where most investigators envisioned the greatest potential for HFV. Here, results of clinical studies were initially perplexing. Animal HFV-RDS studies almost uniformly show that pulmonary air leaks and ventilator-related lung injuries decrease and overall survival improves.[51–53,56,60,61,73] The results of clinical trials in human RDS have been contradictory, although recent trials have been more encouraging. Initial human RDS trials comparing HFJV and CMV show neither clear benefit nor detriment to HFJV, even though gas exchange is maintained at

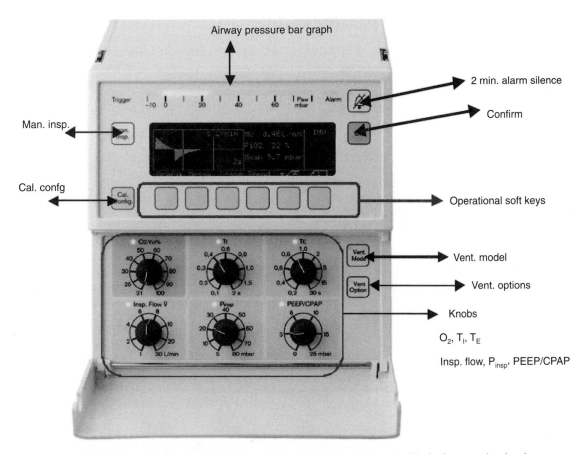

Airway pressure bar graph

2 min. alarm silence

Confirm

Man. insp.

Cal. confg

Operational soft keys

Vent. model

Vent. options

Knobs

O_2, T_I, T_E

Insp. flow, P_{insp}, PEEP/CPAP

Figure 11-8. The Dräger Babylog 8000 neonatal ventilator. This ventilator provides both conventional and high-frequency ventilation using the same platform. Frequency is adjustable from 0 to 1200 breaths/min (0 to 20 Hz). Mean airway pressure is adjusted using the positive end-expiratory pressure/continuous positive airway pressure (PEEP/CPAP) control knob. Amplitude is set from 0% to 100%, with the resulting delivered pressures and tidal volumes displayed. Pressures, respiratory cycle timing, tidal and minute volumes, and basic respiratory system mechanics are measured or calculated during ventilation and displayed. Peak pressure is adjustable from 1 to 80 cm H_2O; PEEP from 0 to 25 cm H_2O. Ventilator functions are selected using the vent mode, vent option, and operational soft keys.

lower proximal airway pressures.[33–39] The results of the first large multicenter RDS clinical trial comparing HFO and CMV were disheartening. In this NIH-directed effort (the HIFI trial), 673 infants with RDS weighing between 750 and 2000 g received either HFO or CMV.[59] Not only was there no benefit to HFO, but infants treated with HFO had more severe intraventricular hemorrhages, more periventricular leukomalacia, and more pneumoperitoneum of pulmonary origin, and they showed a trend toward more pulmonary air leaks. There were no significant differences in the incidence of bronchopulmonary dysplasia or in posttreatment pulmonary mechanics measurements.[77–79] The most alarming finding of this trial was that neurologic outcomes at 1-year follow-up were significantly worse in the HFO-treated infants.[80] It is important to note that this trial was completed before the introduction of surfactant replacement therapy.

What happened? During the initial phase of clinical evaluation, the assumption (implicit or stated) underlying most HFV-RDS projects was that the main attribute of HFV was its ability to provide ventilation at lower peak and mean airway pressures. This was in large part due to the clinical milieu of the early 1980s, in which acute barotrauma was a frequent and often deadly complication of treatment. However, in RDS or other conditions where atelectasis and ventilation-perfusion (V/Q) mismatch predominate, this assumption is incorrect. In such situations low proximal airway pressures, no matter how they are delivered, will be clinically ineffective and may, in fact, exaggerate underlying pathologies. In these situations, alveolar recruitment and lung volume maintenance appear to be the keys to improved ventilation and decreased lung injuries.[51,57,81–85]

When the HIFI trial was performed, the clinical understanding of the interplay between airway pressures and lung volumes was incomplete at best. Although pioneering work by Froese and coworkers demonstrated the necessity of adequate lung volume recruitment during HFV, this was not well translated into the clinical setting.[6,57,81–83] In 1989 Meredith et al.[86] showed in baboons that the use of high tidal volume–low PEEP CMV contributed to the pattern of lung injury recognized as hyaline membrane disease in these animals. In other words, they demonstrated that the ventilator itself was responsible for much of the lung injury previously thought to be the result of surfactant deficiency. They also showed that HFO, using low tidal volumes, prevented the development of similar pathology. What was not clearly understood from this work, as well as from the investigations by Froese et al., was that low tidal volume HFV could not be effective without adequate lung volume recruitment. Today the concept of ventilator-induced lung injury (VILI) is well established.[87–89] VILI can occur in the lung treated with too much pressure (barotrauma), too much volume (volutrauma), or too little volume (atelectrauma).[90]

The key to the successful use of HFV, with the potential of reducing VILI, is matching the type of lung problem being treated to an appropriate lung protective strategy (see Chapters 13 and 15). We still are not completely able to identify these strategies with certainty, but we have made substantial progress since 1989, when the HIFI trial was reported. Clearly, careful attention must be paid to lung volume during HFV, with volume recruitment strategies integrated into treatment. In 1987 Froese et al.[57] reported a small neonatal clinical trial in which a sustained inflation (SI) technique was successfully used for lung volume recruitment. Newer studies of babies with RDS have used a different strategy during HFV designed to recruit lung volume, that of stepwise increases in mean airway pressure. In the laboratory, the SI technique is almost exclusively used. Because assessment of lung volume at the bedside is indirect, the most effective clinical technique has not been clearly defined.

It now appears that HFV can achieve two distinctly different clinical goals. The first is to provide adequate ventilation at the lowest possible proximal airway pressure. This approach, designed to *minimize pressure,* should be considered in the face of restrictive lung disorders, such as air leak syndromes or pulmonary hypoplasia; obstructive lung disorders, such as meconium aspiration syndromes; mixed conditions, such as pneumonia associated with atelectasis; or in persistent pulmonary hypertension, either as an isolated condition or in association with other problems. The second is to *optimize lung volume.* Here, peak and mean airway pressures should actually be higher than those used during CMV, at least initially.[81–84] This technique is used in conditions where diffuse atelectasis predominates, the most common being neonatal RDS. As is true in other areas of medical treatment, different conditions require different approaches.

Pulmonary Air Leaks

Today, HFV is generally accepted as a relatively safe and effective treatment for severe pulmonary air leaks. Barringer et al.[69] and Carlon et al.[70] compared the effects of HFJV and CMV in dogs with large bronchopleural fistulae. HFJV improved gas exchange and, in some cases, hyperventilated the animals. The animals treated with CMV became progressively hypercapnic and acidotic. Humans with airway defects that are as large in cross-sectional area as lobar bronchi have been successfully supported for prolonged periods of time.[91]

Frantz et al.[55] first reported the successful treatment of neonatal pulmonary air leaks using HFO. Pokora et al.[33] noted similar successes using HFJV (Fig. 11-9). These studies were followed by a series of reports all suggesting that HFV was more effective than CMV in the treatment of most neonatal pulmonary air leaks.[34,40,92] Later, several randomized clinical trials examined the effects of various forms of HFV on the incidence of ventilator associated pulmonary air leaks. A British trial compared the incidences of pulmonary air leaks in 346 neonates treated with either HFPPV or CMV. Twenty-six percent of the infants treated with CMV developed air leaks compared to 19% of those who received HFPPV.[13] Mortalities, durations of ventilation, and incidences of CLD and intraventricular hemorrhage were similar. Keszler et al.[40] compared HFPPV and HFJV in 144 infants with severe PIE. Sixty-one percent of those treated with HFJV improved compared to only 37% treated with HFPPV. Forty-five percent of those who did not respond to HFPPV and were transferred to HFJV improved, whereas only 9% of the infants who did not respond to HFJV and were transferred to HFPPV improved. In addition, HFJV appeared to ventilate patients using lower proximal airway pressures. In another multicenter HFO-RDS trial (the HiFO study), the effect of HFO in air leak was examined.[92] Air leaks, either PIE or pneumothorax, were present in 26 (30%) of 86 patients randomized to HFOV and in 22 (24%) of 90 patients randomized to CMV. Although a low-pressure strategy might be presumed in a study of this type, HFOV patients still required higher airway pressures for gas exchange. Air leaks occurred in 42% of HFO patients who entered the study without air leak compared to 63% of CMV patients ($P < 0.05$). Although HFO patients who entered the study with air leaks tended to do better than their counterparts treated with CMV, the differences were not significant. All things considered, most forms of HFV appear to lessen the incidence of ventilator-associated pulmonary air leaks and improve the outcome of preexisting pulmonary air leaks. Of all the forms of HFV considered thus far, HFJV has been the most successful with respect to the incidence and treatment of air leak syndromes.

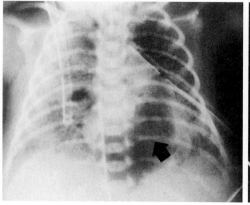

A

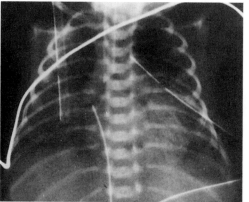

B

Figure 11-9. Chest roentgenogram of a 1300-g infant with severe hyaline membrane disease before (A) and 4 hours after (B) high-frequency jet ventilation (HFJV). Pulmonary interstitial emphysema and air trapped within the pulmonary ligament (arrow) markedly decreased after HFJV. (From Pokora T, Bing D, Mammel M, et al: Neonatal high-frequency jet ventilation. Pediatrics 72:27, 1983.)

Why do pulmonary air leaks improve during HFV? Perhaps because HFV produces smaller pressure fluxes within the distal airways. Pressures in the upper airway equilibrate and gas is delivered distally at a more constant distending pressure. Pressure differentials between airway and intrapleural space lessen. There is less stretching of the injured tissue. Less gas escapes during peak inspiration and there are greater opportunities for self-repair (Fig. 11-10).

Pulmonary Hypoplasia

Infants with various forms of pulmonary hypoplasia may derive at least some short-term benefit from HFV. Some of these infants have associated, equally lethal, abnormalities. In such situations, HFV may provide a brief respite for diagnostic studies to identify potential survivors or confirm diagnoses for family members. In diaphragmatic hernia, HFV may be a useful "bridge" therapy. In the hypoplastic lung, because the number of gas-exchanging units is small, it is only logical to assume that ventilation at rapid rates using low tidal volumes would be most effective. Because of the variety of conditions associated with pulmonary hypoplasia and their relative rarity, controlled studies are difficult to design or perform, and clear evidence-based guidelines simply are not available.

Infants with pulmonary hypoplasia associated with CDH may derive some benefit from HFV. To date there are no controlled studies, only clinical anecdotes. There are 25 early reports of infants with pulmonary hypoplasia associated with CDH treated with HFV. Most of the patients improved initially but had poor long-term outcomes.[34,93–95] In most of the patients, arterial blood gas measurements improved at lower proximal airway pressures; however, few patients survived. These reports predated ECMO. Carter et al.[74] studied 50 infants referred for ECMO who first were treated with HFO. Forty-six

percent improved and did not require ECMO. Four infants had pulmonary hypoplasia associated with CDH. None responded positively to HFO. All required ECMO. Baumgart et al.[76] reviewed results of 73 neonatal ECMO candidates who first were treated with HFJV. Nine infants had pulmonary hypoplasia associated with CDH; only three survived. DeLemos et al.[75] reviewed the outcomes of 122 neonatal ECMO candidates first treated with HFO. Fifty-three percent did not require ECMO; however, only 5 of 20 patients who had pulmonary hypoplasia associated with CDH responded positively to HFO and did not require ECMO. A more recent report of 12 infants with CDH treated with HFO showed much better outcomes.[96] Eleven of the 12 did not require ECMO and ultimately survived. Despite this report's impressive success, overall, HFV has not been terribly successful in the treatment of pulmonary hypoplasia associated with CDH, at least as an independent treatment. As with other forms of pulmonary hypoplasia, however, HFV often can stabilize critically ill patients until their ultimate prognosis becomes clear. HFV also may be used with inhaled nitric oxide (iNO) in patients with pulmonary hypoplasia to lessen the effects of pulmonary hypertension, decrease the need for ECMO, and improve outcomes (see Chapter 14).

Neonatal Respiratory Distress Syndrome

Neonatal RDS continues to be a major cause of long-term morbidity despite advances in perinatal care and the general use of artificial surfactant therapy. The optimal use of HFV in an attempt to improve these outcomes continues to be an elusive goal. Bland et al.[12] described the successful use of HFPPV in RDS in 1980. Since then, many clinical studies have attempted to achieve in the nursery benefits suggested by work in the laboratory. The initial HFV-RDS studies were brief interventions in tightly controlled clinical settings. Under these conditions, HFV provided adequate respiratory support at lower proximal airway pressures[35,36,39]; however, these studies were short term and by design could not address possible complications, such as gas trapping and airway trauma. In 1992, Clark et al.[62] performed a single-center trial comparing HFO to CMV in 83 babies with RDS. Artificial surfactant therapy was not yet available, and the study was small. They evaluated the impact of three different ventilatory treatment strategies: HFO alone, CMV alone, and the combination of 72 hours of HFO followed by CMV. Chronic lung disease, defined as persistently abnormal findings on chest x-ray films and supplemental oxygen required for longer than 30 days, was significantly reduced in infants receiving HFO alone. All other outcomes were similar. The authors concluded that HFO was as safe as CMV and might lead to a decrease in the incidence of CLD; however, they did not go as far as to recommend the routine use of HFV in neonatal RDS.

Exogenous surfactant therapy forever changed the course of neonatal RDS. Mortalities and morbidities associated with CMV decreased dramatically and now are extremely low.[97,98] This encouraging fact mandated a new wave of studies in which surfactant therapy became an integral part of the design. Davis et al.[41] studied 28 newborns who received surfactant during HFJV. These infants showed sustained improvements superior to that seen during HFJV alone or during surfactant treatment without HFJV. Unfortunately, this study was neither randomized nor controlled. A similar controlled study by Heldt

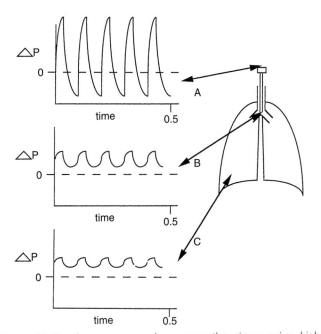

Figure 11-10. Airway pressure drop across the airway using high-frequency oscillatory ventilation, adapted from unpublished observations using the Sensor Medics 3100A. *A,* Pressure measured at the proximal endotracheal tube. *B,* Pressure measured at the carina. *C,* Pressure measured in the distal airways.

et al.[99] suggested that surfactant administered to rabbits in association with HFPPV took longer to reach the distal air spaces. In 1996 Gerstmann et al.[85] performed a prospective multicenter trial comparing HFO to CMV in 125 neonates. All babies were treated with exogenous surfactant therapy. They found a reduction in CLD in HFO-treated babies; however, the infants in this study were generally larger than those in previous studies. Thome et al.[14] performed a larger study involving very small babies, most of whom received prenatal steroids and surfactant treatment. This study used the Infant Star for HFV and the Dräger for CMV (actually HFPPV), making this work different than those using true oscillators. No advantages to this type of HFV were seen. Recently two new multicenter randomized, controlled trials of HFO have been published. One, from the United Kingdom by Johnson et al., included 797 23–28 week newborns randomized to CV or HFO within one hour of birth. The primary outcome variable, death or chronic lung disease (CLD), at 36 weeks postmenstrual age, was similar in the two groups, both numerically and proportionately for death and CLD, as were other secondary outcomes.[100] The second, performed in the United States by Courtney et al., compared HFO to tidal volume-targeted synchronized intermittent mandatory ventilation in 500 babies between 601 and 1200 grams at birth.[101] The chosen strategy was initiated by 4 hours of age in infants who had received one dose of surfactant and continued to require ventilation. Duration of ventilation was shorter in the HFO treated babies. The primary outcome, survival without CLD at 36 weeks postmenstrual age, was 56% in the HFO group vs. 47% in the CV group ($P = .046$). Other secondary outcomes were again similar with the exception of pulmonary hemorrhage, slightly lower in the HFO group, and pulmonary interstitial emphysema, slightly lower in the CV group. In an editorial, Stark commented on similarities and differences in these two large trials, and concluded that "for most preterm infants, conventional mechanical ventilation with low tidal volumes and reasonable ventilation goals remains the appropriate choice."[102] Other works compare use of lung protective strategies during conventional ventilation to HFV.[103–106] With the "open lung" approach during CMV, it may be possible to produce pulmonary outcomes similar to those observed during HFV, which suggests that at least part of the improvement observed in the laboratory and in the neonatal intensive care unit are the result of inadequate conventional techniques rather than superiority of HFV. Taken together, these studies suggest that HFV may be safely applied in neonates with RDS with the potential for reduction in chronic lung injury. The findings also suggest that we may substantially improve conventional outcomes by applying lessons learned with HFV.

The final verdict regarding HFV and RDS is not yet in. Recent reviews from the Cochrane Database conclude that HFV cannot yet be recommended as the primary form of mechanical ventilation for the preterm infant with RDS for a number of reasons. (1) Although studies using a high lung volume strategy have shown benefit in short-term measures of CLD without evidence of increased neurologic injury, treatments cannot be blinded, and outcome assessments have not consistently been blinded. (2) Careful assessment at different gestational ages is incomplete. (3) Long-term outcomes are inadequately studied. (4) Results from groups with large experiences in the use of HFV may not be generalizable.[107]

Persistent Pulmonary Hypertension

Today, persistent pulmonary hypertension often is treated by aggressive mechanical ventilation in conjunction with iNO therapy. While severe hyperventilation is avoided, carbon dioxide levels are lowered and pH levels are raised into the high-to-normal range to dilate the pulmonary vascular bed (see Chapters 2 and 23). Here, HFV may have a theoretical advantage. HFVs remove CO_2 more effectively than CMVs and do so at lower proximal airway pressures. Carlo et al.[37] compared ventilator settings and outcomes in 37 neonates with persistent pulmonary hypertension. Both $PaCO_2$ levels and proximal airway pressures were lower in the infants treated with HFJV; however, the outcomes of the two groups were similar. There was a trend toward fewer air leaks in the infants treated with HFJV, but the difference was not significant.[37] Use of iNO (see Chapter 14) during mechanical ventilation has been shown to improve outcomes in term infants with persistent pulmonary hypertension.[106] For iNO to be effective, it must reach the alveolus. HFV with adequate lung volume recruitment may help achieve this goal.

CLINICAL GUIDELINES

Most clinical guidelines are, by their nature, arbitrary. They reflect the experiences, biases, and, at times, idiosyncrasies of their authors. What follows is a description of HFV use in a variety of situations, using two different HFV strategies: (1) *limiting pressure exposure,* which is used in air leaks and most other rescue situations; and (2) *optimizing lung volume,* which is used in RDS or other conditions where diffuse atelectasis is a major issue. Many clinicians do not consider HFV first-line therapy; however, many quickly move to it when problems develop during CMV. Some practitioners use HFV early in the course of uncomplicated RDS. Likewise, some wean to extubation from HFV. Others choose a return to CMV prior to extubation. Because of these many clinical variations and the lack of data from which to generalize, the following guidelines must be tempered by experience and modified as new information becomes available.

Limiting Pressure Exposure

High-Frequency Jet Ventilators

The only HFJV currently in general use for neonates is the Bunnell Life Pulse. With this machine, initiating HFJV is always the same, regardless of the clinical condition. First, patients are reintubated with Hi-Lo jet triple-lumen endotracheal tubes or the hub is replaced by an adapter. The outer diameter of this tube is 0.8 mm larger than a tube with the same internal diameter. Thus, a 2.5-mm internal-diameter conventional tube has an outer diameter of 3.5 mm; the outer diameter of a similar triple-lumen tube is 4.3 mm, which limits its use in infants weighing less than 900 g. After verifying the position of the endotracheal tube tip, patients are reconnected to the CMV at their previous settings. The jet ventilator is activated and set in its standby mode. The jet injector and pressure monitoring lines are connected to their respective ports on the endotracheal tube. The ventilator's internal pressure transducers now measure airway pressures at the endotracheal tube tip. These values appear on the ventilator's front panel. They are the baseline CMV settings. When CMV rates and airway pressures are not extremely high, pressures measured at the proximal and distal ends of patients' endotracheal tubes usually are similar. During HFJV, however, these pressures often are quite different. Airway pressures should be measured at the endotracheal tube tip. Once baseline airway pressures are established, arterial blood gases should be analyzed. The HFJV rate initially is set at 420 breaths/min, using the shortest possible inspiratory time of 0.02 seconds (these are the default settings programmed into the ventilator). PIP is set at the same level used during CMV. End-expiratory pressure is controlled by the PEEP control and background flow of the CMV circuit. Many use a CMV background or "sigh" rate of 5 to 10 breaths/min to maintain lung volume and prevent atelectasis, which is a common problem during low tidal volume–constant airway pressure ventilation. Little information is available regarding the effectiveness of this strategy. During HFO with the Dräger Babylog in an animal model, "sigh" breaths were useful during lung recruitment but not after recruitment was complete.[107] The PIP of the CMV background breaths should be lower than the PIP of the HFJV breaths. If it is not, these background breaths will interrupt the cycling of the HFJV. When treating respiratory failure unaccompanied by significant air leaks, we set PEEP at the same level or higher than that used during CMV. When treating air leak syndromes, we use low PEEP levels, usually 2 to 5 cm H_2O, and do not use CMV background rates. Once HFJV settings are established, mean airway pressures should be 10% to 20% less than noted during CMV.

After initiating HFJV, some patience is required. During HFJV, airway pressures equilibrate more slowly than during CMV. One must allow adequate time for the system's servo-mechanisms to adjust HFJV driving pressure to achieve the desired pressures measured at the endotracheal tube tip. Patients usually stabilize within 15 to 30 minutes. After this initial equilibration period, interval arterial blood gases are measured. Usually CO_2 elimination improves, and it does so at lower mean airway pressures. Oxygen requirements may transiently increase. Because this strategy is designed to minimize pressure exposure, increases in FIO_2 may be necessary to eliminate air leaks. HFJV is generally a rescue therapy; relatively short-term exposure to HFJV (generally a few days) often will result in substantial clinical improvement. As patients improve, HFJV-PIP can be decreased in increments of 1 to 2 cm H_2O while normal pH and $PaCO_2$ values are maintained. Decrease FIO_2 levels as arterial oxygen saturation values allow. As weaning progresses, expect to see radiographic evidence of losses in lung volume. There is often an HFJV-PIP "threshold" usually 8 to 10 cm H_2O below previous maximum HFJV-PIP values, where blood gas values progressively deteriorate, likely reflecting a loss in lung volume. If this occurs, a CMV background "sigh" rate of 5 to 10 breaths/min with an increase in HFJV-PIP levels 2 to 4 cm H_2O may help resolve this problem. After stabilization for several hours, HFJV-PIP level may again be decreased. When HFJV-PIP values approach 20 cm H_2O and FIO_2 values fall below 0.5, consider returning to total CMV support.

The mechanics of returning to CMV are simple. Set the jet ventilator to standby mode. Set the CMV rate to 60 breaths/min (an arbitrary number). Adjust CMV-PIP levels to deliver tidal volumes of 4 to 6 mL/kg. Adjust FIO_2 levels as necessary to maintain arterial oxygen saturation values greater than 85%. If, after returning to CMV, the patient's general condition worsens or FIO_2 or $PaCO_2$ levels increase significantly, consider a return to HFJV for at least another 24 hours. The response to a variety of clinical situations is summarized in Table 11-2.

High-Frequency Oscillatory Ventilators

Today the most commonly used neonatal HFO is the SensorMedics 3100A. With this device, in contrast to HFJV, reintubation is not necessary. Infants receive HFO and CMV through the same endotracheal tube. HFO frequency is set between 10 and 15 Hertz. This ventilator's "Power" control sets the amplitude of its airway pressure oscillations (ΔP), the prime determinant of CO_2 removal. Increasing airway pressure amplitude increases chest wall movement and decreases $PaCO_2$ values. Decreasing airway pressure amplitude decreases chest wall movement and increases $PaCO_2$ values. Initially set this control at 35 to 40 cm H_2O, then adjust it as necessary to produce normocarbia. During HFO, airway pressures are measured within the oscillator circuit, not in the endotracheal tube or proximal airway. These pressures may or may not reflect the actual pressures within the patients' airways. Airway pressures are rapidly damped across the HFO circuit and further within the airways (Fig. 11-9). Once the desired oscillatory amplitude is established, adjust mean airway pressures to equal that used during CMV. Once patients stabilize and/or start to improve, begin to decrease airway pressures: mean airway pressure, if $PaCO_2$ values are normal and arterial oxygenation is adequate at

TABLE 11-2.   Gas Exchange and Ventilator Adjustment During High-Frequency Ventilation

Problem	HFOV	HFJV
Inadequate oxygenation; atelectasis; poor lung expansion	Increase mean airway pressure in 1–2 cm H_2O increments or SI, then decrease after improvement	Increase PEEP. Add background IMV (5–10 breaths/min). Increase PIP during IMV.
Inadequate oxygenation; ±hypercarbia; lung overexpansion noted on x-ray film, poor cardiac output	Decrease mean airway pressure in 1–2 cm H_2O steps until improved. Repeat x-ray film	Decrease IMV rate and PEEP until mean airway pressure falls in 1–2 cm H_2O steps as needed. Increase HFJV PIP if necessary.
Hypercarbia without lung overexpansion	Increase power to optimize tidal volume delivery. Decrease rate if power at maximum	Increase PIP during HFJV. Increase rate if PIP at maximum.
Hypocarbia	Decrease power to decrease tidal volume. Increase rate if power already at minimum	Decrease PIP during HFJV. Increase PEEP. Decrease rate.
Hyperoxia	Decrease FIO_2, mean airway pressure	Decrease FIO_2, PEEP. Decrease IMV rate and PIP.

HFJV, high-frequency jet ventilation; HFOV, high-frequency oscillatory ventilation; HFV, high-frequency ventilation; IMV, intermittent mandatory ventilation; PEEP, positive end-expiratory pressure; PIP, peak inspiratory pressure; SI, sustained inflation.

FIO₂ levels less than 0.4 to 0.5; and ΔP, if PacO₂ levels are subnormal. During HFO, mean airway pressure is the main determinant of lung volume. Small changes in mean airway pressure can produce large changes in lung volume, either overdistention or atelectasis. During HFO weaning, there often is a mean airway pressure threshold, similar to the PIP threshold seen during HFJV, at which patients suddenly develop respiratory acidosis or show labile oxygen requirements. This threshold usually appears when mean airway pressures reach between 8 and 10 cm H₂O. When this occurs, consider a 1 to 2 cm H₂O increase in mean airway pressures to stabilize lung volume. If things do not improve, a brief (15- to 30-second) increase in mean airway pressure of 5 to 10 cm H₂O simulates an SI maneuver as used in the laboratory. When continuously measured SaO₂ or PaO₂ increases, pressures are returned to baseline. When using either HFO and HFJV, the problem likely stems from a loss of lung volume and atelectasis. Although some clinicians extubate patients directly from HFO, there is little published experience regarding this technique. Most physicians return patients to CMV and wean to the point of extubation using conventional techniques. Responses to a variety of clinical situations are summarized in Table 11-2.

Optimizing Lung Volume

The strategy for optimizing lung volume is critical. Initially demonstrated by Hamilton et al., adequate recruitment of lung volume may be the key to protection and preservation of lung architecture.[81,83] Recruiting and maintaining adequate lung volume during HFV improves the effectiveness of exogenous surfactant therapy.[110] Recruitment is needed not only as ventilation is initiated but also periodically during treatment. When

ventilation is interrupted and volume is acutely lost, such as with suctioning and disconnection of the ventilator circuit for patient position change, re-recruitment of the lung is less contributory to lung injury than a low lung volume ventilation strategy.[111] Currently there are two established techniques for optimizing lung volume during HFV. The first strategy uses sustained lung inflations (15 to 30 seconds in duration) at varied intervals.[57,81] The second strategy involves gradual stepwise increases in mean airway pressures until arterial oxygen saturation values increase significantly.[60,62,85,100,101] The SI technique for lung recruitment, which has been studied extensively in the laboratory during HFO and found to be extremely effective, has not been widely introduced into clinical practice. A number of reasons may account for this clinical reluctance. Because the SI rapidly recruits volume, which is difficult to measure at the bedside, the lung might be inadvertently overdistended. The increase in intrathoracic pressure could impair cardiac output or adversely alter intracranial blood flow. Stepwise gradual pressure increases may prevent these problems. Still, the SI technique offers the potential to best exploit the physiologic advantages of lung hysteresis. With SI, the lung may be maximally inflated, moving ventilation onto the expiratory limb of the pressure-volume (P-V) relationship. This then allows maximal preservation of lung volume at lower pressures, with the potential for the greatest protection from VILI. The lung changes rapidly during the course of illness; theoretically, providing ventilation on the descending limb of the P-V relationship offers potential protection from these rapids changes. Figure 11-11 schematically demonstrates this using basic physiologic principles. A study in lambs reported direct estimation of lung volume change during HFV using respiratory inductive plethysmography. If this technique proves

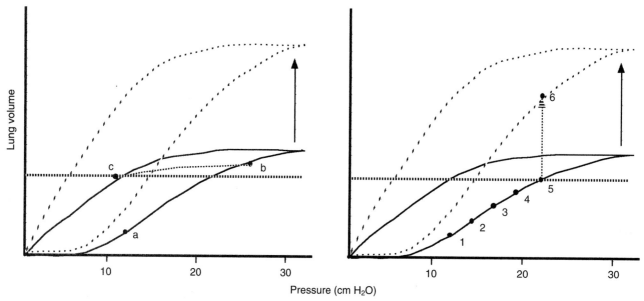

Figure 11-11. Schematic representation of two different approaches to achieving alveolar expansion and the theoretical effect of a sudden improvement in lung compliance. The *horizontal dashed line* indicates the desired mean lung volume. The *solid curve* is a pressure-volume (P-V) relationship of a surfactant-deficient lung prior to the development of structural injury. The *dashed line* shows the P-V curve of the lung after some recovery has occurred. In the left panel, a brief sustained inflation from opening pressure (point *a*) to pressure point *b* inflates the lung to the desired volume. Pressure is then decreased to point *c*, moving to the deflation limb of the curve. In the improved lung, volume at point *c* is still maintained within the desired range at low pressure. In the right panel, progressive increases in mean airway pressure occur on the inflation limb (points *1–5*). Target volume is achieved but at higher pressure. If the lung then improves, rapid overdistention could occur when pressure is maintained but volume increases (point *6*). (Adapted from Froese AB: Neonatal and pediatric ventilation: Physiological and clinical perspectives. In Marini JJ, Slutsky AS (eds): Physiological Basis of Ventilatory Support. New York, Marcel Dekker, 1998, p. 1346.)

clinically applicable, lung volume recruitment may become easier and safer.[112]

Techniques for lung volume recruitment have been primarily studied during HFO. There are little published data on lung volume recruitment during HFJV. Keszler et al.[43] described stepwise pressure increases for lung volume recruitment during a randomized trial of HFJV use in RDS. There are no reports of an SI approach during HFJV or HFPPV; however, with some modification, what works during HFO also should work during HFJV.[111]

High-Frequency Jet Ventilators

HFJV is initiated as previously described. The only difference in this strategy from the previous pressure-limiting strategy is the higher PEEP levels used, usually 6 to 10 cm H_2O. CMV background "sigh" rates at 2 to 5 breaths/min can be used to recruit lung volume. Surfactant is administered either immediately after intubation or during CMV. At this time, there is no convincing evidence that surfactant administration is either more efficient or safer during any form of HFV, although adequate volume recruitment clearly improves surfactant function.[110] Again, patients are reintubated with triple-lumen endotracheal tubes or a triple-lumen adapter is attached to the existing endotracheal tube. The jet ventilator is activated and set to its standby mode. Inspired oxygen concentrations are maintained at the same level used during CMV. Set HFJV rates at 420 breaths/min and inspiratory times at 0.02 seconds. Initially, HFJV-PIP levels are the same as those used during CMV. PEEP levels are set at 6 to 8 cm H_2O to produce mean airway pressures 2 to 3 cm H_2O higher than those used during CMV. PEEP levels are increased in increments of 1 to 2 cm H_2O until arterial oxygen levels no longer increase. When initial recruitment is complete, PIP levels must be weaned rapidly to avoid hypocarbia. When oxygen saturation levels are satisfactory, make an initial decrease in PEEP by 2 cm H_2O to prevent overdistention and to shift the P-V relationship to the expiratory portion of the curve. Then begin decreasing FIO_2 rather than PEEP to prevent atelectasis. When FIO_2 levels fall to 0.4 or less, begin to further decrease PEEP and PIP. HFJVs remove CO_2 very efficiently, possibly more so than HFO.[44,45] If hypocarbia and alkalosis develop, decreasing PIP seems to be the best remedy. If FIO_2 needs increase, it is likely a consequence of diminished lung volume. Remedies here include stepwise increases in PEEP, a brief SI, or adding a CMV background "sigh" rate. A technique for finding optimal PEEP levels is shown in Table 11-3. When mean airway pressures fall to 8 to 10 cm H_2O and PIP levels to 15 to 20 cm H_2O, attempt to return to CMV in the fashion previously described.

High-Frequency Oscillatory Ventilators

Although the goal of treatment is different, use of HFO is similar to the techniques described for minimizing pressure exposure. The key difference is that higher, not lower, mean airway pressures are applied early. Set the ventilator frequency at 10 to 12 Hz for infants weighing more than 1500 g or when $PaCO_2$ is elevated; use 15 Hz for smaller babies. Amplitude is set at 35 to 40 cm H_2O and adjusted to produce visible vibration in the chest and abdomen; mean airway pressures initially are 2 to 3 cm H_2O higher than those used during CMV. Recruitment of lung volume may be accomplished by mean airway pressure increases in increments of 1 to 2 cm H_2O until oxygen saturations rise to greater than 95% (or measured arterial oxygen levels no longer rise), or by increasing mean airway pressure by 5 to 10 cm H_2O above baseline for 10 to 30 seconds as an SI. HFO is continued during the SI. Using either technique, mean airway pressure should be reduced after improvement in oxygenation is seen. As noted earlier, this will maximize the effects of lung hysteresis. If stepwise pressure increases are used, move downward in increments of 1 to 2 cm H_2O every 1 to 2 minutes. Just as the initial pressure increases begin to show effect above the lung's opening pressure, oxygenation should be easily maintained as long as pressures remain above the lung's closing pressure. Because neither of these can be accurately predicted and lung volume changes can only be estimated, careful clinical observation at the bedside is the only solution today. After lung recruitment and pressure adjustment, decrease FIO_2 to less than 0.4, then continue to wean mean airway pressure. Amplitude is adjusted upward, then rate downward, for CO_2 retention, and vice versa for hypocarbia. Increasing oxygen requirements suggest either impaired cardiac output or loss of lung volume. When mean airway pressures fall to 8 to 10 cm H_2O, consider returning to CMV in the fashion previously described or proceeding to extubation from HFO as pressures continue to fall.

PROBLEMS, COMPLICATIONS, AND QUESTIONS WITHOUT ANSWERS

Will HFV become the preferred means of support for neonates with respiratory failure? To date, there is inadequate information to make this leap. Although we have the beginnings of a better understanding of VILI, prevention of neurologic injury during HFV, and ways to establish and monitor lung volumes during therapy, much is left to do. There are a number of practical problems associated with the clinical use of any HFV. Although approved for general use, HFVs are still, in

---

TABLE 11-3. Optimal Positive End-Expiratory Pressure During High-Frequency Jet Ventilation

Operation	Impact of Change	
	Sao₂ goes up or unchanged	Sao₂ goes down
Add IMV (if no IMV in use)	PEEP is inadequate. Raise PEEP 1–2 cm H_2O; wait for Sao₂ to stabilize level, then stop IMV again to test new PEEP level.	PEEP adequate; may be impeding cardiac output or producing lung overdistention
Stop IMV (if IMV in use)	PEEP is adequate; maintain IMV = 0, or go to 1–3 breaths/min with smaller tidal volume and modest I-time.	PEEP is inadequate. Raise PEEP 1–2 cm H_2O; return to IMV = 5–10 if necessary to stop Sao₂ decline. Wait for Sao₂ to return to previous level, then stop IMV again to test new PEEP level.

IMV, intermittent mandatory ventilation; PEEP, positive end-expiratory pressure.

many respects, experimental devices. Each HFV system is different. Generalizations and recommendations developed for one system may or may not apply to the next.[67,114] There are few standards. HFV, whether in the form of HFPPV, HFO, or HFJV, is used in virtually all neonatal intensive care units today. There is no clear HFV "standard of practice." Many different HFV systems are in use around the world; a "best" device has not been identified. HFJV and HFO can be extremely effective in many different clinical situations. Both systems have their complications and their limitations.

In the absence of a good technique for monitoring lung volumes at the bedside, can HFV produce lung overdistention by quietly trapping gas? We know HFV produces higher end-tidal volumes at lower proximal airway pressures.[115] Increased end-tidal lung volumes would seem to mean increased end-tidal alveolar pressures. Under such circumstances, mean alveolar pressures exceed mean proximal airway pressures. Such silent distending pressure is commonly referred to as *inadvertent PEEP* (see Chapter 2). Because this pressure cannot be easily measured, the extent to which it produces problems is a conundrum. In some circumstances it probably causes substantial difficulty with ventilation. In the HIFI trial and other studies, pulmonary air leaks increased or stayed the same during HFO as compared to CMV.[43,59,66,85,92,100,101] As yet there is no convincing evidence that any form of HFV decreases the incidence of acute air leak in humans.

Does HFV produce lung underdistention? Under normal circumstances, small monotonous tidal volumes delivered at relatively constant pressures result in progressive atelectasis. Early HFO primate studies document that this does occur. To combat this problem, many clinicians periodically vary tidal volumes using either manual or mechanical breath "sighs," or periodic SI maneuvers. These sighs recruit alveoli and prevent atelectasis. What is the best way to vary tidal volume during HFV? Are SIs better than gradual increases in mean airway pressure? A bedside technique for rapid accurate assessment of changes in lung volume is needed to resolve these issues.

New therapies often produce new, previously unsuspected complications. A number of early reports linked tracheal inflammation and tracheal obstructions to various forms of HFV.[33,34,116–118] The obstructions were serious and at times fatal. They occurred in both adults and neonates. Initially these lesions were believed to result from inadequate humidification of respiratory gases. This no longer appears to be the entire answer. Ophoven et al.[121] compared the tracheal histopathology seen in animals following CMV and HFJV using different humidity systems. Although humidity was important, regardless of the humidity system, HFJV always produced more inflammation and damage in the proximal trachea than did CMV. The histologic injury patterns observed in these animals were virtually identical to those seen in human patients exposed to HFJV. Similar animal studies compared the tracheobronchial histopathology seen following HFPPV, HFJV, and CMV.[122] HFJV and HFPPV produced nearly identical tracheal lesions. This unique tracheal injury now is referred to as *necrotizing tracheobronchitis* (NTB; Fig. 11-12). This problem has been extensively studied in the laboratory. It now appears that NTB is associated with a number of factors and occurs during all forms of HFV. Ventilator rates and ventilatory strategies, airway humidification, FIO_2 levels, the severity of the underlying illness, durations of ventilation, alterations in epithelial permeability, and infections all seem to play roles.[45,123–131] Current

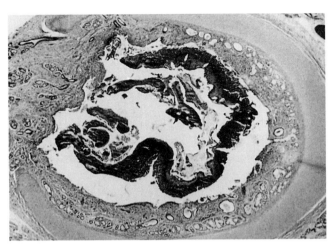

Figure 11-12. Photomicrograph of fatal necrotizing tracheobronchitis. This section was obtained from the trachea just above the carina. The entire mucosal surface has become necrotic and completely obstructs the tracheal lumen.

evidence suggests that between 2% and 4% of HFV-treated patients have either clinical or microscopic evidence of NTB.[121] Although it also occurs during CMV, NTB continues to be more likely during HFV. Acute hypercapnia, respiratory acidosis, and a sudden decrease in chest wall movement during HFV signal possible NTB until proven otherwise. Aggressive airway suctioning, at times using bronchoscopy and sometimes in conjunction with reintubation, can be life saving.[119,120,123]

The most serious potential side effect of HFV is an increase in long-term neurologic injury resulting from early periventricular leukomalacia or severe intraventricular hemorrhage. This finding, originally reported in the HIFI trial,[59] was also seen in a study of HFJV reported by Wiswell et al.[42] These injuries seem to be linked to the strategy of ventilation used in these studies. In neither study was there a standardized technique for lung volume recruitment, and alkalosis during treatment was common. Meta-analysis of randomized trials of HFV has concluded that, in studies using a "high lung volume" strategy, there is no evidence of increased neurologic injury.[132,133] Clearly, the dictum of *primum non nocere* holds here.

SUMMARY

HFV is an exciting and useful form of mechanical ventilation. In some circumstances it can produce gas exchange at lower airway pressures than during CMV, and it allows safer application of high mean airway pressures when necessary for oxygenation. This technique is clearly superior to CMV in airway disruption syndromes and may be a useful rescue technique and/or bridge to ECMO. It has clear but limited usefulness as a rescue or temporizing measure in pulmonary hypoplasia, persistent pulmonary hypertension, and other forms of neonatal respiratory failure unresponsive to CMV. In neonatal RDS, HFV, perhaps in association with surfactant therapy, may yet play a major role in improving long-term pulmonary outcomes. Today, HFV is no longer a treatment in search of a disease, but neither is it the panacea for all forms of neonatal respiratory failure that many initially hoped it would be.

REFERENCES

1. Slutsky AS, Kamm RD, Rossing TH, et al: Effects of frequency, tidal volume and lung volume on CO_2 elimination in dogs by high frequency (2-30 Hz.), low tidal volume ventilation. J Clin Invest 68:1475, 1981.
2. Slutsky AS, Drazen JM, Kamm RD, et al: Effective pulmonary ventilation with small-volume oscillations at high frequency. Science 209:609, 1980.
3. Kamm RD, Slutsky AS, Drazen JM: High-frequency ventilation. CRC Rev Biomed Eng 9:347, 1984.
4. Drazen JM, Kamm RD, Slutsky AS: High-frequency ventilation. Physiol Rev 64:505, 1984.
5. Venegas JG, Fredberg JJ: Understanding the pressure cost of high-frequency ventilation: Why does it work? Crit Care Med 22(Suppl 9): S49–S57, 1994.
6. Froese AB, Bryan AC: High frequency ventilation. Am Rev Respir Dis 135:1363, 1987.
7. Bloom BT, Delmore P, Park YI, et al: Respiratory distress syndrome and tracheoesophageal fistula: Management with high frequency ventilation. Crit Care Med 18:447, 1990.
8. Cavanaugh K, Bloom B: Combined HFV and CMV for neonatal air leak. Respir Manage 20:43, 1990.
9. Randel RC, Manning FL: One lung high frequency ventilation in the management of an acquired neonatal pulmonary cyst. Am J Perinatol 9:66, 1989.
10. Sjostrand V: Review of the physiological rational for and development of high-frequency positive-pressure ventilation—HFPPV. Acta Anaesthesiol Scand Suppl 64:7, 1977.
11. Sjostrand V: Development of high-frequency positive-pressure low-compression ventilation. Int Anesthesiol Clin 21:11, 1983.
12. Bland RD, Kim MH, Light MJ, et al: High frequency mechanical ventilation in severe hyaline membrane disease: An alternative treatment? Crit Care Med 8:275, 1980.
13. Oxford Region Controlled Trial of Artificial Ventilation (OCTAVE) Study Group: Multicentre randomised controlled trial of high against low frequency positive pressure ventilation. Arch Dis Child 66:770, 1991.
14. Thome U, Kössel H, Lipowski G, et al: Randomized controlled trial of high-frequency ventilation with high-rate intermittent positive pressure ventilation in preterm infants with respiratory failure. J Pediatr 135:39, 1999.
15. Boros SJ, Bing DR, Mammel MC, et al: Using conventional infant ventilators at unconventional rates. Pediatrics 74:487, 1984.
16. Gonzalez F, Richardson P, Carlstrom JR, et al: Rapid mechanical ventilation effects on tracheal airway pressure, lung volume, and blood gases of rabbits. Am J Perinatol 3:347, 1986.
17. Fontan JJP, Heldt GP, Gregory GA: Dynamics of respiration during rapid rate mechanical ventilation in anesthetized and paralyzed rabbits. Pediatr Res 8:750, 1986.
18. Fontan JJP, Heldt GP, Targett RC, et al: Dynamics of expiration and gas trapping in rabbits during mechanical ventilation at rapid rates. Crit Care Med 14:39, 1986.
19. Greenough A, Greenall F: Performance of respirators at fast rates commonly used in neonatal intensive care units. Pediatr Pulmonol 3:357, 1987.
20. Hird M, Greenough A, Gamsu H: Gas trapping during high frequency positive pressure ventilation using conventional ventilators. Early Hum Dev 22:51, 1990.
21. Mammel MC, Bing DR: Mechanical ventilation of the newborn: An overview. Clin Chest Med 17:603, 1996
22. Binda RE, Cook DR, Fischer CG: Advantages of infant ventilators over adapted adult ventilators in pediatrics. Anesth Analg 55:769, 1976.
23. Schreiner RL, Kisling JA: Practical Neonatal Respiratory Care. New York, Raven Press, 1982, p 1.
24. Mushin WW, Rendell-Baker L, Thompson PW, et al: Automatic Ventilation of the Lungs. Oxford, Blackwell Scientific Publications, 1980, p. 66.
25. Fisher JB, Mammel MC, Coleman JM, et al: Identifying lung overdistention during mechanical ventilation by using volume-pressure loops. Pediatr Pulmonol 5:10–14, 1988.
26. Mammel MC, Boros SJ, Bing DR, et al: Determining optimum inspiratory time during intermittent positive pressure ventilation in surfactant-depleted cats. Pediatr Pulmonol 7:223, 1989.
27. Mammel MC, Fisher JB, Bing DR, et al: Effect of spontaneous and mechanical breathing on dynamic lung mechanics in hyaline membrane disease. Pediatr Pulmonol 8:222, 1990.
28. Rosen WC, Mammel MC, Fisher JB, et al: The effects of bedside pulmonary mechanics testing during infant mechanical ventilation: A retrospective analysis. Pediatr Pulmonol 16:147, 1993.
29. Smith R: Ventilation at high respiratory frequencies. Anaesthesia 37:1011, 1982.
30. Weisberger SA, Carlo WA, Fouke JM, et al: Measurement of tidal volume during high-frequency jet ventilation. Pediatr Res 20:45, 1986.
31. Carlon GC, Howland WS, Ray C, et al: High-frequency jet ventilation: A prospective randomized evaluation. Chest 84:551, 1983.
32. Sladen A, Guntupalli K, Marquez J, et al: High-frequency jet ventilation in the postoperative period: A review of 100 patients. Crit Care Med 12:782, 1984.
33. Pokora T, Bing D, Mammel M, et al: Neonatal high-frequency jet ventilation. Pediatrics 72:27, 1983.
34. Boros SJ, Mammel MC, Coleman JM, et al: Neonatal high-frequency ventilation: 4 years' experience. Pediatrics 75:657, 1985.
35. Carlo WA, Chatburn RL, Martin RJ, et al: Decrease in airway pressure during high-frequency jet ventilation in infants with respiratory distress syndrome. J Pediatr 104:101, 1984.
36. Carlo WA, Chatburn RL, Martin RJ: Randomized trial of high-frequency jet ventilation versus conventional ventilation in respiratory distress syndrome. J Pediatr 110:275, 1987.
37. Carlo WA, Beoglos A, Chatburn RL, et al: High-frequency jet ventilation in neonatal pulmonary hypertension. Am J Dis Child 143:233, 1989.
38. Spitzer AR, Butler S, Fox WW: Ventilatory response to combined high frequency jet ventilation and conventional mechanical ventilation for the rescue treatment of severe neonatal lung disease. Pediatr Pulmonol 7:244, 1989.
39. Carlo WA, Siner B, Chatburn RLL, et al: Early randomized intervention with high-frequency jet ventilation in respiratory distress syndrome. J Pediatr 117:765, 1990.
40. Keszler M, Donn SM, Bucciarelli RLL, et al: Multicenter controlled trial comparing high-frequency jet ventilation and conventional mechanical ventilation in newborn infants with pulmonary interstitial emphysema. J. Pediatr 119:85, 1991.
41. Davis JM, Richter SE, Kendig JW, et al: High-frequency jet ventilation and surfactant treatment of newborns with severe respiratory failure. Pediatr Pulmonol 13:108, 1992.
42. Wiswell TE, Graziani LJ, Kornhauser MS, et al: High-frequency jet ventilation in the early management of respiratory distress syndrome is associated with a greater risk for adverse outcomes. Pediatrics 98:1035, 1996.
43. Keszler M, Modanlou HD, Brudno DS, et al: Multicenter controlled trial of high-frequency jet ventilation in preterm infants with uncomplicated respiratory distress syndrome. Pediatrics 100:593, 1997.
44. Boros SJ, Mammel MC, Coleman JM, et al: Comparison of high-frequency oscillatory ventilation and high-frequency jet ventilation in cats with normal lungs. Pediatr Pulmonol 7:35, 1989.
45. Mammel MC, Ophoven JP, Lewallen PK, et al: Acute airway injury during high-frequency jet ventilation and high-frequency oscillatory ventilation. Crit Care Med 19:394, 1991.
46. Bhuta T, Henderson-Smart DJ: Elective high frequency jet ventilation versus conventional ventilation for respiratory distress syndrome in preterm infants. Cochrane Database Syst Rev CD00438, 2000.
47. Butler WJ, Bohn DJ, Bryan AC, et al: Ventilation by high-frequency oscillation in humans. Anesth Analg 59:577, 1980.
48. Fredberg JJ, Keefe DH, Glass GM, et al: Alveolar pressure nonhomogeneity during small-amplitude high-frequency oscillation. J Appl Physiol 57:788, 1984.
49. Allen JL, Fredberg JJ, Keefe DH, et al: Alveolar pressure magnitude and asynchrony during high-frequency oscillations of excised rabbit lungs. Am Rev Respir Dis 132:343, 1985.
50. Gerstmann DR, Fouke JMM, Winter DC, et al: Proximal, tracheal, and alveolar pressures during high-frequency oscillatory ventilation in a normal rabbit model. Pediatr Res 28:367, 1990.
51. Thompson WK, Marchak BE, Froese AB, et al: High frequency oscillation compared with standard ventilation in pulmonary injury model. J Appl Physiol 52:543, 1982.
52. Truog WE, Standaert TA, Murphy J, et al: Effect of high-frequency oscillation on gas exchange and pulmonary phospholipids in experimental hyaline membrane disease. Am Rev Respir Dis 127:585, 1983.
53. Bell RE, Kuehl TJ, Coalson JJ, et al: High-frequency ventilation compared to conventional positive-pressure ventilation in the treatment of hyaline membrane disease in primates. Crit Care Med 12:764, 1984.
54. Marchak BE, Thompson WK, Duffy MB, et al: Treatment of RDS by high frequency oscillatory ventilation. A preliminary report. J Pediatr 99:287, 1982.
55. Frantz ID, Werthammer J, Stark AR: High-frequency ventilation in premature infants with lung disease: Adequate gas exchange at low tracheal pressure. Pediatrics 71:483, 1983.

56. Truog WE, Standaert TA, Murphy JH, et al: Effects of prolonged high-frequency oscillatory ventilation in premature primates with experimental hyaline membrane disease. Am Rev Respir Dis 130:76, 1984.

57. Froese AB, Butler PO, Fletcher WA, et al: High-frequency oscillatory ventilation in premature infants with respiratory failure: A preliminary report. Anesth Analg 66:814, 1987.

58. Traverse JH, Korvenranta H, Adams EM, et al: Impairment of hemodynamics with increasing mean airway pressure during high-frequency oscillatory ventilation. Pediatr Res 23:628, 1988.

59. The HIFI Study Group: High-frequency oscillatory ventilation compared with conventional mechanical ventilation in the treatment of respiratory failure in preterm infants. N Engl J Med 320:88, 1989.

60. Kinsella JP, Gerstmann DR, Clark RH, et al: High-frequency oscillatory ventilation versus intermittent mandatory ventilation: Early hemodynamic effects in the premature baboon with hyaline membrane disease. Pediatr Res 29:160, 1991.

61. Jackson JC, Truog WE, Standaert TA, et al: Effect of high-frequency ventilation on the development of alveolar edema in premature monkeys at risk for hyaline membrane disease. Am Rev Respir Dis 143:865, 1991.

62. Clark, RH, Gerstmann DR, Null DM, et al: Prospective randomized comparison of high-frequency oscillatory and conventional ventilation in respiratory distress syndrome. Pediatrics 89:5, 1992.

63. Chan V, Greenough A, Milner AD: The effect of frequency and mean airway pressure on volume delivery during high frequency oscillation. Pediatr Pulmonol 15:183, 1993.

64. Chan V, Greenough A: Determinants of oxygenation during high frequency oscillation. Eur J Pediatr 152:350, 1993.

65. Hoskyns EW, Milner AD, Hopkin IE: Dynamic lung inflation during high frequency oscillation in neonates. Eur J Pediatr 151:846, 1992.

66. Ogawa Y, Miyasaka K, Kawano T, et al: A multicenter randomized trial of high frequency oscillatory ventilation as compared with conventional mechanical ventilation in preterm infants with respiratory failure. Early Hum Dev 32:1, 1993.

67. Jouvet P, Hubert P, Isabey D, et al: Assessment of high-frequency neonatal ventilator performances. Intensive Care Med 23:208, 1997.

68. Lucking SE, Fields AI, Mahfood S, et al: High-frequency ventilation versus conventional ventilation in dogs with right ventricular dysfunction. Crit Car Med 14:798, 1986.

69. Barringer M, Meredith J, Prough D, et al: Effectiveness of high-frequency jet ventilation in management of an experimental bronchopleural fistula. Am Surg 48:610, 1982.

70. Carlon GC, Griffin J, Ray C, et al: High frequency jet ventilation in experimental airway disruption. Crit Car Med 11:353, 1983.

71. Orland III R, Gluck EH, Cohen M, et al: Ultra-high-frequency jet ventilation in a bronchopleural fistula model. Arch Surg 123:591, 1988.

72. Walsh MC, Carlo WA: Determinants of gas flow through a bronchopleural fistula. J Appl Physiol 67:1591, 1989.

73. Clark RH, Gerstmann DR, Null DM, et al: Pulmonary interstitial emphysema treated by high-frequency oscillatory ventilation. Crit Care Med 14:926, 1986.

74. Carter JM, Gerstmann DR, Clark RH, et al: High-frequency oscillatory ventilation and extracorporeal membrane oxygenation for the treatment of acute neonatal respiratory failure. Pediatrics 85:159, 1990.

75. deLemos R, Yoder B, McCurnin D, et al: The use of high-frequency oscillatory ventilation (HFOV) and extracorporeal membrane oxygenation (ECMO) in the management of the term/near term infant with respiratory failure. Early Hum Dev 29:299, 1992.

76. Baumgart S, Hirschl RB, Butler SZ, et al: Diagnosis-related criteria in the consideration of extracorporeal membrane oxygenation in neonates previously treated with high-frequency jet ventilation. Pediatrics 89:491, 1992.

77. Gerhardt T, Reifenberg L, Goldberg RN, et al: Pulmonary function in preterm infants whose lungs were ventilated conventionally or by high-frequency oscillation. J Pediatr 115:121, 1989.

78. HIFI Study Group: High-frequency oscillatory ventilation compared with conventional mechanical ventilation in the treatment of respiratory failure in preterm infants: Assessment of pulmonary function at 9 months of corrected age. J Pediatr 116:933, 1990.

79. Abbasi S, Bhutani VK, Spitzer AR, et al: Pulmonary mechanics in preterm neonates with respiratory failure treated with high-frequency oscillatory ventilation compared with conventional mechanical ventilation. Pediatrics 87:487, 1991.

80. The HIFI Study Group: High-frequency oscillatory ventilation compared with conventional intermittent mechanical ventilation in the treatment of respiratory failure in preterm infants: Neurodevelopmental status at 16-24 months of postterm age. J Pediatr 117:939, 1990.

81. Hamilton PP, Onayemi A, Smyth JA, et al: Comparison of conventional and high-frequency ventilation: Oxygenation and lung pathology. J Appl Physiol 131, 1983.

82. Froese AB: Role of lung volume in lung injury: HFO in the atelectasis-prone lung. Acta Anaesthesiol Scand 33(Suppl 90):126, 1989.

83. McCulloch PR, Forkert PG, Froese AB: Lung volume maintenance prevents lung injury during high frequency oscillatory ventilation. Am Rev Respir Dis 137:1185, 1988.

84. Bryan AC, Froese AB: Reflections on the HIFI Trial. Commentaries. Pediatrics 87:565, 1991.

85. Gerstmann DR, Minton SD, Stoddard RA, et al: The Provo early high-frequency oscillatory ventilation trial: Improved pulmonary and clinical outcome in respiratory distress syndrome. Pediatrics 98:1044, 1996.

86. Meredith KS, deLemos RA, Coalson JJ, et al: Role of lung injury in the pathogenesis of hyaline membrane disease in premature baboons. J Appl Physiol 66:2150–2158, 1989.

87. Hudson LD: Progress in understanding ventilator-induced lung injury. JAMA 282:77, 1999.

88. Ranieri VM, Suter PM, Tortorella C, et al: Effect of mechanical ventilation on inflammatory mediators in patients with acute respiratory distress syndrome: A randomized controlled trial. JAMA 282:54, 1999.

89. Tremblay LN, Slutsky AS: Ventilator-induced lung injury: From barotrauma to biotrauma. Proc Assoc Am Physicians 110:482, 1998.

90. Jobe AH, Ikegami M: Mechanisms initiating lung injury in the preterm. Early Hum Dev 53:81, 1998.

91. Carlon GC, Ray C Jr, Klain M, et al: High pressure positive pressure ventilation in management of a patient with bronchopleural fistula. Anesthesiology 52:160, 1980.

92. HiFO Study Group: Randomized study of high-frequency oscillatory ventilation in infants with severe respiratory distress syndrome. J Pediatr 122:609, 1993.

93. Harris TR, Christensen RD, Matlak ME, et al: High-frequency jet ventilation treatment of neonates with congenital left diaphragmatic hernia [abstract]. Clin Res 32:123A, 1984.

94. Bohn D, Tamura M, Bryan C: Respiratory failure in congenital diaphragmatic hernia: Ventilation by high-frequency oscillation [abstract]. Pediatr Res 18:387A, 1984.

95. Karl SR, Ballantine TVN, Snider MT: High-frequency ventilation at rates of 375 to 1800 cycles per minute in four neonates with congenital diaphragmatic hernia. J Pediatr Surg 18:822, 1983.

96. Stoddard R, Meredith K, Minton S, et al: Treatment of congenital diaphragmatic hernia (CDH) with high frequency oscillatory ventilation (HFOV). Pediatr Pulmonol 15:367, 1993.

97. Corbet A, Bucciarelli R, Goldman S, et al: Decreased mortality rate among small premature infants treated at birth with a single dose of synthetic surfactant: A multicenter controlled trial. J Pediatr 118:277, 1991.

98. Hoekstra RE, Jackson JC, Myers TF, et al: Improved neonatal survival following multiple doses of bovine surfactant in very premature neonates at risk for respiratory distress syndrome. Pediatrics 88:10, 1991.

99. Heldt GP, Merrit TA, Golembeski D, et al: Distribution of surfactant, lung compliance, and aeration of preterm rabbit lungs after surfactant therapy and conventional and high frequency oscillatory ventilation. Pediatr Res 31:270, 1992.

100. Johnson AH, Peacock JL, Greenough A, et al: High-frequency oscillatory ventilation for the prevention of chronic lung disease of prematurity. N Engl J Med 347:633, 2002.

101. Courtney SE, Durand DJ, Asselin JM, et al: High-frequency oscillatory ventilation versus conventional mechanical ventilation for very-low-birth-weight infants. N Engl J Med 347:643, 2002.

102. Stark AR: High-frequency oscillatory ventilation to prevent bronchopulmonary dysplasia—are we there yet? N Engl J Med 347:682, 2002.

103. Vasquez de Anda GF, Gommers D, Verbrugge SJ, et al: Mechanical ventilation with high positive end expiratory pressure. Crit Care Med 28:2921, 2000.

104. Rimensberger P, Pache JC, McKerlie C, et al: Lung recruitment and lung volume maintenance: A strategy for improving oxygenation and preventing lung injury during both conventional mechanical ventilation and high frequency oscillation. Intensive Care Med 26:745, 2000.

105. Rimensberger PC, Cox PN, Frndova H, et al: The open lung during small volume ventilation: Concepts of recruitment and "optimal" positive end expiratory pressure. Crit Care Med 27:1946, 1999.

106. Rimensberger PC, Pristine G, Mullen JBM, et al: Lung recruitment during small tidal volume ventilation allows minimal positive end-expiratory pressure without augmenting lung injury. Crit Care Med 27:1940, 1999.

107. Henderson-Smart DJ, Bhuta T, Cools F, Offringa M: Elective high frequency oscillatory ventilation versus conventional ventilation for acute pulmonary dysfunction in preterm infants. Cochrane Database Syst Rev CD 000104, 2000.

108. Clark RH, Kueser TJ, Walker MW, et al: Low-dose nitric oxide therapy for persistent pulmonary hypertension of the newborn. N Engl J Med 342:469, 2000.

109. Manaligod JM, Meyers PA, Worwa CT, et al: Decreased mean airway pressure requirements for lung volume recruitment during high frequency ventilation with superimposed IMV breaths [abstract 1567]. Pediatr Res 49:274A, 2001.

110. Froese AB, McCulloch PR, Sugiura M, et al: Optimizing alveolar expansion prolongs the effectiveness of exogenous surfactant therapy in the adult rabbit. Am Rev Respir Dis 148:569, 1993.

111. Bond DM, Froese AB: Volume recruitment maneuvers are less deleterious than persistent low lung volumes in the atelectasis-prone rabbit lung during high-frequency oscillation. Crit Care Med 21:402, 1993.

112. Gothberg S, Parker TA, Griebel J, et al: Lung volume recruitment in lambs during high-frequency oscillatory ventilation using respiratory inductive plethysmography. Pediatr Res 49:38, 2001.

113. Sugiura M, Nakabayashi H, Vaclavik S, et al: Lung volume maintenance during high frequency jet ventilation (HFJV) improves physiological and biochemical outcome of lavaged rabbit lung [abstract]. Physiologist 33:A123, 1990.

114. Fredberg JJ, Glass GMM, Boynton BR, et al: Factors influencing mechanical performance of neonatal high-frequency ventilators. Special Communications. J Appl Physiol 62:2485, 1987.

115. Kolton M, Cattram C, Kent G, et al: Oxygenation during high-frequency ventilation compared with conventional mechanical ventilation in two models of lung injury. Anesth Analg 61:323, 1987.

116. Carlon G, Kahn R, Howland W, et al: Clinical experience with high-frequency jet ventilation. Crit Care Med 9:1, 1981.

117. Kirpalani H, Higa T, Perlman M, et al: Diagnosis and therapy of necrotizing tracheobronchitis in ventilated neonates. Crit Care Med 13:792, 1985.

118. Pietsch JB, Nagaraj HS, Groff DB, et al: Necrotizing tracheobronchitis: A new indication for emergency bronchoscopy in the neonate. J Pediatr Surg 20:391, 1985.

119. Boros SJ, Mammel MC, Lewallen PK, et al: Necrotizing tracheobronchitis: A complication of high-frequency ventilation. J Pediatr 109:95, 1986.

120. Wilson KS, Carley RB, Ophoven JP, et al: Necrotizing tracheobronchitis: A newly recognized cause of acute obstruction in mechanically ventilated neonates. Laryngoscope 97:1017, 1987.

121. Ophoven JP, Mammel MC, Gordon MJ, et al: Tracheobronchial histopathology associated with high-frequency jet ventilation. Crit Care Med 12:829, 1984.

122. Mammel MC, Ophoven JP, Lewallen PK, et al: High-frequency ventilation and tracheal injuries. Pediatrics 77:608, 1986.

123. Mammel MC, Boros SJ: Airway damage and mechanical ventilation: A review and commentary. Pediatr Pulmonol 3:443, 1987.

124. Clark RHH, Wiswell TE, Null DM, et al: Tracheal and bronchial injury in high-frequency oscillatory ventilation compared with conventional positive pressure ventilation. J Pediatr 111:114, 1987.

125. Wiswell TE, Clark RH, Null DM, et al: Tracheal and bronchial injury in high-frequency oscillatory ventilation and high-frequency flow interruption compared with conventional positive-pressure ventilation. J Pediatr 112:249, 1988.

126. Polak MJ, Donnelly WH, Bucciarelli RL: Comparison of airway pathologic lesions after high-frequency jet or conventional ventilation. Am J Dis Child 143:228, 1989.

127. Coalson JJ, deLemos RA: Pathologic features of various ventilatory strategies. Acta Anaesthesiol Scand 33(Suppl 90):108, 1989.

128. Wiswell TE, Wiswell SH: The effect of 100% oxygen on the propagation of tracheobronchial injury during high-frequency and conventional mechanical ventilation. Am J Dis Child 144:560, 1990.

129. Wiswell TE, Bley JA, Turner BS, et al: Different high-frequency ventilator strategies: Effect on the propagation of tracheobronchial histopathologic changes. Pediatrics 85:70, 1990.

130. Muller WJ; Gerjarusek S, Scherer PW: Studies of wall shear and mass transfer in a large scale model of neonatal high-frequency jet ventilation. Ann Biomed Eng 18:69, 1990.

131. Maynard RC, Wangensteen OD, Connett JE, et al: Alterations in feline tracheal permeability after mechanical ventilation. Crit Care Med 21:90, 1993.

132. Bhuta T, Henderson-Smart DJ: Elective high frequency oscillatory ventilation versus conventional ventilation in preterm infants with pulmonary dysfunction: Systematic review and meta-analyses. Pediatrics 100:1, 1997.

133. Cools F, Offringa M: Meta-analysis of elective high frequency ventilation in preterm infants with respiratory distress syndrome. Arch Dis Child Fetal Neonatal Ed 80:F15, 1999.

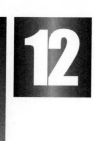

SPECIAL VENTILATORY TECHNIQUES AND MODALITIES I
Patient-Triggered Ventilation

STEVEN M. DONN, MD
MICHAEL A. BECKER, RRT

Advances in ventilator technology have extended the application of techniques that were not previously available in the neonatal intensive care unit to newborns who require mechanical ventilation for respiratory support. This chapter reviews two of these techniques: synchronized ventilation and pressure-support ventilation (PSV). These new neonatal ventilatory modalities have become popular for the management of infants with respiratory failure.

SYNCHRONIZED VENTILATION

The development and implementation of mechanical ventilation are the events most closely associated with the emergence of modern neonatal intensive care. Although assisted ventilation has been the mainstay of treatment for patients with respiratory failure of all causes, it has not been free of complications in the newborn. Although the term *assisted* ventilation has been used, mechanical ventilators that have been available since the mid-1960s have utilized intermittent mandatory ventilation (IMV) and they essentially function independently of the infant. Time-cycled, pressure-limited (TCPL) ventilators deliver a mechanical breath at a preset interval, irrespective of the spontaneous ventilatory effort of the infant. It is therefore not surprising that infants often exhibit asynchronous or dyssynchronous breathing, during which their own spontaneous breaths are out of phase with the mechanically delivered breaths.

Asynchrony may result in several deleterious effects. Efficiency of gas exchange may be impaired, when an infant attempts to exhale against positive pressure or, alternatively, when an infant attempts to inhale during the exhalation phase of the mechanical cycle.[1] Asynchrony has been shown to contribute to air trapping and pneumothorax, thus increasing pulmonary morbidity and prolonging recovery.[2] Even central nervous system function may be adversely impacted.[3] Perlman et al.[4] demonstrated that preterm infants who were breathing asynchronously with mechanical ventilation displayed tremendous variability and irregularity of both arterial blood pressure waveforms and cerebral blood flow velocity, which were associated with a high incidence of intraventricular hemorrhage. They also reported that these abnormalities could be ablated with the use of pancuronium, presumably because they prevent the infant from "fighting" against the ventilator.

Until recently, clinicians have had limited means to deal with asynchrony. One mechanical method is to reduce the arterial carbon dioxide tension ($PaCO_2$) with an increase in ventilator parameters (especially ventilatory rate and pressure) in an attempt to "capture" the infant. Alternatively, pharmacologic agents, such as sedatives, analgesics, and even anesthetics, are used to alter spontaneous breathing. Ultimately, agents such as pancuronium or curare sometimes are used to induce pharmacologic paralysis. Each of these maneuvers is not without potential risks to the infant, including barotrauma, drug toxicity, and even skeletal muscle atrophy.[5]

It seems intuitive that asynchrony might be correctable if the patient's spontaneous effort and the onset of mechanical inspiration could be coordinated. Indeed, *patient-triggered ventilation* (PTV), which achieves synchronization between spontaneous and mechanical breaths, has been in use for many years in adult and older pediatric populations. Technologic limitations precluded its use in the neonatal population until only the last decade.

Advances in microprocessor technology and ventilator design have overcome the obstacles in detecting and responding to the spontaneous effort of even the smallest preterm infants. These advances have enabled clinicians to use synchronized ventilation in the neonatal intensive care unit and have allowed the prospect of reducing pulmonary morbidity and improving outcomes for newborns who require mechanical ventilation. Synchronized ventilatory modes are characterized by the delivery of mechanical breaths in response to a signal derived from the patient representing spontaneous respiratory effort. Collectively, these modes have been referred to as PTV and include *synchronized intermittent mandatory ventilation* (SIMV), *assist/control* (A/C) *ventilation*, and PSV. Hybrid forms of ventilation are also being introduced into clinical practice.

Intermittent Mandatory Ventilation

Figure 12-1 shows the relationship between spontaneous and mechanical breaths during IMV. When synchrony occurs, it is merely a random event. Even if the infant initiates a breath simultaneously with mechanical inspiration, differing inspiratory times may result in the development of asynchrony during the expiratory phase. After only a few breaths, the infant may be exhaling against the full pressure of a mechanical inspiration.

Synchronized Intermittent Mandatory Ventilation

In SIMV, the mechanically delivered breaths are synchronized to the onset of spontaneous patient breaths. In TCPL SIMV, the patient may breathe spontaneously between mechanical breaths from the continuous bias flow in the ventilatory circuit. Figure 12-2 shows the improvement SIMV offers over IMV. Each mechanical breath is initiated in response to the onset of the patient's own respiratory effort; this results in full inspiratory synchrony. However, unless the inspiratory times are identical, the patient may terminate his or her own effort and begin exhalation while the ventilator is still in the inspiratory phase. This again results in partial asynchrony.

Assist/Control Ventilation

Additional improvement in synchronized ventilation is achieved through the use of A/C ventilation. This modality involves either the delivery of a synchronized mechanical breath each time a spontaneous patient breath meeting threshold criteria is detected (assist) or the delivery of a mechanical breath at a regular rate in the event that the patient fails to exhibit spontaneous effort (control). This is shown schematically in Figure 12-3. Note that spontaneous and mechanical breaths have been completely synchronized to the onset of inspiration; however, once again, the possibility exists that expiratory dyssynchrony will occur. This problem has been overcome with the introduction of a second signal detection system that determines when patient inspiratory effort is about to cease and then synchronizes the termination of the mechanical breath to this event. A flow-derived signal can also be used to terminate inspiration and to permit the total synchronization of spontaneous and mechanical breaths throughout the entire respiratory cycle (Fig. 12-4). The patient and ventilator are completely in phase for every breath. Breaths in which the changeover from inspiration to expiration occurs this way are said to be *flow cycled.*

Inspiration

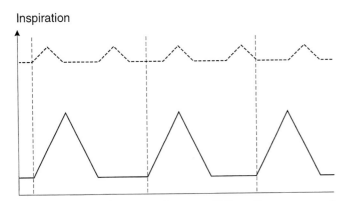

Figure 12-1. Intermittent mandatory ventilation. The *upper graph* represents spontaneous patient breaths, and the *lower graph* represents mechanical ventilator breaths. Note the random occurrence of synchrony, because patient and ventilator essentially function independently of one another. (Courtesy of David Durand, MD.)

Inspiration

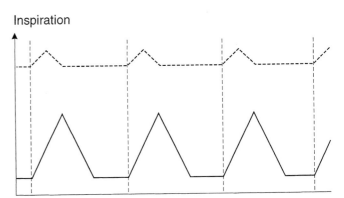

Figure 12-3. Assist/control ventilation. The *upper graph* represents spontaneous patient breaths, and the *lower graph* represents mechanical ventilator breaths. Each spontaneous breath that meets threshold criteria results in the delivery of a nearly simultaneous mechanical breath; however, expiratory asynchrony occurs when inspiratory times for the patient and ventilator are not identical. (Courtesy of David Durand, MD.)

Inspiration

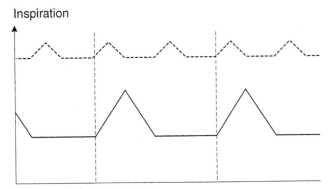

Figure 12-2. Synchronized intermittent mandatory ventilation. The *upper graph* represents spontaneous patient breaths, and the *lower graph* represents mechanical ventilator breaths. The onset of mechanical inspiration is synchronized to the onset of patient inspiration; the patient breathes spontaneously between mechanical breaths. Note that dyssynchrony can develop during the expiratory phase because the inspiratory times of the patient and ventilator differ. (Courtesy of David Durand, MD.)

Inspiration

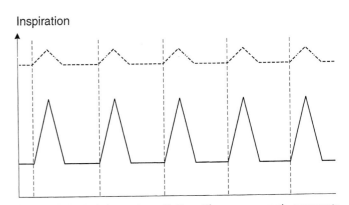

Figure 12-4. Assist/control ventilation. The *upper graph* represents spontaneous patient breaths, and the *lower graph* represents mechanical ventilator breaths. This system (such as the one incorporated in the V.I.P. BIRD infant/pediatric ventilator) synchronizes inspiration by sensing patient effort. It also synchronizes expiration by terminating inspiration in response to a decline in airway flow. This results in complete synchronization of the functioning of the baby and ventilator throughout the entire respiratory cycle. (Courtesy of David Durand, MD.)

Signal Detection

The key element involved in the success of any synchronized system is the ability to detect the onset of the spontaneous inspiratory effort of the patient and to respond immediately with the delivery of a mechanical breath. The signal "event" needs to be an accurate measure of respiratory effort, but it should minimize any artifacts that may result from other sources.

Signals have been derived from abdominal movement, thoracic impedance, and airway pressure or flow changes. Each of these has unique advantages and disadvantages, which are summarized in Table 12-1.

Detection of abdominal movement requires the use of an applanation transducer, such as the Graseby capsule, which is affixed to the abdominal wall.[6] The placement of the transducer is critical to its proper performance and often requires replacement if the patient's position changes. In addition to being subject to movement artifact (such as hiccups), this system may not work in all infants, especially those who lack paradoxical chest and abdominal movements. It is not possible to measure tidal volumes directly, and there is no expiratory synchronization. However, autocycling does not occur (see later), and the technique is relatively easy to master. The Infant Star (Infrasonics, Inc., San Diego, CA, USA) utilizes this system for its STAR SYNCH SIMV mode.

Recording of thoracic impedance signals requires placement of electronic leads on the chest wall.[7] Drying of the electrode gel and erroneous lead placement may interfere with appropriate signal detection, and tidal volume measurement is not possible. The Sechrist SAVI ventilator (Sechrist Industries, Anaheim, CA, USA) detects thoracic impedance signals.

Two methods for processing flow-derived signals presently are available. The first, incorporated into devices such as the Babylog 8000 (Dräger, Inc., Lübeck, Germany), involves the use of a hot wire anemometer to convert temperature differences to flow volumes.[8] Another method utilizes a variable orifice differential pressure transducer (pneumotachograph) for detection of minute changes in airway flow (as little as 0.2 L/min).[9] This enables the measurement of tidal volume, use of flow changes to synchronize expiration, and adjustment of trigger sensitivity to compensate for endotracheal tube leaks. The last of these features is particularly desirable because one disadvantage of flow-derived signals is autocycling, in which endotracheal tube leaks may be erroneously interpreted by the system as spontaneous effort, and this error can result in false triggering. This methodology is used in the V.I.P. BIRD Gold infant/pediatric ventilator (BIRD Products Corp., Viasys Healthcare, Palm Springs, CA, USA) shown in Figure 12-5. Use of the flow-derived signal also allows for complete inspiratory and expiratory synchronization by flow cycling. A feature referred to as *Termination Sensitivity* measures the decline in inspiratory airway flow. The clinician can adjust termination sensitivity to end a mechanical breath when flow declines to 0% to 25% of peak flow (Fig. 12-6). This is clinically advantageous in preventing air trapping and inversion of the inspiratory/expiratory ratio when a baby is breathing very rapidly; conversely, it ensures an adequate inspiratory time when the infant is breathing slowly. Clinicians should be aware of the distinction between flow triggering (in which changes in airway flow initiate a mechanical breath) and flow cycling (in which changes in airway flow terminate the inspiratory phase of a mechanical breath).

Changes in airway pressure may create a signal that can be used to trigger ventilation.[10] One such system is incorporated in the Newport Wave E200 ventilator (Newport Medical Instruments, Inc. Newport Beach, CA, USA). This device also offers SIMV and A/C ventilation. Triggering occurs as a result of the patient's spontaneous effort, which decreases airway pressure to the selected sensitivity level (0 to +5 cm H_2O).

Clinical Problems

Although PTV represents a major advance in technology, several potential clinical problems may arise with its use. False triggering may occur under several circumstances. Systems utilizing abdominal movement, for instance, may inappropriately respond to nonrespiratory motion, such as hiccups (which also can be problematic for flow and pressure triggering). Systems that use changes in airway pressure or flow to detect inspiratory effort are prone to autocycling, which results in the inadvertent delivery of a mechanical breath. Autocycling may result from the presence of water in the ventilator circuit or from endotracheal tube leaks. Among the three flow-triggered ventilators, the V.I.P. BIRD has the lowest rate of autocycling from endotracheal tube leaks.[11] Autocycling also can occur with detection of cardiac impulses by systems that trigger from changes in thoracic impedance.[7]

TABLE 12-1.   Patient-Triggered Ventilation: Trigger Signals

Signal	Detector	Typical Response Times (msec)	Advantages	Disadvantages
Abdominal motion	Applanation transducer (Graseby capsule)	40–60	Ease of use; no autocycling; one sensitivity setting only	Placement critical; requires paradoxic chest/abdomen movement; artifactual triggering; no tidal volume measurements
Airway flow	Differential variable orifice	25–50	Ease of use; expiratory synchrony; measures tidal volumes and minute ventilation	Autocycling (lower); patient must exceed trigger pressure transducer
	Heated wire anemometer	5–100	Ease of use; measures tidal volumes and minute ventilation	Autocycling (higher); patient must exceed trigger threshold
Airway pressure	Pressure transducer	40–100	Ease of use	Higher trigger threshold
Thoracic impedance	Electrocardiogram leads	40–80	Ease of use; active expiration terminates inspiratory cycle	Erroneous lead placement; drying of contact gel; no tidal volume measurements

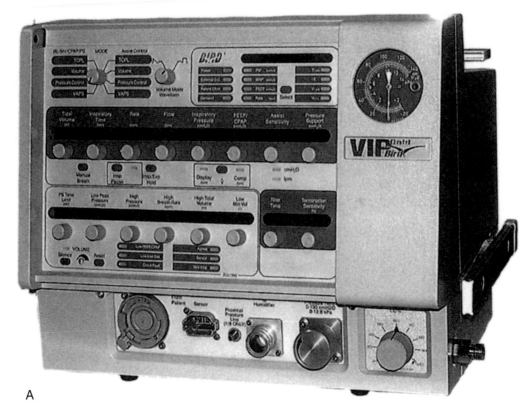

A

VIP GOLD BIRD

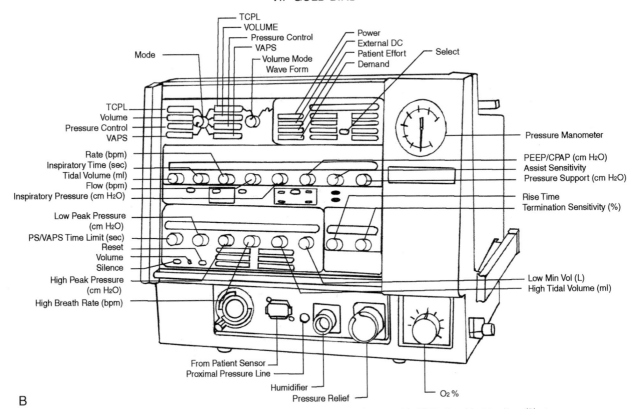

B

Figure 12-5. *A,* V.I.P. BIRD Gold infant/pediatric ventilator shown with BIRD Graphic Monitor. (Photo Courtesy of Bird Products Corp., Viasys Healthcare, Palm Springs, CA, USA.) *B,* Diagram of front panel.

More important, failure of a ventilator to trigger represents a significant clinical problem. It can occur under any circumstance in which the patient does not achieve threshold sensitivity, or it may be a system mechanical problem. Improper placement of the Graseby capsule or chest leads, failure of detection of very small spontaneous breaths, or obstruction or occlusion of transducers all may result in failure to detect patient effort.

Some of the current ventilators appear to perform better in one mode than another. The Babylog 8000, for example, was shown to have a higher reliability of triggering in SIMV than in A/C ventilation. However, it also produces more asynchronous breathing in SIMV than either the Bear Cub/CEM (Bear Medical Systems, Viasys Healthcare) or the Infant Star with STAR SYNCH SIMV.[8] Refinements in computer software may overcome many of these problems in the near future.

Patient-triggered infant ventilators are listed in Table 12-2. In addition to available modes and type of signal detector, other features are described.

Clinical Applications

Virtually every form of SIMV or A/C ventilation has been shown to improve gas exchange and eliminate or markedly decrease asynchronous ventilation in the newborn infant. Figure 12-7 shows the impact of synchronization on pulmonary mechanics testing. Note that during IMV (Fig. 12-7A), pressure-volume and flow-volume loops demonstrate tremendous breath-to-breath variability in delivered tidal volumes, despite relatively constant peak inspiratory pressures. During SIMV (Fig. 12-7B), there is considerable improvement in the consistency of the mechanical breaths. When the ventilatory mode is switched to A/C (Fig. 12-7C) on the V.I.P. BIRD, complete synchronization is achieved, and each breath is nearly identical. These mechanical changes have been shown to result in improved oxygenation, but without concomitant increases in mean airway pressure and without adverse effects on ventilation. In addition, some ventilators now offer PSV combined with pressure-targeted and volume-targeted SIMV to attain full synchronization during spontaneous breathing that is mechanically supported.

Early clinical experience with PTV suggested that prolonged support of the very-low-birthweight infant (gestational age less than 28 weeks) might not be feasible because of patient fatigue. Mitchell et al.[12] reported a clinical observation of 22 preterm infants treated consecutively with the

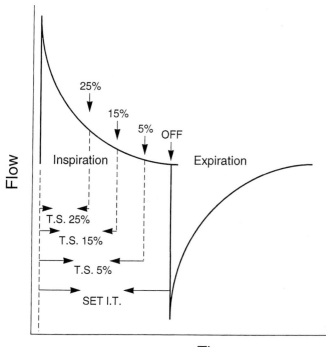

Figure 12-6. Termination sensitivity feature of the V.I.P. BIRD ventilator. The graph represents relationship between flow and time for one ventilator cycle. Termination sensitivity (T.S.) refers to a point on the inspiratory flow curve at which expiration is triggered. The higher the termination sensitivity setting, the shorter the inspiratory time (I.T.); conversely, the lower the termination sensitivity setting, the longer the inspiratory time.

TABLE 12-2.   Patient-Triggered Infant Ventilators

Ventilator	Manufacturer	Modes	Signal	Comments
Babylog 8000	Dräger (Lübeck, Germany)	A/C, SIMV	Airway flow	Heated wire anemometer; graphic displays
Bear Cub/CEM	Bear Medical Systems (Riverside, CA, USA)	A/C, SIMV	Airway flow	Heated wire anemometer; backup ventilation for continuous positive airway pressure mode; requires ventilation monitor
Infant Star/STAR SYNC	Infrasonics (San Diego, CA, USA)	A/C, SIMV	Abdominal motion	Graseby capsule; no trigger sensitivity adjustment; audible placement signal
Newport Wave E200	Newport Medical Instruments (Newport Beach, CA, USA)	A/C, SIMV	Airway pressure	Volume-control and pressure-control modes; pressure support ventilation; sigh function; Compass monitor
Sechrist/SAVI	Sechrist Industries (Anaheim, CA, USA)	A/C	Thoracic impedance	Uses chest leads of Hewlett-Packard 78801-8 cardiorespiratory monitor; maximum control rate of 30 breaths/min
SLE HV2000	Specialized Laboratory Equipment (Surrey, England)	A/C, SIMV	Airway pressure	Airway transducer (not yet available in the United States)
V.I.P. BIRD	Bird Products Corp. (Palm Springs, CA, USA)	A/C, SIMV	Airway flow	Variable orifice differential pressure transducer; volume-controlled ventilation; pressure-support ventilation; requires partner monitor; optional graphic display monitor

A/C, assist/control; SIMV, synchronous intermittent mandatory ventilation.

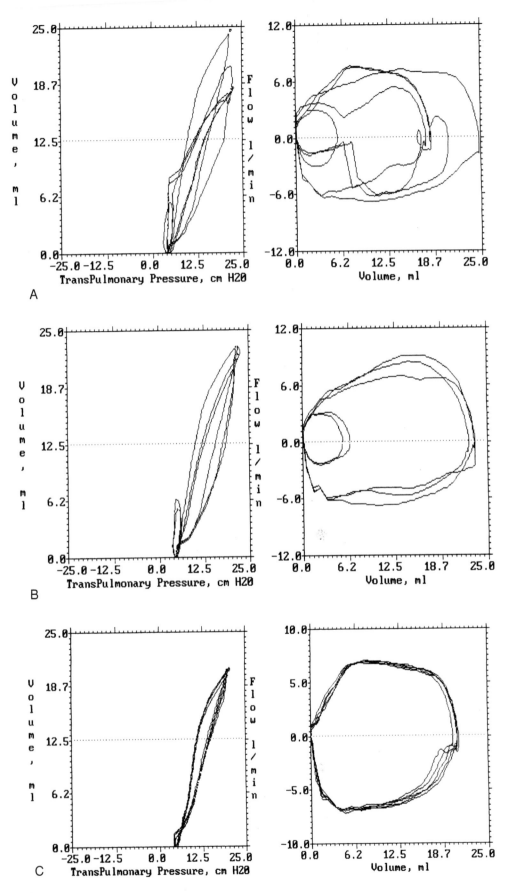

Figure 12-7. Impact of synchronization on pulmonary mechanics. *A,* Pressure-volume and flow-volume relationships during intermittent mandatory ventilation. Note the inconsistency of tidal volume delivery despite nearly identical peak inspiratory pressures for each breath. This demonstrates an effect of asynchrony. *B,* Pressure-volume and flow-volume relationships during synchronized intermittent mandatory ventilation. Note the differences between spontaneous (smaller) and mechanical (larger) breaths. Mechanical breaths are nearly identical to one another as a result of synchrony. *C,* Pressure-volume and flow-volume relationships during assist/control ventilation. Because each spontaneous breath results in the simultaneous delivery of a mechanical breath, a single reproducible loop representing total synchrony between infant and ventilator is created.

SLE 250 Newborn ventilator in the patient-triggered mode. The trigger threshold of the device was a change in flow exceeding 0.4 L/min. A control breath was delivered in the event of the occurrence of apnea lasting 7 seconds (thus, an effective control rate of only 8.5 breaths/min). Eight of the 22 infants could not tolerate PTV. The median gestational age was 27 weeks and the median birthweight was 1080 g in this group compared with 32 weeks and 1600 g, respectively, in the successfully treated group.[12] In a follow-up study by Hird and Greenough,[13] 56 infants with a median gestational age of 29 weeks were examined for the causes of failure of PTV. Factors found to affect PTV adversely included development of expiratory asynchrony, long trigger delays, very short inspiratory times, and use of PTV early in the course of disease.[13] These investigators also compared the Dräger Babylog 8000 ventilator with the SLE 250 Newborn system and found a shorter trigger delay in the former. Again, difficulty was encountered in maintaining support of infants with a gestational age less than 28 weeks because of a lack of sustained spontaneous breathing during the acute phases of respiratory distress syndrome.[14]

More recent technologic advances appear to have solved the problem of providing adequate support for the extremely preterm infant. Improvements in trigger sensitivity and provision of an adequate control rate during A/C ventilation have extended the benefits of synchrony to even the smallest patients. Visveshwara et al.[7] summarized a 3-year experience with PTV using a prototype of the Sechrist SAVI, which utilizes thoracic impedance to both initiate and terminate mechanical breaths. Although this experience was nonrandomized and historically controlled, PTV was associated with a shorter duration of mechanical ventilation and oxygen therapy. It also was associated with a decreased incidence of severe intraventricular hemorrhage. Infants who were included in this observation had birthweights that ranged from 450 to 1250 g. Among the six infants who could not be maintained on PTV, two had apnea (one from sepsis and one from grade IV intraventricular hemorrhage), one had seizures, and three had insufficient respiratory effort.[7]

Servant et al.[9] investigated the prototype flow synchronizer that eventually was incorporated into the V.I.P. BIRD infant/pediatric ventilator.[9] This study examined the safety and feasibility of applying flow-synchronized A/C ventilation to a group of preterm infants in the recovery phase of respiratory distress syndrome. Patients weighing 480 to 1400 g were studied during consecutive 1-hour periods of IMV, A/C ventilation, and IMV and were compared for multiple variables. During flow-synchronized A/C ventilation, infants exhibited a higher rate of mechanical breaths (as a result of triggering) and improved oxygenation (at the same mean airway pressure); no adverse effects on ventilation, tidal volume, or vital signs were seen. The study also evaluated the function of an expiratory trigger, which stopped the inspiratory phase of a mechanical breath when inspiratory flow decreased to 25% of peak flow. This enabled complete synchronization, even in expiration. When the expiratory trigger function is utilized, the patient sets his or her own inspiratory time.

A significant observation of this study was the relatively short inspiratory times exhibited by the patients. The smaller a baby was, the shorter the inspiratory time he or she demonstrated. The 480 g infant consistently triggered expiration after inspiratory times of only 0.15 to 0.18 seconds. The flow syn-

chronizer used in this study responded to changes in airway flow of 0.2 L/min; the transducer weighed only 11.8 g and increased ventilatory dead space by only 0.5 to 0.8 mL.[9]

The prototype flow synchronizer subsequently was incorporated into the currently available V.I.P. BIRD ventilator with one modification. Termination sensitivity, fixed at 25% on the prototype, was made adjustable from 0% to 25% in 5% increments. This enables the clinician to tailor inspiratory times to each individual patient's needs. For instance, if an infant is breathing rapidly, longer inspiratory times increase the risk of air trapping and inversion of the inspiratory/expiratory ratio. By selecting a higher termination sensitivity, inspiration is shortened. Figure 12-6 shows the relationship between termination sensitivity and inspiratory time.

Several randomized controlled trials have examined the impact of PTV on preterm infants with respiratory distress syndrome. The first study, conducted by Chan and Greenough,[15] randomized 40 infants to either PTV (SLE HV 2000 ventilator, Specialized Laboratory Equipment, Surrey, England) or IMV *after* the acute phase of respiratory distress syndrome to determine which modality provided more rapid weaning. Infants were randomized after they had been weaned to a ventilatory rate of 40 breaths/min (from 60 breaths/min) at constant peak pressure and inspiratory time. Further weaning was accomplished with a reduction in peak inspiratory pressure in the PTV group and with a reduction in ventilatory rate in the IMV group. PTV resulted in a 50% reduction in the duration of time from weaning to the first extubation. Three patients, all less than 28 weeks of gestation, did not tolerate PTV and were switched to IMV. The investigators concluded that PTV is more advantageous than IMV for weaning preterm infants with a gestational age greater than 27 weeks.[15]

A similar study performed by Donn et al.[16] examined the impact of PTV and IMV on 30 infants weighing from 1100 to 1500 g who were randomized at the *start* of treatment for respiratory distress syndrome. Entry criteria included the need for mechanical ventilation and severity of disease sufficient to warrant surfactant replacement therapy. After enrollment, patients were randomized to PTV using the V.I.P. BIRD in the A/C mode or to conventional IMV. Groups were demographically and medically comparable. Infants randomized to PTV had a much shorter time to extubation (mean 119 hours; range 15 to 650 hours) than those randomized to conventional IMV (mean 271 hours; range 17 to 746 hours) ($P = .0152$, Mann-Whitney U-test). Although the sample sizes were small, trends suggested a decreased incidence of chronic lung disease in the PTV group. Further study is necessary to confirm this. In the studies by Chan et al. and Donn et al., no increases in acute ventilator complications were observed in the groups that received the new PTV therapy. Donn et al. also reported a statistically significant reduction of approximately $4400 per patient in hospital costs for infants assigned to PTV.[16]

A large, multicenter, open trial of PTV was conducted by Baumer.[17] Although the results of this trial did not show benefits of PTV compared to conventional TCPL IMV, the study had numerous methodologic design flaws, limited investigator experience, and variable devices. The higher incidence of pneumothorax in the group treated with PTV further suggests that an inappropriate weaning strategy was used.[18] A single center study performed by Beresford et al.,[19] using the SLE ventilator, did not report an increased incidence of air leak.

Whereas most of the studies have demonstrated short-term benefits of synchronized ventilation, the onus of future investigation will be to show long-term advantages, particularly improved pulmonary and neurologic outcomes. Other issues will need to be addressed first, including the optimal triggering system and weaning strategy.[20]

PRESSURE-SUPPORT VENTILATION

Since before the mid-1970s, continuous-flow TCPL ventilation has been the primary method of ventilation for newborns. Interestingly, however, the first ventilator designed specifically for infants was a volume-cycled ventilator that probably was patterned after adult ventilators. Even at that time, there was an awareness that infants had specific ventilation needs that could not be met with the use of existing adult ventilators, despite many attempts by clinicians to modify these devices. The design of an infant volume ventilator addressed some of the problems that previously existed, effecting improvement in response time, greater respiratory rates, and reduction in system and circuit compliance. However, technologic limitations included triggering difficulties, inadequate monitoring, and inability to wean with a slow consistent approach. Further attempts at volume-cycled ventilation were abandoned in favor of a system (TCPL) that did not require triggering and delivered a constant pressure, which was easier to control and monitor than the small tidal volumes needed by the newborn. TCPL IMV provided continuous bias flow from which the infant could breathe spontaneously, allowing a consistent approach to weaning.

The 1990s began a "new era" in infant ventilation. The V.I.P. BIRD infant/pediatric ventilator was introduced, which not only provided TCPL but also allowed the clinician to select volume-targeted ventilation modes. The difference between volume ventilation in the late 1960s and the 1990s is remarkable. The development of microprocessor technology and the availability of accurate flow and pressure transducers have made significant improvements possible in ventilator design and performance. In conjunction with engineering developments, enhancements in ventilator modalities included SIMV and PSV, which were first introduced in 1981.[21] Several ventilators using these newer modes of ventilation currently are available for neonatal application. Discussion of volume-controlled ventilation is beyond the scope of this chapter (see Chapter 10); however, PSV, another form of PTV, is addressed in the following section.

Description and Classification

Pressure support is a patient-triggered, pressure-limited, flow-cycled mode of ventilation designed to assist a patient's spontaneous effort with a pressure "boost." Pressure support can be used in conjunction with other techniques, such as volume-targeted SIMV, or it can be applied independently. If PSV is the only form of ventilation, a reliable intrinsic respiratory drive is essential because there is no true backup system on most ventilators. Pressure support is applied during weaning to reduce the imposed work of breathing created by resistive endotracheal tubes, the ventilator circuit, and the demand valve. At the highest level of pressure support, known as PS$_{MAX}$, complete ventilatory support (i.e., a full tidal volume breath) is provided and respiratory muscle work is reduced to almost zero.[22]

The usual pressure-support system is flow or pressure triggered. The patient initiates an inspiratory effort that results in an acceleration of airway flow or a deflection of pressure below the baseline. The trigger sensitivity is set by the clinician to the lowest possible level so that autocycling can be avoided. In ventilators that monitor pressure proximally, triggering sensitivity may be improved; this is in contrast to ventilators that sense pressure from within the ventilator, on either the inspiratory or expiratory side.[23] Further improvement in triggering can be achieved if pressure is sensed at the distal tip of an endotracheal tube.[24] Another factor that can affect trigger sensitivity is the stability of the baseline pressure or positive end-expiratory pressure (PEEP). In pressure-triggered systems, if an airway leak is present, the baseline may drift. This could result in autocycling and necessitates setting the trigger sensitivity to a higher level. Ventilators that incorporate a leak compensation system have improved sensitivity. Flow triggering, available with some ventilators, is thought to reduce the lag time for the delivery of pressure support.[21] Although the baseline may not drift, trigger sensitivity may need to be adjusted to avoid autocycling.

Once the breath is triggered, flow is delivered to the patient airway and pressure rises rather quickly to the selected pressure-support setting. The patient's effort is the primary determinant of the amount of flow delivery that affects the increased time of pressure. Other factors that are controlled by the ventilator include peak flow availability, the pressure-support setting, and the specific pressure-support algorithm applied by the ventilator. Earlier pressure-support systems proved inadequate when applied to patients who had low compliance, high resistance, or who required smaller endotracheal tubes. Problems associated with pressure overshoot and premature termination have been addressed, especially with ventilators designed for use on small infants and children. Flow acceleration of pressure-support breaths has even been modified in newer systems. Algorithms have been incorporated for matching flow delivery for low-compliance, high-resistance applications. A feature on some newer ventilators is an adjustable inspiratory rise time.[21] An increase in inspiratory rise time lessens the flow/pressure increase and may be especially beneficial for neonatal patients. The end of a pressure-support breath can also be determined by the patient because of predetermined variables incorporated within the ventilator. The breath is flow-cycled, meaning that when the inspiratory flow decreases by a certain percentage (usually 75% of peak), inspiration ends. This flow percentage varies among different ventilators; for those designed to be used in the infant population, the endpoint may need to be higher (e.g., 90% to 95%). The occurrence of a very short inspiratory time secondary to an early termination may result in ineffective tidal volume delivery. Every ventilator that has pressure-support capabilities has another mechanism for breath termination in addition to flow (usually an adjustable inspiratory time limit). If an airway leak is present, it may not be possible for breaths to be flow-terminated.

Some of the most recent ventilator designs have incorporated pressure support with a guaranteed minimum tidal volume. The terminology and algorithms for this capability vary; examples include volume-assured pressure support (VAPS, BIRD Products Corp., Viasys Healthcare, Palm Springs, CA, USA) and volume support (Servo 900C, Siemens-Elema AB, Solna, Sweden). These variations in pressure support have been designed to improve patient safety by maintaining a minimum tidal volume while satisfying the patient's demand. Another important safety feature available with some systems is backup mandatory ventilation in the event of apnea, when pressure support is the only form of ventilation.

Volume-Assured Pressure Support

VAPS, a very recent development in neonatal ventilation, is available on the V.I.P. BIRD Gold infant/pediatric ventilator. This is a hybrid form of ventilation that combines features of PSV and volume-targeted ventilation. VAPS can be used alone or in conjunction with other mechanical modes. VAPS breaths begin as pressure-supported breaths. These breaths may be patient-initiated or mechanically-initiated and have all the features of a PSV breath. When inspiratory flow decelerates to the minimal set flow, delivered tidal volume is measured. If it matches or exceeds the minimal desired tidal volume, the breath will be terminated according to the usual pressure-support algorithm. If the minimal desired tidal volume has not been met, however, the breath will transition to a volume-targeted breath by prolonging the inspiratory phase at a constant flow rate, creating the typical square wave flow pattern until the desired tidal volume is delivered (Fig. 12-8). This technique enables full tidal volume delivery in the face of decreasing pulmonary compliance, patient effort, or patient fatigue. It holds great potential for use in weaning or in patients with irregular respiratory drive or rapidly changing compliance.[25]

Early Clinical Experience

Pressure support appears to be attracting increased attention, not only as an alternative weaning mode but also as a primary modality in the treatment of patients with acute and chronic ventilatory failure. PSV was introduced in the early 1980s to the European medical community. The Servo 900C was one of the first ventilators to incorporate this mode of ventilation. Clinical and technical research on PSV was reported somewhat later; the first case report of its use appeared in 1985. This study reported improved mixed venous blood oxygen saturation and decreased oxygen consumption in patients receiving SIMV with pressure support compared with those receiving only SIMV.[24] Other studies have reported reductions in spontaneous respiratory rates,[26] an increase in minute volumes,[27] a decrease in the time to extubation in postoperative thoracic surgery patients,[27] and patient preference for pressure support over SIMV (in communicative patients).[26] Lower work of breathing with PSV is thought to be the reason for improvement. It has been reported that work of breathing through an artificial airway increases by 34% to 154% for each 1-mm reduction in internal diameter in the airway, depending on the minute ventilation.[28] It also has been proved that PSV counteracts the effects of work of breathing imposed by artificial airways, ventilator circuits, and demand systems.[29–32] Furthermore, interest in system design has increased. Two professional conferences, held in 1990 and 1991, focused exclusively on triggering and pressure-support delivery mechanisms.[33,34] As a result of improvement in ventilator design in the last several years, many clinicians are interested in the role pressure support might play in the neonatal intensive care unit. Neonatal specialists are applying pressure support to infants and achieving some success.

Clinical Applications

The application of PSV can accomplish one of two things: a patient may either (1) acquire a greater tidal volume with the same amount of effort or (2) achieve a similar tidal volume with less effort.[35] One physiologic advantage to this alternative

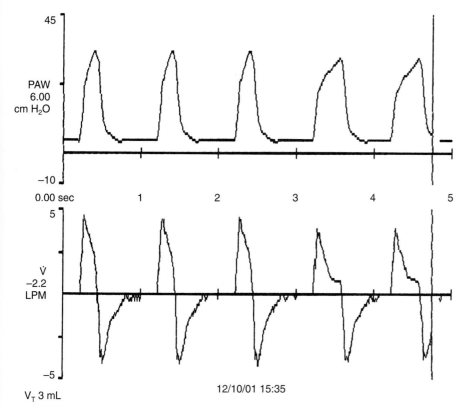

Figure 12-8. Volume-assured pressure support (VAPS). The first three breaths are pure pressure support breaths and show pattern of flow cycling on the flow waveform. The peak inspiratory pressure was reduced slightly for the last two breaths, where VAPS occurs. Because minimal desired tidal volume has not been delivered by the time flow decelerates to 3.0 LPM (liters per minute) (set level), the breath transitions to a volume-targeted breath by prolongation of inspiratory time at this minimal flow rate until additional volume is delivered. Note transitional "shoulder" as flow waveform changes to square wave.

ventilatory modality is that it more closely mimics a spontaneous breath. The patient initiates inspiration and has control of flow, volume, and inspiratory time. With SIMV, the patient may initiate inspiration, but flow, tidal volume, and inspiratory time are preset. Figure 12-9 shows the impact of PSV on respiratory waveforms. Figure 12-9A displays a series of breaths while the patient is receiving volume-cycled SIMV. Figure 12-9B shows visible improvement in flow and tidal volume delivery during spontaneous breaths with the addition of PSV. It is understandable that the breathing pattern may appear to be more comfortable when it more closely matches the patient's own ventilatory drive.

Tidal volumes that provide full support and require a minimum of work can be delivered, usually in the range from 8 to 10 mL/kg. Weaning is accomplished by progressively decreasing the level of pressure support. For endurance conditioning of the respiratory muscles without excessive work, tidal volumes of 4 to 8 mL/kg may be more appropriate. In the neonatal patient, it probably is not necessary to decrease pressure-support levels below 10 cm H_2O. At this point, the work of breathing caused by the highly resistive airway is considerably reduced, and the tidal volume that is generated is the result of patient effort rather than of pressure delivery.

With the application of PSV to the newborn, several important factors must be observed, including triggering and synchrony, inspiratory time, and tidal volume. Reliable patient effort is very important, but of equal concern is the ability of the infant to consistently trigger the system and synchronize his or her breathing with the ventilator. Because of lower compliance and greater resistance, the breath may be prematurely terminated. This could result in an inspiratory time that is too short for adequate tidal volume delivery. Continuous breath-to-breath display of inspiratory time and tidal volume also are important. Tidal volume measurement is more accurate if it is done at the proximal airway. Also, pressure triggering may be more consistent if the pressure is measured at the proximal airway.

There are still limitations in neonatal PSV, usually because of triggering and the breath delivery algorithm. In most cases, pressure support is used as a weaning mode once volume-targeted SIMV has been initiated. A series of successful cases of neonatal volume-cycled ventilation followed by PSV has been reported. Patient profiles included birthweights from 2480 to 4300 g, gestational ages of 36 to 40 weeks, diagnoses of respiratory distress syndrome, streptococcal (group B) sepsis, meconium aspiration syndrome, and persistent pulmonary

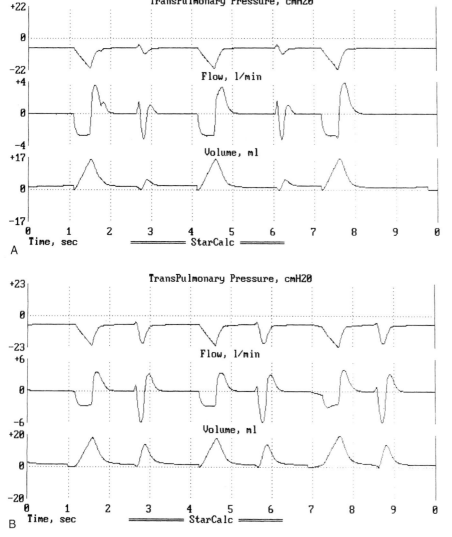

Figure 12-9. Pressure-support ventilation. *A,* Patient is receiving volume-cycled synchronous intermittent mandatory ventilation. *B,* Pressure-support ventilation is added. Note the improvement in flow and in the delivery of tidal volume during spontaneous breaths.

hypertension of the newborn. Each infant required high ventilatory support [mean airway pressure >12 cm H_2O; fraction of inspired oxygen (FIO_2) range 0.7 to 1.0)]. Initially, the indication for volume-targeted ventilation was a rescue approach; TCPL was not providing effective oxygenation. The oxygenation index was significantly reduced when patients were switched from TCPL (23.6) to volume-controlled ventilation (13.6) at virtually identical airway pressures. The infants were placed on volume-targeted SIMV with PSV as soon as the effects of elective paralytics were no longer evident and spontaneous respiratory effort was exhibited. Each patient was promptly weaned in this modality; none developed air leaks or radiographic signs of chronic lung changes.[36] PSV was also used during the weaning phases of a clinical trial that compared the efficacy of volume-targeted ventilation with pressure-limited ventilation in 50 infants with respiratory distress syndrome who weighed more than 1200 g. Infants assigned to volume-targeted A/C and weaned in volume-targeted SIMV and PSV met the success criteria significantly faster than infants kept in pressure-limited A/C, although it is not clear whether the difference is attributable to the acute phase, the chronic phase, or both.[37]

Other applications of PSV include the treatment of infants who are chronically ventilator dependent and the management of infants with bronchopulmonary dysplasia. As long as the infant has a reliable respiratory effort, this mode of ventilation seems to satisfy the greater flow demands imposed by these disease entities.

Equipment

The features of three ventilators with pressure-support capabilities and the capacity for neonatal ventilation are summarized in Table 12-3.

V.I.P. BIRD Gold

The V.I.P. BIRD Gold ventilator (Fig. 12-5) was designed specifically for use in the infant and pediatric populations. Incorporation of both pressure-targeted and volume-targeted modes provides the neonatal clinician with a choice of options that previously was not available on a single infant ventilator. All modes, including PSV, are flow triggered at the proximal airway when the neonatal sensor is used. For more consistent triggering, the clinician can adjust trigger sensitivity to the minimum setting without the fear of autocycling, even when an airway leak is present.

Pressure support is available with various SIMV applications and is adjustable to 50 cm H_2O above the baseline. The peak inspiratory pressure, measured at the proximal airway, is equal to the sum of the pressure support and PEEP. A flow rate of up to 120 L/min is available in PSV. This ventilator now has a clinician-adjustable inspiratory rise time. The pressure-support system on the V.I.P. BIRD Gold adapts flow acceleration to reduce the incidence of pressure overshoot and premature termination in patients with low compliance and high resistance. It can be adjusted further by manipulating the inspiratory rise time. Termination criteria of a pressure-support breath have also been enhanced for the neonatal population. The percentage at which a breath is terminated varies with the expiratory tidal volume measurement at the proximal airway, as shown in Table 12-4. This algorithm reduces the occurrence

of premature termination in neonatal patients, resulting in an appropriate inspiratory time and improved tidal volume delivery. The V.I.P. BIRD Gold also has a variable inspiratory time limit, adjustable from 0.1 to 3.0 seconds, in the event that a leak prevents flow from decreasing to the termination criteria. Inspiratory time can be continuously displayed and is updated on a breath-to-breath basis. Proximal tidal volume and minute ventilation also are displayed.

Newport Wave E200

The Newport Wave E200 ventilator (Fig. 12-10) is designed to be used in the neonatal, pediatric, and adult populations. Ventilation modes include volume and pressure control; pressure support is available in SIMV with either of these modes. Breaths are triggered by pressure changes at the proximal airway. Pressure support is adjustable from 0 to 60 cm H_2O above the PEEP setting. The maximum flow availability of a pressure-support breath is 150 L/min. The Newport Wave E200 has been designed to overcome some of the previous problems associated with pressure support, including those related to improvement of triggering and response time, baseline stability, "educated" inspiratory flow delivery, and appropriate breath termination.

Bias flow, which is adjustable from 0 to 30 L/min, is activated between mechanical breaths. A mechanical breath is delivered only when the patient's effort exceeds the bias flow, deflecting the pressure below the sensitivity threshold. When adjusting the proper setting for bias flow, triggering capability must be considered. When set appropriately, bias flow offers two advantages: (1) it decreases the response time of the servoid valve by 75%, which improves patient-ventilator synchrony and may provide greater patient comfort; and (2) it stabilizes the baseline, helping to prevent autocycling.

Another feature incorporated into the Newport Wave E200 is Learning Logic and Predictive Control. Because patients have a wide variation in compliance, resistance, and inspiratory flow demands as a result of disease process, weight, and endotracheal tube diameter, it is important for the ventilator to interact with the patient. Work of breathing may be excessive because of inadequate or excessive flow delivery. With Learning Logic and Predictive Control, the flow and pressure transducers, microprocessor, and servoid valve interact dynamically, adjusting flow delivery to meet the patient's needs.

The termination criteria for a pressure-support breath are based on a complex calculation that takes into consideration peak flow and inspiratory time. The function of the built-in algorithm is the prevention of premature termination or the prolonged delivery of pressure-support breaths in the event of an airway leak. Other backup parameters that may end a pressure-support breath are an inspiratory time longer than 3.0 seconds, an airway pressure exceeding the set pressure level by greater than 2.0 cm H_2O, or a tidal volume greater than 4.0 L. The Newport Wave E200 monitors inspiratory tidal volume (calculated from flow and inspiratory times) and peak inspiratory flow. There is no form of backup ventilation; however, alarms for high and low inspiratory minute ventilation are included. An optional monitor, called the Compass, also is available. This monitor measures exhaled tidal volume, FIO_2, and peak expiratory flow and includes alarms for FIO_2 and exhaled minute volume.

TABLE 12-3.   Infant Ventilators That Provide Pressure-Support Ventilation

Ventilator	PSV Modes	Trigger Signal	PSV Range (cm H_2O)	Flow Range	Cycling Criteria (L/min)	Alarms	Ventilation Guarantee	Monitoring	Other
V.I.P. BIRD	SIMV volume	Proximal pressure	0–50	0–120	Flow cycling; varies with set Vt; adjustable Ti backup	Apnea; low/high pressure; minute volume	No	I/E Vt; Ve; peak flow; Ti; Paw	Leak compensation; rise time auto-adjusted for low compliance and high resistance
V.I.P. BIRD Gold	SIMV volume, SIMV TCPL, SIMV pressure control, VAPS	Distal flow or proximal pressure (pediatric flow sensor)	0–50	0–120	Flow cycling; varies with exhaled Vt (see Table 12-4); The user sets a maximum inspiratory time limit	High pressure; high breath rate; high tidal volume; low minute ventilation	No, except in VAPS, where a minimal Vt and rate is guaranteed	Peak inspiratory pressure, mean airway pressure, PEEP, rate, inspiratory time, I/E, Vt (mL), minute ventilation (L)	Rise time is set by the user to adjust the acceleration of flow
Newport Wave	SIMV volume/ pressure control	Proximal pressure	0–60	0–150	Flow cycling (a function of peak flow and Ti); backup cycling: Ti > 3.0 sec, >2 cm H_2O over set pressure	Low/high pressure; minute volume	No	I/E Vt; minute volume; peak flow, Paw	Bias flow for leaks; Learning Logic and Predictive Control for control improved flow delivery
Servo 300	SIMV volume/ pressure control	Pressure/flow	0–100	0–200	Flow cycles at 5% of peak flow; backup is 80% of total cycle time	Apnea; low pressure; Pressure; low/high minute volume	Yes, in volume support	I/E; Vt; Ve; Paw	Bias flow; adjustable rise time

I/E, inspiratory-to-expiratory ratio; Paw, mean airway pressure; PEEP, positive end-expiratory pressure; PSV, pressure-support ventilation; SIMV, synchronized intermittent mandatory ventilation; TCPL, time-cycled pressure-limited; Ti, inspiratory time; VAPS, volume-assured pressure support; Ve, expired minute ventilation; Vt, tidal volume.

TABLE 12-4. Termination Criteria for Pressure-Support Ventilation with the V.I.P. BIRD Infant/Pediatric Ventilator

Exhaled VT (mL)	Termination Criteria
0–50	5% of peak flow
50–200	5%–25% of peak flow*
>200	25% of peak flow

*Percentage increases linearly with delivered VT.
Data from Bird Products Corp., Viasys Healthcare, Palm Springs, CA, USA.

Servo 300A

The Servo 300A (Siemens-Elema AB) is a ventilator designed to be used in patients of all ages. Pressure support may be activated in SIMV using either volume control or pressure control. In addition, the pressure-support mode can be used alone. Breaths may be triggered by either flow or pressure. The sensitivity varies with the range setting (neonatal, pediatric, or adult). The flow trigger sensitivity for the neonate ranges from 0.17 to 0.5 L/min, and for the pediatric patient ranges from 0.3 to 1.0 L/min. The clinician can make adjustments in flow sensitivity by rotating the sensitivity control knob within a specific area. If a leak is present, flow triggering may result in autocycling. For situations in which decreased sensitivity is required, the sensitivity selector may be set to a specific pressure (e.g., 1.0 cm H_2O); the patient must draw through the continuous flow the amount of pressure that is below PEEP. Sensing of patient effort, using either flow or pressure signals, occurs within the machine on the expiratory side.

The pressure-support level is adjustable from 0 to 100 cm H_2O, with a maximum peak flow availability dependent on the patient: 13 L/min for newborns, 33 L/min for children, and 200 L/min for adults. Continuous flow is available during expiration so that a stable baseline can be maintained in the presence of an airway leak. The amount of flow present also depends on the range selection, which is 0.5 L/min for newborns, 1.0 L/min for children, and 2.0 L/min for adults.

The Servo 300A has a rise time adjustment that alters the flow and pressure delivery of a breath given in any mode, including PSV. When the rise time is set at zero, the flow and pressure increase instantaneously at the start of inspiration. The rise time can be increased in 1% increments to a maximum of 10% of the preset breath cycle time. This may improve patient comfort by slowing the flow and pressure delivery, thereby preventing overshoot.

Flow termination occurs for pressure-support breaths when the inspiratory flow decreases to 5% of the peak flow. The breath also may be terminated if the inspiratory time reaches 80% of the total cycle time. Inspiratory and expiratory tidal volumes are monitored by pneumotachographs within the ventilator. Alarms for high and low minute volumes, as well as for apnea, are included.

Another spontaneous breathing mode similar to pressure support, called *volume support,* is available on the Servo 300A. A preset tidal/minute volume is selected, as is an expected spontaneous rate. The inspiratory pressure is regulated to a specific level on the basis of the pressure/volume calculation for the previous breath compared with the preset tidal/minute volume. If the patient breathes above or below the preset volume, the inspi-

ratory pressure changes accordingly. If the breathing frequency drops below the apnea alarm limit, the ventilator switches to a controlled ventilation mode; an apnea alarm, indicated by an audible and visual signal, is activated. The controlled ventilation mode is continued until the clinician resets the apnea alarm.

CONCLUSION

With the advancement of ventilator technology, modes of ventilation that have been successful in the pediatric and adult populations for many years are now being applied to the neonatal population. Ventilators designed for neonatal use now offer various modes, including volume ventilation and pressure support. These ventilators have incorporated some of the latest enhancements in pressure support, which have resulted in increased triggering sensitivity, shortened response times, reduced flow acceleration, and improved breath termination parameters. These improvements are important when ventilating with small uncuffed endotracheal tubes and in the management of patients with diseases in which compliance is low and resistance is high. Other improvements being explored include guaranteed volume delivery in different modes, proportional assist ventilation, and availability of adequate alarms to meet the needs of the newborn. Another area that has improved dramatically since the inception of infant ventilation is monitoring.[38] In addition to mean airway pressure monitoring, which has provided valuable information since its introduction in the 1980s, tidal volume monitoring is becoming a common practice largely as a result of the accuracy of available monitors. It also enables calculation of minute ventilation and provides the clinician the ability to assess spontaneous breathing during mechanical ventilation.[39] From 1970 to the early 1990s, neonatal ventilation did not change significantly. Now, the expansion of technology provides neonatal clinicians with exciting new opportunities for research and application of these different modalities of infant ventilation.

FUTURE DIRECTIONS

Introduction of PTV, whether it is SIMV or A/C mode ventilation, has been an exciting breakthrough in the management of newborns with respiratory failure. Early experience has demonstrated the benefits of synchronization in improving gas exchange and pulmonary mechanics and in shortening the duration of mechanical ventilation in some populations. With the addition of flow cycling, mechanical ventilation of the newborn is coming increasingly closer to matching spontaneous breathing. Perhaps even more important, *control* of ventilation now is patient driven rather than ventilator driven. There is a striking similarity between A/C breaths and PSV breaths, as shown in Figure 12-11. During the first 5 seconds of the recording (encompassing the first six breaths), the patient is receiving flow-synchronized A/C ventilation. Thereafter, the breaths are spontaneous PSV delivered at the same pressure. No differences in flow and volume are detectable because each of these parameters is essentially patient controlled.

Numerous infant ventilators that offer synchronization options are now commercially available. All of them have

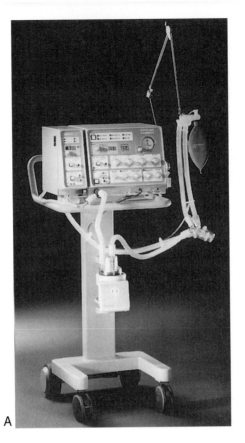

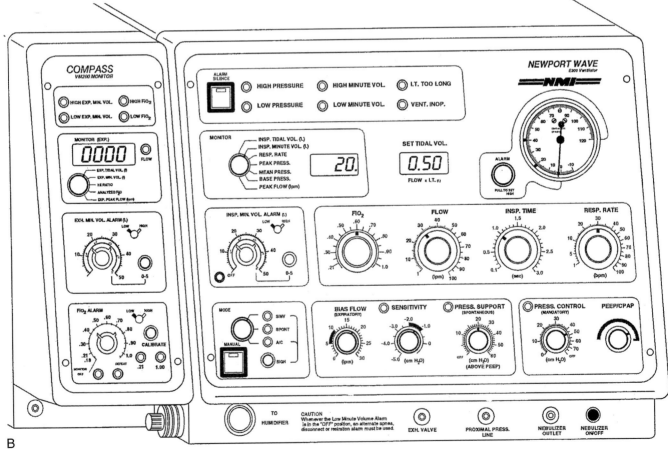

Figure 12-10. *A,* Newport Wave ventilator and Compass monitor. (Courtesy of Newport Medical Instruments, Newport Beach, CA, USA.) *B,* Diagram of the front panel.

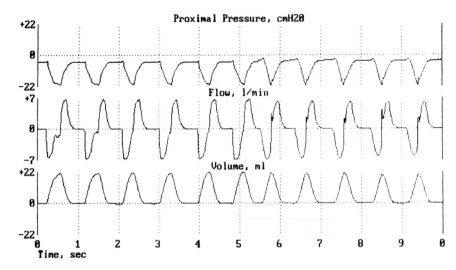

Figure 12-11. Comparison of patient-triggered, flow-synchronized assist/control breaths (first six) and spontaneous pressure support breaths (last five). The similarity of pressure, flow, and delivered tidal volume waveforms is striking.

been demonstrated to be advantageous over conventional IMV. What is yet to be determined, however, is which ventilatory mode is best in different clinical circumstances. Although it may seem intuitive that A/C ventilation should decrease the work of breathing when compared with SIMV, it is unclear what price an infant may ultimately have to pay. For instance, do spontaneous unsupported breaths interspersed with mechanical breaths result in lower mean thoracic pressures, thus promoting venous drainage, cardiac output, and cerebral blood flow? Alternatively, could A/C ventilation speed resolution of respiratory disease states, thus decreasing bronchopulmonary dysplasia and its attendant respiratory and neurologic sequelae?

Although clinicians are experiencing a technologic revolution in the neonatal intensive care unit, they must not embrace the new techniques without close clinical scrutiny. Clearly, enthusiasm should be tempered by continued investigation and refinement. At the same time, the future of neonatal respiratory care has never been brighter.

REFERENCES

1. Greenough A: Patient triggered ventilation. In Lafeber H (ed): Fetal and Neonatal Physiological Measurements. Amsterdam, Excerpta Medica, 1991, p. 247.
2. Lipscomb AP, Thorburn RJ, Reynolds EO, et al: Pneumothorax and cerebral haemorrhage in preterm infants. Lancet 1:414, 1981.
3. Rennie JM, South M, Morley CJ: Cerebral blood flow velocity in infants receiving assisted ventilation. Arch Dis Child 62:1247, 1987.
4. Perlman JM, Goodman S, Kreusser KL, et al: Reduction in intraventricular hemorrhage by elimination of fluctuating cerebral blood-flow velocity in preterm infants with respiratory distress syndrome. N Engl J Med 312:1353, 1985.
5. Rutledge ML, Hawkins EP, Langston C: Skeletal muscle growth failure induced in premature newborn infants by prolonged pancuronium treatment. J Pediatr 109:883, 1986.
6. Mehta A, Callan K, Wright BM, et al: Patient-triggered ventilation in the newborn. Lancet 2:17, 1986.
7. Visveshwara N, Freeman B, Peck M, et al: Patient-triggered synchronized assisted ventilation of newborns: Report of a preliminary study and three years' experience. J Perinatol 11:347, 1991.
8. Bernstein G, Cleary JP, Heldt GP, et al: Response time and reliability of three neonatal patient-triggered ventilators. Am Rev Respir Dis 148:358, 1993.
9. Servant GM, Nicks JJ, Donn SM, et al: Feasibility of applying flow-synchronized ventilation to very low birthweight infants. Respir Care 37:249, 1992.
10. Greenough A, Hird MF, Chan V: Airway pressure triggered ventilation versus high frequency positive pressure ventilation in acute respiratory distress. J Perinatal Med 19:379, 1991.
11. Bernstein G, Heldt GP, Knodel E: Rate of autocycling of flow triggered neonatal patient triggered ventilators. Pediatr Res 33:317A, 1993.
12. Mitchell A, Greenough A, Hird M: Limitations of patient triggered ventilation in neonates. Arch Dis Child 64:924, 1989.
13. Hird M, Greenough A: Causes of failure of neonatal patient triggered ventilation. Early Hum Dev 23:101, 1990.
14. Hird M, Greenough A: Gestational age: An important influence on the success of patient triggered ventilation. Clin Phys Physiol Meas 11:307, 1990.
15. Chan V, Greenough A: Randomised controlled trial of weaning by patient triggered ventilation or conventional ventilation. Eur J Pediatr 152:51, 1993.
16. Donn SM, Nicks JJ, Becker MA: Flow synchronized ventilation of preterm infants with respiratory distress syndrome. J Perinatol 14:90, 1994.
17. Baumer JH: International randomised controlled trial of patient triggered ventilation in neonatal respiratory distress syndrome. Arch Dis Child Fetal Neonatal Ed 82:F5–F10, 2000.
18. Donn SM, Greenough A, Sinha SK: Patient triggered ventilation. Arch Dis Child Fetal Neonatal Ed 83:F225-F226, 2000.
19. Beresford MW, Shaw NJ, Manning D: Randomised controlled trial of patient triggered and conventional fast ventilation in neonatal respiratory distress syndrome. Arch Dis Child Fetal Neonatal Ed 82:F14-F18, 2000.
20. Greenough A: Update on patient-triggered ventilation. Clin Perinatol 28:533–546, 2001.
21. Campbell RS, Branson RD: Ventilatory support for the 90's: Pressure support ventilation. Respir Care 38:526, 1993.
22. Pilbeam SP, Shelleday D: Discontinuation of and weaning from mechanical ventilation. In Pilbeam SP (ed): Mechanical Ventilation: Physiological and Clinical Applications. St. Louis, Mosby-Year Book, 1992, p. 469.
23. Banner MJ, Blanch PB, Kirby RR: Imposed work of breathing and methods of triggering a demand-flow, continuous airway pressure system. Crit Care Med 21:183, 1993.
24. Kanak R, Fahey PJ, Vanderwarf C: Oxygen cost of breathing: Changes dependent upon mode of mechanical ventilation. Chest 87:126, 1985.
25. Sinha SK, Donn SM: Pressure support ventilation. In Sinha SK, Donn SM (eds): Manual of Neonatal Respiratory Care. Armonk, NY, Futura Publishing Co., 2000, pp. 157-160.
26. MacIntyre NR: Respiratory function during pressure support ventilation. Chest 89:677, 1986.
27. Prakash O, Meij S: Cardiopulmonary response to inspiratory pressure support during spontaneous ventilation versus conventional ventilation. Chest 88:403, 1985.
28. Bolder PM, Healy TEJ, Bolder AR, et al: The extra work of breathing through adult endotracheal tubes. Anesth Analg 65:853, 1986.
29. Fiastry JF, Quan BF, Habib MP: Pressure support compensation for inspiratory work due to endotracheal tubes and demand CPAP. Chest 89:441S, 1986.
30. Forrette TL, Cook EW, Jones LE: Determining the efficacy of inspiration assist during mechanical ventilation. Respir Care 30:864, 1985.

31. Nagy RS, MacIntyre NR: Patient work during pressure support ventilation. Respir Care 30:860, 1985.

32. Linn CR, Gish GB, Mathewson HS: The effect of pressure support on the work of breathing. Respir Care 30:861, 1985.

33. MacIntyre NR, Nishimura M, Usada Y, et al: The Nagoya conference on system design and patient-ventilator interactions during pressure support ventilation. Chest 97:1463, 1990.

34. Kacmarek RK, Shimada Y, Ohmura A, et al: The second Nagoya Conference: Triggering and optimizing mechanical ventilatory assist. Respir Care 36:45, 1991.

35. Shelledy DC, Mikles SP: Newer modes of mechanical ventilation part I: Pressure support. Respir Manage July–August:14, 1988.

36. Bandy KP, Nicks JJ, Donn SM: Volume-controlled ventilation for severe neonatal respiratory failure. Neonat Intensive Care 5:70, 1992.

37. Sinha SK, Donn SM, Gavey J, et al: Randomised trial of volume controlled versus time cycled, pressure limited ventilation in preterm infants with respiratory distress syndrome. Arch Dis Child Fetal Neonatal Ed 77:F202–F206, 1999.

38. Donn SM (ed): Neonatal and Pediatric Pulmonary Graphics. Principles and Clinical Applications. Armonk, NY, Futura Publishing Co., 1998.

39. Wilson BJ Jr, Becker MA, Linton ME, Donn SM: Spontaneous minute ventilation predicts readiness for extubation in mechanically ventilated preterm infants. J Perinatol 18:436–439, 1998.

13 SPECIAL VENTILATORY TECHNIQUES AND MODALITIES II
Lung Protective Strategies and Liquid Ventilation

ALAN R. SPITZER, MD
JAY S. GREENSPAN, MD
WILLIAM W. FOX, MD
THOMAS SHAFFER, PHD

HISTORICAL AND MODERN APPROACHES TO POSITIVE-PRESSURE VENTILATOR SUPPORT AND THE EVOLUTION OF LUNG PROTECTIVE STRATEGIES

Despite the many advances in respiratory techniques for the neonate during the past several decades, lung injury remains a significant complication in the care of the critically ill neonate. Managing pulmonary limitations in the chronically affected infant and preventing further injury remain challenges for the clinician. As our understanding of the pathophysiology of neonatal lung disease progresses, so does our appreciation of the potential entry points of therapy. Because chronic lung disease is multifactorial in origin, virtually all aspects of neonatal care can be viewed as subjects for preventative strategies. There is no question that issues such as infection, fluid management, patent ductus arteriosus, nutrition, pulmonary air leaks, anemia, and many others all impact on pulmonary outcome. Consequently, prevention of chronic lung disease will only occur when a global approach, which includes attention to the prenatal and perinatal environment, neonatal nutrition, and thermoregulatory, antioxidant, inflammatory, and other health issues of the infant, is developed. For the purposes of this chapter, however, we focus on preventative pulmonary strategies, although the neurodevelopmental consequences are described where appropriate.

Although preterm infants can have structural or developmental lung problems, the prematurely delivered infant typically has normal lungs with immature structure and function. This immaturity includes anatomic immaturity of the lung parenchyma and airways, surfactant deficiency, immature lung fluid maintenance, and increased chest wall compliance. Managing their pulmonary needs involves the provision of support to maintain adequate gas exchange while minimizing the risk for iatrogenic trauma or intercurrent illness. The preterm infant who progresses to chronic lung disease often does so because of ventilator-induced injury, which may be preventable, at least in part.

Some chronic lung injury is inescapable with current technology. It is clear from studies of preterm infants, however, that certain management techniques and styles appear to be associated with a decreased incidence of chronic lung disease, even when rigid statistical analysis for confounding factors is used.[1,2] Some of these potential strategies are discussed.

Protective Strategies for the Fetus and Management of Ventilation in the Delivery Room

Effective pulmonary management of the infant with respiratory failure begins during prenatal care and in the delivery room. Evidence suggests that a majority of premature infant deliveries are the result of maternal chorioamnionitis, which often is accompanied by elevated cytokine production.[3,4] Because tocolytic therapy is required frequently in premature labor and a conservative approach often is taken with premature rupture of membranes, the premature neonate may be exposed in utero to high levels of cytokines or other vasoactive substances, which may make subsequent resuscitation and ventilatory management more difficult.[5,6] The obstetrician therefore has the complex and unenviable task of attempting to decide when a fetus will do better outside of the uterus than remaining inside. To date, there are few data that can successfully answer this thorny question. Clearly, in the face of evolving infection and fever or with worsening preeclampsia, delivery of the fetus is essential. In the afebrile mother who has repeatedly threatened premature labor, however, there currently are no answers. Is the fetus better with aggressive tocolysis at 25 to 26 weeks, or is the long-term risk actually less ex utero? What about the baby who is beyond 27 to 28 weeks? Where can the line to deliver be successfully drawn, and what are the resulting pulmonary and neurodevelopmental consequences? It is likely that this research issue will be aggressively pursued in the near future.

The development of adequate pulmonary blood flow, functional residual capacity (FRC), and ventilation-perfusion matching with uniform distribution of lung surfactant can be affected by the management in the first few minutes of life. Animal studies demonstrate that airway and lung parenchymal injury can occur with only a few large breaths at the time of birth.[7–10] This potential injury is exacerbated in the preterm infant in whom the immature airway structure can be easily disrupted by pressure deformation. The resulting loss in airway integrity can lead to an escalating cycle of airway collapse and distal atelectasis, the need for increased inflation pressures, and further airway injury. Bjorklund et al.[10] demonstrated in an animal model that manual ventilation with only six large tidal breaths after birth can alter lung function. In addition to airway injury, tidal breathing in the delivery room can cause alterations in surfactant function. These changes may be due to parenchymal disruption with protein leak and surfactant inactivation.[11,12] Hence, tidal breaths in the delivery room can reduce the efficacy of exogenous surfactant administration while simultaneously disrupting the integrity of the airway structure and the pulmonary parenchyma. As a result, from even shortly after birth, the physician attempting to reduce pulmonary trauma in the neonate may be fighting a losing battle.

The early instillation of exogenous surfactant appears to reduce the lung injury and protein leak associated with preterm delivery.[13] This protection is diminished if therapy is delayed beyond 30 minutes.[14] Although distribution of exogenous surfactant is improved with instillation during the first few minutes of life, the outcome of very-low-birthweight infants probably is improved if instillation is delayed until adequate respiration is established.[15] Our ability to predict infants who will develop respiratory distress syndrome (RDS) is limited in later-gestation (>32 weeks) preterm infants, so most practices limit the use of prophylactic exogenous surfactant administration to early-gestation premature infants (see Chapter 20).

The optimal delivery room management of the preterm neonate would include the gentle establishment of an FRC and matched pulmonary blood flow, with even distribution of pulmonary surfactant. These events might be accomplished by the early institution of continuous positive airway pressure or by delivery room initiation of mechanical ventilation with low tidal volumes. The instillation of exogenous surfactant can be given once the infant is stabilized. Although the institution of mechanical ventilation in the very preterm infant may be necessary, delaying intubation in this population and observing if the infant needs ventilation may not necessarily be detrimental.[16] Newer technology may allow for the early institution of controlled continuous positive airway pressure or high-frequency ventilation (HFV) soon after birth, necessitating the presence of ventilators in the delivery room. It is becoming increasingly clear, however, that the use of hand ventilation with nonhumidified gas at high inflation pressures in the delivery room is not optimal and may provoke substantial airway injury during neonatal resuscitation. Furthermore, the uncontrolled use of oxygen, a long-term mainstay of resuscitation, has been questioned by studies indicating that room air resuscitation may be advantageous for long-term outcome.[17] To date, no studies have examined room-air resuscitation in the low-birthweight infant, particularly with respect to pulmonary injury.

Conventional Ventilation

The management of neonatal respiratory failure has changed dramatically over the past several decades. Some therapies, such as the use of endogenous surfactant, HFV, and inhaled nitric oxide (iNO), have been shown to decrease mortality or the need for more invasive therapy such as extracorporeal life support.[14,18] Defining specific management strategies to improve outcomes has been less well documented. It is clear that slightly different pulmonary approaches, even when utilizing similar medications and ventilators, can result in different outcomes. As a result, the incidence of chronic lung disease varies among different intensive care nurseries.[1,2] Because there are many variables that affect the pulmonary outcome of

an infant, determining which factors primarily contribute to these differences is difficult. The multivariate analyses of Van Marter et al.[2] suggested that most of the increased risk for chronic lung disease among very-low-birthweight infants was explained simply by the decision to initiate mechanical ventilation. Using regression analysis, Graziani et al.[19] also showed that the decision to initiate mechanical ventilation had significant neurologic implications for the very-low-birthweight infant. Horbar et al.[20] demonstrated that strategies could be effectively changed through a multidisciplinary collaborative quality improvement program, with resultant diminished chronic lung disease.

Optimizing neonatal management includes reducing ventilator-related lung injury. The specific ventilator variable that induces the greatest injury has remained controversial. As can be seen from the earlier discussion about the various ventilator approaches in the chapter on positive-pressure ventilation (see Chapter 9), the attempt to completely eliminate lung injury in the neonate has been less than successful. Because it is possible to achieve the same tidal volume, minute ventilation, and gas exchange with different ventilator settings, it becomes important to try to determine which variable achieves adequate gas exchange with the least potential iatrogenic injury. Animal studies suggest that tidal breathing (volutrauma), as well as ventilating the atelectatic lung (atelectrauma), causes injury.[21–26] The size of the breath, therefore, may be more important than the inflating pressure in determining the risk for chronic lung disease. In the atelectatic lung, adequate minute ventilation is achieved by overinflating already expanded lung regions, thereby causing damage to those ventilated regions. Using an adequate amount of end-expiratory pressure or mean airway pressure to optimize alveolar volume recruitment may diminish lung injury.

Although less information is available on other ventilator controls, for conventional ventilators used to support infants with restrictive lung disease, shorter inspiratory times with more rapid rates and low flow rates (to prevent turbulent gas flow in the airways) appears to be preferable.[27–30] In addition, the use of a disease-specific ventilator approach that changes as the lung mechanics change may be most beneficial. Hence, the concept of patient-triggered ventilation, especially proportional assist ventilation, may prove increasingly useful as experience is gained with these modalities (see Chapter 12).

Recent advances in technology have allowed the introduction of patient-triggered ventilation and online lung mechanics from conventional ventilators. These new technologies allow for more accurate monitoring of the infant's status and permit a wide array of new ventilator modalities, such as synchronized, pressure-support, proportional assist, and assist/control (A/C) ventilation. In addition, the clinician can use the graphics information from several new ventilators to make more rapid changes, thereby reducing injury (see Chapter 18). These techniques may improve outcomes of infants, although further work on these techniques needs to be pursued.[31,32] New techniques of reducing trauma during conventional ventilation, such as tracheal gas insufflation, continue to be introduced and need more widespread evaluation.[33]

Once an infant is being treated with mechanical ventilation and is stabilized, weaning the infant from the ventilator is always challenging. Mechanical breaths, even at low ventilator settings, can induce lung injury. When the infant finally begins to wean progressively, the decision to finally remove the mechanical ventilator is difficult. Both nasal synchronized intermittent mandatory ventilation (SIMV) and variable-flow nasal continuous positive airway pressures may be approaches that will permit the clinician to successfully wean small infants off of the ventilator more quickly.[34,35]

Approaches to Neonatal Ventilation

The general strategy that we use for mechanical ventilation of the neonate discussed in the chapter on positive-pressure ventilation (see Chapter 9) is only one of the many approaches to respiratory support of the newborn infant. Numerous other methods that work equally well in the hands of experienced clinicians have been described in the literature. In recent years, the number of different strategies has seemingly expanded exponentially, although the evidence supporting one approach compared to another is sparse at the present time. All such techniques are guided by certain basic physiologic principles and consistency of management in an individual nursery. Table 13-1 lists some alternative styles of mechanical ventilation of the newborn and the basic principles on which the techniques are based. These techniques of neonatal ventilation are discussed briefly. For more extensive reviews of HFV and patient-triggered ventilation, the reader is referred to Chapters 11 and 12.

TABLE 13-1. Historical and New Approaches to Neonatal Mechanical Ventilation

Approach	Rationale	Technique
Slow rate ventilation (Reynolds)	Improve oxygenation; decrease barotrauma.	Rate at 20–30 bpm. Increase MAP with longer T_I, or reversal of I/E ratio.
"Gentle ventilation" or permissive hypercapnia (Wung)	Accept higher $Paco_2$ and lower pH in order to reduce airway and lung injury. Focus on adequate oxygenation.	Rate of 20–40 bpm, but increase rate preferentially to PIP. Keep PIP low; accept $Paco_2$ up to 60 torr, occasionally higher. pH can be as low as 7.15–7.20 for brief periods.
Rapid-rate ventilation (Bland)	Use rapid rate and hand ventilation to achieve oxygenation at lower PIP. Reduce barotrauma; accept some inadvertent PEEP.	Rate of 60–80 bpm, higher at times, to maximum of 120–150. Keep low PIP; use shortened T_I.
Hyperventilation (Fox and Peckham)	Use rapid rate and PIP as necessary to reduce $Paco_2$ to the *highest* level at which oxygenation occurs. Reduce right-to-left shunting by decreasing pulmonary artery pressure. In general, used to treat PPHN. Should be used cautiously in other diseases because of risk of air leak.	Rate of 60–150 bpm. Use PIP to reduce $Paco_2$ to 35 torr or less. Achieve the *highest* $Paco_2$ that allows oxygenation. Periodically challenge infant by decreasing support to see if PPHN has resolved or transition phase has begun.
High-frequency jet ventilation (Spitzer)	Use rate of 400–500 bpm at reduced pressure in the treatment of severe lung disease or pulmonary air leak. Extremely low tidal volume. Background sigh used to improve oxygenation.	Rate of 400–500 bpm. T_I of 0.02. Background sigh rate by conventional ventilator of 5–10 bpm with T_I of 0.5 sec. Avoid excessively low $Paco_2$, common in HFJV. Maintain alveolar volume with PEEP.
High-frequency oscillatory ventilation–high-volume strategy (Friese, Bryan, deLemos)	Use rate of 600–900 bpm with alveolar recruitment technique to increase lung volume. Allows use of HFOV with decreased tidal volume and reduces lung injury.	Rate of 600–900 bpm. Give prolonged inflation periodically with bag and mask or ventilator control to recruit volume in lung. Wean by decreasing oscillatory pressure.
Patient-triggered ventilation: SIMV and A/C (Donn)	Allow patient to trigger and self-regulate (to some extent) level of ventilatory support that is required, thereby reduced barotrauma. With SIMV, patient breaths and ventilator breaths are synchronized to avoid "stacking" of pressures and simultaneous patient and ventilator breath. With A/C, patient triggers ventilator to deliver all breaths. Both forms have backup rate if patient becomes apneic.	SIMV: set ventilator rate at about 40–45 to start. Use approach similar to conventional IMV, keeping pressures at a minimum to exchange gas adequately, while reducing barotrauma. With A/C ventilation, set PIP and PEEP for adequate gas exchange; allow patient to increase rate of breathing to blow off CO₂. In both cases give adequate FIO_2 to keep Pao_2 at 60–80 mm Hg.
Tidal volume-guided ventilation or volume-guarantee ventilation	Consistent delivery of a uniform minimum tidal volume while maintaining the ability to set pressure limits.	Clinician sets upper limit of pressure and desired V_T. Ventilator attempts to deliver guaranteed volume with lowest possible pressure. If pressure is inadequate to deliver volume, unit alarms to alert physician to increase pressure limit or lower V_T.
PAV and RMU (Schulze, Bancalari)	Microprocessor-controlled feedback loop to assist mechanical ventilation. Process allows clinician to provide support throughout the ventilatory cycle to ease work of breathing for the infant. Ventilator senses flows throughout respiratory cycle.	With PAV, desired assist flow above baseline is generated during inspiration to overcome airway and ventilator resistance. During RMU, the reverse occurs as circuit pressure falls below baseline and respiratory muscles are unloaded, further easing work of breathing.
Tracheal gas insufflation	Provision of fresh gas into the distal endotracheal tube reduces anatomic dead space and lowers tidal volume and pressure requirements.	Small continuous gas injection into the distal endotracheal tube is given at 0.5 L/min with another form of ventilation simultaneously being used, or with spontaneous breathing on CPAP.

A/C, assist/control; bpm, breaths per minute; CPAP, continuous positive airway pressure; I/E, inspiratory-to-expiratory; HFJV, high-frequency jet ventilation; HFOV, high-frequency oscillatory ventilation; MAP, mean airway pressure; PAV, proportional assist ventilation; PEEP, positive end-expiratory pressure; PIP, peak inspiratory pressure; PPHN, persistent pulmonary hypertension of the neonate; RMU, respiratory muscle unloading; SIMV, synchronized intermittent mandatory ventilation; T_I, inspiratory time; V_T, tidal volume.

Slow-Rate Ventilation

The first systematic approach to mechanical ventilation was devised by Reynolds and Tagizadeh[36] during the early 1970s. This technique, commonly referred to as *slow-rate ventilation*, used a ventilator rate of 20 to 30 breaths/min and a reversed inspiratory-to-expiratory (I/E) ratio (2:1 to 4:1) to improve oxygenation. This method improved oxygenation by increasing mean airway pressure, but it had associated problems. Air trapping and elevated $PaCO_2$ levels were common, and the incidence of intraventricular hemorrhage was much higher than that reported by other investigators. Consequently, this approach fell out of favor and is rarely used today, except for rare instances of oxygenation difficulty.

Rapid-Rate Ventilation

In the mid-1970s, Bland et al.[37] reported on a series of infants treated with more *rapid-rate ventilation,* in whom hand ventilation was often used to improve gas exchange. Bland et al. used lower pressures but rates over 100 breaths/min in an attempt to decrease the risk of chronic lung disease. This approach was one of the first to emphasize the potential of higher rates and lower pressures in reducing lung injury in neonates. The results, although favorable, were likely due to inadvertent positive end-expiratory pressure (PEEP), and the inconsistency of hand ventilation was unsatisfactory in many nurseries. It did suggest, however, that rapid rates could be used successfully in some infants.

Hyperventilation

Several years later, Peckham and Fox[38] explored the possibility of using higher rates and pressures to lower $PaCO_2$ and decrease pulmonary vascular resistance intentionally. This *hyperventilation* technique is still used in some nurseries for treatment of persistent pulmonary hypertension of the neonate (PPHN). Initially, the authors advocated rates as high as 150 breaths/min, but they subsequently suggested that some of the complications of hyperventilation could be prevented through the use of slower rates (60 breaths/min) and sufficient peak inspiratory pressure (PIP) to lower the $PaCO_2$ to the point at which oxygenation improves. This technique has been criticized as being "overly aggressive" by some clinicians, many of whom fail to understand the goals of therapy. This treatment is designed to ventilate an infant only to the highest $PaCO_2$ at which adequate oxygenation is seen (the "critical $PaCO_2$"). Many physicians mistakenly believe that simply "cranking up the ventilator" to achieve the lowest $PaCO_2$ is the primary goal, but this results in needless barotrauma. More importantly, recent evidence has indicated that neurologic injury, especially cerebral palsy and hearing loss, may be more common in infants who are hyperventilated.[39] Because of these risks, we have attempted in recent years to use approaches to ventilatory assistance that are less likely to provoke neurologic injury. It cannot be stressed enough that continued use of high pressures for prolonged periods of ventilatory support are associated with pulmonary and central nervous system injury and should be avoided whenever possible. It may be preferable in many instances, for example, to refer an infant for extracorporeal membrane oxygenation (ECMO) rather than continue high-pressure ventilation.

If hyperventilation is used at all, it should be initiated cautiously in PPHN. Once the rate of 60 breaths/min is set, the PIP should be increased until the $PaCO_2$ begins to fall. At some point, oxygenation suddenly improves. This level is the critical $PaCO_2$. The PaO_2 should be kept at approximately 100 to 120 mm Hg to assist in pulmonary vasodilation. PEEP usually is maintained at 2 to 5 cm H_2O unless the patient also has pneumonitis and volume recruitment within the lung is necessary to sustain oxygenation. Paralysis is sometimes necessary during this phase of illness, although it should be used judiciously. Paralysis removes the work of breathing contributed by the patient and may result in sudden deterioration of blood gases. If patients appear to be "fighting the ventilator," it usually is the result of hypoxemia or hypercarbia. Improvement in gas exchange through an alternative ventilatory approach will often reduce the agitation of the baby while avoiding paralysis. In addition, external stimulation should be kept to a minimum. Vasopressor agents (dopamine or dobutamine) often are beneficial, and intravenous administration of sodium bicarbonate may help in alkalization. Tolazoline is not generally beneficial, and its use has been abandoned by many clinicians, especially now with the availability of iNO therapy. The adverse effects of systemic vasodilation and hypotension with tolazoline usually outweigh any pulmonary benefits. Recently, the manufacturer has seemed to agree with this concept and has announced that tolazoline is being removed from the market.

Once the child has been stable for 12 to 24 hours, it is appropriate to challenge the infant by allowing $PaCO_2$ to increase slightly (3 to 5 mm Hg) by decreasing PIP by 1 to 2 cm H_2O. Excessively large decreases in PIP in the early phases of this disease can often result in sudden marked deterioration ("flip-flop") from which recovery is difficult. If oxygenation remains adequate, it is likely that the child has entered the transitional phase of PPHN, and slow cautious weaning can proceed. Weans of PIP and FIO_2 should always be small (1 cm H_2O or 2% FIO_2) and infrequent to avoid flip-flop. The goal should be to have the child receive below 50% O_2 and a PIP of 25 cm H_2O within 48 hours. Once these levels are reached, management usually poses few difficulties. Additional management strategies are discussed in Chapter 23.

High-Frequency Ventilation

The concept of minimizing volutrauma and atelectrauma is best seen in the use of *high-frequency ventilation*, which often reduces $PaCO_2$ with less barotrauma to the airways and lungs. HFV has been well established as an effective rescue tool for infants with RDS who require high levels of respiratory support or infants with pulmonary air leaks.[40,41] It has been our approach for the past 10 to 15 years to use this ventilatory strategy rather than conventional ventilation with hyperventilation because of the reduced barotrauma and the improved outcomes. HFV is effective in only 38% of patients with PPHN and meconium aspiration, however, which suggests a need for either iNO or ECMO in 60% of patients.[41] It is possible, however, to learn in 6 hours or less which infant will respond to HFV and which probably will not.[41] It does not appear that conventional ventilation in such circumstances is preferable to HFV or likely to produce better outcomes. The benefit of prophylactic HFV has been demonstrated in several different preterm animal models,[42] but translating this animal work to show effectiveness as a preventative lung injury strategy in infants has been difficult. This technique has become more complicated by the recent advances in respiratory therapies that are improving conventional ventilation outcomes. HFV, both high-frequency jet ventilation (HFJV) and high-frequency oscillatory ventilation (HFOV), is extremely useful in limiting barotrauma in tiny premature infants. It has been our experience that HFJV is more useful when air leaks (pneumothorax or pulmonary interstitial emphysema) are present, whereas HFOV may be slightly more advantageous in situations of oxygenation difficulties. Both ventilator units are extremely effective, however, when used appropriately. It is as yet unclear whether HFV is the treatment of choice in early uncomplicated RDS in extremely-low-birthweight infants. Some studies have suggested a greater likelihood of neurologic injury when HFV is used early in the course of illness rather than as a rescue therapy for air leak or high levels of conventional ventilator support, although the results of a more recent trial have been far more encouraging in this respect.[43,44] At present, we prefer to use HFV primarily as a rescue modality for complications of more standard positive-pressure ventilation (see Chapter 11).

Inhalational Nitric Oxide

With the introduction and United States Food and Drug Administration (FDA) approval of iNO as an adjunct to therapy in PPHN, iNO has been shown to be beneficial in some cases of PPHN (see Chapters 14 and 23), but it does not appear to have a significant lung protective role, as it typically is used only when there is already some evidence of airway and lung injury.[45] Nitric oxide acts as a direct pulmonary vasodilator when it is given through a separate circuit to the patient on a ventilator. It appears to work most effectively in PPHN syndromes where there is little debris in the airway. Meconium aspiration syndrome with PPHN seems to respond less well than the "pure" forms of pulmonary hypertension. Approximately 30% to 40% of infants with PPHN will respond to this therapy, and ECMO may be avoided in a number of situations. Some studies have suggested a benefit in oxygenation for the premature infant with RDS, a lung disease that always has some element of increased pulmonary vascular resistance.[46] In premature infants, however, there may be some adverse consequences in terms of cerebral vasodilation and intracranial hemorrhage, although long-term outcome does not appear to be adversely influenced in any way in the few studies described to date.[47,48] Currently iNO is not approved for any use in the neonate other than PPHN, and further studies in the premature population are needed before any clear recommendation can be made regarding its use. Arterial oxygenation appears to improve rapidly, even at nitric oxide concentrations as low as 1 to 2 ppm. The treatment currently is very expensive, however, and is not approved for use in the infant with RDS or in any form of prophylactic care. As a result, iNO has little role as a lung protective strategy in the very-low-birthweight infant. Of perhaps greater concern is the excessively prolonged use of iNO in an attempt to avoid ECMO in the most severely affected larger patients. In these instances, iNO may actually increase exposure to high ventilator pressures, prolong the ultimate length of stay, increase the risk of bronchopulmonary dysplasia (BPD), and be associated with a higher likelihood of neurologic injury. Infants should respond rapidly to iNO or they should be referred to an experienced ECMO center in order to prevent these injuries.

Gentle Ventilation

In contrast to hyperventilation, Wung et al.[49] at Babies Hospital in New York introduced the concept of *gentle ventilation* in the mid-1980s. They advocated the use of ventilator rates of 20 to 40 breaths/min and sufficient pressures to allow adequate oxygenation while tolerating a $Paco_2$ that was as high as 60 to 70 mm Hg rather than injure the lung by using higher pressures. If $Paco_2$ could not be controlled, they recommended the use of more rapid rates (120 to 140 breaths/min) in an attempt to decrease $Paco_2$. If this attempt failed, they suggested returning to the previous lower rates. The pH in this system was accepted at low levels (to 7.15) for periods of time as long as 24 hours. Weaning was accomplished with reduction in pressures as the infant's status improved. The results appear to be comparable with those from hyperventilation but with the added benefit of less chronic lung injury in the patient with PPHN. The use of this technique in premature infants with RDS has been reported, with a very low incidence of BPD (approximately 5%).[1] Furthermore, Wung has suggested that the use of this approach may decrease the need for ECMO in PPHN. The number of infants described in the medical literature to date who were managed with this approach has been small, and follow-up data on the results of this approach are limited. In certain nurseries, however, it appears that "gentle ventilation" is a valuable tool for some infants with severe respiratory disease. What Wung has demonstrated, however, is that the lungs of a critically ill neonate are fragile and need to be treated as such. In addition, his approach has shown neonatologists that tolerance of slightly higher CO_2 levels is preferable to continued battering of the lung with high-pressure ventilation.

The concept of "gentle ventilation" illustrates one of the most confusing aspects of managing respiratory distress in the newborn, namely, when, and to what degree, to intervene. The introduction of mechanical ventilation is potentially detrimental, and deciding to place an infant on mechanical ventilator support remains a difficult decision. In addition, determining what measurements (blood gases, graphics monitoring) should guide ventilator changes remains unclear. Permissive hypercapnia in preterm infants seems safe and may reduce the duration of assisted ventilation.[50] This strategy has particular appeal in that hypocarbia may be related to brain injury.[19,51] Severe hypercapnia may cause brain injury, however, which strongly suggests that there are excellent physiologic reasons why nature has seen fit to establish eucapnic ventilation as the normal range.[52] When using a strategy of permissive hypercapnia, it is important to minimize atelectasis because the recruitment and de-recruitment of lung regions are not optimal. In addition, although the data look promising when this strategy is implemented, long-term follow-up of infants managed with high levels of carbon dioxide has not been explored.

Patient-Triggered Ventilation

Patient-triggered ventilation, as previously indicated, has now become a standard part of the repertoire of neonatologists (see Chapter 12). In general, patient-triggered ventilation consists of two forms of mechanical ventilation: *SIMV and A/C ventilation.* With SIMV, the ventilator is synchronized to the infant's breathing pattern. If the patient triggering threshold is met within a specific time window (depending on the preset ventilator rate), a ventilator breath is not delivered and the infant breathes spontaneously. On the other hand, a ventilator breath is delivered if the infant fails to breathe. Examination of the baby's breathing pattern with SIMV will reveal both spontaneous breaths and ventilator breaths. The value of this form of support is that pressures within the airway are not stacked, so airway and lung injury theoretically is reduced and gas is not inadvertently "dumped" from the ventilator because airway pressures are reached prematurely. Although many neonatologists will use SIMV as their primary mode of ventilator support for neonates, it appears to have greater benefit as a weaning tool or if overdistention is present with A/C ventilation, particularly in the extremely-low-birthweight infant with either RDS or pulmonary insufficiency of prematurity.

A/C ventilation is also a form of patient-triggered support. With A/C ventilation, each infant breath that reaches the trigger threshold will initiate a full ventilator breath. If the infant is apneic or the effort is inadequate to trigger a ventilator breath, the ventilator will deliver a preset backup rate to the baby. All breaths in this form of ventilation appear similar and are entirely ventilator derived. No spontaneous infant breaths ever occur on A/C support, unless the generated pressure is so low that it fails to trigger the ventilator. With A/C ventilation, the infant is fully synchronized to the ventilator. With the use of termination sensitivity as an adjunct, inspiratory time will be limited to a percentage of maximum flow, and air trapping usually can be reduced or eliminated.

A/C ventilation is an effective form of initial treatment for many babies with a variety of neonatal lung diseases in the early stages of their illness. It has been our experience that the use of A/C ventilation will limit pressure exposure for the infant, and the infant often will spontaneously select a rate that is optimal for gas exchange, with a lower pressure than would usually be set on SIMV. Minute ventilation is higher on A/C ventilation than on SIMV.[53] It is more difficult, however, to wean babies who are on A/C ventilation. Occasionally some overdistention will occur if there is excessive neural drive to breathe, and prolonged use of A/C may lead to some diaphragmatic muscle atrophy and further weaning difficulty. Consequently, we often move an infant from A/C ventilation to SIMV when he or she begins to show signs of recovery from the lung disease. With A/C ventilation, one must be cautious of "autocycling" of the ventilator. This problem can occur when there is erroneous triggering of the ventilator from leaks in the system, buildup of humidity in the circuit, or sensing of cardiac pulsations as breaths. Frequent breaths are delivered unnecessarily to the baby. We have also seen an occasional infant on A/C support who does well while he or she is awake, with good gas exchange, but who has inadequate blood gases while he or she is sleeping or sedated. In such cases, it would be helpful to have the capability of using two separate ventilator settings, one for waking periods and one during apneic support when slightly more pressure may be necessary for gas exchange. To date, however, no neonatal ventilator has the capability of selecting multiple ventilator settings simultaneously that could automatically trigger under selected conditions.

Pressure-Support Ventilation

An adjunct therapy during patient-triggered ventilation is *pressure-support ventilation,* in which spontaneous infant breaths are partially or full augmented by an inspiratory pressure assist above baseline PEEP. This modification eases the work of breathing for the infant by allowing additional pressure delivery to overcome the various sources of resistance encountered by the infant, such as the endotracheal tube, circuitry, and valves. This form of therapy can be used alone or, more commonly, in association with SIMV. Because it is fully synchronized with the infant's ventilation, it can be used to treat babies who are becoming fatigued from work of breathing, for sedated infants, and for infants who are in a weaning phase of ventilation who are first beginning to reuse their respiratory musculature. When used in conjunction with SIMV, it is important that the SIMV rate not be set too high, which may reduce the baby's impetus to breathe and would nullify one of the primary purposes of pressure support.

Volume-Guarantee Ventilation

Tidal volume-guided ventilation or *volume-guarantee ventilation* is a new approach to therapy in which the clinician sets a mean tidal volume to be delivered by the ventilator while still allowing management of ventilator pressures. In essence it is a variation of pressure-support ventilation in which volume, not pressure, guides the delivery of an augmented breath. The goal in this form of ventilation is to minimize variation in delivery of tidal volume, which is thought to be the cause of pulmonary barotrauma in many infants. Volume guarantee is available on the Draeger Babylog 8000 ventilator and is used in conjunction with patient-triggered modalities. When the physician sets the upper limit of PIP during patient-triggered support, the ventilator attempts to deliver the set guaranteed tidal volume using the lowest airway pressure possible. When the expired tidal volume exceeds the upper limit PIP, the ventilator will use a lower PIP on the next breath. If the set tidal volume cannot be delivered within the PIP set by the clinician, an alarm alerts the operator to reset the PIP to a higher level or adjust the guaranteed tidal volume to a lower level. Although data to date are not substantial, it appears that volume guarantee can achieve similar levels of gas exchange with slightly lower mean levels of PIP.[54] Further refinement of this patient-triggered approach is likely in the near future. Additional modifications may occur, such as guaranteed minute ventilation, in which a desired minute ventilation is designated, with the ventilator providing a mix of guaranteed tidal volume and frequency to provide the desired minute ventilation.

Proportional Assist Ventilation

Proportional assist ventilation (PAV) and *respiratory muscle unloading (RMU)* require even more sophisticated computer assistance to achieve their effects. These innovative approaches servocontrol ventilator pressure throughout inspiration (in the case of PAV) or throughout the entire respiratory cycle (during RMU). With both forms of ventilator support, the infant's respiratory effort is continuously monitored. During inspiration, as with pressure-support ventilation, pressure rises above baseline to produce the desired inspiratory resistive unloading, thereby easing work of breathing. During exhalation, circuit pressure falls below baseline end-distending pressure, facilitating elastic and resistive unloading throughout that phase of the respiratory cycle (Figs. 13-1 and 13-2). With this form of support, the resulting airway pressure is a moving variable that changes with the needs of the infant at any point during the respiratory cycle and is a weighted summation of a combination of air flow and tidal volume above the baseline (usually PEEP) level. Although human infant studies with PAV/RMU are somewhat limited at the present time, results of work by Schulze and Bancalari appear very encouraging.[55,56] In a trial that examined the relative effects of low-birthweight infants treated with IMV, A/C, and PAV, PAV appeared to maintain equivalent arterial oxygenation at lower airway and transpulmonary pressures than the other two modalities. During PAV, the oxygenation index was reduced by 28%, with no evidence of more frequent apnea or other complications. Intriguingly, there was also a decrease in both systolic and diastolic beat-to-beat variability with PAV, suggesting that there is additional overall cardiovascular stability offered to infants treated with this form of support. Furthermore, a more recent study indicated that there was less thoracoabdominal synchrony during PAV in preterm infants.[57] Few centers are using this form of ventilatory support because it is still in early trials, yet the concepts appear promising. Additional larger-scale trials will unquestionably be seen in the near future.

Tracheal Gas Insufflation

The added space of the ventilator adapter and the endotracheal tube result in a significant amount of anatomic dead space during mechanical ventilation, particularly to the airway of an extremely-low-birthweight (<1000 g) infant. Through a mechanism of tracheal gas insufflation, fresh gas is delivered to the more distal part of the endotracheal tube and aids in washing out CO_2 from the airway (Fig. 13-3). PIP and tidal volume usually can be decreased.[33] These factors may reduce barotrauma and volutrauma in these infants, and results of early trials appear promising.

Commentary

Respiratory insufficiency remains a frequently occurring and challenging complication of birth. Managing the pulmonary status of a sick neonate is a great responsibility. The decision to place an infant on respiratory support and the selection of appropriate ventilator settings should be made with an understanding of the ramifications of those decisions. When many breaths are imposed on an infant each minute, even small deviations from perfection can be significant and potentially catastrophic in terms of lung injury and long-term neurologic impairment. Evidence suggests that, despite recent advances in technology, length of hospital stay for the preterm population has begun to increase, and BPD remains a significant complication in every nursery.

As is evident from much of this discussion, the technologic innovations in positive-pressure ventilation during the past several years have been substantial and, no doubt, confusing to many neonatologists. There is likely to be even more innovation in the future, as computer technology becomes even faster in execution speed. Many of these techniques may offer theoretical benefits to infants, but actual demonstration of substantial clinical value has been sparse in many cases. Moreover, some approaches are so new that they have been limited to small pilot trials. The clinician should always keep in mind that the large majority of infants with lung disease can be successfully ventilated with standard positive-pressure ventilators without all the investigative modifications or all the bells and whistles. When one is caring for an extremely premature infant whose lungs are never supposed to be subject to positive-pressure ventilation (or even air breathing) at such an early

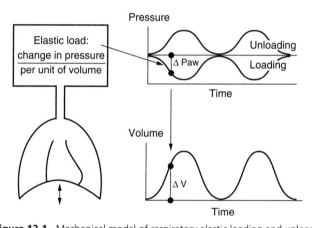

Figure 13-1. Mechanical model of respiratory elastic loading and unloading during the respiratory cycle. Air flow increases during inspiratory to augment the breath and reduce the work of breathing for the infant. (From Schulze A, Bancalari E: Proportional assist ventilation in infants. Clin Perinatol, 28:561–578, 2001.

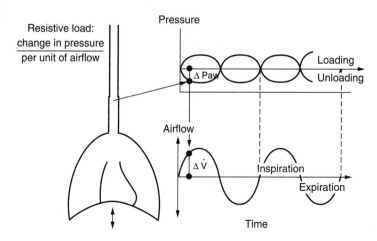

Figure 13-2. Mechanical model of resistive loading and unloading during the respiratory cycle. (From Schulze A, Bancalari E: Proportional assist ventilation in infants. Clin Perinatol, 28:561–578, 2001.

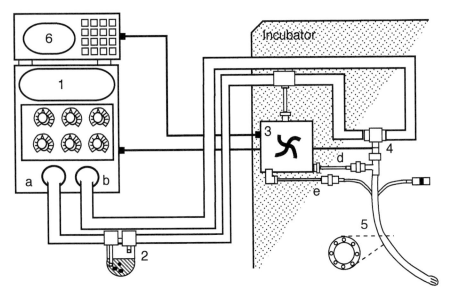

Figure 13-3. Diagram of assembly for controlled positive-pressure ventilation and continuous tracheal gas insufflation (CTGI). 1, Ventilator; 2, heater/humidifier; 3, CTGI pump; 4, flow sensor holder; 5, endotracheal tube; 6, monitoring and safety module; a, inspiratory circuit; b, expiratory circuit; c, CTGI circuit (inlet); d, CTGI circuit (outlet); e, tracheal pressure transducer. (From Dassieu G, Brochard L, Agudze E, et al: Continuous tracheal gas insufflation enables a volume reduction strategy in hyaline membrane disease: Technical aspects and clinical results. Intensive Care Med 24:1076–1082, 1998.)

stage of development, it simply may not be possible to limit the pulmonary injury that occurs in many babies. In addition, no approach to ventilatory support should ever be used unless the physician is well aware of the potential risks, both acute and long-term, especially with respect to neurologic injury and neurodevelopmental handicap. In our own work over many years, the follow-up of our patients over time has been instrumental in allowing us to work to improve outcomes. Although this information occasionally was disappointing to us at first, the obligation to publish this work and consider alternatives has been important in our own education and, we hope, to other clinicians. We believe that all neonatologists have an obligation to examine their infants carefully and publish their findings so that others can benefit from their accomplishments, as well as from their errors. No approach to respiratory support is complete without such information.

Although studies ultimately will help to frame a preferred sequence of ventilators, modalities, and therapies that provide optimal lung protection for a general population of infants, the care will always need to be individualized. No neonate is supposed to have gas forced into the lung under positive pressure; therefore, all ventilators are two-edged swords. Ventilators keep babies alive, but at some cost to the infant. As we continue to undertake the care of ever tinier and more fragile babies, as well as larger infants with pulmonary insufficiency, we will continue to see infants who manifest many long-term problems. Ultimately, optimal pulmonary outcomes can be achieved only when we can guarantee that neurodevelopmental outcomes will be as good as possible.

LIQUID VENTILATION

Despite the advances in mechanical ventilation and respiratory therapy of infants since the mid-1970s, injury of the neonatal airway and pulmonary parenchyma remains a major problem. Because of the frequency of respiratory-related morbidity and mortality, investigators explored liquid ventilation as an alternative approach to gas breathing.[58] This technique is based on sound physiologic and developmental principles that were shown in early animal studies to offer potential benefits for the neonate in respiratory failure.[59–62] Initial human clinical trials suggested safety and efficacy, but delays have occurred in progressing to clinical approval. At the present time, we await the results of pivotal randomized trials in adults that should guide the next steps of this technology.

As discussed later in this chapter, respiratory morbidity is caused, in part, by tidal lung inflation and ventilation of the atelectatic lung. With liquid instillation of the lung, alveolar volumes can be gently recruited and the air–fluid interface eliminated, thereby reducing the high surface forces that are present in the air-filled, surfactant-deficient lung. In addition to reduced surface forces, however, a liquid solution must be able to hold sufficient oxygen to permit adequate gas delivery within the air spaces. Saline solubility for O_2 is only 3 mL per 100 mL of fluid at 1 atm, or about 5% of that needed by the infant. As a result, if liquid breathing is contemplated, an alternative solution capable of dissolving and exchanging far greater concentrations of O_2 must be used.

Solutions for Liquid Ventilation

The first reports of mammalian survival during breathing of oxygenated perfluorocarbon (PFC) liquids came from Clark and Gollan[63] in 1966. Additional work has demonstrated that mammals can successfully breathe these liquids and subsequently return to air-breathing conditions.[64,65] Much of the work in liquid ventilation has, therefore, focused on PFCs.

PFCs have a high solubility for respiratory gases and are formed by the replacement of all carbon-bound hydrogen atoms on organic compounds with fluorine. They are commonly produced with a variety of techniques from benzene through the use of electrochemical fluoridation techniques, heating or agitation with cobalt trifluoride, or direct fluorination by careful addition of fluorine gas under controlled conditions.[66] Oxygen dissolves in PFCs approximately 20 times more readily than in saline. Carbon dioxide (CO_2) solubility also is high, although more variable, and depends on the specific perfluorochemical.[67] In addition to demonstrating excellent solubility of O_2 and CO_2, these liquids are odorless and colorless, have low surface tension properties, and are generally immiscible in lipids, alcohol, and water. They generally are biologically inert and are absorbed systemically in low concentrations. They typically evaporate rapidly in room air.

Although their attributes tend to make PFCs an ideal respiratory medium for gas exchange, these substances have high density, viscosity, and diffusion coefficients, which make the work of breathing during spontaneous respiration with them significantly greater than that needed for gas breathing.[68] In particular, the higher viscosity markedly increases resistance to flow, prolonging both inspiratory and expiratory time constants. In addition, the diffusion coefficient is prolonged so that the inspiratory time requirement is further increased. Because expiratory flow rates are reduced markedly in the PFC-filled lung compared with the gas-filled lung and because they are inversely proportional to lung volume, expiratory time is substantially greater than that seen during gas breathing. One can, therefore, conceive of PFC breathing as a process in which respiratory rate is reduced, inspiratory and expiratory times are more prolonged, and an exchange period or "dwell" time is required for adequate gas exchange to occur.

Some of the physical properties of PFCs that have been used in liquid breathing are listed in Table 13-2. In animal trials, these liquids have been used for periods as long as 30 hours with no apparent ill effects.[69] At the present time, there do not appear to be any physiologic limitations to the duration of exposure of mammals to PFCs in liquid breathing. The long-term toxicities remain unknown. Following liquid ventilation in animals, some species have shown a transient mild deterioration in pulmonary mechanics after return to gas breathing.[70,71] Surface tension has been shown to be somewhat increased in such situations (15 dyne/cm compared with the normal 2 dyne/cm), possibly due to the presence of residual PFCs in the lung.

Histologic evaluation of prematurely delivered animals ventilated with PFCs and recovered to air respiration demonstrates decreased hyaline membrane formation, reduced injury to airway epithelium and distal air spaces, and clearance of alveolar debris.[69,72] Lung ultrastructure appears to remain intact following liquid breathing. In longer-term evaluations, no changes on either light or electron microscopic examinations (except for a slight increase in the number of alveolar macrophages) have been noted in dogs, and adult monkeys have had normal pulmonary function for as long as 3 years after treatment.[73-75]

Systemically, PFCs appear to be eliminated almost entirely through the lungs, with small amounts excreted through the skin. Little PFC is absorbed by the pulmonary circulation during therapy, although small amounts may remain stored in fat cells for years after liquid breathing.[76-78] PFCs appear to be biologically inert and do not undergo transformation; therefore, toxicity seems unlikely. Elimination in these conditions appears to be dependent on subsequent reentry into the circulation, with ultimate excretion occurring through the usual routes of the lungs and skin. Perflubron, a brominated perfluorochemical used during magnetic resonance imaging, has been shown to be safe when it is administered intratracheally.[78] Fluosol-DA, an artificial blood substitute that consists of a 20% perfluorochemical emulsion, has been extensively studied and been found to have few adverse effects.[79] Clearly, extensive additional work must be performed in humans before the ultimate safety of these agents can be determined for pulmonary use.

PFCs other than those mentioned can be used for removal of airway debris, as seen in meconium aspiration syndrome[62]; drug delivery (antibiotics, bronchodilators, cancer chemotherapeutics, surfactants, vasopressors, vasodilators) to the lung[80]; and radiologic applications. The PFC-filled organ has low acoustic attenuation; thus, PFCs are ideal for ultrasound applications, and the presence of fluorine is valuable in magnetic resonance imaging. Furthermore, perfluorochemicals are radiopaque and consequently of value in standard radiographic applications.

Techniques and Results of Liquid Breathing in Animals

In their initial studies of liquid breathing, Clark and Gollan[63] used simple immersion techniques: animals were suspended in the liquid medium and allowed to breathe spontaneously. Although the animals demonstrated their ability to survive, the high viscosity of the liquid indicated that fatigue would likely become a prominent factor with prolonged spontaneous liquid breathing. Later efforts included a gravity-assisted approach in which the oxygenated PFCs were suspended above the animal and allowed to drain into the lung.[72] By altering infusion and emptying cycles, O_2 can be delivered and CO_2 removed. The

TABLE 13-2.   Physical Properties of Selected Perfluorocarbon Liquids Used for Liquid Ventilation

	Water*	FC-77[†]	RM-101[†]	FC-75[†]	Perfluorodecalin[†]	Perflubron[†]
Boiling point (°C)	100	97	101	102	142	143
Density, 25°C (g/mL)	1.00	1.78	1.77	1.78	1.95	1.93
Kinematic viscosity (centistokes, 25°C)	1.00	0.80	0.82	0.82	2.90	1.10
Vapor pressure (mm Hg, 37°C)	47	85	64	63	14	11
Surface tension (dyne/cm, 25°C)	72	15	15	15	15	18
Oxygen solubility, 25°C (mL gas/100 mL liquid)	3	50	52	52	49	53
Oxygen solubility, 37°C (mL gas/100mL liquid)	57	198	160	160	140	210

*Water properties given for comparison.
[†]Industrial perfluorocarbons FC-77 and FC-75 manufactured by 3M Corporation, St. Paul, MN, USA; RM-101 manufactured by Miteni Milan, Milan, Italy; perflubron is the generic name for perfluorooctylbromide, developed for medical applications by Alliance Pharmaceutical Corp., San Diego, CA, USA; perfluorodecalin manufactured by Green Cross Corp., Japan, and others.
From Shaffer TH, Wolfson MR: Principles and applications of liquid breathing-water babies revisited. In Fanaroff AA, Klaus MH (eds): Year Book of Neonatal-Perinatal Medicine 1992. St. Louis, Mosby-Year Book, 1992, p. XV.

awkwardness and expense of this approach for prolonged treatment due to the inability to reuse the PFCs are readily apparent. As a result, most studies to date have focused on alternative cyclic support techniques to deliver oxygenated PFCs to the lung for gas exchange.[81]

Several techniques for mechanically supported liquid breathing are in use. Most commonly, a time-cycled apparatus is used to deliver and recycle the preoxygenated heated liquid (Fig. 13-4). In such devices, either pressure or volume limits can be set for delivery of the desired fluid volume. Because of the expense of the PFCs, reclamation and readministration of the scrubbed fluid are essential. The majority of published studies to date have used this technology, which permits cautious regulation of desired ventilation. With these ventilators, optimal breathing rates usually are between 3 and 6 breaths/min, a rate determined more by the characteristics of the liquid than by lung mechanics. Carbon dioxide levels are managed primarily by changing tidal volume, although gas exchange can be manipulated further by altering the frequency of liquid infusion or I/E ratios, as determined on the basis of pulmonary mechanics. Changing the O_2 content of the PFC or altering the FRC can control arterial oxygenation.

For clinical trials, modification of the prolonged total liquid ventilation approach has been used. Rather than continuous liquid ventilation, a brief filling and cycling of the lungs with oxygenated perfluorochemical is performed for 3 to 5 minutes, and the infants are returned to gas ventilation. This procedure was designed to recruit atelectatic regions of the lung and to take advantage of the surface properties of the perfluorochemical liquids. Several studies have explored this technology for application in patients with other lung injuries.[80-84] A further modification of this technique has been developed in which perfluorochemical is gradually replaced once the subject is returned to gas ventilation with the liquid-filled lung.[85] With this technique, PFCs were replaced as necessary to maintain visible PFCs in the trachea when PEEP was stopped. However, the effects of chronic displacement of the liquid volume within the airway and the risks of airway injury with this technique are uncertain at present. Clearly, the technique of liquid ventilation should not increase the likelihood of airway injury; if this were the case, its utility in the treatment of neonatal pulmonary disease would be limited.

Numerous animal studies have established the effectiveness of gas exchange during liquid breathing. In 1983, Shaffer et al.[60] delivered lambs at 132 days of gestation by cesarean section. The animals were treated with liquid breathing as a rescue therapy before they were returned to gas breathing. During treatment, the animals had decreased inflating pressures, yet the alveolar-arterial difference in O_2 tension and compliance both improved (Fig. 13-5). Furthermore, arterial

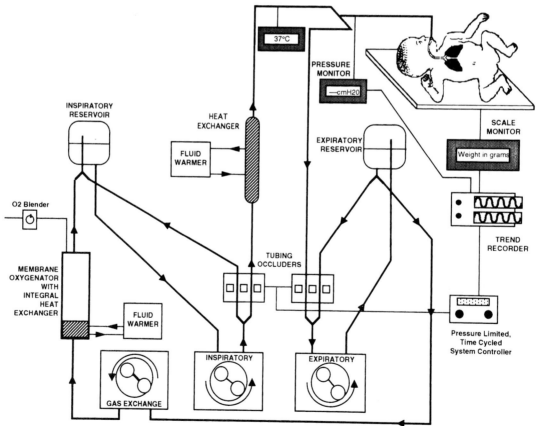

Figure 13-4. Technique for administration of perfluorocarbons at Thomas Jefferson University Hospital (Philadelphia, PA, USA). The system shown is used for infants, but the same circuit can be used for animal studies. Active inspiration and expiration are generated by two roller pumps; fluid is recycled (cleansed, oxygenated, and heated) by a third roller pump. Online infant weight and airway pressure measurements allow for continuous monitoring of driving pressures, tidal volume, functional residual capacity, respiratory mechanics, and alveolar pressure. *Arrows* demonstrate the flow of perfluorocarbons through the circuit.

carbon dioxide tension remained lower after the return to gas ventilation, especially in the youngest animals, which suggested an improvement in alveolar recruitment and stability. The following year, the same investigators treated a series of preterm lambs with meconium aspiration and obtained similarly beneficial results. In addition, the presence of meconium was evident in the liquid expired during treatment, indicating the "scrubbing" effect of the PFCs used in this protocol.[62]

More recently, studies of prematurely delivered animals treated with liquid breathing have revealed some significant differences between liquid breathing and gas ventilation, especially when the former was used prophylactically shortly after birth.[67,86] Prophylactic liquid ventilation provides excellent gas exchange, improves compliance, enhances acid–base balance and cardiovascular stability, and improves survival. During the same study period, gas-ventilated animals demonstrate progressive deterioration and limited survival. As described previously, preterm animals have been maintained with liquid ventilation for as long as 30 hours, with no apparent ill effects.

Recent efforts to use liquid breathing have focused on the improvement of clinical applicability through better interfacing with gas ventilation. During initiation of liquid ventilation following gas breathing, which is likely to be the most common clinical situation, the potential exists for gas trapping between the liquid and the terminal air spaces. Because liquid ventilation must be established by forming an FRC of PFCs, residual gas must be removed by thoracic manipulation and repositioning. Unfortunately this transition may take several minutes, during which gas exchange may deteriorate. Such circum-

stances would not be well tolerated clinically in a sick neonate. Possible solutions in the initiation phase might involve the introduction of several small boluses or a slow infusion. Thus, a strategy that combines gas ventilation during the period of liquid FRC establishment is required, and the optimal technique remains to be determined.

Clinical Applications of Liquid Breathing

Attempts to move PFC technologies into the clinical setting have met with limited success. Although some fluids have been approved for use (for imaging, limited application as an artificial blood product, and replacement fluid for the eye), to date approval, acceptance, and clinical exploration have been limited.

Respiratory Applications

Liquid ventilation seems most applicable in assisting the surfactant and structural deficiencies of the preterm lung. Surface tension forces are reduced or eliminated and lung recruitment can be optimized and atelectasis gently reexpanded, while the fluid environment of the developing fetal lung can be reproduced.[87,88]

Application to the term infant with structural lung disease [e.g., congenital diaphragmatic hernia (CDH)] or lung disease associated with airway or lung parenchymal debris (e.g., aspiration syndromes, pneumonia) has been supported by animal data. Investigation of a lamb preparation of CDH supported with partial liquid ventilation (PLV), either prophylactically at birth or rescued after a period of gas ventilation, showed improved gas exchange and compliance compared to conventional gas ventilation.[89] Many laboratory studies have shown the ability of liquid-assisted ventilation to improve gas exchange, mechanics, and cardiopulmonary stability in both large animal models and neonatal animal models of pneumonia, aspiration syndromes, and acute RDS.[90] In lambs with meconium aspiration, improvements were noted during total liquid ventilation and PLV in Pao_2, alveolar-arterial (A-a) oxygen gradient, and pulmonary compliance and pulmonary blood flow.

Nonrespiratory Applications

In addition to respiratory application, liquid techniques offer other clinically applicable benefits. PFC liquids can be an effective medium for drug delivery, particularly in the lung.[91–94] The physiologic properties of the lung as an exchanger for biologic agents include its large surface area, thin walls, and accessibility to the entire cardiac output. Liquid-assisted drug therapy may be beneficial for both the lung with pathology (i.e., administering an antibiotic or chemotherapeutic agent directly to an affected region of the lung) and for the healthy lung for improved distribution (i.e., delivery of adenovirus for gene therapy, or anesthetic agents).

Radiographic Imaging

PFC liquids have been explored as contrast media, particularly in the lung and the gastrointestinal tract.[95,96] The presence of bromine atoms in a PFC (perflubron, LiquiVent, Alliance Pharmaceutical Corporation, San Diego, CA, USA) can confer

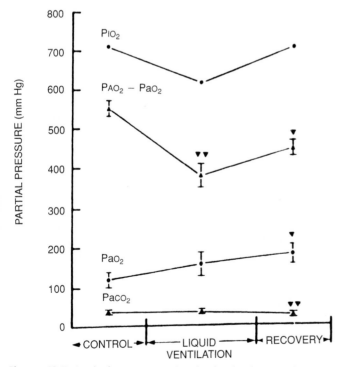

Figure 13-5. Inspired oxygen tension (Pio_2), alveolar-arterial oxygen gradient ($PAo_2 - Pao_2$), arterial oxygen tension (Pao_2), and arterial carbon dioxide tension ($Paco_2$) during control, liquid ventilation, and recovery to gas ventilation after liquid ventilation. (From Shaffer TH, Douglas PR, Lowe CA, et al: Liquid ventilation: Improved gas exchange and lung compliance in preterm lambs. Pediatr Res 17:303, 1983. © 1983, The Williams & Wilkins Company, Baltimore.)

relatively greater radiopacity. In the PFC-filled lung, conventional radiography and high-resolution computed tomography can be used not only to illustrate lung structures with great clarity but also to qualitatively and quantitatively evaluate PFC lung distribution and elimination. Radiographic studies of the perflubron-filled lungs of animals and humans with CDH have proved informative to delineate qualitatively the degree of pulmonary hypoplasia and volume recruitment.[97]

Virtual bronchoscopy is a relatively new technique that allows four-dimensional imaging of the inside of hollow viscera.[95] The PFC liquid perflubron has been used as a bronchographic contrast agent to markedly enhance navigation of substantially more distal airways. PFC liquids also can be used for nuclear magnetic resonance imaging because PFCs are devoid of hydrogen atoms. No magnetic resonance imaging signal is produced and the PFC-filled body cavities appear dark. In addition, because oxygen dissolved in PFC affects the nuclear magnetic resonance signal, regional differences in oxygen tension can be evaluated and gas exchange monitored.

Antiinflammatory Effects

It was shown in several in vivo animal models of acute lung injury that liquid ventilation can reduce alveolar hemorrhage, pulmonary permeability, edema, and neutrophil infiltration.[96] This antiinflammatory effect may be due to clearance of lung debris and improved tissue oxygenation; however, there is also a direct antiinflammatory effect of perfluorochemical liquid.[98,99] It is hypothesized that this antiinflammatory effect could inhibit the development of chronic lung disease.

Lung Recruitment

Recent studies have shown the potential of liquid ventilation as an alternative treatment in supporting gas exchange and lung mechanics in the presence of pulmonary hypoplasia.[100,101] PLV studies of CDH in a lamb showed improved gas exchange and compliance compared to conventional gas ventilation support. These studies demonstrated that animals treated early, prior to gas ventilation, demonstrated improved function and histology compared with rescue treatment. Lung expansion techniques, particularly when used in conjunction with ECMO, may provide a mechanism to stimulate lung growth in term infants with lethal pulmonary hypoplasia.

Partial Liquid Ventilation with Other Therapies

Initial trials of PLV in infants and children were complicated by the availability of newer therapies such as HFV, iNO, and exogenous surfactant. The interaction of these therapies with perfluorochemicals and PLV has been explored recently through animal protocols. Combining PLV with iNO may have a positive effect because the gas may be effectively distributed to the recruited lung units.[102,103] More work is required to explore potential enhancement of toxicity because oxygen and nitric oxide may dwell longer together when placed in perfluorochemicals. The interaction of exogenous surfactant with PLV is less clear. Surfactant administered before initiating PLV appears to diminish lung injury and improve mechanics, but PLV does not appear to improve the function of exogenous surfactant when the surfactant is given after PLV is initiated.[104,105]

The combination of HFV and PLV has been explored in several animal models. The combination of HFOV and PLV may improve lung recruitment, gas exchange, and hemodynamics in both term and preterm respiratory distress animal models.[106,107] Animal models suggest that liquid ventilation may facilitate the efficacy of other modalities that have been used to improve gas exchange with gas ventilation. Future clinical trials will assess the safety and efficacy of these combination therapies in humans.

Clinical Trials

The initial liquid ventilation study enrolled premature human infants who were near death at the time of treatment.[108,109] A gravity-assisted approach was used and tidal volumes of liquid were given in brief cycles. The infants tolerated the procedure, showed improvement in several physiologic parameters including lung compliance and gas exchange, and maintained some improvement after liquid ventilation was discontinued. The protocol used a form of total liquid ventilation, but it also reported on the sustained benefit of gas ventilating the liquid-filled lung: PLV. Subsequent protocols have used a PLV technique.

Several studies of PLV using the PFC sterile perflubron LiquiVent have been completed or are ongoing in humans. Leach et al.[110] reported on 13 premature infants with severe RDS who had not responded to conventional treatment. The infants were treated with PLV for up to 96 hours by protocol (maximal time on PLV for any infant was 76 hours). The infants' lungs were filled with LiquiVent, and supplemental doses were given frequently, generally hourly (Fig. 13-6). The study was not randomized or blinded. The arterial oxygen tension and dynamic compliance increased significantly (Fig. 13-7), and the oxygenation index was reduced within 1 hour of initiating PLV. The authors concluded that there was clinical improvement and survival in some infants who had not been predicted to survive.

Pranikoff et al.[111] reported their results on four patients with CDH who were managed by ECMO. PLV was performed in a phase I/II trial for up to 6 days with daily dosing. They concluded that this technique was safe and possibly associated with improvement in gas exchange and pulmonary compliance.

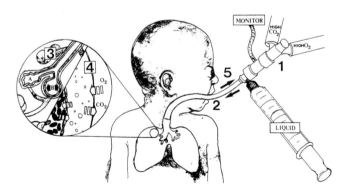

Figure 13-6. Schematic representation of partial liquid ventilation. Conventional gas ventilation (1) is delivered on the liquid-filled lung. Perfluorocarbon liquid is instilled on inspiration via a side port of the endotracheal tube (2). The liquid recruits potential air spaces (3), and gas exchange occurs through the liquid medium (4). Carbon dioxide-enriched gases then escape on exhalation (5).

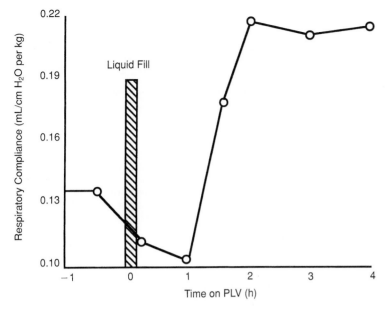

Figure 13-7. Change in respiratory compliance before and during the 4 hours of partial liquid ventilation in a term neonate with a congenital diaphragmatic hernia on extracorporeal membrane oxygenation. Increased compliance occurred after some debris was removed and effective delivery of perfluorocarbon to the distal lung sacs was achieved. The 57% increase in compliance due to volume recruitment and reduction of surface tension is less than that typically observed in preterm animals receiving liquid ventilation.

Greenspan et al.[112] reported on six term infants with respiratory failure whose status was not improving while they were receiving ECMO. The infants were treated with PLV using LiquiVent for up to 96 hours, with hourly dosing. Dynamic pulmonary compliance increased significantly and lung volume was recruited. The authors concluded that the technique appeared to be safe and improved lung function in these critically ill term infants.

The results of these initial studies of PLV in neonates are encouraging and suggest the feasibility of this technique in neonates with severe RDS and acute respiratory distress syndrome (ARDS). It has been observed that the underlying pathophysiology influences the impact of liquid-assisted ventilation. The response of the sick term infant to PLV frequently is more gradual than is typically observed in the preterm infant with RDS. The preterm infant often experiences improvement in lung compliance and gas exchange within hours of PLV initiation, most likely due to reduction in surface tension and volume recruitment. Improving lung function in the term infant on PLV often requires debris removal, which occurs gradually.

Other studies have evaluated PLV in children,[113–117] but none of these studies used a control group. Gauger et al.[113] reported on six pediatrics patients with ARDS who required extracorporeal life support (ECLS). These patients were treated with LiquiVent PLV for 3 to 7 days with daily dosing. They observed some improvement in gas exchange and pulmonary compliance over the 96 hours from the initial dose, and all patients survived. Hirschl et al.[115] treated seven pediatric patients with ARDS who required ECMO. They also found improvement in gas exchange and pulmonary compliance during PLV for 1 to 7 days. Toro-Figueroa et al.[116] presented their results on 10 children up to 17 years old with ARDS treated with PLV for up to 96 hours. Nine of 10 patients tolerated initial dosing, and all nine experienced improvement in gas exchange over the 48-hour treatment period. Lung function did not improve in their patients. The authors concluded that PLV may be safe and efficacious in the treatment of pediatric ARDS.

Several phase I/II studies of PLV using LiquiVent in adults have been reported. Hirschl et al.[114,115] treated 10 adult patients who had ARDS and were on ECLS with PLV for up to 7 days. Patients were dosed daily. The authors reported a decrease in the physiologic shunt from a median of 0.72 to 0.46 over the 72 hours following initiation of PLV and an increase in pulmonary compliance over the same time period. Fifty percent of the patients survived. The authors concluded that PLV may be safe in these patients and may be associated with improvement in gas exchange and pulmonary compliance. Bartlett et al.[117] reported a phase II, randomized controlled trial of PLV in adult patents with acute hypoxemic respiratory failure. Sixty-five adults received PLV with LiquiVent for 5 days. Twenty-five patients served as controls. Ventilator-free days and mortality did not differ between groups, but the investigators reported a statistically significant improvement in ventilator-free days in subjects younger than 55 years treated with PLV. The authors concluded that PLV can be accomplished with safety in this population, and they suggested that larger trials be initiated.

These clinical reports have described few adverse effects. Filling and subsequent ventilation have generally been well tolerated, even in these unstable populations. One noteworthy phenomenon has been the appearance during treatment of tenacious debris, which causes endotracheal tube occlusion and interferes with gas exchange. It has not been determined whether this represents alveolar and deep pulmonary secretions that otherwise would not be mobilized or an exudative response to the liquid.

Although the results of the initial phase I/II trials demonstrate potential safety and efficacy, particularly in younger populations of sick patients, an understanding of the utility of this technique awaits the results of phase III trials. The complications and economics associated with drug approval have limited this pivotal trial to adults. As of the writing of this manuscript, a large randomized PLV trial (phase III, FDA) in adults with ARDS has been completed in North America and Europe. Several liquid ventilation trials in infants and children are under design but await the results of the adult trial.

Future of Liquid Breathing

Although the results of initial studies of perfluorochemical respiration appear encouraging, many questions remain. The long-term efficacy and safety of these substances need to be defined in further trials. The optimal PFC for specific clinical situations is uncertain, and much work still is required for the establishment of an optimal delivery system for therapy of the human infant. The spectrum of drugs that can be effectively delivered by perfluorochemicals must be determined, as well as the efficacy of combination therapies. Liquid breathing appears to be an important therapy, however, and the work that will be done over the next few years unquestionably will be of great value for the critically ill neonate.

REFERENCES

1. Avery ME, Tooley WH, Keller JB, et al: Is chronic lung disease in low birth weight infants preventable? Pediatrics 79:26, 1987.
2. Van Marter LJ, Allred EN, Pagano M, et al: Do clinical markers of barotrauma and oxygen toxicity explain interhospital variation in rates of chronic lung disease? Pediatrics 105:1194, 2000.
3. Vigneswaran R: Infection and preterm birth: Evidence of a common causal relationship with bronchopulmonary dysplasia and cerebral palsy. J Paediatr Child Health 36:293, 2000.
4. Krohn MA, Hitti J: Characteristics of women with clinical intra-amniotic infection who deliver preterm compared with term. Am J Epidemiol 147:111, 1998.
5. Kashlan F, Smulian J, Shen-Schwarz S, et al: Umbilical vein interleukin 6 and tumor necrosis factor alpha plasma concentrations in the very preterm infant. Pediatr Infect Dis J 19:238, 2000.
6. Baud O, Emilie D, Pelletier E, et al: Amniotic fluid concentrations of interleukin-1beta, interleukin-6 and TNF-alpha in chorioamnionitis before 32 weeks of gestation: Histological associations and neonatal outcome. Br J Obstet Gynaecol 106:72, 1999.
7. Panitch HB, Deoras KS, Wolfson MR, et al: Functional changes in airway smooth muscle structure-function relationships. Pediatr Res 31:151, 1992.
8. Bhutani VK, Rubenstein D, Shaffer TH: Effect of positive pressure on the mechanical behavior of the developing rabbit trachea. Pediatr Res 15:829, 1981.
9. Shaffer TH, Bhutani VK, Wolfson MR, et al: In-vivo mechanical properties of the developing airway. Pediatr Res 25:143–146, 1989.
10. Bjorklund LJ, Ingimarsson J, Curstedt T, et al: Manual ventilation with a few large breaths at birth compromises the therapeutic effect of subsequent surfactant replacement in immature lambs. Pediatr Res 42:348–355, 1997.
11. Berry D, Jobe A, Ikegami M: Leakage of macromolecules in ventilated and unventilated segments of preterm lamb lungs. J Appl Physiol 70:423, 1991.
12. Nilsson R, Grossmann G, Robertson B: Lung surfactant and the pathogenesis of neonatal bronchiolar lesions induced by artificial ventilation. Pediatr Res 12:249, 1978.
13. Seidner SR, Ikegami M, Yamada T, et al: Decreased surfactant dose-response after delayed administration to preterm rabbits. Am J Respir Crit Care Med 152:113, 1995.
14. Kendig JW, Notter RH, Cox C, et al: A comparison of surfactant as immediate prophylaxis and as rescue therapy in newborns of less than 30 weeks gestation. N Engl J Med 324:865–871, 1991.
15. Soll RF. Clinical trials of surfactant therapy in the newborn. In Robertson B, Taeusch HW (eds): Surfactant Therapy for Lung Disease. New York, Marcel Dekker, 1995, p. 407.
16. Linder W, Vofsbeck S, Hummler H, et al: Delivery room management of extremely low birth weight infant: Spontaneous breathing or intubation? Pediatrics 103:961–967, 1999.
17. Vento M, Asensi M, Sastre J, et al: Resuscitation with room air instead of 100% oxygen prevents oxidative stress in moderately asphyxiated term neonates. Pediatrics 107:642, 2001.
18. Hintz SR, Suttner DM, Sheehan AM, et al: Decreased use of neonatal extracorporeal membrane oxygenation (ECMO): How new treatment modalities have affected ECMO utilization. Pediatrics 106:1339–1343, 2000.
19. Graziani LJ, Spitzer AR, Mitchell DG, et al: Mechanical ventilation in preterm infants: Neurosonographic and developmental studies. Pediatrics 90:515–522, 1992.
20. Hobar JD, Rogowski J, Plsek PE, et al: Collaborative quality improvement for neonatal intensive care. Pediatrics 107:14–22, 2001.
21. Jobe A, Ikegami M: Mechanisms initiating lung injury in the preterm. Early Hum Dev 53:81–94, 1998.
22. Dreyfuss D, Saumon G: Role of tidal volume, FRC, and end-inspiratory volume in the development of pulmonary edema following mechanical ventilation. Am Rev Respir Dis 148:1194, 1993.
23. Slutsky AS: Lung injury caused by mechanical ventilation. Chest 116(Suppl):9S, 1999.
24. Muscedere JG, Mullen JB, Gan K, et al: Tidal ventilation at low airway pressures can augment lung injury. Am J Respir Crit Care Med 149:1327, 1994.
25. Heicher DA, Kasting DS, Harrod JR: Prospective clinical comparison of two methods for mechanical ventilation of the neonate: Rapid rate and short inspiratory time versus slow rate and long inspiratory time. J Pediatr 98:957–959, 1981.
26. Clark RH, Slutsky AS, Gerstmann DR: Commentary: Lung protective strategies of ventilation in the Neonate: What are they? Pediatrics 105:112, 2000.
27. Oxford Region Controlled Trial of Artificial Ventilation (OCTAVE). Multi-centre randomised controlled trial of high versus low frequency positive pressure ventilation in 346 newborn infants. Arch Dis Child 66:770–777, 1991.
28. Greenough A, Pool J, Gamsu H: Randomized controlled trial of two methods of weaning from high frequency positive pressure ventilation. Arch Dis Child 64:834, 1989.
29. Spahr RC, Klein AM, Brown DR, et al: Hyaline membrane disease: A controlled study of inspiratory to expiratory ratio in its management by ventilator. Am J Dis Child 134:373, 1980.
30. Bernstein G, Marnnion FL, Heldt GP, et al: Randomized multicenter trial comparing synchronized conventional intermittent mandatory ventilation in neonates. J Pediatr 128:453, 1996.
31. DeBoer RC, Ansari NA, Baumer JH, et al: Mode of ventilation in neonatal RDS: Effect on the stress response. Prenatal Neonatal Med 1:266, 1996.
32. Nicks JJ, Becker MA, Donn SM: Bronchopulmonary dysplasia: Response to pressure support ventilation. J Perinatol 14:495–500, 1994.
33. Oliver RE, Rozycki HJ, Greenspan JS, et al: Tracheal gas insufflation (TGI) as a lung protective strategy: Physiologic, histologic, and biochemical markers. Pediatr Res 49:272A, 2001.
34. Barrington KJ, Bull D, Finer N: Randomized trial of nasal synchronized intermittent mandatory ventilation compared to continuous positive airway pressure after extubation of very low birth weight infants. Pediatrics 107:638, 2001.
35. Courtney SE, Pyon KH, Saslow JG, et al: Lung recruitment and breathing pattern during variable versus continuous flow nasal continuous positive airway pressure in premature infants: An evaluation of three devices. Pediatrics 107:304–308, 2001.
36. Reynolds EOR, Tagizadeh A: Improved prognosis of infants mechanically ventilated for hyaline membrane disease. Arch Dis Child 49:505, 1974.
37. Bland RD, Kim MH, Light MJ, et al: High frequency mechanical ventilation in severe hyaline membrane disease. An alternative treatment? Crit Care Med 8:275, 1980.
38. Peckham GJ, Fox WW: Physiologic factors affecting pulmonary artery pressure in infants with persistent pulmonary hypertension. J Pediatr 93:1005, 1978.
39. Graziani LJ, Desai S, Baumgart S, et al: Clinical antecedents of neurologic and audiologic abnormalities in survivors of neonatal ECMO—A group comparison study. J Child Neurol 12:415, 1997.
40. Keszler M, Donn SM, Bucciarelli RL, et al: Multicenter controlled trial comparing high-frequency jet ventilation and conventional mechanical ventilation in newborn infants with pulmonary interstitial emphysema. J Pediatr 119:85, 1991.
41. Spitzer AR, Butler S, Fox WW: Ventilatory response of combined high frequency jet ventilation and conventional mechanical ventilation for the rescue treatment of severe neonatal lung disease. Pediatr Pulmonol 7:244, 1989.
42. Delemos RA, Coalson JJ, Gerstmann DR, et al: Ventilatory management of infant baboons with hyaline membrane disease: The use of high frequency ventilation. Pediatr Res 21:594, 1987.
43. The HIFI Group: A collaborative randomized trial of high frequency oscillatory ventilation versus conventional mechanical ventilation in the

treatment of respiratory failure in preterm infants. N Engl J Med 320:88, 1989.

44. Courtney SE, Durand DJ, Asselin JM, The Neonatal Ventilation Study Group: Early high frequency oscillatory ventilation (HFV) vs synchronized intermittent mandatory ventilation (SIMV) in very low birth weight (VLBW) infants. Pediatr Res 49:387A, 2001.

45. Finer NN, Barrington KJ: Nitric oxide for respiratory failure in infants born at or near term (Cochrane Review). Cochrane Database Syst Rev 2:CD000399, 2001.

46. Hoehn T, Krause MF, Buhrer C: Inhaled nitric oxide in premature infants—A meta-analysis. J Perinat Med 28:7, 2000.

47. Barrington KJ, Finer NN: Inhaled nitric oxide for respiratory failure in preterm infants. Cochrane Database Syst Rev CD000509.

48. Bennett AJ, Shaw NJ, Gregg JE, et al: Neurodevelopmental outcome in high-risk preterm infants treated with inhaled nitric oxide. Acta Paediatr 90:573, 2001.

49. Wung JT, James LS, Kilchevsky E, et al: Management of infants with severe respiratory failure and persistence of the fetal circulation, without hyperventilation. Pediatrics 76:488, 1985.

50. Mariani G, Cifuentes J, Carlo W: Randomized trial of permissive hypercapnia in preterm infants. Pediatrics 104:1082–1088, 1999.

51. Wiswell TE, Graziani LJ, Kornhauser MS, et al: Effects of hypocarbia on the development of cystic periventricular leukomalacia in premature infants treated with high-frequency ventilation. Pediatrics 98:918–924, 1996.

52. Vannucci RC, Towfighi J, Brucklacher RM, et al: Effect of extreme hypercapnia on hypoxic-ischemic brain damage in the immature rat. Pediatr Res 49:799, 2001.

53. Mrozek JD, Bendel-Stenzel EM, Meyers PA, et al: Randomized controlled trial of volume-targeted synchronized ventilation and conventional intermittent mandatory ventilation following initial exogenous surfactant therapy. Pediatr Pulmonol 29:11, 2000.

54. Cheema IU, Ahluwahia JS: Feasibility of tidal volume-guided ventilation in newborn infants: A randomized, crossover trial using the volume guarantee modality. Pediatrics 107:1323, 2001.

55. Schulze A, Gerhardt T, Musante G, et al: Proportional assist ventilation in low birth weight infants with acute respiratory disease: A comparison to assist/control and conventional mechanical ventilation. J Pediatr 135:339, 1999.

56. Schulze A: Enhancement of mechanical ventilation of neonates by computer technology. Semin Perinatol 24:429, 2000.

57. Musante G, Schulze A, Gerhardt T, et al: Proportional assist ventilation decreases thoracoabdominal asynchrony and chest wall distortion in preterm infants. Pediatr Res 49:175, 2001.

58. Shaffer TH, Wolfson MR: Principles and applications of liquid breathing: Water babies revisited. In Fanaroff AA, Klaus MH (eds): Year Book of Neonatal-Perinatal Medicine 1992. St. Louis, Mosby-Year Book, 1992, p. XV.

59. Shaffer TH, Moskowitz GD: Demand controlled liquid ventilation of the lungs. J Appl Physiol 36:208, 1974.

60. Shaffer TH, Douglas PR, Lowe CA, et al: Liquid ventilation: Improved gas exchange and lung compliance in preterm lambs. Pediatr Res 17:303, 1983.

61. Shaffer TH, Tran N, Bhutani VK, et al: Cardiopulmonary function in very preterm lambs during liquid ventilation. Pediatr Res 17:680, 1983.

62. Shaffer TH, Lowe CA, Bhutani VK, et al: Liquid ventilation: Effects on pulmonary function in meconium stained lambs. Pediatr Res 19:49, 1984.

63. Clark LC, Gollan F: Survival of mammals breathing organic liquids equilibrated with oxygen at atmospheric pressure. Science 152:1755, 1966.

64. Schwieler GH, Robertson B: Liquid ventilation in immature newborn rabbits. Biol Neonate 29:343, 1976.

65. Modell JH, Calderwood HW, Ruiz BC: Long-term survival of dogs after breathing oxygenated fluorocarbon liquid. Fed Proc 29:1731, 1970.

66. Sargent JW, Seffl RJ: Properties of perfluorinated liquid. Fed Proc 29:1699, 1970.

67. Shaffer TH, Wolfson MR, Clark LC: Liquid ventilation. Pediatr Pulmonol 14:102, 1992.

68. Moskowitz GD, Shaffer TH, Dubin SE: Liquid breathing trials and animal studies with a demand-regulated liquid breathing system. Med Instrum 9:28, 1973.

69. Shaffer TH, Wolfson MR, Greenspan JS, et al: Animal models and clinical studies of liquid ventilation in neonatal respiratory distress syndrome. In Robertson B (ed): Surfactant in Clinical Practice. Geneva, Harwood Academic Publications, 1992, pp. 187–198.

70. Saga S, Modell JH, Calderwood HW, et al: Pulmonary function after ventilation with fluorocarbon liquid P12-f (Caroxin-F). J Appl Physiol 34:160, 1973.

71. Wolfson MR, Shaffer TH: Liquid ventilation during early development: Theory, physiologic processes, and application. J Dev Physiol 13:1, 1990.

72. Shaffer TH, Rubinstein SD, Moskowitz GD, et al: Gaseous exchange and acid-base balance in premature lambs during liquid ventilation since birth. Pediatr Res 10:227, 1976.

73. Salman NH, Fuhrman BP, Papo ML, et al: Oxygenation and lung mechanics during 24 hour trials of perfluorocarbon associated gas exchange (PAGE) in piglets. Pediatr Res 33:40A, 1993.

74. Matthews WH, Bolzer RH, Shelburne JD, et al: Steady-state gas exchange in normothermic, anesthetized, liquid ventilated dogs. Undersea Biomed Res 5:341, 1978.

75. Modell JH, Calderwood HW, Ruiz BC, et al: Liquid ventilation of primates. Chest 69:79, 1976.

76. Clark LC, Hoffmann RE, Davis SL: Response of the rabbit lung as a criterion of safety for fluorocarbon breathing and blood substitutes. Biomat Artif Immobil Biotechnol 20:1085, 1992.

77. Shaffer TH, Wolfson MR, Greenspan JS, et al: Liquid ventilation: Uptake, biodistribution, and elimination of perfluorochemical (PFC) liquid. Pediatr Res 31:223A, 1992.

78. Liu MS, Long DM: Biological distribution of perfluoroctylbromide: Tracheal administration in alveolography and bronchography. Invest Radiol 11:479, 1976.

79. Keipert PE, Otto S, Flaim SF, et al: Influence of perflubron emulsions particle size on blood half-life and febrile response in rats. Artif Cells Blood Substit Immobil Biotechnol 22:1169, 1994.

80. Wolfson MR, Greenspan JS, Shaffer TH: Pulmonary administration of vasoactive drugs (PAD) by perfluorocarbon liquid ventilation. Pediatr Res 29:336A, 1991.

81. Moskowitz GD: A mechanical respirator for control of liquid breathing. Fed Proc 29:1751, 1970.

82. Shaffer TH, Ferguson JD, Koen PA, et al: Pulmonary lavage in preterm lambs. Pediatr Res 12:695, 1978.

83. Richman PS, Wolfson MR, Shaffer TH, et al: Lung lavage with oxygenated fluorocarbon improves gas exchange and lung compliance in rats with acute lung injury. Crit Care Med 21:768, 1993.

84. Tutuncu AS, Faithfull NS, Lachmann B: Intratracheal perfluorocarbon administration combined with mechanical ventilation in experimental respiratory distress syndrome: Dose-dependent improved gas exchange. Crit Care Med 21:962, 1993.

85. Fuhrman BP, Paczan PR, DeFrancisis M: Perfluorocarbon associated gas exchange. Crit Care Med 19:712, 1991.

86. Wolfson MR, Greenspan JS, Deoras KS, et al: Comparison of gas and liquid ventilation: Clinical, physiological, and histological correlates. J Appl Physiol 72:1024, 1992.

87. Greenspan JS, Wolfson MR, Rubinstein SD, et al: Liquid ventilation in human preterm neonates. J Pediatr 117:106, 1990.

88. Greenspan JS, Cleary GM, Wolfson MR: Is liquid ventilation a reasonable alternative? In Goldsmith JP, Spitzer AR (eds): Clinics in Perinatology: Controversies in Neonatal Pulmonary Care. Philadelphia, W.B. Saunders, 1998, p. 137.

89. Wilcox DT, Glick PL, Karamanoukian H L, et al: Perfluorocarbon associated gas exchange (PAGE) and nitric oxide in the lamb with congenital diaphragmatic hernia model. Pediatr Res 35:260A, 1994.

90. Foust R, Tran NN, Cox C, et al: Liquid-assisted ventilation: An alternative ventilatory strategy for acute meconium aspiration injury. Pediatr Pulmonol 21:316, 1996.

91. Wolfson MR, Greenspan JS, Shaffer TH: Pulmonary administration of vasoactive drugs (PAD) by perfluorocarbon liquid ventilation. Pediatrics 97:449, 1996.

92. Lisby DA, Ballard PL, Fox WW, et al: Enhanced distribution of adenoviral mediated gene transfer to lung parenchyma by perfluorochemical liquid. Hum Gene Ther 8:919, 1997.

93. Kimless-Garber DB, Wolfson MR, Carlsson C, et al: Halothane administration during liquid ventilation. Respir Med 91:255, 1997.

94. Cullen AB, Cox CA, Hipp SJ, et al: Intra-tracheal delivery strategy of gentamicin with partial liquid ventilation. Respir Med 93:770, 1999.

95. Stern RG, Wolfson MR, McGuckin JF, et al: High-resolution computed tomographic bronchiolography using perfluoroctylbromide (PFOB): An experimental model. J Thorac Imaging 8:300, 1993.

96. Smith TM, Steinhorn DM, Thusu K, et al: Liquid perfluorochemical decreases the in vitro production of reactive oxygen species by alveolar macrophages. Crit Care Med 23:1533, 1995.

97. Gross GW, Greenspan JS, Fox WW, et al: Use of liquid ventilation with perflubron during extracorporeal membrane oxygenation: Chest radiographic appearances. Radiology 194:717, 1995.

98. Baba A, Kim YK, Zhang H, et al: Perfluorocarbon blocks tumor necrosis factor-α-induced interleukin-8 release from alveolar epithelial cells in vitro. Crit Care Med 28:1113, 2000.

99. Steinhorn DM, Papo MC, Rotta AT, et al: Liquid ventilation attenuates pulmonary oxidative damage. J Crit Care 14:20, 1999.

100. Major D, Cloutier R, Fournier L, et al: Improved pulmonary function after surgical reduction of congenital diaphragmatic hernia in lambs. J Pediatr Surg 34:426, 1999.

101. Major D, Cardenas M, Cloutier R, et al: Combined ventilation and perfluorochemical (PFC) tracheal instillation as alternative treatment for near-death congenital diaphragmatic hernia. J Pediatr Surg 30:1178, 1995.

102. Barrington KJ, Singh AJ, Etches PC, et al: Partial liquid ventilation with and without inhaled nitric oxide in a newborn piglet model of meconium aspiration. Am J Respir Crit Care Med 160:1922, 1999.

103. Uchida T, Nakazawa K, Yokoyama K, et al: The combination of partial liquid ventilation and inhaled nitric oxide in the severe oleic acid lung injury model. Chest 113:1658, 1998.

104. Mrozek JD, Smith KM, Bing DR, et al: Exogenous surfactant and partial liquid ventilation. Physiologic and pathologic effects. Am J Respir Crit Care Med 156:1058, 1997.

105. Mrozek JD, Smith KM, Simonton SC, et al: Perfluorocarbon priming and surfactant: Physiologic and pathologic effects. Crit Care Med 27:1916, 1999.

106. Sukumar M, Bommaraju M, Fisher JE, et al: High-frequency partial liquid ventilation in respiratory distress syndrome: Hemodynamics and gas exchange. J Appl Physiol 84:327, 1998.

107. Doctor A, Mazzoni MC, Delbalzo U, et al: High-frequency oscillatory ventilation of the perfluorocarbon-filled lung: Preliminary results in an animal model of acute lung injury. Crit Care Med 27:2500, 1999.

108. Greenspan JS, Wolfson MR, Rubenstein SD, et al: Liquid ventilation of human preterm neonates. J Pediatr 117;106, 1990.

109. Greenspan JS, Wolfson MR, Rubenstein SD, et al: Liquid ventilation of preterm baby [letter]. Lancet Nov:1095, 1989.

110. Leach CL, Greenspan JS, Rubenstein SD, et al: Partial liquid ventilation with perflubron in premature infants with severe respiratory distress syndrome. N Engl J Med 335:761, 1996.

111. Pranikoff T, Gauger PG, Hirschl RB: Partial liquid ventilation in newborn patients with congenital diaphragmatic hernia. J Pediatr Surg 31:613, 1996.

112. Greenspan JS, Fox WW, Rubenstein SD, et al: Partial liquid ventilation in critically ill infants receiving extracorporeal life support. Pediatrics 99:1, 1996.

113. Gauger PG, Pranikoff T, Schreiner RJ, et al: Initial experience with partial liquid ventilation in pediatric patients with the acute respiratory distress syndrome. Crit Care Med 24:16–22, 1996.

114. Hirschl RB, Pranikoff T, Gauger P, et al: Liquid ventilation in adults, children and neonates. Lancet 346:1201, 1995.

115. Hirschl RB, Parent A, Tooley R, et al: Lung management with perfluorocarbon liquid ventilation improves pulmonary function and gas exchange during extracorporeal membrane oxygenation (ECMO). Artif Cells Blood Substit Immobil Biotechnol 22:1389, 1994.

116. Toro-Figueroa LO, Meliones JN, Curtis SE, et al: Perflubron partial liquid ventilation (PLV) in children with ARDS: A safety and efficacy pilot study. Crit Care Med 24:150A, 1996.

117. Bartlett R, Croce M, Hirschl R, et al: A phase II randomized controlled trial of partial liquid ventilation (PLV) in adult patients with acute hypoxemic respiratory failure (AHRF). Crit Care Med 25:25A, 1997.

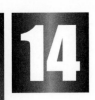

14 SPECIAL VENTILATORY TECHNIQUES AND MODALITIES III
Inhaled Nitric Oxide Therapy

JOHN KINSELLA, MD
STEVEN H. ABMAN, MD

Inhaled nitric oxide (iNO) therapy causes potent, selective, sustained pulmonary vasodilation and improves oxygenation in term newborns with severe hypoxemic respiratory failure and persistent pulmonary hypertension.[1-6] Multicenter randomized clinical studies have demonstrated that iNO therapy reduces the need for extracorporeal membrane oxygenation (ECMO) treatment in term neonates with hypoxemic respiratory failure.[7,8]

Since the last edition of this textbook, the role of iNO therapy has been extensively studied, leading to regulatory approval by the United States Food and Drug Administration for the treatment of near-term and term newborns with hypoxemic respiratory failure. In this chapter, we review an approach to the initial evaluation of the hypoxemic newborn for treatment with iNO, summarize the clinical experience with iNO in near-term and term newborns, and propose guidelines for the use of iNO in this population. The potential role of iNO in the premature newborn is controversial, and its use remains investigational in this population.[9]

BACKGROUND

The physiologic rationale for iNO therapy in the treatment of neonatal hypoxemic respiratory failure is based upon its ability to achieve potent and sustained pulmonary vasodilation without decreasing systemic vascular tone[10] (Fig. 14-1). Persistent pulmonary hypertension of the newborn (PPHN)[11] is a syndrome associated with diverse neonatal cardiac and pulmonary disorders that are characterized by high pulmonary vascular resistance (PVR) causing extrapulmonary right-to-left shunting of blood across the ductus arteriosus and/or foramen ovale[12,13] (see Chapter 23) (Fig. 14-2). Extrapulmonary shunting due to high PVR in severe PPHN can cause critical hypoxemia that is poorly responsive to inspired oxygen or pharmacologic vasodilation. Vasodilator drugs administered intravenously, such as tolazoline and sodium nitroprusside, often are unsuccessful due to systemic hypotension and an inability to achieve or sustain pulmonary vasodilation.[14,15] Thus, the ability of iNO therapy to selectively lower PVR and decrease extrapulmonary venoarterial admixture accounts for the acute improvement in oxygenation observed in newborns with PPHN.[16]

As described in children[17] and adults with severe respiratory failure,[18] oxygenation can improve during iNO therapy in some newborns who do not have extrapulmonary right-to-left shunting. Hypoxemia in these cases is primarily due to intrapulmonary shunting caused by continued perfusion of lung units that lack ventilation (e.g., atelectasis), with variable contributions from ventilation-perfusion (V/Q) inequality. Distinct from its ability to decrease extrapulmonary right-to-left shunting by reducing PVR, low-dose iNO therapy can improve oxygenation by redirecting blood from poorly aerated or diseased lung regions to better aerated distal air spaces ("microselective effect").[19]

In addition to its effects on vascular tone and reactivity, other physiologic targets for iNO therapy in hypoxemic respiratory failure may include direct effects of NO on lung inflammation, vascular permeability, and thrombosis in situ. Although some laboratory studies have suggested that NO can potentiate lung injury by promoting oxidative or nitrosative stress,[20] inactivating surfactant, and stimulating inflammation,[21] other studies have demonstrated striking antioxidant and antiinflammatory effects in models of lung injury.[22-24] Thus, clinical benefits of low-dose iNO therapy may include reduced lung inflammation and edema, as well as potential protective effects on surfactant function,[25] but these effects remain clinically unproven (Table 14-1).

Finally, the diagnostic value of iNO therapy is important because failure to respond to iNO raises important questions about the specific mechanism of hypoxemia. Poor responses to iNO should lead to further diagnostic evaluation for "unsuspected" anatomic cardiovascular or pulmonary disease (see later).

TABLE 14-1. Potential Beneficial Effects of Low-Dose Inhaled Nitric Oxide in Hypoxemic Respiratory Failure

1. Pulmonary vasodilation → decreased extrapulmonary right-to-left shunting
2. Enhanced matching of alveolar ventilation with perfusion
3. ↓ Inflammation (↓ lung neutrophil accumulation)
4. ↓ Vascular leak and lung edema
5. Preservation of surfactant function
6. ↓ Oxidant injury (inhibition of lipid oxidation)
7. Preservation of vascular endothelial growth factor expression
8. Altered proinflammatory gene expression

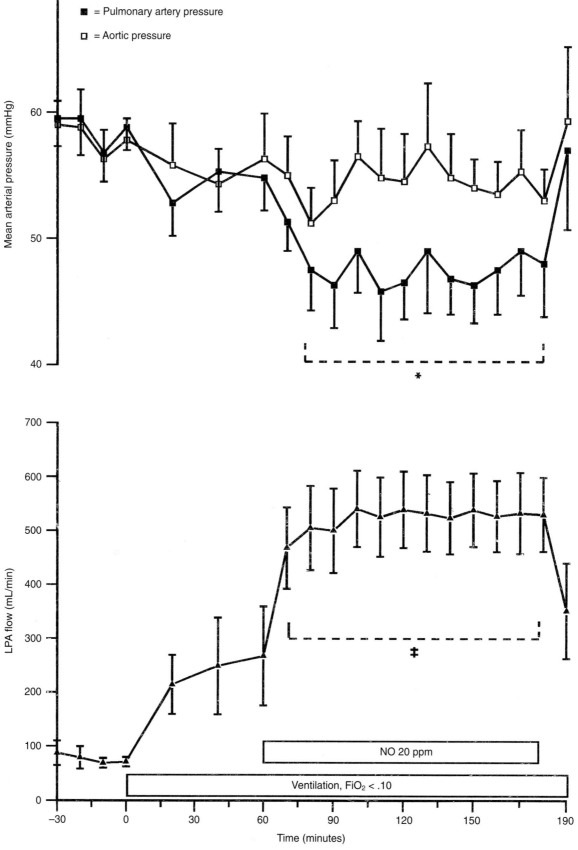

Figure 14-1. Inhaled nitric oxide causes selective and sustained pulmonary vasodilation. (From Kinsella JP, Abman SH. Clinical approach to inhaled nitric oxide therapy in the newborn. J Pediatr 136:717–726, 2000.)

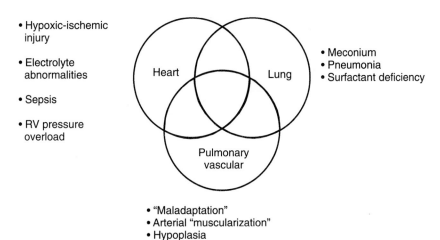

- Hypoxic-ischemic injury
- Electrolyte abnormalities
- Sepsis
- RV pressure overload

- Meconium
- Pneumonia
- Surfactant deficiency

Heart

Lung

Pulmonary vascular

- "Maladaptation"
- Arterial "muscularization"
- Hypoplasia

Figure 14-2. Disorders associated with persistent pulmonary hypertension in the newborn (PPHN).

PHYSIOLOGY OF NITRIC OXIDE IN THE PULMONARY CIRCULATION

The fetal circulation is characterized by high PVR. Pulmonary blood flow accounts for less than 10% of combined ventricular output in the late-gestation ovine fetus.[26] Mechanisms responsible for maintaining high fetal PVR and causing sustained pulmonary vasodilation at birth are incompletely understood; however, studies in fetal and transitional pulmonary vasoregulation have led to increased understanding of the normal physiologic control of PVR. Fetal and neonatal pulmonary vascular tone is modulated through a balance between vasoconstrictor and vasodilator stimuli, including mechanical factors (e.g., lung volume) and endogenous mediators.

The pharmacologic activity of nitrovasodilators derives from the release of NO, which was recognized as a potent vascular smooth muscle relaxant as early as 1979.[27] In 1987 investigators from two separate laboratories reported that the endothelium-derived relaxing factor was NO or an NO-containing substance.[28,29] NO modulates basal pulmonary vascular tone in the late-gestation fetus; pharmacologic NO blockade inhibits endothelium-dependent pulmonary vasodilation and attenuates the rise in pulmonary blood flow at delivery, implicating endogenous NO formation in postnatal adaptation after birth.[30] Increased fetal oxygen tension augments endogenous NO release,[31,32] and the increases in pulmonary blood flow in response to rhythmic distention of the lung and high inspired oxygen concentrations are mediated in part by endogenous NO release.[33] However, in these studies the pulmonary circulation was structurally normal. Studies using a model of PPHN in which marked structural pulmonary vascular changes are induced by prolonged fetal ductus arteriosus compression demonstrated that the *structurally* abnormal pulmonary circulation also was *functionally* abnormal.[34,35] Despite the progressive loss of endothelium-dependent (acetylcholine) vasodilation with prolonged ductus compression in this model, the response to endothelium-independent (ANP [atrial natriuretic peptide], NO) vasodilation was intact.

Exogenous (inhaled) NO causes potent, sustained, selective pulmonary vasodilation in the late-gestation ovine fetus.[36] Based on the chronic ambient levels considered to be safe for adults by regulatory agencies in the United States,[37] studies were performed in near-term lambs using inhaled NO at doses of 5, 10, and 20 ppm. Inhaled NO caused a dose-dependent increase in pulmonary blood flow in mechanically ventilated newborn lambs.[38] Inhaled NO at 20 ppm did not decrease coronary arterial or cerebral blood flow in this model.

Roberts et al.[39] studied the effects of inhaled NO on pulmonary hemodynamics in mechanically ventilated newborn lambs. Inhaled NO reversed hypoxic pulmonary vasoconstriction, and maximum vasodilation occurred at doses greater than 80 ppm. They also found that the vasodilation caused by inhaled NO during hypoxia was not attenuated by respiratory acidosis in this model. Berger et al.[40] investigated the effects of inhaled NO on pulmonary vasodilation during group B streptococcal sepsis in piglets. Inhaled NO at 150 ppm for 30 minutes caused marked pulmonary vasodilation but was associated with physiologically significant increases in methemoglobin concentrations. Corroborating studies in other animal models support the observations that inhaled NO is a selective pulmonary vasodilator at low doses (<20 ppm).[41–43]

INITIAL EVALUATION OF THE TERM NEWBORN FOR INHALED NITRIC OXIDE THERAPY

Although extensive reference material is available to the clinician when a specific diagnosis has been determined for the hypoxemic term newborn, an approach to the initial evaluation of the cyanotic newborn has received less attention. In this section, we propose an approach to the evaluation of the hypoxemic newborn that may be useful in clarifying the etiology of hypoxemia and in assessing the need for iNO treatment (Fig. 14-3).

History

Evaluation of the newborn with cyanosis begins with an approach designed to assess the primary cause of hypoxemia. Marked hypoxemia in the newborn can be caused by parenchymal lung disease with V/Q mismatch or intrapulmonary shunting, pulmonary vascular disease causing *extrapulmonary*

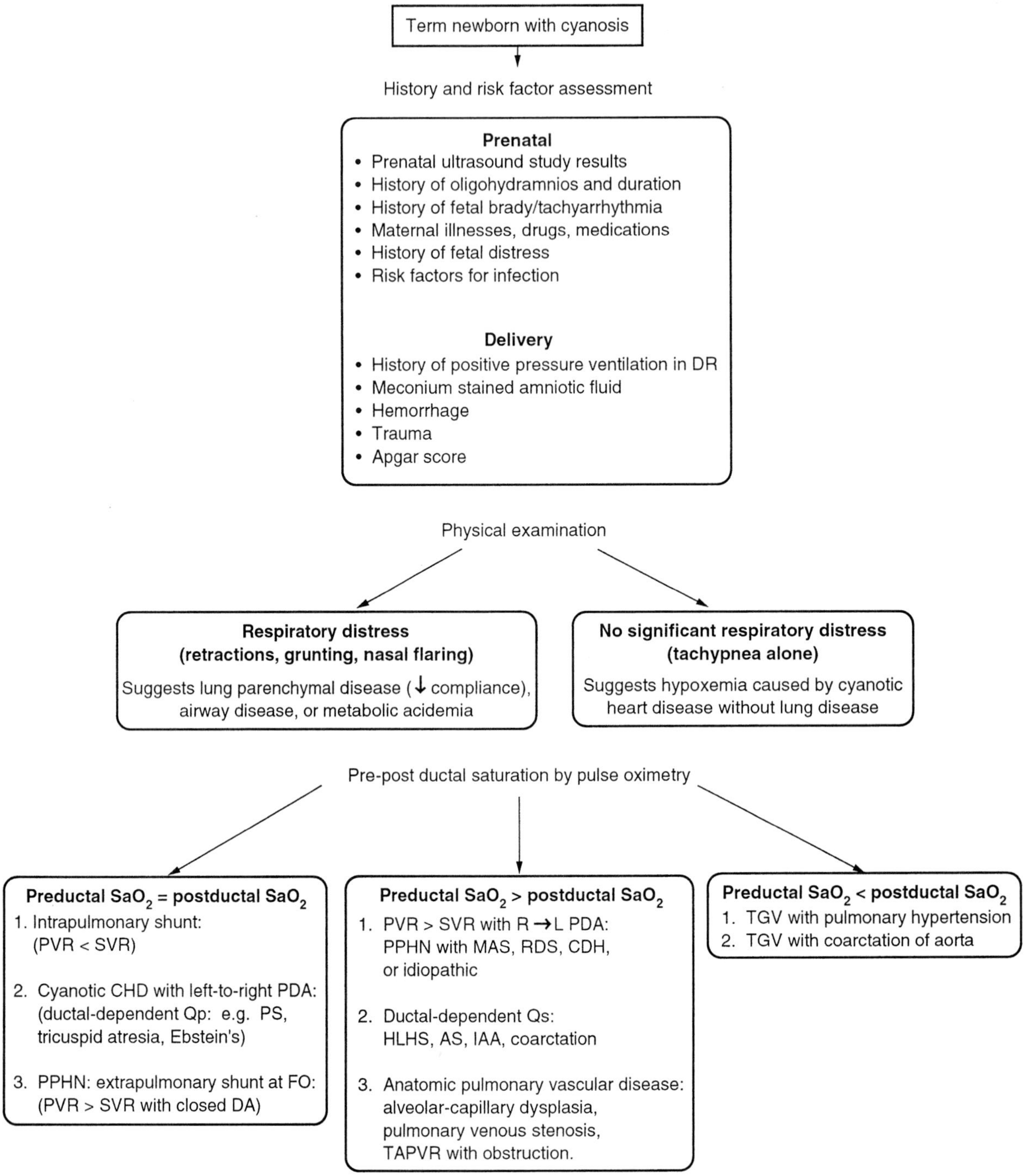

Figure 14-3. An approach to evaluation for inhaled nitric oxide therapy in the cyanotic newborn. AS, aortic stenosis; CDH, congenital diaphragmatic hernia; DA, ductus arteriosus; DR, delivery room; FO, foramen ovale; HLHS, hypoplastic left heart syndrome; IAA, interrupted aortic arch; MAS, melonium aspiration syndrome; PDA, patent ductus arteriosus; PPHN, persistent pulmonary hypertension of the newborn; PVR, pulmonary vascular resistance; RDS, respiratory distress syndrome; SVR, systemic vascular resistance; TAPVR, total anomalous pulmonary venous return; TGV, transposition of the great vessels.

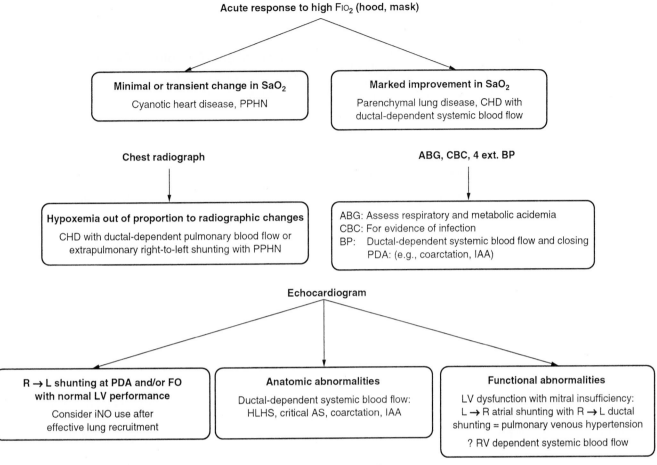

Figure 14-3. *Continued*

right-to-left shunting (PPHN), or anatomic right-to-left shunting associated with congenital heart disease. Evaluation should begin with the history and assessment of risk factors for hypoxemic respiratory failure. Relevant history may include the results of prenatal ultrasound studies. Lesions such as congenital diaphragmatic hernia (CDH) and congenital cystic adenomatoid malformation are diagnosed prenatally with increasing frequency. Although many anatomic congenital heart diseases can be diagnosed prenatally, vascular abnormalities (e.g., coarctation of the aorta, total anomalous pulmonary venous return) are more difficult to diagnose with prenatal ultrasound. A history of a structurally normal heart by fetal ultrasonography should be confirmed by echocardiography in the newborn with cyanosis (see later).

Other historical information that may be important in the evaluation of the cyanotic newborn includes a history of severe and prolonged oligohydramnios causing pulmonary hypoplasia. Prolonged fetal bradyarrhythmia and/or tachyarrhythmia and marked anemia (caused by hemolysis, twin–twin transfusion, or chronic hemorrhage) may cause congestive heart failure, pulmonary edema, and respiratory distress. Maternal illness (e.g., diabetes mellitus), medication use (e.g., aspirin or medications containing nonsteroidal antiinflammatory drugs causing premature constriction of the ductus arteriosus, association of Ebstein malformation with maternal lithium use), and drug use may contribute to acute cardiopulmonary distress in the newborn. Risk factors for

infection that cause sepsis/pneumonia should be considered, including premature or prolonged rupture of membranes, fetal tachycardia, maternal leukocytosis, uterine tenderness, and other signs of intraamniotic infection.

Events at delivery may provide clues to the etiology of hypoxemic respiratory failure in the newborn. For example, if positive-pressure ventilation is required in the delivery room, the risk of pneumothorax increases. A history of meconium-stained amniotic fluid, particularly if meconium is present below the cords, is the *sine qua non* of meconium aspiration syndrome. Birth trauma (e.g., clavicular fracture, phrenic nerve injury) or acute fetomaternal or fetoplacental hemorrhage may cause respiratory distress in the newborn.

Physical Examination

The initial physical examination provides important clues to the etiology of cyanosis. Marked respiratory distress in the newborn (retractions, grunting, nasal flaring) suggests the presence of pulmonary parenchymal disease with decreased lung compliance. However, it is important to recognize that upper airway obstruction (e.g., Pierre Robin sequence or choanal atresia) and metabolic acidemia also can cause severe respiratory distress. In contrast, the newborn with cyanosis alone or cyanosis plus tachypnea ("nondistressed tachypnea") typically has cyanotic congenital heart disease, most commonly transposition of the great vessels (TGV) or idiopathic PPHN.

The presence of a heart murmur in the first hours of life is an important sign in the newborn with cyanosis or respiratory distress. In this setting, it is unusual for the common left-to-right shunt lesions (patent ductus arteriosis, atrial septal defect, ventricular septal defect) to produce an audible murmur because PVR remains high and little turbulence is created across the defect. A murmur that sounds like a ventricular septal defect in the first hours of life is most commonly caused by tricuspid regurgitation (associated with PPHN or asphyxiated myocardium).

Interpretation of Pulse Oximetry Measurements

The interpretation of preductal (right hand) and postductal (lower extremity) saturation by pulse oximetry provides important clues to the etiology of hypoxemia in the newborn. Right-to-left shunting across the ductus arteriosus (but not the patent foramen ovale) causes postductal desaturation (i.e., >5% difference). However, it is important to recognize that variability in oximetry readings may be related to differences in available devices and affected by local perfusion. If the measurements of preductal and postductal SaO_2 are equivalent, this suggests either that the ductus arteriosus is patent and PVR is subsystemic (i.e., the hypoxemia is caused by parenchymal lung disease with intrapulmonary shunting or cyanotic heart disease with ductal-dependent pulmonary blood flow) or that the ductus arteriosus is closed (precluding any interpretation of pulmonary artery pressure without echocardiography). It is uncommon for the ductus arteriosus to close in the first hours of life in the presence of systemic or suprasystemic pulmonary artery pressures.

The most common cause of preductal–postductal gradients in oxygenation is suprasystemic PVR in PPHN causing right-to-left shunting across the ductus arteriosus (associated with meconium aspiration syndrome, surfactant deficiency/dysfunction, CDH, non-CDH pulmonary hypoplasia, or idiopathic). However, ductal-dependent systemic blood flow lesions (hypoplastic left heart syndrome, critical aortic stenosis, interrupted aortic arch, coarctation) may also present with postductal desaturation. Moreover, anatomic pulmonary vascular disease (alveolar-capillary dysplasia, pulmonary venous stenosis, anomalous venous return with obstruction) can cause suprasystemic PVR with right-to-left shunting across the ductus arteriosus and postductal desaturation.

Finally, the unusual occurrence of markedly lower preductal SaO_2 compared to postductal measurements suggests one of two diagnoses: TGV with pulmonary hypertension or TGV with coarctation of the aorta.

Laboratory and Radiologic Evaluation

One of the most important tests to perform in the evaluation of the newborn with cyanosis is the chest radiograph (CXR). The CXR can demonstrate the classic findings of respiratory distress syndrome (air bronchograms, diffuse granularity, underinflation), diffuse parenchymal lung disease in pneumonia, meconium aspiration syndrome, and CDH. Perhaps the most important question to ask when viewing the CXR is whether the severity of hypoxemia is out of proportion to the radiographic changes (Table 14-2). In other words, marked hypoxemia despite supplemental oxygen in the absence of severe pulmonary parenchymal disease radiographically suggests the presence of an extrapulmonary right-to-left shunt (idiopathic PPHN or cyanotic heart disease).

Other essential measurements include an arterial blood gas to determine the blood gas tensions and pH, a complete blood count to evaluate for signs of infection, and blood pressure measurements in the right arm and a lower extremity to determine aortic obstruction (interrupted aortic arch, coarctation).

Response to Supplemental Oxygen

Marked improvement in SaO_2 (increase to 100%) with supplemental oxygen (100% oxygen by hood, mask, or endotracheal tube) suggests the presence of intrapulmonary shunt or V/Q mismatch due to lung disease or reactive PPHN. The response to mask continuous positive airway pressure is also a useful discriminator between severe lung disease and other causes of hypoxemia. Most patients with PPHN have at least a transient improvement in oxygenation in response to interventions such as high inspired oxygen and/or mechanical ventilation. If the preductal SaO_2 never reaches 100%, the likelihood of cyanotic heart disease is high.

Echocardiography

Echocardiography has become a vital tool in the clinical management of newborns with hypoxemic respiratory failure. The initial echocardiographic evaluation is important to rule out structural heart disease causing hypoxemia (e.g., coarctation of the aorta, total anomalous pulmonary venous return). Moreover, it is critically important to diagnose congenital heart

---

TABLE 14-2.   Mechanisms of Hypoxemia in the Term Newborn with Respiratory Failure

Mechanism	Associated Conditions	Response to 100% Oxygen
Ventilation-perfusion (V/Q) disturbances (high V/Q ratios = increased dead space; low V/Q ratios = alveolar underventilation)	Meconium aspiration, retained lung fluid, pulmonary interstitial emphysema, effects of positioning on gas exchange (i.e., decreased ventilation in dependent lung)	Pao_2 ↑
Intrapulmonary right-to-left shunt (V/Q = 0, blood that passes through nonventilated segments of lung)	Atelectasis, alveolar filling (meconium, blood), bronchial collateral circulation	Little change in Pao_2
Extrapulmonary right-to-left shunt	PPHN (right-to-left shunting at FO and DA), cyanotic heart disease	Little change in Pao_2

DA, ductus arteriosus; FO, foramen ovale; PPHN, persistent pulmonary hypertension of the newborn.

lesions for which iNO treatment would be contraindicated. In addition to the lesions mentioned earlier, congenital heart diseases that can present with hypoxemia unresponsive to high inspired oxygen concentrations (i.e., dependent on right-to-left shunting across the ductus arteriosus) include critical aortic stenosis, interrupted aortic arch, and hypoplastic left heart syndrome. Decreasing PVR with iNO in these conditions could lead to systemic hypoperfusion, worsening the clinical course and delaying definitive diagnosis.

Echocardiographic evaluation is an essential component in the initial evaluation and ongoing management of the hypoxemic newborn. Not all hypoxemic term newborns have echocardiographic signs of PPHN. As noted earlier, hypoxemia can be caused by intrapulmonary right-to-left shunting or V/Q disturbances associated with severe lung disease. In unusual circumstances, right-to-left shunting can occur across pulmonary-to-systemic collaterals. However, extrapulmonary right-to-left shunting at the foramen ovale and/or ductus arteriosus (PPHN) also complicates hypoxemic respiratory failure and must be assessed in order to determine initial treatments and evaluate the response to those therapies.

PPHN is defined by the echocardiographic determination of extrapulmonary venoarterial admixture (right-to-left shunting at the foramen ovale and/or ductus arteriosus), not simply evidence of increased PVR (i.e., elevated PVR without extrapulmonary shunting does not directly cause hypoxemia). Echocardiographic signs suggestive of pulmonary hypertension (e.g., increased right ventricular systolic time intervals, septal flattening) are less helpful (Table 14-3).

Doppler measurements of atrial and ductal level shunts provide essential information when managing a newborn with hypoxemic respiratory failure. For example, left-to-right shunting at the foramen ovale and ductus arteriosus with marked hypoxemia suggests predominant intrapulmonary shunting, and interventions should be directed at optimizing lung inflation.

Finally, the measurements made with echocardiography can be used to predict or interpret the response or lack of response to various treatments. For example, in the presence of severe left ventricular dysfunction with pulmonary hypertension, pulmonary vasodilation alone may be ineffective in improving oxygenation. The echocardiographic findings in this setting include right-to-left ductal shunting (caused by suprasystemic PVR) and mitral insufficiency with *left-to-right* atrial shunting. In this setting, efforts to reduce PVR should be accompanied by targeted therapies to increase cardiac performance and decrease left ventricular afterload.

This constellation of findings suggests that left ventricular dysfunction may contribute to *pulmonary venous hypertension,* such as occurs in congestive heart failure. In this setting, pulmonary vasodilation alone (without improving cardiac performance) will not cause sustained improvement in oxygenation. Careful echocardiographic assessment will provide invaluable information about the underlying pathophysiology and help guide the course of treatment.

The initial echocardiographic evaluation determines both structural and functional (i.e., extrapulmonary right-to-left shunting in PPHN, left ventricular performance) causes of hypoxemia. *Serial* echocardiography is important to determine the response to interventions (e.g., pulmonary vasodilators) and to reevaluate cases where specific interventions have not resulted in improvement or with progressive clinical deterioration. For example, in a patient with extrapulmonary right-to-left shunting and severe lung disease, pulmonary vasodilation might reverse the right-to-left venous admixture with little improvement in systemic oxygenation. These observations unmask the critically important contribution of intrapulmonary shunting to hypoxemia.

WHOM TO TREAT

Guidelines for the use of iNO therapy are given in Table 14.4.

Diseases

Due to its selective pulmonary vasodilator effects, iNO therapy is an important adjunct to available treatments for term newborns with hypoxemic respiratory failure. However, hypoxemic respiratory failure in the term newborn represents a heterogeneous group of disorders, and disease-specific responses have clearly been described.[3]

TABLE 14-3. Echocardiographic Findings in Persistent Pulmonary Hypertension of the Newborn

Measurement	Findings in PPHN
Estimate of PA pressure using Doppler estimate of tricuspid regurgitation jet: 4 (V^2) + CVP, where V = peak velocity of tricuspid regurgitation jet (in m/sec), and CVP = central venous pressure	Elevated PA pressure reliably estimated (mm Hg); compare with simultaneous systemic pressure
Direction of PDA shunt (by pulsed and color Doppler)	Right-to-left or bidirectional PDA shunting
Direction of atrial shunt (by pulsed and color Doppler)	Right-to-left or bidirectional shunting through PFO

PA, pulmonary artery; PDA, patent ductus arteriosus; PFO, patent foramen ovale.

TABLE 14-4. Guidelines for Use of Inhaled Nitric Oxide Therapy

Patient profile	Near-term/term newborn ≥34 weeks of gestation in the first week of life with echocardiographic evidence of extrapulmonary right-to-left shunting and OI >25 after effective lung recruitment
Starting dose	20 ppm (decrease to <10 ppm by 4 hours)
Monitoring for methemoglobinemia	Monitor percentage methemoglobin by co-oximetry within 4 hours of starting iNO and at 24-hour intervals
Duration of treatment	Typically <5 days
Discontinuation	FIO_2 <0.60 with increase in FIO_2 <0.15 after discontinuation
ECMO availability	If used in a non-ECMO center, arrangements should be in place to continue iNO during transport

ECMO, extracorporeal membrane oxygenation; iNO, inhaled nitric oxide; OI, oxygenation index.

Several pathophysiologic disturbances contribute to hypoxemia in the newborn infant, including cardiac dysfunction, airway and pulmonary parenchymal abnormalities, and pulmonary vascular disorders. In some newborns with hypoxemic respiratory failure a single mechanism predominates (e.g., extrapulmonary right-to-left shunting in idiopathic PPHN), but more commonly several of these mechanisms contribute to hypoxemia. For example, in a newborn with meconium aspiration syndrome, meconium may obstruct some airways, decreasing V/Q ratios and increasing intrapulmonary shunting. Other lung segments may be overventilated relative to perfusion and increase physiologic dead space. Moreover, the same patient may have severe pulmonary hypertension with extrapulmonary right-to-left shunting at the ductus arteriosus and foramen ovale. Not only does the overlap of these mechanisms complicate clinical management, but time-dependent changes in the relative contribution of each mechanism to hypoxemia requires continued vigilance as the disease progresses. Therefore, understanding the relative contribution of these different causes of hypoxemia becomes critically important as the inventory of therapeutic options expands.

Considering the important role of parenchymal lung disease in many cases of PPHN, pharmacologic pulmonary vasodilation alone would not be expected to cause sustained clinical improvement. The effects of inhaled NO may be suboptimal when lung volume is decreased in association with pulmonary parenchymal disease.[44] Atelectasis and air space disease (e.g., pneumonia, pulmonary edema) will decrease effective delivery of iNO to its site of action in terminal lung units, and PVR increases at lung volumes above and below functional residual capacity. In PPHN associated with heterogeneous ("patchy") parenchymal lung disease, inhaled NO may be effective in optimizing V/Q matching by preferentially causing vasodilation within lung units that are well ventilated. The effects of inhaled NO on V/Q matching appear to be optimal at low doses (<20 ppm).[17,45] However, in cases complicated by homogeneous (diffuse) parenchymal lung disease and underinflation, pulmonary hypertension may be exacerbated because of the adverse mechanical effects of underinflation on

PVR. In this setting, effective treatment of the underlying lung disease is essential (and sometimes sufficient) to resolve the accompanying pulmonary hypertension (Fig. 14-4).

Clinical Criteria

Gestational and Postnatal Age

Available evidence from clinical trials supports the use of iNO in near-term (>34 weeks of gestation) and term newborns.[7,8] The use of iNO in infants less than 34 weeks of gestation remains investigational (see later). Clinical trials of iNO in the newborn have incorporated ECMO treatment as an endpoint. Most patients were enrolled in the first few days of life. Although one of the pivotal studies used to support the new drug application for iNO therapy included as an entry criterion a postnatal age up to 14 days, the average age at enrollment in that study was 1.7 days.[7] Currently, clinical trials support the use of iNO before treatment with ECMO, usually within the first week of life. However, clinical experience suggests that iNO may be of benefit as an adjuvant treatment after ECMO therapy in patients with sustained pulmonary hypertension (e.g., CDH). Thus, postnatal age alone should not define the duration of therapy in cases where prolonged treatment could be beneficial.

Severity of Illness

Studies support the use of iNO in infants who have hypoxemic respiratory failure with evidence of PPHN and require mechanical ventilation and high inspired oxygen concentrations. The most common criterion used has been the oxygenation index (OI). Although clinical trials commonly allowed for enrollment of patients with OI levels greater than 25, the mean OI at study entry in multicenter trials was approximately 40.[3,7] It is unclear whether infants with less severe hypoxemia would benefit from iNO therapy. Davidson et al.[6] reported a controlled clinical trial in which the average OI at study entry was 249. Unlike other trials, however, iNO treatment in this study did not

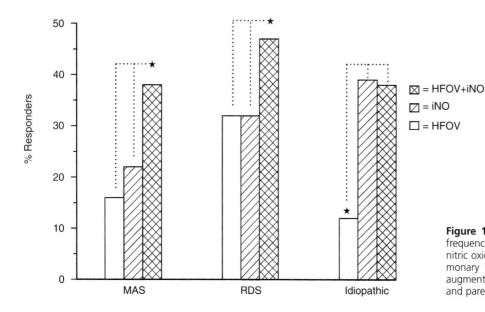

Figure 14-4. Effects of combined therapy with high-frequency oscillatory ventilation (HFOV) and inhaled nitric oxide (iNO) in term newborns with persistent pulmonary hypertension of the newborn (PPHN). HFOV augments the response to iNO in newborns with PPHN and parenchymal lung disease.

reduce ECMO utilization. In addition, although entry criteria for this trial included echocardiographic evidence of pulmonary hypertension, only 9% of the patients had clinical evidence of right-to-left ductal shunting. Because of the mechanism of action of iNO as a selective pulmonary vasodilator, it is likely that acute improvement in oxygenation caused by decreased PVR and reduced extrapulmonary right-to-left shunting would be most predictive of clinical improvement.[7] Current multicenter studies suggest that indications for treatment with iNO may include an OI greater than 25 with echocardiographic evidence of extrapulmonary right-to-left shunting.

Treatment Strategies

Delivery of Nitric Oxide During Mechanical Ventilation

Early studies of NO treatment in newborns used simple two-stage regulators with low-flow meters that were manually adjusted to deliver finely regulated flow rates of NO gas into the circuit of continuous-flow neonatal ventilators. Monitoring of NO/NO_2 was performed using chemiluminescence analyzers.[2] This configuration was inexpensive and reliable but lacked an alarm system to detect high/low delivered gas errors. Currently, gas for NO therapy in the United States is provided by a single manufacturer (INO Therapeutics Inc., Clinton, NJ, USA) and is linked to a single delivery system (INOvent, Datex-Ohmeda. (A second system that is available for use during transport is described later).

The INOvent delivery system (Fig. 14-5) uses an inline sensor to detect flow rates of gas through the ventilator circuit and a mass-flow controller for delivery of NO gas to yield the desired NO concentration. This device allows for stable NO delivery in ventilator systems that do not use continuous flow throughout the inspiratory/expiratory cycle. The range of NO delivery is 0 to 80 ppm, and the system includes NO/NO_2 alarms that use electrochemical sensors. This device also has a manual NO delivery unit for use during bag ventilation; it delivers 20 ppm NO when set at 15 L/min with an 800 ppm NO source tank.

Dose

The first studies of iNO treatment in term newborns reported initial doses that ranged from 80 ppm[1] to 6–20 ppm.[2] The rationale for doses used in these clinical trials was based on

concentrations that previously had been found to be effective in animal experiments by the same investigators.[10,46] Roberts et al.[1] reported that brief (30 minutes) inhalation of NO at 80 ppm improved oxygenation in patients with PPHN, but this response was sustained in only one patient after NO was discontinued. In the second report, rapid improvement in oxygenation in neonates with severe PPHN also was demonstrated, but this was achieved at lower doses (20 ppm) for 4 hours.[2] This study also reported that decreasing the iNO dose to 6 ppm for the duration of treatment provided sustained improvement in oxygenation. The relative effectiveness of low-dose iNO in improving oxygenation in patients with severe PPHN was corroborated in a study by Finer et al.[47] Acute improvement in oxygenation during treatment was not different with doses of iNO ranging from 5 to 80 ppm.

These laboratory and clinical studies established the boundaries of iNO dosing protocols for subsequent randomized clinical trials in newborns.[3–5] Increasing the dose to 40 ppm does not generally improve oxygenation in patients who do not respond to the lower dose of 20 ppm.[3] The initial dose in the Neonatal Inhaled Nitric Oxide Study (NINOS) trial was 20 ppm, but the dose was increased to 80 ppm if the improvement in PaO_2 was less than 20 torr.[7] In this study, only 3 (6%) of 53 infants who had little response to 20 ppm had an increase in PaO_2 greater than 20 torr when treated with 80 ppm iNO. Whether a progressive increase in PaO_2 would have occurred with continued exposure to 20 ppm could not be determined with this study design. Roberts et al.[4] initiated treatment with 80 ppm NO and subsequently weaned the iNO concentration if oxygenation improved; thus, the effects of lower initial iNO doses could not be evaluated and the effects on ECMO utilization were not evaluated.

The effects of sustained exposure to different doses of iNO in separate treatment groups of newborns were evaluated by Davidson et al.[6] These investigators reported the results of a randomized, controlled, dose-response trial in term newborns with hypoxemic respiratory failure. In this study, patients were randomized to treatment with 0 (placebo), 5, 20, or 80 ppm NO. Each iNO dose improved oxygenation compared to placebo, but there was no difference in responses between groups. However, at 80 ppm, methemoglobinemia (blood levels >7%) occurred in 13 (35%) of 37 patients and high inspired NO_2 concentrations (>3 ppm) were reported in 7 (19%) of 37 patients. Thus, iNO at a dose of 80 ppm was not more effective in improving oxygenation than 5 or 20 ppm and was associated with adverse effects.

The available evidence supports the use of doses of iNO beginning at 20 ppm in term newborns with PPHN, because this strategy decreased ECMO utilization without an increased incidence of adverse effects. Although brief exposures to higher doses (40 to 80 ppm) appear to be safe, sustained treatment with 80 ppm NO increases the risk of methemoglobinemia.

Duration of Treatment

In multicenter clinical trials of iNO therapy, the typical duration of iNO treatment has been less than 5 days, which parallels the clinical resolution of PPHN. However, individual exceptions occur, particularly in cases of pulmonary hypoplasia.[48] If iNO is required for more than 5 days, investigations into other causes of pulmonary hypertension should be considered (e.g., alveolar capillary dysplasia), particularly if discontinuation of iNO results in suprasystemic elevations of pulmonary artery pressure

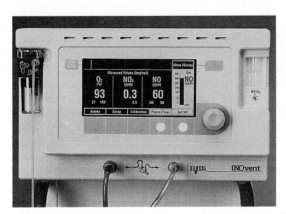

Figure 14-5. Photo of the INOvent delivery system. (Courtesy of INO Therapeutics, Inc.)

noted by echocardiography. In our practice, we discontinue iNO if F_{IO_2} is less than 0.60 and PaO_2 is greater than 60 without evidence of rebound pulmonary hypertension or an increase in F_{IO_2} greater than 15% after iNO withdrawal.

In the pre-iNO era, concerns were raised about delaying ECMO therapy if conventional treatment was prolonged. However, these retrospective data do not account for recent changes in management strategies, which include newer ventilator devices and exogenous surfactant therapy. Moreover, decreased ECMO utilization with iNO treatment in recent multicenter controlled trials has not been associated with an increased incidence of chronic lung disease.[7] In the most recent trial, iNO treatment was associated with improved pulmonary outcomes.[8] No controlled data are available to determine the maximal safe duration of iNO therapy.

Weaning

After improvement in oxygenation occurs with the onset of iNO therapy, strategies for weaning the iNO dose become important. Numerous approaches have been used, and little differences have been noted until final discontinuation of iNO treatment. In one study, iNO was reduced from 20 to 6 ppm after 4 hours of treatment without acute changes in oxygenation. In another trial, iNO was reduced in a stepwise fashion to as low as 1 ppm without changes in oxygenation.[49] Weaning iNO is a different process than discontinuation of iNO therapy (see later).

Discontinuation of Inhaled Nitric Oxide Therapy

Early clinical studies reported rapid and sometimes dramatic decreases in oxygenation and increases in PVR after abrupt withdrawal of iNO during prolonged therapy.[14] These responses often are mild and transient, and many patients with decreased oxygenation after iNO withdrawal will respond to brief elevations of F_{IO_2} and careful observation. In patients with a persistent need for treatment with higher inspired oxygen concentrations or increased pulmonary hypertension after iNO withdrawal, restarting iNO treatment will generally cause rapid clinical improvement. Clinical experience with postoperative cardiac patients suggests that children with higher pulmonary artery pressure at the time of iNO withdrawal may be at greatest risk for adverse hemodynamic effects. In general, this so-called rebound response appears to decrease over time after more prolonged therapy. However, iNO withdrawal can be associated with life-threatening elevations of PVR, profound desaturation, and systemic hypotension due to decreased cardiac output.

Mechanisms that contribute to these "rebound" effects are uncertain but include several factors. First, exogenous NO may down-regulate endogenous NO production, which contributes directly to the severity of vasospasm after iNO withdrawal. For example, exposure of normal adult rats to iNO (40 ppm) for 2 days potentiated the pressor response to angiotensin II and hypoxia and selectively impaired endothelium-dependent vasodilation.[50] This response also occurred at low doses of iNO (1 ppm) and reversed after discontinuation of iNO for 8 hours. Because lung endothelial NO synthase (NOS) protein content was unchanged, these authors speculated that iNO decreased NOS activity by an alternate mechanism. Second, decreased vascular sensitivity to NO due to alterations in other components of the NO-cyclic guanosine monophosphate (cGMP) pathway, such as decreased soluble guanylate cyclase (sGC) or enhanced phosphodiesterase (PDE5) activities, may contribute

to vasospasm after NO withdrawal. For example, in a prospective study of postoperative cardiac patients with marked hemodynamic changes after iNO withdrawal, dipyridamole (a cGMP-specific PDE type V inhibitor) inhibited the adverse effects of acute iNO withdrawal.[51] These findings led to the speculation that dipyridamole may sustain smooth muscle cGMP content and that persistent PDE5 activity may contribute to rebound pulmonary hypertension after iNO withdrawal.

Alternatively, the rise in PVR and drop in oxygenation after iNO withdrawal may simply represent the presence of more severe underlying pulmonary vascular disease with loss of treatment effect of iNO. Increasing pulmonary blood flow into a hypertensive vascular bed with decreased NOS activity may augment myogenic responses or stimulate vasoconstrictor products (such as endothelin) that increase vascular tone.[52] The sudden increase in pulmonary artery pressure after rapid withdrawal of vasodilator therapy is not unique to iNO; it has been observed in other clinical settings, such as prostacyclin withdrawal in adults with primary pulmonary hypertension and in postoperative cardiac patients.

Monitoring

Early experience suggested that careful monitoring of NO and NO_2 levels should be done with chemiluminescence devices. It now has become clear that NO_2 levels remain low at delivered iNO doses within the recommended ranges and that electrochemical devices are reliable. The currently available systems use electrochemical cells and appear to be reliable when they are used appropriately. However, the response time of electrochemical sensors is relatively slow, and these devices are not accurate when measurement of acute changes in NO concentrations is desired.

Methemoglobinemia occurs after exposure to high concentrations of iNO (80 ppm).[6] This complication has not been reported at lower doses of iNO (<20 ppm). Because methemoglobin reductase deficiency may occur unpredictably, it is reasonable to measure methemoglobin levels by co-oximetry within 4 hours of starting iNO therapy and subsequently at 24-hour intervals.

Ventilator Management

Along with iNO treatment, other therapeutic strategies have emerged for the management of the term infant with hypoxemic respiratory failure. Considering the important role of parenchymal lung disease in specific disorders included in the syndrome of PPHN, pharmacologic pulmonary vasodilation alone should not be expected to cause sustained clinical improvement in many cases.[53] Moreover, patients who do not respond to iNO can show marked improvement in oxygenation with adequate lung inflation alone.[22] High success rates in early studies were achieved by withholding iNO treatment until aggressive attempts were made to optimize ventilation and lung inflation with mechanical ventilation. These early studies demonstrated that the effects of iNO may be suboptimal when lung volume is decreased in association with pulmonary parenchymal disease, for several reasons. First, atelectasis and air space disease (pneumonia, pulmonary edema) may decrease the effective delivery of iNO to its site of action in terminal lung units. Second, in cases complicated by severe lung disease and underinflation, pulmonary hypertension may be exacerbated because of the adverse mechanical effects of underinflation on PVR. Third, attention must be given to minimize overinflation to avoid inadvertent positive end-expiratory pressure and gas trapping that may elevate PVR from vascular compression. This commonly complicates the management of infants with asymmetric lung disease or airways obstruction as observed in meconium aspiration syndrome.

In newborns with severe lung disease, high-frequency oscillatory ventilation (HFOV) frequently is used to optimize lung inflation and minimize lung injury.[54] In clinical pilot studies using iNO, we found that the combination of HFOV and iNO resulted in the greatest improvement in oxygenation in some newborns who had severe PPHN complicated by diffuse parenchymal lung disease and underinflation (e.g., respiratory distress syndrome, pneumonia).[55,56] A randomized multicenter trial demonstrated that treatment with HFOV+iNO often was successful in patients who failed to respond to HFOV alone or iNO with conventional mechanical ventilation in severe PPHN, and differences in responses were related to the specific disease associated with the complex disorders of PPHN[3] (Fig. 14-4). For patients with PPHN complicated by severe lung disease, response rates for HFOV+iNO were better than with HFOV alone or iNO with conventional ventilation. In contrast, for patients without significant parenchymal lung disease, both iNO and HFOV+iNO were more effective than HFOV alone. This response to combined treatment with HFOV+iNO likely reflects both improvement in intrapulmonary shunting in patients with severe lung disease and PPHN (using a strategy designed to recruit and sustain lung volume rather than to hyperventilate) and augmented NO delivery to its site of action. Although iNO may be an effective treatment for PPHN, it should be considered only as part of an overall clinical strategy that cautiously manages parenchymal lung disease, cardiac performance, and systemic hemodynamics.

Use in Non-Extracorporeal Membrane Oxygenation Centers and Transport with Inhaled Nitric Oxide

Published reports on the use of iNO in ECMO centers have not substantiated early concerns that iNO would adversely affect outcome by delaying ECMO utilization. In one study, the median time from randomization to treatment with ECMO was 4.4 hours for the control group and 6.7 hours for the iNO group.[17] Although this difference was statistically significant, there were no apparent adverse consequences caused by the delay. Indeed, iNO treatment may play an important role in stabilizing patients before ECMO is initiated, thus improving the chances that ECMO cannulation can proceed without progressive clinical deterioration.[5]

The potential dissemination of iNO therapy to non-ECMO centers warrants a cautious approach. Whether the use of iNO for PPHN in non-ECMO centers will cause undue delays in initiation of transport to an ECMO center, increase the risks of transport, or significantly delay ECMO cannot be determined from the currently available evidence from clinical trials. It is likely that promising new therapies for severe hypoxemic respiratory failure will not be limited to centers that provide all modes of rescue treatment. Although marked improvement in oxygenation occurs in many term newborns with severe PPHN, sustained improvement may be compromised in some patients by the nature of the underlying disease leading to progressive changes in lung compliance or cardiovascular dysfunction.[57] When the clinical course is complicated by progression in severity of the cardiopulmonary disease, withdrawal of iNO during transport to an ECMO center may lead to acute deterioration. In such cases, iNO provides an important therapeutic bridge assuring stability during transport. When progressive deterioration in oxygenation occurs during iNO treatment in institutions that cannot offer more advanced rescue therapy, provisions must be in place to accomplish transport to the ECMO center without interruption of iNO treatment.[58] Hospitals that are not ECMO centers and cannot guarantee uninterrupted iNO deliver during transport to an ECMO center should not begin an iNO therapy program.

Three systems are available for administration of iNO during transport. The two-stage regulator/low-flow meter and INOvent systems were described earlier. A third system is the Aeronox device (Pulmonox Medical Inc., Tofield, Alberta, Canada; Fig. 14-6). This is a portable system (5 kg) that monitors NO/NO_2 using electrochemical cells and is appropriate for use with continuous-flow ventilator devices.

Based on our clinical experience with iNO in emergency medical transport, we have developed local guidelines for the transport use of iNO that may be applicable to other regions.[59] These guidelines include at least five points. First, it is important that communications between referral hospitals and ECMO centers be established prior to initiating iNO therapy. Non-ECMO centers should have an iNO transport system available and be prepared to initiate early referral in the event of a suboptimal response to iNO therapy. Second, prior to initiation of iNO therapy at a non-ECMO center, attention should be given to optimizing hemodynamic stability and lung inflation using conventional mechanical ventilation strategies, as previously described.[9] Moreover, for infants who require emergency medical transport and have not been treated with iNO, the use of iNO should be considered only after careful echocardiographic examination to rule out structural and functional contraindications (anatomic defects with ductal-dependent systemic blood flow or severely diminished left ventricular performance). Third, for near-term and term newborns who have been treated with iNO at a non-ECMO center and subsequently require transport to an ECMO center, iNO should be continued on transport unless withdrawal of iNO can be safely accomplished for at least 1 hour prior to transport. Fourth, newborns treated with HFOV (Sensormedics 3100A) who require transport pose a uniquely difficult challenge. This ventilator has not been configured for use in fixed-wing or helicopter transport, and it is cumbersome in ground transport; thus, conversion to conventional mechanical ventilation often is necessary prior to initiation of transport. The use of iNO may blunt pulmonary vasoreactivity and pulmonary hypertensive episodes, potentially reducing the risk of transport for these infants. Finally, there is insufficient evidence to support the safety of iNO in the stabilization during emergency medical transports of premature newborns (<34 weeks of gestation).

The Federal Aviation Administration (FAA) has not developed a uniform policy to guide the use of iNO on fixed-wing or rotary flights. Currently, recommendations must be based upon policies determined by each of nine FAA regions within the United States. In the Rocky Mountain region, requirements for the use of iNO in transport include the following: (1) the carrier must have approval to handle iNO under a hazardous materials program; (2) proper storage is required and is guided by rules for transported compressed gas; (3) a material safety data sheet (MSDS) must be carried aboard the aircraft; and (4) the pilot must be aware that NO is being carried aboard the aircraft.

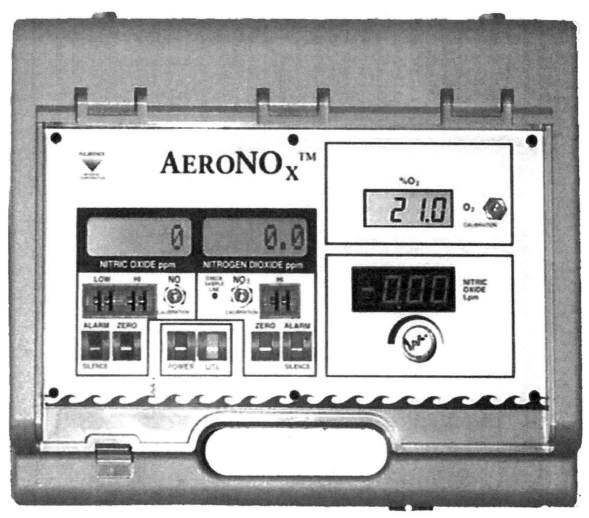

Figure 14-6. Photo of the Aeronox delivery system. (Courtesy of Pulmonox Medical, Inc.)

Continuing iNO delivery during transport sustains acute improvements in oxygenation and diminishes the oxygenation lability characteristic of PPHN. Several delivery systems are available to provide iNO during transport and can be easily incorporated into transport modules. Considering the proliferation of iNO use in non-ECMO centers, prudent integration of functional iNO transport systems within the catchment area of an ECMO center should be a priority. Finally, the use of HFOV and iNO in non-ECMO centers may pose undue risk for infants who subsequently need to be transported. However, iNO may facilitate these transport missions by decreasing vasolability and stabilizing oxygenation en route.

FUTURE APPLICATIONS OF INHALED NITRIC OXIDE THERAPY

Congenital Diaphragmatic Hernia

The cause of hypoxemic respiratory failure in patients with CDH is complex and includes pulmonary hypoplasia, surfactant dysfunction, functional and structural abnormalities of the pulmonary vascular bed, and left ventricular dysfunction.

Early experience with iNO in CDH showed that some patients had sustained improvement in oxygenation.[17] However, Karamanoukian et al.[60] found little improvement in oxygenation with iNO treatment in patients with CDH before treatment with ECMO, despite treatment with surfactant. The only randomized controlled trial of iNO treatment in patients with CDH found no difference in ECMO utilization between NO-treated and control infants. Although iNO may be an effective therapy in some patients with CDH and pulmonary hypertension, patients with CDH as a group are poor responders.[61] The lack of apparent efficacy in CDH may be related, in large measure, to the complexity of this disorder.

The Premature Newborn

Another area of investigation that is of vital clinical importance involves the role of iNO therapy in premature newborns with hypoxemic respiratory failure. Preliminary studies in human premature neonates with severe hypoxemic respiratory failure support the potential role of low-dose iNO as adjuvant therapy. In a small, unmasked, randomized trial of iNO (20 ppm) and dexamethasone treatment, no differences were found in survival, chronic lung disease, or intracranial hemorrhage (ICH) between iNO-treated infants and controls.

To begin to address the potential safety and efficacy of iNO in premature newborns, we conducted a randomized controlled trial of iNO in premature neonates with severe hypoxemic respiratory failure.[62] We randomized 80 premature newborns of gestational age less than 34 weeks with severe hypoxemic respiratory failure in 12 perinatal centers that provide tertiary care. Forty-eight patients were treated with iNO (5 ppm) and 32 served as controls. Treatment assignment was masked. The primary outcome variable was survival to discharge. Secondary outcome variables included incidence and severity of ICH, pulmonary hemorrhage, duration of mechanical ventilation, and chronic lung disease at 36 weeks of postconceptional age. In this study, there were no differences in baseline characteristics or severity of disease between iNO treatment and control groups. Inhaled NO acutely improved oxygenation after 60 minutes of treatment. Survival to discharge was 52% in the iNO group and 47% in controls (P = NS). Total ventilator days for survivors were fewer for the iNO group (P = 0.046). In contrast to uncontrolled pilot studies, we found no difference in the incidence of ICH between the control and iNO-treated groups (Fig. 14-7). The incidence of periventricular leukomalacia also was not different between groups (8% of iNO patients and 13% of controls).

Thus, low-dose iNO caused acute improvement in oxygenation in premature newborns with severe hypoxemic respiratory failure, without increasing the risk of bleeding complications, including ICH. Low-dose iNO may be effective as a lung-specific antiinflammatory therapy to diminish lung neutrophil accumulation and the attendant inflammatory injury that contributes to the evolution of chronic lung disease. Currently, three multicenter clinical trials are underway to test the safety and efficacy of iNO in premature newborns with respiratory failure.

SUMMARY

Inhaled NO improves oxygenation and decreases ECMO utilization in term newborns with PPHN. From the available information, a reasonable recommendation for starting dose of iNO in the term infant is 20 ppm, with reductions in dose over time. Toxicity is apparent at a dose of 80 ppm, which causes increases in methemoglobinemia and inspired NO_2. High doses (>20 ppm) of iNO may prolong bleeding time, but clinically significant increases in bleeding complications have not been reported in term newborns. The use of iNO in non-ECMO centers must be done cautiously, with arrangements in place for transport to an ECMO center without interruption of iNO delivery in patients with suboptimal acute responses. Finally, there is increasing evidence for the potential role of low-dose iNO (5 ppm) in premature newborns with hypoxemic respiratory failure. Low-dose iNO causes acute improvement in oxygenation and may prove to be useful as a lung-specific antiinflammatory therapy. Clinical application currently should be limited to controlled trials that target outcomes of both safety and efficacy.

ACKNOWLEDGMENT

This work was supported in part by Grant MO1 RR00069 from the General Clinical Research Centers Program, National Center for Research Resources, National Institutes of Health.

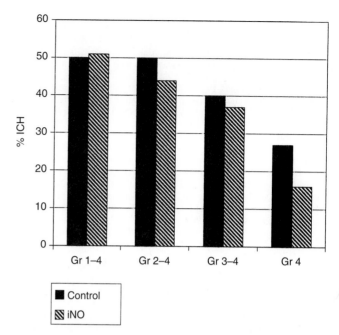

Figure 14-7. Incidence of intracranial hemorrhage (ICH) in premature newborns treated with inhaled nitric oxide (iNO) versus controls.

REFERENCES

1. Roberts JD, Polaner DM, Lang P, et al: Inhaled nitric oxide in persistent pulmonary hypertension of the newborn. Lancet 340:818–819, 1992.
2. Kinsella JP, Neish SR, Shaffer E, et al: Low-dose inhalational nitric oxide in persistent pulmonary hypertension of the newborn. Lancet 340:819–820, 1992.
3. Kinsella JP, Truog WE, Walsh WF, et al: Randomized, multicenter trial of inhaled nitric oxide and high frequency oscillatory ventilation in severe persistent pulmonary hypertension of the newborn. J Pediatr 131:55–62, 1992.
4. Roberts JD, Fineman JR, Morin FC, et al: Inhaled nitric oxide and persistent pulmonary hypertension of the newborn. N Engl J Med 336:605–610, 1997.
5. Wessel DL, Adatia I, Van Marter LJ, et al: Improved oxygenation in a randomized trial of inhaled nitric oxide for persistent pulmonary hypertension of the newborn. Pediatrics 100:e7, 1997.
6. Davidson D, Barefield ES, Kattwinkel J, et al: Inhaled nitric oxide for the early treatment of persistent pulmonary hypertension of the term newborn: A randomized, double-masked, placebo-controlled, dose-response, multicenter study. Pediatrics 101:325–334, 1998.
7. Neonatal Inhaled Nitric Oxide Study Group: Inhaled nitric oxide in full-term and nearly full-term infants with hypoxic respiratory failure. N Engl J Med 336:597–604, 1998.
8. Clark RH, Kueser TJ, Walker MW, et al: Low-dose inhaled nitric oxide treatment of persistent pulmonary hypertension of the newborn. N Engl J Med 342:469–474, 2000.
9. Kinsella JP, Abman SH: Clinical approach to inhaled nitric oxide therapy in the newborn. J Pediatr 136:717–726, 2000.
10. Kinsella JP, McQueston JA, Rosenberg AA, et al: Hemodynamic effects of exogenous nitric oxide in ovine transitional pulmonary circulation. Am J Physiol 262:H875–H880, 2000.
11. Levin DL, Heymann MA, Kitterman JA, et al: Persistent pulmonary hypertension of the newborn. J Pediatr 89:626, 2000.
12. Gersony WM: Neonatal pulmonary hypertension: Pathophysiology, classification and etiology. Clin Perinatol 11:517–524, 1984.
13. Kinsella JP, Abman SH: Recent developments in the pathophysiology and treatment of persistent pulmonary hypertension of the newborn. J Pediatr 126:853–864, 1995.
14. Stevenson DK, Kasting DS, Darnall RA, et al: Refractory hypoxemia associated with neonatal pulmonary disease: The use and limitations of tolazoline. J Pediatr 95:595–599, 1979.
15. Drummond WH, Gregory G, Heymann MA, et al: The independent effects of hyperventilation, tolazoline, and dopamine on infants with persistent pulmonary hypertension. J Pediatr 98:603–611, 1981.

16. Kinsella JP, Neish SR, Ivy DD, et al: Clinical responses to prolonged treatment of persistent pulmonary hypertension of the newborn with low doses of inhaled nitric oxide. J Pediatr 123:103–108, 1993.

17. Abman SH, Griebel JL, Parker DK, et al: Acute effects of inhaled nitric oxide in severe hypoxemic respiratory failure in pediatrics. J Pediatr 24:881–888, 1994.

18. Gerlach H, Rossaint R, Pappert D, et al: Time-course and dose-response of nitric oxide inhalation for systemic oxygenation and pulmonary hypertension in patients with adult respiratory distress syndrome. Eur J Clin Invest 23:499–502, 1993.

19. Rossaint R, Falke KJ, Lopez F, et al: Inhaled nitric oxide for the adult respiratory distress syndrome. N Engl J Med 328:399–405, 1993.

20. Beckman JS, Beckman TW, Chen J, et al: Apparent hydroxy radical production by peroxynitrite: Implications for endothelial injury from nitric oxide and superoxide. Proc Natl Acad Sci USA 87:1620–1624, 1990.

21. Robbins CG, Davis JM, Merritt TA, et al: Combined effects of nitric oxide and hyperoxia on surfactant function and pulmonary inflammation. Am J Physiol 269:L545–L550, 1995.

22. Issa A, Lappalainen U, Kleinman M, et al: Inhaled nitric oxide decreases hyperoxia-induced surfactant abnormality in preterm rabbits. Pediatr Res 45:247–254, 1999.

23. Collet-Martin S, Gatecel C, Kermarrec N, et al: Alveolar neutrophil functions and cytokine levels in patients with the adult respiratory distress syndrome during nitric oxide inhalation. Am J Respir Crit Care Med 153:985–990, 1996.

24. O'Donnell VB, Chumley PH, Hogg N, et al: Nitric oxide inhibition of lipid peroxidation: Kinetics of reaction with lipid peroxyl radicals and comparison with alpha-tocopherol. Biochemistry 36:15216–15223, 1997.

25. Hallman M: Molecular interactions between nitric oxide and lung surfactant. Biol Neonate 71:44–48, 1997.

26. Rudolph AM, Heymann MA: Circulation changes during growth in the fetal lamb. Circ Res 26:289–299, 1970.

27. Gruetter CA, Barry BK, McNamara DB, et al: Relaxation of bovine coronary artery and activation of coronary arterial guanylate cyclase by nitric oxide, nitroprusside and a carcinogenic nitrosoamine. J Cyclic Nucleotide Res 5:211–224, 1979.

28. Palmer RMJ, Ferrige AG, Moncada S: Nitric oxide release accounts for the biological activity of endothelium-derived relaxing factor. Nature 327:524–526, 1987.

29. Ignarro LJ, Buga GM, Wood KS, et al: Endothelium-derived relaxing factor produced and released from artery and vein in nitric oxide. Proc Natl Acad Sci USA 84:9265–9269, 1987.

30. Abman SH, Chatfield BA, Hall SL, et al: Role of endothelium-derived relaxing factor activity during transition of pulmonary circulation at birth. Am J Physiol (Heart Circ Physiol 28) 259:H1921–H1927, 1990.

31. Tiktinsky MH, Morin FC: Increasing oxygen tension dilates fetal pulmonary circulation via endothelium-derived relaxing factor. Am J Physiol 265:H376–H380, 1993.

32. McQueston JA, Cornfield DN, McMurtry IF, et al: Effects of oxygen and exogenous L-arginine on EDRF activity in fetal pulmonary circulation. Am J Physiol (Heart Circ Physiol) 264:865–871, 1993.

33. Cornfield DN, Chatfield BA, McQueston JA, et al: Effects of birth related stimuli on L-arginine-dependent vasodilation in the ovine fetus. Am J Physiol (Heart Circ Physiol 31) 262:H1474–H1481, 1992.

34. McQueston JA, Kinsella JP, Ivy DD, et al: Chronic intrauterine pulmonary hypertension impairs endothelium-dependent vasodilation in fetal lambs. Am J Physiol 268:H288–H294, 1995.

35. Zayek M, Cleveland D, Morin FC: Treatment of persistent pulmonary hypertension in the newborn lamb by inhaled nitric oxide. J Pediatr 122:743–750, 1993.

36. Kinsella JP, McQueston JA, Rosenberg AA, et al: Hemodynamic effects of exogenous nitric oxide in ovine transitional pulmonary circulation. Am J Physiol 262:H875–H880, 1992.

37. Centers for Disease Control: Recommendations for occupational safety and health standards. MMWR Morb Mortal Wkly Rep 37:S7–S21, 1988.

38. Kinsella JP, McQueston JA, Rosenberg AA, et al: Hemodynamic effects of exogenous nitric oxide in ovine transitional pulmonary circulation. Am J Physiol 262:H875–H880, 1992.

39. Roberts JD, Chen TY, Kawai N, et al: Inhaled nitric oxide reverses pulmonary vasoconstriction in the hypoxic and acidotic newborn lamb. Circ Res 72:246–254, 1993.

40. Berger JI, Gibson RL, Redding GJ, et al: Effect of inhaled nitric oxide during group B streptococcal sepsis in piglets. Am Rev Respir Dis 147:1080–1086, 1993.

41. Zayek M, Wild L, Roberts JD, et al: Effect of nitric oxide on the survival rate and incidence of lung injury in newborn lambs with persistent pulmonary hypertension. J Pediatr 123:947–952, 1993.

42. Etches PC, Finer NN, Barrington KJ, et al: Nitric oxide reverses acute hypoxic pulmonary hypertension in the newborn piglet. Pediatr Res 35:15–19, 1994.

43. Nelin LD, Moshin J, Thomas C, et al: The effect of inhaled nitric oxide on the pulmonary circulation of the neonatal pig. Pediatr Res 35:20–24, 1994.

44. Antunes MJ, Greenspan JS, Holt WJ, et al: Assessment of lung function pre-nitric oxide therapy: A predictor of response? Pediatr Res 35:212A, 1994.

45. Gerlach H, Rossaint R, Pappert D, et al: Time-course and dose-response of nitric oxide inhalation for systemic oxygenation and pulmonary hypertension in patients with adult respiratory distress syndrome. Eur J Clin Invest 23:499–502, 1993.

46. Roberts JD, Chen TY, Kawai N, et al: Inhaled nitric oxide reverses pulmonary vasoconstriction in the hypoxic and acidotic newborn lamb. Circ Res 72:246–254, 1993.

47. Finer NN, Etches PC, Kamstra B, et al: Inhaled nitric oxide in infants referred for extracorporeal membrane oxygenation: Dose response. J Pediatr 124:302–308, 1994.

48. Goldman AP, Tasker RC, Haworth SG, et al: Four patterns of response to inhaled nitric oxide for persistent pulmonary hypertension of the newborn. Pediatrics 98:706–713, 1996.

49. Davidson D, Barefield ES, Kattwinkel J, et al: Safety of withdrawing inhaled nitric oxide therapy in persistent pulmonary hypertension. Pediatrics 104:231–236, 1999.

50. Oka M, Ohnishi M, Takahishi H, et al: Altered vasoreactivity in lungs isolated from rats exposed to NO gas. Am J Physiol 271:L419–L424, 1996.

51. Ivy DD, Kinsella JP, Ziegler JW, et al: Dipyridamole attenuates rebound pulmonary hypertension after inhaled nitric oxide withdrawal in postoperative congenital heart disease. J Thorac Cardiovasc Surg 115:875–882, 1998.

52. Storme L, Rairigh RL, Parker TA, et al: In vivo evidence for a myogenic response in the fetal pulmonary circulation. Pediatr Res 45:425–431, 1999.

53. Kinsella JP, Abman SH: Recent developments in the pathophysiology and treatment of persistent pulmonary hypertension of the newborn. J Pediatr 126:853–864, 1995.

54. Clark RH: High-frequency ventilation. J Pediatr 124:661–670, 1994.

55. Kinsella JP, Abman SH: Efficacy of inhalational nitric oxide therapy in the clinical management of persistent pulmonary hypertension of the newborn. Chest 105:92S–94S, 1994.

56. Kinsella JP, Abman SH: Clinical approach to the use of high frequency oscillatory ventilation in neonatal respiratory failure. J Perinatol 16:S52–S55, 1996.

57. Abman SH, Kinsella JP: Inhaled nitric oxide for persistent pulmonary hypertension of the newborn: The physiology matters! Pediatrics 96:1147–1151, 1995.

58. Kinsella JP, Schmidt JM, Griebel J, et al: Inhaled nitric oxide treatment for stabilization and emergency medical transport of critically ill newborns and infants. Pediatrics 95:773–776, 1995.

59. Kinsella JP, Schmidt JM, Griebel J, et al: Inhaled nitric oxide during interhospital transport of newborns. Pediatrics 95:773–776, 1995.

60. Karamanoukian HL, Glick PL, Zayek M, et al: Inhaled nitric oxide in congenital hypoplasia of the lungs due to diaphragmatic hernia or oligohydramnios. Pediatrics 94:715–718, 1994.

61. Neonatal Inhaled Nitric Oxide Study Group: Inhaled nitric oxide and hypoxic respiratory failure in infants with congenital diaphragmatic hernia. Pediatrics 99:838–845, 1997.

62. Kinsella JP, Walsh WF, Bose CL, et al: Inhaled nitric oxide in premature neonates with severe hypoxaemic respiratory failure: A randomised controlled trial. Lancet 354:1061–1065, 1999.

VENTILATORY STRATEGIES

NAMASIVAYAM AMBALAVANAN, MD
ROBERT L. SCHELONKA, MD
WALLY CARLO, MD

Less than 2 decades ago, survival of extremely premature infants was rare. Smaller, more immature neonates survive today,[1] in part due to improved mechanical ventilation. The increased survival of these vulnerable newborns results in more infants at risk for various respiratory morbidities associated with mechanical ventilation, including bronchopulmonary dysplasia (BPD) and air leak syndromes. Improved ventilatory strategies may result in decreased respiratory morbidities in these vulnerable infants.

Infants treated with mechanical ventilation are at risk for acute and chronic lung injury. Pneumothorax and pulmonary interstitial emphysema are common forms of acute lung injury in infants with respiratory distress syndrome (RDS). Air leaks occur in many critically ill infants who require mechanical ventilation. Chronic lung injury, called *BPD,* is a major cause of mortality and long-term morbidity, and its nomenclature has been simplified.[2] The smallest and most immature neonates are at highest risk for BPD following treatment for RDS, although BPD also has been described in neonates requiring ventilatory assistance for other causes of respiratory distress. The risk of BPD increases with decreasing birthweight and gestational age (see Chapter 21).

Evidence suggests that lung injury is partially dependent on the ventilatory strategies used. There is an emerging consensus that mechanical ventilation leads to lung injury,[3,4] and this subject has been reviewed.[5] Various ventilation strategies with the aim of reducing lung injury in neonates have been subjected to clinical trials.[6–13] Based on these data and animal studies, it has been recommended that clinicians use ventilatory strategies that prevent extremes in tidal volume, minimize gas trapping, and prevent alveolar overdistention. Blood gas targets are modified to accept higher than "normal" $Paco_2$ values. This ventilatory strategy is under the rubric of "gentle ventilation."[9,14–16]

Optimal ventilatory strategies should promote adequate gas exchange with minimum lung injury and other adverse effects. Every patient requires an individualized ventilatory approach based on the underlying lung pathophysiology. Objective measures of lung function, such as flow-volume relationships and blood gas data, coupled with the chest radiograph and physical examination findings should identify the disease state and guide decisions regarding ventilator mode and the magnitude of support. The goal of mechanical ventilation is to provide gas exchange while preventing or ameliorating ventilator-associated lung injury. This chapter reviews assisted ventilation strategies of the newborn with an emphasis on the prevention of lung injury.

COMPONENTS OF POSITIVE-PRESSURE VENTILATION

A discussion of six components of conventional mechanical ventilation and their physiologic impacts follows.

Positive End-Expiratory Pressure

Adequate positive end-expiratory pressure (PEEP) or continuous distending pressure prevents alveolar collapse and improves functional residual capacity (FRC) and ventilation-perfusion (V/Q) matching.[17] Increasing PEEP raises the mean airway pressure and increases oxygenation by improving V/Q matching. PEEP levels in excess of 6 to 7 cm H_2O may overdistend the lung and decrease pulmonary compliance. Overdistention of the lung reduces venous return and cardiac output and leads to decreased oxygen transport.

While raising PEEP levels increases FRC, there is a concomitant reduction in tidal volume. Unless peak inspiratory pressure (PIP) is increased, alveolar hypoventilation may result. Furthermore, elevated FRC alters pulmonary mechanoreceptor-mediated prolongation of expiratory time (TE) and may decrease the infant's spontaneous respiratory rate. A decrease in the patient's respiratory rate reduces the contribution of spontaneous ventilation to total gas exchange and may lead to hypoventilation. Another potential hazard of high PEEP is air leak. Optimal PEEP prevents alveolar collapse without overdistention of the lung. For most infants, PEEP levels between 3 and 6 cm H_2O improve oxygenation and are well tolerated.

Peak Inspiratory Pressure

PIP affects the pressure gradient ($\Delta P = PIP–PEEP$), which determines the tidal volume delivered to the infant. Tidal volume is proportional to the pressure gradient. Therefore, tidal volume, alveolar ventilation, and carbon dioxide elimination are strongly dependent on PIP. An increase in PIP normally increases carbon dioxide elimination and oxygenation (Pao_2). Changes in PIP affect oxygenation by altering mean airway pressure and V/Q matching. However, high levels of PIP increase tidal volume and thus increase the risk of "volutrauma," air leak syndromes, and lung injury. Very high PIP may result in hyperinflation and lower lung perfusion and cardiac output, leading to a decrease in oxygen transport despite an adequate Pao_2.

The level of PIP required to deliver the desired tidal volume depends mainly on the compliance of the respiratory system. The compliance in turn depends on the pathophysiology of the underlying disease process. A useful clinical indicator of adequate PIP is gentle chest rise with every ventilator-delivered breath. Chest rise of ventilator-delivered breaths should be similar to the chest expansion with unlabored spontaneous breathing. The degree of observed chest wall movement during the ventilator-delivered breaths indicates the compliance with fair accuracy.[18] The quality of breath sounds on auscultation is not helpful in determining optimal PIP; however, the absence of breath sounds may indicate inadequate PIP, displacement or obstruction of the endotracheal tube, or ventilator malfunction. It is advisable to use the minimum effective PIP that maintains adequate gas exchange but minimizes volutrauma.

Although estimation of the airway resistance and time constant are useful to identify if pressure equilibration is occurring, they are more important in adjusting inspiratory time (T_I) and expiratory time (T_E) and ventilatory rates; they are not directly involved in the adjustment of PIP. An increase in PIP and tidal volume when airway resistance is increased and the time constant is prolonged may result in volutrauma and gas trapping.

Ventilator Rate

The ventilator rate (frequency) and tidal volume determine alveolar minute ventilation according to the following relationship: alveolar minute ventilation = frequency × (tidal volume − dead space). Changes in ventilator rate alter alveolar minute ventilation and thereby $Paco_2$.

As ventilator rate is increased beyond physiologic and T_I decreases below three time constants, tidal volume delivery is impaired. With ventilator rates above certain levels, minute ventilation plateaus and later falls.[19] The threshold frequency at which tidal volume decreases with increasing rate depends on the time constant of the respiratory system. Lungs with longer time constants will achieve the threshold frequency at lower ventilator rates, and tidal volume with each breath delivered will be reduced. In disease states with short pulmonary time constants, higher respiratory rates can be tolerated without compromising tidal volume delivered. This problem rarely occurs with rates less than 60 per minute in preterm infants.

Very rapid rates may lead to inadvertent PEEP and gas trapping due to inadequate time for exhalation, leading to CO_2 retention, elevation of mean airway pressure, and impaired cardiac output. Analysis of chest wall movement may help detect the adequacy of T_I and T_E. The absence of a brief pause in chest wall movement at end-inspiration or at end-expiration may indicate an inadequate T_I (with decreased tidal volume delivery) or an inadequate T_E (with gas trapping), respectively. Maneuvers that increase T_E, such as reducing the ventilator frequency or shortening the T_I, may be necessary to allow adequate time for exhalation and to avoid inadvertent PEEP. As compliance is low and resistance is typically not elevated in RDS, higher rates (≥60/min) can be used in the acute and resolving phase of RDS.[20] In BPD or obstructive airway disease the time constant is prolonged. With a prolonged time constant, rapid ventilatory rates may cause gas trapping, decreased tidal volume, and carbon dioxide retention. As compliance is not corrected for lung size in the calculation of

time constant, larger infants have a longer time constant than smaller infants. Gas trapping is also more common in larger infants.

Mechanical ventilation supplements spontaneous respiratory effort, when present, and does not replace it completely. Sedated infants require increased ventilatory support. Apneic and paralyzed infants require full ventilatory support. In spontaneously breathing infants, adjustments to the ventilator may not impact arterial blood gases to the degree anticipated, in view of the variable respiratory contribution by the neonate. In infants with minimal lung disease who are mechanically ventilated for recurrent apnea, there does not seem to be a benefit to higher mechanical ventilatory rates in reducing energy expenditure[21]; hence, low rates (about 10/min) may be sufficient.

Inspiratory Time, Expiratory Time, or Inspiratory-to-Expiratory Ratio

The respiratory system time constant determines optimal T_I and T_E. The ventilator T_I and T_E must be at least three to five times longer than the T_I and T_E constants of the lung for adequate inhalation and exhalation. T_I and T_E time constants are not necessarily equal. The time constant is longer in exhalation because expiratory airway resistance is higher during exhalation. Normally, once the ventilatory rate and T_I are set, the other dependent variables [T_E and inspiratory-to-expiratory (I/E) ratio] are automatically determined. It is preferable to avoid extremes in T_I (<0.2 seconds or >0.7 seconds) as a T_I of 0.3 to 0.5 seconds suffices for most neonates. Infants with BPD often have a prolonged time constant and may need longer T_I and T_E; infants with acute RDS may do better with short T_I and T_E and rapid rates.[7,8]

The main effect of changes in the I/E ratio is on mean airway pressure and thus on oxygenation. When corrected for mean airway pressure, changes in the I/E ratio are not as effective in improving oxygenation as changes in PIP or PEEP.[22] Reversed I/E ratios (with inspiration longer than expiration) may improve V/Q matching and oxygenation, but at the expense of impaired venous return, decreased cardiac output, gas trapping, and air leaks. Low ventilator rates (30 to 40/min) with reversed I/E ratios (I/E =1:1) were once suggested as a means to avoid high PIP and reduce the incidence of BPD,[23] but subsequent studies have shown that reversed I/E ratios do not reduce mortality or morbidity.[24] Higher ventilatory rates combined with a short T_I decrease air leaks and BPD.[7,8]

Inspired Oxygen Concentration

Changes in the fraction of inspired oxygen (Fio_2) alter oxygenation directly by changing the alveolar pressure of oxygen. Because both Fio_2 and mean airway pressure affect oxygenation, it is important to balance their relative contributions. Although there are insufficient data to compare the roles of oxygen-induced versus pressure-associated (or volume-associated) lung injury in the neonate, it is generally believed that the risk of oxygen toxicity is less than that of volutrauma when Fio_2 is less than 0.6 to 0.7. It usually is necessary to wean or increase Fio_2 based on pulse oximetry or transcutaneous oximetry rather than occasional blood gases, as frequent changes in Fio_2 often are required. A change in the anticipated trend of Fio_2 or other ventilator adjustments should prompt reevaluation of the clinical situation.

Flow Rate

An adequate flow rate is required for the ventilator to deliver the desired PIP and waveform. As long as a sufficient flow is used, there is minimal effect of flow rate on gas exchange. A higher flow leads to a more "square wave" pressure waveform, increasing PIP to the desired value in a shorter period of time. Shortening the time to peak pressure with high flow may cause a small increase in mean airway pressure. However, with higher flow rates, more turbulent flow is created, especially with small endotracheal tubes. High flows may be required when TI values are short, in order to maintain tidal volume delivery. A minimum flow rate of about three times the infant's minute ventilation usually is required, and flows of 6 to 10 L/min are sufficient for most neonates.

VENTILATORY STRATEGIES IN NEONATES WITH RESPIRATORY DISTRESS SYNDROME

The premature infant is at risk for respiratory failure because of surfactant deficiency and inactivation, as well as structural immaturity of the lungs. Relative surfactant deficiency leads to alveolar collapse, decreased pulmonary compliance, and low FRC. Pulmonary time constants are characteristically short (0.05 to 0.1 seconds).[25] Surfactant deficiency, altered lung mechanics, and structural immaturity increase the risk of lung injury and air leak syndromes. Lung injury, which is accentuated in infants with RDS, may predispose to subsequent development of BPD. Table 15-1 lists suggested ventilatory strategies for common neonatal respiratory disorders.

Initiating Positive-Pressure Ventilation

The most common indications for assisted ventilation in the newborn infant are respiratory distress, cyanosis unresponsive to supplemental oxygen therapy, and apnea of prematurity that is refractory to medical management (Table 15-2). Clinical presentation of neonatal pulmonary insufficiency is variable. Some infants present in the immediate newborn period with severe distress or inadequate respiratory effort and require intubation and mechanical ventilation. Infants with RDS may show rapid deterioration with increasing oxygen requirement and need for continuous positive airway pressure (CPAP) or mechanical ventilation within the first few hours of life. Other neonates may require little or no respiratory support in the first postnatal days but subsequently may develop respiratory failure from sepsis, necrotizing enterocolitis, intracranial hemorrhage, or severe apnea.

TABLE 15-1.   Suggested Ventilatory Strategies for Common Neonatal Respiratory Disorders

Disease	Initial Strategy	Blood Gas Targets
RDS	1. Rapid rates (≥60/min) 2. Moderate PEEP (4–5 cm H_2O) 3. Low PIP (10–20 cm H_2O) 4. TI 0.3–0.4 sec 5. Tidal volume 4–6 mL/kg body weight	pH 7.25–7.35 Pao_2 50–70 mm Hg $Paco_2$ 45–55 mm Hg
Bronchopulmonary dysplasia	1. Slow rates (20–40/min) 2. Moderate PEEP (5–6 cm H_2O) 3. Lowest PIP required (20–30cm H_2O) 4. TI 0.4–0.7 sec 5. Tidal volume 5–8 mL/kg body weight	pH 7.25–7.30 Pao_2 50–70 mm Hg $Paco_2$ 55+ mm Hg
Meconium aspiration syndrome (without PPHN)	1. Relatively rapid rate (40–60/min) 2. Low-to-moderate PEEP (4–5 cm H_2O) 3. Adequate TE (0.5–0.7 sec) 4. If gas trapping occurs, increase TE to 0.7–1.0 sec and decrease PEEP to 3–4 cm H_2O	pH 7.3–7.4 Pao_2 60–80 mm Hg $Paco_2$ 40–50 mm Hg
PPHN	1. Higher rates from 50–70/min 2. PIP from 15–25 cm H_2O 3. PEEP 3–4 cm H_2O 4. TI 0.3–0.4 sec 5. High Fio_2 (80–100% O_2)	pH 7.4–7.6 Pao_2 70–100 mm Hg $Paco_2$ 30–40 mm Hg
Congenital diaphragmatic hernia	1. Relatively rapid rates (40–80/min) 2. Lowest PIP sufficient for chest excursion (20–24 cm H_2O) 3. Moderate PEEP (4–5 cm H_2O) 4. Short TI (0.3–0.5 sec)	pH >7.25 Pao_2 80–100 mm Hg $Paco_2$ 40–65 mm Hg (sicker neonates may need less aggressive goals for oxygenation, as long as preductal Spo_2 is >85%)
Apnea of prematurity	1. Relatively slow rates (10–15/min) 2. Minimal peak pressures (7–15 cm H_2O) 3. PEEP 3 cm H_2O 4. Fio_2 usually <0.25	pH 7.25–7.30 Pao_2 50–70 mm Hg $Paco_2$ 55+ mm Hg
Hypoxic-ischemic encephalopathy	1. Rates 30–45/min or slower, depending on spontaneous rate 2. PIP 15–25 cm H_2O 3. Low-to-moderate PEEP (3–4 cm H_2O) 4. Fio_2 to maintain Spo_2 92%–96%	pH 7.35–7.45 Pao_2 60–90 mm Hg $Paco_2$ 35–45 mm Hg

PEEP, positive end-expiratory pressure; PPHN, persistent pulmonary hypertension of the newborn; PIP, peak inspiratory pressure; RDS, respiratory distress syndrome.

TABLE 15-2. Indications for Neonatal Mechanical Ventilation

Clinical Criteria	Laboratory Criteria

Respiratory distress:
  Severe retractions: intercostal, subcostal, and suprasternal
  Tachypnea (respiratory rate >60–70/min)
	Severe hypercapnia: arterial carbon dioxide tension ($Paco_2$) >60 mm Hg in early RDS > 70–80 mm Hg in resolving RDS, accompanied by pH <7.20

Central cyanosis:
  Cyanosis of oral mucosa or
  Oxygen saturation <85% on O_2 by hood (head box) or CPAP at Fio_2 >0.60–0.70
Refractory apnea:
  Apnea unresponsive to medical management (e.g., theophylline, caffeine, CPAP)
	Severe hypoxemia:
	  Arterial oxygen tension (Pao_2) <40–50 mm Hg on O_2 by hood (head box) or CPAP at Fio_2 >0.60–0.70
	Adequate methylxanthine levels

CPAP, continuous positive airway pressure; RDS, respiratory distress syndrome.

Intubation and mechanical ventilation are indicated for infants with respiratory failure. Indications for intubation include respiratory or mixed acidosis with pH less than 7.20 and $Paco_2$ greater than 55 mm Hg, and hypoxemia (Pao_2 <50 mm Hg) despite treatment with supplemental oxygen. However, decisions to provide assisted ventilation for critically ill neonates frequently must be made after only clinical assessment. Signs of respiratory failure include cyanosis, deep intercostal and sternal retractions, or apnea and require prompt immediate evaluation and intervention.

Although assisted ventilation may be life saving for infants with established respiratory failure, not all extremely premature infants require mechanical ventilation. Increased use of mechanical ventilation may lead to a higher incidence of BPD.[26] Reducing the intubation and mechanical ventilation rates of very-low-birthweight neonates may decrease the incidence of BPD.[27] Furthermore, individualized airway management in the delivery room that limits endotracheal intubation and mechanical ventilation only to those extremely-low-birthweight infants with respiratory failure does not appear to increase mortality or morbidity.[28] Although observational and retrospective data suggest lower rates of BPD with a selective approach to the initiation of intubation and assisted ventilation, this strategy of airway management has not been tested in randomized controlled trials.

Surfactant treatment combined with early nasal CPAP, initiated after the onset of respiratory distress, decreases the need for mechanical ventilation and reduces mortality, but this strategy may possibly increase the risk of pneumothorax.[29,30]

Early Respiratory Distress Syndrome

Optimal management of mechanical ventilation requires astute bedside clinical assessment and accurate interpretation of blood gas data and chest radiographs. Blood gas analysis performed soon after initiation of mechanical ventilation and at regular intervals thereafter will facilitate decisions regarding ventilator management. However, pulmonary mechanics change rapidly in infants with RDS, and it may be necessary to make ventilator adjustments frequently, based on changes in chest excursion, oxygen saturation, and transcutaneous oxygen and carbon dioxide tension measurements. Meticulous attention to the pulmonary status and rational ventilator management will prevent the potential hazards of hyperventilation and hypoventilation of infants with RDS.

Recommended initial settings for pressure-limited, time-cycled ventilation of neonates with RDS are a respiratory rate of at least 60 breaths/min, PIP set to achieve minimal chest excursion during inspiration (10 to 20 cm H_2O), moderate PEEP (4 to 5 cm H_2O), and Ti of 0.3 to 0.4 seconds. Rationale for these settings are derived from clinical trials and physiologic principles.

Rapid ventilator rates and short Ti values are generally tolerated because of the characteristically low pulmonary compliance and short time constant in neonatal RDS. Clinical trials comparing rapid versus slow respiratory rates and short versus long Ti have been conducted. Strategies that use rapid respiratory rate and short Ti are associated with a lower incidence of air leaks.[6–8] The optimal ventilator rate for any given neonate will depend not only on the pathophysiology of the underlying disorder but also on the target $Paco_2$. Generally, it is preferable to increase minute ventilation by increasing rate rather than using other maneuvers such as elevating PIP. Although minute ventilation can improve by increasing PIP, this maneuver increases tidal volume and is more likely to induce volutrauma of the lung. Likewise, if a mechanically ventilated infant is hypocapneic, the PIP rather than ventilator rate should be reduced first to decrease minute ventilation.

In pressure-limited ventilation, changes in alveolar airway pressure and lung volume are closely linked. Changes in PIP determine the pressure gradient between the onset and end of inspiration and thus affect alveolar ventilation. Tidal volume, then, is a function of the pressure gradient between PIP and PEEP. The required tidal volume for infants with RDS is generally less than 5 to 6 mL/kg body weight. Animal models have demonstrated that a strategy of rapid shallow ventilation produces less lung injury than slow deep breaths.[31] Although animal studies demonstrate that small tidal volume ventilation reduces lung injury, human data in neonates are less definitive and generally inferential.

Overventilation, as indicated by low $Paco_2$ levels in infants receiving mechanical ventilation, has been associated with adverse pulmonary and neurologic outcomes. In one retrospective analysis, ventilated infants whose highest $Paco_2$ levels at 48 or 96 hours were less than 40 mm Hg were 1.45 times as likely to develop BPD as those whose highest $Paco_2$ levels were higher than 50 mm Hg [95% confidence interval (CI) 1.04 to 2.01].[12] Similarly in another study, infants with hypocarbia before the first dose of surfactant had a higher risk for development of BPD, with an odds ratio for BPD of 5.6 (CI 2.0 to 15.6) for $Paco_2$ level 29 or less versus 40 mm Hg or more.[13] Using multiple logistic regression analysis, these studies independently concluded that ventilator strategies that lead to hypocapnia during the early neonatal course increase the risk of BPD.[12,13] Furthermore, hypocarbia has been shown to predispose to periventricular leukomalacia[32,33] and cerebral palsy.[34]

A prospective randomized trial has shown that ventilatory strategies that maintained mild hypercapnia ($Paco_2$ 45 to 55 mm Hg) were safe and reduced the need for assisted ventilation in the first 96 hours after randomization.[9] A larger, multicenter, randomized trial reported that use of "minimal ventilation" (target Pa_{CO_2} >52 mm Hg) resulted in a reduction in ventilatory need at 36 weeks (16% vs 1%, $P < 0.01$) but did not decrease death and/or the need for supplemental oxygen at 36 weeks (68% vs 63%).[10] Further trials of ventilatory strategies that may prevent ventilator-associated lung injury seem warranted.

Although mild hypercapnia is thought to be safe in neonates, Pa_{CO_2} greater than 60 mm Hg may be an indication for mechanical ventilation in preterm infants because of concerns of altered cerebral blood flow and the potential increased risk for intraventricular hemorrhage.[9,35] In the early phase of RDS, it is appropriate to maintain a Pa_{CO_2} of 45 to 55 mm Hg with a pH above 7.20 to 7.25. By postnatal day 3 to 4, metabolic compensation gradually develops, which permits a higher Pa_{CO_2} for the same pH.

The initial level of PIP should be determined by the extent of chest excursion. The PIP required cannot be predicted based on the neonate's birthweight, gestational age, or postnatal age. A good starting point for the first few breaths in infants with RDS is a PIP of 15 to 20 cm H_2O. The PIP level can be adjusted in increments of 1 to 2 cm H_2O until adequate chest movement is obtained. If there is excessive chest rise with the initial PIP, the PIP should be reduced rapidly. Frequent adjustments in PIP may be required as pulmonary mechanics can change rapidly, as occurs after administration of exogenous surfactant.

In the acute phase of RDS, when alveolar atelectasis due to surfactant deficiency predominates, PEEP levels of 4 to 5 cm H_2O may be necessary. During the latter stages of RDS, PEEP levels of 3 to 4 cm H_2O may be adequate to prevent alveolar collapse. Reduction of PEEP levels below 2 to 3 cm H_2O is not recommended because the endotracheal tube eliminates the infant's physiologic maintenance of FRC by continuous vocal cord adduction.

During the period of increasing ventilatory support, F_{IO_2} can be first increased to 0.6 to 0.7 before increasing mean airway pressure. During weaning, once the PIP has been brought down to relatively safer levels, F_{IO_2} can be decreased to 0.4 to 0.5. Maintenance of an adequate mean airway pressure and V/Q matching may permit a substantial reduction in F_{IO_2}. Mean airway pressures should be reduced before a very low F_{IO_2} (<0.3) is reached, in order to reduce the likelihood of lung injury.

Weaning Ventilator Support

Discontinuation of ventilatory support may be attempted when there is spontaneous breathing and mechanical ventilation contributes only minimally to total ventilation. Weaning can be attempted when ventilator settings are relatively low. Weaning may be successful when the ventilator rate is 15/min or less, when the delivered PIP minimally moves the chest, and when F_{IO_2} is less than 0.40. The small endotracheal tubes used in premature neonates add a high resistive load, and most infants can be extubated from a low ventilator rate, without a period of endotracheal CPAP. A meta-analysis showed that extubation from low rates is more successful than extubation after a period of endotracheal CPAP.[36] Techniques such as patient triggered ventilation, synchronized intermittent mandatory ventilation (SIMV), pressure support, and breath termination sensitivity may facilitate weaning, as there may be less patient agitation and "fighting the ventilator" due to ventilator synchrony and termination of ventilator breaths during the infant's attempts to exhale.[37,38] A meta-analysis demonstrated

that SIMV and patient triggered ventilation shortened the duration of mechanical ventilation by almost 32 hours in preterm infants (95% CI 10 to 54 hours).[39]

Neonates can be extubated to an oxygen hood, to nasal CPAP (NCPAP), or to NCPAP with synchronized ventilator breaths (NCPAP+SIMV). The elective use of NCPAP after extubation reduces the need for additional ventilatory support in preterm infants [relative risk 0.62 (0.49–0.79)].[40,41] Clinical trials suggest that a combination of NCPAP with SIMV may increase the likelihood of successful extubation by 30%.[42,43]

Methylxanthines (theophylline, caffeine) may aid the weaning and extubation process, resulting in a reduction in failed extubations [relative risk 0.44 (0.27–0.72)], especially in extremely-low-birthweight infants.[44]

VENTILATORY STRATEGIES IN NEONATES WITH RESPIRATORY DISORDERS OTHER THAN RESPIRATORY DISTRESS SYNDROME

Table 15-1 lists suggested ventilatory strategies for common neonatal respiratory disorders.

Persistent Pulmonary Hypertension of the Newborn

Persistent pulmonary hypertension of the newborn (PPHN) is characterized by severe hypoxemia that is out of proportion to clinically evident lung disease. Elevated pulmonary arterial pressure due to increased pulmonary vascular resistance exceeds systemic arterial pressure and drives a pulmonary-to-systemic shunt through a patent ductus arteriosus or a right-to-left shunt at the atrial level in a structurally normal heart. Increased pulmonary vascular resistance may result from hypoxemia, sepsis, meconium aspiration syndrome (MAS), asphyxia, maternal drug therapy (e.g., nonsteroidal antiinflammatory agents that inhibit vasodilator prostaglandin synthesis), or various other causes. Many cases are idiopathic (see Chapter 23).

There is little evidence from controlled clinical trials to guide conventional ventilator management. Treatment principles are primarily based on lung pathophysiology. Strategies for mechanical ventilation in PPHN should decrease pulmonary vasoconstriction and improve pulmonary blood flow. Hypoxemia and acidosis are known to elevate pulmonary arterial pressure in the neonatal pulmonary circulation.[45] Therefore, ventilator adjustments are made to prevent hypoxemia and produce alkalosis. Hypoxemia can be prevented by maintaining the arterial P_{O_2} in the range from 70 to 100 mm Hg. If oxygenation is extremely labile, a higher target range of Pa_{O_2} (>100 mm Hg) may be attempted, although the benefits and risks of such a strategy have not been evaluated. Alkalosis can be achieved by hyperventilation (to maintain arterial P_{CO_2} in the range from 30 to 40 mm Hg) and infusion of sodium bicarbonate (0.25 to 1 mEq/kg/hour) to maintain a pH in the range from 7.5 to 7.6. Retrospective clinical data suggest that alkalosis induced by hyperventilation may be more beneficial than that induced by infusions of alkali alone. In a multicenter retrospective study in which hyperventilation was used by almost two thirds of the neonates, hyperventilation reduced the risk of extracorporeal membrane oxygenation (ECMO) without increasing the need for oxygen at 28 days of age. In contrast, the use of alkali infusion was associated with increased use of ECMO (odds ratio: 5.03, compared with those treated with hyperventilation).[46] Although hyperventilation has been shown to reduce pulmonary pressures and improve oxygenation,[47] there are concerns regarding the possible risks of induced respiratory alkalosis. Very low $PaCO_2$ in the range from less than 20 to 25 mm Hg causes cerebral vasoconstriction and may lead to long-term neurologic morbidity. In a small study, the need for prolonged hyperventilation in infants with PPHN was associated with poorer neurodevelopmental outcome.[48] The volutrauma associated with hyperventilation may lead to air leaks.[49]

It is important to remember that increasing ventilator rates much higher than usual (approximately >60 to 80/min) may actually decrease, rather than increase, minute ventilation, depending on the ventilator used (see Fig. 11-2*A* and *B*).[19] Therefore, although the ventilator rate is relatively high, subsequent attempts to increase minute ventilation must aim at increasing tidal volume, usually by increasing PIP, decreasing PEEP, or optimizing the I/E ratio.

Alternatively, some clinicians prefer a more "gentle" approach to ventilation and tolerate mild hypoxemia and/or hypercapnia in order to diminish lung injury. In this strategy, ventilator settings and FIO_2 are selected to maintain a PaO_2 between 50 and 70 mm Hg and $PaCO_2$ is allowed to increase as high as 60 mm Hg.[50] Hyperventilation and muscle relaxants typically are not used, although vasodilators such as inhaled nitric oxide (iNO) may be used. Gentle ventilatory strategies for treatment of PPHN are used infrequently at present.[46,51]

Inhaled NO has been shown to improve oxygenation in neonates with PPHN.[52–56] If hypoxemia or acidosis persists despite conventional ventilator therapy, iNO with or without high-frequency ventilation (HFV) often is attempted. Treatment with high-frequency oscillatory ventilation (HFOV) combined with iNO may be more often successful than treatment with either HFOV or iNO used alone in severe PPHN (see Figs. 14-3 and 14-4).[55]

After the initial 3 to 5 days, there typically is a transition period when oxygenation stabilizes. During the transition period, there are fewer fluctuations in PaO_2 as the pulmonary vasculature becomes less responsive to changes in arterial pH and $PaCO_2$.[57] Hyperventilation usually can be discontinued gradually (over 1 to 2 days) and ventilatory settings adjusted to "normalize" blood gases until extubation. If the infant has received HFV or iNO, they also can be gradually reduced and withdrawn. Rapid weaning of ventilator and vasodilator support occasionally results in recurrence of shunting.

Meconium Aspiration Syndrome

Airway obstruction, pneumonitis, surfactant inactivation, and increased pulmonary vascular resistance characterize MAS. Meconium partially obstructs airways, resulting in a ball valve phenomenon. The ball valve phenomenon leads to gas trapping and airway distention and increases risk of pneumothorax. A chemical pneumonitis of variable severity results from direct toxicity of meconium and release of inflammatory mediators. Surfactant is inactivated directly by meconium and by mediators of inflammation. Surfactant inactivation predisposes the lungs to atelectasis. Atelectasis, gas trapping, and

pneumonitis lead to V/Q mismatch, causing hypoxemia, hypercapnia, and acidosis. Hypoxemia and acidosis, coupled with antenatal pulmonary vascular remodeling that occurs in utero due to chronic hypoxemia, may lead to hypoxic pulmonary vasoconstriction and pulmonary hypertension.

There is little evidence from controlled clinical trials to guide conventional ventilator management and treatment principles are primarily based on lung pathophysiology. Infants with hypoxemia (PaO_2 <50 mm Hg) without significant evidence of right-to-left shunting either at the ductal or atrial level probably have severe V/Q mismatch and intrapulmonary shunting of blood past poorly ventilated or nonventilated areas of the lung. Ventilator management of the neonate with MAS is challenging due to the conflicting demands of areas of atelectasis and hyperinflation. Meconium-stained infants who have hypoxemia (PaO_2 <50 mm Hg), hypercapnia ($PaCO_2$ >60 mm Hg), or acidosis (pH <7.25) in an oxygen environment with FIO_2 greater than 0.80, often are considered candidates for mechanical ventilation.

In infants with MAS without associated PPHN, it is sufficient to maintain a pH of 7.3 to 7.4, with PaO_2 60 to 80 mm Hg and $PaCO_2$ 40 to 50 mm Hg. A relatively rapid rate (40 to 60/min), the minimum effective PIP for chest rise, a low-to-moderate PEEP (3 to 5 cm H_2O), and an adequate TE (usually 0.5 to 0.7 seconds) are required to prevent gas trapping and air leaks. If gas trapping is noticed, TE should be increased (0.7 to 1.0 seconds) and PEEP decreased (3 to 4 cm H_2O). If oxygenation is borderline (PaO_2 50 to 60 mm Hg) despite moderate ventilator settings and a high FIO_2, it may be appropriate to conservatively manage the infant without further increases in ventilator settings that may increase volutrauma and the risk of air leaks. Some infants with MAS, especially those whose spontaneous respirations or activity oppose the ventilator, may benefit from sedation with narcotics or muscle relaxants.

Ventilator strategies differ in infants with MAS and concomitant PPHN. Hypoxemia should be prevented by maintaining the arterial PO_2 at greater than 60 to 80 mm Hg. Poor oxygenation secondary to V/Q mismatch may improve with increased inhaled oxygen concentration. It is preferable to increase FIO_2 before increasing ventilatory pressures. Compared to premature neonates, there is less concern about the risks of hyperoxemia because neonates with MAS generally are term or post term.

If hypoxemia or hypercapnia does not respond adequately to conventional mechanical ventilation, HFV in the form of either HFOV or high-frequency jet ventilation may be effective.[58–60]

Congenital Diaphragmatic Hernia

The pathophysiology of impaired gas exchange in congenital diaphragmatic hernia (CDH) results from lung hypoplasia with decreased surface area for gas transfer complicated by pulmonary hypertension. The current surgical approach in most centers is one of cardiopulmonary stabilization and delayed surgical repair of the diaphragmatic hernia.

The ventilatory management of neonates with CDH often is challenging. Prospective randomized trials in this population have not been done. Preliminary evidence from retrospective studies suggests that gentle ventilation with the avoidance of hyperventilation and alkalosis may be associated with improved survival.[61–64] Early ventilatory management focuses on avoidance of bag-and-mask ventilation or CPAP that may increase gaseous distention of the herniated loops of bowel and impair pulmonary gas exchange. The objectives of mechanical ventilation in CDH should be to attain sufficient oxygenation (Pao_2 50 to 60 mm Hg) and a pH greater than 7.25. Very low pH values (<7.20) may increase pulmonary vascular resistance. It usually is sufficient to achieve a $Paco_2$ of 40 to 65 mm Hg, unless the presence of pulmonary hypertension requires it to be lower (30 to 40 mm Hg). Relatively rapid rates (40 to 80/min) with low peak pressures sufficient for chest excursion (20 to 24 cm H_2O), short TI values (0.3 to 0.5 seconds), and moderate PEEP (4 to 5 cm H_2O) in combination with mild sedation usually are indicated to attain these objectives.[62] For critically ill patients who do not meet these goals, marginal pulmonary gas exchange can be tolerated as long as there is good perfusion and adequate cerebral oxygen delivery indicated by preductal saturations of at least 85%. Postductal Pao_2 as low as 30 mm Hg or $Paco_2$ greater than 65 mm Hg can be tolerated if the patient is otherwise stable. Patients who do not maintain preductal saturations greater than 85% or postductal Pao_2 greater than 30 mm Hg or who show evidence of inadequate oxygen delivery based on rising serum lactate levels can be given a trial of iNO. Some infants will not respond to these measures and require treatment with ECMO.[62] Severe pulmonary hypoplasia associated with CDH may result in respiratory death despite all interventions.

Inhaled NO does not improve outcomes significantly in CDH.[56,65,66] Clinicians in some centers follow a policy of elective HFOV, followed by surfactant or iNO, and ECMO for preoperative stabilization if HFOV alone is not sufficient.[67–69] However, no controlled trials have concluded that HFOV is superior to conventional mechanical ventilation in neonates with CDH.

Refractory Apnea of Prematurity

Infants born prematurely may have apneic episodes that are of central (central nervous system), obstructive, or mixed (central + obstructive) etiology. Apnea in neonates is often due to immature control of breathing; however, other causes of apnea must be excluded. Apnea may be due to anemia, infection, hypoxemia, metabolic disturbances such as hypoglycemia, and central nervous system disorders such as intraventricular hemorrhage and hydrocephalus (see Chapter 3). Infants without a specific treatable cause of apnea may be given a trial of methylxanthines (theophylline or caffeine) and/or CPAP. In premature infants, CPAP reduces apnea by relieving upper airway obstruction, possibly via splinting of the pharyngeal airway. CPAP can decrease the incidence of both mixed and obstructive apnea episodes but usually is ineffective for central apnea.[70] High-flow nasal cannulae (flows 1 to 2.5 L/min) also generate positive distending pressure and may be as effective as CPAP for apnea.[71] However, the delivered pressure is not measured and is variable. Infants with persistent apnea on CPAP can be given a trial of nasal intermittent positive-pressure ventilation (CPAP+IMV or NIPPV),[72] although more studies are required to evaluate the benefits and risks of this technique in infants with refractory apnea.

Infants who are unresponsive to CPAP or NIPPV may require intubation and positive-pressure ventilation. Because the lungs are generally healthy or are in the healing phase following the initial respiratory disorder, it is important to avoid ventilator-associated lung injury. The ventilator rate usually is set between 10 and 15 per minute, with minimal peak pressures (7 to 15 cm H_2O), enough to produce minimal chest rise. A physiologic PEEP (2 to 3 cm H_2O) and low Fio_2 (usually <0.25) often are sufficient. Planned attempts of extubation to CPAP or NIPPV should be considered when the infant shows regular spontaneous breathing patterns while on the ventilator.

Asphyxia with Hypoxic-Ischemic Encephalopathy

Neonates with hypoxic-ischemic encephalopathy (HIE) may present with mild-to-severe lung pathology and impaired control of breathing. Infants may be tachypneic secondary to acidosis or apneic due to severe cerebral insult. Lung pathology can be seen secondary to meconium aspiration, pulmonary hypertension, pulmonary edema, or acute RDS. Some infants, especially those with meconium aspiration, may have pulmonary hypertension as a result of acute hypoxia or due to abnormal pulmonary vascular remodeling secondary to chronic intrauterine hypoxia. Infants with severe HIE may have cardiac or renal failure that may result in pulmonary edema.

The ventilatory management strategy for neonates with asphyxia and HIE but no other pulmonary pathology targets maintenance of arterial blood gases in the normal range (pH 7.35 to 7.45, Pao_2 60 to 90 mm Hg, $Paco_2$ 35 to 45 mm Hg). Hyperventilation and hypoventilation should be avoided, as cerebral blood flow is in part dependent on $Paco_2$. Hypoxemia must be avoided to reduce accentuation of the hypoxic-ischemic damage, and hyperoxia must be avoided to reduce free radical production and potentiation of cerebral injury. If minimal or no spontaneous respiratory efforts are present due to encephalopathy or because high doses of anticonvulsants were administered, a ventilator rate of 30 to 45 per minute with low peak pressures (8 to 15 cm H_2O), physiologic PEEP (2 to 3 cm H_2O), and Fio_2 adjusted to maintain normal oxygen saturation usually is appropriate. If the infant is spontaneously breathing, the ventilator rate may be reduced accordingly.

The ventilator management for infants with PPHN due to asphyxia or MAS is based on the underlying lung pathophysiology. The goal should be to maintain normocapnia with adequate oxygenation; therefore, hyperventilation, alkalosis, or permissive hypercapnia strategies may not be suitable for infants with concurrent HIE.

Bronchopulmonary Dysplasia

BPD was the term originally used by Northway et al.[73] to describe lung injury as a result of oxygen and mechanical ventilation in preterm infants. The term BPD now usually is used for infants with oxygen or ventilator dependence at a postnatal age of 28 days. BPD is considered moderate or severe if oxygen or ventilator dependence persists at a postmenstrual age of 36 weeks. BPD is a heterogeneous lung disease characterized by airway, alveolar, and vascular abnormalities.[2,74,75] Over the last two decades, the pathology has changed as smaller and more premature infants have survived. Prior to the era of exogenous surfactant, airway injury, inflammation, and parenchymal fibrosis were prominent findings in BPD. More recently, lungs of infants who died of BPD show more uniform inflation. The small airways are relatively free of epithelial metaplasia, smooth muscle hypertrophy, and fibrosis. Early pathologic descriptions of BPD included epithelial metaplasia and fibrosis, but the "new BPD" is characterized by more disturbance of alveolar septation and development and less epithelial metaplasia or fibrosis (see Chapter 21).[2,76]

The main objective of ventilatory management in BPD is to maintain adequate gas exchange while minimizing ventilator-associated lung injury. In view of the prolonged time constant in portions of the lungs, rapid ventilatory rates may not be optimal and may lead to gas trapping or inadequate tidal volume delivery. Older infants with BPD often tolerate higher levels of PEEP (5 to 7 cm H_2O) with improvements in oxygenation without CO_2 retention,[77] although higher levels of PEEP have not been systematically investigated in this population. Infants with the noncystic form of BPD, which is characterized by a predominantly homogeneous hazy appearance of the lungs on chest radiograph, and minimal or no cysts or coarse reticulation may tolerate faster rates and higher PEEPs. Infants with the cystic form of BPD, who have a tendency for gas trapping, are less likely to tolerate rapid rates and high PEEP. Pulmonary function in infants with BPD shows short-term variability despite apparent clinical stability[78]; therefore, ventilatory parameters may require frequent modifications. The emphasis should be on gradual weaning despite fluctuation in the clinical condition. Some neonates with marked variability in compliance and resistance over time may benefit from volume-controlled ventilation or patient-initiated, pressure-regulated, volume-controlled ventilation, which is an attempt to deliver adequate tidal volume with the least pressures. Although these modes of ventilation have theoretical benefits and many experienced clinicians use these modes routinely, there is insufficient evidence from randomized controlled trials or other studies to identify the superiority of one technique over another. Management of these neonates is empirical, based on pathophysiologic considerations and the experience of the clinician.

Newer ventilators with sensitive patient-triggered modes may benefit older infants with BPD who have a tendency to become agitated and "fight the ventilator." The term *fighting the ventilator* usually is applied to infants who actively exhale against a ventilator-delivered breath. In addition to patient-triggered ventilation, sedation may be required to calm the infant in this situation.

Many neonates with BPD do not have indwelling arterial catheters. Ventilator adjustments often are made on the basis of pulse oximetry and venous or capillary pH and Pco_2. If the infant is on low ventilator settings, attempts should be made to extubate the infant after optimizing fluid and pulmonary status. If the infant continues to require high ventilator settings, $Paco_2$ may be allowed to rise to high levels, as long as the arterial pH continues to stay above 7.25 (or venous/capillary pH >7.20). It is important to maintain Pao_2 higher than 50 mm Hg and oxygen saturation higher than 90%, in order to prevent or treat pulmonary hypertension and cor pulmonale. Weaning can be continued as long as pH and oxygenation are adequate.

Inhaled NO may have a therapeutic effect on infants with ventilator-dependent BPD. In a small nonrandomized trial, iNO improved oxygenation but not carbon dioxide elimination in some infants with severe BPD.[79] The role of iNO in BPD is unclear and should be considered experimental until further data are available.

Tracheobronchomalacia may complicate BPD[80] and is associated with the occurrence of *BPD spells*, which are sudden episodes of respiratory deterioration usually associated with

expiratory air flow limitation due to tracheobronchial narrowing following agitation and vigorous diaphragmatic and abdominal muscle activity.[81] Infants with BPD spells may require sedation and occasionally pharmacologic muscle paralysis[82] if they do not respond to a transient increase in ventilator settings.

HFV is unlikely to have a major role in the management of established moderate-to-severe BPD because high airway resistance in the lungs decreases the efficacy of gas exchange during HFV. No randomized controlled trials of HFV in the management of BPD have been reported.

Consideration should be given to tracheotomy in infants with BPD who have been ventilated for prolonged periods of time. Often ventilatory settings can be decreased secondary to reduced airway resistance, and the movement of the artificial airway to the neck may enhance developmental aspects of the infant's hospitalization. Nutritional support must be optimized in these chronically ill infants (see Chapter 24). Often placement of a gastrostomy tube and a fundoplication procedure improve enteral nutritional and prevent chronic microaspiration from impairing pulmonary recovery in BPD infants.

NEWER MODALITIES OF VENTILATORY SUPPORT

Newer techniques such as continuous tracheal gas insufflation, proportional assist ventilation (PAV), and perfluorocarbon-assisted gas exchange may help in improving respiratory outcomes in preterm neonates with RDS. When used as an adjunct to IMV, continuous tracheal gas insufflation may reduce tidal volume and peak pressures or increase carbon dioxide elimination at the same settings by continuous flushing of the dead space (Fig. 15-1; see also Fig. 13-3).[83] PAV, also called *resistive and elastic unloading* or *negative ventilator impedance,* is a mode of assisted mechanical ventilation wherein the applied airway pressure is servocontrolled and increases in proportion to the magnitude of the patient's respiratory effort. This allows the patient to fully control frequency, timing, and amplitude of lung inflation with his or her own control of breathing mechanisms. In pilot studies in premature infants, PAV has been shown to maintain similar oxygenation at lower airway and transpulmonary pressures as compared to IMV.[84] Perfluorocarbon-assisted gas exchange or partial liquid ventilation (PLV) is a technique in which a perfluorocarbon liquid instilled into the lung assists in gas transport in combination with mechanical ventilation.[85] Combinations of techniques may prove to be useful. HFV combined with partial liquid ventilation has been shown to be successful in a lamb model of RDS,[86] and PAV combined with partial liquid ventilation has been shown to be useful in a rabbit model of RDS, compared to PAV alone.[87]

High-Frequency Ventilation

HFV has become an established and effective modality for treatment of a variety of respiratory disorders (see Chapter 11). There is a trend for use of smaller tidal volumes and higher PEEP levels to optimize lung inflation and minimize volutrauma. Available controlled trials of HFV versus tidal ventilation do not clearly differentiate whether improved outcomes

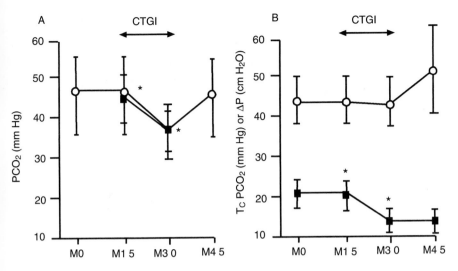

Figure 15-1. Continuous tracheal gas insufflation (CTGI) clinical tests. **A,** Pco₂ reduction test (n = 30). After an observation period M0 to M15, CTGI at 0.5 L/min was initiated at M15 for 15 minutes and discontinued at M30. All ventilator settings were kept constant. TcPco₂ (open circles) and Paco₂ (closed squares) are shown. *P < 0.0001. **B,** Pressure reduction test (n = 14). During the CTGI period, peak inspiratory pressure (PIP) was reduced in order to keep TcPco₂ constant. At M30, CTGI was removed and PIP was not modified during the following 15 minutes. TcPco₂ (open circles) and ÄP (PIP–positive end-expiratory pressure; closed squares) are shown. *P < 0.0001. (From Dassieu G, Brochard L, Agudze E, et al: Continuous tracheal gas insufflation enables a volume reduction strategy in hyaline membrane disease: Technical aspects and clinical results. Intensive Care Med 24:1076–1082, 1998.)

are the result of HFV per se or are a reflection of the effects of optimizing lung volume, a benefit that may not be unique to HFV. Much investigation has focused on whether HFV can reduce BPD when it is started relatively early before chronic lung disease is well established. In an immature baboon model, it was shown that early prolonged (for 1 to 2 months) HFOV significantly improved pulmonary mechanics and produced more uniform lung inflation compared to low tidal volume positive-pressure ventilation.[88] Although meta-analysis demonstrated that HFV decreases BPD, this observation is confounded by several earlier trials that found some benefit and more recent larger trials that showed no improvement in BPD even with a lung recruitment strategy.[89–93] The routine use of HFV in RDS cannot therefore be recommended, although "rescue" HFV in infants with air leak syndromes such as pulmonary interstitial emphysema and pneumothorax may be beneficial.[94,95] In conditions in which it is difficult to deliver adequate tidal volume, such as RDS with severe abdominal distention or hypoplastic lungs, HFV may be of benefit.[69,96,97]

SUMMARY

Small premature infants survive today in large part due to advances in mechanical ventilation. These surviving infants are at high risk for ventilator-induced lung injury. The degree of lung injury is partially dependent on the ventilatory strategies used. Ventilatory strategies that prevent high tidal volume, minimize gas trapping, and prevent alveolar overdistention may lead to improved outcomes.

REFERENCES

1. Lemons JA, Bauer CR, Oh W, et al: Very low birth weight outcomes of the National Institute of Child health and human development neonatal research network, January 1995 through December 1996. NICHD Neonatal Research Network. Pediatrics 107:E1, 2001.
2. Jobe AH, Bancalari E: Bronchopulmonary dysplasia. Am J Respir Crit Care Med 163:1723–1729, 2001.
3. Slutsky AS: Mechanical ventilation. American College of Chest Physicians' Consensus Conference. Chest 104:1833–1859, 1993.
4. Artigas A, Bernard GR, Carlet J, et al: The American-European Consensus Conference on ARDS, part 2: Ventilatory, pharmacologic, supportive therapy, study design strategies, and issues related to recovery and remodeling. Acute respiratory distress syndrome. Am J Respir Crit Care Med 157:1332–1347, 1998.
5. Auten RL, Vozzelli M, Clark RH: Volutrauma. What is it, and how do we avoid it? Clin Perinatol 28:505–515, 2001.
6. Heicher DA, Kasting DS, Harrod JR: Prospective clinical comparison of two methods for mechanical ventilation of neonates: Rapid rate and short inspiratory time versus slow rate and long inspiratory time. J Pediatr 98:957–961, 1981.
7. Multicentre randomised controlled trial of high against low frequency positive pressure ventilation. Oxford Region Controlled Trial of Artificial Ventilation OCTAVE Study Group. Arch Dis Child 66:770–775, 1991.
8. Pohlandt F, Saule H, Schroder H, et al: Decreased incidence of extra-alveolar air leakage or death prior to air leakage in high versus low rate positive pressure ventilation: Results of a randomised seven-centre trial in preterm infants. Eur J Pediatr 151:904–909, 1992.
9. Mariani G, Cifuentes J, Carlo WA: Randomized trial of permissive hypercapnia in preterm infants. Pediatrics 104:1082–1088, 1999.
10. Carlo WA, Stark AR, Wright LL, et al: Minimal ventilation to prevent bronchopulmonary dysplasia in extremely-low-birth-weight infants. J Pediatr 141:370–374, 2002.
11. Rhodes PG, Graves GR, Patel DM, et al: Minimizing pneumothorax and bronchopulmonary dysplasia in ventilated infants with hyaline membrane disease. J Pediatr 103:634–637, 1983.
12. Kraybill EN, Runyan DK, Bose CL, et al: Risk factors for chronic lung disease in infants with birth weights of 751 to 1000 grams. J Pediatr 115:115–120, 1989.
13. Garland JS, Buck RK, Allred EN, et al: Hypocarbia before surfactant therapy appears to increase bronchopulmonary dysplasia risk in infants with respiratory distress syndrome. Arch Pediatr Adolesc Med 149:617–622, 1995.
14. Carlo WA: Gentle ventilation. In Bancalari E (ed): Perspectives in Neonatology. St. Louis, Mosby, 2000, pp. 4–15.
15. Wung JT, James LS, Kilchevsky E, et al: Management of infants with severe respiratory failure and persistence of the fetal circulation, without hyperventilation. Pediatrics 76:488–494, 1985.
16. Dreyfuss D, Saumon G: Role of tidal volume, FRC, and end-inspiratory volume in the development of pulmonary edema following mechanical ventilation. Am Rev Respir Dis 148:1194–1203, 1993.
17. Thome U, Topfer A, Schaller P, et al: The effect of positive end-expiratory pressure, peak inspiratory pressure, and inspiratory time on functional residual capacity in mechanically ventilated preterm infants. Eur J Pediatr 157:831–837, 1998.
18. Aufricht C, Huemer C, Frenzel C, et al: Respiratory compliance assessed from chest expansion and inflation pressure in ventilated neonates. Am J Perinatol 10:139–142, 1993.
19. Boros SJ, Bing DR, Mammel MC, et al: Using conventional infant ventilators at unconventional rates. Pediatrics 74:487–492, 1984.

20. Chan V, Greenough A, Hird MF: Comparison of different rates of artificial ventilation for preterm infants ventilated beyond the first week of life. Early Hum Dev 26:177–183, 1991.

21. Locke RG, Greenspan J: Effects of different intermittent mandatory ventilation rates on oxygen consumption in premature infants recovering from respiratory distress syndrome. J Am Osteopath Assoc 95:366–369, 1995.

22. Stewart AR, Finer NN, Peters KL: Effects of alterations of inspiratory and expiratory pressures and inspiratory/expiratory ratios on mean airway pressure, blood gases, and intracranial pressure. Pediatrics 67:474–481, 1981.

23. Herman S, Reynolds EO: Methods for improving oxygenation in infants mechanically ventilated for severe hyaline membrane disease. Arch Dis Child 48:612–617, 1973.

24. Spahr RC, Klein AM, Brown DR, et al: Hyaline membrane disease. A controlled study of inspiratory to expiratory ratio in its management by ventilator. Am J Dis Child 134:373–376, 1980.

25. Reynolds EO: Pressure waveform and ventilator settings for mechanical ventilation in severe hyaline membrane disease. Int Anesthesiol Clin 12:259–280, 1974.

26. Van Marter LJ, Allred EN, Pagano M, et al: Do clinical markers of barotrauma and oxygen toxicity explain interhospital variation in rates of chronic lung disease? The Neonatology Committee for the Developmental Network. Pediatrics 105:1194–1201, 2000.

27. Poets CF, Sens B: Changes in intubation rates and outcome of very low birth weight infants: A population-based study. Pediatrics 98:24–27, 1996.

28. Lindner W, Vossbeck S, Hummler H, et al: Delivery room management of extremely low birth weight infants: Spontaneous breathing or intubation? Pediatrics 103:961–967, 1999.

29. Ho JJ, Subramaniam P, Henderson-Smart DJ, et al: Continuous distending pressure for respiratory distress syndrome in preterm infants. Cochrane Database Syst Rev 2:CD002271, 2000.

30. Verder H, Albertsen P, Ebbesen F, et al: Nasal continuous positive airway pressure and early surfactant therapy for respiratory distress syndrome in newborns of less than 30 weeks' gestation. Pediatrics 103:E24, 1999.

31. Albertine KH, Jones GP, Starcher BC, et al: Chronic lung injury in preterm lambs. Disordered respiratory tract development. Am J Respir Crit Care Med 159:945–958, 1999.

32. Okumura A, Hayakawa F, Kato T, et al: Hypocarbia in preterm infants with periventricular leukomalacia: The relation between hypocarbia and mechanical ventilation. Pediatrics 107:469–475, 2001.

33. Liao SL, Lai SH, Chou YH, et al: Effect of hypocapnia in the first three days of life on the subsequent development of periventricular leukomalacia in premature infants. Acta Paediatr Taiwan 42:90–93, 2001.

34. Ambalavanan N, Carlo WA: Hypocapnia and hypercapnia in respiratory management of newborn infants. Clin Perinatol 28:517–531, 2001.

35. Wallin LA, Rosenfeld CR, Laptook AR, et al: Neonatal intracranial hemorrhage: II. Risk factor analysis in an inborn population. Early Hum Dev 23:129–137, 1990.

36. Davis PG, Henderson-Smart DJ: Extubation from low-rate intermittent positive airways pressure versus extubation after a trial of endotracheal continuous positive airways pressure in intubated preterm infants. Cochrane Database Syst Rev 4:CD001078, 2000.

37. Baumer JH: International randomised controlled trial of patient triggered ventilation in neonatal respiratory distress syndrome. Arch Dis Child Fetal Neonatal Ed 82:F5–F10, 2000.

38. Beresford MW, Shaw NJ, Manning D: Randomised controlled trial of patient triggered and conventional fast rate ventilation in neonatal respiratory distress syndrome. Arch Dis Child Fetal Neonatal Ed 82:F14–F18, 2000.

39. Greenough A, Milner AD, Dimitriou G: Synchronized mechanical ventilation for respiratory support in newborn infants (Cochrane Review). Cochrane Database Syst Rev 1:CD000456, 2001.

40. Davis PG, Henderson-Smart DJ: Nasal continuous positive airways pressure immediately after extubation for preventing morbidity in preterm infants. Cochrane Database Syst Rev 3:CD000143, 2000.

41. Dimitriou G, Greenough A, Kavvadia V, et al: Elective use of nasal continuous positive airways pressure following extubation of preterm infants. Eur J Pediatr 159:434–439, 2000.

42. Khalaf MN, Brodsky N, Hurley J, et al: A prospective randomized, controlled trial comparing synchronized nasal intermittent positive pressure ventilation versus nasal continuous positive airway pressure as modes of extubation. Pediatrics 108:13–17, 2001.

43. Barrington KJ, Bull D, Finer NN: Randomized trial of nasal synchronized intermittent mandatory ventilation compared with continuous positive airway pressure after extubation of very low birth weight infants. Pediatrics 107:638–641, 2001.

44. Henderson-Smart DJ, Davis PG: Prophylactic methylxanthine for extubation in preterm infants. Cochrane Database Syst Rev 1:CD000139, 2000.

45. Lyrene RK, Philips JB III: Control of pulmonary vascular resistance in the fetus and newborn. Clin Perinatol 11:551–564, 1984.

46. Walsh-Sukys MC, Tyson JE, Wright LL, et al: Persistent pulmonary hypertension of the newborn in the era before nitric oxide: Practice variation and outcomes. Pediatrics 105:14–20, 2000.

47. Drummond WH, Gregory GA, Heymann MA, et al: The independent effects of hyperventilation, tolazoline, and dopamine on infants with persistent pulmonary hypertension. J Pediatr 98:603–611, 1981.

48. Bifano EM, Pfannenstiel A: Duration of hyperventilation and outcome in infants with persistent pulmonary hypertension. Pediatrics 81:657–661, 1988.

49. Hageman JR, Adams MA, Gardner TH: Pulmonary complications of hyperventilation therapy for persistent pulmonary hypertension. Crit Care Med 13:1013–1014, 1985.

50. Wung JT, James LS, Kilchevsky E, et al: Management of infants with severe respiratory failure and persistence of the fetal circulation, without hyperventilation. Pediatrics 76:488–494, 1985.

51. Walsh-Sukys MC, Cornell DJ, Houston LN, et al: Treatment of persistent pulmonary hypertension of the newborn without hyperventilation: An assessment of diffusion of innovation. Pediatrics 94:303–306, 1994.

52. Inhaled nitric oxide in full-term and nearly full-term infants with hypoxic respiratory failure. The Neonatal Inhaled Nitric Oxide Study Group. N Engl J Med 336:597–604, 1997.

53. Wessel DL, Adatia I, Van Marter LJ, et al: Improved oxygenation in a randomized trial of inhaled nitric oxide for persistent pulmonary hypertension of the newborn. Pediatrics 100:E7, 1997.

54. Davidson D, Barefield ES, Kattwinkel J, et al: Inhaled nitric oxide for the early treatment of persistent pulmonary hypertension of the term newborn: A randomized, double-masked, placebo-controlled, dose-response, multicenter study. The I-NO/PPHN Study Group. Pediatrics 101:325–334, 1998.

55. Kinsella JP, Truog WE, Walsh WF, et al: Randomized, multicenter trial of inhaled nitric oxide and high-frequency oscillatory ventilation in severe, persistent pulmonary hypertension of the newborn. J Pediatr 131:55–62, 1997.

56. Finer NN, Barrington KJ: Nitric oxide for respiratory failure in infants born at or near term (Cochrane Review). Cochrane Database Syst Rev 4:CD000399, 2001.

57. Sosulski R, Fox WW: Transition phase during hyperventilation therapy for persistent pulmonary hypertension of the neonate. Crit Care Med 13:715–719, 1985.

58. McDougall PN, Loughnan PM, Campbell NT, et al: High frequency oscillation in newborn infants with respiratory failure. J Paediatr Child Health 31:292–296, 1995.

59. Hintz SR, Suttner DM, Sheehan AM, et al: Decreased use of neonatal extracorporeal membrane oxygenation (ECMO): How new treatment modalities have affected ECMO utilization. Pediatrics 106:1339–1343, 2000.

60. Davis JM, Richter SE, Kendig JW, et al: High-frequency jet ventilation and surfactant treatment of newborns with severe respiratory failure. Pediatr Pulmonol 13:108–112, 1992.

61. Frenckner B, Ehren H, Granholm T, et al: Improved results in patients who have congenital diaphragmatic hernia using preoperative stabilization, extracorporeal membrane oxygenation, and delayed surgery. J Pediatr Surg 32:1185–1189, 1997.

62. Kays DW, Langham MR Jr, Ledbetter DJ, et al: Detrimental effects of standard medical therapy in congenital diaphragmatic hernia. Ann Surg 230:340–348, 1999.

63. Wilson JM, Lund DP, Lillehei CW, et al: Congenital diaphragmatic hernia—A tale of two cities: The Boston experience. J Pediatr Surg 32:401–405, 1997.

64. Wung JT, Sahni R, Moffitt ST, et al: Congenital diaphragmatic hernia: Survival treated with very delayed surgery, spontaneous respiration, and no chest tube. J Pediatr Surg 30:406–409, 1995.

65. Inhaled nitric oxide and hypoxic respiratory failure in infants with congenital diaphragmatic hernia. The Neonatal Inhaled Nitric Oxide Study Group (NINOS). Pediatrics 99:838–845, 1997.

66. Mercier JC, Lacaze T, Storme L, et al: Disease-related response to inhaled nitric oxide in newborns with severe hypoxaemic respiratory failure. French Paediatric Study Group of Inhaled NO. Eur J Pediatr 157:747–752, 1998.

67. Somaschini M, Locatelli G, Salvoni L, et al: Impact of new treatments for respiratory failure on outcome of infants with congenital diaphragmatic hernia. Eur J Pediatr 158:780–784, 1999.

68. Reyes C, Chang LK, Waffarn F, et al: Delayed repair of congenital diaphragmatic hernia with early high-frequency oscillatory ventilation during preoperative stabilization. J Pediatr Surg 33:1010–1014, 1998.

69. Desfrere L, Jarreau PH, Dommergues M, et al: Impact of delayed repair and elective high-frequency oscillatory ventilation on survival of antenatally diagnosed congenital diaphragmatic hernia: First application of these strategies in the more "severe" subgroup of antenatally diagnosed newborns. Intensive Care Med 26:934–941, 2000.

70. Miller MJ, Carlo WA, Martin RJ: Continuous positive airway pressure selectively reduces obstructive apnea in preterm infants. J Pediatr 106:91–94, 1985.

71. Sreenan C, Lemke RP, Hudson-Mason A, et al: High-flow nasal cannulae in the management of apnea of prematurity: A comparison with conventional nasal continuous positive airway pressure. Pediatrics 107:1081–1083, 2001.

72. Davis PG, Lemyre B, de Paoli AG: Nasal intermittent positive pressure ventilation (NIPPV) versus nasal continuous positive airway pressure (NCPAP) for preterm neonates after extubation (Cochrane Review). Cochrane Database Syst Rev 3:CD003212, 2001.

73. Northway WH Jr, Rosan RC, Porter DY: Pulmonary disease following respirator therapy of hyaline-membrane disease. Bronchopulmonary dysplasia. N Engl J Med 276:357–368, 1967.

74. Erickson AM, de la Monte SM, Moore GW, et al: The progression of morphologic changes in bronchopulmonary dysplasia. Am J Pathol 127:474–484, 1987.

75. Van Lierde S, Cornelis A, Devlieger H, et al: Different patterns of pulmonary sequelae after hyaline membrane disease: Heterogeneity of bronchopulmonary dysplasia? A clinicopathologic study. Biol Neonate 60:152–162, 1991.

76. Jobe AJ: The new BPD: An arrest of lung development. Pediatr Res 46:641–643, 1999.

77. Greenough A, Chan V, Hird MF: Positive end expiratory pressure in acute and chronic respiratory distress. Arch Dis Child 67:320–323, 1992.

78. Nickerson BG, Durand DJ, Kao LC: Short-term variability of pulmonary function tests in infants with bronchopulmonary dysplasia. Pediatr Pulmonol 6:36–41, 1989.

79. Banks BA, Seri I, Ischiropoulos H, et al: Changes in oxygenation with inhaled nitric oxide in severe bronchopulmonary dysplasia. Pediatrics 103:610–618, 1999.

80. Miller RW, Woo P, Kellman RK, et al: Tracheobronchial abnormalities in infants with bronchopulmonary dysplasia. J Pediatr 111:779–782, 1987.

81. McCoy KS, Bagwell CE, Wagner M, et al: Spirometric and endoscopic evaluation of airway collapse in infants with bronchopulmonary dysplasia. Pediatr Pulmonol 14:23–27, 1992.

82. Greenough A: Chronic lung disease. In Greenough A, Milner AD, Roberton NRC (eds): Neonatal Respiratory Disorders. London, Arnold, 1996, pp. 393–425.

83. Dassieu G, Brochard L, Agudze E, et al: Continuous tracheal gas insufflation enables a volume reduction strategy in hyaline membrane disease: Technical aspects and clinical results. Intensive Care Med 24:1076–1082, 1998.

84. Schulze A, Gerhardt T, Musante G, et al: Proportional assist ventilation in low birth weight infants with acute respiratory disease: A comparison to assist/control and conventional mechanical ventilation. J Pediatr 135:339–344, 1999.

85. Wolfson MR, Greenspan JS, Shaffer TH: Liquid-assisted ventilation: An alternative respiratory modality. Pediatr Pulmonol 26:42–63, 1998.

86. Sukumar M, Bommaraju M, Fisher JE, et al: High-frequency partial liquid ventilation in respiratory distress syndrome: Hemodynamics and gas exchange. J Appl Physiol 84:327–334, 1998.

87. Thome UH, Schulze A, Schnabel R, et al: Partial liquid ventilation in severely surfactant-depleted, spontaneously breathing rabbits supported by proportional assist ventilation. Crit Care Med 29:1175–1180, 2001.

88. Yoder BA, Siler-Khodr T, Winter VT, et al: High-frequency oscillatory ventilation: Effects on lung function, mechanics, and airway cytokines in the immature baboon model for neonatal chronic lung disease. Am J Respir Crit Care Med 162:1867–1876, 2000.

89. Thome UH, Carlo WA: High-frequency ventilation in neonates. Am J Perinatol 17:1–9, 2000.

90. Thome U, Kossel H, Lipowsky G, et al: Randomized comparison of high-frequency ventilation with high-rate intermittent positive pressure ventilation in preterm infants with respiratory failure. J Pediatr 135:39–46, 1999.

91. Moriette G, Paris-Llado J, Walti H, et al: Prospective randomized multicenter comparison of high-frequency oscillatory ventilation and conventional ventilation in preterm infants of less than 30 weeks with respiratory distress syndrome. Pediatrics 107:363–372, 2001.

92. High-frequency oscillatory ventilation compared with conventional mechanical ventilation in the treatment of respiratory failure in preterm infants. The HIFI Study Group. N Engl J Med 320:88–93, 1989.

93. Bhuta T, Henderson-Smart DJ: Elective high frequency jet ventilation versus conventional ventilation for respiratory distress syndrome in preterm infants. Cochrane Database Syst Rev 2:CD000328, 2000.

94. Keszler M, Donn SM, Bucciarelli RL, et al: Multicenter controlled trial comparing high-frequency jet ventilation and conventional mechanical ventilation in newborn infants with pulmonary interstitial emphysema. J Pediatr 119:85–93, 1991.

95. Gaylord MS, Quissell BJ, Lair ME: High-frequency ventilation in the treatment of infants weighing less than 1,500 grams with pulmonary interstitial emphysema: A pilot study. Pediatrics 79:915–921, 1987.

96. Fok TF, Ng PC, Wong W, et al: High frequency oscillatory ventilation in infants with increased intra-abdominal pressure. Arch Dis Child Fetal Neonatal Ed 76:F123–F125, 1997.

97. Revillon Y, Sidi D, Chourrout Y, et al: High-frequency ventilation in newborn lambs after intra-uterine creation of diaphragmatic hernia. Eur J Pediatr Surg 3:132–138, 1993.

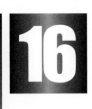

16 EXTRACORPOREAL MEMBRANE OXYGENATION

FAWN C. LEWIS, MD
MARLETA REYNOLDS, MD
ROBERT MASON ARENSMAN, MD

Despite advances made in assisted ventilation, including therapies such as high-frequency oscillatory ventilation (HFOV) and nitric oxide, some neonates fail to improve and die of respiratory insufficiency without alternate therapy. Extracorporeal membrane oxygenation (ECMO) or extracorporeal life support (ECLS) is a method of placing patients on heart-lung bypass in the intensive care unit. This pulmonary and cardiac support allows time (generally as much as 3 weeks) for neonates to improve so they can be returned to conventional ventilatory and minimal cardiac support.

The therapy of ECMO is an extension of cardiopulmonary bypass used for cardiac operations. John Gibbon[1] developed the first mechanical heart-lung bypass machine in 1937, but it was not until the 1950s that the machine was used to permit successful cardiac surgery. Severe protein denaturation limited early therapy because it occurred after only 2 hours. Further research led to a series of improvements in the gas exchange device or oxygenator. Factors limiting therapeutic use involved (1) direct exposure of blood to oxygen that caused cellular and protein damage, and (2) thrombosis in the circuit from blood exposure to foreign materials and exacerbated by stasis in the large reservoir component of the circuit. Evolution of the modern ECMO circuit (Figs. 16-1 to 16-3) had to address these and other problems. The major advance was the membrane oxygenator, described in 1956, that more physiologically exchanged gases by diffusion rather than direct exposure.[2] When Kammermeyer[3] reported the better gas transfer properties of dimethylsiloxane polymer (silicone), membranes allowed adequate oxygenation over a smaller surface area. This improvement in efficiency and alteration of the circuit reservoir allowed the first infant trials.[4]

As the pulmonary component of the ECMO circuit evolved, so did the cardiac component. Initially, roller pumps gained popularity due to ease of operation and reliability. Rollerhead pumps use rollers to compress the blood-filled circuit tubing against the circular wall of the pumping chamber. Blood cannot flow backward in the circuit, and as the rollers roll forward, significant pressure is generated inside the tubing: positive pressure ahead of the pump and negative pressure behind. Problems associated with the rollerhead pumps include trauma to the circuit tubing from repeated compression and the possibility of tubing rupture or air embolism in the circuit. The other pump in common use is the centrifugal pump. In this system the magnetic cone of the pump head is incorporated into the circuit and coupled with the magnetic base on the pump. As the base magnet turns, the cone inside the circuit tubing turns, causing forward flow of the blood around the pump head. In this system

there is less danger of tubing rupture or air embolism. If the tubing on either side of the pump is clamped, the pump head continues to turn without generating flow. This creates turbulence and leads to severe hemolysis. Servoregulators on both systems now minimize high negative or positive pressures and reduce the frequency of hemolysis or tubing rupture.[5] The characteristic that both systems have in common is that they create continuous nonpulsatile output.

As development of the cardiac and pulmonary components of the ECMO circuit progressed, the remaining critical issue was inflow and outflow. As in the native heart where cardiac output cannot exceed venous return, adequate circuit flow and pump output depend upon adequate venous inflow. Initial investigators of neonatal ECMO used umbilical vessels for venous and arterial access; however, these vessels were not large enough to provide sufficient flow for adequate oxygenation. There was inadequate therapeutic benefit. Utilization of the internal jugular vein for outflow and the common carotid artery for inflow allowed sufficient circuit flow for therapeutic benefit and enabled Bartlett et al.[6] to complete the first successful application of ECMO for neonatal respiratory failure in 1975.

PHYSIOLOGY OF EXTRACORPOREAL CIRCULATION

The membrane lung currently used has two compartments, one on either side of the gas-permeable silicone polymer membrane (Fig. 16-4). The ventilating gas flows on one side of the membrane (gas phase), and blood flows on the other (blood phase) in a countercurrent fashion. Oxygen and carbon dioxide diffuse across the membrane at a rate based on the diffusion gradient and the diffusion coefficient of each gas. The inherent potential for O_2 diffusion across silicone is 1210 mL O_2/m^2 per minute per mil thickness when the oxygen gradient is 760 mmHg across the membrane (1 mil = 0.001 inch = 25 μm). The Avecor 0800 silicone membrane lung (the standard neonatal oxygenator) has a surface area of 0.8 m^2 and a thickness of 1.5 mil; therefore, the maximum O_2 transfer across this membrane is 645 mL O_2/min. Oxygen diffusion through the blood phase is 100 mL O_2/m^2 per minute per 100-μm film thickness (blood thickness between two layers of membrane). Transmembrane pressure is defined as the sum of the pressures on either side of the membrane. When the transmembrane pressure exceeds 750 mmHg, the membrane alters its geometric configuration resulting in

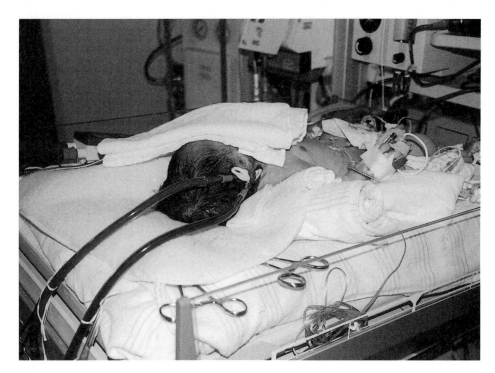

Figure 16-1. Photograph of a neonate on venovenous extracorporeal membrane oxygenation.

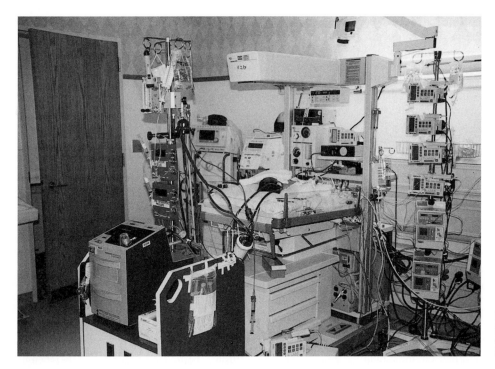

Figure 16-2. Photograph of the bed space for infant on extracorporeal membrane oxygenation (ECMO) showing a centrifugal ECMO pump in the foreground.

decreased O_2 transfer. ΔP is the difference between the pressure of the blood entering and leaving the oxygenator. When ΔP exceeds 350 mmHg, the blood film thickness widens, thus increasing the time needed for O_2 diffusion. Under usual conditions, the transmembrane pressure should not exceed 400 mmHg and ΔP should be 100 to 200 mmHg. This yields the thinnest blood film possible, which in the Avecor 0800 is 200 μm. The maximum diffusion of O_2 into the blood phase for an 0.8-m² membrane is approximately 40 mL O_2/min (compared to the potential 645 mL O_2/min for the silicone membrane itself). The

potential of the membrane is limited by diffusion of O_2 through the blood film (Fig. 16-5).

For any given membrane lung, the amount of venous blood that can be completely saturated with oxygen is a function of the O_2 content of the venous blood and the time spent along the membrane. As flow increases, oxygen transfer increases proportionally until limitation to O_2 transfer is imposed by the thickness of the blood film. When venous blood entering the membrane is 75% saturated, the flow rate at which exiting blood is 96% saturated is termed the *rated flow* of that device. This

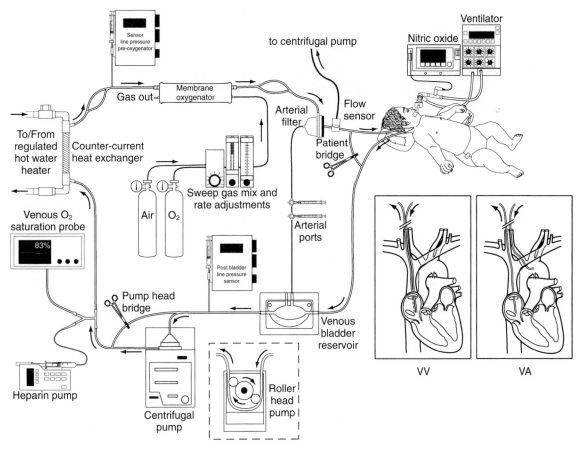

Figure 16-3. Extracorporeal membrane oxygenation circuit diagram. VA, venoarterial; VV, venovenous.

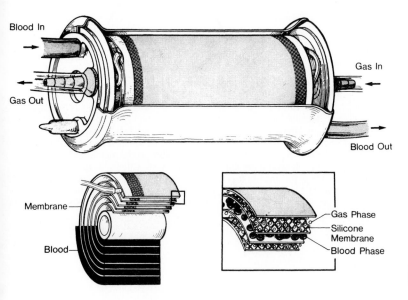

Figure 16-4. The SciMed Kolobow spiral silicone membrane lung.

number allows for standardization and comparison of membrane lungs. If the membrane is large enough, the amount of O_2 that can be transferred across the membrane depends on blood flow, not on the membrane's capacity to transfer O_2 (Fig. 16-6).

As in the body, CO_2 is more diffusible than O_2 through plasma. CO_2 transfer is limited by its diffusion rate across the membrane. For the 0.8-m^2 Avecor silicone membrane oxygenator, the potential for CO_2 transfer is 160 mL/min, or about

four times that of O_2. Carbon dioxide transfer is so efficient that many centers mix inlet gas (sweep gas) for the gas phase of the oxygenator with carbon dioxide to decrease the diffusion gradient and allow greater sweep gas flow without respiratory alkalosis. Because CO_2 transfer is relatively independent of blood flow along the membrane but dependent upon membrane surface area, an increasing partial pressure of CO_2 in the outlet blood is a sensitive indicator of loss of surface area and oxygenator function, usually caused by blood clot formation in the blood phase or accumulation of water along the membrane in the gas phase.

Blood flow in the circuit and to the membrane is limited by the patient's total circulating blood volume and the length and diameter (resistance) of the venous catheter. The system should allow 120 mL/kg/min of flow for near-total cardiorespiratory support, and the selected membrane should have a greater rated flow. ECMO with inadequate flow is of no benefit.

DISEASE STATES

The goal in ECMO is to identify patients with a severe but treatable or reversible disease process and to provide support to allow time for physiologic recovery. Because ECMO is not a specific therapy, it provides no assistance to patients with irreversible or progressive disease processes. The National Cooperative ECMO Study in adults showed that most forms of acute end-stage respiratory failure are not reversible even with prolonged extracorporeal support; ECMO did not improve survival.[7] As the adult lung heals, resolution is accompanied by pulmonary fibrosis, preventing normal lung function. Some improvement in adult survival rates (up to 60%) has been reported with narrower selection criteria and earlier ECMO therapy (Fig. 16-7).

In contrast to adults, much of the respiratory failure that occurs in the newborn period is potentially reversible, and 90% of lung growth occurs after the neonatal period. In term infants, the major underlying causes of profound hypoxia are meconium aspiration and persistent pulmonary hypertension of the newborn (PPHN). With a neonate's first few breaths, the high pulmonary vascular resistance present in the fetal lung normally decreases dramatically, allowing pulmonary arterial pressures to fall to levels lower than aortic pressure. Blood following the path of least resistance flows through the lungs instead of through the ductus arteriosus, and often flow in the ductus reverses. Over the next few days, the ductus arteriosus normally closes, thus completing the stages through "transitional" circulation to the normal adult circulation pattern. In some stressed infants, persistently high pulmonary vascular resistance leads to right-to-left shunting through the ductus

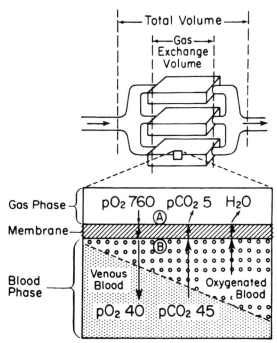

Figure 16-5. Principles of gas transfer in a membrane oxygenator. This expanded view shows interactions across the gas exchange membrane. Venous blood enters from the left and becomes arterialized as O_2 diffuses through the membrane and blood film and as CO_2 diffuses from the blood film into the gas phase. (From Bartlett RH, Gazzaniga AB: Extracorporeal circulation for cardiopulmonary failure. Curr Prob Surg 15:9, 1978.)

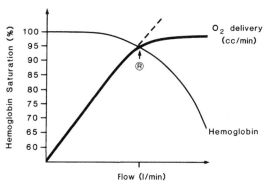

Figure 16-6. Rated flow. As flow through the membrane increases, actual O_2 transfer increases proportionally until the residence time of the venous return prevents complete hemoglobin saturation. At this point, the absolute O_2 transfer becomes fixed, but as the flow continues to increase, a smaller percentage of the venous return to the membrane becomes saturated. ® represents the rated flow, which is the flow at which the blood leaving the membrane is 95% saturated. (Adapted from Galletti PM, Richardson PD, Snider MT: A standardized method for defining the overall gas transfer performance of artificial lungs. Trans Am Soc Artif Intern Organs 18:359, 1972.)

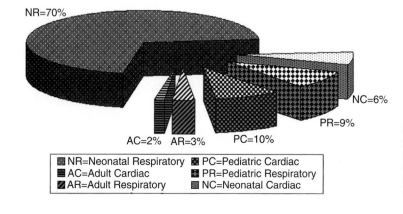

Figure 16-7. Pie chart showing percentage of extracorporeal membrane oxygenation (ECMO) patients by category. Neonatal respiratory causes are the most common ECMO diagnoses. Data are from the ECMO Registry of the Extracorporeal Life Support Organization (ELSO), Ann Arbor, Michigan, 1980–2001. Data from 2001 are incomplete.

arteriosus, foramen ovale, or via intrapulmonary vasculature. The resulting hypoxia and acidosis can be severe and lead to a worsening cycle of pulmonary vasoconstriction, hypoxia, and acidosis. Additionally, pulmonary vasoconstriction may lead to hyperplasia of the pulmonary arterial smooth muscle, making PPHN even more resistant to therapy. Persistent high-pressure, high-oxygen ventilation in these infants exacerbates fibrosis, leading to chronic lung disease and bronchopulmonary dysplasia (see Chapter 23).[8,9]

PPHN can be idiopathic or can be associated with a variety of stressful processes, including meconium aspiration syndrome (MAS), congenital diaphragmatic hernia (CDH), sepsis, perinatal asphyxia, and total anomalous pulmonary venous return (TAPVR). TAPVR is different from the other conditions in that the PPHN associated with TAPVR is not reversible without surgery. In TAPVR, the heart may be structurally normal internally on transthoracic echocardiography, but some or all of the pulmonary veins may not return blood to the left atrium but instead to systemic vessels. If these veins are obstructed, as commonly they are, PPHN results.[10,11] ECMO can be used to stabilize TAPVR patients preoperatively, but the condition ultimately requires surgical correction. ECMO is used as a short-term adjunct to support cardiac failure in neonates whose native function is expected to recover or in those who await heart transplant. In this way, ECMO is commonly used as a ventricular assist device to assist cardiotomy patients in coming off cardiopulmonary bypass.

PATIENT SELECTION/SELECTION CRITERIA

In general, a therapeutic intervention is offered when the potential benefit outweighs the potential risks and when the intervention outweighs the benefit and risks of alternative treatments. Therapy that increases mortality, has unacceptable morbidity, or is futile—the therapy adds no survival benefit or the patient's disease process is nonsurvivable—is contraindicated. Because complications during and after ECMO can be severe, ECMO usually is not offered unless there is a predicted mortality of 80% or greater with conventional therapy. Because it is difficult to measure any infant's predicted mortality, specific criteria reflecting such mortality are used as indications for ECMO, in addition to clinical judgment (Table 16-1).

Evaluation Before Extracorporeal Membrane Oxygenation

When an infant is considered for ECMO, the patient's history and hospital course are reviewed to evaluate the treatment received to date and to assess whether the infant is failing to respond to optimal conventional support. A physical examination is performed to screen for congenital anomalies, and cardiac echocardiography is performed to evaluate for possible structural heart defects that might contribute to the infant's symptoms. Cardiac echocardiography also indirectly evaluates PPHN by demonstrating right-to-left shunting through a patent ductus arteriosus or patent foramen ovale). A tricuspid regurgitation jet also provides indirect evidence of PPHN. The echocardiogram frequently documents poor ventricular function in babies with severe hypoxia; this is not a contraindication to ECMO because function usually recovers with adequate oxygenation over time.

It is important to estimate the degree of possible ischemic neurologic damage that may be present. Apgar scores are used to evaluate the overall status of a neonate in the first minutes of life. However, depressed Apgar scores are not always due to asphyxia, and ischemic damage can occur after good Apgar scores are recorded. Therefore, the predictive value of Apgar scores on neurologic outcome is limited, and they are not used to determine candidacy for ECMO. Most infants who are being considered for ECMO are sedated and many are pharmacologically paralyzed; thus, seizure activity or focal neurologic deficits are difficult to detect. In such infants, the most reliable bedside indicator of ischemic encephalopathy is the electroencephalogram. The presence of low-voltage burst suppression or isoelectric patterns is associated with poor neurologic outcome. The presence of seizure activity in and of itself does not preclude ECMO. In practice, obtaining an electroencephalogram takes valuable time in a patient who is not very stable. Without findings on physical examination or a history consistent with development of severe or global ischemic damage, the screening test of choice is the bedside cranial ultrasound. As the skull is incompletely calcified, cranial ultrasound through the fontanelles is used to evaluate the brain for evidence of congenital anomalies, intracranial hemorrhage (ICH), intraventricular

---

TABLE 16-1.   ECMO Selection Criteria

Indications
- Aa_{DO_2} >610 × 8 hours or >605 × 4 hours, if PIP >38 cm H_2O
- Oxygen index >40
- Acute deterioration with Pa_{O_2} <40 × 2 hours and/or pH <7.15 × 2 hours
- Unresponsive to treatment: Pa_{O_2} <55 and pH <7.4 × 3 hours
- Barotrauma (any four concurrently)
    Pneumothorax
    Pneumopericardium
    Pneumoperitoneum
    Pulmonary interstitial emphysema
    Persistent air leak >24 hours
    MAP >15 cm H_2O and subcutaneous emphysema
- Postoperative cardiac dysfunction
- Bridge to cardiac transplantation

Relative Contraindications
- Prolonged severe hypoxia
- Prolonged mechanical ventilation >7 days
- Structural cardiac disease
- History or evidence of ischemic neurologic damage
- Lack of parental consent

Absolute Contraindications
- Lack of parental consent
- Inadequate conventional therapy
- Weight <2000 g
- Gestational age <35 weeks
- Contraindication to anticoagulation
    Severe pulmonary hemorrhage
    IVH grade II or greater
    Gastrointestinal hemorrhage
    Head trauma
- Prolonged mechanical ventilation >7–14 days
- History of severe asphyxia or severe global cerebral ischemia
- Lethal genetic condition or unrelated fatal diagnosis (trisomy 13, trisomy 18, untreatable malignancy)
- Untreatable nonpulmonary disease, significant non treatable congenital cardiac malformation or disease

ECMO, extracorporeal membrane oxygenation; IVH, intraventricular hemorrhage; MAP, mean airway pressure; PIP, peak inspiratory pressure.

hemorrhage (IVH), edema, or periventricular leukomalacia. It is intuitive that systemic anticoagulation after an intracranial hemorrhage might easily cause rapid extension of the hematoma. However, von Allmen et al.[12] showed that patients with grade I IVH can be anticoagulated without significant risk of complications. Such patients are anticoagulated for ECMO using lower amounts of heparin and slightly lower target activated clotting times (ACTs). Von Allmen et al. also confirmed that more severe IVH has a high risk of rapid extension, and patients with edema or periventricular leukomalacia have a 63% incidence of major intracranial complications.

Parental Consent

Once a patient is a candidate for ECMO, it is necessary to obtain consent for cannulation, therapy, and decannulation. The mother usually is immediately postpartum and possibly is at a different facility but available by phone; the father may be present with the neonate. Effort is made to involve both parents and to communicate in the parents' primary language. The concept of ECMO is described, and it is made clear that ECMO is not a specific therapy but a way of providing time for healing or directed therapy. Data are given regarding outcomes for the patient's specific disease with and without ECMO therapy. Risks of major complications from anticoagulation (such as cerebral hemorrhage or other hemorrhage) and risks associated with hypoxia, hypotension, or mechanical ventilation (such as hearing loss and developmental delay) are discussed. It is generally made clear that the timing of decannulation is a decision made by the physicians and that if ECMO therapy is provided for 3 to 4 weeks without improvement, the risks of bleeding, infection, or other complication outweigh any further expected benefit. At that time, the baby is removed from ECMO and returned to conventional or high-frequency ventilation. Many ECMO centers provide parents with handbooks that further explain ECMO and the purpose of all the equipment and blood drawing.

Mode of Extracorporeal Membrane Oxygenation

There are two modes of ECMO: venovenous (V-V) and venoarterial (V-A) (Table 16-2). In V-V ECMO, a double-lumen catheter is placed into the right atrium, usually via the right internal jugular vein (Fig. 16-8). Blood flows from the right atrium into side holes of the cannula, through the pump, through a warmer, and through the membrane before being returned to the right atrium via the end of the double-lumen catheter. In this mode, the blood still travels through the patient's heart and lungs; the cardiac output is completely dependent upon native heart function. In the usual neonate with PPHN but without structural cardiovascular anomalies, the flow of highly oxygenated blood through the lungs assists in dilation of the vascular bed, improves cardiac function, and decreases the right-to-left shunt. This type of bypass allows the native circulation to provide physiologic pulsatile flow to the end organs in the usual fashion. However, complete reliance upon native cardiac function for cardiac output can be problematic in certain circumstances, especially when depressed cardiac function is severe. Other disadvantages to V-V ECMO include flow limitation due to the smaller lumen of the double-lumen cannula and decreased end-organ oxygen delivery due to admixture of blood from the native circulation bypassing the pump. If measured by radial or umbilical artery oxygen saturation (SaO_2) and partial pressures of oxygen and carbon dioxide (PaO_2, $PaCO_2$), V-V ECMO is very good at removing CO_2 from the circulation, but it is not as good as V-A ECMO at oxygenation. However, in the absence of hypotension or acidosis there is no evidence that hypoxia, even to a PaO_2 of 40, has undesirable sequelae in the neonate.

V-A ECMO involves a single-lumen catheter placed into the right atrium via the right internal jugular vein and another cannula typically placed into the right carotid artery with its tip pointed downstream in the aortic arch. Blood removed from the right atrium flows through the circuit and is returned to the aortic arch. The largest venous cannula that can be safely placed is used to maximize the potential flow achievable through the circuit. Because preload on the native cardiopulmonary system is decreased, the heart and lungs have a decreased workload and function with minimal strain. Oxygenated blood is returned via the aortic cannula to the aortic arch for delivery to the coronary arteries, arch vessels, and periphery.

Cannulation

When the decision is made to proceed with ECMO, the first call goes to the ECMO specialist who will prime the circuit. The operating room team is also notified of the impending procedure and estimated incision time. At this time, cross-matched packed red blood cells (pRBCs), fresh-frozen plasma

---

TABLE 16-2.   Comparison of V-V and V-A ECMO

V-V ECMO	V-A ECMO
Advantages	**Advantages**
• Requires venous access only	• Good oxygenation and CO_2 removal
• Pulsatile flow to organs preserved via native cardiac function in series with ECMO circuit	• ECMO circuit both in parallel and in series with native cardiopulmonary circuit. The fraction of blood flowing in parallel is dependent upon the ECMO pump velocity.
• Good CO_2 removal	• Can provide partial cardiac bypass and cardiac rest
• Easy to wean off ECMO support	• Rapid wean of ventilator, inotropes, and pressors
Disadvantages	**Disadvantages**
• Dependence on native cardiac function for cardiac output	• Nonpulsatile pump flow
• Flow through circuit may be limited by smaller cannula compared to single-lumen V-A venous cannula	• Cannulation of right carotid artery
• Decreased oxygen delivery to periphery compared to V-A ECMO	• Somewhat more difficult to wean off ECMO support
• Decreased flow if mediastinum is displaced	

ECMO, extracorporeal membrane oxygenation; V-A, venoarterial; V-V, venovenous.

(FFP), and circuit medications are ordered. Timing of the incision depends upon the readiness of the circuit. A fully assembled but unprimed (dry) neonatal circuit is always available, and in higher volume centers a partially primed (wet) circuit often is kept available to speed the preparation time. After dry assembly, circuits are stored covered by a sterile drape in a controlled, low-traffic area.

To prime the circuit, the tubing is first flushed with CO_2 that is circulated for 15 to 30 minutes. The circuit then is filled with lactated Ringer's solution. Continuous fluid circulation provides an opportunity to control any leakage from connectors or ports and identifies any visible air pockets or bubbles. At this point, a circuit could be stored as a "wet-primed" circuit. Institutions that store partially primed circuits have protocols regarding antibiotic use in the stored circuit and longevity of partially primed circuits. About half of institutions that allow stored circuits add a dose of a first-generation cephalosporin to the crystalloid priming solution; maximum storage intervals vary from 2 weeks to 2 months.

When the circuit is bubble-free, one unit of FFP is added to the circuit while the same volume of crystalloid solution is withdrawn into the reservoir bag. The plasma proteins in the FFP circulate to coat the internal surfaces of the circuit and decrease the amount of the patient's plasma proteins that will adhere to the circuit. Once the patient is on ECMO, an equilibrium is achieved between the proteins of the circulating blood and those on exposed circuit surfaces. After addition of the FFP, the circuit volume is replaced with red blood cells (approximately 1.5 units pRBCs). The pump medications, which consist of 800 units heparin, 600 mg calcium gluconate, and 15 mEq sodium bicarbonate, are added before cannulation.

The cannulation operation begins in the neonatal intensive care unit (NICU) as the FFP circulates in the pump; this allows the ECMO specialist to continue with the blood prime at the bedside as the operation is underway. For the operation itself, the surgeons require the assistance of a scrub nurse and circulating nurse, a sterile table with appropriate equipment, a headlight or other bright, directable light source, electrocautery, and suction. The patient is positioned with the head out toward the room on the padded mattress of a radiant warming bed. It is important to have a tray underneath the bed for radiograph cassettes. When all is ready, a small transverse incision is made in the right neck at the anterior or posterior border of the sternocleidomastoid muscle 1 cm above the clavicle. The right internal jugular vein is exposed first, as V-V cannulation proceeds with this vessel alone. After the right internal jugular vein is exposed and controlled, the right carotid artery is similarly prepared. In the event V-V ECMO is planned, the carotid artery is simply encircled with a short length of permanent suture so that the vessel can be easily located should a conversion to V-A ECMO become necessary. After the vessels are exposed and controlled, heparin (100 units/kg) is given to the patient and allowed to circulate for 2 to 3 minutes. The depth of catheter insertion is measured externally on the infant's chest, and the venous catheter inserted to a depth equal to the distance from the venotomy to the xiphoid. The arterial catheter is placed to a depth equal to the distance from the arteriotomy to the estimated location of the aortic arch (Fig. 16-9).

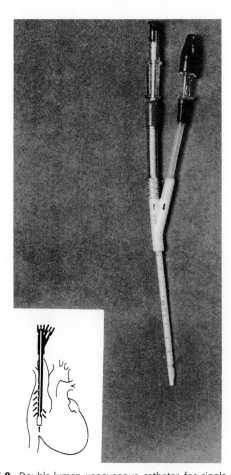

Figure 16-8. Double-lumen venovenous catheter for single-site access. The indwelling obturator seen in the venous drainage lumen. The two lumens, separated by an eccentrically located septum, allow both venous blood drainage and reinfusion of warmed oxygenated blood. The catheter is inserted through a venotomy in the internal jugular vein such that the tip of the catheter, and thus the reinfusion port, is located in the right atrium (*inset*). (From Anderson HL, Snedecor SM, Otsu T, et al: Multicenter comparison of conventional venoarterial access versus venovenous double-lumen catheter access in newborn infants undergoing extracorporeal membrane oxygenation. J Pediatr Surg 28:530, 1993.)

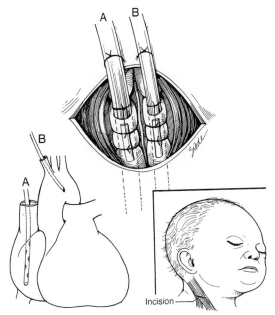

Figure 16-9. Vessel cannulation for venoarterial extracorporeal membrane oxygenation. Both the internal jugular vein (*A*) and the carotid artery (*B*) are ligated. The cannulae are then secured in the vessels with two ligatures over a small piece of vessel loop. When these ligatures are removed, they are cut over the vessel loop without risking damage to the vessels or the cannulae. Both cannulae are also secured to the skin of the neck.

After the catheters are in position and the pump is completely primed and air-free, ECMO pump flow is decreased to about 20 to 30 cc/kg/min and the loop of circuit tubing for connection to the patient is delivered to the surgical field in a sterile manner. The tubing loop is clamped and divided while the ECMO specialist unclamps the patient bridge to preserve pump flow. The appropriate patient cannulae are carefully attached to the proper ends of the tubing, and clamps are removed while the connection sites are inspected for missed air bubbles trapped in the circuit. The patient bridge clamp is replaced, and after flow is instituted the pump velocity is gradually increased in order to achieve adequate flow. The optimal flow is the lowest velocity greater than 200 cc/min that provides adequate oxygenation and carbon dioxide removal.

Another component of the circuit that requires adjustment is the sweep gas that flows in a countercurrent fashion through the gas phase of the membrane. The sweep gas is a normal oxygen-nitrogen mixture that is blended with oxygen to an adjustable FIO_2. Because the membrane is so highly efficient at removing carbon dioxide from the blood phase, some centers add carbogen (95% oxygen and 5% carbon dioxide) to the sweep gas to provide for more independent adjustment of oxygenation and carbon dioxide removal. If carbogen is used, the PCO_2 in the circuit must be adjusted to a normal physiologic level (35 to 45 mm Hg) before the circuit is connected to the patient. If the nitrogen-oxygen mixture is used without carbogen, the sweep begins at 1 to 2 L/min with the FIO_2 beginning at 100%; the rate is titrated as indicated by blood gas analysis after the infant is on ECMO. It is common to decrease the sweep rate substantially after a short time on the pump. The Avecor 0800 neonatal oxygenator has minimum (0.1 L/min) and maximum (2.4 L/min) sweep rates printed on the membrane casing.

After the circuit is flowing smoothly, the infant's blood pressure usually rises quickly and SaO_2 increases. Hemostasis in the neck wound is achieved, and the wound is closed with a few interrupted sutures. Cannula position is verified by portable chest radiograph (CXR) (Fig. 16-10). After the CXR is evaluated, the cannulas are secured to the skin, the wound is dressed with sterile gauze and an occlusive dressing, the sterile field is disassembled, and the operating room team released. In V-A ECMO, echocardiography is requested if the aortic cannula position is in question based upon the plain radiograph. The aortic cannula should be in the arch or descending aorta but not through or directed toward the aortic valve.

MANAGEMENT

Once ECMO is established with good flow, the patient generally becomes much more stable. Any cardioactive or inotropic drips are discontinued as tolerated, usually quickly as cardiac function responds to the increased oxygen delivery and decreased work requirement. Hypertension, whether natural or drug induced, is dangerous in these anticoagulated infants. If HFOV is in use, it is converted back to conventional ventilation. Ventilator support is then weaned to "rest settings" that maximize lung recovery by minimizing barotrauma and oxygen toxicity while maintaining positive end-expiratory pressure (PEEP) to prevent atelectasis. The patient's last full-effort ventilation settings are recorded and posted prominently on the ventilator as "Emergency Vent Settings" in case of a

sudden problem with the circuit and acute need to return to full ventilatory support. Patients who have been on HFOV will have settings for the conventional ventilator posted. These "rest settings" have not been specifically described, but most centers use targets similar to these: pressure control [= peak inspiratory pressure (PIP)] 20 cm H_2O, PEEP 10 cm H_2O, FIO_2 21%, and rate 10 breaths/min. If the infant has pneumothoraces and/or an air leak, then PEEP is reduced as far as 4 cm H_2O until the leak substantially decreases or stops. When there has been no leak for 24 hours, PEEP is cautiously increased to the resting level, near 10 cm H_2O. In V-A ECMO these "rest settings" are generally achieved within hours. During V-V ECMO, the PIP and ventilator rate are quickly decreased, but it may take several days to fully achieve "rest settings."

Pulmonary care while the patient is on ECMO is modified from conventional routines. All suctioning is omitted until the ACT is below 250 seconds. Gentle suctioning with a soft catheter is then allowed every 4 hours, but the length of the catheter is measured against the endotracheal tube. The maximum depth of suctioning, which is not to extend past the endotracheal tube by more than 3 to 4 mm, is clearly posted on the bed. Nasal and oral suctioning is with a soft bulb syringe only. Gentle chest physical therapy is allowed, as is postural drainage with the caveat that extreme care is taken to move the patient's body, head, and cannulae as one unit. Many centers allow patient movement only by a physician.

To assure complete and optimal daily ECMO care, it is useful to have preprinted orders with which all the ECMO specialists are familiar. These include routine orders that allow the nurses to act to maintain platelet counts above 50,000/mL, hemoglobin above 10 mg/dL, and potassium above 3.5 mEq/L. The patient has both a bedside nurse to monitor the patient, and an ECMO specialist to monitor the pump. The ECMO specialist carefully inspects the entire circuit several times per shift and opens clamps on all stagnant portions of the circuit every

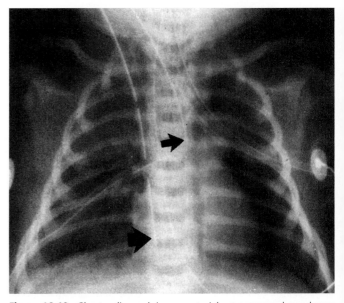

Figure 16-10. Chest radiograph in venoarterial extracorporeal membrane oxygenation patient showing the venous cannula *(large arrow)* in the right atrium, with the tip at the right atrium–inferior vena cava junction, and the arterial cannula *(small arrow)* in the aortic arch, with the tip directed down the descending aorta.

15 minutes or as needed to prevent clot formation in any portion of the circuit. One specialist might monitor two pumps if they are in easy reach and eyesight of each other and the patients are stable. In most institutions, ECMO patients are placed in close or adjacent beds to promote efficient utilization of personnel and assure high-quality care.

Full sets of blood gases (pump arterial, pump venous, and right radial or umbilical artery) are evaluated soon after institution of ECMO flow, and every 4 hours for the first 24 hours. The frequency then is usually decreased to every 8 hours. Other laboratory test values obtained immediately include a complete blood count (CBC) with platelets and measurement of serum potassium. Additionally, the effect of heparin anticoagulation is measured frequently. One of the most common methods is bedside ACT measurement. There have been many studies evaluating the different methods of bedside ACT measurement and methods of directly measuring heparin concentrations. Several investigators have described the differences in the standard measured ACT among different machines in neonates and suggest that the target therapeutic range be adjusted to the equipment used.[13,14] Typically, an institution will choose one or two target therapeutic ACT ranges (such as 180 to 200 or 200 to 220 seconds) and then choose the specific desired range for the given infant. The lower range is chosen if there is a concern about IVH or other hemorrhage, especially in lower-gestational-age infants. In infants who are placed on ECMO intraoperatively or immediately postoperatively (usually for cardiac support after surgical repair of congenital cardiac abnormalities), there is a neonatal circuit that is heparin bonded and operates with minimal or no systemic anticoagulation. This circuit is expensive and requires more frequent circuit changes, so it is not used frequently.

An orogastric tube is placed to gravity drainage. If there was no orogastric tube present before cannulation, the ACT should be below 250 seconds before one is placed.

Extracorporeal Membrane Oxygenation Routine

After the initial flurry of studies and laboratory tests, the ECMO routine settles into something similar to the following:

Early morning daily: CBC, platelets, sodium, potassium, chloride, carbon dioxide, blood urea nitrogen (BUN), creatinine, glucose, prothrombin time (PT), partial thromboplastin time (PTT), fibrinogen, fibrin split products, plasma free hemoglobin, portable CXR
Early morning on alternating days: Albumin, magnesium, phosphate, total and direct bilirubin
Every 6 hours: Potassium, platelets
Every 12 hours: CBC
Once daily: Blood cultures
Every morning for 5 days: Head ultrasound
Every 3 days: Endotracheal tube culture
Once stable: Daily physical therapy

Fluids and electrolytes: Normal intravenous maintenance fluids are given to the infant, with attention to possibly increased insensible loss via the membrane oxygenator. This increased loss is proportional to the sweep gas velocity. Most patients on ECMO have a variable degree of capillary leak due to a systemic inflammatory stress response and become edematous. Infants are placed on parenteral nutrition that is incrementally increased to goal levels as in the usual term or near-term NICU infant.

Oxygenation and ventilation monitoring: Blood gas measurements are performed on blood from the patient (umbilical artery catheter or radial artery catheter) and from the ECMO circuit preoxygenator (pump venous) and postoxygenator (pump arterial) sides. All samples are sent every 4 hours for the first 24 hours and then every 8 hours thereafter. As the ECMO course proceeds, the number of simultaneous blood gases is often decreased.

Sedation, pain control, and paralysis: These critically ill infants are often already on sedative, narcotic, and paralytic drips. If not, it is customary to order doses of a benzodiazepine and a narcotic as needed for pain or agitation. The ECMO surgical site is a source of pain that should not be ignored. As in the usual NICU infant, tachycardia, hypotension, hypertension, desaturation, or shunting are all symptoms of agitation and should be treated with an anxiolytic such as a benzodiazepine. The need for frequent dosing suggests that a continuous drip might better achieve the desired therapeutic effect. The infant is given at least one dose of a paralytic for the cannulation procedure and, unless the infant remains unstable, the paralytic is allowed to wear off, which allows more accurate evaluation of the infant's neurologic status. While the infant is pharmacologically paralyzed, continuous sedation as well as seizure prophylaxis, such as phenobarbital, is provided because the more apparent signs of seizure activity have been masked.

Anticoagulation monitoring: After cannulation, the ACT is measured every 15 to 30 minutes until the ACT is below 300 seconds. A continuous heparin infusion then is begun at a rate usually near 10 units/kg/hour. ACT measurements are continued at short (15 to 30 minutes) intervals until the ACT is stable. The heparin infusion is then titrated to keep the ACT within the ordered target range. No endotracheal tube suctioning, gastric tube suction, or placement or adjustment of indwelling catheters is allowed until the ACT has decreased below 250 to 300 seconds.

Daily Evaluation

Daily evaluation of the infant on ECMO involves evaluating pulmonary status by hand ventilation while listening to breath sounds, noting the amount of pressure delivered by the ventilation and the presence or degree of chest movement. The daily CXR is inspected for effusions and degree of pulmonary aeration. During the first few days, the patient's pulmonary status often worsens as evidenced by opacification of the lung fields on CXR and decreased pulmonary compliance. As the infant improves, the aeration returns, hand ventilation becomes easier, and chest movement is seen with lessening amounts of inspiratory pressure. Sites of cannulation and catheter placement are inspected, and all laboratory data are evaluated. Results of the head ultrasound are reviewed. The infant's volume status is measured by evaluating blood pressure, heart rate, capillary refill, peripheral perfusion, urine output, venous return to the pump, and venous blood gas analysis as an indicator of both perfusion and oxygen delivery. Intravascular hypovolemia can be corrected by adding aliquots of 10 mL/kg of blood or lactated Ringer's solution to the patient's intravenous line or directly to the pump. Caution is exercised in the evaluation of decreased venous return to the pump. It may indicate intravascular hypovolemia, but it also may reflect poor cannula position or pump flows too high for the cannula size or position. Repeated problems with the bladder collapsing and low preoxygenator circuit pressures, which indicate poor venous return to the pump, trigger an evaluation of the cannula position and perhaps gentle adjustment of the infant's head position in order to find a position that allows better flow. Other causes of poor venous return to the pump include a venous catheter that is too small or too long for the required flow, improper catheter position, or inadequate height of the patient relative to the pump. Because venous drainage into the pump is assisted by gravity, raising the patient's height relative to the pump can augment venous drainage. In V-A ECMO, the pump venous blood gas is used as usual to estimate the status of the patient's oxygen delivery and consumption. In V-V ECMO, however, high pump venous Svo_2 is usually an indication of recirculation, in which blood just returned to the atrium by the arterial side of the cannula is then sucked directly back into the pump through the venous side of the cannula. If the pump venous Svo_2 is greater than 95% in V-V ECMO, a decrease in the pump flow may decrease the fraction of blood that is recirculating, improve the efficiency of the system, and thus raise the cardiac output and Sao_2. If there are continued problems with recirculation or venous flow, the cannula may need to be repositioned.

Total flow through the circuit and membrane oxygenator controls the patient's mixed Pao_2 by varying the relative flow through the pump and through the infant's heart and lungs. Pump adjustments are made in response to the measured blood gas values, with the pump flow adjusted for necessary changes in oxygenation. $Paco_2$ is related to minute ventilation as in the conventionally ventilated neonate. Minute ventilation is a function of the tidal volume and respiratory rate. In the membrane lung, minute ventilation is controlled by the velocity of sweep gas in the gas phase of the membrane. When mixed gas systems including carbogen are used, the diffusion of CO_2 across the membrane is altered by changing the CO_2 gradient between the blood and the gas phases. In V-V ECMO, the sweep Fio_2 can be lowered as tolerated to 21%, allowing the blood then to travel through the pulmonary circulation for further oxygenation. In V-A ECMO, however, blood that is delivered directly to the aortic arch must be oxygenated. The pump flow can be weaned, as can the sweep velocity, but the sweep Fio_2 should be weaned cautiously in order to avoid creating a shunt. Changes are targeted toward normalizing the radial artery or umbilical artery values while minimizing pump flow to minimize platelet activation and hemolysis.

Daily measurement of hemoglobin levels, platelet count, fibrinogen, fibrin split products, and plasma free hemoglobin and evaluation of urine for gross hematuria allow monitoring of the level of hemolysis occurring in the circuit. As stated earlier, the plasma proteins equilibrate with the protein coat adherent to the internal surfaces of the circuit. After a variable duration of use, the circuit begins to "age," with increased protein deposition, blood clot formation, platelet activation, decreased fibrinogen, and increased fibrin split products. This has the appearance of a consumptive coagulopathy and is termed disseminated intravascular coagulopathy of the pump or *pump DIC*. This generally occurs every 4 to 14 days during an ECMO run, and the treatment is a circuit change. In order to change the circuit, an entire new circuit with a new oxygenator and a second pump is primed. The ventilator is turned up to emergency vent settings for about 30 minutes. When the new circuit is ready, the patient arterial and venous cannulae are clamped and divided; new connectors are placed in the tubing ends; and the ends of the new circuit tubing are quickly connected. Times

off bypass for this maneuver range from 30 seconds to 2 minutes. Flow on the new pump, which is decreased to about 20 mL/kg/min as at the initial cannulation, is quickly increased to the prechange settings. A circuit change restarts the timing schedule for all the laboratory tests. A circuit change also stresses the infant and exposes the infant's circulation to a new set of tubing. This usually triggers a systemic inflammatory response as seen at the initial cannulation. The pulmonary compliance may worsen and the lung fields may again opacify on CXR, setting the patient's progress back by several days. For this reason, a circuit change may be cautiously delayed a day or so for an infant who is close to decannulation with the understanding that there is an increasing risk of sudden thrombosis or embolism within the circuit.

Hemolysis also occurs within the circuit as the blood is driven by the mechanical pump. There is more hemolysis associated with the centrifugal pump system, but it occurs in both systems. The hemoglobin levels, the serum level of plasma-free hemoglobin, and the presence of hemoglobinuria indicate increasing levels of hemolysis. The best way to reduce and delay hemolysis is to maintain pump flow at the minimum velocity adequate for oxygenation and perfusion. When hemolysis worsens, increasing hemoglobinuria or a plasma-free hemoglobin level that rises from a baseline of 5 to 30 mg/dL to over 60 mg/dL generally indicates the need for either a circuit change or a pump head change. When using centrifugal pumps, the pump head is the greatest source of turbulence and hemolysis.

The pump head can be quickly changed without changing the rest of the circuit tubing or equipment. In this case, after the ventilator has been turned to emergency settings, the pump bridge is painted with povidone iodine (Betadine) and covered with sterile drapes. The bridge (usually clamped in the middle) is clamped at each end and then divided. The new pump head, which is primed with lactated Ringer's solution and carefully inspected for any bubbles, is spliced into the pump bridge. After the new pump head is inline, pump flow is rapidly decreased to zero, the old pump head is removed from the magnetic plate, and the new pump head is put in place. The clamps are removed from the new pump head and placed on either side of the old pump head. Flow is rapidly restored to prechange settings. Time off ECMO is approximately 6 to 15 seconds. The old pump head is then removed from the circuit and a bridge restored. When only the pump head is changed, the infant does not usually exhibit the systemic inflammatory response seen when changing the whole circuit.

Another potential management problem is pulmonary hemorrhage, which usually is evidenced by pink-tinged secretions noted upon suctioning of the endotracheal tube but occasionally is seen as frank hemorrhage into the lungs and airway. Management is adjusted to the severity of the hemorrhage. Response to minimal bleeding is to limit endotracheal suctioning, decrease the target ACT range by about 20 seconds (usually to 180 to 200), and increase PEEP slightly to help tamponade the bleeding site. The target platelet count also can be increased from 50,000/mL to 75,000/mL or even 100,000/mL if necessary. More severe hemorrhage warrants repeated transfusions of RBCs and platelets, higher increases in PEEP, or intratracheal epinephrine at 0.1 to 0.2 mL/kg of 1:10,000 concentration. Further efforts at pulmonary hemorrhage control are targeted toward limiting pulmonary vascular pressures by augmenting cardiac output and minimizing both left ventricular end-diastolic pressure and left ventricular afterload. Use of agents such as milrinone, which increase contractility without much increase in heart rate or myocardial oxygen demand, can be considered. Other important actions are aggressive transfusions as necessary to maintain a hemoglobin of 12 mg/dL, replacement platelets, judicious use of FFP to replace clotting factors, and willingness to treat what can be substantial and spectacular hemorrhage without allowing thrombosis within the circuit.

As a response to hypoxia and acid–base disturbances, there is often substantial cardiac dysfunction. When V-A ECMO is begun, the right and left ventricular preloads are substantially decreased by diverting flow through the circuit. Left ventricular afterload is increased by return of pump blood directly into the aortic arch. This situation can cause "cardiac stun" in which the pulse pressure is substantially decreased, and contractility and ejection fraction are noted to be depressed by echocardiogram. In this instance, aortic cannula position is verified by echocardiography as being directed toward the descending aorta and not toward the aortic valve. Other management consists of maintaining normovolemia and tailoring pump flow to the minimum output that provides adequate tissue perfusion and oxygen delivery to the periphery. Decreasing pump flow allows a larger fraction of the circulation to transit the native cardiopulmonary circulation and decreases left ventricular afterload. Cardiac stun generally begins to resolve within a day or two when a stronger pulse waveform is seen on the arterial line tracing and greater contractility is seen on echocardiogram. In the most severe cases, the arterial waveform is completely flat, and the patient essentially has pulseless electrical activity.

Many of the other severe events or complications in neonatal ECMO patients are neurologic (Fig. 16-11). Global neurologic deficits are generally related to the degree and length of hypoxia and acidosis sustained prior to ECMO. ICH is related to sudden changes in blood pressure, pH, or $Paco_2$ that occur as

ECMO therapy is instituted or at any time during therapy. Very tight control of hypertension, especially at the start of ECMO, as well as frequent surveillance of platelets, ACT, and $Paco_2$ are maintained. Many programs routinely perform a head ultrasound daily for 3 to 5 days and at any sudden change in mental status, decrease in oxygenation, tachycardia, decrease in platelet count, or rise in blood pressure. Studies have shown that the majority of cerebral hemorrhage in infants on ECMO occurs within the first 5 days.[15] If an IVH is detected, those designated grade I are followed with daily ultrasounds, the target platelet count is raised to 75,000, and the ACT target range is lowered to 180 to 200 seconds. In patients with IVH grades II to IV, the same measures are instituted, but continued anticoagulation as required on ECMO often results in extension of the hemorrhage with devastating results. These patients are evaluated for decannulation and return to conventional or high-frequency ventilation or withdrawal of support.

WEANING AND DECANNULATION

As the infant improves, a diuresis occurs. This can be assisted with gentle doses of a loop diuretic, but regular use of diuretics increases the infant's risk of hearing loss. As the lung fields clear, pulmonary compliance and pulmonary vascular resistance improve. At this time, the patient's Sao_2 may decrease, reflecting a relative increase in the percentage of circulation flowing through the normal cardiopulmonary circuit instead of the pump. Pump flow can be decreased as tolerated, to a minimum of 200 mL/min. This much flow is preserved to prevent stasis and coagulation in the circuit. As pump flows are decreased, the ventilator support is gently increased, both

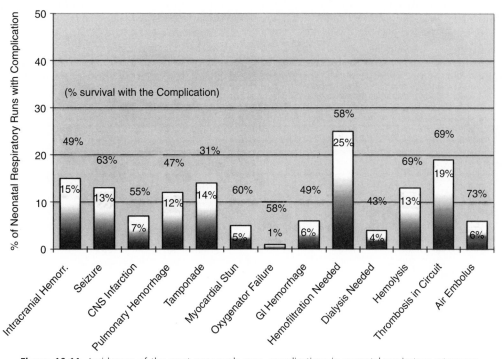

Figure 16-11. Incidences of the most commonly seen complications in neonatal respiratory extracorporeal membrane oxygenation (ECMO). Data are from the ECMO Registry of the Extracorporeal Life Support Organization (ELSO), Ann Arbor, Michigan, 1980–2001. Data from 2001 are incomplete.

to help pulmonary fluid clearing and to prepare the lungs to resume full function. Some centers increase the PIP for 8 to 12 hours a day and then return to rest settings for a day or two, but once pump flows are decreased enough to require native pulmonary function, the normal ventilator settings are maintained to compensate. In V-V ECMO, the sweep velocity and FIO_2 are weaned, as is the pump flow. Once the sweep is at 21% FIO_2 and the sweep velocity is weaned to zero, the cannula is simply removing and replacing blood from and to the right atrium without altering it. To prove that the infant is completely in charge of his or her own oxygenation and ventilation, the oxygenator is "capped off." This means that the oxygenator sweep inflow and outflow ports are connected directly to one another using oxygen tubing so that even entrained air entering the oxygenator is excluded. Umbilical artery or radial blood gases are obtained immediately, at 30 minutes, and at 1 hour. If the baby is doing well, decannulation proceeds. In V-A ECMO, sweep velocity can be weaned, as can pump flow, but sweep FIO_2 should remain high as described previously. When the infant is doing well on minimal settings and the ventilator is on acceptable settings, a "Trial Off" is performed. The arterial and venous cannulae are clamped near the baby's head, and the bridge is opened to maintain flow in the circuit. A blood gas from the infant is measured immediately and at 15-minute intervals for 1 hour. During this time, the cannulae are unclamped ("flashed") every 15 minutes after the sample is drawn to maintain patency of the cannulae should they still be needed. The maximum decannulation ventilator settings allow for the infant to worsen slightly after cannulation, allowing room to adjust the PIP and FIO_2. Decannulation ventilator settings should not be much higher than PIP 25 cm H_2O, PEEP 5 to 6 cm H_2O, FIO_2 40%, and rate 40 breaths/min.

If the infant passes these tests, he or she is ready for decannulation. The infant is given intravenous sedation and pain control medications, a paralytic medication, and a dose of perioperative antibiotics if he or she is not receiving antibiotic coverage. The surgeon and assistant need a table with sterile drapes for the instruments, a headlight, electrocautery, and suction, as well as an appropriately sized Broviac catheter to provide further intravenous access after decannulation. In V-A ECMO, the venous cannula is removed first, followed by the arterial cannula after ensuring proximal and distal control of each vessel. If there is blood loss during removal of the venous cannula and Broviac placement, the patient can be transfused using the aortic cannula. There are many opinions regarding the benefit of either simply ligating the neonatal common carotid artery or repairing it (Table 16-3). There has been no definitive study showing that either path has clear benefit, but one study looking at the condition of the vessels described a 25% success rate in reconstruction without tension.[16]

No study has shown a difference in neurodevelopmental outcome in neonates with ligated versus repaired carotid arteries over time.[17,18] In V-V ECMO, any vessel loops left around the carotid at the original operation are removed. A Broviac catheter is placed into the venotomy after the ECMO catheter is removed from the internal jugular vein. Whether the catheter is tunneled or placed directly into the venotomy and brought straight out through the cannulation wound, it is trimmed to the proper length. After the venous cannula is removed, proximal control of the vessel is loosened slightly to allow the Broviac to be inserted. Flow in the Broviac is tested and the wound loosely closed with a few interrupted sutures. Great care is taken whenever changing the dressing over the Broviac catheter, because it is easily adherent to the dressing and will pull out of the vein when the dressing is removed. Some centers allow only physicians to change these dressings. A CXR is ordered to evaluate the lung fields and Broviac position.

FOLLOW-UP

After decannulation, therapy returns to normal for the given diagnosis. Umbilical and arterial lines are removed as soon as possible after the heparin has metabolized, usually the next morning. Any chest tubes left in place due to anticoagulation are removed as soon as possible. Enteral nutrition is gently advanced to goal as tolerated, and total parenteral nutrition weaned when possible. For infants placed quickly on ECMO for MAS, it is not uncommon for the ECMO run to last 3 to 6 days, and the infant is ready for discharge home only 3 to

---

TABLE 16-3. Rationale for Carotid Artery Repair vs Ligation

Carotid Ligation	Carotid Artery Repair
Benefits	**Benefits**
• Faster decannulation procedure	• Restore normal flow to vessel
• No worry about future stenosis, aneurysm, or leak	• No need to rely on collateral perfusion from circle of Willis or vertebrobasilar system
• No vascular repair in contaminated wound	
• No risk of air or thrombus embolism during repair	
• No evidence that repair has clear benefit	
• No need for follow-up vascular studies	
• As child grows, remaining vasculature will compensate and deliver needed flow	
Risks	**Risks**
• Permanently remove right carotid artery from circulation	• Blowout at repair site from ischemic vessel at arteriotomy or rupture of repair from tension after segmental resection
• Risk of relative ischemia of right cerebral hemisphere	• Future stenosis or aneurysm, with alteration of flow or showers of emboli
	• Need for serial follow-up vascular studies to evaluate flow and rule out stenosis

7 days after decannulation. Infants with other diagnoses usually have more prolonged ECMO runs and more complex hospital courses. Before discharge, all infants have a developmental evaluation, a computed tomographic (CT) scan of the brain, and audiology screening in the form of auditory brainstem response testing as screening tools. CT scan is a more sensitive and specific evaluator of intracranial abnormalities than the head ultrasound performed while the infant was on ECMO[19] and is more accurate for future comparison. The infant is seen in a multidisciplinary ECMO clinic 1 week after discharge to evaluate progress and coordinate any necessary follow-up specialty care. Long-term follow-up consists of physical therapy and serial developmental and audiologic screening, at which time medical checkups focusing on any ongoing problems, nutrition, weight gain, and growth are performed. Developmental screening evaluations at 4, 8, 12, 18, and 24 months and then annually to around 8 years of age are appropriate to identify and initiate treatment of any problems through early development and to provide assistance as the child begins to attend school. Audiology screening is performed at 6-month intervals until at least 6 years of age in order to identify and initiate treatment for any hearing deficit or progressive hearing loss that can occur in these patients despite initially normal screening tests. In patients with carotid artery repairs, physical examination may reveal evidence of aneurysm, pseudoaneurysm, or bruit. Doppler duplex flow studies are performed initially and annually for several years to evaluate the vessel for evidence of stenosis. Repaired arteries have a stenosis rate of approximately 50% at 1 to 4 years, but only 5% to 10% were hemodynamically significant.[20,21] There are no compelling reports supporting any specific length or frequency of follow-up evaluations for carotid arteries repaired after neonatal ECMO cannulation. Some centers utilize magnetic resonance imaging, vision screening, electroencephalograms, and cerebral blood flow studies as part of their routine post-ECMO outpatient care. These additional tests may be helpful in children with specific indications but probably are not cost effective as general screening tools.

RESULTS

ECMO outcomes vary both by diagnosis and by the timing of ECMO initiation. The earlier an infant with respiratory insufficiency is placed on ECMO, the sooner the lungs are allowed to rest and heal.[22] Improved survival for infants with severe PPHN has been clearly established,[23-26] but survival rates and outcomes vary by diagnosis (Figs. 16-12 and 16-13). Overall survival for ECMO neonates at age 2 years has been reported to be 70%, with survival by diagnosis in one cohort as follows: MAS 100%, sepsis 79%, CDH 52%, and other diagnoses 63%. Another factor affecting ECMO mortality is the need for precannulation cardiopulmonary resuscitation, which decreases survival from 82% to 61%.[27] Fifteen years ago, initial studies led to the development of our current age and weight criteria by finding dismal rates of survival (25%) and ICH (100%) in infants less than 35 weeks of gestational age. More recent studies have shown improvement in survival (63%) and ICH (37%) in these patients, but ECMO remains less successful in these patients who do not meet currently accepted ECMO candidate criteria.[28] Furthermore, one study separated infants less than 34 weeks of gestation, 34 to 36 weeks of gestation, and 36 to 38 weeks of gestation and determined the relative odds ratio of ICH in each group to be 12.1, 4.1, and 2.1, respectively.[29] Separately, infants weighing 2 to 2.5 kg had a higher mortality (relative risk 3.45) than those weighing more than 2.5 kg. Infants of lower gestational age also had higher mortality, more frequent ICH, and more developmental delay at 1 to 2 years.[30]

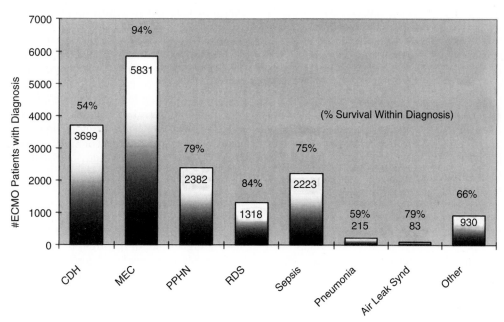

Figure 16-12. Distribution of extracorporeal membrane oxygenation (ECMO) between neonatal respiratory diagnoses and survival rates to hospital discharge with each diagnosis. Data are from the ECMO Registry of the Extracorporeal Life Support Organization (ELSO), Ann Arbor, Michigan, 1980–2001. Data from 2001 are incomplete.

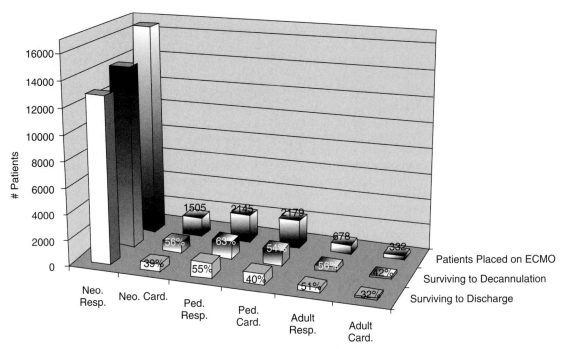

Figure 16-13. Distribution of extracorporeal membrane oxygenation (ECMO) between patient categories and survival rates to decannulation and discharge within each category. Data are from the ECMO Registry of the Extracorporeal Life Support Organization (ELSO), Ann Arbor, Michigan, 1980–2001. Data from 2001 are incomplete.

Other factors that affect ECMO patient outcome are lowest pH before ECMO, hypocapnia, severe hypotension, and prolonged mechanical ventilation before ECMO. Interestingly, when not associated with hypotension, hypoxemia did not confer an increased risk of future neurodevelopmental problems.[31] Overall studies of varying size and design report that anywhere from 6% to 30% of neonatal ECMO survivors show evidence of developmental disability, mental retardation, or neurologic deficit at 3 to 5 years, and 42% to 49% of patients are reported to have behavioral or school problems.[32–35] The most prevalent statistics, however, show ECMO survivors are in the 11% to 20% range for developmental disability at 2 to 5 years. One study that compared ECMO survivors to near-miss ECMO patients reports no differences between these groups in terms of cognitive outcome, adaptive skills, behavior problems, and risk of school failure at 5 years.[36] In terms of predictive value, there is a clear association between presence of a neuroimaging abnormality and future risk of neurodevelopmental abnormality that is proportional to the severity of the CT, magnetic resonance imaging, or head ultrasound abnormality. Of patients with no, mild, moderate, or severe neuroimaging abnormality, the reported (neurologic, motor, or developmental) disability at age 5 years was 10%, 13%, 33%, or 57%, respectively.[37,38] Although survival correlates with initial diagnosis, developmental outcome was not associated with initial diagnosis.[20]

Addressing overall ICH in ECMO patients, the reported rate varies from 9% to 20%, including those patients placed on ECMO with IVH grade I.[15,27,28,39] Differences in target ACT ranges and average gestational age may account for the wide variation in reports. Some authors propose that adding a cephalic venous drainage catheter can significantly decrease the frequency of IVH[40] and improve cerebral blood flow,[41] but other investigators have reported no difference. Another study promotes regular use of aminocaproic acid (Amicar) to decrease the rate of ICH.[42]

Auditory abnormalities are of great concern in survivors. Up to 25% of ECMO survivors are reported to have abnormal auditory brainstem-evoked response evaluations by discharge,[43] and reported rates in follow-up of sensorineural hearing loss (SNHL) are 16.7% to 24%, with high frequencies more impaired than low frequencies. Statistically similar numbers of non-ECMO neonates treated with HFOV have SNHL.[44–47] Audiometry evaluations are continued after discharge and into the early school years because of a documented incidence of progressive hearing loss over time in these populations[45,48] and a 5% requirement for bilateral amplification by age 5 years.[49] Profound hypocarbia was identified in one study as being associated with an increased risk of SNHL,[31] and patients with CDH have significantly higher rates of SNHL (37% to 60%) than infants with other diagnoses.[44,48]

In addition to higher rates of SNHL, CDH ECMO survivors show an increased incidence of respiratory and feeding problems.[20] Results are mixed regarding increased neuromotor and cognitive delay.[50,51] Both CDH and trisomy 21 infants have a higher rate of recurrent or refractory PPHN, and case reports describe successful nitric oxide use to prevent need for ECMO recannulation.[52] Survival after a second cannulation and ECMO run for CDH patients is reported to be 47%, but for other PPHN patients the survival was only 8%.[53] Trisomy 21 infants placed on a primary ECMO run have equivalent survival to decannulation, but reported survival to discharge was 65.9% compared to 75.6% in infants without trisomy 21.[54]

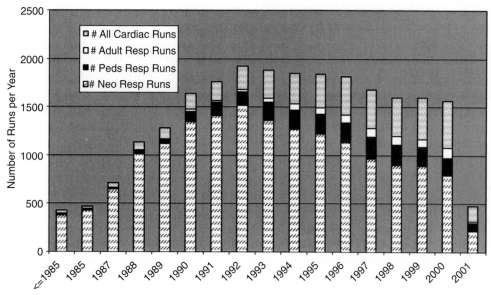

Figure 16-14. Number of extracorporeal membrane oxygenation (ECMO) runs each year by patient category. There is a steady decline over the past 9 years in neonatal respiratory ECMO cases. Data are from the ECMO Registry of the Extracorporeal Life Support Organization (ELSO), Ann Arbor, Michigan, 1980–2001. Data from 2001 are incomplete.

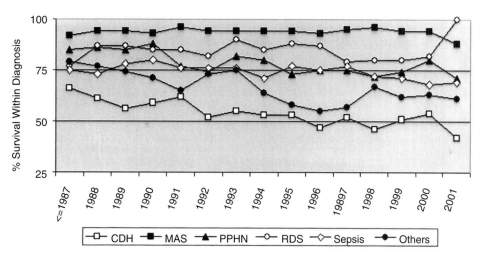

Figure 16-15. Trends in survival to hospital discharge over time for extracorporeal membrane oxygenation (ECMO) patients with neonatal respiratory diagnoses. There is decrease in survival over the last year in survival for ECMO infants with meconium aspiration and persistent pulmonary hypertension in the neonate (PPHN). There is also a steady decline in survival for ECMO infants with congenital diaphragmatic hernia (CDH). Selection of patients with more severe disease or patients with longer pre-ECMO mechanical ventilation may explain these trends. The success of high-frequency oscillatory ventilation, permissive hypercapnia, nitric oxide, and other intensive strategies also selects the more severely ill patients for ECMO therapy. Data are from the ECMO Registry of the Extracorporeal Life Support Organization (ELSO), Ann Arbor, Michigan, 1980–2001. Data from 2001 are incomplete. MAS, meconium aspiration syndrome; RDS, respiratory distress syndrome.

SUMMARY

ECMO is no longer an experimental therapy but is a valid tool that improves survival for certain diseases, decreases hospital time, and decreases long-term morbidity. There is no question that an ECMO run lasting 3 to 5 days with discharge home on day 7 of life in a neonate with MAS is more desirable than weeks of oscillator, nitric oxide, and ventilator therapy with associated pulmonary long-term morbidity. The critical issue in these babies is to tread the path between overaggressive ECMO use when

ECMO and its attendant risks perhaps are unnecessary and reticence to use ECMO in babies who clearly meet criteria. The success and recent increased availability of nitric oxide therapy in conjunction with HFOV use has decreased the number of PPHN and MAS infants meeting ECMO criteria (Fig. 16-14), but there is concern that the occasionally temporary improvement provided by these therapies may cause the infant to become an ECMO candidate only after days of ventilation, barotrauma, and high oxygen exposure or may cause the infant to be excluded as a candidate due to prolonged mechanical ventilation (Fig. 16-15).

It has been suggested that ECMO criteria be changed in these populations to consider infants with an oxygenation index of 25 or greater after 72 hours of treatment.[55] It certainly is true that early referral for ECMO can minimize ventilator trauma and allow more rapid and complete pulmonary recovery.

Investigators continue to push the age and weight limits accepted for clinical ECMO use. Premature and low-birthweight infants currently have greater survival than they did 10 years ago. As improvements are made in the surface characteristics of the membrane oxygenator and the circuit tubing, the need for anticoagulation will decrease, and smaller and younger infants will achieve greater ECMO success. Research on the inflammatory cascade may help to achieve this end. Moderation of the systemic inflammatory response to ECMO or cardiopulmonary bypass may help speed pulmonary recovery, lengthen the lifespan of the ECMO circuit, improve neurologic or renal morbidity, and decrease the cost of ECMO and the overall hospital course. Other technical improvements that might decrease morbidity are percutaneous cannula insertion techniques using the Seldinger method that some centers use in pediatric or adult ECMO patients, new pumping devices that allow single lumen/single-cannula tidal flow ECMO, and supersaturated oxygen solutions that may allow for more efficient ECMO and more complete bypass using cannulae previously inadequate to the task.

ECMO is one area of medicine where the world of research and technology interfaces directly with the world of clinical patient care. As such, advancements must be embraced by both sides with equal enthusiasm and caution. An overabundance of either will severely limit the utility of this clinical tool, and patient survival will be affected.

REFERENCES

1. Gibbon JH: Artificial maintenance of circulation during experimental occlusion of pulmonary artery. Arch Surg 34:1105, 1937.
2. Clowes GH, Hopkins AL, Neville WE: An artificial lung dependent on diffusion of oxygen and carbon dioxide through plastic membranes. J Thorac Cardiovasc Surg 32:630, 1956.
3. Kammermeyer K: Silicone rubber as a selective barrier. Ind Eng Chem 49:1685, 1957.
4. Doreson W, Baker E, Cohen ML, et al: A perfusion system for infants. Trans Am Soc Artif Intern Organs 15:155, 1969.
5. Pedersen TH, Videm V, Svennevig JL, et al: Extracorporeal membrane oxygenation using a centrifugal pump and a servo regulator to prevent negative inlet pressure. Ann Thorac Surg 63:1333–1339, 1997.
6. Bartlett RH, Gazzaniga AB, Jefferies MR, et al: Extracorporeal membrane oxygenation (ECMO) cardiopulmonary support in infancy. Trans Am Soc Artif Intern Organs 22:80, 1976.
7. Zapol WM, Snider MT, Hill JD, et al: Extracorporeal membrane oxygenation in severe acute respiratory failure: A randomized prospective study. JAMA 242:2193, 1979.
8. Markestad T, Fitzhardinge PM: Growth and development in children recovering from bronchopulmonary dysplasia. J Pediatr 98:597, 1981.
9. Schwendeman, CA, Clark RH, Yoder BA, et al: Frequency of chronic lung disease in infants with severe respiratory failure treated with high-frequency ventilation and/or extracorporeal membrane oxygenation. Crit Care Med 2:372, 1992.
10. Haworth SG, Ried L: Structural study of pulmonary circulation and of heart in total anomalous venous return in early infancy. Br Heart J 39:80, 1977.
11. Fyde D, Moodie DS, Gill LC: Resistant pulmonary hypertension complicating diagnosis and treatment of total anomalous pulmonary venous return in the neonate. Cleve Clin J Med 49:173, 1981.
12. von Allmen D, Babcock D, Matemoto J, et al: The predictive value of head ultrasound n the ECMO candidate. J Pediatr Surg 27:36, 1992.
13. Wallock M, Jeske WP, Bahkos M, et al: Evaluation of a new point of care heparin test for cardiopulmonary bypass: The TAS heparin management test. Perfusion 16:147–153, 2001.
14. Seay RE, Uden DL, Kriesmer PJ, et al: Predictive performance of three methods of activated clotting time measurement in neonatal ECMO patient. ASAIO J 39:39–42, 1993.
15. Khan AM, Shabarek FM, Zwischenberger JB, et al: Utility of daily head ultrasonography for infants on extracorporeal membrane oxygenation. J Pediatr Surg 33:1229–1232, 1998.
16. Levy MS, Share JC, Fauza DO, et al: Fate of the reconstructed carotid artery after extracorporeal membrane oxygenation. J Pediatr Surg 30:1046–1049, 1995.
17. Baumgart S, Streletz LJ, Needleman L, et al: Right common carotid artery reconstruction after extracorporeal membrane oxygenation: Vascular imaging, cerebral circulation, electroencephalographic, and neurodevelopmental correlates to recovery. J Pediatr 125:295–304, 1994.
18. Lohrer RM, Bejar RF, Simko AJ, et al: Internal carotid artery blood flow velocities before, during, and after extracorporeal membrane oxygenation. Am J Dis Child 146:201–207, 1992.
19. Bulas DI, Taylor GA, O'Donnell RM, et al: Intracranial abnormalities in infants treated with extracorporeal membrane oxygenation: Update on sonographic and CT findings. AJNR Am J Neuroradiol 17:287–294, 1996.
20. Jaillard S, Pierrat V, Truffert P, et al: Two years' follow-up of newborn infants after extracorporeal membrane oxygenation (ECMO). Eur J Cardiothorac Surg 18:328–333, 2000.
21. Cheung PY, Vickar DB, Hallgren RA, et al: Carotid artery reconstruction in neonates receiving extracorporeal membrane oxygenation: A 4-year follow-up study. Western Canadian ECMO follow-up Group. J Pediatr Surg 32:560–564, 1997.
22. Kornhauser MS, Cullen JA, Baumgart S, et al: Risk factors for bronchopulmonary dysplasia after extracorporeal membrane oxygenation. Arch Pediatr Adolesc Med 148:820, 1994.
23. Bartlett RH, Roloff DW, Cornell RG, et al: Extracorporeal circulation in neonatal respiratory failure; a prospective randomized study. Pediatrics 76:479–487, 1985.
24. O'Rourke PP, Crone RK, Vacanti JP, et al: Extracorporeal membrane oxygenation and conventional medical therapy in neonates with persistent pulmonary hypertension of the newborn: Prospective randomized study. Pediatrics 84:957–963, 1989.
25. UK Collaborative ECMO Trial Group: UK collaborative randomised trial of neonatal extracorporeal membrane oxygenation. Lancet 13:75–82, 1996.
26. Bartlett RH, Andrews AF, Toomasian JM, et al: Extracorporeal membrane oxygenation for newborn respiratory failure: Forty-five cases. Surgery 92:425–433, 1982.
27. Doski JJ, Butler TJ, Louder DS, et al: Outcome of infants requiring cardiopulmonary resuscitation before extracorporeal membrane oxygenation. J Pediatr Surg 32:1318–1321, 1997.
28. Hirschl RB, Schumacher RE, Snedecor SN, et al: The efficacy of extracorporeal life support in premature and birth weight newborns. J Pediatr Surg 29:186–190, 1994.
29. Hardart GE, Fackler JC: Predictors of intracranial hemorrhage during neonatal extracorporeal membrane oxygenation. J Pediatr 134:156–159, 1999.
30. Revenis ME, Glass P, Short BL: Mortality and morbidity rates among lower birth weight infants (2000 to 2500 grams) treated with extracorporeal membrane oxygenation. J Pediatr 121:452–458, 1992.
31. Graziani LJ, Baumgart S, Desai S, et al: Clinical antecedents of neurologic and audiologic abnormalities in survivors of neonatal extracorporeal membrane oxygenation. J Child Neurol 12:415–422, 1997.
32. Glass P, Wagner AE, Papero PH, et al: Neurodevelopmental status at age five years of neonates treated with extracorporeal membrane oxygenation. J Pediatr 127:447–457, 1995.
33. Hofkosh D, Thompson AE, Nozza RJ, et al: Ten years of extracorporeal membrane oxygenation; neurodevelopmental outcome. Pediatrics 87:549–555, 1991.
34. Adolph V, Ekeluno C, Smith C, et al: Developmental outcome of neonates treated with extracorporeal membrane oxygenation. J Pediatr Surg 25:43–46, 1990.
35. Dodge NN, Engle WA, West KW, et al: Outcome of extracorporeal membrane oxygenation Survivors at age two years: Relationship to status at one year. J Perinatol 16(3 Pt. 1):191–196, 1996.
36. Rais-Bahrami K, Wagner AE, Coffman C, et al: Neurodevelopmental outcome in ECMO vs near-miss ECMO patients at 5 years of age. Clin Pediatr 39:145–152, 2000.
37. Glass P, Bulas DI, Wagner AE, et al: Severity of brain injury following neonatal extracorporeal membrane oxygenation and outcome at age 5 years. Dev Med Child Neurol 39:441–448, 1997.
38. Lazar EL, Abramson SJ, Weinstein S, et al: Neuroimaging of brain injury in neonates treated with extracorporeal membrane oxygenation: Lessons learned from serial examinations. J Pediatr Surg 29:186–190, 1994.

39. Radack DM, Baumgart S, Gross GW: Subependymal (grade 1) intracranial hemorrhage in neonate extracorporeal membrane oxygenation. Frequency and patterns of evolution. Clin Pediatr 33:583–587,1994.

40. O'Connor TA, Haney BM, Grist GE, et al: Decreased incidence of intracranial hemorrhage using cephalic jugular venous drainage during neonatal extracorporeal membrane oxygenation. J Pediatr Surg 28:1332–1335, 1993.

41. Weber TR, Kountzman B: The effects of venous occlusion on cerebral blood flow characteristics during ECMO. J Pediatr Surg 31:1124–1127, 1996.

42. Wilson JM, Bower LK, Fackler JC, et al: Aminocaproic acid decreases the incidence of intracranial hemorrhage and other hemorrhagic complications of ECMO. J Pediatr Surg 28:536–540, 1993.

43. Desai S, Stanley C, Graziani L, et al: Brainstem auditory evoked potential screening (BAEP) unreliable for detecting sensori-neural hearing loss in ECMO survivors: A comparison of neonatal BAEP and follow-up behavioral audiometry. CNMC ECMO Symposium 62, 1994.

44. Lasky RE, Wiorek L, Becker TR: Hearing loss in survivors of neonatal extracorporeal membrane oxygenation (ECMO) therapy and high-frequency oscillatory (HFO) therapy. J Am Acad Audiol 9:47–58, 1998.

45. Mann T, Adams K: Sensorineural hearing loss in ECMO survivors. Extracorporeal membranous oxygenation. J Am Acad Audiol 9:367–370, 1998.

46. Sweitzer RS, Lowry JK, Georgeson KE, et al: Hearing loss associated with neonatal ECMO: A clinical investigation. Int J Pediatr Otorhinolaryngol 18;339–345, 1997.

47. Paccioretti DC, Haluschak MM, Finer NN, et al: Auditory brain-stem responses in neonates receiving extracorporeal membrane oxygenation. J Pediatr 120:464–467, 1992.

48. Robertson CM, Cheung PY, Haluschak MM, et al: High prevalence of sensorineural hearing loss among survivors of neonatal congenital diaphragmatic hernia. Western Canadian ECMO Follow-up Group. Am J Otol 19:730–736, 1998.

49. Glass P, Wagner AE, Coffman C: Outcome and followup of neonates treated with ECMO. In Zwischenberger JB, Steinhorn RH, Bartlett RH (eds): ECMO Extracorporeal Cardiopulmonary Support in Critical Care, 2nd ed. Extracorporeal Life Support Organization, 2000, p. 413.

50. Rasheed A, Tindall S, Cueny DL, et al: Neurodevelopmental outcome after congenital diaphragmatic hernia: Extracorporeal membrane oxygenation before and after surgery. J Pediatr Surg 36:539–544, 2001.

51. Bernbaum J, Schwartz IP, Gerdes M, et al: Survivors of extracorporeal membrane oxygenation at 1 year of age: The relationship of primary diagnosis with health and neurodevelopmental sequelae. Pediatrics 96:907–913, 1995.

52. Dillon PW, Cilley RE, Hudome SM, et al: Nitric oxide reversal of recurrent pulmonary hypertension and respiratory failure in an infant with CDH after successful ECMO therapy. J Pediatr Surg 31:462, 1996.

53. Lally KP, Breaux CW Jr: A second course of extracorporeal membrane oxygenation in the neonate–Is there a benefit? Surgery 117:175–178, 1995.

54. Southgate WM, Annibale DJ, Hulsey TC, et al: International experience with trisomy 21 infants placed on extracorporeal membrane oxygenation. Pediatrics 107:549–552, 2001.

55. Kossel H, Bauer K, Kewitz G, et al: Do we need new indications for ECMO in neonates pretreated with high-frequency ventilation and/or inhaled nitric oxide? Intensive Care Med 26:1489–1495, 2000.

17

BLOOD GASES
Technical Aspects and Interpretation

DAVID J. DURAND, MD
BARRY PHILLIPS, MD
JUDD BOLOKER, MD

Arterial blood gas measurements are the "gold standard" by which the adequacy of oxygenation and ventilation is assessed. Arterial blood gas values can be directly measured from indwelling arterial catheters or estimated from intermittent peripheral artery punctures, arterialized capillary bed samples, and central venous blood samples. Continuous monitoring devices, particularly the pulse oximeter, play an essential role in the respiratory management of the newborn by giving ongoing estimates of blood gas values. Other continuous monitoring devices, such as indwelling oxygen and carbon dioxide electrodes, indwelling saturation monitors, transcutaneous oxygen and carbon dioxide electrodes, and end-tidal carbon dioxide monitors, can be used to provide estimates of blood gas values. The relative advantages and disadvantages of these techniques are discussed here and summarized in Table 17-1.

TECHNIQUES FOR OBTAINING BLOOD SAMPLES

The most accurate arterial blood gas values are obtained from indwelling arterial catheters. Although it is possible to manage a sick newborn without arterial access, the presence of an arterial catheter often simplifies care significantly. Not only does it allow the accurate measurement of arterial blood gases without disturbing the patient, but it also allows direct

TABLE 17-1. Blood Gas Monitoring Techniques

Technique	Advantages	Disadvantages
Indwelling umbilical artery catheterization	1. Steady-state gases 2. Usually easily placed 3. Easy access once catheter placed 4. Can be used for fluid and medication infusion 5. Can be used for continuous blood pressure monitoring	1. Potential for major complications 2. Catheter cannot be placed in 10%–15% of patients
Indwelling peripheral artery catheterization	1. Steady-state gases 2. Easy access once catheter placed 3. Can be used for continuous blood pressure monitoring	1. Potential for major complications 2. Catheter cannot be placed in 25% of patients 3. Cannot be used for medication or blood infusion
Intermittent arterial puncture	1. Allows access when no catheter in place	1. Potential for major complications although less than with indwelling catheters 2. Patient may not be in a steady state
Arterialized capillary sampling	1. Can be performed easily 2. Low complication rate 3. Good for chronically ill patients 4. Fair estimates of pH, P_{CO_2}	1. Patient may not be in a steady state 2. Not reliable for P_{O_2} 3. Not reliable when perfusion is poor
Transcutaneous monitoring	1. Noninvasive 2. Continuous record of P_{O_2} and P_{CO_2} or in older BPD patients	1. Expensive equipment 2. May be unreliable if perfusion is decreased 3. May cause burns at electrode site
Pulse oximetry	1. Noninvasive 2. Continuous record of O_2 saturation 3. No burns	1. Works less well in active patients 2. May not work in hypotensive or edematous patients
End-tidal CO_2 monitoring	1. Noninvasive 2. Continuous record of end-tidal CO_2 3. Rapid assessment of tracheal intubation	1. More useful in larger ventilated patients 2. Adds significant dead space 3. Only rough estimate of Pa_{CO_2} in infants with significant lung disease

BPD, bronchopulmonary dysplasia.

279

measurement of arterial blood pressure and provides a route for obtaining other blood samples.

Umbilical Artery Catheters

Umbilical artery catheters are the preferred route for arterial access in most intensive care nurseries, particularly for infants in the first few days of life. They usually can be quickly and easily placed, with small risk of complications. The umbilical arteries are readily accessible during the first several days of life and often can be cannulated in patients as old as 2 weeks.

An umbilical catheter should be flexible, nonkinking, radiopaque, transparent, and nonthrombogenic; it should have an end hole but no side hole.[1,2] There are two common catheter sizes: 3.5-French and 5.0-French. Some clinicians believe that the larger catheter should be used whenever possible to minimize problems with thrombus formation within the catheter; the larger size makes it less prone to "clotting off." Others believe that the smaller catheter is better because it minimizes the changes in aortic blood flow that occur when a catheter is in place. Because there are almost no published data about the relative merits of the two catheter sizes, the decision about catheter size usually is based on personal preference. Our approach is to use a 3.5-French catheter in infants who weigh less than 1250 g and a 5.0-French catheter in infants who weigh more than 1250 g.

Prior to insertion, the catheter is attached to a three-way stopcock and syringe containing a heparinized saline solution and flushed thoroughly. When the catheter has been inserted and is functioning adequately, the stopcock should be attached to a continuous infusion of heparinized fluid and to a pressure transducer. The syringe, three-way stopcock, and catheter can be taped to a tongue blade to minimize accidental disconnection (Fig. 17-1).

The catheter is inserted while the infant is under a radiant warmer or in a heated isolette where the infant's temperature can be maintained and the vital signs monitored. The infant's legs should be loosely restrained. It may be helpful to also loosely restrain the arms. Insertion of the catheter should be done under sterile conditions, after the umbilical cord is cleaned with povidone iodine or chlorhexidine. A sterile umbilical tie is placed around the lower portion of the cord and tied

loosely with a single knot. The tie is placed so it can be either tightened if bleeding occurs when the cord is cut or loosened if it prevents passage of the catheter. Next, the cord is cut approximately 0.5 cm above the skin. Severing the cord with a scalpel in a single cut, rather than with a sawing motion, results in a flat umbilical surface from which the umbilical arteries usually protrude. The two thick-walled arteries and the single, larger thin-walled vein can easily be identified.

The most important step in the insertion of an umbilical arterial catheter is dilation of the arterial lumen. Failure to dilate carefully is the most common cause of catheter insertion failure. The goal of dilation is to open the lumen enough to allow smooth catheter passage without tearing the intima of the vessel. If the catheter tip tears the intima and creates a "false lumen" within the vessel, it will not reenter the lumen and successful catheter passage is nearly impossible. Dilation of the vessel should begin by placing one arm tip of a small forceps into the lumen. If this is done gently, the vessel will dilate, which will allow placement of both arms of the forceps into the lumen (Fig. 17-2). Once both arms have been placed, they can be slowly spread, gradually dilating the vessel to the caliber of the catheter. As the vessel lumen dilates, the forceps should be advanced with the goal of dilating at least 5 to 8 mm of the vessel. Once the vessel has been adequately dilated, the catheter can be inserted. It is easier to pass the catheter if the vessel is stabilized with one or two small curved forceps. Usually the catheter passes smoothly. When the catheter meets significant resistance, it usually means that the catheter has dissected through the intima and has created a false lumen within the wall of the vessel. When this occurs, the catheter should be removed. Forcing the catheter at this point more likely will result in damage to the vessel than success.

On occasion, a catheter will travel down into the iliac artery rather than up into the aorta. If this occurs, a second catheter usually can be inserted into the same umbilical artery, without removing the first catheter. With the first catheter lodged in the iliac artery, the second is often directed into the aorta.[3]

Once the catheter enters the aorta, the ideal tip position is either between the level of the third and fourth lumbar vertebrae (low position) or between the level of the sixth and tenth thoracic vertebrae (high position). In the low position, the tip is

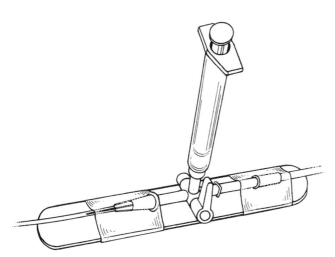

Figure 17-1. Taping method for preventing disconnection of a catheter system.

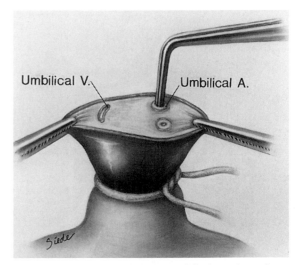

Figure 17-2. Umbilical stump with two umbilical arteries and one vein. A small forceps is used to gently dilate one artery.

below the renal and mesenteric arteries; in the high position, the tip is above the origin of the celiac plexus. Both positions are commonly used. Several prospective randomized studies comparing low versus high catheter placement found a greater rate of peripheral vascular complications in infants with catheters in the low position, although most of the complications were minor.[4,5] A recent meta-analysis of the data on catheter position concluded that the lower incidence of peripheral vascular complications associated with high catheters made this the preferable position.[6] Although one might postulate that catheters in the high position would be more likely to cause disturbances in renal, mesenteric, or cerebral blood flow, this has not been borne out by clinical studies.[7–9a]

Several published graphs are useful for estimating the distance a catheter must be inserted for it to be correctly placed in the lower position.[10,11] The simplest method is based on the infant's weight.[12] For a 1-kg infant the catheter should be inserted approximately 7 cm, for a 2-kg infant approximately 8 cm, and for a 3-kg infant approximately 9 cm. For a catheter to be placed in the high position, the formula "3 × weight (in kilograms) + 9" gives a rough estimate of the required catheter insertion length in centimeters. For either method, the catheter position should be checked radiographically (Fig. 17-3).

Once the correct position is confirmed, the catheter should be sutured and taped in place. We use a 3-0 or 4-0 silk suture tied in a "pursestring" around the circumference of the umbilical cord, then tied to the catheter. The catheter is secured with a tape bridge (Fig. 17-4).

Subumbilical Cutdown

If attempts to cannulate both umbilical arteries are unsuccessful and the patient cannot be adequately managed without an umbilical catheter, the arteries can be cannulated via sub-

umbilical cutdown.[13] This procedure was commonly performed in the 1970s and 1980s, but it is rarely needed now because cannulation of peripheral arteries is performed more frequently. This is a surgical procedure that should not be attempted by anyone without previous experience with the technique.

With a subumbilical cutdown, the arteries are exposed through an incision approximately 1 cm below the umbilical stump. The subcutaneous tissues are dissected to the anterior rectus sheath, then the sheath is incised and the rectus muscles are retracted laterally from the midline. The arteries are identified and separated from the urachus (Fig. 17-5). Two

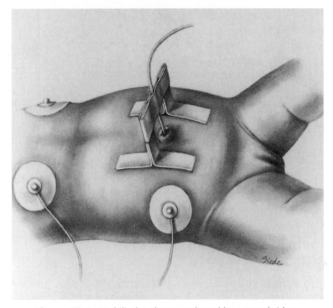

Figure 17-4. Umbilical catheter anchored by a tape bridge.

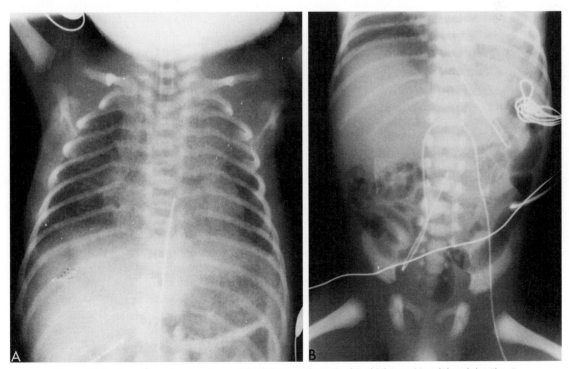

Figure 17-3. X-ray films showing the umbilical artery catheter in the "high" position *(A)* and the "low" position *(B)*.

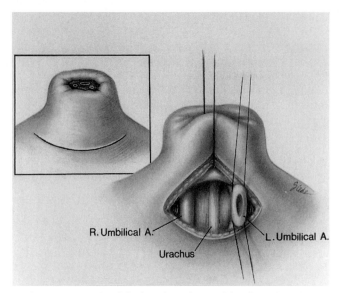

Figure 17-5. Subumbilical cutdown for arterial catheter insertion.

sutures are placed around one artery, and a small arteriotomy is made between the sutures. The catheter is inserted, and the distal suture is secured around the catheter and artery. The artery is tied off with the proximal suture, and the fascia and skin are closed.

Complications of Umbilical Artery Catheterization

Although umbilical artery catheterization is safe and well tolerated in most patients, it is important to remember that it is not without risks. Occasionally, catheter placement is associated with severe thrombotic complications, including frank gangrene and necrosis of the buttocks or leg. Studies from the early days of umbilical artery catheterization found a significant number of thrombi at autopsy in babies who had umbilical artery catheters.[14,15] An aortographic study revealed small thrombi in 95% of catheterized patients,[16] and an echocardiographic study found intracardiac thrombi in 5% of infants with umbilical catheters.[17]

Infants with umbilical artery catheters occasionally will develop dusky or purple discoloration of their toes, presumably from microemboli or vasospasm. In some cases, warming of the contralateral leg may cause reflex vasodilation and increased perfusion in the compromised leg. In contrast to this longstanding practice of warming the contralateral foot, a study in normal infants without vasospasm found local warming has no effect on peripheral blood flow to the contralateral heel.[18] Regardless of whether there is any value in warming the contralateral foot, the compromised leg probably should not be warmed because of the risk of increased hypoxic tissue injury as a result of the increased metabolic rate of the warmed tissues.

Although the majority of patients with dusky toes have adequate perfusion and suffer no ill effects, there is the risk that this represents potential significant vascular compromise. Failure to recognize worsening perfusion may result in necrosis and loss of a portion of the foot. If the toes remain dusky and have poor capillary filling, the catheter should be removed. Similarly, if the dusky discoloration involves more of the foot

or leg, the catheter should be removed. In rare instances, an infant with an umbilical catheter will develop blanching of the entire leg or part of the leg. Because blanching represents severely compromised arterial blood flow, the catheter should be immediately removed.

If perfusion to the limb does not immediately improve with withdrawal of the catheter, the infant should be evaluated for possible severe thrombotic complications. Evaluation in this case usually includes some combination of ultrasound or Doppler assessment, or even angiography. Both systemic and topical vasodilators have been described as having some efficacy in this situation.[19,20] When a significant clot is identified, there may be a role for treatment with tissue plasminogen activator, either infused directly into the affected vessel or systemically.[17,21] The potential advantages of thrombolytic therapy must be weighed against the theoretical risks of such therapy, particularly in the infant with a preexisting intracranial hemorrhage that could extend. Unfortunately, there is little literature available regarding the optimal approach to infants with severe vascular obstruction.

The incidence of infection from umbilical artery catheterization is difficult to assess. A retrospective review of patients from one center suggested that the incidence of umbilical catheter sepsis, primarily due to staphylococci, was 5%.[22] Interestingly, the duration of catheterization was not found to be a predictor of the rate of infection.

Although many centers avoid feeding infants with an umbilical artery catheter in place because of the theoretical concern that the catheter may interfere with mesenteric blood flow, at least one small study suggests that this is not a problem.[23]

One of the most concerning side effects of umbilical artery catheters is the effect of blood sampling on cerebral blood flow. At least two studies have suggested that routine blood sampling alters cerebral hemodynamics and oxygenation.[24,25] This effect seems to be less with catheters in the low position than in the high position.[24] Although the long-term effect, if any, on cerebral hemodynamics is unclear, it seems advisable to be cautious about rapidly withdrawing from or infusing into any umbilical catheter.

Other unusual complications associated with umbilical artery catheters include air embolism,[26] paraplegia,[27] hypertension,[28] perforation of the bladder,[29] aortic aneurysm,[30] and pelvic exsanguination, which may occur if the umbilical artery is perforated during catheter insertion.[31] If the catheter is inadvertently pulled out or a connection loosens, the baby may suffer rapid severe blood loss.

We have been impressed with the wide range of attitudes about the duration of umbilical artery catheter use. In some institutions they are rarely used, and if the catheters are placed they almost always are removed within several days. Other institutions maintain them in place for as long as 3 weeks. As with all therapies, the potential risks of umbilical artery catheterization must be balanced against the potential advantages for each infant. This balance must be continually reassessed as the infant's clinical course evolves.

Other Indwelling Catheter Sites

Umbilical artery catheterization is unsuccessful in approximately 10% of infants. In these cases, percutaneous cannulation of a peripheral artery may be the best alternative. Other techniques, such as umbilical artery or peripheral artery

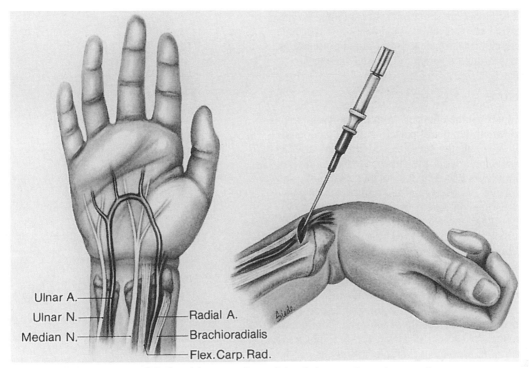

Figure 17-6. Anatomy of the hand demonstrating radial and ulnar arteries and surrounding structures.

cutdown, are more difficult to perform and involve more risk to the patient. Although percutaneous cannulation of a peripheral artery is technically challenging, especially in infants weighing less than 1 kg, cannulation of the radial, ulnar, dorsalis pedis, or posterior tibial artery usually is possible. One should avoid cannulating the temporal artery because cerebral emboli have been reported in patients with temporal artery catheters.[32,33]

If the radial artery is to be cannulated, an Allen test should be performed to ensure ulnar artery patency. Conversely, if the ulnar artery is to be cannulated, radial artery patency should be assessed. Begin the Allen test by gently squeezing the hand to empty it of blood. Apply pressure to both the radial and ulnar arteries, then remove pressure from the hand and the artery that will not be cannulated. If the entire hand flushes and fills with blood, then it is safe to proceed with cannulation.

The artery can be localized by either palpation or transillumination. If the radial or ulnar artery is to be cannulated, the hand should be restrained in mild hyperextension. We usually administer an analgesic dose of morphine or fentanyl before beginning the cannulation. Local anesthesia with lidocaine is less effective and leaves a wheal over the area where the pulse must be felt.

Prior to cannulation, the insertion site should be cleaned with an iodine or chlorhexidine solution. The radial artery is usually most easily cannulated at the point of maximal pulsation over the distal portion of the radius, proximal to the superficial palmar branch of the artery. In this position, the artery lies between two tendons, superficial and lateral to the median nerve (Fig. 17-6).

The catheter can be used dry or flushed with a heparinized saline solution. The catheter and needle are advanced at an angle of approximately 30 degrees until the vessel is entered and a pulsatile blood return is encountered. The needle is held stationary and the catheter is threaded into the artery. The needle is then withdrawn.

An alternative technique is to puncture the artery through both the anterior and posterior walls and then withdraw the needle. The catheter is withdrawn until its tip reenters the vessel lumen and a brisk blood return is obtained, at which point it is threaded into the vessel. We have found that in some cases where there is blood return but the catheter cannot be advanced, insertion of a small guidewire through the catheter into the vessel lumen will help guide the catheter into the vessel.

Once the catheter is in place, it should be taped securely and connected to an infusion of heparinized saline with a T-connector and a three-way stopcock. The tape securing the catheter must allow for unobstructed view of all five digits because hypoperfusion, potentially leading to ischemic necrosis, is the major complication of peripheral arterial catheters.

Infusion of Fluids Through Arterial Catheters

Patency of central and peripheral arterial catheters should be maintained with a heparinized solution. In most centers, heparin concentrations range from 0.25 to 1.0 unit/mL. Differences in heparin concentration do not appear to affect the incidence of intracranial hemorrhage.[34] We use 1 unit/mL for catheters infusing at a rate of 0.5 to 1.0 mL/hour and 0.5 unit/mL for catheters running at a higher rate. We never run arterial catheters at rates less than 0.5 mL/hour.

Although saline, glucose, and hyperalimentation solutions all can be infused into an umbilical artery catheter, a recent study suggests that infusing an amino-acid-containing solution of normal osmolarity causes less hemolysis than does a quarter normal saline solution.[35] In contrast to umbilical arteries where we have infused a wide range of solutions, we are concerned about the irritant effects of anything other than a physiologic saline solution infused into a peripheral artery. In small infants for whom 1 mL/hour of a physiologic saline solution provides an excessive sodium load, we sometimes infuse 0.45% saline. In cases where extra base is required, we infuse sodium acetate rather than sodium chloride. Medications or blood products are never administered through a peripheral arterial catheter.

Arterial Puncture

Blood gas samples can be obtained from intermittent puncture of the radial, ulnar, temporal, posterior tibial, or dorsalis pedis arteries. In general, the femoral and brachial arteries should not be used for arterial puncture because significant thrombus formation could lead to loss of the extremity, and median nerve damage has been reported with brachial puncture.[36] As noted earlier, an Allen test should be performed before the radial or ulnar artery is punctured.

After the exact location of the desired artery has been determined by transillumination or palpation, the skin should be prepared with a povidone iodine or chlorhexidine solution. A 25-gauge needle is inserted in the bevel-up position at a 45-degree angle through the skin, against the direction of arterial flow. Blood should flow into the tubing spontaneously or with gentle suction. After the needle is removed, continuous pressure should be applied to the artery for 5 minutes. If hematoma formation is prevented, multiple specimens can be obtained from the same artery.

The main drawback to arterial puncture is that the procedure can rarely be done without disturbing the patient. One study showed that venipuncture, generally regarded as less traumatic than arterial puncture, caused a 6 mm Hg decrease in $Paco_2$ and a 17 mm Hg decrease in Pao_2.[37] Although subcutaneous administration of lidocaine (without epinephrine) over the artery before arterial puncture will provide partial analgesia, most infants still become agitated during the puncture. For this reason, we rarely use arterial puncture to obtain blood gases.

Arterialized Capillary Blood

Arterialized capillary blood can provide a crude estimate of arterial blood values. In theory, there is little time for O_2 and CO_2 exchange to occur in blood flowing through a dilated peripheral capillary bed; therefore, capillary blood gas values approximate those in arterial blood.

Capillary samples can be obtained from a warmed heel or from the sides of the distal phalanges. To arterialize the capillary blood, the extremity should be warmed for several minutes. Warming should be performed with an exothermic chemical pack specifically designed for arterializing capillary blood rather than with warm compresses, which provide poor control over temperature. The site should be carefully cleaned, and a small lancet should be used to puncture the skin. When obtaining blood from the heel, the puncture should be made on the medial or lateral aspect of the plantar surface. The posterior curvature should not be used (Fig. 17-7).

Mistakes made in obtaining capillary blood include inadequate warming of the site, which results in inadequate arterialization of the blood; excessive squeezing, which causes contamination with venous blood or interstitial fluid; and exposure of blood to air during collection. Calcaneal osteochondritis and calcified heel nodules may result from heel punctures.[38] These calcified nodules may persist for several months to years, but they do not seem to cause problems for the infant.

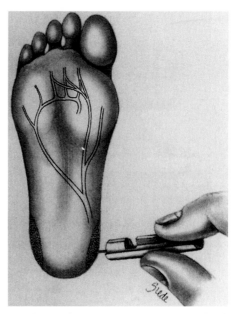

Figure 17-7. Technique for obtaining arterialized capillary heel sample. Stippled sections denote correct areas for sampling.

Capillary puncture can only rarely be done without disturbing the infant. This, plus the fact that arterialized capillary blood is not the same as true arterial blood, means that a capillary blood gas represents only an approximation of the infant's baseline arterial blood gas status. One study and review of the literature on capillary blood gases concluded that capillary blood gases are "at best, only gross predictors of arterial values and, at worst, misleading assessments that may result in inappropriate management decisions."[39] We find that they sometimes are useful for tracking gross changes in pH and Pco_2. In an era of routine pulse oximetry, we find no value in tracking capillary Po_2.

Continuous Invasive Monitoring

Over the last 2 decades, a number of devices have been developed for the direct intravascular measurement of hemoglobin saturation, Po_2, and Pco_2. One of the most intriguing of these is a catheter that is threaded through an umbilical catheter directly into the bloodstream and provides a continuous reading of blood gas values.[40] Although this technology is promising and has a number of advocates, the advantages must be weighed against the cost and risks associated with placing them.

Errors in Blood Gas Measurements

Even small air bubbles in a blood gas sample can cause significant errors. Room air has a Pco_2 of essentially zero and a Po_2 of approximately 150 mm Hg. If air bubbles contaminate a blood gas sample, they lower the Pco_2 and can either raise or lower the Po_2, depending on whether the Po_2 is below or above 150 mm Hg.[41] One study showed that the amount of air that comes in contact with arterial blood drawn through a butterfly infusion set is enough to alter the Po_2 measurement.[42]

Dilution of a blood sample with intravenous fluids lowers Pco_2 and increases the base deficit without affecting pH. This effect probably is due to the diffusion of CO_2 from blood into the intravenous fluid, which contains no CO_2.[41,43,44] Because of the buffering capacity of the blood, pH changes little despite the decrease in Pco_2, giving the appearance of a combined metabolic acidosis and respiratory alkalosis. Dilution of a blood gas sample with a lipid emulsion does not appear to have any effect on blood gas measurements.[45] Dry heparin does not appear to affect blood gas results.[44]

After blood is withdrawn from an artery, it continues to consume oxygen and produce carbon dioxide. Blood gas results may be inaccurate if the specimen is not processed promptly. Placing the sample in ice minimizes these changes. Immediate measurement, as with "point of care" techniques, also minimizes these changes.

Most blood gas analyzers measure Po_2 and then calculate the saturation, assuming that the blood sample is from an adult. However, if the sample contains a significant amount of fetal hemoglobin, the calculated saturation will be inappropriately low. If it is important to exactly measure the patient's saturation, this should be done with a co-oximeter rather than with a standard blood gas analyzer.

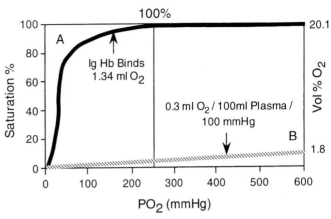

Figure 17-8. Comparison between the dissociation curve of hemoglobin (curve A) and the amount of oxygen dissolved in plasma (curve B). Note that the hemoglobin is almost 100% saturated at Po_2 80 mm Hg. When fully saturated, 15 g Hb will bind 20.1 mL O_2. (From Duc G: Assessment of hypoxia in the newborn: Suggestions for a practical approach. Pediatrics 48:469, 1971.)

NONINVASIVE ESTIMATION OF BLOOD GASES

The development of techniques for simply and safely obtaining continuous noninvasive estimates of blood gases was one of the most important advances in neonatal care in the last 25 years. Pulse oximeters have become so ubiquitous in intensive care nurseries that many believe oxygen saturation is as important a vital sign as heart rate or blood pressure. Although less commonly used than pulse oximeters, both transcutaneous monitoring and end-tidal CO_2 monitoring have a role in some situations.

Pulse Oximetry

Pulse oximeters work on the principle that saturated hemoglobin is a different color than desaturated hemoglobin and thus absorbs light at a different frequency.[46–49] A sensor, which consists of a light source and a photosensor, is placed so that the light source and photosensor are on opposite sides of an artery. As light passes through the artery and the surrounding tissues, the saturated and desaturated hemoglobin absorb different frequencies. By measuring the difference between light absorbed during systole and diastole, the amount absorbed due to arterial flow can be calculated. By comparing the absorption at the two appropriate frequencies, the percentage of saturated hemoglobin can be calculated. Refinements of this system include complex algorithms for calculating exact saturation and separating arterial pulsations from motion artifact. The calculation of saturation is dependent on sensing light, so ambient light striking the sensor can lead to a false reading.

In general, pulse oximeters provide excellent data about oxygenation in the physiologic range. However, the values they provide must not be accepted without caution. Poor perfusion, ambient light, and motion all interfere with an adequate signal. Also, different manufacturers use different algorithms for calculating saturation, which may give slightly different results. Manufacturers are constantly updating the software in their

devices, so many published articles on the limitations of specific devices are of minimal use.

Pulse oximeters are dependent on an adequate arterial pulse. They may not function reliably in situations such as shock or severe edema obscuring pulsatile arterial flow. Similarly, in patients on total support from a venoarterial extracorporeal membrane who have minimal arterial pulsations, we have found that pulse oximeters rarely function if the pulse pressure is less than 10 mm Hg.

The shape of the oxygen-hemoglobin dissociation curve (Fig. 17-8) makes it impossible for pulse oximeters to differentiate between degrees of hyperoxia. Pao_2 of 80 mm Hg and Pao_2 of 180 mm Hg both represent essentially 100% saturation in a preterm neonate. Pulse oximeters are also less accurate in the low end of the saturation range (e.g., <70% saturation) than in the normal physiologic range. Fortunately, this does not usually pose a clinically significant problem because the exact degree of severe desaturation is less important than the desaturation itself.

One major advantage of pulse oximetry is that oxygen saturation is a more physiologically relevant measure than is Pao_2. Also, because fetal and adult hemoglobin have significantly different oxygen dissociation curves, it often is impossible to determine an "ideal" Pao_2. In an extremely preterm infant with a large percentage of fetal hemoglobin, Pao_2 of 40 mm Hg may be adequately saturated, whereas in an older infant, especially after multiple transfusions of adult blood and relatively little fetal hemoglobin, the same Pao_2 may represent significant desaturation.

Transcutaneous Monitoring

Transcutaneous oxygen and carbon dioxide electrodes allow continuous indirect estimation of Pao_2 and $Paco_2$. Pulse oximetry has largely replaced transcutaneous monitoring as a tool for estimating oxygenation, but some centers still find an important role for transcutaneous CO_2 monitoring.

There are several good reviews of the theory of transcutaneous monitoring.[46,48,50] In summary, transcutaneous Po_2 (tcPo_2) measures the Po_2 of skin. The Po_2 of skin usually is lower than the Pao_2, but local cutaneous vasodilation causes the skin Po_2 to approach Pao_2. This cutaneous vasodilation is accomplished by heating the area directly under the $tcPO_2$ electrode. Although heating the skin causes several effects other than vasodilation, these effects on the oxygen dissociation curve, tissue oxygen consumption, and electrode oxygen consumption cancel out for most patients so that $tcPO_2$ approximates PaO_2. In most neonates, when PaO_2 is less than 100 mm Hg, $tcPO_2$ will be within 10 mm Hg of PaO_2. If PaO_2 is greater than 100 mm Hg, $tcPO_2$ often significantly underestimates PaO_2.[51] In patients with poor perfusion or in older infants with chronic lung disease, $tcPO_2$ underestimates PaO_2.[52]

The relationship between $PaCO_2$ and transcutaneous PCO_2 ($tcPCO_2$) is more complex than that between PaO_2 and $tcPO_2$. Transcutaneous PCO_2 is always greater than $PaCO_2$ because of the combination of several effects. Heating causes increased production of CO_2 by blood and skin cells; there is a significant arterial-cellular CO_2 gradient; and the skin has a cooling effect on the electrode. These effects are fairly uniform at a given temperature and combine to create a linear relationship between $tcPCO_2$ and $PaCO_2$.[53] Severe hypotension causes the $tcPCO_2$ electrode to overestimate $PaCO_2$.[54] The $tcPCO_2$ electrode also overestimates $PaCO_2$ in older patients with bronchopulmonary dysplasia.[52]

Capnography

Capnography, also known as *end-tidal CO_2 monitoring,* is the measurement of exhaled CO_2. This is a technique that has found widespread use in adult and pediatric intensive care units, as well as in operating rooms. It is an attractive technology because it is relatively inexpensive, portable, noninvasive, and easy to use. However, it has not been as widely accepted into intensive care nurseries, primarily because it gives only a rough estimate of $PaCO_2$ in patients with significant lung disease.

Because alveolar PCO_2 approximates $PaCO_2$, if one can sample pure alveolar gas, one can get a good estimate of $PaCO_2$. Capnographs measure the concentration of CO_2 in exhaled gas and display this concentration as a function of time. If there is a good end-tidal plateau in exhaled PCO_2, this usually represents the alveolar PCO_2. In adult and pediatric patients with relatively large tidal volumes and relatively low respiratory rates, this alveolar plateau is readily measured. However, ill newborns frequently are too tachypneic to obtain an end-tidal sample of alveolar gas. In addition, animal studies suggest that alveolar disease interferes with end-tidal CO_2 versus $PaCO_2$ correlation, independent of respiratory rate and tidal volume.[55]

Clinical studies in newborns demonstrate that capnography is an accurate method of estimating $PaCO_2$ in healthy infants, but it provides only a rough estimate of $PaCO_2$ in infants with significant lung disease.[8,56,57] However, before dismissing the role of capnography in infants with lung disease, it should be remembered that it is not necessarily worse than transcutaneous monitoring or capillary blood gas monitoring.[57] Certainly capnography is easier to apply than transcutaneous monitoring and is less traumatic than capillary blood gas sampling.

In addition to using capnography to estimate $PaCO_2$, some investigators have tried to tease more information about lung function from the capnogram.[58] Although this is an intriguing concept, it has not gained widespread use. We suspect that with the gradual increase in the use of capnography in nurseries, we soon will see more novel ways of using capnogram data.

One of the most useful applications of exhaled CO_2 monitoring is a colorimetric qualitative determination of whether an endotracheal tube is actually in the trachea.[59] We have used this approach in our nursery for several years and have found it to be an extremely useful tool for determining successful intubation.

CHOICE OF MONITORING METHODS

Over the last decade several factors have led to a gradual decline in the reliance on arterial blood gas samples. The heightened awareness of blood transfusion risks has led to a general decrease in the number of blood tests, including blood gases. The "permissive hypercapnia strategy" has led most institutions to accept a wider range of $PaCO_2$ values and therefore to feel less compelled to perform frequent blood gas measurements (see Chapter 15). The increased use of ventilator modes, such as assist/control and pressure support, where the patient controls his or her respiratory rate and minute ventilation, has gradually led many neonatologists to believe that blood gases need not be measured as frequently as previously.

There is still a need for reliable arterial blood gas sampling in unstable infants. Our approach is to place an umbilical catheter into any newborn with respiratory distress that is significant enough to require arterial blood sampling. We routinely place an umbilical artery catheter in any infant who requires intubation, most infants who weight less than 1.25 kg and require nasal continuous positive airway pressure (CPAP), and all infants on nasal CPAP who have severe respiratory distress and/or significant oxygen requirement. We usually remove umbilical artery catheters by 5 to 7 days, although we sometimes leave them in place for as long as 2 to 3 weeks in extremely unstable infants who weigh less than 1 kg. For other infants who are critically ill and need arterial monitoring, we place peripheral arterial catheters.

Infants without arterial access are monitored primarily with pulse oximetry, although we believe there is some role for capillary blood gases. In our nursery, capillary blood gases usually are performed every 24 to 48 hours in stable ventilated infants but as frequently as two to three times per day in less stable infants. In critically ill infants without arterial access, we sometimes use samples drawn from an umbilical venous catheter to provide a crude estimate of PCO_2. Although venous PCO_2 is at least several millimeters of mercury higher than arterial (and may be significantly higher), we believe it is preferable to use this crude measure than to perform repeated arterialized capillary blood gas samples or intermittent arterial punctures.

Continuous pulse oximeter monitoring is our standard for tracking oxygenation, mainly because it provides much more information than do measurements of PaO_2 with intermittent arterial blood gases. Because blood gases provide information about the status of the patient at only a discrete time, they do not provide adequate information about the ongoing respiratory status of the patient. The patient with an "acceptable" arterial blood gas but with substantial minute-to-minute lability in saturation is quite different from a patient with the same blood gas values and stable saturation. In our nursery, any infant on supplemental oxygen, nasal CPAP, or mechanical ventilation or any infant with apnea is monitored with continuous pulse oximetry.

We occasionally use transcutaneous CO_2 monitoring, particularly for term and near-term infants during periods of potential instability or rapidly changing ventilatory needs, such as are seen with surfactant administration or with conversion from one type of ventilation to another. Although we are intrigued with the theoretical potential of capnography, we have not yet used it as a primary method of tracking Pco_2. We suspect that the newer capnographs, which impose minimal dead space, will prove to be a useful tool, at least in some patient populations.

PHYSIOLOGY OF BLOOD GASES

As blood flows past ventilated alveoli, oxygen is added to the blood and carbon dioxide is removed. In simplest terms, the amount of oxygen in blood leaving the left heart reflects the matching of perfusion to ventilation. Any condition that causes blood to emerge from the left heart without passing ventilated alveoli will decrease arterial oxygen content. This occurs if blood passes from the right heart to the left heart without going through the pulmonary circulation (extrapulmonary shunt) or if blood passes atelectatic or underventilated alveoli (intrapulmonary shunt). Similarly, the amount of carbon dioxide removed from the blood reflects the adequacy of alveolar ventilation. As alveolar ventilation decreases, less CO_2 is removed from the blood flowing through the lungs, and the Pco_2 in blood leaving the left heart increases. Arterial blood gases therefore provide information about the matching of ventilation to perfusion and the adequacy of alveolar ventilation. However, they do not provide direct information about the adequacy of oxygen delivery to the systemic vascular bed and peripheral tissues.

The cells of the body use oxygen for aerobic metabolism of glucose. When aerobically metabolized to CO_2 and water, glucose produces adenosine triphosphate (ATP). If sufficient oxygen does not reach the cells, tissue hypoxia occurs. In this case, glucose is metabolized anaerobically to pyruvate, which also produces ATP. Pyruvate is then metabolized to lactic acid. As lactic acid accumulates in the blood, it is reflected by an increased base deficit (or decreased base excess) of arterial blood. Lactic acid is buffered in the blood by three major components: hemoglobin, serum proteins, and bicarbonate. The normal or ideal buffering capacity of blood is 48 mEq/L. Base excess is defined as the difference between the actual buffer capacity and the ideal buffer capacity.

To more accurately estimate whether an adequate amount of oxygen has been delivered to tissues, one must look at blood returning from the systemic circulation to the lungs.[60] Although mixed venous blood should ideally be sampled from the pulmonary artery, this is impractical in most neonates. Instead, blood sampled from the right atrium is assumed to closely approximate mixed venous blood. Monitoring mixed venous oxygenation is an extremely useful tool for assessing adequacy of tissue oxygen delivery and is widely used in adult intensive care units and in neonatal extracorporeal membrane oxygenation (ECMO).

Oxygen Transport

The amount of oxygen that can be delivered to the tissues is dependent upon two major factors: cardiac output and the oxygen content of the blood. In most neonates, cardiac output is approximately 120 to 150 mL/kg/min. The oxygen content of arterial blood (Cao_2) is dependent upon several factors. Because blood carries both oxygen bound to hemoglobin and free dissolved oxygen, the Cao_2 of blood can be thought of as follows:

$$Cao_2 = (Hb\ O_2) + (Dissolved\ O_2)$$

where Cao_2 is oxygen content, $Hb\ O_2$ is oxygen bound to hemoglobin, and Dissolved O_2 is oxygen in solution.

The amount of oxygen carried in the blood by hemoglobin depends upon both the hemoglobin concentration and the percent saturation of the hemoglobin. The relationship between Po_2 and amount of oxygen combined with hemoglobin, or hemoglobin saturation, is sigmoidal over the physiologic range. Hemoglobin is almost fully saturated at Po_2 of 80 to 100 mm Hg (Fig. 17-8, curve A.) The amount of oxygen combined with hemoglobin at a given Po_2 is dependent upon the position of the hemoglobin dissociation curve. The position of the dissociation curve depends mainly on two factors: the concentration of red blood cell diphosphoglycerate (DPG) and the ratio of adult hemoglobin (A) to fetal hemoglobin (F). With increasing age, the concentration of DPG and the proportion of hemoglobin A increase, shifting the curve to the right (Fig. 17-9). Temperature, Pco_2, and hydrogen ion concentration play smaller roles in determining the position of the curve.

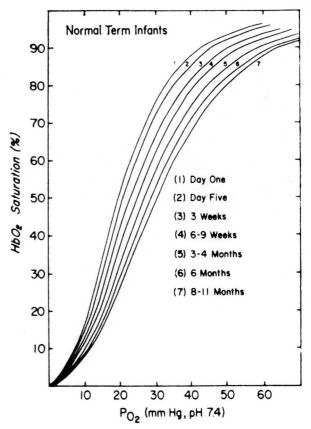

Figure 17-9. Oxygen dissociation curves from term infants at different postnatal ages. (From Delivoria-Popadopoulos M, Roncevic NP, Oski FA: Postnatal changes in oxygen transport of term, premature, and sick infants. Pediatr Res 5:235, 1971.)

As temperature, Pco_2, or hydrogen ion concentration increase (i.e., pH decreases), the curve is shifted to the right. As the curve shifts to the right, hemoglobin releases oxygen more easily to the tissues.

Only a small amount of oxygen is dissolved in the plasma. This amount is directly proportional to Po_2. At 38°C, 0.3 mL of oxygen is dissolved in 100 mL of plasma per 100 mm Hg of oxygen. This relationship is linear over the entire range of Po_2 (Fig. 17-6, curve B). Because the amount of oxygen that is dissolved in the blood is much less than the amount that is bound to hemoglobin, we can simplify the earlier equation to an approximation:

$$Cao_2 = (Hb\ O_2).$$

The amount of oxygen that is bound to hemoglobin, and therefore the approximate oxygen content of the blood, is dependent upon three factors: concentration of hemoglobin in blood, percent hemoglobin saturation, and oxygen capacity of hemoglobin. Mathematically this is expressed as:

$$Cao_2 = (Hb\ O_2) = (gm\ \%\ Hb) \times (O_2\ capacity) \times (\%\ Saturation).$$

O_2 capacity is a constant that represents the maximum amount of O_2 that can be carried by a gram of hemoglobin that is fully saturated. This value is 1.34 mL O_2 per gram of 100% saturated hemoglobin.

Assuming that a normal infant has a hemoglobin of 15 g per 100 mL blood and that arterial blood is normally 100% saturated, and ignoring the small amount of O_2 that is dissolved in blood, the oxygen content of normal arterial blood is approximately:

$$Cao_2 = (15) \times (1.34) \times (1.0)$$
$$= 20\ mL\ O_2\ per\ 100\ mL\ arterial\ blood.$$

Assuming that the normal newborn cardiac output is approximately 120 mL/kg/min, the amount of O_2 that can be delivered to the systemic circulation is calculated:

$$O_2\ delivered = (CO) \times (Cao_2)$$
$$= (120\ mL\ blood/kg/min) \times (0.2\ mL\ O_2/mL\ blood)$$
$$= 24\ mL\ O_2/kg/min.$$

Under normal circumstances, oxygen consumption for a neonate is approximately 6 mL/kg/min. Under normal circumstances, the body extracts O_2 at a rate of 6 mL/kg/min from the approximately 24 mL/kg/min that is delivered to the systemic circulation. Therefore, approximately 25% of the oxygen has been removed from the blood by the time it returns to the heart. The mixed venous blood will be approximately 75% saturated. In general, a measured mixed venous saturation of 70% to 75% represents adequate tissue oxygen delivery. In patients in whom mixed venous saturation can be directly monitored (usually patients on ECMO), we try to maintain mixed venous saturation in the normal physiologic range of 70% to 75%.

Hypoxemia and Hypoxia

Hypoxia exists when there is inadequate delivery of oxygen to tissue. Hypoxemia exists when there is a low arterial blood oxygen content. Although hypoxemia and hypoxia frequently occur together, they are not synonymous.

Hypoxemia occurs in any situation where blood reaches the aorta without perfusing adequately ventilated alveoli. Blood can bypass adequately ventilated alveoli by extrapulmonary shunts, intrapulmonary shunts, or some combination of the two. With cyanotic congenital heart disease, a structurally abnormal heart leads to some blood entering the aorta without passing through the lungs (extrapulmonary shunt). Similarly, patients with pulmonary artery hypertension can have extrapulmonary shunting through the foramen ovale and/or ductus arteriosus. A right-to-left shunt across the ductus arteriosus often can be detected by comparing the Pao_2 or oxygen saturation of preductal and postductal blood (Fig. 17-10). If the saturation of the preductal blood is significantly higher (5% difference) than the saturation of the postductal blood, clinically significant right-to-left shunt exists. However, equal preductal and postductal saturations do not exclude the possibility of pulmonary hypertension with a shunt through the foramen ovale. The hypoxemia associated with lung diseases that are characterized by atelectasis (e.g., respiratory distress syndrome, pneumonia) is caused primarily by intrapulmonary shunting. In any condition where alveoli are inadequately ventilated, the blood flowing past those alveoli will not be fully saturated. Thus, the greater the degree of atelectasis, the greater the intrapulmonary shunt and the greater the degree of hypoxemia.

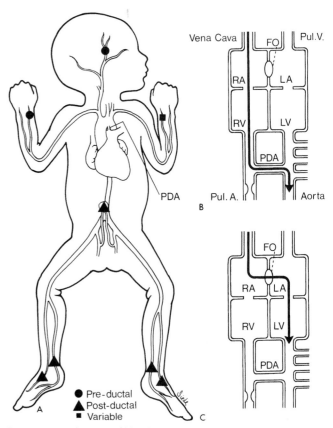

Figure 17-10. Shunting of blood in pulmonary hypertension. *A,* Sampling sites. *B,* Right-to-left shunt across the ductus arteriosus. *C,* Right-to-left shunt across the foramen ovale. FO, foramen ovale; LA, left atrium; LV, left ventricle; PDA, patent ductus arteriosus; RA, right atrium; RV, right ventricle.

Tissue hypoxia can occur despite adequate Pao_2. This will occur in any situation where there is inadequate tissue perfusion (e.g., severe myocardial dysfunction) or insufficient oxygen-carrying capacity (e.g., severe anemia). It also will occur in rare cases where abnormal hemoglobin (e.g., methemoglobin) fails to release oxygen to the tissues.

Carbon Dioxide Transport

Carbon dioxide transport is significantly less complicated than oxygen transport. Carbon dioxide is produced in tissues during the aerobic metabolism of glucose and is transported in the blood to the lungs where it is exhaled. Eighty-five percent of the carbon dioxide in blood is transported as bicarbonate ion, 10% is carried by hemoglobin as carbamate, and 5% is transported as either dissolved gas or carbonic acid. Due to the equilibrium between dissolved carbon dioxide and the bicarbonate ion, the relationship between CO_2 content and Pco_2 in blood is essentially linear over the physiologic range (Fig. 17-11).

Because carbon dioxide diffuses rapidly from blood into alveolar gas, the Pco_2 in blood leaving the lungs is essentially the same as the Pco_2 in alveolar gas. Increasing minute alveolar ventilation decreases the Pco_2 in alveolar gas and decreases the $Paco_2$, which is the reason $Paco_2$ is dependent on alveolar ventilation.

Metabolic Acidosis

Anaerobic metabolism of glucose leads to accumulation of lactic acid, resulting in metabolic acidosis. Lactic acid reacts with bicarbonate, causing the serum bicarbonate to fall and resulting in a base deficit. This usually is caused by inadequate tissue oxygen delivery as a result of some combination of hypoxemia, anemia, and inadequate cardiac output. Other less common causes of metabolic acidosis in the newborn include inborn errors of metabolism and renal bicarbonate wasting.

The most important approach to treating metabolic acidosis is correcting the underlying problem, usually by improving circulating blood volume and/or cardiac output. In cases of significant metabolic acidosis (base deficit >10–12), it may be useful to give exogenous base to help correct the pH, most commonly by giving sodium bicarbonate. The number of milliequivalents of bicarbonate needed to half correct a base deficit can be approximated from the following equation:

$$\text{Milliequivalents of bicarbonate} = (\text{Base deficit}) \times (\text{Body weight in kg}) \times 0.3.$$

Because it is so hypertonic, sodium bicarbonate (1 mEq/mL) should be diluted 1:1 with sterile water and administered slowly, preferably over 30 to 60 minutes. Rapid administration, with subsequent hyperosmolarity of the blood and resulting fluid shifts, has been associated with intraventricular hemorrhage.[61] Bicarbonate should be administered with care in the infant with combined respiratory and metabolic acidosis, because the $Paco_2$ may increase further as the bicarbonate is metabolized.

Metabolic Alkalosis

If too much bicarbonate is given in an attempt to correct metabolic acidosis, the serum bicarbonate will rise and a base excess results. Other causes of metabolic alkalosis in the newborn include hypokalemia and hypochloremia from chronic vomiting, drainage of gastric secretions, and diuretic therapy. Mild metabolic alkalosis can occur following an exchange transfusion, when the citrate in the anticoagulant is metabolized. Metabolic alkalosis will occur if a compensated respiratory acidosis is corrected by rapidly lowering the Pco_2. It is rarely necessary to aggressively correct metabolic alkalosis with drugs such as ammonium chloride.

CLINICAL INTERPRETATION OF BLOOD GASES

Understanding the physiology of gas exchange makes the interpretation of blood gases a relatively straightforward process. Hypoxemia is the result of ventilation-perfusion mismatch or shunting, usually due to atelectasis and/or extrapulmonary shunting. It is treated by reversing atelectasis and/or decreasing pulmonary vascular resistance. Hypercapnia is the result of inadequate alveolar minute ventilation and is treated with some maneuver that results in increased minute ventilation. Despite decades of experience with mechanical ventilatory support for newborns, there are still a number of questions about what blood gas values are acceptable.

Most healthy infants, including preterm infants, have arterial saturation values in the 90s.[62,63] It is not clear where arterial saturation should be maintained in infants with lung disease, other than that tissue hypoxia should be avoided. In all infants, we attempt to keep arterial saturation (as well as hemoglobin level and cardiac output) high enough to avoid metabolic acidosis from anaerobic metabolism. In most infants, we attempt to maintain arterial oxygen saturation in the 88% to 95% range. This provides nearly maximal arterial oxygen content but prevents high Pao_2 values, which may be seen if the saturation is allowed to go as high as 98% to 100%. In a study of the impact of low versus high saturation (Spo_2 89% to 94% vs 96% to 99%) on infants with retinopathy of prematurity, infants in the high-saturation group had an increased incidence

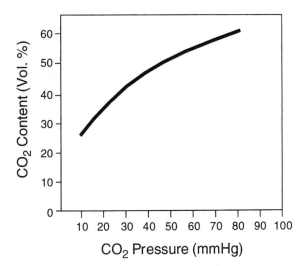

Figure 17-11. Curve describing the relationship between CO_2 content and Pco_2 in blood. (From Comroe JH: The Lung. Chicago, Year Book Medical Publishers, 1962, pp. 44–49.)

of adverse pulmonary outcomes, including more pneumonia and/or exacerbation of chronic lung disease and an increased need for prolonged oxygen therapy.[64] This study provides some support for continuing to avoid saturation above 95%, particularly in preterm infants.

It is important to remember that many patients with cyanotic cardiac disease tolerate long periods of time with SpO_2 in the 70% to 80% range without developing signs of tissue hypoxia. This suggests that, in the presence of adequate cardiac output and hemoglobin level, much lower arterial saturations than are usually considered ideal can be safe. At least one retrospective study has suggested that preterm infants may benefit from management with relatively low SpO_2,[65] an idea that is at marked variance from the more traditional assumption that infants, particularly those with chronic lung disease, should have SpO_2 levels at least in the mid-90s.[66] We agree with those who have stated that we really do not know the optimal level of oxygenation, particularly for very preterm infants, and that this is an area that urgently needs carefully designed clinical trials.[67]

There is considerable uncertainty about the acceptable range of $PaCO_2$ values for neonates. Over the last decade, there has been a steady trend toward *permissive hypercapnia,* where progressively higher $PaCO_2$ values are accepted. This strategy is based on the assumption that maintaining $PaCO_2$ in the "normal" range often requires an unacceptable degree of ventilation and associated ventilator-induced injury. Although this strategy seems reasonable and has been widely accepted, it has not been thoroughly studied. One small study of infants weighing less than 1200 g showed that patients who were managed with $PaCO_2$ 45 to 55 mm Hg required fewer days of ventilation that did those who were managed with $PaCO_2$ 34 to 45 mm Hg, but the study did not show any difference in longer-term outcomes.[68] Unfortunately, the large multicenter trial that was designed to test the impact of permissive hypercapnia (as well as the impact of steroid treatment) on the incidence of chronic lung disease was terminated before the permissive hypercapnia question could be answered.[69] Subsequent analysis of the infants who completed this trial suggested that there was no definite benefit to a strategy of permissive hypercapnia, except possibly in infants of birthweight between 500 and 750 g.[70] As pointed out by several reviews, we are left with attractive arguments in favor of permissive hypercapnia, theoretical concerns about its side effects, and relatively few strong data supporting its benefits.[71,72]

There is a growing body of information suggesting that hyperventilation and hypocapnia are potentially dangerous.[71] It is well known that acute hyperventilation and hypocapnia lead to a significant decrease in cerebral blood flow.[73,74] At least one study suggests that severe hypocapnia ($PaCO_2$ <25 mm Hg) is associated with an increased risk of cystic periventricular leukomalacia.[75] There also appears to be an association between degree of hyperventilation and hearing loss.[76] Both anecdotal experience and retrospective studies support the belief that it is possible to obtain good outcomes in infants with pulmonary hypertension while avoiding hyperventilation.[77–79] Although deliberate hyperventilation to a target $PaCO_2$ in the 20s or 30s was once the standard of care for treating pulmonary hypertension, we believe this practice can no longer be justified, particularly when there is ready access to inhaled nitric oxide and to ECMO.

Avoiding wide swings in $PaCO_2$ probably is at least as important as maintaining $PaCO_2$ within a specified range, because abrupt changes in $PaCO_2$ can have significant effects on systemic blood pressure and cerebral blood flow. Furthermore, abrupt changes in $PaCO_2$ values often reflect significant mechanical issues, such as evolving atelectasis, airway obstruction from secretions, and endotracheal tube malposition. Reflexively escalating ventilator settings in this situation often will increase potential ventilator-related toxicity but fail to correct the underlying problem.

The acceptable range of arterial base deficit values remains unclear. In most healthy newborns, the base deficit is between 0 and 5. Although it makes sense to provide bicarbonate to infants who have a metabolic acidosis from bicarbonate loss, there is essentially no evidence that bicarbonate therapy is beneficial in patients with metabolic acidosis from tissue hypoxia. To the contrary, studies in adults have shown that bicarbonate administration may actually be deleterious to the patient with hypoxia and metabolic acidosis.[80–82] Regardless of whether bicarbonate is used to treated metabolic acidosis, the diagnosis and treatment of hypoxemia and tissue hypoxia are of paramount importance. If the infant is not hypoxic, we tend to avoid treating pure metabolic acidosis with bicarbonate unless the base deficit approaches the −10 range. We similarly try to avoid administering multiple fluid boluses to treat metabolic acidosis unless the clinical history is consistent with volume loss (e.g., hemorrhage or sepsis with associated capillary leak).

Despite the many unanswered questions about the ideal range for SpO_2, $PaCO_2$, and pH, we must constantly make decisions about the risks and benefits of escalating therapies to maintain our patients within specific ranges. With each successive edition of this text, we have acknowledged acceptance of higher $PaCO_2$ values and lower pH values. Our current approach emphasizes avoiding both hypocapnia and rapid changes in $PaCO_2$ and accepting modest permissive hypercapnia. In most infants with acute pulmonary disease, we maintain $PaCO_2$ in the range from 45 to 55 mm Hg. In more chronic patients who have had time to compensate for respiratory acidosis, we often maintain $PaCO_2$ in the range from 55 to 65 mm Hg. For the unusual infant with severe disease for whom the cost of escalating ventilation may be unacceptable (e.g., infants with pulmonary interstitial emphysema), we will hesitantly tolerate even higher $PaCO_2$ values. For premature infants we now consider a pH greater than 7.25 acceptable, but we will often tolerate pH values in the 7.20 to 7.25 range. In patients with pulmonary hypertension, we aim for a pH between 7.30 and 7.40 (Table 17-2).

TABLE 17-2.   Target Blood Gas Values

	<28 Weeks' Gestation	28–40 Weeks' Gestation	Term Infant with Pulmonary Hypertension	Infant with BPD
PaO_2	45–65	50–70	80–120	50–80
$PaCO_2$	45–55 (60)	45–55 (60)	30–40	55–65
pH	≥7.25 (≥7.20)	≥7.25 (≥7.20)	7.30–7.50	7.35–7.45

Parentheses indicate value may be accepted in certain strategies.
BPD, bronchopulmonary dysplasia.

Although arterial blood gas values frequently are invaluable in managing patients with respiratory distress, they should not be interpreted in the absence of other clinical data. A blood gas result that is significantly different than previous results may indicate a major change in the patient's status or may represent an error in blood gas measurement. Similarly, if the blood gas results do not correlate with the results of the patient's physical examination, further evaluation is needed. Neither a blood gas laboratory test nor the most sophisticated noninvasive monitors can replace careful clinical observation.

REFERENCES

1. Barrington KJ: Umbilical artery catheters in the newborn: Effects of catheter design (end vs side hole) (Cochrane Review). In: The Cochrane Library, Issue 2, 2002. Oxford, Update Software.
2. Kitterman JA, Phibbs RH, Tooley WH: Catheterization of umbilical vessels in newborn infants. Pediatr Clin North Am 17:895, 1970.
3. Schreiber MD, Perez CA, Kitterman JA: A double-catheter technique for caudally misdirected umbilical arterial catheters. J Pediatr 104:768, 1984.
4. Mokrohisky ST, Levine RL, Blumhagen JD, et al: Low positioning of umbilical-artery catheters increases associated complications in newborn infants. N Engl J Med 299:561, 1978.
5. Umbilical Artery Catheter Trial Study Group: Relationship of intraventricular hemorrhage or death with the level of umbilical artery catheter placement: A multicenter randomized clinical trial. Pediatrics 90:881, 1992.
6. Barrington KJ: Umbilical artery catheters in the newborn: Effects of position of the catheter tip (Cochrane Review). In: The Cochrane Library, Issue 2, 2002. Oxford, Update Software.
7. Kempley ST, Gamsu HR: Randomized trial of umbilical arterial catheter position: Doppler ultrasound findings. Arch Dis Child 67:855, 1992.
8. Hagerty JJ, Kleinman ME, Zurakowski D, et al: Accuracy of a new low-flow sidestream capnography technology in newborns: A pilot study. J Perinatol 22:219, 1992.
9. Shah JB, Bracero LA, Gewitz MD, et al: Umbilical artery catheters and blood flow velocities in the superior mesenteric artery: Effect of insertion, removal, aspiration, and bolus infusion. J Clin Ultrasound 26:73, 1992.
9a. Roll C, Hanssler L: Effect of umbilical arterial catheters on intestinal blood supply. Acta Paediatr 87:955, 1998.
10. Dunn P: Localization of the umbilical catheter by post mortem measurement. Arch Dis Child 41:69, 1966.
11. Rosenfeld W, Estrada R, Jhaveri R, et al: Evaluation of graphs for insertion of umbilical artery catheters below the diaphragm. J Pediatr 98:627, 1981.
12. Shukla H, Ferrara A: Rapid estimation of insertional length of umbilical catheters in newborns. Am J Dis Child 140:786, 1986.
13. Clark JM, Jung AL: Umbilical artery catheterization by a cutdown procedure. Pediatrics 59:1036, 1977.
14. Goetzmann BW, Stadalnik RC, Bogren HG, et al: Thrombotic complications of umbilical artery catheters: A clinical and radiographic study. Pediatrics 56:374, 1975.
15. Harris MS, Little GA: Umbilical artery catheters: High, low, or no. J Perinat Med 6:15, 1975.
16. Neal WA, Reynolds JW, Jarvis CW, et al: Umbilical artery catheterization: Demonstration of arterial thrombosis by aortography. Pediatrics 50:6, 1972.
17. Ferrari F, Vagnarelli F, Gargano G, et al: Early intracardiac thrombosis in preterm infants and thrombolysis with recombinant tissue type plasminogen activator. Arch Dis Child Fetal Neonatal Ed 85:F66, 2001.
18. Dollberg S, Atherton H, Hoath S: Changes in skin blood flow over the foot with warming of the contralateral heel. Acta Paediatr 87:416, 1998.
19. Heath RE: Vasospasm in the neonate: Response to tolazoline infusion. Pediatrics 77:405, 1986.
20. Varughese M, Koh TH: Successful use of topical nitroglycerine in ischaemia associated with umbilical arterial line in a neonate. J Perinatol 21:556, 2001.
21. Kennedy LA, Drummond WH, Knight ME, et al: Successful treatment of neonatal aortic thrombosis with tissue plasminogen activator. J Pediatr 116:798, 1990.

22. Landers S, Moise AA, Fraley JK, et al: Factors associated with umbilical catheter-related sepsis in neonates. Am J Dis Child 145:675, 1991.
23. Davey AM, Wagner CL, Cox C, et al: Feeding premature infants while low umbilical artery catheters are in place: A prospective, randomized trial. J Pediatr 124:795, 1994.
24. Lott JW, Conner GK, Phillips JB: Umbilical artery catheter blood sampling alters cerebral blood flow velocity in preterm infants. J Perinatol 16:341, 1996.
25. Roll C, Huning B, Kaunicke M, et al: Umbilical artery catheter blood sampling decreases cerebral blood volume and oxygenation in very low birthweight infants. Acta Paediatr 89:862, 2000.
26. Gwinn JL, Lee FA, Weinberg HD: Radiological case of the month. Am J Dis Child 126:63, 1973.
27. Aziz EM, Robertson AF: Paraplegia: A complication of umbilical artery catheterization. J Pediatr 82:1051, 1973.
28. Bauer SB, Feldman SM, Gellis SS, et al: Neonatal hypertension. A complication of umbilical-artery catheterization. N Engl J Med 293:1032, 1975.
29. Dmochowski RR, Crandell SS, Corriere JN: Bladder injury and uroascites from umbilical-artery catheterization. Pediatrics 77:421, 1986.
30. Mendeloff J, Stallion A, Hutton M, et al: Aortic aneurysm resulting from umbilical artery catheterization: Case report, literature review, and management algorithm. J Vasc Surg 33:419, 2001.
31. Miller D, Kirkpatrick BV, Kodroff M, et al: Pelvic exsanguination following umbilical artery catheterization in neonates. J Pediatr Surg 14:264, 1979.
32. Prian GW, Wright GB, Rumack CM, et al: Apparent cerebral embolization after temporal artery catheterization. J Pediatr 93:115, 1978.
33. Simmons MA, Levine RL, Lubchenco LO, et al: Warning: Serious sequelae of temporal artery catheterization. J Pediatr 92:284, 1978.
34. Barrington KJ: Umbilical artery catheters in the newborn: Effects of heparin (Cochrane Review). In: The Cochrane Library, Issue 2, 2002. Oxford, Update Software.
35. Jackson J, Biondo DJ, Kilbride H, et al: Can an alternative umbilical arterial catheter solution and flush regimen decrease iatrogenic hemolysis while enhancing nutrition. Pediatr Res 51:373A, 2002.
36. Pape KE, Armstrong DL, Fitzhardinge PM: Peripheral median nerve damage secondary to brachial arterial blood gas sampling. J Pediatr 93:852, 1978.
37. Kim EH, Cohen RS, Ramachandran P: Effect of vascular puncture on blood gases in the newborn. Pediatr Pulmonol 10:287, 1991.
38. Sell EJ, Hansen RC, Struck-Pierce S: Calcified nodules on the heel: A complication of neonatal intensive care. J Pediatr 96:473, 1980.
39. Courtney SE, Weber KR, Breakie LA, et al: Capillary blood gases in the neonate: A reassessment and review of the literature. Am J Dis Child 144:168, 1990.
40. Meyers PA, Worwa C, Trusty R, et al: Clinical validation of a continuous intravascular neonatal blood gas sensor introduced through an umbilical artery catheter. Respir Care 47:682, 2002.
41. Fan LL, Dellinger KT, Mills AL, et al: Potential errors in neonatal blood gas measurements. J Pediatr 97:650, 1980.
42. Thelin OP, Karanth S, Pourcyrous M, et al: Overestimation of neonatal PO_2 by collection of arterial blood gas values with the butterfly infusion set. J Perinatol 13:65, 1993.
43. Dennis RC, Ng R, Yeston NS, et al: Effect of sample dilutions on arterial blood gas determinations. Crit Care Med 13:1067, 1985.
44. Gayed AM, Marino ME, Dolanski EA: Comparison of the effects of dry and liquid heparin on neonatal arterial blood gases. Am J Perinatol 9:159, 1992.
45. Quartin AA, Papale JJ, Marchant D, et al: Effects of exogenous lipids on blood gas measurements. Crit Care Med 21:1041, 1993.
46. Clark JS, Votteri B, Ariagno RL, et al: Noninvasive assessment of blood gases. Am Rev Respir Dis 145:220, 1992.
47. Lindberg LG, Lennmarken C, Vegfors M: Pulse oximetry: Clinical implications and recent technical developments. Acta Anaesthesiol Scand 39:279, 1995.
48. Poets CF, Southall DP: Noninvasive monitoring of oxygenation in infants and children: Practical considerations and areas of concern. Pediatrics 93:737, 1994.
49. Sinex JE: Pulse oximetry: Principles and limitations. Am J Emerg Med 17:59, 1999.
50. Hess D: Detection and monitoring of hypoxemia and oxygen therapy. Respir Care 45:65, 2000.
51. Martin RJ, Robertson SS, Hopple MM: Relationship between transcutaneous and arterial oxygen tension in sick neonates during mild hyperoxemia. Crit Care Med 10:670, 1982.

52. Rome ES, Stork EK, Carlo WA, Martin RJ: Limitations of transcutaneous PO₂ and PCO₂ monitoring in infants with bronchopulmonary dysplasia. Pediatrics 74:217, 1984.

53. Monaco F, McQuitty JC, Nickerson BG: Calibration of a heated transcutaneous carbon dioxide electrode to reflect arterial carbon dioxide. Am Rev Respir Dis 127:322, 1983.

54. Brunstler I, Enders A, Versmold HT: Skin surface PCO₂ monitoring in newborn infants in shock: Effect of hypotension and electrode temperature. J Pediatr 100:454, 1982.

55. Hopper AO, Nystrom GA, Deming DD, et al: Infrared end-tidal CO₂ measurement does not accurately predict arterial CO₂ values or end-tidal to arterial PCO₂ gradients in rabbits with lung injury. Pediatr Pulmonol 17:189, 1994.

56. Meredith KS, Monaco FJ: Evaluation of a mainstream capnometer and end-tidal carbon dioxide monitoring in mechanically ventilated infants. Pediatr Pulmonol 9:254, 1990.

57. Rozycki HJ, Sysyn GD, Marshall MK, et al: Mainstream end-tidal carbon dioxide monitoring in the neonatal intensive care unit. Pediatrics 101:648, 1998.

58. Hsieh KS, Lee CL, Lin CC, et al: Quantitative analysis of end-tidal carbon dioxide during mechanical and spontaneous ventilation in infants and young children. Pediatr Pulmonol 32:453, 2001.

59. Aziz HF, Martin JB, Moore JJ: The pediatric disposable end-tidal carbon dioxide detector role in endotracheal intubation in newborns. J Perinatol 19:110, 1999.

60. Dudell G, Cornish JD, Bartlett RH: What constitutes adequate oxygenation? Pediatrics 85:39, 1990.

61. Simmons MA, Adcock EW, Bard H, et al: Hypernatremia and intracranial hemorrhage in neonates. N Engl J Med 291:6, 1974.

62. Ng A, Subhedar N, Primhak RA, et al: Arterial oxygen saturation profiles in healthy preterm infants. Arch Dis Child Fetal Neonatal Ed 79:F64, 1998.

63. O'Brien LM, Stebbens VA, Poets CF, et al: Oxygen saturation during the first 24 hours of life. Arch Dis Child Fetal Neonatal Ed 83:F35, 2000.

64. The STOP-ROP Multicenter Study Group: Supplemental therapeutic oxygen for prethreshold retinopathy of prematurity (STOP-ROP), a randomized, controlled trial. I: Primary outcomes. Pediatrics 105:295, 2000.

65. Tin W, Milligan DWA, Pennefather P, et al: Pulse oximetry, severe retinopathy, and outcome at one year in babies of less than 28 weeks gestation. Arch Dis Child Fetal Neonatal Ed 84:F106, 2001.

66. Poets CF: When do infants need additional inspired oxygen? A review of current literature. Pediatr Pulmonol 26:424, 1998.

67. Saugstad OD: Is oxygen more toxic than currently believed? Pediatrics 108:1203, 2001.

68. Mariani G, Cifuentes J, Carlo WA: Randomized trial of permissive hypercapnia in preterm infants. Pediatrics 104:1082, 1999.

69. Stark AR, Carlo WA, Tyson JE, et al: Adverse effects of early dexamethasone in extremely-low-birth-weight infants. N Engl J Med 344:95, 2001.

70. Carlo WA, Stark AR, Bauer C, et al: Effects of minimal ventilation in a multicenter randomized controlled trial of ventilator support and early corticosteroid therapy in extremely low birth weight infants. Pediatrics 104:S738, 1999.

71. Ambalavanan N, Carlo WA: Hypocapnia and hypercapnia in respiratory management of newborn infants. Clin Perinatol 28:517, 2001.

72. Varughese M, Patole S, Shama A, et al: Permissive hypercapnia in neonates: The case of the good, the bad, and the ugly. Pediatr Pulmonol 33:56, 2002.

73. Gleason CA, Short BL, Jones MD: Cerebral blood flow and metabolism during and after prolonged hypocapnia in newborn lambs. J Pediatr 115:309, 1989.

74. Kusuda S, Shishida N, Miyagi N, et al: Cerebral blood flow during treatment for pulmonary hypertension. Arch Dis Child Fetal Neonatal Ed 80:F30, 1999.

75. Wiswell TE, Graziani LJ, Kornhauser MS, et al: Effects of hypocarbia on the development of cystic periventricular leukomalacia in premature infants treated with high-frequency jet ventilation. Pediatrics 98:918, 1996.

76. Graziani LJ, Baumgart S, Desai S, et al: Clinical antecedents of neurologic and audiological abnormalities in survivors of neonatal extracorporeal membrane oxygenation. J Child Neurol 12:415, 1997.

77. Kays DW, Langham MR Jr, Ledbetter DJ, et al: Detrimental effects of standard medical therapy in congenital diaphragmatic hernia. Ann Surg 230:340, 1999.

78. Marron MJ, Crisafi MA, Driscoll JM, et al: Hearing and neurodevelopmental outcome in survivors of persistent pulmonary hypertension of the newborn. Pediatrics 90:392, 1992.

79. Wilson JM, Lund DP, Lillehei CW, et al: Congenital diaphragmatic hernia—A tale of two cities: The Boston experience. J Pediatr Surg 32:401, 1997.

80. Ayus JC, Krothapalli RK: Effect of bicarbonate administration on cardiac function. Am J Med 87:5, 1989.

81. Cooper DJ, Walley KR, Wiggs BR, et al: Bicarbonate does not improve hemodynamics in critically ill patients who have lactic acidosis: A prospective, controlled clinical study. Ann Intern Med 112:492, 1990.

82. Howell JH: Sodium bicarbonate in the perinatal setting—Revisited. Clin Perinatol 14:807, 1987.

PULMONARY FUNCTION AND GRAPHICS

VINOD K. BHUTANI, MD, FAAP
EMIDIO M. SIVIERI, MS

Clinical access to measurements of neonatal pulmonary function, previously only feasible in a research setting, have been made possible by the technologic enhancements of neonatal ventilators. Bedside technologies of the past decade and reports on uses of neonatal pulmonary function tests provided a glimpse of pulmonary graphics. Pulmonary function data were collected for analysis and subsequent interpretation. Limitations in technology prevented the continuous visualization of real-time data and the clinician had to cope with "spot" measured values of respiratory vectors and with calculated measures of dynamic pulmonary mechanics. The current use of advanced microprocessor and sensor technologies has allowed manufacturers and designers of ventilatory equipment to provide the clinician with continuous and real-time analysis of ventilatory function. When combined with known physiologic principles and clinical judgment, the clinician can gain access to a rich source of previously untapped information on the respiratory status of the sick newborn.

Pulmonary graphics refers to the direct and online visualization of the three fundamental parameters of the respiratory system, namely, driving pressure, air flow, and tidal volume. These parameters are continuously displayed on a monitor either as scalar waveforms along a time axis or as X-Y plots of one variable versus another. The graphic displays may be accompanied by running average calculated values of pulmonary function parameters, such as compliance and resistance, as well as the more basic respiratory measurements, such as tidal volume and minute ventilation. Visualization of pulmonary gas exchange, a graphic assessment of blood gases and their relationship to respiratory support settings, also may be considered an extension of pulmonary graphics. The clinician's ability to use these technologies to advantage will transform this available information to relevant knowledge that assesses neonatal pulmonary status. This new data source can then be used along with blood gas data, chest radiographs, and other clinical data as another input in the decision-making process for determining ventilator settings and overall ventilatory management of neonates with respiratory failure.

In this chapter, we provide an overview as to how we utilize pulmonary graphics in our clinical management. The reader is referred to classic descriptions of physiologic principles that have led to our understanding of neonatal pulmonary function and graphics (see Chapter 2).

BACKGROUND

BACKGROUND

Signals of Respiration

Respiratory cycles are described by three fundamental signals: driving pressure (P), flow ($\dot{V}$), and volume (V). The first two signals are directly measurable; volume usually is derived from integration of the flow signal, which is simply the rate of change of volume. Thus, the usual mode of evaluating physiologic changes in respiration is by studying the standard scalar interrelationships of pressure, flow, volume, and time (Fig. 18-1). Breathing requires the generation of a driving pressure. For inspiration to occur, alveolar pressure must be less than the pressure at the mouth. For expiration to occur, alveolar pressure must be higher than the mouth pressure. During spontaneous breathing, this pressure gradient is generated by the respiratory muscles. In mechanical ventilation the ventilator produces the driving pressure. In either case, the driving pressure initiates a flow that overcomes the elastic, resistive, and inertial properties of the entire respiratory system resulting in a volume change in the lungs. This relationship has been best described by Röhrer[1] using an equation of motion in which the driving pressure is equal to the sum of elastic (P_E), resistive (P_R), and inertial (P_I) pressure components, or:

$$P = P_E + P_R + P_I \tag{1}$$

In this relationship, the elastic pressure is assumed to be proportional to volume change by a constant (E) representing the elastance (or elastic resistance) of the system. The resistive pressure component is assumed proportional to air flow by a constant (R) representing inelastic airway and tissue resistances. The inertial component of pressure is assumed to be proportional to gas and tissue acceleration $\ddot{V}$) by an inertial constant (I). Thus:

$$P = EV + R\dot{V} + I\ddot{V} \tag{2}$$

This linear model of respiratory system mechanics has become one of the fundamental principles used in respiratory physiology for the study of pulmonary function. Based on an ideal single-compartment model, this equation assumes linear relationships between pressure and volume and pressure and flow, such that the coefficients E, R, and I remain constant

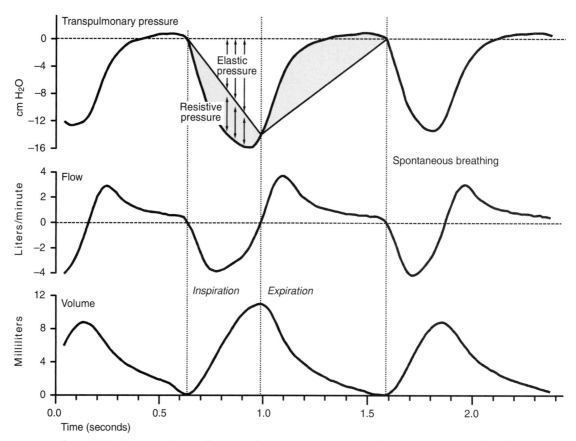

Figure 18-1. Scalar monitoring of pressure, flow, and volume signals during spontaneous breathing. The pressure signal has been divided (as demarcated by a *straight line* connecting points of zero flow) to differentiate the elastic pressure from the resistive pressure *(shaded portion)*.

throughout the ventilatory cycle. The assumption of linearity breaks down at extremes of ventilation or in infants with abnormal elastic and resistive pulmonary characteristics, as frequently is the case during mechanical ventilation. Although more complex multicompartment and nonlinear models of the respiratory system have been investigated,[2–4] the simple linear model with its inherent limitations has remained the most widely used for general pulmonary function measurements because of its simplicity.

The interrelationships between the components of the Röhrer equation can be easily visualized using two-dimensional graphic plots of its variables, that is, pressure versus volume (P-V), flow versus volume ($\dot{V}$-V), and pressure versus flow (P-$\dot{V}$). Such simple X-Y plots provide valuable insight into pulmonary status and the pattern of breathing and are the basis of pulmonary graphics. Physiologic interpretations of pulmonary function can be further enhanced by mathematical evaluations of compliance (inverse of elastance) and resistance based on the Röhrer equation. Because of the inherent nature of respiratory signals to be variable, it is important to evaluate the signals during resting conditions and over a sufficient period of time to avoid artifacts and to allow averaging of random variations, thus providing a more representative time-averaged sample.

SIGNAL COMPONENTS OF BEDSIDE PULMONARY GRAPHICS: PRESSURE, VOLUME, AND FLOW

Pressure Signal

Pulmonary Graphic Representation of Driving Pressure

As described earlier, driving pressure (or compression pressure) is the net pressure change required to overcome elastic, air flow resistive, and inertial properties of the respiratory system during inspiration. During spontaneous breathing, it is the gradient between the mouth and intrapleural pressures and is defined as the transpulmonary pressure (see Fig. 18-1). During positive-pressure ventilation the driving pressure usually is measured as the gradient between the peak inflating pressure (PIP) and the positive end-expiratory pressure (PEEP). The driving pressure at the end-inspiratory portion of the ventilation cycle, as indicated in Figure 18-2, provides a close estimate of elastic pressure as described by the Röhrer equation. It is in this context that the ratio of tidal volume to driving pressure provides an indirect approximation of total respiratory compliance. In the absence of overinflation or

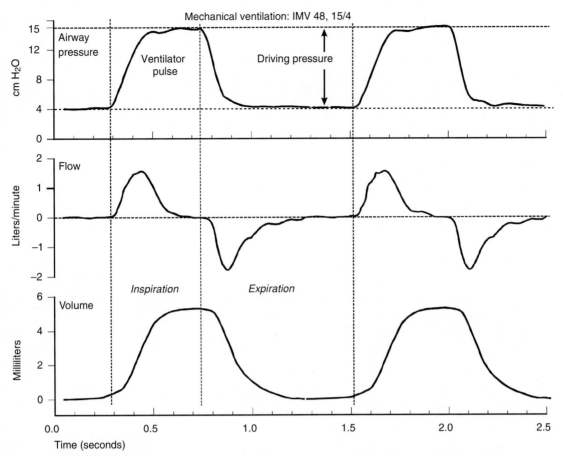

Figure 18-2. Scalar monitoring of pressure, flow, and volume signals during mechanical ventilation. Driving pressure can be approximated as peak inflating pressure minus positive end-expiratory pressure = 11 cm H_2O. IMV, intermittent mandatory ventilation.

underinflation and when ventilation is being administered in the most linear portion of the respiratory pressure-volume relationship, this value of respiratory compliance (in mL/cm H_2O) provides an estimation of the volume change (in milliliters) per 1 cm H_2O change in driving pressure. These estimated data can provide a crucial understanding of the anticipated change in tidal volume for a given incremental change in ventilator driving pressure. Based on this observation the clinician can differentiate between the effects of overdistending or underdistending the lung. As demonstrated in Figure 18-3, when ventilation is shifting *away from* the linear portion of the P-V loop, actual tidal volume becomes smaller than anticipated. Likewise, when ventilation is moving *into* the linear portion of the P-V loop, actual tidal volume becomes larger than anticipated.

The driving pressure should be distinguished from the mean airway pressure, which is a function of inspiratory time flow, PIP, end-distending pressure, and respiratory rate (see Chapter 2). Mean airway pressure has a direct relationship to oxygenation; driving pressure provides an insight to respiratory elastic status.

Instrumentation for Pressure Measurement

The pressure sensor used for monitoring of airway pressure (PIP and PEEP) in ventilated neonates is an integral ventilator component. The measurement is obtained from a side port where the ventilator circuit connects to the endotracheal tube adapter. This type of pressure sensing is adequate for basic waveform monitoring and for real-time display of pressure-volume loops. Measurement of pulmonary function requires a more dedicated pressure sensor placed close to the measurement point of interest. This can be a differential type that can be used to measure a pressure difference between two points, such as between mouth and pleural pressure (via esophageal balloon or catheter) to yield transpulmonary pressure or between mouth and atmospheric pressure to yield transthoracic pressure for use in calculating combined lung and chest wall mechanics. Two independent transducers, instead of a single differential transducer, are also commonly used for this purpose. A typical measurement range for such pressure transducers is ±50 cm H_2O (±4.9 kPa).

Instrumentation also includes pressure transducer measurements of airway pressure (Paw) and esophageal pressure (Pes). Paw is measured at the proximal airway. Mechanical breaths generate a positive Paw. Conversely, spontaneous breaths generate both negative Paw and negative intrapleural pressure. Direct measurement of intrapleural pressure requires placement of catheters within the pleural space. An indirect means of approximating intrapleural pressure is the measurement of changes in Pes. When a catheter or esophageal balloon is positioned within the lower third of the esophagus, continuous Pes

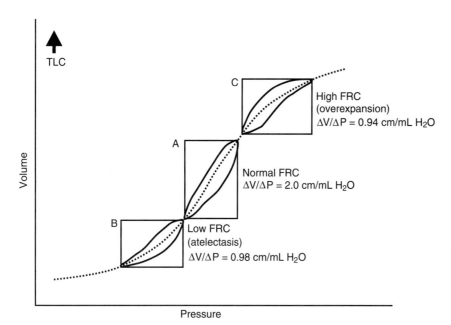

Figure 18-3. Pressure-volume loops superimposed on the overall pressure-volume relationship of the respiratory system *(dotted line)*. Relationship of positive end-expiratory pressure, peak inflating pressure, functional residual capacity (FRC), and lung compliance. The linear portion *(A)* is the optimal ventilation point.

readings can be obtained. The sum of Paw and Pes is the Ptp, which is essential in the calculation of the pulmonary functions of compliance and resistance. However, studies have shown that the correlation between intrapleural pressure and Pes in very small infants is poor. Therefore, calculations based on estimates of intrapleural pressure determined with the use of Pes measurements should be considered suspect in extremely small infants.

Volume and Flow Signals

Pulmonary Graphic Representation of Tidal Volume

Tidal volume is the volume of each breath as measured during inspiration, expiration, or averaged for the entire respiratory cycle. The value should be normalized to body weight or length. During spontaneous breathing, normal values in healthy neonates range from 5 to 10 mL/kg.[5–9] Based on a database of ventilatory parameters measured in our clinical laboratory, the 10th, 50th, and 90th percentile values for these parameters are listed in Table 18-1. Very small preterm infants may have spontaneous breathing tidal volumes as little as 3.2 mL/kg.[10] When measured while the infant is on respiratory support, the resultant tidal volume is highly dependent on ventilator settings; values >8.5 mL/kg have been considered to suggest volume overdistention.[11] Tidal volume observations during mechanical ventilation of an infant should be considered an important monitoring parameter for infant ventilatory support, along with blood gas values and other clinical data. In addition, tidal volume measurement is essential for the determination of compliance.

Pulmonary Graphic Assessment of Minute Ventilation

The summation of individual tidal volumes over a 1-minute period gives us the minute ventilation. This can also be expressed as the product of tidal volume and respiratory rate. Respiratory rates of most preterm and term infants are 20 to 60 breaths/min. A normal full-term newborn infant at rest breathing at a rate of 40 breaths/min and a tidal volume of 8 mL/kg would have a minute ventilation of 320 (mL/kg)/min. Usual normal values range from 240 to 480 (mL/kg)/min.[12] Minute ventilation minus ventilated dead space equals alveolar ventilation.[13] Alveolar ventilation has a direct inverse relationship to alveolar P_{CO_2} or arterial carbon dioxide tension.[14] Thus, at extremes of infant tachypnea (~100 breaths/min or more), tidal volume is reduced while dead space is unchanged and effective minute ventilation is lost, as in untreated respiratory distress syndrome (RDS).

Pulmonary Graphic Representation of Inspiratory and Expiratory Air Flow

Air flow increases at the initiation of the respiratory cycles, reaches a maximum usually at mid-cycle, and returns to zero flow at the end of each phase (see Figs. 18-1 and 18-2). The

TABLE 18-1.   Basic Respiratory Parameters Observed in Spontaneously Breathing Neonates in Several Weight Ranges

Weight Range (g)	Peak Inspiratory Flow (L/min)			Peak Expiratory Flow (L/min)			Tidal Volume (mL/kg)			Minute Ventilation (mL/min)		
Percentiles	10th	50th	90th	10th	50th	90th	10th	50th	90th	10th	50th	90th
500–1000	0.8	1.3	2.1	0.5	0.9	1.6	3.2	5.4	8.3	230	400	600
1000–2500	1.3	2.3	3.5	1.0	1.8	3.0	3.4	5.7	8.1	250	400	600
2500–5000	1.8	3.2	5.2	1.6	2.9	4.8	2.4	4.7	7.2	170	300	500
5000–15000	4.1	5.9	9.9	3.4	4.9	8.6	5.2	6.9	8.9	180	240	400

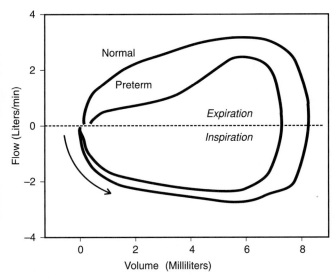

Figure 18-4. Tidal flow-volume loop from a normal term neonate and a preterm neonate with high expiratory resistance, thus the "ski-slope" effect during expiration

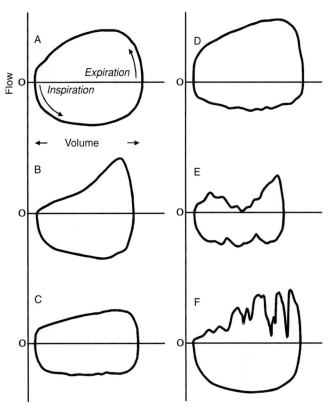

Figure 18-5. Flow-volume loops illustrating different types of flow limitation. *A,* Normal loop. *B,* "Ski-slope" loop observed with expiratory air flow limitation as seen in babies with bronchopulmonary dysplasia. *C,* Extrathoracic airway obstruction with inspiratory and expiratory air flow limitation as seen in babies with subglottic stenosis or narrow endotracheal tubes. *D,* Intrathoracic inspiratory air flow limitation as seen in babies with intraluminal obstruction (close to the carina) or an aberrant vessel compressing the trachea. *E,* Unstable airways or tracheomalacia. *F,* This type of loop usually is suggestive of an erratic air flow limitation as seen with airway secretions.

location of the peak value depends on the site of maximal airway resistance, such that air flow is measured at its peak rather than at mid-respiratory cycles. Typical peak flow ranges for premature infants are listed in Table 18-1. It is important to differentiate ventilator circuit air flow from the inspiratory and expiratory air flow that traverses the endotracheal tube.

Pulmonary Graphic Representation of Tidal Flow-Volume Relationships

The tidal flow-volume relationship describes the pattern of air flow during tidal breathing. It is characterized by the tidal volume and peak inspiratory and expiratory air flow. The location of the flow peaks in relation to the origin of inspiration and expiration and the ensuing pattern provide an insight to subtle changes in flow limitation. Usually, peak inspiratory air flow occurs during mid-inspiration, whereas peak expiratory air flow values precede mid-expiration.

Air flow limitation is described as abrupt downward deviation of the flow signal toward baseline and away from its normal direction. A complete flow limitation is defined as 80% or greater reduction of the air flow signal. Actual visual evidence of flow limitation during a specific phase of the respiratory cycle is an important indication of obstructive airway disease. Preterm neonates, with compliant airways, manifest high expiratory resistance because of expiratory phase airway collapsibility. This accounts for the peak expiratory air flow occurring early in the expiratory cycle and the "ski-slope" effect apparent in the expiratory limb of the tidal flow-volume relationship as shown in Figure 18-4. A characteristic flow-volume profile for various types of intrathoracic and extrathoracic flow limitation is illustrated in Figure 18-5.

Evidence of expiratory flow limitation is best evidenced from flow-volume loops obtained during a maximum effort maneuver as measured in adults via the forced expiratory volume (FEV_1) test. In the neonate this may be simulated by measuring the partial expiratory flow-volume (PEFV) response using the rapid thoracic compression technique (Fig. 18-6).[6,15-18]

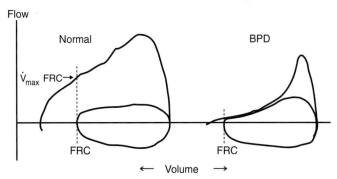

Figure 18-6. Partial expiratory flow-volume curves. The normal curve indicates a substantial flow at functional residual capacity (FRC), while the bronchopulmonary dysplasia (BPD) infant demonstrates significant flow limitation during the forced expiratory maneuver.

Pulmonary Graphic Representation of Pressure-Volume Relationships

The pressure-volume relationship describes the pattern of tidal volume as a function of driving pressure. The slope of the P-V loop represents the elasticity of the lung. Based upon the location of the P-V loop on the total respiratory P-V relationship, the shape of the P-V loop may be altered and

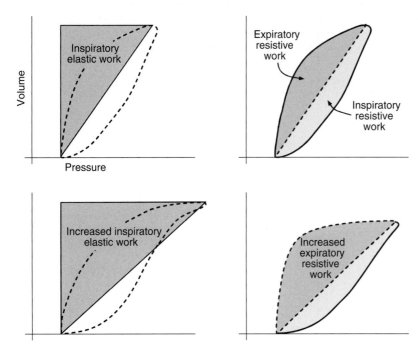

Figure 18-7. Pressure-volume relationships showing components of inspiratory elastic work and inspiratory and expiratory resistive work. *Lower two panels* illustrate examples of increased elastic work (as may be observed with respiratory distress syndrome, pneumonia, or atelectasis) and increased expiratory resistive work (as may be observed with obstructive airway diseases such as meconium aspiration syndrome or bronchopulmonary dysplasia).

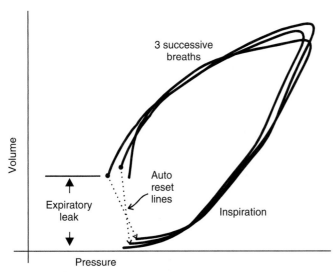

Figure 18-8. Example of endotracheal tube leak during expiration as indicated by failure of the expiratory limb to return to start inspiratory point.

may indicate either pressure or volume overdistention (see Fig. 18-3).

The inspiratory and expiratory portions of the P-V loop describe a hysteresis that represents the resistive work of breathing (Fig. 18-7). During spontaneous breathing, when the absolute intrapleural pressure is not known, the origin of this loop cannot be accurately determined; thus, it is not feasible to calculate the total work of breathing. In babies with air trapping or obstructive airway disease, the expiratory component of the hysteresis is excessively increased. The online display of P-V loops is an ideal indicator of endotracheal tube leakage or as gauged by the inspiratory–expiratory volume discrepancy (Fig.18-8). Generally, any inspiratory–expiratory volume discrepancy should be less than 10%. Large discrepancies may be indicative of a faulty flow signal.

Instrumentation for Flow and Tidal Volume Measurements

Flow measurements. Several flow-sensing technologies have evolved for measurement of air flow for the purpose of monitoring pulmonary graphics and for pulmonary function determination in small neonates. These include the following. (1) *Pneumotachometers.* These are resistive-type devices in which gas flowing through a fixed resistance creates a pressure differential across the resistive element. This pressure difference is easily measured with a sensitive differential pressure transducer. The resistive element can be either a fine mesh screen[19] or a bundle of small capillaries (Fleish type),[20,21] both of which produce a laminar flow that is directly proportional to the measured differential pressure and thus have a linear output over a specific range of air flow. (2) *Nonlinear flow resistive sensors,* such as variable orifice and pitot tube flow sensors. These types of flow sensors also require measurement of a pressure difference produced by gas flowing through a tube, however, the flow-pressure relationship for these devices is nonlinear. (3) A relatively *new type of flow sensor uses a piezo-electric film* to detect the turbulence produced in a gas stream. Vibration of the film results in an electrical output proportional to the flow. (4) *Anemometers.* These operate on the principle of measuring the amount of electrical current needed to maintain a given temperature in a fine heated wire suspended across an air stream. The added current increases as the air flow increases and more heat is dissipated, but the relationship is nonlinear as well as insensitive to flow direction.

In addition to dedicated sensors that measure flow at the airway opening, air flow can be measured by plethysmography.[22,23] A computerized and self-calibrating whole-body plethysmograph-incubator has been developed for use with mechanically ventilated infants (Fig. 18-9).[24] A sealed incubator acts as constant pressure flow-type plethysmograph where ventilator tubing and other support lines are passed through special seals to the infant. A sensitive pneumotach in the wall of the incuba-

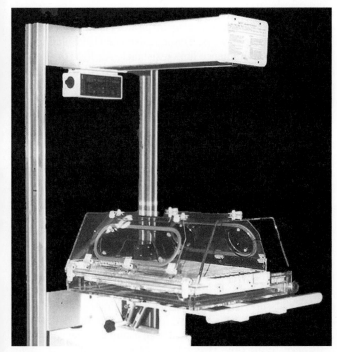

Figure 18-9. Plethysmograph/incubator. (Courtesy of Vital Trends Technology, Inc., NY, NY, USA.)

tor measures tidal air flow as air is displaced due to chest expansion during inspiration and chest contraction during expiration either spontaneously or mechanically. This is a truly non-invasive pulmonary monitoring system because no dead space or resistive loading is added to the neonate's breathing circuit, which is left undisturbed.

Whereas the conventional pneumotachometer is a simple device having very linear input-output characteristics and can be easily and precisely calibrated, it is also a relatively large instrument and creates a significant dead space for neonatal use. Thus, the pneumotach is appropriate when performing discrete pulmonary function tests, but it is inappropriate for continuous air flow monitoring. The alternative flow-sensing devices mentioned earlier have the disadvantage of being either nonlinear, nondirectional, or both; thus, they require more sophisticated signal conditioning and calibration techniques. Nonetheless, these sensors have the advantage of generally being lighter and smaller than pneumotachometers and having less dead space; thus, they are more suitable for continuous monitoring of mechanically ventilated babies. In these infants, the air flow sensor is placed between the endotracheal tube connector and the ventilator circuit connection. Usually a heater is incorporated in the sensor to prevent condensation of water vapor, which can otherwise affect system response and accuracy. For spontaneous breathing measurements the flow sensor is commonly attached to a snug-fitting face mask. To avoid tidal volume augmentation and changes in breathing pattern due to increased dead space and resistance, as well as the effect of facial stimulation[25] of the typical face mask and pneumotachometer apparatus, some investigators have used nasal prongs or nasal masks, although neonates are not necessarily obligate nasal breathers.[26] The specified measurement range of the flow sensor should be close to the expected flow range to be measured. Flow ranges can be as low as ±20 mL/sec for small prematures, up to ±400 mL/sec for ventilated infants depending on

the ventilator waveform, and ±200 mL/sec for spontaneously breathing newborn infants.[27] To maintain accuracy, all flow sensors should be periodically checked for buildup of secretions and cleaned and recalibrated regularly. It should be noted that gas composition, temperature, and humidity can have significant effects on flow sensor accuracy if they are not properly corrected or compensated.[28–30]

Volume measurement. For continuous monitoring, volume can be easily measured indirectly as the integral (i.e., area under the curve) of the flow signal. The integration can be performed electronically or digitally in computerized systems. The inspiratory and expiratory portions of measured tidal volume signal will necessarily be different because inspiratory gas differs from expiratory gas in O_2 and CO_2 composition, water vapor, temperature, and viscosity.[29,30] In addition, flow sensors do not always have perfectly symmetrical inspiratory and expiratory response characteristics. Because of these reasons, the volume signal typically demonstrates a small baseline drift. However, differences in inspiratory and expiratory tidal volumes larger than 10% could be indicative of air flow leakage around the endotracheal tube. Large differences could indicate faulty flow sensor readings due to factors such as water vapor condensation, buildup of secretions, calibration drift, and integrator drift and should be investigated.

Signal calibration. All monitoring or testing instruments require calibration for maintenance of accuracy and reproducibility. Reproducibility can be hampered by changes in the observed condition between tests, by errors of measurement, or by errors of calibration. Calibration, which determines the relationship between the output signal of a transducer and a known input signal, should be performed under both static and dynamic conditions and over the frequency and amplitude ranges of infant ventilation. For this purpose, only calibration reference standards that have certifiable accuracy should be used. In clinical practice, graduated or calibrated syringes, precise ball-in-tube flow meters, water column manometers, and reference transducers are generally used. Linearity is a measure of how well the output-to-input ratio is maintained over a given measurement range for a transducer. Operation of an instrument outside its linear calibration range results in erroneous measurements. Use of the properly ranged flow sensor is crucial for accurate measurement of infant flow dynamics. Finally, it is important to carefully follow manufacturer's procedure and guidelines for maintenance and calibration of a device or system.

Pulmonary Mechanics

Lung compliance. If pressure is sequentially decreased (made more subatmospheric) around the outside of an excised lung, the lung volume increases. When the pressure is removed from the lung, it deflates along a pressure-volume curve that is different from that during inflation. The difference between the inflation and deflation levels of the pressure-volume curve is called *hysteresis*. The elastic behavior of the lungs is characterized by this pressure-volume curve (see Fig. 18-3). More specifically, the ratio of change in lung volume to change in distending pressure defines the compliance of the lungs. Although the pressure-volume relationship of the lung is not linear over the entire range, the compliance (of slope $\Delta V/\Delta P$) is linear over the normal range of tidal volumes beginning at functional residual capacity (FRC). Thus, for a given change in driving pressure, tidal volume will increase in proportion to lung compliance, or $\Delta V = C/\Delta P$. As lung compliance is decreased, the lungs are stiffer and more difficult to expand. When lung compliance is increased, the lung becomes easier to distend and is more compliant. Lung compliance and pressure-volume relationships are determined by the interdependence of elastic tissue elements and alveolar surface tension. Tissue elasticity is dependent on elastin and collagen content of the lung. A typical value for lung compliance in a young healthy newborn is 1.5 to 2.0 mL/cm H_2O/kg. This value is dependent on the size of the lung (mass of elastic tissue). As can be expected, the compliance of the lung increases with development as the tissue mass of the lung increases. Based upon where we measure the driving pressure, we can describe the compliance of that structure. Thus:

$$\text{Total Compliance (chest + lung) = Tidal Volume/} \quad (3)$$
$$\text{Change in}$$
$$\text{Driving Pressure}$$

where the change in driving pressure is the net driving pressure for the entire respiratory system. In ventilated neonates the driving pressure can be measured as the airway pressure at the mouth while the infant is connected to a mechanical ventilator. During respiratory cycles of consecutive breaths, the equilibration of changes in pressure and volume may have yet to be completed at the termination of air flow. Thus, the respiratory mechanics are probably still in a dynamic state. Therefore:

$$\text{Dynamic Lung Compliance = Tidal Volume/} \quad (4)$$
$$\text{Change in}$$
$$\text{Driving Pressure}$$

where driving pressure is the gradient between PIP and PEEP, or the *peak-to-peak pressure*. This is the net driving pressure used to expand the lungs. The dynamic compliance overestimates the actual "static" compliance when the pressure measurements are underestimated. On the other hand, a slower equilibration of tidal volume may result in underestimation of dynamic compliance. From a clinical perspective, the dynamic compliance is likely to be overestimated when there is an impaired surface activity, as with RDS. In babies with bronchopulmonary dysplasia (BPD), the areas of fibrosis, scarring, and the associated resistive load may lead to underestimation of tidal volume and thereby of lung compliance. In both of these conditions, the baby has to generate a higher driving pressure to achieve a similar tidal volume, otherwise hypoventilation would occur. Estimation of dynamic compliance is a poor measurement of the "stiffness" of lung and not an objective index of its elasticity. Its clinical usefulness is that it provides the clinician with an index of the volume change that is likely to occur for every 1 cm H_2O change in driving pressure, provided the lungs are operating in a linear pressure-volume relationship. This assumption should be valid and anticipated during tidal breathing at optimal FRC.

Resistive properties. Nonelastic properties of the respiratory system characterize its resistance to motion. Because motion between two surfaces in contact usually involves friction or loss of energy, resistance to breathing occurs in any moving part of the respiratory system. These resistances include frictional resistance to air flow, tissue resistance, and inertial forces. Lung resistance is predominantly (80%) attributed to frictional resistance to inspiratory and expiratory air flow in the larger airways. Tissue resistance (19%) and inertial forces (1%) also influence lung resistance. Air flow through the airways requires a driving pressure resulting from changes in alveolar pressure. When alveolar pressure is less than atmospheric pressure (during spontaneous inspiration), air flows into the lung. When alveolar pressure is greater than atmospheric pressure, air flows out of the lung. By definition, resistance to air flow is equal to the resistive component of driving pressure (P_R) divided by air flow ($\dot{V}$). Thus:

$$\text{Resistance} = P_R/\dot{V}. \quad (5)$$

When determining lung resistance the resistive component of the measured transpulmonary pressure is used as the driving pressure (see Fig. 18-1). To measure airway resistance the differential between alveolar pressure and atmospheric pressure is used as the driving pressure. Under normal tidal breathing conditions, there is a linear relationship between air flow and driving pressure. The slope of the flow versus pressure curve changes as the airways narrow, indicating that the patient with airway obstruction has a greater resistance to air flow. The resistance to air flow is greatly dependent on the size of the airway lumen. According to Poiseuille's law the resistive pressure (ΔP) required to achieve a given flow ($\dot{V}$) for a gas of viscosity μ and flowing through a rigid and smooth cylindrical tube of specific length L and radius r is given as:

$$\Delta P = 8\mu L\dot{V}/\pi r^4. \quad (6)$$

According to this relationship, resistance to air flow increases by a power of four with any decrease in airway radius. Because the newborn airway lumen is approximately half that of the adult, the neonatal airway resistance is about 16-fold that of the adult. Normal airway resistance in a term newborn is approximately 20 to 40 cm H_2O/L/sec, which is about 16-fold the value observed in adults (1 to 2 cm H_2O/L/sec). Also, the hysteresis of the pressure-volume relationship represents the resistive work of breathing and can be separated into inspiratory and expiratory components. In babies with obstructive airway disease, the expiratory component of resistive work of breathing is increased (see Fig. 18-3). Nearly 80% of the total resistance to air flow occurs in large airways up to about the fourth to fifth generation of bronchial branching. The patient usually has large airway disease when resistance to air flow is increased. Because the smaller airways contribute a small proportion of total airway resistance, they have been designated as the *silent zone* of the lung in which airway obstruction can occur without being readily detected. Unlike babies with RDS, babies with BPD (because of the associated airway barotrauma) have higher values of airway resistance with an associated increased resistive work of breathing.

Synchronous and asynchronous breathing. Real-time evaluation of synchronous respiratory cycles allows for visualization of successive P-V and $\dot{V}$-V loops as they superimpose neatly over each preceding loop. Asynchrony of respiratory cycles may be evident during airway obstruction (secretions, bronchospasm), "bucking" (during mechanical ventilation or involuntary valsalva maneuvers), and during agitation (pain, excessive handling, impaired gas exchange). Objective evaluation of asynchrony is difficult to quantify. On the other hand, synchronous ventilation is easily observed.

Relationship of oxygenation to mean airway pressure. Other manifestations of pulmonary graphics include the visual interpretation of the relationship of arterial oxygenation to changes in mean airway pressure. Enhancements in bedside ventilatory software can easily provide the clinician with such data.

Relationship of carbon dioxide elimination to alveolar ventilation. The relationship of arterial carbon dioxide tension to alveolar ventilation is feasible, provided no change in dead space has occurred during the phase of evaluation. The relationship between the driving pressure and alveolar ventilation and then to arterial carbon dioxide tension is feasible but requires a specially designed software program.

ROLE OF PULMONARY FUNCTIONS IN BEDSIDE VENTILATOR MANAGEMENT

Bedside evaluation of history, clinical assessment, blood gas, and acid-base profiles and the interaction of the baby to any supportive respiratory devices enhance the bedside application of pulmonary physiologic principles, especially for a neonate with respiratory distress. The noninvasive assessment of the three respiratory signals provides objective, valuable online data that may be used in an adjunctive manner to monitor, interpret, and define the severity of dysfunction. These data do not provide a clinical diagnosis, but they can be useful in the following situations: (1) evaluation of alteration and/or limitation in inspiratory/expiratory air flow; (2) evaluation of driving pressure, work, and effort to maintain minute ventilation; (3) evaluation and calculation of the elastic and resistive components of pulmonary dysfunction; (4) calculation of the inspiratory, expiratory, and total lung time constants; (5) evaluation of the interaction between spontaneous breathing and conventional mechanical ventilation, including continuous positive airway pressure (CPAP); (6) evaluation of the degree of response to a therapeutic intervention; and (7) evaluation of the evolution and resolution of the respiratory disease.

Optimizing Peak Inflating Pressure

If a baby is being managed on a pressure-limited ventilatory support, visualizing the concomitant tidal volume may corroborate the selection of a chosen PIP. A suggested goal would be to initially ventilate at the low "normal" value of tidal volume (such as 5 to 6 mL/ kg). This provides for a more objective approach than choosing the PIP on the basis of auscultation for adequate breath sounds during manual ventilation. Similarly, the tidal volume actually delivered to a neonate can be measured when setting the volume support during volume-controlled ventilation.

Optimizing Positive End-Expiratory Pressure

It is feasible to define an optimal end-distending pressure using pulmonary graphics; however, the process is complex and at present not user friendly. Using a combination of the effects of driving pressure on tidal volume and visual changes in P-V relationships, one can ascertain whether incremental changes in PEEP lead to pulmonary overdistention or underdistention or moving to a linear component of the P-V relationship (see

example in Fig. 18-10). Because the clinical goal is to ventilate at the linear portion of the P-V loop, bedside incremental changes in PEEP should only be done by experienced clinicians who can accurately assess the changes in measured data and thereby calculate the impact of PEEP manipulation.

Optimizing Circuit Air Flow

Usually the circuit air flow of the ventilator has not been an active decision of the clinician and has been based upon manufacturer's guidelines. It is well known that excessive circuit air flow can lead to overdistention (Fig. 18-11) and inadvertent excessive PEEP. Both of these effects would lead to hypoventilation and subsequent hypercapnia. The pulmonary graphic manifestations would be lower tidal volumes, wider pulmonary hysteresis, pressure overdistention, and perhaps turbulence in the air flow signal. These would be immediately corrected by a bedside maneuver to reduce the circuit air flow. Another option to set the circuit air flow is to base the setting on eightfold of the desired minute ventilation (tidal volume and respiratory frequency).

Optimizing Inspiratory Time

Inspiratory time can be increased or decreased (and thereby the expiratory time) by the physician as a response to change the mean airway pressure and oxygenation. These clinical decisions usually are made based on the physiologic understanding of respiratory time constants (product of compliance and resistance). In addition to the impact on oxygenation, the concomitant and often indirect beneficial or deleterious effects of the new inspiratory time can be assessed by pulmonary graphics. These include the effects on tidal volume, inspiratory and expiratory hysteresis, pressure-volume relationship (such as overdistention from excessive mean airway pressure), and flow-volume relationships (such as expiratory flow limitation from excessive and inadvertent PEEP) as sequelae of shortened expiratory time.

Optimizing Synchrony and Rate of Ventilatory Support

Real-time evaluation of synchronous ventilation on the graphic displays is helpful for nurses, respiratory therapists, and physicians to assess nonventilatory means to correct asynchronous ventilation. The clinical value of the visual display allows for early response to a neonate's discomfort. Babies who continue to "buck" the ventilator and are not amenable to bedside comforting and nursing measures may demonstrate their response to ventilatory technologies such as patient-triggered ventilation.

Optimizing Tidal Volume

The tidal volume is evident with placement of the pneumotachometer, and the digital readout provides the variability that is evident among spontaneous, mechanical, and augmented breaths. In fact, the optimal PIP can be ascertained by adjusting to appropriate tidal volume (thereby providing a more objective assessment to auscultation). In a clinical condition when the baby is breathing synchronously or when spontaneous breathing has been diminished or abolished, the steady measures of

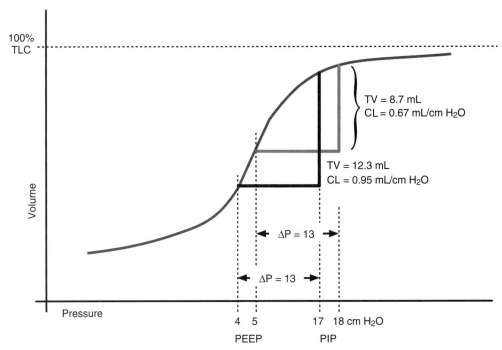

Figure 18-10. Deflation limb of the respiratory pressure-volume curve (deflation from total lung capacity to residual volume) is shown on an X-Y plot. In this simulated example, tidal volume ventilation is occurring at the functional residual capacity (FRC, or the lung volume at end-expiration) that is governed by the positive end-expiratory pressure (PEEP). Thus, for a baby who is being administered a peak inflating pressure (PIP) of 18 cm H_2O and PEEP of 5 cm H_2O and the recorded tidal volume (TV) is 8.7 mL, then the estimated compliance (CL) is 8.7 divided by 13 (difference of 18 and 5), which is 0.67 mL/cm H_2O. If the baby is dual weaned to 17/4 driving pressure, the tidal volume is now being ventilated at a more optimal FRC and the estimated compliance is improved (0.95 mL/cm H_2O).

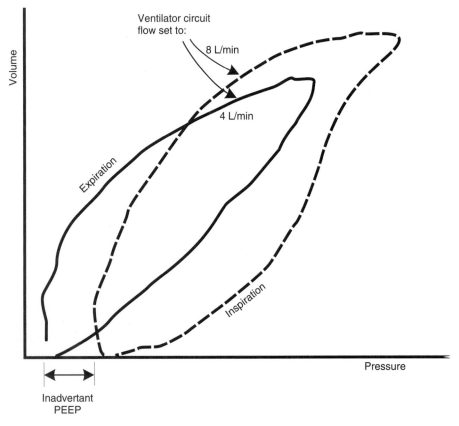

Figure 18-11. Effect of excessive ventilator circuit air flow settings on pressure-volume characteristic. Overdistention due to increased peak inflating pressure and inadvertent increase in positive end-expiratory pressure (PEEP).

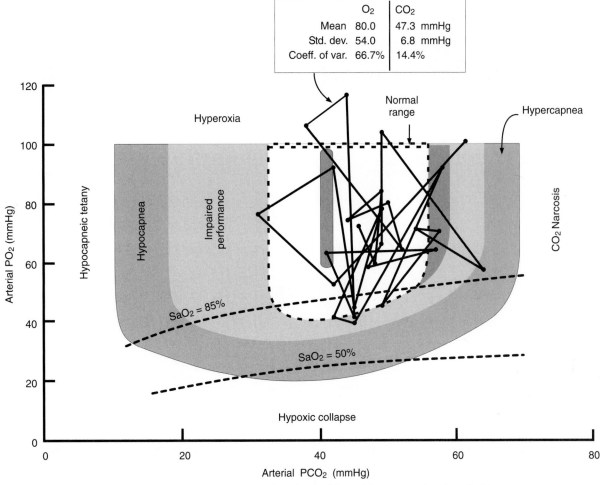

	O₂	CO₂
Mean	80.0	47.3 mmHg
Std. dev.	54.0	6.8 mmHg
Coeff. of var.	66.7%	14.4%

Figure 18-12. Arterial Po_2-CO_2 nomogram that plots serial arterial oxygen and carbon dioxide gas tensions. The "normal" range is demarcated by *dashed lines*. *Dotted lines* define the ranges of oxygen saturation. *Solid lines* connect serial values of blood gases. Mean values, standard deviations, and coefficients of variance for both arterial oxygen and carbon dioxide tensions are shown in the *inset*. These variations may be due to disease-related or operator-induced effects and may be interpreted by clinical review.

tidal volume provide clinically useful information. First, when the tidal volume value is between 5 to 8 mL/kg and there are no signs of pressure-volume overdistention, the clinician may ascertain that ventilation is at optimal FRC. Incremental changes (by 1 cm H_2O) in PEEP and PIP (such that the driving pressure is unchanged) should not result in an appreciable change in tidal volume. The rationale for this observation is that if the baby is being ventilated at optimal FRC (at the linear component of the respiratory PV curve: see Fig. 18-3), slight movements along the curve should maintain the tidal volume. Second, if the tidal volume is less than 5 mL/kg, the baby is being ventilated at either a low lung volume (increase in PIP would improve the tidal volume) or a high lung volume (decrease in PIP would actually improve the tidal volume). Finally, if the tidal volume is in excess of 8 mL/kg, both P-V and flow-volume curves should be evaluated for pulmonary overdistention and increased resistive work of breathing.

Optimizing Inspired Oxygen

The process of plotting serial arterial blood gases on the Po_2-Pco_2 nomogram (Fig. 18-12) provides the clinician a perspective on the extent of variation induced by either the disease or the operator. Operator-driven swings in oxygenation may be minimized by prospective decisions (such as use of the alveolar gas equation) or by invoking changes in a cautious and incremental manner.

Optimizing Ventilatory Strategies for Permissive Hypercapnia

The relationship between alveolar ventilation and arterial carbon dioxide tension is incredibly linear and can be used as an advantage in defining desired goals for "permissive" hypercapnia. Selection of Pco_2 value of 50 torr in lieu of the "normal" 40 torr is a choice of defining a 25% deviation; this may indicate hypoventilation by 25%. This decision could be an elective clinical maneuver, but the clinician needs to ensure that the decision is not a passive one such that atelectatic lungs are being ventilated. Again, the plotting of serial blood gases on a Po_2-Pco_2 nomogram (Fig. 18-12) provides the clinician with a direct visual impact of the recent gas exchange history such that prospective decisions are made consciously and conscientiously.

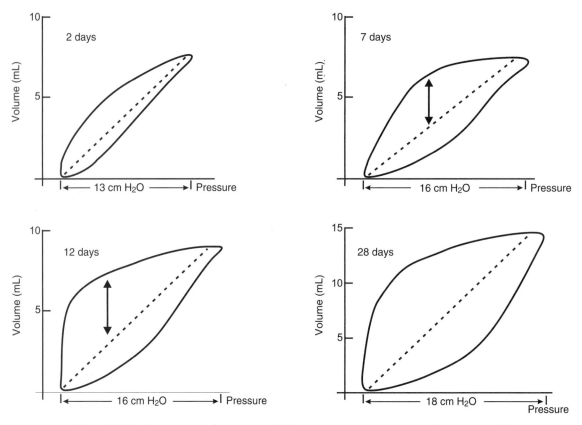

Figure 18-13. Clinical case 1 of a newborn with bronchopulmonary dysplasia and airway instability.

Clinical Case Studies: Bedside Application of Pulmonary Graphics

Case 1 of a Newborn with Bronchopulmonary Dysplasia and Airway Instability (Possible Tracheobronchomalacia)

Baby boy AS was born at 26 weeks of gestation with a birthweight of 740 g. The mother delivered by cesarean section because of pregnancy-induced hypertension, and she was treated with one dose of betamethasone. The infant had been treated with surfactant in the delivery room, with follow-up doses at 12 and 24 hours of age. Mechanical ventilatory support was initiated with PIP = 16 cm H_2O, PEEP = 4 cm H_2O, and a synchronized intermittent mandatory ventilation (SIMV) = 40/min. The baby was extubated to CPAP at approximately 4 days of age and reintubated at day 7 for intractable apnea for 10 days. By 4 weeks of age, the baby was oxygen dependent and had increased work of breathing and radiographic changes of BPD. Serial pressure-volume loops at days 2, 7, 12, and 28 showed increased expiratory resistive work with a widened pulmonary hysteresis (Fig. 18-13). By 4 weeks of age, the baby had increased resistive work with both elastic and resistive load.

Case 2 of a Newborn with "Bronchopulmonary Dysplasia Spells" (Bronchopulmonary Dysplasia and Possible Airway Reactivity)

Baby girl RJ was born at 27 weeks of gestation with a birthweight of 852 g. The mother delivered by spontaneous vaginal delivery with presumed maternal chorioamnionitis, and she

was treated with parenteral antibiotics and one dose of betamethasone. The baby was treated with surfactant in the delivery room, with follow-up doses at 12 and 24 hours of age. Mechanical ventilatory support was initiated with PIP = 18 cm H_2O, PEEP = 5 cm H_2O, and SIMV = 40/min for congenital pneumonia. The baby was extubated to CPAP at approximately 5 days of age and reintubated at day 8 for nosocomial sepsis for 7 days. Subsequently the baby had frequent episodes of "BPD" spells with desaturations and bradycardia that were responsive to albuterol inhalation. By 4 weeks of age the baby was oxygen dependent and had increased work of breathing and radiographic changes of BPD. Serial pressure-volume loops at days 3, 8, 15, and 30 show increased inspiratory resistive work with a widened pulmonary hysteresis (Fig. 18-14). By 4 weeks of age the baby had increased resistive work with both elastic and resistive loads.

Case 3 of a Newborn with Respiratory Distress Syndrome Treated with End-Distending Pressure and Surfactant

Baby boy GW was born at 28 weeks of gestation with a birthweight of 1040 g. He was delivered emergently by cesarean section because of placental abruption. Following resuscitation, the baby was placed on ventilatory support: PIP = 18 cm H_2O, PEEP = 5 cm H_2O, and SIMV = 40/min. Surfactant was administered at about 1 hour of age. Pulmonary graphics (P-V loops) were recorded and FRC measurements were made as the baby was placed on ventilatory support and prior to changes in PEEP at 3, 4, and 5 cm H_2O (Fig. 18-15). Pre-PEEP and pre-surfactant FRC = 10.1 mL (~11 mL/kg). Post-PEEP (5 cm H_2O) and

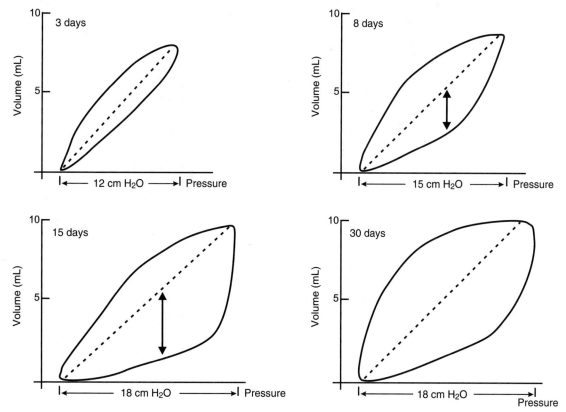

Figure 18-14. Clinical case 2 of a newborn with bronchopulmonary dysplasia spells.

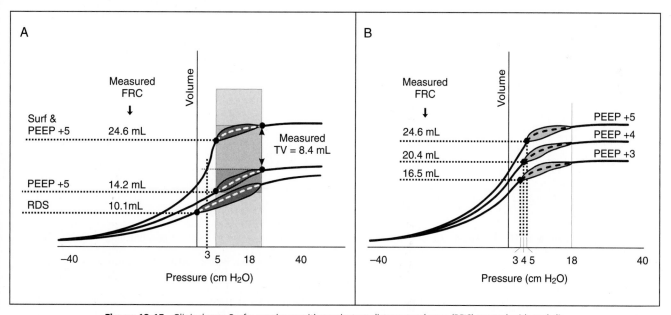

Figure 18-15. Clinical case 3 of a newborn with respiratory distress syndrome (RDS) treated with end-distending pressure and surfactant. FRC, functional residual capacity; PEEP, positive end-expiratory pressure.

presurfactant FRC = 14.2 mL (~14 mL/kg) with slight improvement in tidal volume and pulmonary compliance (steeper slope of the P-V loop). Postsurfactant FRC = 24.6 mL (~24 mL/kg), but the improvement in tidal volume and compliance were masked by the PEEP as evidenced by a flatter (overdistended)

P-V loop. Serial reduction of PEEP to 3 and 4 cm H_2O showed FRC = 16.5 and 20.4 mL, respectively, and improvement in compliance (as evidenced by steeper and less overdistended P-V loops). Note that the selection of optimal PEEP value also depends on its effect on oxygenation.

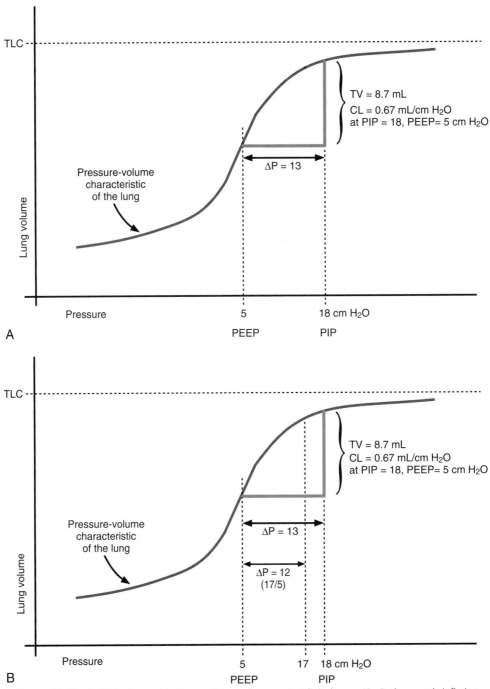

Figure 18-16. *A,* Clinical case 4A. No ventilatory changes. *B,* Clinical case 4B. Reduce peak inflating pressure (PIP).

Figure continued on following page

Case 4 Study of Weaning Strategy in a Newborn with Respiratory Distress Syndrome on Ventilatory Support

At 6 hours of age, this 1350-kg male neonate with RDS was treated with surfactant and was on ventilatory support of PIP = 18 cm H_2O, PEEP = 5 cm H_2O, SIMV = 35 breaths/min, and FIO_2 = 0.55. Arterial gas: pH = 7.32, Pao_2 = 82 torr, and $Paco_2$ = 54 torr. Measured tidal volume (by pneumotachography) = 8.7 mL (6.4 mL/kg). By calculation, driving pressure was 18 (PIP)–5 (PEEP) = 13 cm H_2O; thus, the effective compliance of the baby on a ventilator = $\ddot{A}V/\ddot{A}P$ or 8.7/13 mL/cm H_2O = 0.67 mL/cm H_2O. Therefore, any 1 cm H_2O change in driving pressure leads to a change in volume of 0.67 mL.

Bedside weaning options could include the following: (1) make no changes (Fig. 18-16*A*); (2) reduce PIP by 1 cm H_2O (to 17 cm H_2O) and the driving pressure (at 17–5) = 12 cm H_2O (Fig. 18-16*B*); (3) reduce PEEP by 1 cm H_2O (to 4 cm H_2O) and the driving pressure (at 18/4) = 14 cm H_2O (Fig. 18-16*C*); or (4) change SIMV and thus alter minute ventilation and alveolar ventilation. The impact on tidal volume can be calculated and confirmed by actual measure-

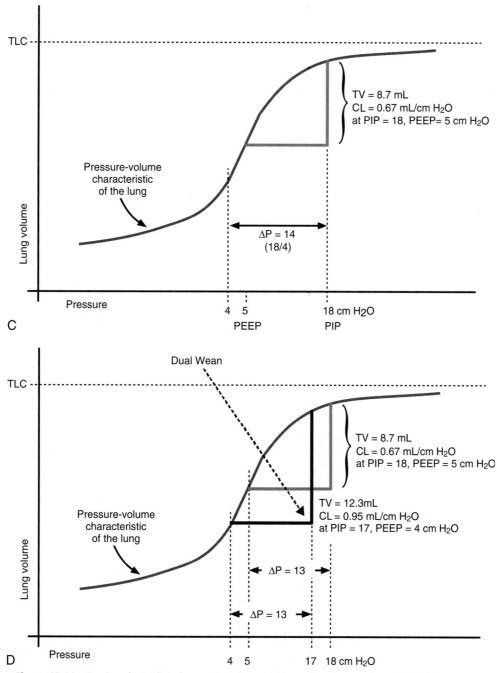

Figure 18-16. *Continued.* *C,* Clinical case 4C. Reduce positive end-expiratory pressure (PEEP). *D,* Clinical case 4D. Dual weaning. CL, compliance; TV, tidal volume.

ment. If the baby is being overventilated at the upper and flatter ends of the P-V slope (as shown in the schematic), the change in the actual tidal volume will be disproportionate to the expected change (as determined from the "effective compliance").

An alternative option could be a *dual wean:* reduce PIP/PEEP (wean both from 18/5 to 17/4 cm H_2O) such that the driving pressure is unchanged = 13 cm H_2O. If the baby is being ventilated at the upper and flatter ends of the P-V slope

(as shown in Fig. 18-16*D*), a dual wean will result in "moving" down to a more linear part of the P-V slope and a marked improvement in the tidal volume, disproportionate to that anticipated as there is now is a change in the driving pressure and no change in tidal volume is expected. Based on bedside calculations ("alveolar algebra" for pulmonary mechanics) the baby could be subsequently and effectively weaned to a lower driving pressure. Note that the weaning of PEEP is to be monitored by its effect on oxygenation.

Alveolar Algebra: Mechanics

Compliance = Δ volume/Δ pressure
Δ of 1 cm H_2O leads to a Δ in volume
Compliance = 12.3 mL/13 cm H_2O = 0.95 mL/cm H_2O
Δ of 1 cm H_2O leads to Δ in volume = 0.95 mL
Δ of 1 cm H_2O to 16/4 will decrease tidal volume (TV) to ~11.3 mL
Δ of 1 cm H_2O to 15/4 will decrease TV to ~10.3 mL
Δ of 1 cm H_2O to 14/4 will decrease TV to ~9.3 mL
Thus, effective driving pressure = 10 cm H_2O

Case 5 of a Very Preterm Newborn with Respiratory Distress Syndrome Being Ventilated with Excessive Circuit Air Flow

Baby boy RS was a 540-g neonate who at 16 hours of age had received two doses of surfactant and was on ventilatory support for RDS with PIP = 20 cm H_2O, PEEP = 5 cm H_2O, SIMV = 60/min, and FIO_2 = 0.66. Arterial blood gases were PO_2 = 72 torr, PCO_2 = 58 torr, and pH = 7.29. Chest radiograph showed evidence of pulmonary interstitial emphysema. Clinicians were considering increasing the level of support or using high-frequency ventilation and an additional dose of surfactant. Another option was to reduce the circuit air flow (which was generally adjusted to eightfold of minute ventilation). In this baby, a reduction of the circuit air flow from 8 to 4 L/min led to an appreciable reduction of the inadvertent PEEP such that subsequent reductions in PIP and PEEP (dual wean, as described earlier) allowed for lowered levels of driving pressure. The resultant reduction in volutrauma/barotrauma possibly was related to the "flow" overdistention. In such a clinical situation, the hypercapnia and the pulmonary air leak usually are iatrogenic.

Outcome Measures for Using Online Pulmonary Functions

Presently there are no evidence-based studies indicating that optimization of ventilatory support, reduction in pressure-related barotrauma, volume, or air flow overdistention, or reduction in alveolar hyperoxemia would reduce the severity or incidence of chronic lung disease. Even though this effect may be conjectured based on the fundamental principles of pulmonary physiology and clinical acumen, such evidence needs to be gathered. Limitations in designing such studies may be attributed to ability to achieve clinical consensus, define appropriate monitoring endpoints for respiratory and alveolar barotrauma, and shift the emphasis from the ventilator (equipment) to the Ventilator (the clinician at the bedside). In the meantime, a clinician needs to be guided to a fundamental principle of neonatal ventilation: "First, use the least level of support to maintain adequate gas exchange."

REFERENCES

1. Röhrer F: Der stromungswiderstand in den mencschlichen atemwegen und der einflus der unregelmassigen verzweigung des bronchialsystems auf den atmingswelauf in verschiedenen lung enberzirken. Arch Ges Physiol 162:225–299, 1915.
2. Peslin R, Felicio da Silva J, Chabot F, et al: Respiratory mechanics studied by multiple linear regression in unsedated ventilated patients. Eur Respir J 5:871–878, 1992.
3. Fisher JB, Mammel MC, Coleman JM, Bing DR, Boros SJ: Identifying lung overdistention during mechanical ventilation by using volume-pressure loops. Pediatr Pulmonol 5:10–14, 1988.
4. Rousselot JM, Peslin R, Duvivier C: Evaluation of multiple linear regression method to monitor respiratory mechanics in ventilated neonates and young children. Pediatr Pulmonol 13:161–168, 1992.
5. Taussig LM, Harris TR, Lebowitz MD: Lung function in infants and young children. Am Rev Respir Dis 116:233, 1977.
6. Tepper RS, Morgan WJ, Cota K, et al: Physiologic growth of the lung during the first year of life. Am Rev Respir Dis 134:513–519, 1986.
7. Gaultier C: Lung volumes in neonates and infants. Eur Respir J Suppl 4:130S–134S, 1989.
8. Abbasi S, Bhutani VK: Pulmonary mechanics and energetics of normal, non-ventilated low birthweight infants. Pediatr Pulmonol 8:89, 1990.
9. Hanrahan JP, Tager IB, Castile RG, et al: Pulmonary function measures in healthy infants. Variability and size correction. Am Rev Respir Dis 141 (5 Pt 1):1127–1135, 1990.
10. Kaiserman KB, Cunningham MD, Martin G, et al: Optimal tidal volume for the mechanical ventilation of the neonate. Pediatr Res 31:311A, 1992.
11. Davis JM, Veness-Meehan K, Notter RH, et al: Changes in pulmonary mechanics after the administration of surfactant to infants with respiratory distress syndrome. N Engl J Med 319:476–479, 1988.
12. Joint Committee of the ATS Assembly on Pediatrics and the ERS Pediatrics Assembly: Respiratory mechanics in infants: Physiologic evaluation in health and disease. Am Rev Respir Dis 147:474–496, 1993.
13. Scarpelli EM: Pulmonary mechanics and ventilation. In Scarpelli EM (ed): Pulmonary Physiology: Fetus, Newborn, Child and Adolescent, 2nd ed. Philadelphia, Lea & Febiger, 1990, p. 276.
14. West JB: Respiratory Physiology: The Essentials, 4th ed. Baltimore, Williams & Wilkins, 1990, p. 16.
15. Taussig LM, Landau LI, Godfrey S, et al: Determinants of forced expiratory flows in newborn infants. J Appl Physiol 53:1220–1227, 1982.
16. Tepper RS, Cota KA, Wilcox EL, Taussig LM, et al: Tidal expiratory flow-volume curves: A simple noninvasive test of pulmonary function in sick and healthy infants. Am Rev Respir Dis 127:217, 1983.
17. Tepper RS, Morgan WJ, Cota K, et al: Expiratory flow-limitation in infants with bronchopulmonary dysplasia. J Pediatr 109:1040–1046, 1986.
18. Tepper RS, Reister T: Forced expiratory flows and lung volumes in normal infants. Pediatr Pulmonol 15:357–361, 1993.
19. Silverman L, Whittenberger JL: Clinical pneumotachograph. In Comroe JH (ed): Methods in Medical Research, Vol. 2. Chicago, Year Book Medical Publishers, 1950, pp. 104–112.
20. Fleisch A: Pneumotachograph: Apparatus for recording respiratory flow. Arch Ges Physiol 209:713, 1925.
21. Sullivan W, Peters G, Enright P: Pneumotachographs: Theory and application. Respir Care 29:736–749, 1984.
22. Polgar G, Lacourt G: A method for measuring respiratory mechanics in small newborn (premature) infants. J Appl Physiol 32:555, 1972.
23. Edberg KE, Sandberg K, Silberberg A, et al: A plethysmographic method for assessment of lung function in mechanically ventilated very low birth weight infants. Pediatr Res 30:501, 1991.
24. Cheviot JS: Continuous non-invasive respiratory monitoring with a neonatal workstation. Neonatal Intens Care 5:26–29, 1992.
25. Fleming PJ, Levine MR, Goncalves A: Changes in respiratory pattern resulting from the use of a face mask to record respiration in newborn infants. Pediatr Res 16:1031–1034, 1982.
26. Miller MJ, Martin RJ, Carlo WA, et al: Oral breathing in newborn infants. J Pediatr 107:465–469, 1985.
27. Stocks J, Beardsmore C, Helms P: Infant lung function: Measurement conditions and equipment. Eur Respir J Suppl 4:123S–129S, 1989.
28. Roske K, Foitzik B, Wauer RR, et al: Accuracy of volume measurements in mechanically ventilated newborns: A comparative study of commercial devices. J Clin Monit Comput 14:413–420, 1998.
29. Bates J, Turner M, Lanteri C, et al: Measurement of flow and volume. In Stocks J, Sly P, Tepper R, et al. (eds): Infant Respiratory Function Testing. New York, Wiley-Liss 1996, pp. 97–98.
30. Yeh MP, Adams TD, Gardner RM, et al: Effect of O_2, N_2, and CO_2 composition on nonlinearity of Fleisch pneumotachograph characteristics. J Appl Physiol 56:1423–1425, 1984.

Suggested Readings

1. Polgar G, Promadhat V: Pulmonary Function Testing in Children. Philadelphia, W.B. Saunders, 1971.

2. Comroe JH: Physiology of Respiration, 2nd ed. Chicago, Year Book Medical Publishers, 1974.

3. West JB: Respiratory Physiology: The Essentials. Oxford, Blackwell Scientific Publications, 1974.

4. Bhutani VK, Abbasi S, Sivieri EM, et al: Evaluation of neonatal pulmonary mechanics and energetics: A two factor least mean square analysis. Pediatr Pulmonol 4:150, 1988.

5. Bhutani VK, Shaffer TH, Vidyasagar D (eds): Neonatal Pulmonary Function Testing. Ithaca, NY, Perinatology Press, 1988.

6. Bhutani VK, Sivieri EM, Abbasi S: Evaluation of pulmonary function in the neonate. In Polin RA, Fox WW (eds): Fetal and Neonatal Physiology, 2nd ed. Philadelphia, W.B. Saunders, 1999, Chapter 105, pp. 1143–1164.

PHARMACOLOGIC ADJUNCTS I

MICHAEL D. WEISS, MD
JAY M. MILSTEIN, MD
DAVID J. BURCHFIELD, MD

Pharmacologic agents are frequently used as adjuncts to therapy with mechanical ventilation. Neonates present a special challenge in this regard because knowledge of drug dosage, distribution, metabolism, and side effects for them is often incomplete. Reported experience is frequently anecdotal, and extrapolation of information from adults or older children to the neonate may be inappropriate. Furthermore, many agents must be used off-label because they have not undergone the rigorous testing in this age group required by the United States Food and Drug Administration (FDA) for inclusion in the package insert. The following discussion is limited to those commonly used drugs not discussed elsewhere in this text, and it is not intended to be a complete reference work.

SEDATIVES AND ANALGESICS

In a survey published in 1997, neonatologists and neonatal nurses rated the pain associated with intubation and with endotracheal suctioning at approximately 2 on a scale from 0 to 4 scale (not painful to very painful). Yet, on average, these same clinicians used pharmacologic pain management rated less than 0.5 on a scale from 0 to 4 scale (never to always).[1] Infants with pain and discomfort may struggle against the ventilator, thereby decreasing the effectiveness of ventilation. This often is referred to as *agitation*. Under such circumstances, sedation and analgesia not only improve ventilation but also may make patients more comfortable, hasten recovery, and even decrease the risk of complications such as pneumothorax and intraventricular hemorrhage.[2,3] Anand et al.[4] found that morphine administered prophylactically reduced the incidence of poor neurologic outcomes from 24% in preterm, ventilated, nontreated patients to 4% in the morphine group. In addition, evidence suggests that pain experienced in the neonatal period carries long-term consequences.[5,6] Therefore, one should consider use of analgesics in all ventilated neonates. In addition, environmental strategies such as swaddling, containment, and facilitated tucking may attenuate physiologic responses to ventilation and endotracheal suctioning and should be attempted as well.[7] Typical dosages for sedatives and analgesics are listed in Table 19-1.

Morphine

Morphine is a well-known opium alkaloid whose major effects are on the central nervous system (CNS) and organs containing smooth muscle, such as the gastrointestinal and urinary tracts. Its mechanism of action as an analgesic agent is the stimulation of opiate receptors in the CNS that mimic the effects of natural endorphins.[8] Sedation, analgesia, and respiratory depression and reduction in body temperature are all produced by the administration of morphine in conventional dosages. Respiratory depression, which is due to effects on respiratory centers in the brainstem, may be marked but is not usually of clinical significance in ventilated infants unless weaning from the ventilator is anticipated. Morphine may cause a reduction in peripheral resistance with little or no effect on cardiac index, leading to hypotension, but usually is well tolerated in neonates. Histamine release is common; bronchoconstriction may occur either as an idiosyncratic reaction or from large dosages. Morphine decreases gastric motility and, at the same time, increases anal sphincter tone and urinary tract smooth muscle tone.

Morphine is well absorbed by all routes, including the oral route, but it is usually given parenterally to sick neonates. The onset of action is prompt and peaks at about 1 hour after injection.[9] The duration of action in neonates may be 2 to 4 hours. Morphine is primarily detoxified by hepatic conjugation with glucuronide, which is then excreted in the urine and bile. The elimination half-life may be up to 9 hours in preterm infants.

The usual dose of morphine sulfate in neonates is 0.05 to 0.2 mg/kg. Repeat doses of the same magnitude may be given as necessary, usually every 2 to 6 hours. Morphine can also be given by continuous intravenous infusion at a rate of 10 to 15 μg/kg/hour after an initial loading infusion of 100 μg/kg over the first hour. With prolonged administration, some degree of tolerance develops, necessitating an increase in dosage. Following this, a weaning regimen that reduces the dose by 10% to 20% per day is recommended to prevent withdrawal.

TABLE 19-1. Sedation and Analgesia for Neonates

Agent	Bolus Dose	Dose Frequency	Infusion Dose
Sedation			
Lorazepam	0.05–0.1 mg/kg	4–12 hr	Not recommended
Midazolam	0.05–0.15 mg/kg	2–4 hr	10–60 μg/kg/hr
Analgesia			
Morphine	0.05–0.2 mg/kg	2–4 hr	10–15 μg/kg/hr
Fentanyl	1–4 μg/kg	2–4 hr	1–2 μg/kg/hr

* Slowly, over approximately 5 minutes

Respiratory depression, decreased gastric motility, and urine retention must be anticipated and considered in the management of infants receiving morphine. Morphine effects can be reversed by naloxone 0.1 mg/kg.

Fentanyl

Fentanyl is a synthetic opioid that has been used for anesthesia and is a popular analgesic agent in neonates. It is 80-fold more potent than morphine on a weight basis but has fewer respiratory depressant and cardiovascular effects. The latter characteristic is considered to be a result of its lesser effect on histamine release.[10] It also has been shown to have less gastrointestinal side effects.[11] Disadvantages of fentanyl, with respect to morphine, include a lack of sedative properties and the risk of chest wall rigidity.[12,13] Fortunately, this as well as its other effects can be reversed by naloxone administration. Fentanyl decreases the stress response to surgery and inhibits certain reflexes such as the baroreflex control of heart rate and the irritant receptors in the airway.[14]

Fentanyl has a fast onset of action; however, it has a shorter duration of effect than morphine (1 to 2 hours).[15] Tolerance occurs more readily with fentanyl than with morphine, and a weaning regimen similar to that described for morphine is highly recommended for infants treated for more than a few days.[16] Fentanyl can be given periodically by intravenous bolus, 1 to 4 μg/kg, when short-term analgesia is desired. If prolonged use is anticipated, infusion is begun at a rate of 1 to 2 μg/kg/hour and is increased according to symptom relief. Clearance is directly related to gestational age and birth weight, so adjustment of the infusion should be individualized in preterm infants.[17] Apnea is much less common when fentanyl is administered as an infusion compared to a bolus; however, it may prolong duration of mechanical ventilation,[18] and one should be cognizant of the possibility of withdrawal.[19]

Diazepam

Diazepam has anxiolytic, hypnotic, anticonvulsant, muscle relaxant, and amnesic effects that are characteristic of benzodiazepines and, like other benzodiazepines, has no analgesic properties. Diazepam is absorbed rapidly following oral administration but irregularly after intramuscular administration. The elimination half-life approximates 75 hours in premature newborn infants and 30 hours in full-term infants.[20] It is metabolized in the liver and, along with its metabolites, is slowly excreted in the urine. No simple correlations exist between plasma level and clinical response. Diazepam can cause respiratory depression, which may actually help infants to "settle" on the ventilator. This agent can be useful as a long-acting sedative when given in doses ranging from 0.10 to 0.25 mg/kg every 6 hours.

Midazolam

Midazolam is a benzodiazepine that is water soluble at acid pH. It has a rapid onset of action (5 to 6 minutes) because at physiologic pH it is lipophilic. It is about twice as potent as diazepam, and it has a more rapid onset and shorter duration of action.[21] Because of this, midazolam has become a popular sedative, especially as a continuous infusion. It is metabolized in the liver, and the metabolites are excreted in the urine. Rapid

injection may produce apnea and a decrease in blood pressure; however, with slower infusions, these side effects are less pronounced than with diazepam.[22] In adult patients, midazolam has more amnesic properties than other benzodiazepines. It is not clear what impact the prolonged administration of midazolam has on neonatal development.

Using the Premature Infant Pain Profile scores, neonates treated with midazolam tolerate painful procedures (such as endotracheal suctioning), as do neonates treated with morphine, and both groups tolerate these interventions better than untreated controls.[4] However, in the study by Anand et al.,[4] infants treated with midazolam showed a higher incidence of adverse neurologic events (death, grade III to IV intraventricular hemorrhage, periventricular leukomalacia) compared with the other groups, particularly morphine. In addition, the midazolam group had a statistically significantly longer duration of neonatal intensive care unit stay compared to the placebo group.

Midazolam usually is given intravenously or intramuscularly in a dose of 0.1 mg/kg, which is repeated every 2 to 4 hours as needed or as a continuous infusion.[23] Clearance is directly related to birthweight,[24] and the dose should be titrated to desired effects. In seriously ill neonates, the terminal elimination half-life of midazolam is substantially prolonged (6.5 to 12.0 hours) and the clearance reduced (0.07 to 0.12 L/hour/kg) compared to healthy adults or other groups of pediatric patients.[24] It cannot be determined if these differences are due to age, immature organ function or metabolic pathways, or underlying illness or debility.

Toxicity due to overdosage is unusual and would likely present as excessive somnolence. Poor social interaction and dystonic movements have been reported in some infants after 4 to 11 days of sedation with a combination of midazolam and fentanyl. Symptoms resolve after discontinuation of use of the medications.[25] Some concern exists regarding possible withdrawal following prolonged use.[26] Finally, the usual parenteral preparation contains 1% benzoyl alcohol as a preservative; this may need to be taken into consideration when dosing this drug.[21] Use of the more concentrated 5 mg/mL preparation will reduce exposure to benzoyl alcohol per milligram of midazolam used.

Lorazepam

Lorazepam is a benzodiazepine with potent anticonvulsant activity, and because it is lipophilic it has a rapid onset of action.[27] The sedative effects of lorazepam are variable in duration (3 to 24 hours). It is conjugated in the liver to an inactive glucuronide, which the liver excretes. Apnea, somnolence, and movement disorders may occur.[28,29] The parenteral preparation contains 2% benzoyl alcohol and 18% polyethylene glycol. Propylene glycol has been implicated in serious toxicity when lorazepam was given as a continuous infusion[30,31]; therefore, we do not recommend this practice.

Lorazepam usually is administered parenterally in doses of 0.05 to 0.10 mg/kg, and administration is repeated every 4 to 12 hours, depending on effect. It can be administered in conjunction with morphine or fentanyl.

Chlorpromazine

Chlorpromazine is a dimethylamine derivative of phenothiazine. It has variable absorption when given orally, reaching peak plasma concentration within 2 to 4 hours after administration. Absorption is greater following intramuscular injection, which results in a fourfold to tenfold greater plasma concentration.[32] Frequently, it is used in combination with meperidine and promethazine, the so-called *lytic cocktail* or *DPT*. As a single agent, chlorpromazine has little if any sedative or analgesic properties[33] and toxicity is common, with its antiadrenergic and anticholinergic properties predominating. Because of lack of efficacy, unacceptable complications, and better alternatives, we do not recommend chlorpromazine, or DPT, as a sedative for ventilated newborns.

Chloral Hydrate

Chloral hydrate is a hypnosedative with actions similar to those of the barbiturates. It does not significantly depress respiratory drive[34]; however, it has no analgesic properties and it is a gastrointestinal tract irritant. Chloral hydrate is well absorbed from the gastrointestinal tract and is converted to trichloroethanol by the liver. Both trichloroethanol and an inactive metabolite, trichloroacetic acid, are conjugated and excreted as glucuronides, primarily in the urine and, to some degree, in the bile.[9]

The half-life of trichloroethanol is 9 to 40 hours and that of trichloroacetic acid is even longer, with no appreciable clearance over a 6-day period after a single 50 mg/kg dose of chloral hydrate.[35] With repeated and prolonged use, trichloroethanol can accumulate to toxic levels and cause paradoxical CNS stimulation, cardiac arrhythmias, and hypotension.[36] Although published documentation of clinical toxicity is scant, the prolonged clearance of these metabolites and potential accumulation make repeated dosing of chloral hydrate in neonates undesirable.

Trichloroacetic acid may displace protein-bound drugs and bilirubin in the newborn. Increased incidence of direct hyperbilirubinemia from chloral hydrate also occurs[37]; therefore, it should be used with caution in jaundiced infants.[10] Dosage of 25 mg/kg every 6 hours has been reported to be effective, but caution is warranted if administration is prolonged beyond a few days.[38] Larger, single doses for one-time sedation appear to be well tolerated.

MUSCLE RELAXANTS

Use of muscle relaxants is not routinely indicated during mechanical ventilation of neonates, although it seems to be popular in certain patient populations such as persistent pulmonary hypertension of the newborn (PPHN).[39] Although paralysis may improve oxygenation and ventilation of severely hypoxemic term infants with persistent pulmonary hypertension, it may have adverse effects on premature infants with respiratory distress syndrome (RDS).[40] Use of synchronized ventilation using ventilator rates above the spontaneous rate of the patient frequently will accomplish the goals of paralysis (see Chapter 12).[41] It may be useful in selected premature infants whose own respiratory efforts interfere with ventilation and may reduce the incidence of pneumothorax in this group of infants.[42]

Perlman et al.[43] demonstrated that the elimination of fluctuating cerebral blood flow velocity by muscle paralysis reduced the incidence of intraventricular hemorrhage in selected preterm infants with RDS. It has also been suggested that muscle paralysis may reduce oxygen consumption[44]; this would be advantageous to infants with compromised oxygenation.[45] Prolonged paralysis of 2 weeks' duration has been associated with disuse atrophy and subsequent skeletal muscle growth failure.[46] Importantly, in terms of pulmonary mechanics, Bhutani et al.[47] have shown a decrease in dynamic lung compliance and an increase in total pulmonary resistance after only 48 hours of continuous paralysis with pancuronium. Both parameters improved by 41% to 43% at 6 to 18 hours after discontinuation of paralysis.

Spontaneous respiratory efforts appear to contribute very little to minute ventilation in the severely ill premature infant with low lung compliance.[45] These infants are at risk of dropping their functional residual capacity following paralysis, possibly through loss of upper airway braking mechanisms.[40] In infants with lung compliance that is less compromised and in larger infants, spontaneous respiratory efforts contribute significantly to total ventilation. Thus, ventilator adjustments (usually increases in rate) are necessary to prevent significant hypoventilation when paralysis is instituted. Monitoring of blood gases, end-tidal carbon dioxide tension, or both, is recommended. Although loss of intercostal muscle tone may lead to an increase in intrathoracic pressure, this does not appear to cause an increase in respiratory resistance.[48]

The primary hazard during paralysis appears to be accidental inconspicuous extubation. The paralyzed neonate is entirely dependent on mechanical ventilation, and careful observation is required. Also, paralysis obscures a variety of clinical signs whose expression depends on muscle tone and movement, such as seizures. Finally, paralysis does not alter the sensation of pain; thus, analgesics should be administered under circumstances in which their use would be indicated in a nonparalyzed infant.

In practice, the decision to administer a muscle relaxant is most often based on clinical observation of an infant in combination with arterial blood gas measurements. Muscle relaxants are used frequently to facilitate hyperventilation therapy (see Chapter 9 and the section entitled Persistent Pulmonary Hypertension of the Newborn in Chapter 23). Analysis of ventilator or esophageal pressure waveforms is a more objective method of assessing whether an infant is in phase with the ventilator and whether mean intrathoracic pressure is increased.[42] However, there is no reliable way of predicting which infants in this circumstance will benefit from paralysis. Thus, muscle relaxants should be administered as a therapeutic trial and their use continued if arterial blood gas values improve during the trial, if nursing care is greatly simplified, or if patient comfort is obvious. If the complications of prolonged paralysis are to be prevented, periodic assessment of the infant in the nonparalyzed state is essential.

The short-acting depolarizing muscle relaxant succinylcholine is infrequently used in the care of neonates, except when paralysis for intubation is necessary; therefore, only the commonly used nondepolarizing agents are discussed in this section. Recommended dosages are listed in Table 19-2.

Pancuronium

Pancuronium bromide, a long-acting, competitive neuromuscular blocking agent, is the muscle relaxant most frequently used in neonates. Gallamine and D-tubocurarine are

TABLE 19-2. Neuromuscular Blocking Agents for Neonates

Agent	Initial Dose (mg/kg)	Dose Frequency	Infusion Dose (mg/kg/hr)
Pancuronium	0.04–0.15	1–4 hr	Not recommended
Vecuronium	0.03–0.15	1–2 hr	0.05–0.10

* Incremental doses, 50 to 100% of the initial dose.

seldom used because of significant cardiovascular effects, sympathetic ganglionic blockade, and, in the case of the former, obligatory renal excretion. All of these agents block transmission at the neuromuscular junction by competing with acetylcholine for receptor sites on the postjunctional membrane.[49] Pancuronium has vagolytic effects, and an increase in heart rate is commonly observed during its use. Pancuronium, administered intravenously, produces maximum paralysis within 2 to 4 minutes. The duration of apnea after a single dose is variable and prolonged in neonates and can last from 1 to several hours. Incremental doses increase the duration of respiratory paralysis. In addition, the duration of paralysis is prolonged by acidosis, hypokalemia, use of aminoglycoside antibiotics, and decreased renal function. Alkalosis can be expected to antagonize blockade. Although renal excretion is the major route of elimination of pancuronium, hepatobiliary excretion and metabolism may account for the elimination of a significant portion of an administered dose.[9]

The recommended dosage in neonates varies from 0.06 to 0.10 mg/kg[49] (see Table 19-2). Although it is customary to administer repeat doses that are of the same magnitude as the initial dose, subsequent doses of half the initial dose may be effective in prolonging paralysis when muscular activity or spontaneous respiration returns. Continuous infusion of pancuronium in neonates is associated with the potential for accumulation because of these patients' slow rate of excretion; thus, this method of administration is best avoided unless electrophysiologic monitoring is available.

The long-term benefits of respiratory paralysis need to be balanced with potential complications. Prolonged use of pancuronium bromide has been implicated in sensorineural hearing loss in childhood survivors of congenital diaphragmatic hernia (CDH).[50] In a pediatric intensive care unit setting, head trauma patients treated with and without paralysis were compared. In the 15 patients with isolated intracranial pathology who received continuous paralysis, compliance progressively dropped by 50% over 4 days. This improved to normal following discontinuation of paralysis. No changes in compliance were measured in the 15 patients with isolated intracranial pathology who were ventilated but not paralyzed. The paralyzed patients required mechanical ventilation longer than the nonparalyzed patients, and 26% of these patients developed nosocomial pneumonia, a complication that was not seen in the nonparalyzed patients.

The effects of pancuronium can be rapidly reversed with the use of the anticholinesterase agent neostigmine 0.08 mg/kg intravenously, preceded by the administration of glycopyrrolate 2.5 to 5 µg/kg, which blocks the muscarinic side effects. Although rapid reversal is seldom needed for medical reasons in neonates receiving assisted ventilation, it may occasionally be useful diagnostically in infants considered to have suffered a CNS insult during paralysis.

Vecuronium

Vecuronium is a short-acting nondepolarizing muscle relaxant that is structurally related to pancuronium. Its onset of action is 1.5 to 2.0 minutes after intravenous bolus infusion, but its duration is only 30 to 40 minutes.[49] It has few cardiovascular side effects and is cleared rapidly by biliary excretion. Thus, it is safer than pancuronium in the presence of renal failure. Interference with excretion or potentiation of effect has been suggested for the use of metronidazole, aminoglycosides, and hydantoins. However, no problems have been observed in infants receiving these agents and vecuronium in its usual dosage.[49] Acidosis can be expected to enhance the neuromuscular blockade provided by vecuronium and alkalosis to antagonize it.[9]

Vecuronium usually is given by continuous intravenous infusion at a rate of 0.1 mg/kg/hour after an initial paralyzing bolus dose of 0.1 mg/kg.[51] Intermittent bolus dosing would need to be so frequent (i.e., every 30 to 60 minutes) that this type of regimen usually is impractical (see Table 19-2.) Continuous infusion is preferred for certain postoperative cardiac patients whose respiratory or other muscular movement may jeopardize the success of the repair. The effects of vecuronium can be reversed by neostigmine administration, as described earlier for pancuronium.

CARDIOTONIC AGENTS

Hypotension is common in premature neonates with RDS. In neonates 23 to 27 weeks of gestation, between 47% and 67% will require inotropic support for hypotension.[52] Signs of cardiogenic shock and its precursors also may be recognized in term newborns following perinatal asphyxia, during severe hypoxemia or metabolic derangements, in certain types of congenital heart disease, and during sepsis. When other attempts to reduce oxygen demand and to support the circulation are inadequate, use of cardiotonic agents may prove life saving.

Development of rational and individualized therapy requires knowledge of the important actions of available agents in neonates, as well as of techniques for the assessment and monitoring of the patients' cardiovascular function. Central venous filling pressures and cardiac output can be difficult to determine in neonates and are not routinely measured. When available, these measures should be considered in conjunction with the usual heart rate, systemic blood pressure, and blood gas measurements and can provide a more objective basis for the selection and manipulation of inotropic agents. Echocardiography can provide several indices of cardiac function that may be useful in guiding therapy with inotropes. For instance, Lopez et al.[53] used echocardiography to show that preterm neonates with RDS treated with a combination of dopamine and dobutamine had supranormal cardiac output despite having blood pressure lower than control infants. The clinician should consider echocardiography in deciding when a neonate may need cardiotonic support and in assessing the response to its use.[54,55]

The developmental status of the cardiovascular system and the transition from the fetal to the newborn state further complicate decisions about therapy in newborns, particularly those born prematurely. The immature myocardium has more non-contractile elements than that of the adult, and the orientation of the contractile elements does not appear to be as well organized.[56] Also, cardiovascular receptors for sympathomimetic amines may differ in number, distribution, and sensitivity from those of the adult.[57] Normally, the heart of the newborn appears to function at near-maximum contractile levels; thus, reserve and inotropic response may be limited.[58,59] Afterload appears to be an important determinant of cardiac output in the newborn state.[60] In addition, the reactive pulmonary circulation of the newborn and the potential for shunting via fetal pathways can compromise oxygen delivery and increase the demands placed on the myocardium.

Attempts to increase the cardiac output pharmacologically should be preceded by strategies to correct hypoxemia, acidosis, hypoglycemia, hypocalcemia, and hypovolemia and to reduce metabolic demands. Cardiac output is the product of left ventricular stroke volume and heart rate (cardiac output = stroke volume × heart rate). The latter can be temporarily augmented by vagolysis with atropine or, more commonly, with chronotropic agents such as isoproterenol or epinephrine administered continuously. An increase in heart rate of 30% usually can be obtained with similar increases in cardiac output. Stroke volume can be increased by increasing the preload (venous return), reducing the afterload (systemic vascular resistance), or increasing myocardial contractility. Drugs that have the ability to increase contractility (positive inotropic effect) include certain sympathomimetic amines, cardiac glycosides, glucagon, and xanthines. Only the first of these currently has practical clinical importance in the treatment of shock.

Sympathomimetic amines are the most potent positive inotropic agents available. These agents have complex actions, depending on their interaction with specific receptors and the distribution of these receptors in the host. Extensive studies have led to the classification of receptors as alpha-adrenergic, beta-adrenergic, or dopaminergic. These receptors are located in the heart and blood vessels, as well as in liver, kidney, pancreas, and nerve terminals.[61] Dopaminergic receptors, which mediate dilation of renal, mesenteric, coronary, and cerebral arterioles, have also been characterized.[62] The receptor actions related to sites in the cardiovascular system are listed in Table 19-3.

The available therapeutic agents have a range of activity from almost pure alpha activity to almost pure beta activity.

The pharmacologic actions of the catecholamines epinephrine, norepinephrine, dopamine, dobutamine, and isoproterenol are related to their selectivity and potency with regard to the stimulation of adrenergic receptors, as summarized in Table 19-4. A further discussion of inotropic agents and their use in the postoperative care of neonatal cardiovascular disease can be found in Chapter 26.

The metabolism of all of the catecholamines is similar. Catechol-O-methyltransferase (COMT) is responsible for the degradation of most exogenously administered agents and monoamine oxidase participates to a lesser degree. COMT activity has wide interpatient variability and increases twofold to sixfold during dopamine treatment, but it may not be the rate-limiting step in catecholamine clearance.[63] All catecholamines are thought to have short half-lives of approximately 2 minutes; therefore, continuous infusion is necessary for attainment of prolonged effect. However, in sick premature infants, half-life and clearance can be prolonged and may explain the enhanced responsiveness to the infusion.[64,65] Metabolites, and perhaps 20% of unchanged substances, are excreted in the urine.

Because norepinephrine has limited clinical usefulness in the neonate, only dopamine, dobutamine, isoproterenol, and epinephrine are discussed further. The recommended dosages of these agents for neonates are listed in Table 19-5.

Dopamine

Dopamine is a naturally occurring catecholamine. Administered exogenously, it has complex cardiovascular effects that are dose related (see Table 19-5).[62,66] In low doses (<4 µg/kg/min), it has primarily vasodilator effects on renal[67,68] and perhaps mesenteric, coronary, and cerebral arterioles. However, in premature infants, an enhanced pressor response has been demonstrated even for these low doses, possibly due to decreased clearance.[65] Larger doses (5 to 10 µg/kg/min) exert a positive inotropic effect on the myocardium via the release of norepinephrine from nerve terminals and through a direct effect on beta$_1$-adrenergic receptors in the myocardium.[69] Decreases in norepinephrine stores secondary to immaturity, heart failure, or both could be expected to limit the inotropic response to dopamine.[70] This has been found to be true in most studies on immature animals.[71] Dosages greater than 10µg/kg/min cause increases in systemic vascular resistance

TABLE 19-3. Cardiovascular Actions of Adrenergic Receptors

Adrenergic Receptor	Site	Action
Beta$_1$	Myocardium	Increase atrial and ventricular contractility
	Sinoatrial node	Increase heart rate
	AV conduction system	Enhance conduction
Beta$_2$	Arterioles	Vasodilation
Alpha$_1$	Peripheral arterioles	Vasoconstriction
Dopamine	Renal, cerebral, mesenteric, and coronary arterioles	Vasodilation

TABLE 19-4. Selectivity of Catecholamines for Adrenergic Receptors

Catecholamine	Receptor			
	Alpha$_1$	Beta$_1$	Beta$_2$	Dopamine
Epinephrine	+++	+++	+++	−
Norepinephrine	+++	+++	+	−
Isoproterenol	−	+++	+++	−
Dopamine*	− to +++	− to +++	++	+++
Dobutamine	− to +	+++	+	−

+, Relative degree of stimulation; −, no stimulation.
* Variable, dose-dependent effects. High doses produce predominant alpha$_1$-adrenergic effects.
Adapted from Zaritsky A, Chernow B: Catecholamines, sympathomimetics. In Chernow B, Lake CR (eds): The Pharmacologic Approach to the Critically Ill Patient. Baltimore, Williams & Wilkins, 1983, p. 483.

TABLE 19-5. Inotropic Agents for Shock in the Neonate

Agent	Dosage (μg/kg/min)	Receptor Affected	Action
Dopamine	2–4	Dopaminergic	Increased renal and mesenteric blood flow
	4–10	Beta$_1$	Increased myocardial contractility
	>10	Alpha$_1$ + beta$_1$	Peripheral vasoconstriction accompanies cardiac effect
Dobutamine	<10	Beta$_1$	Increased myocardial contractility
	>10	Alpha$_1$ + beta$_1$	Peripheral vasodilation accompanies cardiac effect
Isoproterenol	0.05–0.50	Beta$_1$ + beta$_2$	Tachycardia usually accompanies contractility and vascular effects

through stimulation of alpha-adrenergic receptors. Dosages greater than 20 µg/kg/min may increase pulmonary vascular resistance.[72]

Dopamine is effective in treating hypotension in premature infants with RDS.[73–79] In this population, doses as low as 2 µg/kg/min tend to increase blood pressure,[65] although studies show a median effective dose range of 7.5 to 12.5 µg/kg/min for treatment of hypotension.[76,79] One should realize that the improvement in blood pressure with dopamine infusion may come at the expense of left ventricular output, which drops about an average of 14%.[76] Intestinal perfusion also may be compromised,[80] but this has not been universally found.[74]

Dopamine is frequently used in the treatment of neonates with myocardial dysfunction, even though its efficacy in these patients has not been well documented.[61,67,81,82] It is commonly used in neonates with renal insufficiency to improve urine output.[83] Studies to show improvement in the renal side effects of indomethacin have reported conflicting results.[84–86] It also is used for the prevention of the hypotensive effects of pulmonary vasodilators in the treatment of pulmonary hypertension of the newborn.[87] Complications such as arrhythmias and gangrenous skin sloughs (due to infiltrated intravenous infusions of dopamine) are infrequently observed.

In summary, the rate of dopamine infusion must be individually determined for each patient, depending on changes in cardiac output, urine output, blood pressure, and peripheral perfusion desired. In premature infants, even low doses of dopamine probably will affect blood pressure through increasing afterload and thus compromise left ventricular output.

Dobutamine

Dobutamine is a derivative of isoproterenol and has a structure similar to that of dopamine. However, it does not have dopaminergic properties and appears to stimulate the heart primarily via beta$_1$-receptors. In larger doses (>10 µg/kg/min), stimulation of vascular receptors occurs, with beta$_2$-stimulation predominating over alpha$_1$-stimulation.[88] Peripheral vasodilation occurs, which is in contrast to the vasoconstriction that results from the use of similar doses of dopamine.

The inotropic effect of dobutamine appears to be similar to that of dopamine in neonatal animals[69] and, probably, in human infants.[89,90] However, in small preterm infants, dobutamine appears to be more effective in increasing left ventricular output, whereas dopamine appears more effective in raising the mean blood pressure.[53,74–76,78] Therapy combining dobutamine with low doses of dopamine has been tried and appears more promising than treatment with either agent alone.[53,91] Arrhythmias appear to be an infrequent side effect, but, appar-

ently, increased intrapulmonary shunting of blood can occur with dobutamine as well as with dopamine and isoproterenol.[92]

Isoproterenol

Isoproterenol is a synthetic catecholamine with nearly pure beta-adrenergic actions. Because beta$_1$- and beta$_2$-adrenergic receptors are stimulated, both increased myocardial activity and peripheral vasodilation occur.[66] Marked tachycardia and low blood pressure have accompanied its use in neonatal animals.[93] As heart rate increases, so does myocardial oxygen consumption; simultaneously, myocardial oxygen delivery may decrease in the presence of hypotension.[61]

For the neonate, isoproterenol appears to be a secondary agent for the treatment of shock. It may have application when afterload reduction is desirable and when an increase in heart rate can be tolerated. It may be of short-term benefit in patients with complete heart block[94] and has been used to lower pulmonary artery pressure in a patient with Ebstein anomaly.[95] Dosage varies between 0.05 and 0.5 µg /kg/min.

Tachycardia and hypotension are the most common adverse effects of isoproterenol administration. Careful monitoring of central venous pressure and attention to circulating blood volume should accompany its use.

Epinephrine

Epinephrine is an endogenous catecholamine with both alpha- and beta-adrenergic action.[66] The relative actions are dose dependent. At low doses, beta-adrenergic activity predominates, resulting in increased cardiac contractility and output.[96] At higher doses, alpha-adrenergic effects develop, and the resultant peripheral vasoconstriction may offset the desired beta-adrenergic effects.[97] Dosages range from 0.05 to 0.50 µg/kg/min.

For inotropic support when pulmonary blood flow is excessive, epinephrine infusion may be beneficial. In a newborn piglet model of first-stage repair of hypoplastic left heart, Riordan et al.[98] showed epinephrine 0.1 µg/kg/minute decreased the ratio of pulmonary-to-systemic blood flow and improved oxygen delivery compared to dopamine and dobutamine.

Summary

Myocardial dysfunction resulting in a decrease in cardiac output may be accompanied by a combination of increases or decreases in peripheral resistance, hypovolemia, or hypervolemia, and by increases or decreases in metabolic rates. Thus, sound clinical judgment and hemodynamic measure-

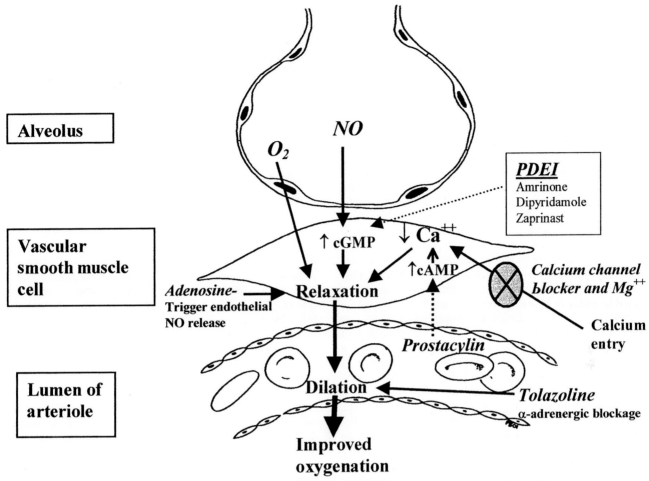

Figure 19–1. Various substances that decrease pulmonary vascular resistance are illustrated graphically. Nitric oxide and phosphodiesterase inhibitors (PDEI) mediate vasodilation by an increase in the amount of cycle guanosine monophosphate (cGMP). Calcium channel blockers and magnesium (by competitive inhibition) block the entry of calcium into the vascular smooth muscle, which decreases the intracellular stores of calcium and leads to vasodilation. Prostacyclin produces a decrease in the amount of cyclic adenosine monophosphate (cAMP), which also decreases intracellular calcium. Adenosine, tolazoline, and oxygen (O_2) mechanisms of action leading to vasodilation also are described.

ments are essential for the selection and dosage of cardiotonic agents. A summary of inotropic agents used in the treatment of shock is given in Table 19-5.

PULMONARY VASODILATORS

PPHN with right-to-left shunting of blood through the ductus arteriosus, foramen ovale, or both can cause severe hypoxemia in newborn infants, both with and without lung disease.[99,100] The diagnosis, clinical course, and causes of PPHN are all discussed in detail in Chapter 23. Although PPHN has numerous etiologies and some of these etiologies, such as CDH, premature closure of the ductus arteriosus, and chronic intrauterine hypoxia, exhibit structural changes in the pulmonary vascular smooth muscle, the common endpoint of increased pulmonary vascular resistance is universal. Agents that decrease pulmonary vascular resistance may be useful therapies for PPHN when hypoxemia proves refractory to mechanical ventilation and O_2 therapy. Substances that

decrease pulmonary vascular resistance are shown graphically in Figure 19-1. Clinical experience with adenosine,[101] magnesium sulfate,[102] calcium channel blockers,[103] prostaglandin E_1,[104] prostaglandin D_2,[105] and prostacyclin[106] is limited. Although tolazoline[100] is still rarely used, it has an undesirable vasodilator effect on the systemic vasculature and recently its production has been stopped by the manufacturer. The use of high concentrations of oxygen and alkalizing agents to increase the blood pH, sometimes combined with hyperventilation, currently remains the front-line vasodilator strategy in neonates with documented PPHN.[39] Recently, inhaled nitric oxide was approved by the FDA for use in neonates. The addition of nitric oxide to the ventilating gas has added a selective pulmonary vasodilator to the clinicians' armamentarium[107,108] and is discussed in detail in Chapter 14.

Alkalosis

Alkalosis to produce a blood pH of 7.50 to 7.60 appears to be the most common vasodilatation therapy, in addition to O_2 therapy, currently used for treatment of PPHN.[39] The mechanism is not clearly established but appears to depend directly on the pH of the blood and not on the release of nitric oxide.[109–111] No critical partial pressure of arterial CO_2 ($Paco_2$) exists, as once thought. Thus, respiratory alkalosis, metabolic alkalosis, or a combination of the two can be used to produce the desired elevation in pH.

Sodium bicarbonate, sodium acetate, and tromethamine (THAM) have all been used to produce alkalosis, with similar results[112,113]; therefore, selection of one of these alkalizing agents often depends on other clinical circumstances. Sodium acetate requires conversion to bicarbonate in the liver and should not be used in the presence of persistent hypoxemia, hypoperfusion, or liver dysfunction.[114] When significant elevation of $Paco_2$ or sodium overload is a concern, some clinicians prefer to use THAM. THAM binds with hydrogen ions, resulting in an increase in bicarbonate ions. Although THAM can change intracellular pH faster than sodium bicarbonate, this characteristic does not appear to be a significant factor in its pulmonary vasodilator effect.[109,110] THAM may cause hyperkalemia and hypoglycemia; therefore its use is not indicated in anuric or hypoglycemic patients.[114]

Treatment usually is initiated with bolus infusions of 1 to 2 mEq/kg of sodium bicarbonate or 1 to 2 mmol/kg of THAM.[114] A continuous infusion is then begun to obtain a desired pH level. Although each infant may have a particular pH at which he or she responds, that pH is routinely between 7.50 and 7.60. After the desired pH has been achieved, it usually is possible to decrease the alkali infusion rate. Often the infusion can be stopped after approximately 48 hours, and the infant remains alkalotic for several more days as the bicarbonate, or THAM, is slowly cleared by the kidneys.

The adverse effects of alkalosis, including an increase in the affinity of hemoglobin for O_2, a decrease in the concentration of ionized calcium, and a decrease in cerebral blood flow, have not been reported to be problems during the treatment of infants with PPHN. A low incidence of neurosensory deafness has been observed in survivors of PPHN, and concern has been raised regarding the role of alkalosis in this sequela.[115] Rapid infusion of hypertonic sodium bicarbonate may play a role in intracranial hemorrhage in premature neonates,[116] and it is recommended that the concentration of sodium bicarbonate not exceed 0.5 mEq/mL and that it not be infused at a rate greater than 1 mEq/mL/min. An infusion of bicarbonate will transiently raise $Paco_2$ but appears to be clinically unimportant in infants receiving effective mechanical ventilation.

All alkalinizing agents, especially THAM, should only be given intravenously, because intra-arterial administration of these solutions has been associated with significant vascular complications, as has administration into the portal system of the liver.[117]

Several reports have drawn attention to the lack of controlled clinical trials in evaluating alkalosis therapy for PPHN. Walsh-Sukys et al.[39] found that systemic alkalosis was not equivalent to respiratory alkalosis in the treatment outcomes of neonates with PPHN. Neonates who were treated with alkali infusions did not show a decrease in mortality and had an increased risk for the use of extracorporeal membrane oxygenation (ECMO) and prolonged oxygen dependency.[39] This is in contrast to neonates treated with hyperventilation who showed a decrease in the use of ECMO without increasing pulmonary morbidity as measured by the use of oxygen at 28 days of age.[39] These same concerns about alkalosis have been raised in particular patient populations, such as neonates with CDH. Based on historical controls, Kays et al.[118] demonstrated decreased mortality in the management of PPHN in neonates with CDH who did not have rigorous management of acidosis or hypercapnia with exogenous alkali infusions or ventilator adjustments. These concerns hopefully will generate a carefully controlled clinical trial of the best management strategy involving alkalosis. Until then, due to the lack of better initial treatment options, alkalosis combined with oxygen will remain a frontline therapy for the treatment of PPHN.

Tolazoline

Tolazoline hydrochloride has been widely used as a pulmonary vasodilator agent in PPHN.[100] Tolazoline, classified as an alpha-adrenergic blocking agent, also has known sympathomimetic, parasympathomimetic, and histamine-like effects.[114] Much of the pulmonary vasodilator action of tolazoline is due to interaction with histamine H_1 and H_2 receptors in the pulmonary circulation[119] and is not mediated through the production of nitric oxide.[120] Tolazoline is excreted unchanged in the urine by means of a combination of glomerular filtration and tubular secretion by the active transport system for organic bases. In neonates, the half-life varies from 3.3 to 33 hours[121] and is highly dependent on urine output.[122]

Tolazoline usually is administered intravenously via vessels returning blood to the superior vena cava. An initial dose of 1 to 2 mg/kg is infused over several minutes, followed by an infusion of 1 to 2 mg/kg/hour. Depending on the response, dosage can be increased to 4 to 6 mg/kg/hour, but caution must be used because of tolazoline's potentially long half-life. It is currently unclear whether continuous infusions of this agent are safe, particularly in the presence of oliguria.[122] A positive response to tolazoline, indicated by an increase in Pao_2 of 15 mm Hg or more within 15 to 60 minutes of administration, occurs in 30% to 60% of infants with PPHN. When the fraction of inspired O_2 has been reduced to 0.6, the tolazoline infusion rate can be reduced every 6 to 12 hours if no deterioration in Pao_2 occurs.

In the presence of myocardial dysfunction or systemic hypotension, a cardiotonic regimen should precede tolazoline infusion. Dopamine infusion, which is continued during tolazoline infusion, appears to be useful in this regard.[123] It should be noted that tolazoline also has cardiac stimulating effects, which may be beneficial when myocardial dysfunction is present.[123]

Adverse effects related to tolazoline infusion are seen in 30% to 80% of infants. The presence of a cutaneous vasodilator response (skin flush) provides evidence that a therapeutic dosage range has been reached. Systemic hypotension responds well to the infusion of blood, colloid solution, or saline. Hypertension is unusual and resolves when the rate of tolazoline infusion is reduced. Abdominal distention is common, and judicious use of nasogastric suction is advised. If gastric bleeding occurs, the use of antacids may be helpful. Oliguria is common; thus, careful fluid administration is recommended. At high dosages (4 to 6 mg/kg/hour), irritability of the CNS has been noted. Because of its multiple side effects, tolazoline should be used with caution after the risks and benefits of therapy have been carefully considered.

Due to the systemic effects of tolazoline and the advent of nitric oxide, the usage of tolazoline has decreased markedly.

Our center, which is a tertiary care ECMO facility, has used this agent eight times in the last 15 years. The last administration was 6 years ago, when our neonatal intensive care unit began using nitric oxide. Tolazoline is no longer commercially available as of 2002.

Endotracheal administration of tolazoline offers an interesting method to circumvent many of the problems associated with systemic administration while gaining the positive pulmonary vasodilator effects. Parida et al.[124] administered endotracheal tolazoline to 12 neonates with gestational ages ranging from 25 to 42 weeks and PPHN. The patients demonstrated a significant increase in arterial oxygen saturation, a decrease in the oxygen index, and no noted drop in systemic blood pressures. However, larger clinical trials should be performed before this is considered an accepted mode of delivery.

Other Agents

Other agents have demonstrated therapeutic value in the treatment of PPHN in small clinical trials. In light of the fact that large randomized trials of nitric oxide have not shown definitive improvements in mortality or a reduction in length of hospitalization, many of these agents may be tried in combination with nitric oxide in the future.[125] This section briefly reviews some of these agents.

Adenosine

Adenosine is a purine nucleoside with a short half-life (<10 seconds) and causes vasodilation by the stimulation of theophylline-sensitive A2 receptors on vascular endothelial cells and subsequent release of nitric oxide by endothelial cells.[101] Endogenous adenosine has been shown to play an important role in facilitating the decrease in pulmonary vascular resistance following birth.[101]

Two small studies examined the effects of adenosine infusion on neonates with PPHN. In a randomized placebo-controlled, masked trial, Konduri and Woodard[101] infused adenosine at a dosage of 25 to 50 µg/kg/min over a 24-hour period and compared the effects on Pao_2 in neonates infused with saline. The results demonstrated an improvement of Pao_2 levels from a baseline of 69 ± 19 to 94 ± 15. The arterial blood pressure and heart rate did not change during the adenosine infusion. Patole et al.[126] used adenosine to treat six neonates with PPHN who did not respond to conventional therapy.[126] A rise in Pao_2 greater than 20 mm Hg occurred in 5 of 6 cases within 30 minutes of commencing infusion. No side effects (bradycardia, hypotension, prolonged bleeding time) were noted. Given the success of these two studies and absence of side effects, larger trials would be of benefit to determine if adenosine alone or in combination with other agents has any bearing on the mortality and/or need for ECMO in neonates with PPHN.

Magnesium Sulfate

Magnesium as a therapeutic drug that produces vasodilation by antagonizing the entry of calcium into smooth muscle cells. It also may act by its effects on the metabolism of prostaglandins, suppression of the release of catecholamines, activation of adenyl cyclase, and reduction of smooth muscle to vasopressors.[127] Magnesium has other potentially desirable effects, including antithrombosis, sedation, muscle relaxation, and the alleviation of oxidant-mediated tissue injury following hypoxia-ischemia.[127]

Several groups have reported beneficial effects of magnesium sulfate therapy in patients with PPHN.[102,127,128] These studies have been small, nonrandomized series of patients. Tolsa et al.[102] administered a loading dose of 200 mg/kg of magnesium sulfate over 20 minutes, followed by an infusion of 20 to 150 mg/kg/hour to maintain a serum concentration between 3.5 and 5.5 mmol/L to neonates with PPHN. Oxygen index and mean airway pressure were significantly reduced after 72 hours of therapy, with no systemic hypotension or other side effects noted.[102] The other two studies had similar findings.[127,128]

Prospective, randomized controlled studies of magnesium sulfate therapy for PPHN have not been performed.[103] Further studies may reveal that magnesium sulfate is a valuable adjunct to other drug therapies for PPHN.

Calcium Channel Blockers

The lack of pulmonary specificity, the high incidence of adverse effects, and the absence of a predictable response in adults suggest caution should be exercised in using calcium channel blockers in newborns with PPHN and related disorders.[103] In spite of these concerns, calcium channel blockers may have a role in certain subsets of patients with PPHN. Islam et al.[129] administered diltiazem hydrochloride to five neonates with recurrent pulmonary hypertension associated with pulmonary hypoplasia refractory to maximal conventional therapy. These neonates demonstrated a significant reduction in right ventricular pressure without overt side effects or systemic hypotension. In conclusion, calcium channel blockers may have a therapeutic value in patients with long-standing pulmonary hypertension.

Prostacyclin (Prostaglandin I₂)

Prostacyclin is an important mediator of pulmonary vasodilation.[130] Increased production of prostacyclin at birth occurs as a result of rhythmic distention of the alveoli.[131] Increased production of prostacyclin results in pulmonary vasodilation, which is an important element in the normal transition to extrauterine life. Patients with severe pulmonary hypertension have demonstrated a deficiency in prostacyclin synthase in pulmonary precapillary vessels.[103] Similarly, transgenic mice overexpressing prostacyclin synthase do not exhibit vascular smooth muscle hypertrophy or pulmonary hypertension when exposed to hypobaric hypoxia.[132]

In humans, a trial of repeated or continuous infusion of prostacyclin via an endotracheal tube to four preterm infants with PPHN demonstrated an improvement in oxygenation.[106] No overt side effects were noted. Other studies have demonstrated a synergy with other pharmacologic agents, including phosphodiesterase inhibitors. Hence, prostacyclin is a promising modality for the treatment of PPHN in neonates.

Nitric Oxide

Nitric oxide therapy has given the clinician a powerful selective pulmonary vasodilating agent. The topic of inhaled NO is discussed in Chapter 14.

BRONCHODILATORS AND MUCOLYTIC AGENTS

For many years, premature infants were thought to have too little bronchiolar smooth muscle to experience bronchospasm. This misconception has been disproved. Subsequently, bronchodilators have been shown to decrease airway resistance and increase compliance in neonates as premature as 28 weeks of gestation with bronchopulmonary dysplasia (BPD), as well as in other infants as young as 2 days of age with RDS.[133] The bronchodilators used have been administered parenterally, enterally, or in aerosol form. In addition to effecting bronchodilation, some agents such as aminophylline have been shown to improve diaphragmatic and inspiratory muscle contractility,[134,135] which may result in both improved ventilation and a greater likelihood of successful extubation. Theophylline and caffeine, methylxanthines that have bronchodilator action, are also used as respiratory stimulants. A more complete discussion and the dosages of these two agents are provided later in this chapter in the section on Respiratory Stimulants. Typical dosages for commonly used aerosolized medications are listed in Table 19-6.

Much of the current literature on bronchodilators has focused on the type of delivery system used for administration.[136] This is discussed in detail at the end of this chapter.

Albuterol (Salbutamol)

Albuterol (also known as *salbutamol*) is a selective beta$_2$-adrenergic agonist. It promotes the production of intracellular cyclic adenosine monophosphate (cAMP), which enhances the binding of intracellular calcium to the cell membrane. This action decreases the calcium concentration within cells and results in the relaxation of smooth muscle and bronchodilation.[137] Denjean et al.[138] studied the effects of albuterol on pulmonary mechanics in premature infants with a mean postnatal age of 13.3 ± 4.9 days and with subacute BPD. Albuterol 100 mg, administered via metered-dose inhaler with a spacer device, resulted in significant improvement in both resistance and compliance in approximately 65% of the infants studied; the remaining patients required 200 mg. The peak responses occurred at 30 minutes and were sustained for approximately 3 hours. Some systemic effects were present as evidenced by an increase in heart rate. In another study involving ventilator-dependent neonates weighing less than 1500 g at birth and between 1 and 4 weeks of age, albuterol improved

compliance; however, airway resistance did not change significantly.[139]

Controversy has arisen over long term beta-agonist stimulation of nonpulmonary tissues, possible adverse effects of long-term bronchodilation on healing lung tissue, and theoretical concerns over the development of tolerance. Therefore, most authors would advocate using beta-agonists in acute symptomatic situations for short periods of time.[140]

Acetylcysteine

Mucolytic agents usually are not required for airway maintenance during mechanical ventilation in the neonate. However, acetylcysteine, a free radical scavenger[141] and potent mucolytic agent, has been useful in some centers. *N*-Acetylcysteine, which has a free sulfhydryl group, liquefies mucus by opening the disulfide bonds in the mucoproteins. It does not affect fibrin, blood clots, or living tissues. At one center, 0.1 or 0.2 mL of acetylcysteine was introduced into the endotracheal tube hourly to maintain airway patency; this was followed by aspiration of the secretions 30 minutes later. No histologic effects were observed on the tracheas or bronchi evaluated on postmortem examination.[142] Bibi et al.[143] showed in 10 ventilator-dependent infants (gestational age 27 weeks; postnatal age 22 days) that treatment with intratracheal *N*-acetylcysteine increased airway resistance significantly. Thus, use of this agent should be undertaken cautiously because its adverse effects may outweigh its benefits. When administered for mucolytic actions, it often is combined with other bronchodilators so that these undesirable effects are offset.

Cromoglycic Acid

Cromoglycic acid (cromolyn sodium) prevents the release of inflammatory mediators from mast cells, inhibits the influx of neutrophils, and inhibits the assembly of an active nicotinamide adenine dinucleotide phosphate (NADPH) oxidase in the neutrophil, thereby preventing tissue damage induced by oxygen radicals.[144] In one study of former premature neonates born at 29 weeks of gestation with recurrent respiratory symptoms, including coughing and wheezing, prophylactic cromoglycic acid aerosol resulted in improvement in both functional residual capacity and "symptom score."[145] Although the results from The Neonatal Cromolyn Study Group did not show a reduction in BPD in the neonates treated with cromolyn sodium,[146] a decrease in inflammatory markers associated with

TABLE 19-6.	Aerosolized Medications for Neonates		
Agent	**Dose**	**Dose Frequency**	**Comments**
Salbutamol	0.20 mg/kg	Every 3–6 hr	With 0.5% solution, dilute 0.04 mL/kg in 1.5 mL NS 18-µg/puff, 1–2 puffs/dose
Ipratropium bromide	0.025 mg/kg	Every 8 hr	with metered-dose inhaler*
N-Acetylcysteine	10–20 mg	Every 6–8 hr	Add bronchodilator if bronchospasm occurs; restricted use advised in view of undesirable effects
Cromoglycic acid (cromolyn sodium)	10 mg	Every 6 hr	Dilute 1 mL of 10 mg/mL solution up to 1.5 mL NS

* Only available metered dose inhaler in the United States
NS; normal saline.

BPD can be demonstrated when sodium cromolyn is used in conjunction with surfactant, diuretics, and steroids.[144,146] Sodium cromolyn may be an important adjunct therapy when used with other agents such as steroids and bears further clinical trials.

Racemic Epinephrine

The subglottis is the narrowest portion of the airway in neonates. The presence of a foreign body, as occurs with prolonged intubation, produces edema in the subglottic region, which can produce further narrowing of the airway when the neonate is extubated. Racemic epinephrine stimulates both alpha- and beta-adrenergic receptors. It acts on vascular smooth muscle to produce vasoconstriction, which markedly decreases blood flow at the capillary level. This shrinks upper respiratory mucosa and reduces edema.[147] Racemic epinephrine is a useful agent in patients with postextubation stridor. The efficacy of racemic epinephrine for prevention of postextubation stridor has not been proven.[147] When using racemic epinephrine, one should be aware of the side effects, which include tachycardia, arrhythmias, hypertension, peripheral vasoconstriction, hyperglycemia, hyperkalemia, metabolic acidosis, and leukocytosis.[147]

DIURETICS

Diuretics are used to treat systemic fluid retention and to decrease edema in the pulmonary interstitium; the latter may cause both oxygenation and ventilation abnormalities and is implicated in the pathogenesis of BPD.[133] Diuretics may help clear the pulmonary interstitial fluid by shifting this fluid into the plasma space following diuresis of intravascular water.

Furosemide

Furosemide is the most common diuretic used in sick neonates. The usual dosage is 1 to 2 mg/kg intravenously. The mode of action is inhibition of chloride reabsorption in the ascending limb of the loop of Henle.[148] The major hazards are electrolyte imbalance, including hyponatremia, hypokalemia, hypochloremia, and alkalosis, as well as dehydration and reduction in blood volume. In addition, hypercalciuria leading to nephrocalcinosis can occur.[149,150] Furosemide is potentially ototoxic and should be used with caution in patients receiving aminoglycosides.[114]

Furosemide therapy has resulted in short-term improvement in airway resistance and dynamic pulmonary compliance in infants with BPD.[151] Furosemide has also been shown to improve lung compliance in infants recovering from RDS. The latter effect appears to result from direct pulmonary effects and is independent of the drug's diuretic actions.[152] In patients with BPD, prolonged therapy has resulted in improvement in mechanical properties of the lung without significant change in gas exchange.[153]

When inhaled, furosemide may have a direct effect on the lung, as the pulmonary effects can occur in the absence of diuresis.[154] In a small series of neonates with BPD, compliance and resistance improved.[155] This mode of delivery offers the advantage of possibly decreasing systemic side effects while maintaining desired pulmonary effects. However, in view of the lack of data from randomized trials on the effects of aerosolized loop diuretics on important clinical outcomes, routine or sustained use of this mode of deliver cannot be justified based on the current evidence.[156]

Furosemide may decrease transvascular fluid flux in the interstitium via nondiuretic mechanisms. These changes may be mediated by prostaglandin E release, which has bronchodilator and pulmonary vasodilator action.[157] The release of prostaglandin E may explain the association of furosemide therapy resulting in an increased risk for patent ductus arteriosis.[158]

Thiazides and Potassium-Sparing Diuretics

Chlorothiazide, a potent oral diuretic, has its major site of action in the proximal portion of the distal tubule[148] by inhibiting chloride reabsorption.[157] In addition, it decreases renal calcium excretion compared to loop diuretics.[148] Spironolactone, a potassium-sparing diuretic, competes with aldosterone in the distal convoluted tubule.[157] Because of the nature of aldosterone's mode of action, which is dependent on protein synthesis, the onset of action of spironolactone is delayed. In combination, these agents increase urinary excretion of sodium, potassium, and phosphorus while decreasing urinary calcium excretion. The usual dosages of chlorothiazide and spironolactone are 10 to 20 mg/kg and 1 to 2 mg/kg, respectively. This combination, given orally, results in improved lung function in infants with chronic lung disease (CLD).[159] Potential electrolyte imbalance (particularly potassium and phosphorus depletion) may occur; thus, monitoring of these electrolytes is necessary.

Because of reports of serious neurologic complications with systemic steroid use, diuretic therapy should be strongly considered as a first-line therapy for early CLD. Chronic administration of thiazide–spironolactone leads to improved lung function and reduces the need for furosemide in neonates older than 3 weeks of age with CLD.[160] Further, thiazide–spironolactone may decrease the risk of death and decrease the incidence of continued intubation beyond 8 weeks in neonates who do not receive corticosteroids, bronchodilators, or aminophylline.[160]

STEROIDS

Corticosteroids have been tried for three distinct respiratory entities in neonatal medicine: acute RDS, post-extubation stridor, and developing CLD. They have not proved useful in treating the RDS in the newborn.[161]

Steroids may be helpful in reducing glottic and subglottic edema during trials of extubation in these infants. The Cochrane Collaborative Review concluded that dexamethasone reduces the need for endotracheal reintubation after a period of mechanical ventilation.[162] However, the review also warns that given the side effects of the medication, dexamethasone usage should be restricted to infants at increased risk for airway edema and obstruction, such as those who have undergone repeated or prolonged intubations.[162]

Despite the use of antenatal corticosteroids and postnatal surfactant treatment, the incidence of CLD has increased.[163]

Two associated points may offer a partial explanation for the increase in the incidence of CLD: the incidence of CLD has an inverse relationship with birthweight and gestational age,[164] and survival of extremely-low-birthweight neonates has increased.[165] Steroids are widely used in the treatment of CLD of prematurity, also known as BPD.[166–169] CLD is a common complication seen in survivors of neonatal intensive care, and inflammation plays an important role in its pathogenesis.[170] Treatment with corticosteroids is an attractive therapy due to its powerful anti-inflammatory properties.

Glucocorticoids have relatively long half-lives (cortisol 8 to 12 hours; prednisone 12 to 36 hours; dexamethasone 36 to 72 hours). These agents are metabolized in the liver to inactive compounds that are excreted by the kidney. High-dose therapy with dexamethasone or prednisone has resulted in rapid reduction in O_2 requirements and ventilator settings[171] and in improvement in lung compliance and gas exchange[172] in over half of the infants treated. In most cases, any improvement occurred during the first 5 days of therapy. The major positive effect has been a shortening of the time to extubation by 1 to 3 weeks.[166–169]

Systemic corticosteroids have potent acute side effects, which include hyperglycemia, hypertension, hypertrophic obstructive cardiomyopathy, gastrointestinal hemorrhage and perforation, growth failure, and hypothalamic-pituitary-adrenal suppression.[163] Animal studies have also demonstrated that steroids can permanently affect brain cell division, differentiation, and myelination, as well as ontogeny of cerebral cortical development.[163] Follow-up studies in humans have added further cause for alarm. Neonates given dexamethasone 12 hours after birth showed a twofold increase in neuromotor impairments compared with controls at 2 years of age.[163,173]

The timing of initiation of therapy has been the subject of analysis in the Cochrane Collaboration, which performed a set of meta-analyses on corticosteroid therapy instigated at three different time points: early (<96 hours in at-risk neonates), moderately early (7 to 14 days in at-risk neonates), and delayed (>3 weeks). At the early time point, the meta-analysis demonstrated benefits with regard to early extubation, decreased risks of CLD, death or CLD at 28 days, patent ductus arteriosis, and pulmonary air leaks.[174] Gastrointestinal bleeding and intestinal perforation were important adverse effects at this time point.[174] Importantly, several adverse neurologic effects were found at follow-up examinations of neonates treated with early steroid therapy: abnormal neurologic examination, cerebral palsy, and developmental delay.[174,175]

Results for the administration at the moderately early time point (7 to 14 days) demonstrated most of the positive effects seen in the early time point.[176] Only one small follow-up study performed at this time point did not reveal any increase in adverse neurologic outcome.[168,176] At the later time point, steroids did not reduce mortality, lung disease at 36 weeks, or the need for late rescue treatment with dexamethasone.[177]

Due to the concerns of neurologic outcomes, we reserve steroid therapy to neonates 12 to 14 days of age who are not actively weaning from the ventilator. A short course of 7 days is given, consisting of 0.25 mg/kg/dose every 12 hours for 4 days followed by 0.05 mg/kg/dose every 12 hours for 3 days. The therapy is then stopped. If the patient experiences a marked increase in ventilator settings after steroid therapy is stopped, the therapy is restarted and a longer weaning course is begun.

Inhaled steroids offer an attractive way to interrupt the inflammatory cascade of CLD while minimizing potential side effects and long-term morbidity. To date, inhaled steroids have shown a reduction in the need for systemic steroids but have not demonstrated a reduction in the incidence of CLD.[163] The results of the various inhaled steroid studies are summarized in Table 19-7.[154] Although no particular study shows a clear benefit over systemic steroids, inhaled steroids offer an attractive therapy for CLD for the reasons stated. The exact dosage, timing of therapy, agent, course, and possible combination with systemic steroids remain to be elucidated before this mode of delivery replaces systemic steroids.

The American Academy of Pediatrics has recently issued a statement reviewing the short- and long-term effects of systemic and inhaled postnatal corticosteroids for the prevention or treatment of CLD. Routine use in very-low-birthweight infants was not recommended.[177a]

RESPIRATORY STIMULANTS

Respiratory stimulants can be useful in the treatment of neonates with apnea of prematurity.[133,178,179] After the evaluation and treatment of these infants for specific, treatable underlying conditions such as infection or hypoglycemia, therapeutic regimens for apnea often include tactile stimulation, reduction in ambient temperature, continuous positive airway pressure, or intermittent mandatory ventilation. Some infants respond favorably to respiratory stimulants as separate or adjunctive therapy. In practice, the decision to administer a respiratory stimulant is dependent on the severity of the apnea and the patient's response to other interventions. If the apnea is severe and frequent, assisted ventilation usually is instituted first. When the apnea is less severe, the stimulant can be used without resorting to mechanical ventilation (see Chapter 3).

Occasionally, babies with severe RDS have recurrent apnea during attempts at weaning from assisted ventilation. Some have been effectively weaned more rapidly while being treated with respiratory stimulants.[180] Weaning from ventilatory support with the use of respiratory stimulants has been reported in small series of infants with BPD[181] and in infants on low ventilatory settings.[152] The benefit of using theophylline prophylactically to reduce the incidence of postextubation respiratory failure and the need for reintubation was shown in an earlier study,[182] but a more recent meta-analysis of the literature could not prove efficacy in this regard.[162] However, in postoperative premature patients, caffeine appears to prevent postoperative apnea/bradycardia and episodes of oxygen desaturation.[183]

The methylxanthines theophylline and caffeine are the most frequently used respiratory stimulants. These agents are respirogenic, primarily because they increase the respiratory center output.[178,184] In addition, they increase chemoreceptor sensitivity to carbon dioxide and strengthen diaphragmatic contractions.[134] The two agents may not have exactly the same mechanism of action. The tidal volume appears to be increased by theophylline, but the drug has minimal effect on respiratory frequency. In contrast, it is the respiratory frequency, not the tidal volume, that is increased by caffeine. Usual dosages for the methylxanthines are listed in Table 19-8. The biochemical and physiologic effects of xanthines are listed in Table 19-9.

TABLE 19-7. Published Randomized Placebo-Controlled Trials of Inhaled Steroids

Reference	Sample Size	Dosage	Recruitment Criteria	Delivery Method	Placebo	Positive Results in Steroid-Treated Infants
Laforce et al	13	Beclomethasone 3 × 50 μg for 28 days	>14 days, CXR BPD, VLBW	Nebulization through ventilator circuit or face mask	No blinded placebo	CRS; R(aw); no difference in infection
Geip et al	19	Beclomethasone 1000 μg daily for 7 days or until extubated	>14 days, VLBW, CXR BPD	MDI + spacer	Double blind	Extubation
Arnon et al	20	Budesonide 600 μg twice daily for 7 days	14 days, BW <2000 g, IPPV	MDI + spacer	Double blind	Significant PIP; no difference in serum cortisol levels
Ng et al	25	Fluticasone propionate 1,000 μg per day for 14 days	First 24 hours, <32 weeks' GA, VLBW	MDI + spacer	Double blind	Basal and post stimulation plasma ACTH and serum plasma cortisol concentrations significantly suppressed
Kovacs et al	60	Dexamethasone 0.5 mg/kg/day for 3 days, then nebulized budesonide 1000 μg for 18 days	>7 days, <30 weeks' GA, VLBW, IPPV	Nebulization	Not double blind	7/30 vs 17/30 required rescue dexamethasone; CRS; similar cortisol levels
Fok	53	Fluticasone 500 μg bid for 14 days	<24 hours, VLBW, IPPV	MDI + spacer	Double blind	17/27 vs 8/26 extubated at 14 days; CRS
Cole et al	253	Beclomethasone 40 μg/kg/day, decreasing to 5 μg/kg over 4 weeks	3–14 days, <33 weeks' GA, ≤1 250 g, IPPV	MDI + spacer neonatal anesthesia bag + ET tube (even when extubated)	Double blind	Rescue dexamethasone, RR 0.6 (0.4–1.0); IPPV at 28 days, RR 0.8 (0.6–1.0) at 28 days

ACTH, adrenocorticotropic hormone; CRS, compliance; CXR BPD, chest radiograph appearance consistent with bronchopulmonary dysplasia, ET, endotracheal; GA, gestational age; IPPV, ventilator dependent (intermittent positive-pressure ventilation; MDI, metered-dose inhaler; PIP, peak inspiratory pressure; R(aw), airway resistance; VLBW, very low birthweight. (From Greenough A: Prevention and management of neonatal chronic lung disease: Short-term gains, but long-term losses. Neonat Respir Dis 10:1–7, 2000.)

TABLE 19-8. Methylxanthines for Neonatal Apnea

Drug	Loading Dose (IV, mg/kg)	Maintenance Dosage (IV)*	Plasma Concentration (mg/L)	Toxicity
Theophylline	5.5–6.0	1 mg/kg every 8 hr, or 2 mg/kg every 12 hr	7–20† (~ 10 ideal)	Cardiovascular: tachycardia CNS stimulation: seizures, jitteriness Gastrointestinal: vomiting, distention
Caffeine	10	2.5–5 mg/kg every 24 hr	7–20†	Unlikely with plasma levels <50 mg/L
Caffeine citrate	20	5–10 mg/kg every 24 hr		As for caffeine

* Oral dosage = IV dosage × 1.25.
† Monitor levels and screen for signs of toxicity.

TABLE 19-9. Effects of Xanthines

Biochemical
Inhibition of phosphodiesterase

Central Adenosine Antagonism
Enhancement of calcium flux across sarcolemma (?)

Physiologic
Increased minute ventilation
Shift of CO_2 response curve to left, with or without increase in slope
Greater efficiency of diaphragmatic contraction
Improved pulmonary mechanics
Decreased hypoxic ventilatory depression

Theophylline

Theophylline (1,3-dimethylxanthine) has a half-life of approximately 30 hours. In the adult, theophylline is eliminated by hepatic biotransformation and urinary excretion. In the newborn, however, the hepatic biotransformation with N-demethylation is absent; instead, the occurrence of N-7-methylation produces caffeine.[178] The therapeutic plasma concentration is about 7 to 20 mg/L. In one study, levels greater than 6.6 mg/L controlled apneic spells, whereas cardiovascular toxicity with tachycardia was noted only at levels greater than 13.0 mg/L.[185] Some newborns manifested toxicity at levels of 9.0 mg/L of transplacentally acquired theophylline. Because of the problems at these lower levels and because of the potential additive effects of the caffeine produced from theophylline, 10 mg/L may be a desirable level. Signs of toxicity may include irritability, diaphoresis, diarrhea, seizures, gastroesophageal reflux, and tachycardia.[133] The usual intravenous loading dose of theophylline is 4.0 to 6.0 mg/kg, with a maintenance dose of 1 mg/kg every 8 hours or 2 mg/kg every 12 hours. Serum trough levels should be evaluated 48 to 72 hours after maintenance therapy has been started.

Caffeine

Caffeine (1,3,7-trimethylxanthine) has a plasma half-life of about 100 hours in the newborn. The extremely long half-life is due primarily to a slow elimination rate. In the adult, most of the caffeine is converted to demethylated xanthines and methyluric acids by the liver. In the neonate, however, most of the caffeine is excreted unchanged in the urine. This may be due to deficiency of the hepatic cytochrome P-450 enzyme system, which may be responsible for methylxanthine metabolism. The therapeutic plasma concentration is about 8 to 20 mg/L. Concentrations as low as 3 to 4 mg/L have controlled apneic spells, and no cardiovascular, CNS, or gastrointestinal toxicity was noted at levels up to 50 mg/L.[178] The usual loading dose of caffeine is 10 mg/kg, with a daily maintenance dose of 2.5 to 5 mg/kg. (The usual form of caffeine, the citrate in a 20-mg/mL solution, is equivalent to a 10-mg/mL solution of the base.)

The toxic manifestations of these agents are related to the relative activity each has on different sites. Theophylline has more cardiovascular than CNS activity. Consequently, early signs of toxicity are cardiovascular in origin, followed by seizure activity. Caffeine has more marked CNS than cardiovascular activity, but toxicity is rarely seen because the levels required for toxic manifestations are extremely high. Although theophylline may have a slight advantage over caffeine in mean number of apnea events during the first 1 to 3 days of treatment, this advantage disappears later.[186] Because of the similar therapeutic profile combined with fewer toxicities,[186] we prefer to use caffeine as a first-line respiratory stimulant.

When methylxanthine therapy fails to prevent apneic spells, other respiratory stimulants, including doxapram, have occasionally been used successfully.[187] Studies of its use have been hampered by small sample sizes, and its long-term benefits are unclear.[188] Doxapram is formulated in sodium benzoate, which is the suspected cause of the "gasping syndrome" in neonates, and thus it is not currently recommended for neonatal use.[189]

Aerosolized Medications

As illustrated in several examples throughout the chapter, aerosol medications offer the theoretical advantage of drug delivery directly to the airways and lungs, often with smaller dose requirements and fewer adverse side effects compared to intravenous or oral therapy.[190] However, aerosol delivery of medications remains a very complicated endeavor. Such issues as host-related factors, the characteristics of the medication (particle size, shape, density), most effective aerosol generator

(nebulizer, pressurized meter dose inhaler), delivery device (face mask, endotracheal tube), and drug dosing remain to be fully evaluated.[190] These issues are discussed briefly in the following paragraphs. For a more thorough review, please consult the review by Cole.[190]

Host-Related Factors

The neonatal pulmonary anatomy (size of airways, nasal breathing, lung development), physiology (breathing pattern, tidal volume, pulmonary mechanics), and pathophysiology (inflammation, mucus, atelectasis, fibrosis) present several unique challenges to aerosolized drug delivery to the distal airway compared to adults.[191,192] The host-related factors often require the clinician to use the following strategies to deliver adequate drug delivery to the neonate: increasing the amount of aerosol, applying meticulous techniques in aerosol delivery, and providing slower breaths with larger inspiratory volumes via face mask or endotracheal tube during aerosol delivery.[190]

Aerosol-Related Factors

Aerosol characteristics include particle size, shape, viscosity, and density.[190] Of these characteristics, particle size is probably the most important. Particles between 2 and 6 μm deposit in the central airway. Smaller, less dense particles are more likely to distribute to the peripheral airways and distal lung regions, thereby reaching desired pulmonary receptors or being absorbed systemically.[193,194]

The aerosol delivery system is the next major variable in ensuring adequate drug delivery using the respiratory route. The advantages and disadvantages of each delivery device are summarized in Table 19-10.[190]

Clinical Applications

Currently, the primary use of aerosolized medications in neonates is for treatment of evolving or established CLD.[190] The medications most commonly used are bronchodilators and anti-inflammatory agents. However, as mentioned in earlier sections, other agents may have a major impact on the neonatal lung when they are delivered via aerosolization while minimizing unwanted systemic side effects.

In spite of the complexities associated with aerosolized drug delivery, the inhaled drug delivery route offers great potential promise for delivery of many medications in the neonate.

SUMMARY

All of the drugs discussed should be dispensed by personnel who are competent in their administration, know their effects, and are aware of the attention required for patient monitoring. Techniques for the monitoring of many serum drug levels now are available in many centers. The information that such monitoring provides may allow the clinician to use these agents with greater accuracy and safety. A list of some drugs commonly used for ventilated infants and their recommended dosages is found in Appendix 32.

TABLE 19-10.   Advantages and Disadvantages of Aerosol Generators in Neonates

Aerosol Generator	Advantages	Disadvantages
Pressurized metered-dose inhaler (pMDI)	• More consistent aerosol particle size and output • Less time consuming to administer • Less preparation time • Less contamination • Less expensive than single-use nebulizers	• Technique problems • Lack of pure medications • Not all medications available in pMDI • New HFA formulations needed for clinical study
Jet nebulizer	• Tidal breathing • Passive cooperation • May be used for long periods to deliver high doses • Wide range of medications output	• Expensive and inconvenient • Inefficient and highly variable aerosol output • Numerous environmental factors affect aerosol particle size and • Poor aerosolization of suspensions and viscous solutions • Preparation time • Time consuming to administer • Contamination potential • Requires compressed gas
Ultrasonic nebulizer	• Potentially more efficient than jet nebulizer and pMDI • Tidal breathing • Passive cooperation • May be used for long periods to deliver high doses	• Expensive and inconvenient • Requires power source • Contamination potential • Limited medications available for use • Preparation time • Time consuming to administer

(From Cole C: Use of aerosolized medicines in neonates. Neonat Respir Dis 10:1–12, 2000.)

REFERENCES

1. Porter FL, Wolf CM, Gold J, et al: Pain and pain management in newborn infants: A survey of physicians and nurses. Pediatrics 100:626–632, 1997.
2. Quinn MW, Otoo F, Rushforth JA, et al: Effect of morphine and pancuronium on the stress response in ventilated preterm infants. Early Hum Dev 30:241–248, 1992.
3. Levene MI, Quinn MW: Use of sedatives and muscle relaxants in newborn babies receiving mechanical ventilation. Arch Dis Child 67 (7 Spec No):870–873, 1992.
4. Anand KJ, Barton BA, McIntosh N, et al: Analgesia and sedation in preterm neonates who require ventilatory support: Results from the NOPAIN trial. Neonatal Outcome and Prolonged Analgesia in Neonates. Arch Pediatr Adolesc Med 153:331–338, 1999.
5. Johnston CC, Stevens BJ: Experience in a neonatal intensive care unit affects pain response. Pediatrics 98:925–930, 1996.
6. Taddio A, Katz J, Ilersich AL, et al: Effect of neonatal circumcision on pain response during subsequent routine vaccination. Lancet 349:599–603, 1997.
7. Anand KJ: Consensus statement for the prevention and management of pain in the newborn. Arch Pediatr Adolesc Med 155:173–180, 2001.
8. Beaumont A, Hughes J: Biology of opioid peptides. Annu Rev Pharmacol Toxicol 19:245–267, 1979.
9. Jaffe JH MW: Opioid analgesics and antagonists. In: The Pharmacologic Basis of Therapeutics, 7th ed. New York, Macmillan Publishing Co., 1985, p. 491.
10. Maxwell GM: Principles of Pediatric Pharmacology. London, Croom Helm, 1984, p. 124.
11. Saarenmaa E, Huttunen P, Leppaluoto J, et al: Advantages of fentanyl over morphine in analgesia for ventilated newborn infants after birth: A randomized trial. J Pediatr 134:144–150, 1999.
12. Wells S, Williamson M, Hooker D: Fentanyl-induced chest wall rigidity in a neonate: A case report. Heart Lung 23:196–198, 1994.
13. Lindemann R: Respiratory muscle rigidity in a preterm infant after use of fentanyl during Caesarean section. Eur J Pediatr 157:1012–1013, 1998.
14. Murat I, Levron JC, Berg A, et al: Effects of fentanyl on baroreceptor reflex control of heart rate in newborn infants. Anesthesiology 68:717–722, 1988.
15. Arnold JH, Truog RD, Scavone JM, et al: Changes in the pharmacodynamic response to fentanyl in neonates during continuous infusion. J Pediatr 19:639–643, 1991.

16. Arnold JH, Truog RD, Orav EJ, et al: Tolerance and dependence in neonates sedated with fentanyl during extracorporeal membrane oxygenation. Anesthesiology 73:1136–1140, 1990.
17. Saarenmaa E, Neuvonen PJ, Fellman V: Gestational age and birth weight effects on plasma clearance of fentanyl in newborn infants. J Pediatr 136:767–770, 2000.
18. Vaughn PR, Townsend SF, Thilo EH, et al: Comparison of continuous infusion of fentanyl to bolus dosing in neonates after surgery. J Pediatr Surg 31:1616–1623, 1996.
19. Katz R, Kelly HW, Hsi A: Prospective study on the occurrence of withdrawal in critically ill children who receive fentanyl by continuous infusion. Crit Care Med 22:763–767, 1994.
20. Yaffe SJ, Back N: Pediatric pharmacology. Postgrad Med 40:193–201, 1966.
21. Reves JG, Fragen RJ, Vinik HR, et al: Midazolam: Pharmacology and uses. Anesthesiology 62:310–324, 1985.
22. Jacqz-Aigrain E, Wood C, Robieux I: Pharmacokinetics of midazolam in critically ill neonates. Eur J Clin Pharmacol 39:191–192, 1990.
23. Jacqz-Aigrain E, Daoud P, Burtin P, et al: Placebo-controlled trial of midazolam sedation in mechanically ventilated newborn babies. Lancet 344:646–650, 1994.
24. Burtin P, Jacqz-Aigrain E, Girard P, et al: Population pharmacokinetics of midazolam in neonates. Clin Pharmacol Ther 56(6 Pt 1):615–625, 1994.
25. Bergman I, Steeves M, Burckart G, et al: Reversible neurologic abnormalities associated with prolonged intravenous midazolam and fentanyl administration. J Pediatr 119:644–649, 1991.
26. Fonsmark L, Rasmussen YH, Carl P: Occurrence of withdrawal in critically ill sedated children. Crit Care Med 27:196–199, 1999.
27. McDermott CA, Kowalczyk AL, Schnitzler ER, et al: Pharmacokinetics of lorazepam in critically ill neonates with seizures. J Pediatr 120:479–483, 1992.
28. Sexson WR, Thigpen J, Stajich GV: Stereotypic movements after lorazepam administration in premature neonates: A series and review of the literature. J Perinatol 15:146–149; quiz 50–51, 1995.
29. Lee DS, Wong HA, Knoppert DC: Myoclonus associated with lorazepam therapy in very-low-birth-weight infants. Biol Neonate 66:311–315, 1994.
30. Arbour RB: Propylene glycol toxicity related to high-dose lorazepam infusion: Case report and discussion. Am J Crit Care 8:499–506, 1999.
31. Reynolds HN, Teiken P, Regan ME, et al: Hyperlactatemia, increased osmolar gap, and renal dysfunction during continuous lorazepam infusion. Crit Care Med 28:1631–1634, 2000.

32. Roberts R: Drug Therapy in Infants. Philadelphia, WB Saunders, 1984, p. 305.
33. American Academy of Pediatrics Committee on Drugs: Reappraisal of lytic cocktail/demerol, Phenergan, and Thorazine (DPT) for the sedation of children. Pediatrics 95:598–602, 1995.
34. Lees MH, Olsen GD, McGilliard KL, et al: Chloral hydrate and the carbon dioxide chemoreceptor response: A study of puppies and infants. Pediatrics 70:447–450, 1982.
35. Mayers DJ, Hindmarsh KW, Sankaran K, et al: Chloral hydrate disposition following single-dose administration to critically ill neonates and children. Dev Pharmacol Ther 16:71–77, 1991.
36. Hartley S, Franck LS, Lundergan F: Maintenance sedation of agitated infants in the neonatal intensive care unit with chloral hydrate: New concerns. J Perinatol 9:162–164, 1989.
37. Lambert GH, Muraskas J, Anderson CL, et al: Direct hyperbilirubinemia associated with chloral hydrate administration in the newborn. Pediatrics 86:277–281,1990.
38. Kuzemko JA, Hartley S: Treatment of cerebral irritation in the newborn: Double-blind trial with chloral hydrate and diazepam. Dev Med Child Neurol 14:740–746, 1972.
39. Walsh-Sukys MC, Tyson JE, Wright LL, et al: Persistent pulmonary hypertension of the newborn in the era before nitric oxide: Practice variation and outcomes. Pediatrics 105(1 Pt 1):14–20, 2000.
40. Miller J, Law AB, Parker RA, et al: Effects of morphine and pancuronium on lung volume and oxygenation in premature infants with hyaline membrane disease. J Pediatr 125:97–103, 1994.
41. Shaw NJ, Cooke RW, Gill AB, et al: Randomised trial of routine versus selective paralysis during ventilation for neonatal respiratory distress syndrome. Arch Dis Child 69(5 Spec No):479–482, 1993.
42. Greenough A, Wood S, Morley CJ, et al: Pancuronium prevents pneumothoraces in ventilated premature babies who actively expire against positive pressure inflation. Lancet 1(8367):1–3, 1984.
43. Perlman JM, Goodman S, Kreusser KL, et al: Reduction in intraventricular hemorrhage by elimination of fluctuating cerebral blood-flow velocity in preterm infants with respiratory distress syndrome. N Engl J Med 312:1353–1357, 1985.
44. Vernon DD, Witte MK: Effect of neuromuscular blockade on oxygen consumption and energy expenditure in sedated, mechanically ventilated children. Crit Care Med 28:1569–1571, 2000.
45. Stark AR, Bascom R, Frantz ID 3rd: Muscle relaxation in mechanically ventilated infants. J Pediatr 94:439–443, 1979.
46. Rutledge ML, Hawkins EP, Langston C: Skeletal muscle growth failure induced in premature newborn infants by prolonged pancuronium treatment. J Pediatr 109:883–886, 1986.
47. Bhutani VK, Abbasi S, Sivieri EM: Continuous skeletal muscle paralysis: Effect on neonatal pulmonary mechanics. Pediatrics 81:419–422, 1988.
48. Burger R, Fanconi S, Simma B: Paralysis of ventilated newborn babies does not influence resistance of the total respiratory system. Eur Respir J 14:357–362, 1999.
49. Costarino AT, Polin RA: Neuromuscular relaxants in the neonate. Clin Perinatol 14:965–989, 1987.
50. Cheung PY, Tyebkhan JM, Peliowski A, et al: Prolonged use of pancuronium bromide and sensorineural hearing loss in childhood survivors of congenital diaphragmatic hernia. J Pediatr 135(2 Pt 1):233–239, 1999.
51. Fitzpatrick KT, Black GW, Crean PM, et al: Continuous vecuronium infusion for prolonged muscle relaxation in children. Can J Anaesth 38:169–174, 1991.
52. Moise AA, Wearden ME, Kozinetz CA, et al: Antenatal steroids are associated with less need for blood pressure support in extremely premature infants. Pediatrics 95:845–850, 1995.
53. Lopez SL, Leighton JO, Walther FJ: Supranormal cardiac output in the dopamine- and dobutamine-dependent preterm infant. Pediatr Cardiol 18:292–296, 1997.
54. Keeley SR, Bohn DJ: The use of inotropic and afterload-reducing agents in neonates. Clin Perinatol 15:467–489, 1988.
55. Driscoll DJ: Use of inotropic and chronotropic agents in neonates. Clin Perinatol 14:931–949, 1987.
56. Spotnitz WD, Spotnitz HM, Truccone NJ, et al: Relation of ultrastructure and function. Sarcomere dimensions, pressure-volume curves, and geometry of the intact left ventricle of the immature canine heart. Circ Res 44:679–691, 1979.
57. Lebowitz EA, Novick JS, Rudolph AM: Development of myocardial sympathetic innervation in the fetal lamb. Pediatr Res 6:887–893, 1972.
58. Klopfenstein HS, Rudolph AM: Postnatal changes in the circulation and responses to volume loading in sheep. Circ Res 42:839–845, 1978.
59. Teitel DF, Sidi D, Chin T, et al: Developmental changes in myocardial contractile reserve in the lamb. Pediatr Res 19:948–955, 1985.
60. Van Hare GF, Hawkins JA, Schmidt KG, et al: The effects of increasing mean arterial pressure on left ventricular output in newborn lambs. Circ Res 67:78–83, 1990.
61. Zaritsky A, Chernow B: Use of catecholamines in pediatrics. J Pediatr 105:341–350, 1984.
62. Broddle O: Vascular dopamine receptors: Demonstration and characterization by in vitro studies. Life Sci 31:289, 1982.
63. Allen E, Pettigrew A, Frank D, et al: Alterations in dopamine clearance and catechol-O-methyltransferase activity by dopamine infusions in children. Crit Care Med 25:181–189, 1997.
64. Bhatt-Mehta V, Nahata MC, McClead RE, et al: Dopamine pharmacokinetics in critically ill newborn infants. Eur J Clin Pharmacol 40:593–597, 1991.
65. Seri I, Rudas G, Bors Z, et al: Effects of low-dose dopamine infusion on cardiovascular and renal functions, cerebral blood flow, and plasma catecholamine levels in sick preterm neonates. Pediatr Res 34:742–749, 1993.
66. Zaritsky A, Chernow B: Catecholamines, sympathomimetics. In Chernow B, Lake CR (eds): The Pharmacologic Approach to the Critically Ill Patient. Baltimore, Williams & Wilkins 1983, p. 483.
67. Tulassay T, Seri I, Machay T, et al: Effects of dopamine on renal functions in premature neonates with respiratory distress syndrome. Int J Pediatr Nephrol 4:19–23, 1983.
68. Seri I, Abbasi S, Wood DC, et al: Regional hemodynamic effects of dopamine in the sick preterm neonate. J Pediatr 133:728–734, 1998.
69. Goldberg LI, Hsieh YY, Resnekov L: Newer catecholamines for treatment of heart failure and shock: An update on dopamine and a first look at dobutamine. Prog Cardiovasc Dis 19:327–340, 1977.
70. Bhatt-Mehta V, Nahata MC: Dopamine and dobutamine in pediatric therapy. Pharmacotherapy 9:303–314, 1989.
71. Driscoll DJ, Gillette PC, Lewis RM, et al: Comparative hemodynamic effects of isoproterenol, dopamine, and dobutamine in the newborn dog. Pediatr Res 13:1006–1009, 1979.
72. Drummond WH, Webb IB, Purcell KA: Cardiopulmonary response to dopamine in chronically catheterized neonatal lambs. Pediatr Pharmacol 1:347–356, 1981.
73. Bourchier D, Weston PJ: Randomised trial of dopamine compared with hydrocortisone for the treatment of hypotensive very low birthweight infants. Arch Dis Child Fetal Neonatal Ed 76:F174–F178, 1997.
74. Hentschel R, Hensel D, Brune T, et al: Impact on blood pressure and intestinal perfusion of dobutamine or dopamine in hypotensive preterm infants. Biol Neonate 68:318–324, 1995.
75. Greenough A, Chan V, Emery EF, et al: Respiratory status and diuresis following treatment with dexamethasone. Early Hum Dev 32:87–91, 1993.
76. Roze JC, Tohier C, Maingueneau C, et al: Response to dobutamine and dopamine in the hypotensive very preterm infant. Arch Dis Child 69(1 Spec No):59–63, 1993.
77. Cuevas L, Yeh TF, John EG, et al: The effect of low-dose dopamine infusion on cardiopulmonary and renal status in premature newborns with respiratory distress syndrome. Am J Dis Child 145:799–803, 1991.
78. Klarr JM, Faix RG, Pryce CJ, et al: Randomized, blind trial of dopamine versus dobutamine for treatment of hypotension in preterm infants with respiratory distress syndrome. J Pediatr 125:117–122, 1994.
79. Gill AB, Weindling AM: Randomised controlled trial of plasma protein fraction versus dopamine in hypotensive very low birthweight infants. Arch Dis Child 69(3 Spec No):284–287, 1993.
80. Zhang J, Penny DJ, Kim NS, et al: Mechanisms of blood pressure increase induced by dopamine in hypotensive preterm neonates. Arch Dis Child Fetal Neonatal Ed 81:F99–F104, 1999.
81. Fiddler GI, Chatrath R, Williams GJ, et al: Dopamine infusion for the treatment of myocardial dysfunction associated with a persistent transitional circulation. Arch Dis Child 55:194–198, 1980.
82. DiSessa TG, Leitner M, Ti CC, et al: The cardiovascular effects of dopamine in the severely asphyxiated neonate. J Pediatr 99:772–776, 1981.
83. Emery EF, Greenough A: Efficacy of low-dose dopamine infusion. Acta Paediatr 82:430–432, 1993.
84. Fajardo CA, Whyte RK, Steele BT: Effect of dopamine on failure of indomethacin to close the patent ductus arteriosus. J Pediatr 121(5 Pt 1):771–775, 1992.
85. Baenziger O, Waldvogel K, Ghelfi D, et al: Can dopamine prevent the renal side effects of indomethacin? A prospective randomized clinical study. Klin Padiatr 211:438–441, 1999.

86. Seri I, Tulassay T, Kiszel J, et al: The use of dopamine for the prevention of the renal side effects of indomethacin in premature infants with patent ductus arteriosus. Int J Pediatr Nephrol 5:209–214, 1984.

87. Hegyi T, Hiatt IM: Tolazoline and dopamine therapy in neonatal hypoxia and pulmonary vasospasm. Acta Paediatr Scand 69:101–103, 1980.

88. Sonnenblick EH, Frishman WH, LeJemtel TH: Dobutamine: A new synthetic cardioactive sympathetic amine. N Engl J Med 300:17–22, 1979.

89. Driscoll DJ, Gillette PC, Duff DF, et al: Hemodynamic effects of dobutamine in children. Am J Cardiol 43:581–585, 1979.

90. Perkin RM, Levin DL: Shock in the pediatric patient. Part II. Therapy. J Pediatr 101:319–332, 1982.

91. Richard C, Ricome JL, Rimailho A, et al: Combined hemodynamic effects of dopamine and dobutamine in cardiogenic shock. Circulation 67:620–626, 1983.

92. Ward RM, Mirkin BL, Singh S: Response of infants with low cardiac output to dobutamine. Pediatr Res 15:686, 1981.

93. Hagen EA, Drummond WH, Shrager HH, et al: Response of newborn lambs to isoproterenol infusion. Pediatr Res 18:122A, 1984.

94. Fukushige J, Takahashi N, Igarashi H, et al: Perinatal management of congenital complete atrioventricular block: Report of nine cases. Acta Paediatr Jpn 40:337–340, 1998.

95. Suzuki H, Nakasato M, Sato S, et al: Management of functional pulmonary atresia with isoproterenol in a neonate with Ebstein's anomaly. Tohoku J Exp Med 181:459–465, 1997.

96. Yeager SB, Horbar J, Lucey JF: Sympathomimetic drugs in the neonate. N Engl J Med 303:1122–1123, 1980.

97. Gow RM, Bohn D, Koren G, et al: Cardiovascular pharmacology. In Radde IC, Mac Leod SM (eds): Pediatric Pharmacology and Therapeutics St. Louis, Mosby-Year Book, 1993, p. 204.

98. Riordan CJ, Randsbaek F, Storey JH, et al: Inotropes in the hypoplastic left heart syndrome: Effects in an animal model. Ann Thorac Surg 62:83–90, 1996.

99. Gersony WM, Duc GV, Sinclair JC: "PFC" syndrome (persistence of the fetal circulation). Circulation 39:111, 1969.

100. Goetzman BW, Sunshine P, Johnson JD, et al: Neonatal hypoxia and pulmonary vasospasm: Response to tolazoline. J Pediatr 89:617–621, 1976.

101. Konduri GG, Woodard LL: Selective pulmonary vasodilation by low-dose infusion of adenosine triphosphate in newborn lambs. J Pediatr 119(1 Pt 1):94–102, 1991.

102. Tolsa JF, Cotting J, Sekarski N, et al: Magnesium sulphate as an alternative and safe treatment for severe persistent pulmonary hypertension of the newborn. Arch Dis Child Fetal Neonatal Ed 72:F184–F187, 1995.

103. Weinberger B, Weiss K, Heck DE, et al: Pharmacologic therapy of persistent pulmonary hypertension of the newborn. Pharmacol Ther 89:67–79, 2001.

104. Kulik TJ, Lock JE: Pulmonary vasodilator therapy in persistent pulmonary hypertension of the newborn. Clin Perinatol 11:693–701, 1984.

105. Soifer SJ, Morin FC 3rd, Heymann MA: Prostaglandin D2 reverses induced pulmonary hypertension in the newborn lamb. J Pediatr 100:458–463, 1982.

106. De Jaegere AP, van den Anker JN: Endotracheal instillation of prostacyclin in preterm infants with persistent pulmonary hypertension. Eur Respir J 12:932–934, 1998.

107. Kinsella JP, Neish SR, Ivy DD, et al: Clinical responses to prolonged treatment of persistent pulmonary hypertension of the newborn with low doses of inhaled nitric oxide. J Pediatr 123:103–108, 1993.

108. Roberts JD, Polaner DM, Lang P, et al: Inhaled nitric oxide in persistent pulmonary hypertension of the newborn. Lancet 340(8823):818–819, 1992.

109. Lyrene RK, Welch KA, Godoy G, et al: Alkalosis attenuates hypoxic pulmonary vasoconstriction in neonatal lambs. Pediatr Res 19:1268–1271,1985.

110. Schreiber MD, Heymann MA, Soifer SJ: Increased arterial pH, not decreased Paco$_2$, attenuates hypoxia-induced pulmonary vasoconstriction in newborn lambs. Pediatr Res 20:113–117, 1986.

111. Fineman JR, Wong J, Soifer SJ: Hyperoxia and alkalosis produce pulmonary vasodilation independent of endothelium-derived nitric oxide in newborn lambs. Pediatr Res 33(4 Pt 1):341–346, 1993.

112. Van Vliet PK, Gupta JM: THAM v. sodium bicarbonate in idiopathic respiratory distress syndrome. Arch Dis Child 48:249–255, 1973.

113. Berg D, Mulling M, Saling E: Use of THAM and sodium bicarbonate in correcting acidosis in asphyxiated newborns. Arch Dis Child 44:318–322, 1969.

114. Young TE, Mangum B: Neofax: A Manual of Drugs Used in Neonatal Care, 13th ed. Raleigh, North Carolina, Acorn Publishing, 2000.

115. Marron MJ, Crisafi MA, Driscoll JM, et al: Hearing and neurodevelopmental outcome in survivors of persistent pulmonary hypertension of the newborn. Pediatrics 90:392–396, 1992.

116. Goldberg RN, Chung D, Goldman SL, et al: The association of rapid volume expansion and intraventricular hemorrhage in the preterm infant. J Pediatr 96:1060–1063, 1980.

117. Goldenberg VE, Wiegenstein L, Hopkins GB: Hepatic injury associated with tromethamine. JAMA 205:81–84,1968.

118. Kays DW, Langham MR, Ledbetter DJ, et al: Detrimental effects of standard medical therapy in congenital diaphragmatic hernia. Ann Surg 230:340–348; discussion 48–51, 1999.

119. Goetzman BW, Milstein JM: Pulmonary vasodilator action of tolazoline. Pediatr Res 13:942–944, 1979.

120. Curtis J, Palacino JJ, O'Neill JT: Production of pulmonary vasodilation by tolazoline, independent of nitric oxide production in neonatal lambs. J Pediatr 128:118–124, 1979.

121. Monin P, Vert P, Morselli PL: A pharmacodynamic and pharmacokinetic study of tolazoline in the neonate. Dev Pharmacol Ther 4(Suppl):124–128, 1982.

122. Ward RM, Daniel CH, Kendig JW, et al: Oliguria and tolazoline pharmacokinetics in the newborn. Pediatrics 77:307–315, 1986.

123. Meadow WL, Meus PJ: Hemodynamic consequences of tolazoline in neonatal group B streptococcal bacteremia: An animal model. Pediatr Res 18:960–965, 1984.

124. Parida SK, Baker S, Kuhn R, et al: Endotracheal tolazoline administration in neonates with persistent pulmonary hypertension. J Perinatol 17:461–464, 1997.

125. Clark RH, Kueser TJ, Walker MW, et al: Low-dose nitric oxide therapy for persistent pulmonary hypertension of the newborn. Clinical Inhaled Nitric Oxide Research Group. N Engl J Med 342:469–474, 2000.

126. Patole S, Lee J, Buettner P, et al: Improved oxygenation following adenosine infusion in persistent pulmonary hypertension of the newborn. Biol Neonate 74:345–350, 1998.

127. Wu TJ, Teng RJ, Tsou KI: Persistent pulmonary hypertension of the newborn treated with magnesium sulfate in premature neonates. Pediatrics 96(3 Pt 1):472–474, 1995.

128. Abu-Osba YK, Galal O, Manasra K, et al: Treatment of severe persistent pulmonary hypertension of the newborn with magnesium sulphate. Arch Dis Child 67(1 Spec No):31–35, 1992.

129. Islam S, Masiakos P, Schnitzer JJ, et al: Diltiazem reduces pulmonary arterial pressures in recurrent pulmonary hypertension associated with pulmonary hypoplasia. J Pediatr Surg 34:712–714, 1999.

130. Terragno NA, Terragno A: Prostaglandin metabolism in the fetal and maternal vasculature. Fed Proc 38:75–77, 1979.

131. Rose F, Zwick K, Ghofrani HA, et al: Prostacyclin enhances stretch-induced surfactant secretion in alveolar epithelial type II cells. Am J Respir Crit Care Med 160:846–851, 1999.

132. Geraci MW, Gao B, Shepherd DC, et al: Pulmonary prostacyclin synthase overexpression in transgenic mice protects against development of hypoxic pulmonary hypertension. J Clin Invest 103:1509–1515, 1999.

133. Blanchard PW, Brown TM, Coates AL: Pharmacotherapy in bronchopulmonary dysplasia. Clin Perinatol 14:881–910, 1987.

134. Aubier M, De Troyer A, Sampson M, et al: Aminophylline improves diaphragmatic contractility. N Engl J Med 305:249–252, 1981.

135. Sigrist S, Thomas D, Howell S, et al: The effect of aminophylline on inspiratory muscle contractility. Am Rev Respir Dis 126:46–50, 1982.

136. Fok TF, Lam K, Ng PC, et al: Randomised crossover trial of salbutamol aerosol delivered by metered dose inhaler, jet nebuliser, and ultrasonic nebuliser in chronic lung disease. Arch Dis Child Fetal Neonatal Ed 79:F100–F104, 1998.

137. Isles AF, Newth CJL: Respiratory pharmacology. In Radde IC, Mac Leod SM (eds): Pediatric Pharmacology and Therapeutics. St. Louis, Mosby-Year Book, 1993.

138. Denjean A, Guimaraes H, Migdal M, et al: Dose-related bronchodilator response to aerosolized salbutamol (albuterol) in ventilator-dependent premature infants. J Pediatr 120:974–979, 1992.

139. Rotschild A, Solimano A, Puterman M, et al: Increased compliance in response to salbutamol in premature infants with developing bronchopulmonary dysplasia. J Pediatr 115:984–991, 1989.

140. Rush MG, Hazinski TA: Current therapy of bronchopulmonary dysplasia. Clin Perinatol 19:563–590, 1992.

141. Langley SC, Kelly FJ: N-acetylcysteine ameliorates hyperoxic lung injury in the preterm guinea pig. Biochem Pharmacol 45:841–846, 1993.

142. King R: Acetylcysteine in airway maintenance. Lancet 1:900–901, 1967.

143. Bibi H, Seifert B, Oullette M, et al: Intratracheal N-acetylcysteine use in infants with chronic lung disease. Acta Paediatr 81:335–339, 1992.

144. Viscardi RM, Hasday JD, Gumpper KF, et al: Cromolyn sodium prophylaxis inhibits pulmonary proinflammatory cytokines in infants at high risk for bronchopulmonary dysplasia. Am J Respir Crit Care Med 156:1523–1529, 1997.

145. Yuksel B, Greenough A: Inhaled sodium cromoglycate for pre-term children with respiratory symptoms at follow-up. Respir Med 86:131–134, 1997.

146. Watterberg K, Murphy S: Failure of cromolyn sodium to reduce the incidence of bronchopulmonary dysplasia: A pilot study. The Neonatal Cromolyn Study Group. Pediatrics 91:803–806, 1993.

147. Davies MW, Davis PG: Nebulized racemic epinephrine for extubation of newborn infants. Cochrane Database Syst Rev 2, 2000.

148. Chemtob S, Kaplan BS, Sherbotie JR, et al: Pharmacology of diuretics in the newborn. Pediatr Clin North Am 36:1231–1250, 1989.

149. Downing GJ, Egelhoff JC, Daily DK, et al: Furosemide-related renal calcifications in the premature infant. A longitudinal ultrasonographic study. Pediatr Radiol 21:563–565, 1991.

150. Ezzedeen F, Adelman RD, Ahlfors CE: Renal calcification in preterm infants: Pathophysiology and long-term sequelae. J Pediatr 113:532–539, 1988.

151. Kao LC, Warburton D, Sargent CW, et al: Furosemide acutely decreases airways resistance in chronic bronchopulmonary dysplasia. J Pediatr 103:624–629, 1983.

152. Najak ZD, Harris EM, Lazzara A, et al: Pulmonary effects of furosemide in preterm infants with lung disease. J Pediatr 102:758–763, 1983.

153. Engelhardt B, Elliott S, Hazinski TA: Short- and long-term effects of furosemide on lung function in infants with bronchopulmonary dysplasia. J Pediatr 109:1034–1039, 1986.

154. Greenough A: Prevention and management of neonatal chronic lung disease: Short-term gains, but long-term losses. Neonat Respir Dis 10:1–7, 2000.

155. Rastogi A, Luayon M, Ajayi OA, et al: Nebulized furosemide in infants with bronchopulmonary dysplasia. J Pediatr 25(6 Pt 1):976–979, 1994.

156. Brion LP, Primhak RA, Yong W: Aerosolized diuretics for preterm infants with (or developing) chronic lung disease. Cochrane Database Syst Rev 2, 2000.

157. Green TP: The pharmacologic basis of diuretic therapy in the newborn. Clin Perinatol 14:951–964, 1987.

158. Green TP, Johnson DE, Bass JL, et al: Prophylactic furosemide in severe respiratory distress syndrome: Blinded prospective study. J Pediatr 112:605–612, 1988.

159. Kao LC, Warburton D, Cheng MH, et al: Effect of oral diuretics on pulmonary mechanics in infants with chronic bronchopulmonary dysplasia: Results of a double-blind crossover sequential trial. Pediatrics 74:37–44, 1984.

160. Brion LP, Primhak RA, Ambrosio-Perez I: Diuretics acting on the distal renal tubule for preterm infants with (or developing) chronic lung disease (Cochrane review). Cochrane Database Syst Rev 3, 2000.

161. Taeusch HW, Wang NS, Baden N, et al: A controlled trial of hydrocortisone therapy in infants with respiratory distress syndrome: II. Pathology. Pediatrics 52:850–854, 1973.

162. Davis PG, Henderson-Smart DJ: Intravenous dexamethasone for extubation of newborn infants. Cochrane Database Syst Rev 2, 2000.

163. Shah V, Ohlsson A, Halliday HL, et al: Early administration of inhaled corticosteroids for preventing chronic lung disease in ventilated very low birth weight preterm neonates. Cochrane Database Syst Rev 2, 2000.

164. Sinkin RA, Cox C, Phelps DL: Predicting risk for bronchopulmonary dysplasia: Selection criteria for clinical trials. Pediatrics 86:728–736, 1990.

165. Shaw N, Gill B, Weindling M, et al: The changing incidence of chronic lung disease. Health Trends 25:50–53, 1993.

166. Ohlsson A, Calvert SA, Hosking M, et al: Randomized controlled trial of dexamethasone treatment in very-low-birth-weight infants with ventilator-dependent chronic lung disease. Acta Paediatr 81:751–756, 1992.

167. Yeh TF, Torre JA, Rastogi A, et al: Early postnatal dexamethasone therapy in premature infants with severe respiratory distress syndrome: A double-blind, controlled study. J Pediatr 117(2 Pt 1):273–282, 1990.

168. Cummings JJ, D'Eugenio DB, Gross SJ: A controlled trial of dexamethasone in preterm infants at high risk for bronchopulmonary dysplasia. N Engl J Med 320:1505–1010, 1989.

169. Harkavy KL, Scanlon JW, Chowdhry PK, et al: Dexamethasone therapy for chronic lung disease in ventilator- and oxygen-dependent infants: A controlled trial. J Pediatr 115:979–983, 1989.

170. Pierce MR, Bancalari E: The role of inflammation in the pathogenesis of bronchopulmonary dysplasia. Pediatr Pulmonol 19:371–378, 1995.

171. Mammel MC, Green TP, Johnson DE, et al: Controlled trial of dexamethasone therapy in infants with bronchopulmonary dysplasia. Lancet 1:1356–1358, 1983.

172. Avery GB, Fletcher AB, Kaplan M, et al: Controlled trial of dexamethasone in respirator-dependent infants with bronchopulmonary dysplasia. Pediatrics 75:106–111, 1985.

173. Whitelaw A, Thoresen M: Antenatal steroids and the developing brain. Arch Dis Child Fetal Neonatal Ed 83:F154–F157, 2000.

174. Halliday HL, Ehrenkranz RA: Early postnatal (<96 hours) corticosteroids for preventing chronic lung disease in preterm infants. Cochrane Database Syst Rev 2, 2000.

175. Yeh TF, Lin YJ, Huang CC, et al: Early dexamethasone therapy in preterm infants: A follow-up study. Pediatrics 101:E7, 1998.

176. Halliday HL, Ehrenkranz RA: Moderately early (7–14 days) postnatal corticosteroids for preventing chronic lung disease in preterm infants. Cochrane Database Syst Rev 2, 2000.

177. Halliday HL, Ehrenkranz RA: Delayed (>3 weeks) postnatal corticosteroids for chronic lung disease in preterm infants. Cochrane Database Syst Rev 2, 2000.

177a. Committee on Fetus and Newborn, American Academy of Pediatrics: Postnatal corticosteroids to treat or prevent chronic lung disease in preterm infants. Pediatrics 109:330–338, 2002.

178. Aranda JV, Turmen T: Methylxanthines in apnea of prematurity. Clin Perinatol 6:87–108, 1979.

179. Martin RJ, Miller MJ, Carlo WA: Pathogenesis of apnea in preterm infants. J Pediatr 109:733–741, 1986.

180. Barr PA: Weaning very low birthweight infants from mechanical ventilation using intermittent mandatory ventilation and theophylline. Arch Dis Child 53:598–600, 1978.

181. Rooklin AR, Moomjian AS, Shutack JG, et al: Theophylline therapy in bronchopulmonary dysplasia. J Pediatr 95(5 Pt 2):882–888, 1979.

182. Viscardi RM, Faix RG, Nicks JJ, et al: Efficacy of theophylline for prevention of post-extubation respiratory failure in very low birth weight infants. J Pediatr 107:469–472, 1985.

183. Henderson-Smart DJ, Steer P: Postoperative caffeine for preventing apnea in preterm infants. Cochrane Database Syst Rev 2, 2000.

184. Gerhardt T, McCarthy J, Bancalari E: Aminophylline therapy for idiopathic apnea in premature infants: Effects on lung function. Pediatrics 62:801–804, 1978.

185. Shannon DC, Gotay F, Stein IM, et al: Prevention of apnea and bradycardia in low-birthweight infants. Pediatrics 55:589–594, 1975.

186. Steer PA, Henderson-Smart DJ: Caffeine versus theophylline for apnea in preterm infants. Cochrane Database Syst Rev 2, 2000.

187. Alpan G, Eyal F, Sagi E, et al: Doxapram in the treatment of idiopathic apnea of prematurity unresponsive to aminophylline. J Pediatr 104:634–637, 1984.

188. Henderson-Smart DJ, Steer PA: Doxapram treatment for apnea in preterm infants. Cochrane Database Syst Rev 2, 2000.

189. Jordan GD, Themelis NJ, Messerly SO, et al: Doxapram and potential benzyl alcohol toxicity: A moratorium on clinical investigation? Pediatrics 78:540–541,1986.

190. Cole C: The use of aerosolized medicines in neonates. Neonat Respir Dis 10:1–12, 2000.

191. Bisgaard H: Delivery options for inhaled therapy in children under the age of 6 years. J Aerosol Med 10(Suppl 1):S37–S40, 1997.

192. Dolovich M: Aerosol delivery to children: What to use, how to choose. Pediatr Pulmonol Suppl 18:79–82, 1999.

193. Dolovich MA: Influence of inspiratory flow rate, particle size, and airway caliber on aerosolized drug delivery to the lung. Respir Care 45:597–608, 2000.

194. Salmon B, Wilson NM, Silverman M: How much aerosol reaches the lungs of wheezy infants and toddlers? Arch Dis Child 65:401–403, 1990.

PHARMACOLOGIC ADJUNCTS II
Exogenous Surfactants

G A U T H A M   K .   S U R E S H ,   M B B S ,   M D ,   D M
R O G E R   F .   S O L L ,   M D

Exogenous surfactant therapy is widely used in the management of respiratory distress syndrome (RDS) in preterm infants who require ventilatory assistance, and its use in the treatment of other neonatal respiratory disorders such as meconium aspiration syndrome is increasing. The introduction of surfactant therapy is widely credited with recent improvements in neonatal mortality.[1–3] In this chapter we present an overview of the current use of exogenous surfactant therapy for neonates, based on currently available evidence.

HISTORY

The development of exogenous surfactant therapy was a significant and historic advance in neonatal intensive care. This discovery was built upon work by pioneers in the field of surfactant research that described the existence and composition of surfactant, the role of surfactant in lowering surface tension, and the role of surfactant in maintaining alveolar stability.[4–6] A landmark in our current understanding of RDS was the demonstration of surfactant deficiency in the lungs of infants dying of hyaline membrane disease.[7] The introduction of surface active substances into the lung was suggested as early as 1947.[8] Initial attempts to provide exogenous surfactant therapy for immature lungs were unsuccessful[9,10] but were followed several years later by successful attempts in animals[11] and in human neonates.[12] Since these initial efforts, numerous animal experiments and human clinical trials were conducted to study the efficacy of surfactant therapy, the relative efficacy of different surfactant preparations, the optimal timing of administration, the optimal dosage, and other aspects of exogenous surfactant therapy. The history and evolution of surfactant therapy have been reviewed in detail elsewhere.[13–15]

SURFACTANT FUNCTION, COMPOSITION, AND METABOLISM

The function, composition, secretion, and metabolism of mammalian surfactant have been reviewed extensively elsewhere[16–18] and are summarized here.

Function

Pulmonary alveoli, where gas exchange occurs, are bubble shaped and have a high curvature. The surface tension of the moist inner surface is due to the attraction between the molecules in the alveolar fluid and tends to make the alveoli contract. Unchecked, this tendency would result in lung collapse. Surfactant greatly reduces the surface tension on the inner surface of the alveoli, thus preventing the alveoli from collapsing during expiration.

Composition

Accurate determination of the composition of pulmonary surfactant is difficult. In order to obtain surfactant for analysis, one must either wash out lungs (with the possible limitation of leaving important components behind) or extract surfactant from minced lungs (with the possible problem of adding cellular contaminants). Mammalian surfactant obtained by lung lavage consists of 80% phospholipids, 8% neutral lipids, and 12% protein. The predominant class of phospholipid (nearly 60%) is dipalmitoylphosphatidylcholine (DPPC), with lesser amounts of unsaturated phosphatidylcholine compounds (25%), phosphatidyl glycerol (PG) (15%), and phosphatidylinositol. Of all the constituents of surfactant, DPPC alone has the appropriate properties to reduce alveolar surface tension; however, DPPC alone is a poor surfactant because it adsorbs very slowly to air–liquid interfaces. Surfactant proteins or other lipids facilitate its adsorption. Approximately half the protein in surfactant consists of contaminating protein from the plasma or lung tissue.[19] The remaining proteins include four unique surfactant-associated apoproteins: SP-A, SP-B, SP-C, and SP-D.[20] SP-A and SP-D are hydrophilic proteins; SP-B and SP-C are hydrophobic. SP-A and SP-D belong to a subgroup of mammalian lectins called *collectins*. They may play important roles in the defense against inhaled pathogens. SP-A may have a regulatory function in the formation of the monolayer that lowers the surface tension.[16] The hydrophobic proteins are required to enhance spreading of phospholipid in the airs paces. SP-B promotes phospholipid adsorption and induces the insertion of phospholipids into the monolayer, thus enhancing the formation of a stable surface film.[16] SP-C enhances phospholipid adsorption, stimulates the insertion of phospholipids out of the subphase into the air–liquid interface, and may increase the resistance of surfactant to inhibition by serum proteins or edema fluid.[16,17]

Secretion and Metabolism

Surfactant is produced in the type II cells of the alveoli (Fig. 20-1). It is assembled and stored in the lamellar bodies, which consist of concentric or parallel lamellae, predominantly

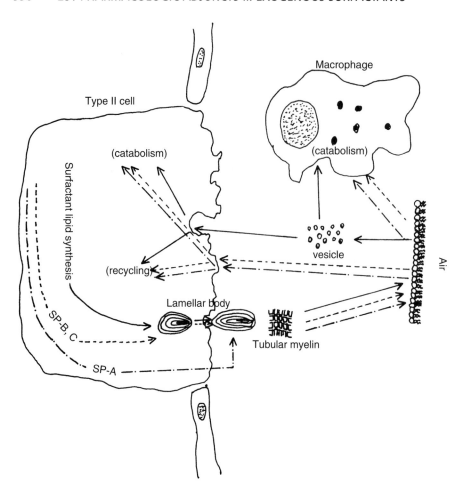

Figure 20-1. Metabolism of surfactant. *Solid line,* surfactant + liquid; *dashed and dotted line,* SP-A; *dashed line,* SP-B, SP-C. (From Jobe AH, Ikegami M: Biology of surfactant. Clin Perinatol 28:655, 2001.)

composed of phospholipid bilayers. Lamellar bodies are extruded into the fluid layer lining the alveoli by exocytosis and form structures known as *tubular myelin.* Tubular myelin consists of long stacked tubes composed mainly of phospholipid bilayers, the corners of which appear fused, resulting in a lattice-like appearance on cross section. Tubular myelin is thought to be the major source of the monolayer surface film lining the air–liquid interface in the alveoli, in which the hydrophobic fatty acyl groups of the phospholipids extend into the air while the hydrophilic polar head groups bind water.[21] This surfactant monolayer lowers the surface tension at the air–liquid interface by replacing water at the surface.[21] The phospholipid from the monolayer eventually reenters the type II cells by endocytosis and forms multivesicular bodies. These multivesicular bodies are either "recycled" by rapid incorporation into the lamellar bodies or degraded in lysosomes. Of note, all critical components (DPPC, PG, SP-A, SP-B, SP-C) are recycled.[18]

TYPES OF SURFACTANT

Two types of surfactant are available for exogenous therapy: (1) surfactant derived from animal sources or "*natural*" surfactant and (2) *synthetic* surfactant.

Types of Natural Surfactant

Currently, commercially available natural surfactants are obtained from either bovine or porcine lungs (Table 20-1). Beractant (Survanta, Abbott Laboratories, North Chicago, IL, USA) and Surfactant TA (Surfacten, Tokyo Tanabe, Tokyo, Japan) are lipid extracts of bovine lung mince with added DPPC, tripalmitoyl glycerol, and palmitic acid. Calf lung surfactant extract (calfactant, Infasurf, ONY, Inc., Amherst, NY, USA), SF-RI1(Alveofact, Thomae GmbH, Biberach/Riss, FGR), and Bovine Lipid Extract Surfactant (BLES; BLES Biochemicals Inc., Ontario, Canada) are bovine lung washes subjected to chloroform-methanol extraction. Porcine surfactant (poractant, Curosurf, Chiesi Farmaceutici, Parma, Italy) is a porcine lung mince that has been subjected to chloroform-methanol extraction and further purified by liquid gel chromatography. It consists of approximately 99% polar lipids (mainly phospholipids) and 1% hydrophobic low-molecular-weight proteins (SP-B, SP-C).[22] All the natural surfactants contain SP-B and SP-C, but the lung mince extracts (Survanta and Curosurf) contain less than 10% of the SP-B that is found in the lung-wash extracts (Infasurf, Alveofact, and bLES).[23] The purification procedure, including extraction with organic solvents, removes the hydrophilic proteins SP-A and SP-D, leaving a material containing only lipids and small amounts of hydrophobic proteins. Poractant (Curosurf), which is further

TABLE 20-1.   Commercially Available Natural (Animal-derived) Surfactants

Trade Name	Generic Name	Preparation	Protein and Major Phospholipid Content*	Manufacturer
Surfacten	Surfactant-TA	Bovine lung mince extract with added DPPC, tripalmitoylglycerol, and palmitic acid	DPPC, PG, SP-B, SP-C	Tokyo Tanabe (Japan)
Survanta	Beractant	Bovine lung mince extract with added DPPC, tripalmitoylglycerol, and palmitic acid	DPPC, PG, SP-B, SP-C	Ross Products Division of Abbott Laboratories (USA)
Curosurf	Poractant	Porcine lung mince subjected to chloroform-methanol extraction; purified by liquid gel chromatography	DPPC, SP-B, SP-C	Chiesi Pharmaceuticals (Italy)
Infasurf	Calf lung surfactant extract	Calf (bovine) lung lavage extract subjected to chloroform-methanol extraction	DPPC, SP-B, SP-C	Forrest Laboratories (USA)
BLES	Bovine lipid extract surfactant	Cow (bovine) lung lavage extract subjected to chloroform-methanol extraction	DPPC, SP-B, SP-C	BLES Biochemicals (Canada)
Alveofact	SF-RI 1	Cow (bovine) lung lavage extract subjected to chloroform-methanol extraction	DPPC, SP-B, SP-C	Boehringer Ingelheim (Germany)

* All natural surfactants contain smaller proportions of other phospholipids, neutral lipids, and fatty acids. The purification processes using organic acids removes hydrophilic proteins. Hence, none of the natural surfactants contain either surfactant protein A (SP-A) or surfactant protein D (SP-D).
From Wiswell TE: Expanded uses of Surfactant Therapy. *Clin Perinat* 28:695, 2001.
DPPC, dipalmitoylphosphatidylcholine; PG, phosphatidylglycerol; (SP-B mimic); SP-B, surfactant protein B; SP-C, surfactant protein C.

TABLE 20-2.   Synthetic Surfactants

Trade Name	Generic Name	Preparation	Protein and Major Phospholipid Content	Manufacturer
Exosurf	Colfosceril plamitate, hexadecanol, tyloxapol	DPPC with 9% hexadecanol and 6% tyloxapol	DPPC, no protein	Burroughs-Wellcome Company (USA and UK)
Pneumactant*	Artificial lung expanding compound (ALEC)	DPPC and PG in a 7:3 ratio	DPPC and PG, no protein	Britannia Pharmaceuticals (UK)
Surfaxin	Lucinactant	Chemically synthesized peptide combined with phospholipids and palmitic acid	Sinapultide, DPPC, POPG, and palmitic acid	Discovery Laboratories (USA)
Venticute	rSP-C surfactant	Recombinant SP-C combined with phospholipids and palmitic acid	rSP-C, DPPC, POPG, and palmitic acid	Byk Gulden (Germany)

* Pneumactant was removed from the market by the manufacturer in the year 2000.
From Wiswell TE: Expanded uses of surfactant therapy. *Clin Perinat* 28:695, 2001.
DPPC, dipalmitoylphosphatidylcholine; PG, phosphatidylglycerol; POPG, palmitoyl-oleoyl phosphatidylglycerol; rSP-C, recombinant surfactant protein C; sinapultide, KL_4-peptide (SP-B mimic); SP-C, surfactant protein C.

purified by liquid gel chromatography, contains only polar lipids and about 1% hydrophobic proteins (SP-B and SP-C in an approximate molar ratio of 1:2).[24] None of the commercial preparations contain SP-A.[23] A surfactant obtained from human amniotic fluid was originally tested in clinical trials[25,26] but is currently not used.

Types of Synthetic Surfactant

The original exogenous products tested in the 1980s were synthetic surfactants composed solely of DPPC; however, DPPC alone will not perform all the functions required of pulmonary surfactant. The currently available synthetic products are mixtures of a variety of surface active phospholipids and spreading agents (Table 20-2). These products include colfosceril and artificial lung-expanding compound. Colfosceril palmitate, hexadecanol, tyloxapol (Exosurf, Glaxo-Wellcome, formerly Burroughs-Wellcome, Research Triangle Park, NC, USA) consists of 85% DPPC, 9% hexadecanol, and 6% tyloxapol (a spreading agent). Artificial lung-expanding compound (Pneumactant, Britannia Pharmaceuticals, Redhill, Surrey, UK) is a 7:3 mixture of DPPC and phosphatidyl glycerol but was removed from the market by the manufacturer in 2000. The principal surface-active agent in the synthetic surfactants is DPPC. The other components facilitate surface adsorption. Neither contains any of the other phospholipids or the apoproteins. The only synthetic surfactant currently available commercially (Exosurf) lacks many of the components of natural surfactant. Two new synthetic surfactants (Surfaxin and Venticute) are currently in clinical trials and discussed later in this chapter.

ACUTE PULMONARY AND CARDIAC EFFECTS OF SURFACTANT THERAPY

Immediate Pulmonary Effects of Surfactant Therapy

In animal models of RDS, administration of exogenous surfactant has been shown to result in improved lung function (Fig. 20-2)[27] and improved alveolar expansion (Fig. 20-3)[28] when compared with controls. Studies in human neonates have also shown that the administration of exogenous surfactant therapy leads to rapid improvement in oxygenation and a decrease in the degree of support provided by mechanical ventilation (Fig. 20-4).[29] These rapid changes are accompanied by an increase in functional residual capacity and followed by a slower and variable increase in lung compliance.[30–32] A decrease in pulmonary ventilation-perfusion mismatch has also been reported.[33–35]

Immediate Effects on Pulmonary Circulation

In three studies, pulmonary blood flow was unchanged with surfactant therapy.[36–38] In contrast, other studies reported a decrease in pulmonary artery pressure or an increase in pulmonary artery flow with surfactant therapy,[39–42] as well as an increase in the ductal flow velocity from the systemic-to-pulmonary circuit.[41] It is uncertain whether these changes in pulmonary circulation are related to ventilation practices, blood gas status, or the surfactant itself.[43]

Radiographic Changes

In addition to the physiologic changes, treatment with exogenous surfactant results in radiologic improvement, with chest radiographs taken after treatment often (but not always) showing a decrease in the signs of RDS. This clearing of the lungs can be uniform, patchy, or asymmetric, sometimes with disproportionate improvement of radiologic changes in the right lung.[44–48]

CLINICAL TRIALS OF SURFACTANT THERAPY

Numerous randomized controlled trials have been conducted in neonatology to study different aspects of surfactant therapy. The findings from these trials, grouped according to the questions the trials addressed, have been reviewed in

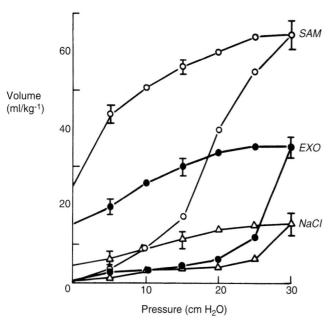

Figure 20-2. Pressure-volume characteristics of lungs from 10 matched prematurely delivered rabbits after treatment with saline (NaCl), Exosurf (EXO), or surface active material obtained by lavaging lungs of young adult rabbits with saline (SAM), plus ventilation for 30 minutes. Measurements were made 10 minutes after the animals died and their lungs were allowed to degas spontaneously. (From Tooley WH, Clements JA, Muramatsu K, et al.: Lung function in prematurely delivered rabbits treated with a synthetic surfactant. Am Rev Respir Dis 136:651, 1987.)

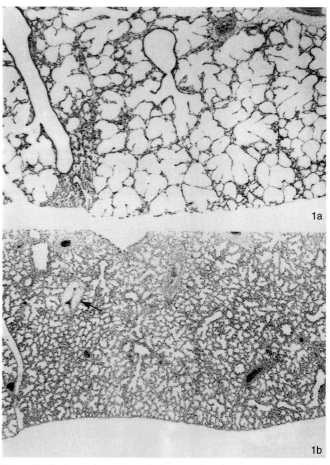

Figure 20-3. Expansion patterns in lung sections from premature rabbits. 1a, Well-expanded area in surfactant-treated fetus. The rounded appearance of the aerated alveoli contrasts with the pattern in 1b and with the wedge of unexpanded parenchyma *(lower left)*. 1b, "Unexpanded" lung in control fetus that did not receive surfactant. The configuration of the alveoli reflects the fluid-filled state. Note abundant interstitial fluid around a pulmonary vein *(arrow)* (hematoxylin and eosin, magnification x27). (From Robertson B, Enhorning G: The alveolar lining of the premature newborn rabbit after pharyngeal deposition of surfactant. Lab Invest 31:54, 1974.)

multiple systematic reviews in the Cochrane Database of Systematic Reviews.[49–54] The findings of these systematic reviews and of other relevant studies are summarized in the following sections. The results of the meta-analyses are presented as the "typical" or "pooled" estimates of relative risk (RR) and absolute risk difference (ARD), with 95% confidence intervals (CI).

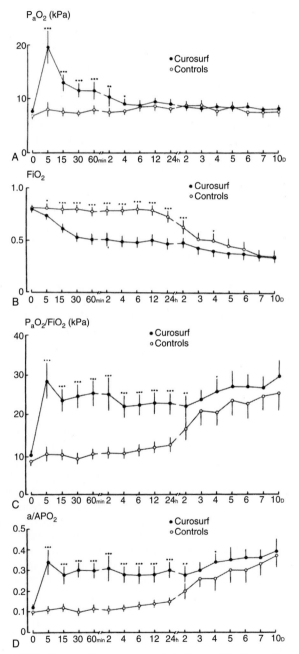

Figure 20-4. Oxygenation measurements in Curosurf-treated and control infants at various intervals after randomization. Results are mean values and 95% confidence intervals. If confidence intervals are overlapping, bars are shown on only one side of data point. Note that the time scale is not linear. Conversion factor: 1 kPa = 7.52 mm Hg. *P <0.05, **P <0.01, ***P <.001. (From Collaborative European Multicenter Study Group: Surfactant replacement therapy for severe neonatal respiratory distress syndrome: An international randomized clinical trial. Pediatrics 82:683, 1988.)

Surfactant Therapy Compared to Placebo or No Therapy

Many of the early trials in the late 1980s and early 1990s studied the effects of surfactant therapy compared to placebo or no therapy. Some of these trials studied the effects of prophylactic administration of surfactant to preterm infants at risk for developing RDS. Others studied the effects of treatment with surfactant in preterm infants with clinical and/or radiologic features of RDS. Some of these studies used natural surfactant and others used synthetic surfactant. Systematic reviews of these trials show that, compared to placebo or no therapy, surfactant treatment or prophylaxis (with either natural or synthetic surfactant) decreases the risk of pneumothorax and decreases mortality.[49–51,55] Estimates from the meta-analyses indicate that there is a 30% to 65% relative reduction in the risk of pneumothorax and up to a 40% relative reduction in the risk of mortality. There were no consistent effects on other clinical outcomes such as chronic lung disease, patent ductus arteriosus, and intraventricular hemorrhage.

Further support for beneficial outcomes following surfactant therapy is derived from comparisons of the outcomes of very-low-birthweight infants before and after the introduction of surfactant therapy. Such studies have demonstrated a decrease in mortality and morbidity for such infants after the introduction of surfactant therapy.[1,3,56–60]

Comparison of Natural and Synthetic Surfactants

Although both synthetic and natural surfactants are effective, their composition differs. Natural surfactant extracts contain surfactant specific proteins that aid in surfactant adsorption and resist surfactant inactivation.[20,61] Eleven randomized trials have compared the effects of natural and synthetic surfactants in the treatment or prevention of RDS.[62–72] A total of more than 4500 infants were studied in these trials. A systematic review of these trials is available.[52] The results of the meta-analysis are summarized in Figure 20-5. Compared to synthetic surfactant, treatment with natural surfactant extracts resulted in a decrease in the frequency of pneumothorax (typical RR 0.63, 95% CI 0.52, 0.76; typical ARD -5%, 95% CI -7%, -3%) and a decreased mortality (typical RR 0.87, 95% CI 0.75, 0.99, typical ARD -2%, 95% CI –5%, 0%). There were no significant differences in chronic lung disease, intraventricular hemorrhage, sepsis, or patent ductus arteriosus. In addition to these benefits, natural surfactants have a more rapid onset of action, which allows ventilator settings and inspired oxygen concentrations to be lowered more quickly than with synthetic surfactant.[65,66,69,73,74] A comparison of physical properties and the results of animal studies also suggest that natural surfactants have advantages over synthetic surfactants.[75] These properties are attributed to the presence of the surfactant proteins SP-B and SP-C in natural surfactants.[76]

The use of natural surfactant preparations should be favored in most clinical situations because their use results in greater clinical benefits than synthetic surfactants. However, all natural surfactants have to be refrigerated for storage. The synthetic surfactant colfosceril (Exosurf) is available as a lyophilized powder that is to be stored at below 30°C in a dry place (not to be frozen) and reconstituted with sterile water before use. Therefore, in situations where refrigeration is a problem (such

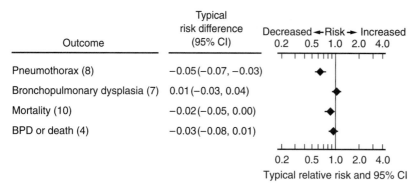

Outcome	Typical risk difference (95% CI)	Decreased ← Risk → Increased
Pneumothorax (8)	−0.05(−0.07, −0.03)	
Bronchopulmonary dysplasia (7)	0.01(−0.03, 0.04)	
Mortality (10)	−0.02(−0.05, 0.00)	
BPD or death (4)	−0.03(−0.08, 0.01)	

Typical relative risk and 95% CI

Figure 20-5. Meta-analysis of 10 randomized trials comparing natural and synthetic surfactant. Numbers in parentheses following the outcomes are the numbers of trials in which that outcome was reported. BPD, bronchopulmonary dysplasia; CI, confidence interval; diamonds, point estimate; horizontal bars, 95% confidence interval of the relative risk. (From Soll RF, Blanco F: Natural surfactant extract versus synthetic surfactant for neonatal respiratory distress syndrome [Cochrane Review]. In: The Cochrane Library, Issue 2, 2001. Oxford: Update Software, 2001.)

as during transport of an outborn infant or in developing countries), it may be more practical to use colfosceril (Exosurf) than natural surfactants.

Comparison of Different Types of Natural Surfactants

Many natural surfactant products are available for clinical use. There is no current evidence establishing the superiority of one or more natural surfactant products over others. Two randomized trials have compared the efficacy and adverse effects of different natural surfactant products. In a comparison of beractant (Survanta) and calf lung surfactant extract (Infasurf),[77] there were no differences detected between the two groups with regard to the frequency of air leaks, complications associated with dosing, complications of prematurity, mortality, or survival without chronic lung disease. However, some differences were noted among subgroups of infants. Among infants treated for established RDS, those who received calf lung surfactant extract (Infasurf) had a significantly longer interval between doses, a lower inspired oxygen concentration, and a lower mean airway pressure in the first 48 hours of life than infants treated with beractant (Survanta). Among infants in whom these surfactants were administered in a preventive manner, mortality in infants with a birthweight less than 600 g was significantly higher with calf lung surfactant extract (Infasurf) than with beractant (Survanta).

In another small unblinded trial comparing poractant (Curosurf) and beractant (Survanta),[78] infants treated with poractant (Curosurf) had more rapid improvement in oxygenation and reduced ventilatory requirements up to 24 hours after start of treatment compared to infants treated with beractant (Survanta). This trial did not have enough power to detect true differences in important clinical outcomes between the two groups. In addition, the apparent superiority of poractant over beractant has two alternative explanations: the trial investigators were more experienced with poractant than beractant, and a higher dose of phospholipids was used with poractant (200 mg/kg) than with beractant (100 mg/kg).

Prophylactic Surfactant Administration Compared to "Rescue" Administration

The rationale for prophylactic administration of surfactant is provided by the observation that, in animal studies, a more uniform and homogenous distribution of surfactant is achieved when it is administered into a fluid-filled lung[79,80] and by the belief that administration of surfactant into a previously unven-

tilated or minimally ventilated lung will diminish acute lung injury. Even brief periods (15 to 30 minutes) of mechanical ventilation prior to surfactant administration have been shown, in animal models, to cause acute lung injury resulting in alveolar capillary damage, leakage of proteinaceous fluid into the alveolar space, and release of inflammatory mediators[81–83] and to decrease the subsequent response to surfactant replacement.[84,85] Surfactant-deficient animals who receive assisted ventilation develop necrosis and desquamation of the bronchiolar epithelium as early as 5 minutes after onset of ventilation.[86]

Eight randomized controlled trials compared the effects of prophylactic surfactant administration to surfactant treatment of established RDS.[26,87–93] All of these trials used natural surfactant preparations.

Trials varied regarding whether surfactant was given before or after the onset of air breathing (preventilatory or postventilatory administration), but all administered surfactant before 15 minutes of age. The average time of administration of surfactant in the selective treatment groups ranged from 1.5 to 7.4 hours. The results of the meta-analysis of these trials from a systematic review[53] are summarized in Figure 20-6. Compared to surfactant treatment of established RDS, prophylactic administration of surfactant resulted in a decrease in the risk of pneumothorax (typical RR 0.62, 95% CI 0.42, 0.89; typical ARD -2%, 95% CI -4%, -1%), a decrease in the risk of pulmonary interstitial emphysema (typical RR 0.54, 95% CI 0.36, 0.82; typical ARD -3%, 95% CI -4%, -1%), a reduction in the risk of neonatal mortality (typical RR 0.61, 95% CI 0.48, 0.77; typical ARD -5%, 95% CI -7%, -2%), and a trend toward a decrease in the risk of intraventricular hemorrhage (typical RR 0.92, 95% CI 0.82, 1.03, typical ARD -3%, 95% CI -6%, 1%). Because of the greater risk of RDS and mortality with decreasing gestational age, the benefits of prophylactic administration compared to selective administration were of greater magnitude. The meta-analysis demonstrates that, compared to selective administration, prophylactic administration of natural surfactant to infants less than 30 weeks of gestation resulted in a greater reduction in neonatal mortality (typical RR 0.62, 95% CI 0.49, 0.78; typical ARD -6%, 95% CI -9%, -3%) and a reduction in the combined outcome of bronchopulmonary dysplasia or death (typical RR 0.87, 95% CI 0.77, 0.97; typical ARD -5%, 95% CI -9%, -1%).

The benefits of prophylactic surfactant must be weighed against the fact that prophylaxis with surfactant will result in the treatment of a proportion of infants who do not require surfactant and, if infants are intubated solely for the purpose of surfactant administration, will result in the intubation of a

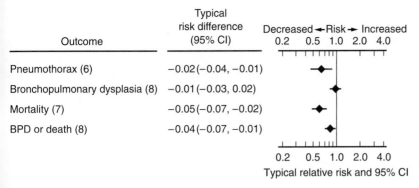

Figure 20-6. Meta-analysis of eight randomized trials comparing prophylactic and rescue treatment with surfactant. Numbers in parentheses following the outcomes are the numbers of trials in which that outcome was reported. BPD, bronchopulmonary dysplasia; CI, confidence interval; diamonds, point estimate; horizontal bars, 95% confidence interval of the relative risk. (From Soll RF, Morley CJ: Prophylactic versus selective use of surfactant for preventing morbidity and mortality in preterm infants [Cochrane Review]. In: The Cochrane Library, Issue 2, 2001. Oxford: Update Software, 2001.)

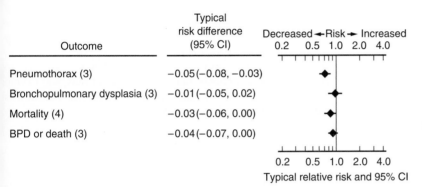

Figure 20-7. Meta-analysis of four randomized trials comparing early and delayed administration of surfactant. Numbers in parentheses following the outcomes are the numbers of trials in which that outcome was reported. BPD, bronchopulmonary dysplasia; CI, confidence interval; diamonds, point estimate; horizontal bars, 95% confidence interval of the relative risk. (From Yost CC, Soll RF: Early versus delayed selective surfactant treatment for neonatal respiratory distress syndrome [Cochrane Review]. In: The Cochrane Library, Issue 2, 2001. Oxford: Update Software, 2001.)

proportion of infants who otherwise would have not been intubated. At what point do the potential benefits of decreased mortality, pneumothorax, and lung injury from prophylactic surfactant exceed the potential risks of endotracheal intubation and the costs of surfactant dosing to infants who would not have required it? Based on the evidence, we believe this threshold is around 30 weeks of gestation. Others have proposed a gestation of 29 weeks[23,94] or 28 weeks.[95] There are no trials comparing the effects of prophylactic surfactant administration to very early selective administration, for example, at 30 to 60 minutes of life; therefore it is uncertain whether very early selective administration is as effective as prophylactic surfactant administration.

Preventilatory Versus Postventilatory Prophylactic Surfactant Administration

The initial studies using prophylactic surfactant administered the drug as an immediate bolus after intubating the infants rapidly after birth (i.e., "before the first breath"). This approach delays the initiation of neonatal resuscitation, including positive-pressure ventilation, and is associated with a risk for surfactant delivery into the right mainstem bronchus or esophagus. It has been shown in a randomized trial that prophylaxis can be administered in small aliquots soon after resuscitation and confirmation of endotracheal tube position, with equivalent or greater efficacy.[96] Based on this trial, prophylactic surfactant should be administered after initial resuscitation of the infant at birth and administration prior to the "first breath" is unnecessary.

Early Versus Late Treatment of Established Respiratory Distress Syndrome

In preterm infants who do not receive prophylaxis, many of the same arguments in support of prophylactic surfactant

administration are also supportive of early surfactant treatment of established RDS. Four randomized controlled trials,[97–100] including the largest randomized trial conducted in neonatology (the OSIRIS trial), evaluated early versus delayed selective surfactant administration. The results of these trials have been summarized in a systematic review.[54] Early administration of surfactant in these trials consisted of administration of the first dose of surfactant within the first 30 minutes, within the first hour, or within the first 2 hours of life. Two of these studies used natural surfactants and two used synthetic surfactant. The results of the meta-analysis of these studies are summarized in Figure 20-7. Early selective treatment resulted in a decrease in the risk of pneumothorax (typical RR 0.70, 95% CI 0.59, 0.82; typical ARD -5%, 95% CI -8%, -3%), a decrease in the risk of pulmonary interstitial emphysema (typical RR 0.63, 95% CI 0.43, 0.93; typical ARD -6%, 95% CI -10%, -1%), a decrease in the risk of chronic lung disease (requirement for supplemental oxygen at 36 weeks of gestation, typical RR 0.70, 95% CI 0.55, 0.88; typical ARD -3%, 95% CI -5%, -1%), and a decrease in the risk of neonatal mortality (typical RR 0.87, 95% CI 0.77, 0.99; typical ARD -3%, 95% CI -6%, 0%). Therefore, in preterm infants who do not receive prophylactic surfactant, the first dose of surfactant should be administered as early as possible. Outborn infants are at highest risk for delayed administration. Tertiary referral units accepting outborn infants should attempt to develop systems to ensure the administration of surfactant as early as possible to these infants, either by the transporting team or, if appropriate, by the referring hospital. In inborn infants, delays in administration of surfactant occur if other admission procedures such as line placement, radiographs, and nursing procedures are allowed to take precedence over surfactant dosing soon after birth. Surfactant administration should be given priority over other admission procedures.

Repeated Administration of Surfactant

Many of the initial trials of surfactant therapy tested a single dose of surfactant; however, surfactant may become rapidly metabolized, and functional inactivation of surfactant can result from the action of soluble proteins and other factors in the small airways and alveoli.[19] The ability to administer subsequent doses of surfactant after the first dose is thought to be useful because multiple dosing can overcome such inactivation. The results of two randomized controlled trials that compared multiple dosing regimens to single-dose regimens of natural surfactant extract for treatment of established RDS[101,102] have been evaluated in a systematic review.[103] In one study,[101] after the initial dose of bovine lipid extract surfactant, infants assigned to the multiple-dose group could receive up to three additional doses of surfactant during the first 72 hours of life if they had a respiratory deterioration, provided they had shown a positive response to the first dose and a pneumothorax had been eliminated as the cause of the respiratory deterioration. In the other study,[102] infants in the multiple-dose group received additional doses of Curosurf at 12 and 24 hours after the initial dose if they still needed supplemental oxygen and mechanical ventilation. Approximately 70% of the infants randomized to the multiple-dose regimen received multiple doses. The meta-analysis supports a decreased risk of pneumothorax associated with multiple-dose surfactant therapy (typical RR 0.51, 95% CI 0.30, 0.88; typical ARD -9%, 95% CI -15%, -2%). There was also a trend toward decreased mortality (typical RR 0.63, 95% CI 0.39, 1.02; typical ARD -7%, 95% CI -14%, 0%). No differences were detected in other clinical outcomes. No complications associated with multiple-dose treatment were reported in these trials. In a third study in which synthetic surfactant was used in a prophylactic manner, the use of two doses of surfactant in addition to a prophylactic dose led to a decrease in mortality, respiratory support, necrotizing enterocolitis, and other outcomes compared to a single prophylactic dose.[103a] In the OSIRIS trial, which used synthetic surfactant, a two-dose treatment schedule was found to be equivalent to a treatment schedule permitting up to four doses of surfactant.

Criteria for Repeat Doses of Surfactant

The use of a higher threshold for re-treatment with surfactant appears to be as effective as a low threshold and can lead to significant savings in costs of the drug. The question of what criteria to use for administration of repeat doses of surfactant has been addressed by two studies, both of which used natural surfactant. In one study[104] the re-treatment criteria compared were an increase in the fraction of inspired oxygen by 0.1 over the lowest baseline value (standard re-treatment) versus a sustained increase of just 0.01 (liberal re-treatment). There were no differences in complications of prematurity or duration of respiratory support; however, short-term benefits in oxygen requirement and ventilatory support were noted in the liberal re-treatment group. In another study,[105] re-treatment at a low threshold (FIO_2 >30%, still requiring endotracheal intubation) was compared to re-treatment at a high threshold (FIO_2 >40%, mean airway pressure >7 cm H_2O). Again, there were minor short-term benefits to using a low threshold with no differences in major clinical outcomes. However, in a subgroup of infants with RDS complicated by perinatal compromise or infection,

infants in the high-threshold group had a trend toward higher mortality than the low-threshold group. Based on current evidence it appears appropriate to use persistent or worsening signs of RDS as criteria for re-treatment with surfactant. It is uncertain whether a low-threshold strategy should be used in certain subgroups of infants or with certain preparations of surfactant.

Methods of Administration of Surfactant

A theoretical model for the transport of exogenous surfactant through the airways has been proposed,[106] consisting of four distinct mechanisms: (1) the instilled bolus may create a liquid plug that occludes the large airways but is forced peripherally during mechanical ventilation; (2) the bolus creates a deposited film on the airway walls, either from the liquid plug transport or from direct coating, which drains under the influence of gravity through the first few airway generations; (3) in smaller airways, surfactant species form a surface layer that spreads due to surface–tension gradients, that is, Marangoni flows; and (4) the surfactant finally reaches the alveolar compartment where it is cleared according to first-order kinetics.

Administration Through Catheter, Side Port, or Suction Valve

According to the manufacturers' recommendations, beractant (Survanta) and poractant (Curosurf) should be administered through a catheter inserted into the endotracheal tube. Colfosceril (Exosurf) should be administered through a side-port adapter attached to the endotracheal tube, and calf lung surfactant extract (Infasurf) can be administered through either a feeding catheter or a side-port adapter. Other methods of administration of surfactant have been tested in randomized trials. In one randomized trial, the administration of beractant (Survanta) through a catheter inserted through a neonatal suction valve without detachment of the neonate from the ventilator was compared to the administration of the dose (with detachment from the ventilator) in two aliquots through a catheter and to the standard technique of administration of the dose in four aliquots through a catheter.[107] Administration through the suction valve led to less dosing-related oxygen desaturation but more reflux of beractant (Survanta) than the two-aliquot catheter technique. In another study,[108] the administration of poractant (Curosurf) as a bolus was compared in a randomized trial to administration via a catheter introduced through a side hole in the tracheal tube adapter without changing the infants' position or interrupting ventilation. The numbers of episodes of hypoxia and/or bradycardia as well as other outcomes were similar in both groups. A slight and transient increase in $PaCO_2$ was observed in the side-hole group.

Administration Through Dual-Lumen Endotracheal Tube

The administration of poractant (Curosurf) through a dual-lumen endotracheal tube without a change in position or interruption of mechanical ventilation was compared to bolus instillation in a randomized trial.[109] The dual-lumen group had fewer episodes of dosing-related hypoxia, a smaller decrease in heart rate and SaO_2, and a shorter total time in supplemental oxygen than the bolus group. The dual-lumen method also has been compared to the side-port method of administration of colfosceril (Exosurf) in a randomized trial.[110] No difference was found between the two methods in terms of dosing-related hypoxemia.

Other Methods

In one randomized clinical trial,[111] the slow infusion of colfosceril (Exosurf) using a microinfusion syringe pump over 10 to 20 minutes was compared to manual instillation over 2 minutes. Pump administration resulted in fewer infants with loss of chest wall movement during dosing, as well as a lesser increase in peak inspiratory pressure than with hand administration. However in animals, slow infusion of surfactant into the endotracheal tube results in nonhomogenous distribution of surfactant in the lung.[112,113] More clinical trials are needed to assess the efficacy of a slow infusion of surfactant. Other methods of administration, such as nebulization or aerosolization[114-117] and in utero administration to the human fetus,[118,119] have been reported. These methods are not currently recommended.

Chest Position During Administration of Surfactant

In a study in rabbits, pulmonary distribution of intratracheally instilled surfactant was largely determined by gravity, and changing the chest position after instillation did not result in any redistribution of the surfactant. For neonates receiving surfactant, keeping the chest in the horizontal position may result in the most even distribution of the surfactant in the two lungs.[120]

In summary, current evidence suggests that the administration of surfactant either using a dual-lumen endotracheal tube or through a catheter passed through a suction valve appears to be effective and may cause less dosing-related adverse events than standard methods. The side-port method of administration and the catheter method of administration appear to be equivalent. More studies are required before firm conclusions can be drawn about the optimal method of administration of surfactant and whether the optimal method is different for different types of surfactant.

ADVERSE EFFECTS OF SURFACTANT THERAPY

Transient hypoxia and bradycardia can occur due to acute airway obstruction immediately following surfactant instillation.[121,122] Other acute adverse effects of surfactant administration include reflux of surfactant into the pharynx from the endotracheal tube, increase in transcutaneous carbon dioxide tension, tachycardia, gagging, and mucous plugging of the endotracheal tube. These complications of surfactant administration generally respond to a slower rate of surfactant administration or to an increase the airway pressure or FIO_2 during administration. Rapid improvement in oxygenation after surfactant administration necessitates close monitoring and appropriate reduction of ventilatory parameters.

Several authors have reported a transient decrease in blood pressure,[123-125] a transient decrease in cerebral blood flow velocity,[126-128] a transient decrease in cerebral oxyhemoglobin concentration,[128] and a transient decrease in cerebral activity on amplitude-integrated electroencephalography (EEG)[123] immediately after surfactant administration. The EEG depression observed after surfactant instillation is not caused by cerebral ischemia,[129] and the EEG suppression is not directly related to alterations in blood gases or systemic circulation.[130] The clinical significance of these findings is uncertain. One study[131] reported an increase in the incidence of intraventricular hemorrhage, and a case report documents a temporal association between the development of intraventricular hemorrhage and the administration of surfactant-TA to improve respiratory failure caused by pulmonary hemorrhage.[132] The meta-analyses of multiple trials do not, however, show an increase in the risk of intraventricular hemorrhage with surfactant therapy compared to placebo.[49-51]

There is a well-described increase in the risk of pulmonary hemorrhage with surfactant therapy.[133,134] The overall incidence of pulmonary hemorrhage was low and the absolute magnitude of the increased risk was small.[133] However, moderate and severe pulmonary hemorrhage is associated with an increased risk of death and short-term morbidity. It is not associated with increased long-term morbidity.[135] Although trials in which natural surfactants were used reported a higher incidence (5% to 6%) of pulmonary hemorrhage than trials of synthetic surfactant (1% to 3%), direct comparison of these two types of surfactants in randomized trials demonstrates no difference in the risk of pulmonary hemorrhage. The occurrence of pulmonary hemorrhage may be related to the presence of a hemodynamically significant patent ductus arteriosus.[136] Seppanen et al.[137] studied the association of neonatal complications with the Doppler-derived aortopulmonary pressure gradient (APPG) across the ductus arteriosus, which reflects pulmonary artery pressure during the first day of life. Infants in whom the APPG decreased after birth had a lower frequency of patent ductus arteriosus and pulmonary hemorrhage than those whose APPG remained low. Another mechanism for pulmonary hemorrhage may be a direct cytotoxicity, which has been demonstrated in in vitro studies and appears to be different for different surfactants and different dosages.[138]

When surfactant initially became available for clinical testing, there was concern that the introduction of foreign proteins from animal-based lung surfactants into the lungs of preterm infants could lead to immunologic responses. Two studies did not find antibodies specific to surfactant protein in the sera of preterm infants treated with bovine surfactant.[139,140] In other studies, immune complexes or antibodies to the protein in exogenous porcine, bovine, or human surfactant have been identified in the sera of neonates with RDS. However, similar immune complexes or antibodies were also noted in control infants who did not receive surfactant-TA, and no significant differences were noted between surfactant-treated and control infants. [141-143] The presence of antibodies in control infants may be the result of leakage of surfactant proteins into the circulation.[141]

With natural surfactants there is a theoretical risk of transmission of infectious agents, including bovine spongiform encephalitis with surfactants derived from bovine sources and other viral infections in swine. Organic solvent processing of phospholipids, terminal sterilization techniques, and screening of animal sources have been used to minimize this risk.

ECONOMIC ASPECTS OF SURFACTANT THERAPY

With the introduction of surfactant therapy there was concern that the increased number of survivors and a possible increase in the length of hospital stay would lead to an increase in the overall cost of neonatal care.[144] These increased costs can by offset to a variable extent by the fact that surfactant therapy can lower hospital charges,[145] reduce the costs or charges per survivor of neonatal intensive care[3,146–148] and reduce the charges for infants who die.[3] In an economic analysis for a hypothetic cohort of infants 700 to 1350 g treated with synthetic surfactant, based on the results of a randomized controlled trial,[149] the total hospital charges through 1-year adjusted age were similar to those for a comparable cohort of infants receiving air placebo, even though more babies in the synthetic surfactant cohort survived and thus required prolonged hospital care during their first year of life. The incremental cost per survivor estimated in this study was $1585 (1995 dollars).

In 1990, the cost per quality-adjusted life-year (QALY) with surfactant therapy was estimated in one study to be $1500[150] and in another study to be 710 pounds.[151] From a societal perspective, the cost effectiveness of surfactant therapy is more favorable than that of health care interventions such as renal transplantation, coronary bypass surgery, and dialysis.[151] In a geographically defined, population-based study from Australia, cost effectiveness and cost-utility ratios in presurfactant and postsurfactant periods were compared for infants of birthweight 500 to 999 g. When costs incurred during the primary hospitalization were considered, both of these ratios were lower (i.e., economically better) in the postsurfactant era than in the presurfactant era (presurfactant vs postsurfactant $7040 vs $4040 per life year gained; $6700 vs $5360 per QALY). Both ratios fell with increasing birthweight. With costs for long-term care of severely disabled children added, both cost ratios were higher in the postsurfactant era.

FACTORS AFFECTING THE RESPONSE TO SURFACTANT THERAPY

Several factors have been reported by various authors to be associated with a poor response to surfactant therapy, in terms of either immediate pulmonary response or later morbidity and mortality. These factors are high total fluid and colloid intake in the first days of life,[152] low mean airway pressure relative to the FIO_2,[152] presence of an additional pulmonary disorder such as infection,[153] perinatal asphyxia, infection, other complications of prematurity,[154] high fraction of inspired oxygen requirement at entry (had a negative impact on mean arterial/alveolar oxygen tension ratio 6 and 24 hours after treatment), lower birthweight, male sex, outborn status, perinatal asphyxia, and high airway pressure requirement at entry.[155] Low birthweight, low Apgar score, and initial disease severity were associated with increased mortality.[156]

A high pulmonary resistance prior to therapy was associated with a poor response to therapy at 24 and 48 hours.[157] In addition, the immediate response to surfactant therapy itself has

been reported to be a significant prognostic indicator for mortality and morbidity.[158] In animal studies, poor response to surfactant has been associated with delayed administration[80] and leakage of proteinaceous fluid into the alveolar spaces. Within some multicenter trials, significant differences in outcomes of surfactant-treated infants have been noted between participating hospitals,[155,156] suggesting that variations in patient care practices have an important influence on the outcomes of surfactant-treated infants.

As noted earlier, observational studies have demonstrated a decrease in mortality and morbidity for such infants after the introduction of surfactant therapy[1,3,56–60]; however, racial differences in this decline in mortality have been reported. In one study, the overall neonatal mortality for black very-low-birthweight (VLBW) infants did not change after the introduction of surfactant therapy.[57] In another study, declines in neonatal mortality risks caused by RDS and all respiratory causes were greater for non-Hispanic white VLBW infants than for black VLBW infants.[159] Although such racial differences have been noted at a population level, the role of racial factors in the response pattern of individual infants with RDS to exogenous surfactant therapy is unknown.

LONG-TERM OUTCOMES AFTER SURFACTANT THERAPY

Long-term outcomes after surfactant therapy have been well studied for synthetic surfactant. Follow-up studies of long-term outcomes after natural surfactant therapy have consisted of small numbers of patients, with a variable proportion of survivors being tested. For both synthetic and natural surfactants, the "long-term" outcomes reported consist of outcomes predominantly in the first 3 years of life, with very few reports of outcomes at school age or higher. Given these limitations, the evidence suggests that not only do more infants survive from surfactant therapy but they are also at no selective disadvantage for neurodevelopmental sequelae due to the surfactant therapy. Most comparisons of long-term outcomes have been between infants treated with surfactant and those treated with placebo. There are few or no comparisons of long-term outcomes between infants treated with different types of surfactant or different regimens of the same surfactant. The following sections mainly address comparisons between infants treated with surfactant and with placebo.

Neurodevelopmental Outcomes

No significant differences have been reported in the long-term neurodevelopmental outcomes of infants treated with surfactant compared to those treated with placebo, either with synthetic surfactant[160–162] or natural surfactant.[58,142,163–166]

Long-Term Respiratory Outcomes

Compared to infants treated with placebo, infants treated with surfactant in the neonatal period have been reported to have either improved[167–169] or equivalent[170–172] results on pulmonary function testing. Some studies have reported a lower frequency of subsequent clinical respiratory disorders in surfactant-treated infants compared to placebo,[173,174] whereas others have reported no difference[142,161,163,167] or a trend toward an increase in allergic manifestations.[166]

Physical growth

No significant differences have been reported in weight or height outcomes between surfactant-treated and placebo-treated infants on follow-up.[142,160,162,166–168,173,175]

Outcomes of Prophylactic Versus Rescue Treatment Strategies

Two studies compared the long-term outcomes of infants treated with prophylactic surfactant to those treated with a "rescue" strategy. In one study, at school age there were no differences in neurodevelopmental outcome or in the results of pulmonary function testing between the two groups, although infants who had received prophylactic surfactant showed fewer clinical pulmonary problems than those who received rescue treatment.[176] In another study in which there was significant number of infants lost to follow-up (and therefore a high likelihood of attrition bias), the mean scores on the Bayley scales of infant development at 12 months adjusted age were higher in the rescue group than in the prophylactic group.[177]

EXOGENOUS SUFACTANT THERAPY FOR CONDITIONS OTHER THAN RESPIRATORY DISTRESS SYNDROME

Meconium Aspiration Syndrome

In vitro studies[178,179] and animal studies[180–182] have demonstrated that meconium inhibits surfactant function and likely is partially responsible for alveolar collapse in meconium aspiration syndrome. Components of meconium that may contribute to altered surfactant function include cholesterol, free fatty acids, bile salts, bilirubin, and proteolytic enzymes.[178–180,183]

In animal models of meconium aspiration syndrome, exogenous surfactant therapy administered as a bolus was shown to have beneficial effects on lung compliance, gas exchange, and alveolar expansion in some studies[184–186] but not in others.[187,188] Treatment of experimental animals with meconium aspiration syndrome by lavage with surfactant has been shown to be beneficial[189,190] and superior to bolus administration.[191,192]

In noncontrolled studies of human infants with meconium aspiration syndrome, improved oxygenation has been reported with exogenous surfactant therapy.[193–195] A randomized trial in infants greater than 34 weeks of gestation with severe respiratory failure on extracorporeal membrane oxygenation (ECMO; including infants with meconium aspiration syndrome) showed that infants treated with beractant (Survanta) had improved lung function, a shorter duration of ECMO, and fewer complications after ECMO.[196]

A systematic review of two randomized controlled trials[197,197a] that evaluated the effect of beractant (Survanta) administration in term infants with meconium aspiration syndrome is available.[197b] In one trial,[197] infants treated with surfactant had fewer pneumothoraces (relative risk 0.09, 95% CI

0.01, 1.54, risk difference -0.25, 95% CI -0.45, -0.05), improved oxygenation, and shorter durations of ventilation and hospitalization. Both trials reported a decrease in the number of infants receiving ECMO. A meta-analysis of these trials supports a significant reduction in the risk of requiring ECMO (typical relative risk 0.64, 95% CI 0.46, 0.91 typical risk difference -0.17, 95% CI -0.30, -0.04). No difference was noted in overall mortality (typical relative risk 1.86, 95% CI 0.35, 9.89, typical risk difference 0.02, 95% CI -0.03, 0.07).

In the randomized trials described earlier, surfactant therapy was administered as a bolus. A number of investigators have attempted to treat meconium aspiration syndrome with diluted surfactant solutions used as a lavage to wash residual meconium from the airway.[198–200] This approach to surfactant treatment remains experimental.

In conclusion, the use of exogenous surfactant therapy in infants with severe meconium aspiration syndrome is likely to be beneficial. Multiple doses usually are required in such infants. Only natural surfactants have been tested in human clinical trials in this setting, and the efficacy of synthetic surfactants is unknown. Each dose should be administered cautiously, with close cardiorespiratory and oxygen saturation monitoring, in case preexisting airway obstruction from meconium is aggravated by surfactant.

Acute Respiratory Distress Syndrome

Because of the success of surfactant replacement therapy in infants with neonatal RDS, surfactant replacement has been proposed as a treatment for patients with acute lung injury and acute RDS. The occurrence of ARDS has been reported in term neonates.[201,202] There are no randomized trials of exogenous surfactant therapy specifically for ARDS in neonates. It often is difficult to reliably distinguish ARDS from RDS due to surfactant deficiency. Because of this, and based on the pathophysiologic, clinical, and radiologic similarities between the two conditions, we believe that it is reasonable to provide exogenous surfactant therapy to term infants with a clinico-radiologic picture of ARDS (severe respiratory failure with pulmonary opacification and air bronchograms on chest radiographs).

In two randomized controlled trials in children (not neonates) with acute hypoxemic respiratory failure,[203,204] patients who received calfactant (Infasurf) demonstrated rapid improvement in oxygenation, were extubated sooner, and spent fewer days in pediatric intensive care than control patients. There was no difference in mortality or overall hospital stay. No serious adverse effects were noted. In another randomized trial in children with respiratory failure due to bronchiolitis, treatment with poractant (Curosurf) resulted in similar short-term improvements.[205] Exogenous surfactant therapy has also been attempted in ARDS in adults but the results of clinical trials have not been promising.[206,207] Further research is required in this area.

Other Conditions

There are reports (anecdotal or case series) of the use of exogenous surfactant therapy in human infants for the management of pulmonary hemorrhage,[208] neonatal pneumonia,[209] and congenital diaphragmatic hernia.[210–212] However, the efficacy of surfactant in these conditions is uncertain and its routine use in these conditions cannot be recommended.

NEWER SURFACTANTS

Two synthetic surfactants are currently in a development and testing phase. Lucinactant (Surfaxin) is a synthetic preparation that contains a peptide called *KL4* (sinapultide), a mimic of SP-B. KL4 is a 21-residue peptide consisting of repeated units of four hydrophobic leucine (L) residues, bounded by basic polar lysine (K) residues. It is combined with dipalmitoyl phosphatidylcholine, palmitoyl oleoylphosphatidyl glycerol, and palmitic acid.[192,213] Another synthetic surfactant, rSP-C surfactant (Venticute), contains a recombinant form of SP-C, along with DPPC, palmitoyl oleoylphosphatidyl glycerol, palmitic acid, and calcium chloride.[214,215] The recombinant surfactant protein C in this preparation (rSP-C) is an analogue of the human surfactant protein SP-C.

CONCLUSION

Exogenous surfactant therapy has been a significant advance in the management of preterm infants with RDS and has become established as a standard part of the management of such infants. Both natural and synthetic surfactants lead to clinical improvement and decreased mortality, with natural surfactants having additional advantages over synthetic surfactants. The use of prophylactic surfactant, administered after initial stabilization at birth, in infants at risk for RDS has benefits over "rescue" surfactant given to treat infants with established RDS. In infants who do not receive prophylaxis, earlier treatment (before 2 hours) has benefits over later treatment. The use of multiple doses of surfactant is a strategy to the use of a single dose, and the use of a higher threshold for re-treatment appears to be as effective as a low threshold. Adverse effects of surfactant therapy are infrequent and usually not serious. Long-term follow-up of infants treated with surfactant in the neonatal period is reassuring. In the future we likely will see the development of new types of surfactants, and further research is required on the optimal use of surfactant in conjunction with other respiratory interventions.

REFERENCES

1. Lee K, Khoshnood B, Wall SN, et al: Trend in mortality from respiratory distress syndrome in the United States, 1970–1995. J Pediatr 134:434–440, 1999.
2. Schoendorf KC, Kiely JL: Birth weight and age-specific analysis of the 1990 US infant mortality drop. Was it surfactant? Arch Pediatr Adolesc Med 151:129–134, 1997.
3. Schwartz RM, Luby AM, Scanlon JW, et al: Effect of surfactant on morbidity, mortality, and resource use in newborn infants weighing 500 to 1500 g. N Engl J Med 330:1476–1480, 1994.
4. Clements JA: Surface tension of lung extracts. Proc Soc Exp Biol Med 95:170–172, 1957.
5. Pattle RE: Properties, function and origin of the alveolar lining layer. Nature 175:1125–1126, 1955.
6. von Neergaard K: Neue auffassungen uber einen grundbegriff der atemmechanik. Die retraktionskraft der lunge, abhangig von der oberflachenspannung in den alveolen. Z Gesamte Exp Med 66:373–394, 1929.
7. Avery ME, Mead J: Surface properties in relation to atelectasis and hyaline membrane disease. Am J Dis Child 97:517–523, 1959.
8. Gruenwald P: Surface tension as a factor in the resistance of neonatal lungs to aeration. Am J Obstet Gynecol 53:996–1007, 1947.
9. Chu J, Clements JA, Cotton EK, et al: Neonatal pulmonary ischemia: Clinical and physiological studies. Pediatrics 40:709–782, 1967.
10. Robillard E, Alarie Y, Dagenais-Perusse P, et al: Microaerosol administration of synthetic dipalmitoyl-L-lecithin in the respiratory distress syndrome: A preliminary report. Can Med Assoc J 90:55–57, 1964.
11. Enhorning G, Robertson B: Lung expansion in the premature rabbit fetus after tracheal deposition of surfactant. Pediatrics 50:58–66, 1972.
12. Fujiwara T, Maeta H, Chida S, et al: Artificial surfactant in hyaline membrane disease. Lancet 1:55–59, 1980.
13. Avery ME: Surfactant deficiency in hyaline membrane disease: The story of discovery. Am J Respir Crit Care Med 161:1074–1075, 2000.
14. Enhorning G: From bubbles to babies: The evolution of surfactant replacement therapy. Biol Neonate 71(Suppl 1):28–31, 1997.
15. McGee RS Jr: Pulmonary surfactant. A historical perspective of how it came to be used in the treatment of respiratory distress syndrome in the neonate. N C Med J 54:447–451, 1993.
16. Creuwels LA, van Golde LM, Haagsman HP: The pulmonary surfactant system: Biochemical and clinical aspects. Lung 175:1–39, 1997.
17. Griese M: Pulmonary surfactant in health and human lung diseases: State of the art. Eur Respir J 13:1455–1476, 1999.
18. Jobe AH, Ikegami M: Surfactant metabolism. Clin Perinatol 20:683–696, 1993.
19. Jobe AH: Pulmonary surfactant therapy. N Engl J Med 328:861–868, 1993.
20. Kuroki Y, Voelker DR: Pulmonary surfactant proteins. J Biol Chem 42:25943–25946, 1994.
21. Possmayer F, Yu SH, Weber JM, et al: Pulmonary surfactant. Can J Biochem Cell Biol 62:1121–1133, 1984.
22. Wiseman LR, Bryson HM: Porcine-derived lung surfactant. A review of the therapeutic efficacy and clinical tolerability of a natural surfactant preparation (Curosurf) in neonatal respiratory distress syndrome [published erratum appears in Drugs 49:70, 1995]. Drugs 48:386–403, 1994.
23. Kattwinkel J: Surfactant. Evolving issues. Clin Perinatol 25:17–32, 1998.
24. Robertson B, Halliday HL: Principles of surfactant replacement. Biochim Biophys Acta 1408:346–361, 1998.
25. Hallman M, Merritt TA, Jarvenpaa AL, et al: Exogenous human surfactant for treatment of severe respiratory distress syndrome: A randomized prospective clinical trial. J Pediatr 106:963–969, 1985.
26. Merritt TA, Hallman M, Berry C, et al: Randomized, placebo-controlled trial of human surfactant given at birth versus rescue administration in very low birth weight infants with lung immaturity. J Pediatr 118:581–594, 1991.
27. Tooley WH, Clements JA, Muramatsu K, et al: Lung function in prematurely delivered rabbits treated with a synthetic surfactant. Am Rev Respir Dis 136:651–656, 1987.
28. Robertson B, Enhorning G: The alveolar lining of the premature newborn rabbit after pharyngeal deposition of surfactant. Lab Invest 31:54–59, 1974.
29. Collaborative European Multicenter Study Group: Surfactant replacement therapy for severe neonatal respiratory distress syndrome: An international randomized clinical trial. Pediatrics 82:683–691, 1988.
30. Bhat R, Dziedzic K, Bhutani VK, et al: Effect of single dose surfactant on pulmonary function. Crit Care Med 18:590–595, 1990.
31. Bhutani VK, Abbasi S, Long WA, et al: Pulmonary mechanics and energetics in preterm infants who had respiratory distress syndrome treated with synthetic surfactant. J Pediatr 120:S18–S24, 1992.
32. Couser RJ, Ferrara TB, Ebert J, et al: Effects of exogenous surfactant therapy on dynamic compliance during mechanical breathing in preterm infants with hyaline membrane disease. J Pediatr 116:119–124, 1990.
33. Billman D, Nicks J, Schumacher R: Exosurf rescue surfactant improves high ventilation-perfusion mismatch in respiratory distress syndrome. Pediatr Pulmonol 18:279–283, 1994.
34. Bowen W, Martin CR, Krauss AN, et al: Ventilation-perfusion relationships in preterm infants after surfactant treatment. Pediatr Pulmonol 18:155–162, 1994.
35. Sandberg KL, Lindstrom DP, Sjoqvist BA, et al: Surfactant replacement therapy improves ventilation inhomogeneity in infants with respiratory distress syndrome. Pediatr Pulmonol 24:337–343, 1997.
36. Alexander J, Milner AD: Lung volume and pulmonary blood flow measurements following exogenous surfactant. Eur J Pediatr 154:392–397, 1995.
37. Bloom MC, Roques-Gineste M, Fries F, et al: Pulmonary haemodynamics after surfactant replacement in severe neonatal respiratory distress syndrome. Arch Dis Child Fetal Neonatal Ed 73:F95–F98, 1995.

38. Halliday HL, McCord FB, McClure BG, et al: Acute effects of instillation of surfactant in severe respiratory distress syndrome. Arch Dis Child 64:13–16, 1989.

39. Hamdan AH, Shaw NJ: Changes in pulmonary artery pressure in infants with respiratory distress syndrome following treatment with Exosurf. Arch Dis Child Fetal Neonatal Ed 72:F176–F179, 1995.

40. Hamdan AH, Shaw NJ: Changes in pulmonary artery pressure during the acute phase of respiratory distress syndrome treated with three different types of surfactant. Pediatr Pulmonol 25:191–195, 1998.

41. Kaapa P, Seppanen M, Kero P, et al: Pulmonary hemodynamics after synthetic surfactant replacement in neonatal respiratory distress syndrome. J Pediatr 123:115–119, 1993.

42. Seppanen M, Kaapa P, Kero P: Acute effects of synthetic surfactant replacement on pulmonary blood flow in neonatal respiratory distress syndrome. Am J Perinatol 11:382–385, 1994.

43. Skinner J: The effects of surfactant on haemodynamics in hyaline membrane disease. Arch Dis Child Fetal Neonatal Ed 76:F67–F69, 1997.

44. Bick U, Muller-Leisse C, Troger J, et al: Therapeutic use of surfactant in neonatal respiratory distress syndrome. Correlation between pulmonary X-ray changes and clinical data. Pediatr Radiol 22:169–173, 1992.

45. Clarke EA, Siegle RL, Gong AK: Findings on chest radiographs after prophylactic pulmonary surfactant treatment of premature infants. AJR Am J Roentgenol 153:799–802, 1989.

46. Dinger J, Schwarze R, Rupprecht E: Radiological changes after therapeutic use of surfactant in infants with respiratory distress syndrome. Pediatr Radiol 27:26–31, 1997.

47. Slama M, Andre C, Huon C, et al: Radiological analysis of hyaline membrane disease after exogenous surfactant treatment. Pediatr Radiol 29:56–60, 1999.

48. Soll RF, Horbar JD, Griscom NT, et al: Radiographic findings associated with surfactant treatment. Am J Perinatol 8:114–118, 1991.

49. Soll RF: Prophylactic natural surfactant extract for preventing morbidity and mortality in preterm infants (Cochrane Review). In: The Cochrane Library, Issue 2, 2001. Oxford: Update Software, 2001.

50. Soll RF: Prophylactic synthetic surfactant for preventing morbidity and mortality in preterm infants (Cochrane Review). In: The Cochrane Library, Issue 2, 2001. Oxford: Update Software, 2001.

51. Soll RF: Synthetic surfactant for respiratory distress syndrome in preterm infants (Cochrane Review). In: The Cochrane Library, Issue 2, 2001. Oxford: Update Software, 2001.

52. Soll RF, Blanco F: Natural surfactant extract versus synthetic surfactant for neonatal respiratory distress syndrome (Cochrane Review). In: The Cochrane Library, Issue 2, 2001. Oxford: Update Software, 2001.

53. Soll RF, Morley CJ: Prophylactic versus selective use of surfactant for preventing morbidity and mortality in preterm infants (Cochrane Review). In: The Cochrane Library, Issue 2, 2001. Oxford: Update Software, 2001.

54. Yost CC, Soll RF: Early versus delayed selective surfactant treatment for neonatal respiratory distress syndrome (Cochrane Review). In: The Cochrane Library, Issue 2, 2001. Oxford: Update Software, 2001.

55. Soll RF: Surfactant treatment of the very preterm infant. Biol Neonate 74(Suppl 1):35–42, 1998.

56. Doyle LW, Gultom E, Chuang SL, et al: Changing mortality and causes of death in infants 23–27 weeks' gestational age. J Paediatr Child Health 35:255–259, 1999.

57. Hamvas A, Wise PH, Yang RK, et al: The influence of the wider use of surfactant therapy on neonatal mortality among blacks and whites. N Engl J Med 334:1635–1640, 1996.

58. Hoekstra RE, Ferrara TB, Payne NR: Effects of surfactant therapy on outcome of extremely premature infants. Eur J Pediatr 153:S12–S16, 1994.

59. Horbar JD, Wright EC, Onstad L: Decreasing mortality associated with the introduction of surfactant therapy: An observational study of neonates weighing 601 to 1300 grams at birth. The Members of the National Institute of Child Health and Human Development Neonatal Research Network. Pediatrics 92:191–196, 1993.

60. Philip AG: Neonatal mortality rate: Is further improvement possible? J Pediatr 126:427–433, 1995.

61. Possmayer F: The role of surfactant associated proteins. Am Rev Respir Dis 142:749–752, 1990.

62. Ainsworth SB, Beresford MW, Milligan DW, et al: Pumactant and poractant alfa for treatment of respiratory distress syndrome in neonates born at 25–29 weeks' gestation: A randomised trial [published erratum appears in Lancet 12:600, 2000]. Lancet 355:1387–1392, 2000.

63. Alvarado M, Hingre R, Hakason D, et al: Clinical trial of Survanta versus Exosurf in infants <1500 g with respiratory distress syndrome. Pediatr Res 33:314A, 1993.

64. da Costa DE, Pai MG, Al Khusaiby SM: Comparative trial of artificial and natural surfactants in the treatment of respiratory distress syndrome of prematurity: Experiences in a developing country. Pediatr Pulmonol 27:312–317, 1999.

65. Horbar JD, Wright LL, Soll RF, et al: A multicenter randomized trial comparing two surfactants for the treatment of neonatal respiratory distress syndrome. J Pediatr 123:757–766, 1993.

66. Hudak ML, Farrell EE, Rosenberg AA, et al: A multicenter randomized, masked comparison trial of natural versus synthetic surfactant for the treatment of respiratory distress syndrome. J Pediatr 128:396–406, 1996.

67. Hudak ML, Martin DJ, Egan EA, et al: A multicenter randomized masked comparison trial of synthetic surfactant versus calf lung surfactant extract in the prevention of neonatal respiratory distress syndrome. Pediatrics 100:39–50, 1997.

68. Kukkonen AK, Virtanen M, Jarvenpaa AL, et al: Randomized trial comparing natural and synthetic surfactant: Increased infection rate after natural surfactant? Acta Paediatr 89:556–561, 2000.

69. Modanlou HD, Beharry K, Padilla G, et al: Comparative efficacy of Exosurf and Survanta surfactants on early clinical course of respiratory distress syndrome and complications of prematurity. J Perinatol 17:455–460, 1997.

70. Pearlman SA, Leef KH, Stefano JL, et al: A randomized trial comparing Exosurf versus Survanta in the treatment of neonatal RDS. Pediatr Res 33:340A, 1993.

71. Sehgal SS, Ewing CK, Richards T, et al: Modified bovine surfactant (Survanta) versus a protein-free surfactant (Exosurf) in the treatment of respiratory distress syndrome in preterm infants: A pilot study. J Nat Med Assoc 86:46–52, 1994.

72. Vermont-Oxford Neonatal Network: A multicenter, randomized trial comparing synthetic surfactant with modified bovine surfactant extract in the treatment of neonatal respiratory distress syndrome. Pediatrics 97:1–6, 1996.

73. Choukroun ML, Llanas B, Apere H, et al: Pulmonary mechanics in ventilated preterm infants with respiratory distress syndrome after exogenous surfactant administration: A comparison between two surfactant preparations. Pediatr Pulmonol 18:273–278, 1994.

74. Rollins M, Jenkins J, Tubman R, et al: Comparison of clinical responses to natural and synthetic surfactants. J Perinat Med 21:341–347, 1993.

75. Halliday HL: Controversies: Synthetic or natural surfactant. The case for natural surfactant. J Perinat Med 24:417–426, 1996.

76. Hall SB, Venkitaraman AR, Whitsett JA, et al: Importance of hydrophobic apoproteins as constituents of clinical exogenous surfactants. Am Rev Respir Dis 145:24–30, 1992.

77. Bloom BT, Kattwinkel J, Hall RT, et al: Comparison of Infasurf (Calf Lung Surfactant Extract) to Survanta (Beractant) in the treatment and prevention of respiratory distress syndrome. Pediatrics 100:31–38, 1997.

78. Speer CP, Gefeller O, Groneck P, et al: Randomised clinical trial of two treatment regimens of natural surfactant preparations in neonatal respiratory distress syndrome. Arch Dis Child Fetal Neonatal Ed 72:F8–13, 1995.

79. Jobe A, Ikegami M, Jacobs H, et al: Surfactant and pulmonary blood flow distributions following treatment of premature lambs with natural surfactant. J Clin Invest 73:848–856, 1984.

80. Seidner SR, Ikegami M, Yamada T, et al: Decreased surfactant dose-response after delayed administration to preterm rabbits. Am J Respir Crit Care Med 152:113–120, 1995.

81. Ikegami M, Wada K, Emerson GA, et al: Effects of ventilation style on surfactant metabolism and treatment response in preterm lambs. Am J Respir Crit Care Med 157:638–644, 1998.

82. Jobe AH, Ikegami M: Mechanisms initiating lung injury in the preterm. Early Hum Dev 53:81–94, 1998.

83. Jobe AH, Ikegami M: Surfactant and acute lung injury. Proc Assoc Am Physicians 110:489–495, 1998.

84. Bjorklund LJ, Ingimarsson J, Curstedt T, et al: Manual ventilation with a few large breaths at birth compromises the therapeutic effect of subsequent surfactant replacement in immature lambs. Pediatr Res 42:348–355, 1997.

85. Rider ED, Jobe AH, Ikegami M, et al: Different ventilation strategies alter surfactant responses in preterm rabbits. J Appl Physiol 76:2089–2096, 1992.

86. Nilsson R, Grossman G, Robertson B: Bronchiolar epithelial lesions induced in the premature rabbit neonate by short periods of artificial ventilation. Acta Pathol Microbiol Scand 88:359–367, 1980.

87. Bevilacqua G, Chernev T, Parmigiani S, et al: Use of surfactant for prophylaxis versus rescue treatment of respiratory distress syndrome: Experience from an Italian-Bulgarian trial. Acta Biomed Ateneo Parmense 68(Suppl 1):47–54, 1997.

88. Bevilacqua G, Parmigiani S, Robertson B: Prophylaxis of respiratory distress syndrome by treatment with modified porcine surfactant at birth: A multicentre prospective randomized trial. J Perinat Med 24:609–620, 1996.

89. Dunn MS, Shennan AT, Zayack D, et al: Bovine surfactant replacement therapy in neonates of less than 30 weeks' gestation: A randomized controlled trial of prophylaxis versus treatment. Pediatrics 87:377–386, 1991.

90. Egberts J, de Winter JP, Sedin G, et al: Comparison of prophylaxis and rescue treatment with Curosurf in neonates less than 30 weeks' gestation: A randomized trial. Pediatrics 92:768–774, 1993.

91. Kattwinkel J, Bloom BT, Delmore P, et al: Prophylactic administration of calf lung surfactant extract is more effective than early treatment of respiratory distress syndrome in neonates of 29 through 32 weeks' gestation. Pediatrics 92:90–98, 1993.

92. Kendig JW, Notter RH, Cox C, et al: A comparison of surfactant as immediate prophylaxis and as rescue therapy in newborns of less than 30 weeks' gestation. N Engl J Med 324:865–871, 1991.

93. Walti H, Paris-Llado J, Breart G, et al: Porcine surfactant replacement therapy in newborns of 25–31 weeks' gestation: A randomized, multicentre trial of prophylaxis versus rescue with multiple low doses. The French Collaborative Multicentre Study Group. Acta Paediatr 84:913–921, 1995.

94. Spafford PS, Kendig JW, Maniscalco WM: Use of natural surfactants to prevent and treat respiratory distress syndrome. Semin Perinatol 17:285–294, 1993.

95. Halliday HL: Prophylactic surfactant for preterm infants. In Cockburn F (ed): Advances in Perinatal Medicine. Lancaster, Parthenon Press, 1997, pp. 360–370.

96. Kendig JW, Ryan RM, Sinkin RA, et al: Comparison of two strategies for surfactant prophylaxis in very premature infants: A multicenter randomized trial. Pediatrics 101:1006–1012, 1998.

97. European Exosurf Study Group: Early or selective surfactant (colfosceril palmitate, Exosurf) for intubated babies at 26 to 29 weeks gestation. A European double-blind trial with sequential analysis. Online J Curr Clin Trials Doc No 28:3886, 1992.

98. Konishi M, Fujiwara T, Chida S, et al: A prospective, randomized trial of early versus late administration of a single dose of surfactant-TA. Early Hum Dev 29:275–282, 1992.

99. Gortner L, Wauer RR, Hammer H, et al: Early versus late surfactant treatment in preterm infants of 27 to 32 weeks' gestational age: A multicenter controlled clinical trial. Pediatrics 102:1153–1160, 1998.

100. The OSIRIS Collaborative Group: Early versus delayed neonatal administration of a synthetic surfactant—The judgment of OSIRIS. (Open study of infants at high risk of or with respiratory insufficiency—the role of surfactant.) Lancet 340:1363–1369, 1992.

101. Dunn MS, Shennan AT, Possmayer F: Single- versus multiple-dose surfactant replacement therapy in neonates of 30 to 36 weeks' gestation with respiratory distress syndrome. Pediatrics 86:564–571, 1990.

102. Speer CP, Robertson B, Curstedt T, et al: Randomized European multicenter trial of surfactant replacement therapy for severe neonatal respiratory distress syndrome: Single versus multiple doses of Curosurf. Pediatrics 89:13–20, 1992.

103. Soll RF: Multiple versus single dose natural surfactant extract for severe neonatal respiratory distress syndrome (Cochrane Review). In: The Cochrane Library, Issue 2, 2001. Oxford: Update Software, 2001.

103a. Corbet A, Gerdes J, Long W, et al: Double-blind, randomized trial of one versus three prophylactic doses of synthetic surfactant in 826 neonates weighing 700 to 1100 grams: Effects on mortality rate. American Exosurf Neonatal Study Groups I and IIa. J Pediatr 126:969–978, 1995.

104. Dunn MS, Shennan AT, Zayack D, et al: Bovine surfactant replacement therapy-a comparison of 2 retreatment strategies in premature infants with RDS. Pediatr Res 29:212A, 1991.

105. Kattwinkel J, Bloom BT, Delmore P, et al: High-versus low-threshold surfactant retreatment for neonatal respiratory distress syndrome. Pediatrics 106:282–288, 2000.

106. Halpern D, Jensen OE, Grotberg JB: A theoretical study of surfactant and liquid delivery into the lung. J Appl Physiol 85:333–352, 1998.

107. Zola EM, Gunkel JH, Chan RK, et al: Comparison of three dosing procedures for administration of bovine surfactant to neonates with respiratory distress syndrome. J Pediatr 122:453–459, 1993.

108. Soler A, Lopez-Heredia J, Fernandez-Ruanova MB, et al: A simplified surfactant dosing procedure in respiratory distress syndrome: The "side-hole" randomized study. Spanish Surfactant Collaborative Group. Acta Paediatr 86:747–751, 1997.

109. Soler A, Fernandez-Ruanova B, Lopez H, et al: A randomized comparison of surfactant dosing via a dual-lumen endotracheal tube in respiratory distress syndrome. The Spanish Surfactant Collaborative Group. Pediatrics 101:E4, 1998.

110. Nelson M, Nicks JJ, Becker MA, et al: Comparison of two methods of surfactant administration and the effect on dosing-associated hypoxemia. J Perinatol 17:450–454, 1997.

111. Sitler CG, Turnage CS, McFadden BE, et al: Pump administration of exogenous surfactant: Effects on oxygenation, heart rate, and chest wall movement of premature infants. J Perinatol 13:197–200, 1993.

112. Ueda T, Ikegami M, Rider ED, et al: Distribution of surfactant and ventilation in surfactant-treated preterm lambs. J Appl Physiol 76:45–55, 1994.

113. Segerer H, van Gelder W, Angenent FW, et al: Pulmonary distribution and efficacy of exogenous surfactant in lung-lavaged rabbits are influenced by the instillation technique. Pediatr Res 34:490–494, 1993.

114. Berggren E, Liljedahl M, Winbladh B, et al: Pilot study of nebulized surfactant therapy for neonatal respiratory distress syndrome. Acta Paediatr 89:460–464, 2000.

115. Dijk PH, Heikamp A, Oetomo SB: Surfactant nebulization versus instillation during high frequency ventilation in surfactant-deficient rabbits. Pediatr Res 44:699–704, 1998.

116. Ellyett KM, Broadbent RS, Fawcett ER, et al: Surfactant aerosol treatment of respiratory distress syndrome in the spontaneously breathing premature rabbit. Pediatr Res 39:953–957, 1996.

117. Fok TF, al Essa M, Dolovich M, et al: Nebulisation of surfactants in an animal model of neonatal respiratory distress. Arch Dis Child Fetal Neonatal Ed 78:F3–F9, 1998.

118. Cosmi EV, La Torre R, Di Iorio R, et al: Surfactant administration to the human fetus in utero: A new approach to prevention of neonatal respiratory distress syndrome (RDS). J Perinat Med 24:191–193, 1996.

119. Petrikovsky BM, Lysikiewicz A, Markin LB, et al: In utero surfactant administration to preterm human fetuses using endoscopy. Fetal Diagn Ther 10:127–130, 1995.

120. Broadbent R, Fok TF, Dolovich M, et al: Chest position and pulmonary deposition of surfactant in surfactant depleted rabbits. Arch Dis Child Fetal Neonatal Ed 72:F84–F89, 1995.

121. Liechty EA, Donovan E, Purohit D, et al: Reduction of neonatal mortality after multiple doses of bovine surfactant in low birth weight neonates with respiratory distress syndrome. Pediatrics 88:19–28, 1991.

122. Zola EM, Overbach AM, Gunkel JH, et al: Treatment investigational new drug experience with Survanta (beractant). Pediatrics 91:546–551, 1993.

123. Hellstrom-Westas L, Bell AH, Skov L, et al: Cerebroelectrical depression following surfactant treatment in preterm neonates. Pediatrics 89:643–647, 1992.

124. Skov L, Bell A, Greisen G: Surfactant administration and the cerebral circulation. Biol Neonate 61(Suppl 1):31–36, 1992.

125. Skov L, Hellstrom-Westas L, Jacobsen T, et al: Acute changes in cerebral oxygenation and cerebral blood volume in preterm infants during surfactant treatment. Neuropediatrics 23:126–130, 1992.

126. Cowan F, Whitelaw A, Wertheim D, et al: Cerebral blood flow velocity changes after rapid administration of surfactant. Arch Dis Child 66:1105–1109, 1991.

127. Murdoch E, Kempley ST: Randomized trial examining cerebral haemodynamics following artificial or animal surfactant. Acta Paediatr 87:411–415, 1998.

128. Edwards AD, McCormick DC, Roth SC, et al: Cerebral hemodynamic effects of treatment with modified natural surfactant investigated by near infrared spectroscopy. Pediatr Res 32:532–536, 1992.

129. Bell AH, Skov L, Lundstrom KE, et al: Cerebral blood flow and plasma hypoxanthine in relation to surfactant treatment. Acta Paediatr 83:910–914, 1994.

130. Lundstrom KE, Greisen G: Changes in EEG, systemic circulation and blood gas parameters following two or six aliquots of porcine surfactant. Acta Paediatr 85:708–712, 1996.

131. Horbar JD, Soll RF, Schachinger H, et al: A European multicenter randomized controlled trial of single dose surfactant therapy for idiopathic respiratory distress syndrome. Eur J Pediatr 149:416–423, 1990.

132. Funato M, Tamai H, Noma K, et al: Clinical events in association with timing of intraventricular hemorrhage in preterm infants. J Pediatr 121:614–619, 1992.

133. Raju TN, Langenberg P: Pulmonary hemorrhage and exogenous surfactant therapy: A metaanalysis. J Pediatr 123:603–610, 1993.

134. Tomaszewska M, Stork E, Minich NM, et al: Pulmonary hemorrhage: Clinical course and outcomes among very low-birth-weight infants. Arch Pediatr Adolesc Med 153:715–721, 1999.

135. Pandit PB, O'Brien K, Asztalos E, et al: Outcome following pulmonary haemorrhage in very low birthweight neonates treated with surfactant. Arch Dis Child Fetal Neonatal Ed 81:F40–F44, 1999.

136. Garland J, Buck R, Weinberg M: Pulmonary hemorrhage risk in infants with a clinically diagnosed patent ductus arteriosus: A retrospective cohort study. Pediatrics 94:719–723, 1994.

137. Seppanen MP, Kaapa PO, Kero PO: Hemodynamic prediction of complications in neonatal respiratory distress syndrome. J Pediatr 127:780–785, 1995.

138. Findlay RD, Taeusch HW, David-Cu R, et al: Lysis of red blood cells and alveolar epithelial toxicity by therapeutic pulmonary surfactants. Pediatr Res 37:26–30, 1995.

139. Bartmann P, Bamberger U, Pohlandt F, et al: Immunogenicity and immunomodulatory activity of bovine surfactant (SF-RI 1). Acta Paediatr 81:383–388, 1992.

140. Whitsett JA, Hull WM, Luse S: Failure to detect surfactant protein-specific antibodies in sera of premature infants treated with Survanta, a modified bovine surfactant. Pediatrics 87:505–510, 1991.

141. Chida S, Phelps DS, Soll RF, et al: Surfactant proteins and anti-surfactant antibodies in sera from infants with respiratory distress syndrome with and without surfactant treatment. Pediatrics 88:84–89, 1991.

142. Robertson B, Curstedt T, Tubman R, et al: A 2-year follow up of babies enrolled in a European multicentre trial of porcine surfactant replacement for severe neonatal respiratory distress syndrome. Collaborative European Multicentre Study Group. Eur J Pediatr 151:372–376, 1992.

143. Strayer DS, Merritt TA, Hallman M: Surfactant replacement: Immunological considerations. Eur Respir J Suppl 3:91s–96s, 1989.

144. Eidelman AI: Economic consequences of surfactant therapy. J Perinatol 13:137–139, 1993.

145. Maniscalco WM, Kendig JW, Shapiro DL: Surfactant replacement therapy: Impact on hospital charges for premature infants with respiratory distress syndrome. Pediatrics 83:1–6, 1989.

146. Mugford M, Piercy J, Chalmers I: Cost implications of different approaches to the prevention of respiratory distress syndrome. Arch Dis Child 66:757–764, 1991.

147. Phibbs CS, Phibbs RH, Wakeley A, et al: Cost effects of surfactant therapy for neonatal respiratory distress syndrome. J Pediatr 123:953–962, 1993.

148. Soll RF, Jacobs J, Pashko S, et al: Cost effectiveness of beractant in the prevention of respiratory distress syndrome. Pharmacoeconomics 4:278–286, 1993.

149. Mauskopf JA, Backhouse ME, Jones D, et al: Synthetic surfactant for rescue treatment of respiratory distress syndrome in premature infants weighing from 700 to 1350 grams: Impact on hospital resource use and charges. J Pediatr 126:94–101, 1995.

150. Mammel M, Mullett M, Derleth DL, et al: Economic impact of two rescue doses of Exosurf neonatal in 700–1350 gram infants [abstract]. Pediatr Res 29:260A, 1991.

151. Tubman TR, Halliday HL, Normand C: Cost of surfactant replacement treatment for severe neonatal respiratory distress syndrome: A randomised controlled trial [published erratum appears in BMJ 302:27, 1991]. BMJ 301:842–845, 1990.

152. Hallman M, Merritt TA, Bry K, et al: Association between neonatal care practices and efficacy of exogenous human surfactant: Results of a bicenter randomized trial. Pediatrics 91:552–560, 1993.

153. Segerer H, Stevens P, Schadow B, et al: Surfactant substitution in ventilated very low birth weight infants: Factors related to response types. Pediatr Res 30:591–596, 1991.

154. Konishi M, Chida S, Shimada S, et al: Surfactant replacement therapy in premature babies with respiratory distress syndrome: Factors affecting the response to surfactant and comparison of outcome from 1982–86 and 1987–91. Acta Paediatr Jpn 34:617–630, 1992.

155. Collaborative European Multicentre Study Group: Factors influencing the clinical response to surfactant replacement therapy in babies with severe respiratory distress syndrome. Eur J Pediatr 150:433–439, 1991.

156. Herting E, Speer CP, Harms K, et al: Factors influencing morbidity and mortality in infants with severe respiratory distress syndrome treated with single or multiple doses of a natural porcine surfactant. Biol Neonate 61(Suppl 1):26–30, 1992.

157. Wallenbrock MA, Sekar KC, Toubas PL: Prediction of the acute response to surfactant therapy by pulmonary function testing. Pediatr Pulmonol 13:11–15, 1992.

158. Kuint J, Reichman B, Neumann L, et al: Prognostic value of the immediate response to surfactant. Arch Dis Child Fetal Neonatal Ed 71:F170–F173, 1994.

159. Ranganathan D, Wall S, Khoshnood B, et al: Racial differences in respiratory-related neonatal mortality among very low birth weight infants. J Pediatr 136:454–459, 2000.

160. Corbet A, Long W, Schumacher R, et al: Double-blind developmental evaluation at 1-year corrected age of 597 premature infants with birth weights from 500 to 1350 grams enrolled in three placebo-controlled trials of prophylactic synthetic surfactant. American Exosurf Neonatal Study Group I. J Pediatr 126:S5–S12, 1995.

161. Morley CJ, Morley R: Follow up of premature babies treated with artificial surfactant (ALEC). Arch Dis Child 65:667–669, 1990.

162. Courtney SE, Long W, McMillan D, et al: Double-blind 1-year follow-up of 1540 infants with respiratory distress syndrome randomized to rescue treatment with two doses of synthetic surfactant or air in four clinical trials. American and Canadian Exosurf Neonatal Study Groups. J Pediatr 126:S43–S52, 1995.

163. Dunn MS, Shennan AT, Hoskins EM, et al: Two-year follow-up of infants enrolled in a randomized trial of surfactant replacement therapy for prevention of neonatal respiratory distress syndrome. Pediatrics 82:543–547, 1988.

164. Ferrara TB, Hoekstra RE, Couser RJ, et al: Effects of surfactant therapy on outcome of infants with birth weights of 600 to 750 grams. J Pediatr 119:455–457, 1991.

165. Wagner CL, Kramer BM, Kendig JW, et al: School-age follow-up of a single-dose prophylactic surfactant cohort. J Dev Behav Pediatr 16:327–332, 1995.

166. Ware J, Taeusch HW, Soll RF, et al: Health and developmental outcomes of a surfactant controlled trial: Follow-up at 2 years [published erratum appears in Pediatrics 87:412, 1991]. Pediatrics 85:1103–1107, 1990.

167. Abbasi S, Bhutani VK, Gerdes JS: Long-term pulmonary consequences of respiratory distress syndrome in preterm infants treated with exogenous surfactant. J Pediatr 122:446–452, 1993.

168. Pelkonen AS, Hakulinen AL, Turpeinen M, et al: Effect of neonatal surfactant therapy on lung function at school age in children born very preterm. Pediatr Pulmonol 25:182–190, 1998.

169. Yuksel B, Greenough A, Gamsu HR: Respiratory function at follow-up after neonatal surfactant replacement therapy. Respir Med 87:217–221, 1993.

170. Couser RJ, Ferrara TB, Wheeler W, et al: Pulmonary follow-up 2.5 years after a randomized, controlled, multiple dose bovine surfactant study of preterm newborn infants. Pediatr Pulmonol 15:163–167, 1993.

171. Gappa M, Berner MM, Hohenschild S, et al: Pulmonary function at school-age in surfactant-treated preterm infants. Pediatr Pulmonol 27:191–198, 1999.

172. Walti H, Boule M, Moriette G, et al: Pulmonary functional outcome at one year of age in infants treated with natural porcine surfactant at birth. Biol Neonate 61(Suppl 1):48–53, 1992.

173. Sell M, Cotton R, Hirata T, et al: One-year follow-up of 273 infants with birth weights of 700 to 1100 grams after prophylactic treatment of respiratory distress syndrome with synthetic surfactant or air placebo. American Exosurf Neonatal Study Group I. J Pediatr 126:S20–S25, 1995.

174. Vaucher YE, Merritt TA, Hallman M, et al: Neurodevelopmental and respiratory outcome in early childhood after human surfactant treatment. Am J Dis Child 142:927–930, 1988.

175. Gappa M, Berner MM, Hohenschild S, et al: Pulmonary function at school-age in surfactant-treated preterm infants. Pediatr Pulmonol 27:191–198, 1999.

176. Sinkin RA, Kramer BM, Merzbach JL, et al: School-age follow-up of prophylactic versus rescue surfactant trial: Pulmonary, neurodevelopmental, and educational outcomes. Pediatrics 101:E11, 1998.

177. Vaucher YE, Harker L, Merritt TA, et al: Outcome at twelve months of adjusted age in very low birth weight infants with lung immaturity: A randomized, placebo-controlled trial of human surfactant. J Pediatr 122:126–132, 1993.

178. Clark DA, Nieman BS, Thompson JE, et al: Surfactant displacement by meconium free fatty acids: An alternative explanation of atelectasis in meconium aspiration syndrome. J Pediatr 110:765–770, 1987.

179. Moses D, Holm BA, Spitale P, et al: Inhibition of pulmonary surfactant function by meconium. Am J Obstet Gynecol 164:477–481, 1991.

180. Sun B, Curstedt T, Robertson B: Surfactant inhibition in experimental meconium aspiration. Acta Paediatr 82:182–189, 1993.

181. Chen TC, Tuong TJK, Rogers MC: Effect of intraalveolar meconium on pulmonary surface tension properties. Crit Care Med. 13:233–236, 1985.

182. Davey AM, Becker JD, Davis JM: Meconium aspiration syndrome: Physiologic and inflammatory changes in a newborn piglet model. Pediatr Res 16:101–108, 1993.

183. Lieberman J: Protolytic enzyme activity in fetal pancreas and meconium. Gastroenterology 50:183–190, 1966.

184. Sun B, Curstedt T, Song GW, et al: Surfactant improves lung function and morphology in newborn rabbits with meconium aspiration. Biol Neonate 63:96–104, 1993.

185. Sun B, Herting E, Curstedt T, et al: Exogenous surfactant improves lung compliance and oxygenation in adult rats with meconium aspiration. J Appl Physiol 77:1961–1971, 1994.

186. Sun B, Curstedt T, Robertson B: Exogenous surfactant improves ventilation efficiency and alveolar expansion in rats with meconium aspiration. Am J Crit Care Med 154:764–770, 1996.

187. Wiswell TE, Peabody SS, Davis JM, et al: Surfactant therapy and high-frequency jet ventilation in the management of a piglet model of the meconium aspiration syndrome. Pediatr Res 36:494–500, 1994.

188. Pauly TH, Berry DD, Whitehead VL, et al: Artificial surfactant in the treatment of meconium aspiration syndrome (MAS) [abstract 1898]. Pediatr Res 31:319A, 1992.

189. Ohama Y, Ogawa Y: Treatment of meconium aspiration syndrome with surfactant lavage in an experimental rabbit model. Pediatr Pulmonol 28:18–23, 1999.

190. Paranka MS, Walsh WF, Stancombe BB: Surfactant lavage in a piglet model of meconium aspiration syndrome. Pediatr Res 31:625–628, 1992.

191. Balaraman V, Sood SL, Finn KC, et al: Physiologic response and lung distribution of lavage vs. bolus Exosurf in piglets with acute lung injury. Am J Respir Crit Care Med 153:1838–1843, 1996.

192. Cochrane CG, Revak SD, Merritt TA, et al: Bronchoalveolar lavage with KL4-surfactant in models of meconium aspiration syndrome. Pediatr Res 44:705–715, 1998.

193. Auten RL, Notter RH, Kendig JW, et al: Surfactant treatment of full-term newborns with respiratory failure. Pediatrics 87:101–107, 1991.

194. Halliday HL, Speer CP, Robertson B: Treatment of severe meconium aspiration syndrome with porcine surfactant. Collaborative Surfactant Study Group. Eur J Pediatr 155:1047–1051, 1996.

195. Khammash H, Perlman M, Wojtulewicz J, et al: Surfactant therapy in full-term neonates with severe respiratory failure. Pediatrics 92:135–139, 1993.

196. Lotze A, Knight GR, Martin GR, et al: Improved pulmonary outcome after exogenous surfactant therapy for respiratory failure in term infants requiring extracorporeal membrane oxygenation. J Pediatr 122:261–268, 1993.

197. Findlay RD, Taeusch HW, Walther FJ: Surfactant replacement therapy for meconium aspiration syndrome. Pediatrics 97:48–52, 1996.

197a. Lotze A, Mitchell BR, Bulas DI, et al: Multicenter study of surfactant (beractant) use in the treatment of term infants with severe respiratory failure. Survanta in Term Infants Study Group. J Pediatr 132:40–47, 1998.

197b. Soll RF, Dargaville P: Surfactant for meconium aspiration syndrome in full term infants (Cochrane Review). In: The Cochrane Library, Issue 2, 2001. Oxford: Update Software, 2001.

198. Ibara S, Ikenoue T, Murata Y, et al: Management of meconium aspiration syndrome by tracheobronchial lavage and replacement of Surfactant-TA. Acta Paediatr Jpn 37:64–67, 1995.

199. Lam BC, Yeung CY: Surfactant lavage for meconium aspiration syndrome: A pilot study. Pediatrics 103:1014–1018, 1999.

200. Ogawa Y, Ohama Y, Itakura Y, et al: Bronchial lavage with surfactant solution for the treatment of meconium aspiration syndrome. J Jpn Med Soc Biol Interface 26:179–184, 1996.

201. Faix RG, Viscardi RM, Dipietro MA, et al: Adult respiratory distress syndrome in full-term newborns. Pediatrics 83:971–976, 1989.

202. Pfenninger J, Tschaeppeler H, Wagner BP, et al: The paradox of adult respiratory distress syndrome in neonates. Pediatr Pulmonol 10:18–24, 1991.

203. Willson DF, Jiao JH, Bauman LA, et al: Calf's lung surfactant extract in acute hypoxemic respiratory failure in children. Crit Care Med 24:1316–1322, 1996.

204. Willson DF, Zaritsky A, Bauman LA, et al: Instillation of calf lung surfactant extract (calfactant) is beneficial in pediatric acute hypoxemic respiratory failure. Crit Care Med 27:188–195, 1999.

205. Luchetti M, Casiraghi G, Valsecchi R, et al: Porcine-derived surfactant treatment of severe bronchiolitis. Acta Anaesthesiol Scand 42:805–810, 1998.

206. Anzueto A, Baughman RP, Guntupalli KK, et al: Aerosolized surfactant in adults with sepsis-induced acute respiratory distress syndrome. N Engl J Med 334:1417–1421, 1996.

207. Gregory TJ, Steinberg KP, Spragg R, et al: Bovine surfactant therapy for patients with acute respiratory distress syndrome. Am J Respir Crit Care Med 155:1309–1315, 1997.

208. Pandit PB, Dunn MS, Colucci EA: Surfactant therapy in neonates with respiratory deterioration due to pulmonary hemorrhage. Pediatrics 95:32–36, 1995.

209. Robertson B: New targets for surfactant replacement therapy: Experimental and clinical aspects. Arch Dis Child Fetal Neonatal Ed 75:F1–F3, 1996.

210. Bos AP, Tibboel D, Hazebroek FW, et al: Surfactant replacement therapy in high-risk congenital diaphragmatic hernia. Lancet 338:1279, 1991.

211. Glick PL, Leach CL, Besner GE, et al: Pathophysiology of congenital diaphragmatic hernia III: Exogenous surfactant therapy for the high-risk neonate with CDH. J Pediatr Surg 27:866–869, 1992.

212. Lotze A, Knight GR, Anderson KD, et al: Surfactant (beractant) therapy for infants with congenital diaphragmatic hernia on ECMO: Evidence of persistent surfactant deficiency. J Pediatr Surg 29:407–412, 1994.

213. Cochrane CG, Revak SD, Merritt TA, et al: The efficacy and safety of KL4-surfactant in preterm infants with respiratory distress syndrome. Am J Respir Crit Care Med 153:404–410, 1996.

214. Hafner D, Germann PG: Additive effects of phosphodiesterase-4 inhibition on effects of rSP-C surfactant. Am J Respir Crit Care Med 161:1495–1500, 2000.

215. Spragg RG, Smith RM, Harris K, et al: Effect of recombinant SP-C surfactant in a porcine lavage model of acute lung injury. J Appl Physiol 88:674–681, 2000.

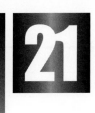

COMPLICATIONS

SHELDON B. KORONES, MD

Complications of assisted ventilation continue to be major causes of troublesome outcomes (Table 21-1). This chapter addresses three entities: bronchopulmonary dysplasia (BPD), extraneous air syndromes (air leaks), and retinopathy of prematurity (ROP). The first two are direct lung injuries, whereas the last is a destructive response of the immature retina to several noxious factors, of which oxygen (O_2) is but one.[1]

BRONCHOPULMONARY DYSPLASIA

History and Incidence

In 1967, Northway et al.[2] first reported the clinical, pathologic, and radiologic features of BPD. The term *bronchopulmonary dysplasia* was chosen "to emphasize the involvement of all the tissues of the lung." Four stages of disease, in graduated degrees of severity, were described in terms of their time of occurrence, tissue changes, radiologic abnormalities, and clinical features (Table 21-2). Although the disease has changed in its clinical and radiologic progressions,[3] the four stages described in 1967 remain as valuable points of reference for an understanding of the disease, even in its altered contemporary manifestations.[4,5]

Before the introduction of mechanical ventilation for the treatment of respiratory distress syndrome (RDS), affected infants often died within 5 days of birth. If they survived, abnormal clinical signs and radiographic findings improved by the fifth postnatal day; complete recovery was apparent by 7 to 10 days. Sequelae suggestive of BPD were not recognized until premature infants survived long enough, largely as a result of the widespread use of mechanical ventilatory support. Mortality from RDS declined after the introduction of respirator therapy, but the price paid was the emergence of BPD as a major cause of severe morbidity and significant mortality. Fundamentally, BPD occurs in immature lungs exposed to pressure-induced trauma, at high concentrations of O_2, usually with endotracheal tubes in place during periods of mechanical ventilatory support.[6,7] Mature lungs are infrequently affected. Babies who have not received mechanical ventilator support are also less frequently affected.

In the majority of instances, RDS precedes the onset of BPD, but other acute pulmonary disorders have been cited as preludes to BPD.[4,8–10] Pneumonia[10] and meconium aspiration have been observed prior to the onset of BPD. In one report, 9 of 23 infants with BPD had antecedent disorders other than RDS, but the illnesses were not described.[8] Whether BPD is preceded by RDS or some other pulmonary disorder, with a few exceptions the appearance of BPD is influenced by (1) respiratory insufficiency in immature lungs, (2) use of high oxygen concentration, and (3) the degree and duration of applied airway pressure and supplemental oxygen. The relative significance of each of these factors has not been clearly defined.

In the 1970s, BPD was estimated to occur in 30% to 40% of infants who were maintained on mechanical ventilation. In his report of a 12-year experience, Edwards[11] identified BPD (stage IV) in 21% of 299 infants who required ventilation with O_2 for at least 24 hours. Johnson[12] suggested that the incidence of the disease in stages III and IV diminished from 25% to 11% as a result of the use of positive end-expiratory pressure (PEEP). Berg et al.[13] noted a diminished incidence that they also attributed to the use of distending pressure.

Estimates and calculations of BPD incidence have varied so widely that they defy comparison.[14,15] Consequently, accurate statements comparing the impact of various management practices, mortality, morbidity, and long-term outcomes have not been accurate. A large number of studies involve populations and diagnostic parameters that vary widely. Farrell and Palta[15] reported a survey of 17 centers at which the diagnosis of BPD was dependent on different durations of mechanical ventilation and O_2 administration. In another study that addressed the therapeutic practices of eight centers, BPD was uniformly diagnosed only when O_2 supplementation was required at 28 days or beyond.[16] In summarizing 18 published studies, Boynton[14] pointed to incidence estimates that varied from 0% to 70%. In

---

TABLE 21-1. Complications of Assisted Ventilation

Upper airway
    Nasal septum necrosis (NCPAP)
    Palatal groove, abnormal dental development
    Nasofacial cellulitis (nasotracheal tube)
    Subglottic edema
    Subglottic tracheal stenosis
    Necrotizing tracheobronchitis
Lower airway
    Bronchopulmonary dysplasia
    Extraneous air syndromes (air leaks)
    Pulmonary hemorrhage
    Atelectasis
    Pneumonia
Extrapulmonary
    Retinopathy of prematurity
    Sepsis
    Periventricular/intraventricular hemorrhage

TABLE 21-2.   Bronchopulmonary Dysplasia

Stage	Time	Pathologic Findings	Radiologic Findings	Clinical Features
I (mild)	2–3 days	Patchy loss of cilia; bronchial epithelium intact; profuse hyaline membranes	Air bronchograms; diffuse reticulogranularity (identical to RDS)	Identical to RDS
II (moderate)	4–10 days	Loss of cilia; fewer hyaline membranes; necrosis of alveolar epithelium; regeneration of bronchial epithelium; ulceration in bronchioles	Opacification; coarse, irregularly shaped densities containing small vacuolar radiolucencies	Increased O_2 requirements and increasing ventilatory support when recovery is expected; rales, retractions
III (severe)	10–20 days	Advanced alveolar epithelial regeneration; extensive alveolar collapse; bronchiolar metaplasia and interstitial fibrosis; bronchial muscle hypertrophy	Small radiolucent cysts in generalized pattern	Prolonged O_2 dependency; $Paco_2$ retention; retractions; early barrel chest; severe acute episodes of bronchospasm
IV (advanced-chronic)	1 mo	Obliterative bronchiolitis; active epithelial proliferation; peribronchial and some interstitial fibrosis; severe bronchiolar metaplasia	Dense fibrotic strands; generalized cystic areas; large or small heart; hyperinflated lungs; hyperlucency at bases	Increased chest anteroposterior diameter; cor pulmonale; frequent respiratory infection; prolonged O_2 dependency; failure to thrive

RDS, respiratory distress syndrome.

Liverpool, Cooke[17] concluded that the incidence of BPD was more significantly associated with early postnatal use of intralipids in infants at younger gestational ages than with any recent changes in population features, survival, or ventilator therapy. Parker et al.[18] considered that an increased incidence of BPD was largely attributable to enhanced rates of survival and to other unidentified variables. There was an obvious need to define BPD, if only for consistent use by reporting investigators. The incidence of BPD has varied widely, and the definitions of the disease have not been uniform.

The original definition by Northway et al.[2] included clinical signs, duration of oxygen therapy, radiologic appearance, and pathology. The most severe form of disease was stage IV, which was said to persist with a need for oxygen and respiratory support beyond 28 postnatal days. Bancalari[19] modified this approach by including the following requirements: (1) ventilatory support at least for the first 3 days; (2) respiratory signs at 28 postnatal days; and (3) oxygen supplementation needed to maintain Pao_2 above 50 torr at 28 postnatal days. Later studies proposed that a need for oxygen supplementation at 28 days was itself sufficient for the diagnosis, with the level of Pao_2 notwithstanding.

Subsequently, Shennan et al.[20] found that very-low-birthweight infants who still needed O_2 at 28 days had only a 37% probability of developing abnormal lung function later in infancy. In contrast, when the point of reference was a need for supplemented oxygen at 36 weeks postmenstrual age (PMA), poor outcome was correctly predicted in 63% of infants. Discrepancies in definition precluded accurate estimations of incidence and outcomes. For purposes of study and evaluation, in most instances the definition now provides homogeneity to the diagnosis of BPD.[21] Most authors consider a need for supplemental oxygen at 36 postmenstrual weeks a reasonable indication of BPD.

As early as 1983, the incidence of BPD was noted to increase, possibly as a result of enhanced survival of very-low-birthweight babies.[18] More recently, the National Institute of Child Health and Human Development (NICHD) Neonatal Research Network reported increased BPD in outcomes of very-low-birthweight infants born between January 1995 and December 1996 compared to those born in 1991.[21] Of all surviving infants, 23% had BPD. At birthweights from 501 to 750 g the incidence was 52%, at 751 to 1000 g it was 34%, at 1001 to 1250 g it was 15%, and at 1251 to 1500 g it was 7%. Contemporary management was used at all 14 participating centers and diagnostic definitions were uniform, yet the incidence of BPD varied from 3% to 43% among the 14 centers. In essence, for birthweights from 501 to 1500 g, the incidence of BPD had increased from 19% in 1991 to 23% in 1996.[21] There is no evidence that the occurrence of BPD has diminished as a result of surfactant therapy.[22] Some investigators speculate that the use of surfactant should lower the incidence of the disease. Jobe[23] reasons that the documented reduced mortality, the increased survival of infants who do not have BPD, and the decreased severity of the disease when it does occur are all supportive of a hypothesis that surfactant treatment does decrease the incidence of BPD. On the other hand, the role of inflammation in the very preterm lung and the occurrence of BPD in infants who have not had RDS suggest that surfactant is of little or no benefit in decreasing the incidence of BPD.[23]

Etiologic Considerations

A "new BPD" has been described recently and with it an expanded perspective on the etiology of BPD is evolving. The new version is notably milder than the more advanced stages of the traditional disease as first reported by Northway et al.[2] BPD apparently is less likely to develop in larger preterm infants (birthweight >1200 g)[24]; rather, it occurs preponderantly in smaller premature infants whose birthweights are 1000 g or less. BPD is still one of the most troublesome chronic diseases of prematurity, contemporary changes notwithstanding. Recent advances in management are thought to contribute significantly to measured outcome improvement and diminished severity in the clinical course of the disorder. Surfactant, gentle respiratory support, and antenatal steroids seem to be largely responsible for a diminished incidence in larger prematures and a less destructive impact on the lungs of the smaller ones.

Fundamentally, BPD may represent an arrest of lung maturation with or without the superimposition of injury by hyperoxia and barotrauma (or volutrauma). The halt in alveolarization that is now seen to characterize BPD[25] is associated with other maturational impediments, such as abnormal capillary bed development, presence of antioxidants, and lack of surfactant. Whereas the primary trigger of progressive chronic inflammation was considered to be the barotrauma of mechanical ventilation, as well as the damage of high oxygen concentrations, it now seems likely that, in many instances, chronic destructive change is initiated in utero by cytokines released during inflammatory processes.[25] The role of intrauterine cytokines and its possible impact on the fetal lung and brain have received considerable attention in recent years.[26]

The role of mechanical ventilation, which entails delivery of high oxygen concentrations under high pressure to vulnerable lungs, is still a pivotal etiologic factor. Van Marter et al.[27] clearly demonstrated in a comparison of three neonatal intensive care units that an increased risk for BPD in two of the hospitals was "explained simply" by their more frequent use of mechanical ventilation. The appearance of BPD in some smaller infants who never received mechanical ventilatory support is noteworthy, but these are events that occur in a distinct minority of affected infants compared to the numbers of babies with BPD who required mechanical ventilatory support at birth.[28] The vulnerability to BPD in premature lungs is in contrast to the much reduced likelihood of BPD in term and near-term infants who, for instance, needed high inspiratory pressures for management of persistent pulmonary hypertension.[29] Some infants born weighing less than 1000 to 1250 g have been shown to have BPD in the absence of mechanical ventilatory support.[28,30] Reports of these apparently spontaneous clinical onsets of BPD have been published for decades.[31–35] In most instances, these infants are asymptomatic until 6 to 9 days of age, when supplemental oxygen needs to be initiated or reinstituted.[28] The diminished frequency of damaging vigorous mechanical support has unmasked BPD to reveal a milder disease that may have been initiated in utero. Use of maternal steroids, surfactant, and more gentle respiratory support has reduced the impact of high pressures and oxygen concentrations. The significance of intrauterine events has become more apparent[26,36] because intensive respiratory support is applied less often. As a consequence, the etiologic roles of intrauterine factors, such as amniotic infection, cytokines, and the "fetal inflammatory response syndrome," can be seen more clearly and in better perspective. There is significant evidence supporting associations between intrauterine infections, release of cytokines, impairment of lung development with subsequent progression to BPD, and occurrence of periventricular leukomalacia and cerebral palsy.[26]

In essence, we are dealing with new clinical manifestations of BPD, which now indicate a far broader concept of etiology than had existed previously. These changes probably are the result of improved management. Intrauterine factors may be fundamental to the development of BPD postnatally, but as long as severe respiratory inadequacy at birth yet prevails, intense respiratory support will be necessary.

The factors that initiate or enhance BPD changes include oxygen toxicity, baro-volutrauma, nutritional insufficiencies, infection (fetal and neonatal), excessive fluids, left-to-right shunting across a patent ductus arteriosus, and fluid management (Table 21-3).

TABLE 21-3. Factors Implicated in the Causation of Bronchopulmonary Dysplasia

In utero
  Cytokines (infection)
Direct cause
  Mechanical ventilation
    O_2 toxicity
    Barotrauma
Contributory factors
  Prematurity
  Primary lung disease
  Race
  Sex
  Family history
  Undernutrition
    Vitamin A
    Vitamin E
  Pulmonary edema
    Patent ductus arteriosus
    Excess fluid load
  Pulmonary air leak syndromes (barotrauma)
  Infection (*Ureaplasma urealyticum*)
  Antioxidant hypoactivity (oxygen radicals)
  Poorly inhibited protease activity

Oxygen Toxicity

In their original description, Northway et al.[2] considered the inspiration of high concentrations of O_2 the most likely cause of BPD. In their experience, affected infants had been given O_2 in concentrations of 80% or higher for at least 6 days. They stated that BPD was probably "the result of oxygen induced lesions in the respiratory mucosa, with subsequent defective drainage, combined with lesions in the alveoli and capillaries induced by oxygen and respiratory distress." They also speculated that intermittent positive-pressure ventilation (IPPV) and endotracheal intubation may have played a role. Now more than 35 years after their original description, speculation still lingers. The individual impact of O_2, IPPV, and endotracheal intubation has yet to be defined despite numerous inquiries. Although contemporary consensus holds that all three of these factors are significant,[4] some clinicians have insisted on the preponderant importance of barotrauma,[37,38] whereas others consider O_2 toxicity as a primary activator.[8,39–41]

In the years that have passed since BPD was first described by Northway et al.,[2] successive investigators have reported toxicity at lower O_2 concentrations and with shorter durations of therapy. As early as 1969, Pusey et al.[10] questioned the contention of Northway et al.[2] that 6 days of therapy at O_2 concentrations of 80% or higher were the essential antecedents of BPD. They cited three affected infants who did not receive "high oxygen concentrations" and two others who did, but for less than 24 hours. In the experience of Rhodes et al.,[41] BPD occurred in babies who had received O_2 concentrations of greater than 60% beyond 72 hours of ventilation through an endotracheal tube. Banerjee et al.[8] failed to identify BPD in any infant whose fraction of inspired O_2 (FIO_2) was less than 0.60; however, above this level, sometimes the disease appeared after only 46 hours of therapy; when therapy exceeded 123 hours, BPD was present invariably. It remained for Philip[9] to describe the appearance of BPD with O_2 concentrations as low as 40% at a minimum of 72 hours. He proposed that BPD developed as a function of "oxygen plus pressure plus time." In a later analysis of data from their 12-year experience, Edwards et al.[40] similarly concluded that the duration of therapy with O_2 concentrations of greater than 40% was the best predictor. They proposed a reciprocal relationship between FIO_2 at any concentration plus duration of administration. Thus, regardless of oxygen concentrations, if therapy is sufficiently protracted, BPD ensues. In support of this contention, Edwards et al. described the disorder in babies whose FIO_2 was only 0.22 to 0.30 for as long as 53 days.

There is no definite FIO_2 at which one can predict the inception of BPD. Immaturity of the lungs is a fundamental variable. Increased vulnerability of lung tissue in smaller premature infants is well known: the more premature the lungs, the more likely it is that BPD will occur. Variability of tissue response is surely related to the degree of immaturity. The impact of O_2 toxicity is closely related to lung immaturity, which entails a limited capacity for O_2 detoxification.[42] In rabbits and other animals, antioxidant enzyme activity seems to develop within a time frame that coincides with the maturation of surfactant synthesis.[43,44] The level of antioxidant enzymes (as well as that of surfactant) in newborn rats is significantly increased in response to maturation stimulated by maternal dexamethasone given 24 and 48 hours before delivery.[45] The capacity to resist damage from oxygen radicals is a function of maturation, and this may partially explain the increased frequency and severity of BPD in the most immature infants. Preterm rabbit neonates are considerably less resistant to airway hyperoxia than are term pups. Antioxidant enzyme responses are almost nonexistent in prematures compared to term pups.[46]

Oxidant and protease activities are destructive, and they may operate synergistically. White[47] has informatively reviewed the subject of pulmonary O_2 toxicity. The levels of O_2 metabolites (superoxide, hydrogen peroxide, hydroxyl radicals, and others) are augmented during periods of hyperoxia; their production in the lung is destructive. Hyperoxia generally incites a profuse inflammatory response; it injures epithelial cells even in the absence of inflammation. Infants with RDS who are destined to progress to BPD have been identified in the first postnatal week by demonstration of increased concentrations of oxyradical markers. Infants with RDS who did not develop BPD showed no such increase.[48,49] Defense mechanisms against toxic O_2 metabolites (radicals) are critical to the prevention or attenuation of oxidant lung damage. Superoxide dismutase is probably the primary substance of this defense; glutathione peroxidase and catalase also play significant protective roles.

Superoxide dismutase promotes elimination of the superoxide radical, and an effective pulmonary response to hyperoxia requires its enhancement. In human premature infants given supplemental O_2, however, superoxide dismutase was not increased in either the lungs or the blood.[50] This lack of response may explain the immature lung's vulnerability to oxidant injury. In a study reported by Rosenfeld,[51] bovine superoxide dismutase was administered subcutaneously to infants with RDS who were receiving mechanical ventilation. A significant reduction in the incidence of BPD was observed, but confirmation has not been reported since publication of this study in 1984. In a later study by Rosenfeld et al.,[52] the results of superoxide dismutase prophylaxis were at best equivocal. There was indication of less injury early in the disease in infants who received superoxide dismutase intratracheally. Davis et al.[53] reported no effect on the incidence of BPD. Welty[54] summarizes the evidence for the significance of oxidant injury and the need for research to identify effective antioxidant therapy.

Other attempts to minimize oxidant damage to the lung have been reported in studies that evaluated the antioxidant activity of vitamin E. Vitamin E is a major antioxidant known to diminish peroxidation of polyunsaturated lipids by virtue of its scavenger activity. Vitamin E deficiency is pervasive among premature infants; supplementation would be logical. However, a summary of the several trials that evaluated vitamin E supplementation has indicated its ineffectiveness in diminishing the incidence of BPD.[55]

Overall, the evidence for O_2 toxicity is impressive. Hyperoxia inhibits lung growth and maturation, resulting in the development of smaller lungs with fewer alveoli and the inhibition of vascular development. It also causes interstitial edema by increasing capillary permeability. Hyperoxia incites profuse inflammation, setting the stage for subsequent fibrosis. Some investigators have been convinced that O_2 toxicity is the principal cause of BPD,[8,39–41,56] but the evidence for this conclusion is largely derived from animal experiments. In human infants, there is a considerable accumulation of evidence that oxygen radicals cause significant injury early in the course of disease. Saugstad[49] and Frank and Sosenko[57] have published excellent reviews of the topic. Davis et al.[58] demonstrated in piglets that a minimum of acute injury follows positive-pressure ventilation in room air; however, when an FIO_2 of 1.0 was added, the severity of lesions increased significantly. Providing for enhanced antioxidant capacity could significantly reduce vulnerability to lung damage. Suggested investigations include antenatal stimulation of antioxidant enzyme production, administration of deficient enzymes, genetic manipulation to enhance production of enzymes, and perhaps a pharmacologic substitute for the enzymes.[57]

Baro-volutrauma

The association of high ventilatory pressures, alveolar rupture (air leak syndromes), and subsequent BPD has long been recognized.[59] Moylan et al.[60] reported a close association between alveolar rupture and BPD. Rhodes et al.[61] and Boynton et al.[62] were convinced of the advisability of using low peak inspiratory pressures and short inspiratory times to minimize barotrauma. Kraybill et al.[37] found in their multicenter retrospective study that lower arterial carbon dioxide ($PaCO_2$) levels were associated with a higher incidence of BPD, suggesting a role for higher ventilatory pressures in the development of BPD. Wung et al.[35] reported a decrease in the incidence of BPD over a 12-month period, which they attributed to early continuous positive airway pressure (CPAP) and low inspiratory pressures. However, no prospective controlled studies have related the occurrence of BPD to airway pressures at specific levels.[3] Taghizadeh and Reynolds[38] emphasized the importance of peak inspiratory pressure. In their series of autopsied infants, they calculated a statistically significant correlation between pressures of over 35 cm H_2O and the presence of "the most serious lesions" of BPD. In animals, exaggerated permeability of epithelial and endothelial tissues quickly follows overdistention of lungs for even short periods of time (volutrauma).[27,35,38,63,64] Because ventilator management of surfactant-deficient infants entails overdistention of small airways, a similar phenomenon may be involved in the early appearance of lung edema among mechanically ventilated infants.[65]

The most immediate and frequent cause of BPD is lung injury imposed by mechanical ventilatory support.[66] Lower incidence of BPD seems to be a function of fewer mechanically ventilated babies.[27,35,64] On the other hand, high inspiratory pressure (and FIO$_2$) enhances both the likelihood and the severity of BPD.[27,38,63] High inspiratory pressure has long been identified as a major cause of BPD (barotrauma), but tissue damage now is attributed to the stretch imposed by excessive alveolar volume (volutrauma).[67,68] Pressure delivers volume, which stretches alveolar walls and capillaries.[69] Volume delivered by any given pressure is modified by compliance and airway resistance. In a study that clearly demonstrated the effect of pressure (barotrauma) compared to the stretch of overinflation (volutrauma), tissue damage in three different rabbit preparations was compared at different peak pressures.[70] In one preparation, expansion of the chest wall was virtually eliminated by a full body cast, thereby restricting lung and alveolar distention. In another preparation, distention was restricted only by the chest wall of intact animals. In a third preparation, the lungs were excised and isolated, thereby allowing unrestricted lung expansion. Microvascular permeability was compared in the three groups and was found to be maximal in the isolated lung preparation and in the intact chest preparation where lung expansion was relatively unrestricted. Minimal changes were noted in the body cast preparation where lung inflation was virtually absent. These data indicate that injury is directly associated with volume distention rather than peak inspiratory pressure in itself.

The importance of the term *volutrauma* is that it conveys the concept that "stretch" is the predominant injury. Stressful alveolar distention is generated by high tidal volume. At birth, high tidal volume in lambs has been observed to cause lowered compliance, less ventilatory efficiency, and high protein recovery.[71] In another study of lambs at birth, only six manual inflations of 35 to 40 mL/kg were observed to cause blunted responses to surfactant that was administered immediately after the six inflations.[72] The lungs of the bagged lambs were poorly expanded compared to controls who were not bagged prior to surfactant insufflation. Inspiratory capacity and deflation compliance in control lambs were much higher, whereas the bagged lambs were more difficult to ventilate. In addition, tissue injury was more extensive in histologic sections of the lungs of bagged lambs. These experimental observations are compatible with clinical studies that demonstrated or suggested that BPD was more frequent and severe with use of mechanical ventilation, particularly with high inspiratory pressures.[27,35,38,63,64]

Injury imposed by ventilators leads to alveolar capillary leak and seepage of fluid, plasma, and blood into airways, alveoli, and interstitial tissue. Preexisting (intrauterine) inflammation and premature birth enhance vulnerability to ventilator injury. The seepage from capillary leak inactivates surfactant, leading to a need for higher ventilator pressures to overcome unopposed surface tension forces. Ventilator pressure also increases the accumulation of inflammatory cells. In ventilated animals, lung lavage has been shown to contain increased quantities of inflammatory mediators, platelet activating factor, thromboxane-β$_2$, and tumor necrosis factor (TNF)-α.[70,73] This has been demonstrated with clarity in a multicenter study of mechanically ventilated adults with RDS.[74] Two different tidal volumes (12 vs 6 mL/kg) were applied and the cytokine content of bronchoalveolar lavage fluid was analyzed. Concentrations of inflammatory mediators in lungs and in plasma were significantly lower in the group that received lower tidal volumes. The study was stopped early because significant survival benefits were demonstrated in the low tidal volume patients.[75]

Inflammatory Response: Infections

The role of inflammatory mediators in the mechanism of premature labor has attracted intense study.[76] Proinflammatory cytokines, including interleukin (IL)-1β, TNF-α, IL-8, IL-6, and substances such as platelet activating factor, prostaglandins, leukotrienes, and others may be significant in the onset of labor. They also have been proposed as likely etiologic factors in the fetal onset of lung injury.[77] Ascending intrauterine infection involves entry of microorganisms from the cervix and below, into the decidua and thence through membranes into the amniotic fluid. This identical ascending route of fetal bacterial infection was described by Benirschke et al.[78,79] in 1960 and by Blanc[80] in 1961. Contemporary advances have shed considerable light on the significance of these inflammatory sites in that the resultant inflammatory response produces cytokines and proinflammatory mediators. Unless premature labor is initiated, microorganisms subsequently penetrate intact membranes to enter the amniotic cavity and thence to the fetus by swallowing or by aspiration into the airway. The "fetal inflammatory response syndrome" is thus initiated. This syndrome involves accumulation and activation of inflammatory cells, largely neutrophils and monocytes, as increased levels of IL-6 and other cytokines are generated.[77,81]

Elevated plasma IL-6 is identified in all cases of fetal inflammatory response syndrome.[26,82] Neonatal complications occur more frequently in affected fetuses; their mothers often have asymptomatic bacterial invasion of the amniotic cavity.[82] In 1961 Blanc[80] reported a series of infants with congenital pneumonia in which chorioamnionitis was seen in virtually all cases. More than 4 decades later, Watterberg et al.[83] reported a series in which chorioamnionitis was associated with a diminished incidence of RDS but with an increased incidence of BPD. Tracheal lavage showed higher concentrations of IL-1β on the first postnatal day in infants who proceeded to develop BPD; thromboxane β$_2$ was higher on days 2 and 4.

Chorioamnionitis was thought by the authors to be a significant initiating factor in the development of BPD. Funisitis is evidence of chorioamnionitis. It is present in all fetuses in whom the inflammatory response syndrome has appeared.[84] Neonates with funisitis are more likely to have neonatal sepsis,[85] cerebral palsy,[86] and BPD.[26] Elevated cytokines in amniotic fluid and in tracheal lavage have been shown in babies who either have BPD or are destined to have it.[26,87–90] Fetal aspiration of amniotic fluid that contains microorganisms or high concentrations or proinflammatory cytokines may lead to arrested development and an inflamed lung that is substantially more vulnerable to postnatal barovolutrauma and oxidant injury.[24,26] Additionally, capillary damage leads to leakage and alveolar destruction.[26] Groneck et al.[91] performed a series of extensive assessments of tracheobronchial aspirates on postnatal days 10 and 15. They concluded that BPD involved an enhanced inflammatory reaction and microvascular permeability with leakage in the presence of a high content of cytokines and proinflammatory mediators. Lung lavage has demonstrated increased IL-6 activity repeatedly. Several reports have described high content of IL-1, IL-6, and TNF-α in amniotic fluid and in lung lavage in advance of clinical recognition of BPD.[36,90–92] In summary, BPD is associated with accumulations of inflammatory cells and the elaboration of cytokines and other inflammatory mediators intrinsic to the lung.[93] The release of these substances may be stimulated by a variety of factors that include prenatal and postnatal infection, ventilator injury, and oxygen toxicity. The immature lung is particularly vulnerable to these insults. Prenatal and postnatal alveolar development is thus markedly impeded when any of these injuries occur, and alveoli are larger but fewer, whether fetal or neonatal, with or without surfactant treatment.[24,94] There are no data indicating whether there is a difference in the inflammatory response to microbes, hyperoxic injury, or ventilator baro-volutrauma.[76]

Attention has been directed to the possible causative significance of *Ureaplasma urealyticum* infection (or colonization) in the lung. This organism colonizes the female genital tract and occasionally of the male. Cervical colonization was observed in 44% of pregnant women who were followed longitudinally during gestation.[95] In another study, at the time of cesarean section 20% of endometrial cultures were positive for the organism, even though membranes had not yet ruptured.[96] Cassell et al.[97] documented *U. urealyticum* as the most common organism associated with chorioamnionitis. Review articles by Holtzman et al.[98] and Wang et al.[99] have summarized several investigations that demonstrated a strong relationship between *U. urealyticum* from tracheal cultures and the subsequent development of BPD. Infants with positive-testing cultures are at least twice as likely to develop BPD as are infants whose culture test results are negative, but this association has been demonstrated only for smaller premature infants whose birthweights were 1250 g or less.

Payne et al.[100] studied 93 infants whose birthweights were 1250 g or less and who were treated with surfactant. Cultures were positive for *U. urealyticum* in 17 infants (18%); in this group, the risk of progression to BPD was 1.66 times greater than that in the group with negative-testing cultures. Crouse et al.[101] studied 292 low-birthweight infants whose tracheal cultures were taken within 7 days of birth. Forty-four infants (15%) had positive results on culture for *U. urealyticum.* Infants with positive culture results for *U. urealyticum* were likely to develop radiographic evidence of pneumonia and a precocious progression to severe chronic lung disease (CLD) at about 2 weeks of age. The authors concluded that the radiographic appearance of "precocious dysplastic lung" and pneumonia were both correlated with isolation of *U. urealyticum* from the trachea within 7 days of birth.

If a causal relationship between *U. urealyticum* and BPD does exist, it most likely involves only a subset of all infants who develop BPD. It is possible that increased vulnerability to CLD is a result of the need for more intense and protracted ventilatory support.[102] Alternatively, infection with *U. urealyticum* may trigger an inflammatory cascade that produces acute tissue destruction and subsequent BPD.[103] A number of studies indicate association between the organism's colonization in the airway and later appearance of BPD, but there is no clear evidence that these findings are independent of prematurity.[104] If the organism is a cause of BPD and not solely a marker, then masked and randomized trials with effective antibiotics should demonstrate reduced incidence of the infection and of BPD.

No data seriously suggest an etiologic role for infections directly caused by other organisms. Several reports describe associations between bacterial, viral, or fungal organisms and BPD. The data are equivocal; a distinct and direct causal relationship between organisms and BPD has not been shown.[104]

A probable indirect effect of infection has been reported by Gonzalez et al.[105] They described a series of bacterial bloodstream infections due to several organisms that were associated with patency of the ductus arteriosus. There was a distinct temporal relationship between the infections and failed ductal closure or late ductal reopening. They postulated that the increased prostaglandin and tumor necrosis factor that were produced by infection was associated with patency of the ductus, which impaired lung mechanics and gas exchange. In addition elevated TNF-α, which was demonstrated in the infected infants, could have sequestered neutrophils in the lungs to increase capillary injury and pulmonary edema. Thus, by a direct effect on patency of the ductus, infection seems to have indirectly increased the likelihood of chronic changes of BPD.

Nutrition

A number of speculations have been made regarding the roles of specific nutritional deficiencies in the pathogenesis of BPD. Undernutrition of the premature infant is often cited as a major factor; however, in most instances, these speculations have not been proved in human infants.[106–109] The relatively high caloric needs of premature infants and their meager nutritional stores at birth have been pointed out repeatedly (see Chapter 24). Furthermore, the aggregate of requirements for growth, overall metabolism, and work of respiration impose unmet nutritional requirements. The combination of high need and meager stores is speculated to cause or contribute to CLD. Inadequate nutrition may well amplify the damage of baro-volutrauma and O_2 toxicity. Theoretically, the deficiency of antioxidant enzymes and, therefore, the extent of hyperoxic lung injury could be prevented or minimized through supplementation with the trace elements that are integral parts of the enzymatic structures of antioxidants (copper, zinc, selenium). These are reasonable speculations but they have not materialized to clinical significance in the management of infants with BPD. No attempts have been made to prevent BPD in human infants by means of specific supplementation of these and other trace elements; however, the preventive roles of vitamin E and vitamin A have been studied. Meta-analysis of eight randomized trials has demonstrated that supplemental vitamin E does not diminish the incidence of BPD.[55] The case for vitamin A supplementation may be more hopeful.

Similar to so many other nutritional components, vitamin A stores in premature infants are lower at birth than they are in adults or in older infants.[106,107] Furthermore, vitamin A deficiency apparently causes changes in the lower respiratory tract that are similar in appearance to those of BPD.[110] Hustead et al.[111] demonstrated that infants who developed BPD had low levels of vitamin A at birth and 28 days after birth compared with babies who did not have BPD. Shenai et al.[112] confirmed these findings and, in a subsequent controlled study,[113] demonstrated diminished incidence and severity of BPD in infants who were given vitamin A supplements for 28 days, beginning with the fourth day after birth. The study of Papagaroufalis et al.[114] identified similar beneficial effects. Two other studies[115,116] did not, perhaps because their populations differed somewhat from those of the earlier successful studies. In a report from the NICHD Neonatal Network, Tyson et al.[117] studied 807 infants whose mean birthweight was 769 g. The primary outcome was death or CLD at 36 weeks PMA. CLD occurred with a significantly reduced frequency in the vitamin A group (55%) compared to controls (62%). The authors calculated that one additional infant survived without BPD for every 14 to 15 infants who received vitamin A prophylactically on Monday, Wednesday, and Friday for 4 weeks beginning 24 to 96 hours after birth. In a meta-analysis from the Cochrane Neonatal Review Group, which involved six eligible trials, the authors suggest that vitamin A supplementation leads to a reduced oxygen requirement at 36 postmenstrual weeks and it trends toward reduction of death or oxygen requirement at 36 postmenstrual weeks and death or oxygen requirement at 1 month of age.[118] The benefits of vitamin A are not firmly established.

Role of Patent Ductus Arteriosus

Left-to-right shunting across the ductus arteriosus increases pulmonary blood flow, which results in pulmonary edema. Lung compliance is reduced and airway resistance is increased; this creates a need for more vigorous and protracted ventilatory support, which then enhances O_2 toxicity and baro-volutrauma. With this in mind, the impact of early closure of the ductus arteriosus in reducing the incidence or severity of BPD has been investigated in several studies. Ehrenkranz and Mercurio[55] reviewed and subjected to meta-analyses a total of 11 studies that sought closure of the ductus arteriosus, either prophylactically or therapeutically. Their meta-analyses did not support the hypothesis that early closure of a patent ductus arteriosus diminishes the incidence of BPD.

Fluid Maintenance

Several retrospective studies have produced evidence for the existence of a relationship between high fluid intake and the development of BPD.[116,119–122] These studies involved fluid management during the first few days of life, and they postulated that excessive volumes caused pulmonary edema and an exaggerated requirement for ventilatory support and thus a higher incidence of BPD. However, two randomized trials have failed to demonstrate a difference in the incidence of BPD in association with higher fluid volumes.[123,124] There is no firm evidence supporting the contention that use of maintenance fluids in high volume contributes to the development of BPD. A Cochrane Review of water intake and its relation to morbidity and mortality in four studies indicated that restricted water intake significantly reduces risks of patent ductus arteriosus, necrotizing enterocolitis, and death; however, there was no significant reduction in the risk for BPD.[125]

Pathology

Table 21-4 lists the most frequently observed structural changes in the "old" version of BPD, according to severity and the anatomic component involved. The pathologic lesions of BPD have been described in numerous communications,[126,127] dating from the original description of Northway et al. Although their description distinctly categorized four stages of the disease and the duration of each (see Table 21-2), changes in the clinical course described in more recent years have blurred the sharp distinctions. This discussion presents histopathologic changes, according to severity of disease, but times of onset or resolution can be neither predicted nor classified. At any given moment, morphologic abnormalities may range from mild to severe. Although details vary among reports, there is general agreement with regard to the morphologic changes that occur. Ultimately, every tissue in the lung is affected. Early, the morphologic changes of BPD comprise cellular necrosis, edema, and inflammation; these changes represent an acute stage that is followed by fibroproliferation, the intensity of which determines the ultimate extent of structural disruption. In the airways, widespread fibroproliferative activity, squamous metaplasia of epithelial linings, accumulation of debris, and hypertrophy of smooth muscle result in maldistribution, obstruction, and trapping of air (atelectasis and emphysema). In the pulmonary vasculature, late reparative responses narrow the lumina of blood vessels, causing maldistribution of blood flow (hypoperfusion and pulmonary hypertension). The cardiac consequences of these late vascular abnormalities include right-sided ventricular hypertrophy and cor pulmonale.

Mild BPD is said to be indistinguishable from RDS. It is characterized by slight septal edema at the alveolar level, patchy loss of cilia with focal loss of epithelium in the bronchi and bronchioles, and slight edema in the interstitial tissue. Hyaline membranes abound.

Moderate BPD is characterized by necrosis of scattered individual alveolar cells, progressive septal edema, small foci of collapsed alveoli, and fewer hyaline membranes than are seen in mild BPD. The lumina of bronchi and bronchioles now contain small quantities of eosinophilic material, inflammatory cells, and mucus. Obstruction of smaller bronchioles probably leads to the appearance of isolated foci of alveolar collapse. Peribronchial, peribronchiolar, and perivascular edema appear, interstitial edema becomes widespread, and interstitial fibrosis is prominent. The interstitial edema is a consequence of leakage through damaged capillary endothelium. With disease of this moderate severity, FIO_2 requirements and inspiratory pressure must be increased at a time when recovery from RDS is anticipated.

Severe BPD is characterized by continuation of the acute responses to injury and by a widespread appearance of reparative processes. Necrosis of alveolar cells is generalized, and previously clear alveolar spaces are now filled with fibrinous exudate, connective tissue overgrowth, macrophages, and debris. Alveolar collapse is more extensive, with the collapsed areas often surrounding spherical foci of trapped air (focal emphysema). Airway obstruction is more pervasive because bronchial and bronchiolar lumina contain larger quantities of debris, denuded necrotic epithelial cells, inflammatory cells, and mucus. The airway mucosa is frankly necrotic. Active chronic inflammation within the walls of the bronchi and bronchioles sometimes extends externally to adjacent tissue. Whereas in earlier stages only patchy areas of squamous metaplasia are present in larger bronchi, in severe disease the metaplastic process becomes widespread to involve the lower airways, causing luminal encroachment and consequent obstruction of airflow due to newly generated cells. Hypertrophy of smooth muscle progresses to cause recurrent episodes of bronchospasm. Edema of the peribronchial and peribronchiolar areas becomes widespread, but fibrosis in these particular areas is negligible, if it occurs at all. Edema is

TABLE 21-4.   Pathology of Bronchopulmonary Dysplasia: Progressive Changes in Major Lung Components

	Mild	Moderate	Severe	Advanced
Alveoli				
Alveolar cells	No necrosis	Necrosis of individual cells	Widespread necrosis	Severe disruption of alveolar architecture due to fibrosis
Alveolar spaces	Clear	Clear	Fibrinous exudates; connective tissue overgrowth; macrophages; debris	
Edema	Mild septal	Septal	Focal intra-alveolar septal	No edema
Atelectasis	None	Small foci	Large areas	Multilobular areas of emphysema interspersed with extensive areas of atelectasis
Emphysema	None	None	Spherical foci surrounded by collapsed alveoli	
Hyaline membranes	Profuse	Fewer	Absent or rare (fragments)	None
Bronchi, Bronchioles				
Lumens	Normal	Small amount of eosinophilic exudate, inflammatory cells, and mucus	Large amount of eosinophilic debris, necrotic epithelial cells, inflammatory cells, mucus	Lumens plugged with dense eosinophilic amorphous debris; distended terminal bronchioles alternating with contracted ones; obstruction by marked squamous metaplasia
Mucosa	Patchy loss of cilia; focal limited loss of epithelium	Extensive loss of cilia; patchy loss of epithelium; inflammation; patchy squamous metaplasia in larger bronchi	Marked necrosis; mural chronic active inflammation occasionally extending beyond walls; marked squamous metaplasia in bronchi and bronchioles	Widespread necrosis; extensive squamous metaplasia extending into and obstructing lumina
Smooth muscle	No hypertrophy	No hypertrophy	Hypertrophy	Marked hypertrophy
Edema	None	Peribronchial, peribronchiolar	Increased peribronchial, peribronchiolar, widespread	Scattered areas of peribronchial, peribronchiolar
Fibrosis	None	None	None to early	Peribronchial and peribronchiolar
Interstitium				
Connective tissue	Slight edema; no fibrosis	Widespread edema; prominent fibrosis	Widespread edema; increased fibrosis	Focal edema, peribronchial, and peribronchiolar
Lymphatics	Slight distention	Moderate distention	Severe distention	Severe distention
Vascular	No changes	Edema perivascular spaces	Early hypertensive changes in arteries and arterioles, including medial hypertrophy and degenerated intima; thrombi in small arterioles; patent ductus arteriosus, right ventricular hypertrophy; pulmonary vasospasm	Severe arterial/arteriolar changes; adventitial fibrosis proliferating endothelium with narrowed lumina; patent ductus arteriosus; severe right ventricular hypertrophy; cor pulmonale

Compiled from Northway WH Jr, Rosan RC, Porter DY: Pulmonary disease following respiratory therapy of hyaline membrane disease: BPD. N Engl J Med 276:357, 1967; Bonikos DS, Bensch KG, Northway WH, et al: Bronchopulmonary dysplasia: The pulmonary pathologic sequel of necrotizing bronchiolitis and pulmonary fibrosis. Hum Pathol 7:643, 1976; and Taghizadeh A, Reynolds EOR: Pathogenesis of bronchopulmonary dysplasia following hyaline membrane disease. Am J Pathol 82:241, 1976.

prominent in the interstitium and perivascular spaces, where fibrosis becomes conspicuous. Alteration of blood vessel structure is rather extensive, giving the appearance of early hypertensive changes (medial hypertrophy, degenerated intima, and thrombi). The ductus arteriosus is often patent, and some degree of right-sided ventricular hypertrophy is almost the rule at this stage of the disease. In the presence of extensive airway obstruction, alveolar collapse, focal emphysema, widespread edema, and vascular damage, oxygenation is increasingly troublesome and CO_2 retention is a significant problem.

Advanced BPD is largely a manifestation of the extensive structural disruption brought by ongoing reparative processes. Alveoli are alternately emphysematous and atelectatic; multilobular involvement pervades. Destruction of alveolar septa results in bullous emphysema. Edema of alveolar structures has disappeared. Lower airways are everywhere plugged by dense eosinophilic debris and extensive squamous metaplasia; lumina are often obliterated. Terminal bronchioles are either distended by trapped air or are constricted. Bronchial and bronchiolar smooth muscles are severely hypertrophic. The interstitium, peribronchial, peribronchiolar, and perivascular tissues are fibrotic. Lymphatics are distended and tortuous. Vascular changes are substantially more severe. Adventitial fibrosis is conspicuous, and continued endothelial proliferation further narrows lumina and sometimes completely obliterates them. Overall, the lungs are severely overexpanded; diaphragms are depressed. In the heart, right-sided ventricular hypertrophy is advanced, and in the sickest babies cor pulmonale supervenes. Advanced involvement progresses inexorably to pulmonary and cardiac failure.

"New BPD" abnormalities differ from the traditional descriptions of "old BPD."[128,129] Severity of airway damage is correlated with the height of peak inspiratory pressures and the overall amount of oxygen administered. In recent years, there has been a reduction of airway pressure and oxygen concentrations in management of ventilatory support. It is likely that the diminution in severity of airway lesions and interstitial fibrosis are related to the less intense approach. With reduced barovolutrauma there is less stretching of alveolar walls.[60,130] Outstanding features of tissue changes are hypoalveolarization and the virtual absence of severe fibrosis.[131] Baro-volutrauma and hyperoxia in the ventilatory support of premature lungs impede alveolarization, thus reducing the number of alveoli and diminishing internal surface area.[132–134] With the current practice of less intense ventilatory support, it now remains to be seen if normal alveolarization can resume after cessation of therapy.[128] In essence, the lesions of "new BPD" are characterized by markedly less or absent fibrosis compared to the "old" version of the disease, but with an almost universal prevalence of diminished numbers of alveoli.

Clinical Course

The First Few Weeks

It often is difficult to designate a precise time for the clinical onset of BPD. In usual circumstances, at approximately 7 days after birth, an infant being treated for RDS has not improved as expected and diminished ventilator support is not feasible. In other circumstances, improvement has occurred and ventilatory support is decreased serially or discontinued, but soon thereafter an abrupt need for increased O_2 supplementation and ventilator pressures arises. In either circumstance, protracted treatment for CLD has begun.[108]

Most BPD is now mild to moderate, characterized by an initial need for mechanical ventilatory support that sometimes must be maintained longer than initially anticipated. This prolonged support is followed by days or weeks of O_2 supplementation in a hood. In infants with mild BPD, radiologic indication of BPD often is uncertain, even though retractions, generally diminished breath sounds, and crepitant rales are prominent.

The early phases of moderate and severe disease are associated with a radiographic appearance that is highly suggestive of BPD, the lack of specificity notwithstanding. During the ensuing days or weeks, O_2 concentrations and ventilatory pressures must be increased relentlessly. Overdistention of lungs is progressive on radiography; barrel chest is obvious clinically. Carbon dioxide retention worsens progressively, causing respiratory acidosis. The acidosis is compensated eventually by renal conservation of bicarbonate, creating a sizable positive base excess.

As a rule, if respiratory support can be diminished in an infant at any time within the first month of life, the subsequent course of BPD is relatively benign. On the other hand, a need for increased support at about this time often portends severe protracted disease. Chest film abnormalities progress as hyperinflation, focal atelectasis, and sometimes cardiac enlargement become evident. Maintenance of adequate oxygenation and control of CO_2 retention require a greater FIO_2 and increased ventilator pressures. Ironically, the disease worsens as a consequence of the more vigorous ventilator support that its treatment requires.

Acute episodes of respiratory deterioration often occur at any time during the course of the disease, whether or not the infant is on mechanical ventilation. These acute episodes of respiratory decompensation usually are troublesome. Mere augmentation of respiratory support from its existing level may be insufficient because the infant often needs more than an increase in ventilator settings; therefore, one must consider that these acute events may be caused by (1) infection; (2) pulmonary edema as a consequence of patent ductus arteriosus, overhydration, or progression of the chronic disease; (3) congestive heart failure; or (4) bronchospasm.

The frequency of severe acute bronchospasm is impressive. It occurs while infants are mechanically supported or when they are simply receiving O_2 in a hood. Cyanosis appears suddenly, and when breath sounds are virtually inaudible, wheezing may not be heard with the stethoscope. An absence of breath sounds is particularly dramatic in infants who had previously breathed spontaneously but who now exert maximum effort to no avail. The absence or marked diminution of breath sounds is generalized, that is, it is not restricted to one area of the lungs. In infants on mechanical support, insufflations are barely audible, if at all. Frequently, a temporary increase in peak inspiratory pressure by 2 or 3 cm H_2O with an increase of FIO_2 to 1.0 may totally eliminate bronchospasm without need of pharmacologic management. If, however, the changed respiratory settings are ineffective after approximately 2 minutes, treatment with bronchodilating agents is mandatory. The mechanism of severe bronchospasm is unknown; however, a significant role for bronchial muscle hypertrophy is presumed. Hypoxia has been noted to cause bronchospastic episodes.[135]

In the infant older than age 1 month, progressive BPD may involve right-sided heart failure (cor pulmonale) as a result of increased pulmonary vascular resistance (pulmonary hypertension). In the autopsy series of Bonikos et al.,[39] right-sided heart failure was considered the immediate cause of death in 30% of infants. Changes seen post mortem in arteriolar intima and media reflect pulmonary hypertension. In a careful study that involved only one infant, the cross-sectional area of pulmonary vasculature was significantly contracted.[136] To some extent, increased pulmonary vascular resistance is caused by parenchymal fibrotic changes; right-sided heart failure develops as vasculature changes progress. Even in the absence of cardiac failure, right-sided ventricular hypertrophy due to increased pulmonary vascular resistance is virtually universal during progressive CLD. These cardiovascular changes are rare in the "new BPD."

Cardiac catheterization of infants with BPD has demonstrated that right-sided ventricular hypertrophy is associated with pulmonary hypertension, as indicated by prolonged right-sided systolic ejection times (right-sided systolic time intervals). The vascular bed is responsive (diminished resistance) to O_2 supplementation; pulmonary artery pressures are significantly lower when continuous O_2 is given via nasal cannula.[137] On the other hand, small decrements of FIO_2 result in diminished PaO_2 and prolongation of right-sided systolic time intervals.[138] These data suggest the advisability of a generous FIO_2 during O_2 supplementation for the sustained treatment of BPD. Catheterization data also indicate a need for appropriately copious FIO_2. When hypoxia occurs, elevation of FIO_2 lowers pulmonary artery pressure.[139–141]

Cardiovascular abnormalities are likely to develop during the months of progressive BPD, and they were major determinants of severe illness and death during the course of "old

BPD." Cardiovascular dysfunction is primarily a consequence of increased resistance to pulmonary blood flow. In the extreme, cor pulmonale appears as a consequence. Pulmonary hypertension is accentuated by chronic and recurrent hypoxemia. In recent years, the frequency of severe cardiovascular dysfunction has diminished considerably, possibly because the disease is milder, the management is more effective, or both. In its most protracted form, BPD requires the application of mechanical ventilation for months and frequently involves high pressures that intensify lung damage. Although cardiovascular dysfunction is common, respiratory failure is the most frequent cause of death.

Growth failure is prominent in CLD. It is not uncommon for affected infants to require up to 25% more calories for satisfactory growth compared with unaffected infants.[142] Increased metabolic rate and O_2 consumption have been described, and a need for more calories is also attributed to work of respiration.[8,142,143]

Osteopenia is common, particularly in smaller premature infants in whom it may develop in the absence of BPD. However, in infants with BPD, vulnerability to osteopenia is enhanced, presumably because of low calcium and vitamin D intake and sometimes because diuretic therapy causes significant calciuria. Fractures of the long bones and ribs result, often noted as unexpected findings on radiography or during routine nursing care.

Extubation frequently is followed by a capricious respiratory course. Inspiratory stridor from tracheal edema, scarring, or both may be evident immediately upon extubation. Tracheal stenosis may be apparent only after several days or weeks, when severe stridor appears as laryngeal scarring progresses. Even if complications of intubation are absent, the course often is undulating. Severe episodes of wheezing due to bronchospasm are frequent. Oxygen requirements wax and wane for no discernible reason. Overproduction of airway secretions requires frequent chest physiotherapy, yet many infants tolerate the procedure poorly. Whether these infants are managed at home or in the hospital, O_2 supplementation is indispensable for weeks or months. In infants who recover from BPD, decrements of inspired O_2 are feasible at a very slow rate; room air is tolerated only after a course of weeks or months. Survival beyond 7 or 8 months of age is associated with an increased likelihood of normal cardiopulmonary function by 5 to 6 years of age[144] and sometimes later.

Systemic hypertension occurs in a significant number of infants with BPD aside from pulmonary hypertension. Anderson et al.[145] described 11 of 87 BPD patients whose systemic hypertension was identified in the nursery or after discharge. In another report, 5 (12%) of 41 infants with BPD were affected.[146] Mean age of onset was 105 days. Clinical risk factors for hypertension included a high incidence of bronchodilator therapy and use of diuretics, as well as the need for a longer course of O_2 therapy at home. The presence of these risk factors may simply indicate that severe disease is more likely to be associated with systemic hypertension. Abman et al.[147] observed systemic hypertension in 13 (43%) of 30 patients who were receiving treatment at home. Three of these patients had left-sided ventricular hypertrophy, and another had a cerebrovascular accident. In the aggregate, the experience in all studies seems to indicate that among survivors, systemic hypertension is benign and amenable to appropriate therapy.[148]

The Later Months and Beyond

Risks to surviving infants continue through the first year or two of life, depending on disease severity. Thereafter, in most instances, the difficulties created by chronic disease diminish gradually. Outcomes vary considerably by virtue of a wide variability in patient characteristics, the inability of investigators to account and control for all significant variables, and the inevitable differences in study designs (see Chapter 28). Added to these confounding factors are lag time between the year that intensive care methodology is being studied and the outcomes reported years later. Among survivors, investigators have been concerned with physical and psychosocial outcomes. Principal hazards include sudden unanticipated death, pneumonia, acute episodes of bronchospasm, and aspiration during feedings. These are the most frequent causes of hospitalization following discharge from the nursery. These hospitalizations are most common during the first year of life; they usually diminish in the second year. Pneumonia, viral or bacterial, often is severe, prompting the need for mechanical ventilatory support. Acute pulmonary edema usually follows indiscrete increments in formula intake, which elevate fluid load beyond tolerance. Because feeding problems at home are frequent, they sometimes result in an inadequate overall state of nutrition.

During the first few postnatal weeks, prediction of outcomes in later childhood is not feasible. Furthermore, the direct impact of BPD on later outcomes, distinct from the role of other risk factors (e.g., prematurity, asphyxia, intraventricular hemorrhage), has not been clearly defined.[149]

Growth is retarded and does not assume a normal rate until after the child is 2 to 5 years old.[150] The child with BPD often resists feeding, is difficult to nourish, and is recurrently beset with acute illness. Feeding problems are particularly frustrating for anxious parents who have been sensitized to the importance of caloric intake. Sound parental counseling often is gratifying; feeding behavior may improve and intake can thereby be augmented. However, the growth of some BPD children is impaired even though caloric intakes apparently are sufficient. With improved respiratory status beyond 2 years of age, growth in height and head circumference is accelerated, as is weight gain but to a lesser degree.[151] With more normal respiratory function, growth pattern differs little from infants without BPD. It has been hypothesized that lung growth in these children consumes an inordinately large fraction of the caloric intake and, as pulmonary difficulties subside, catchup of body growth ensues. Recurrent illness and readmissions to the hospital surely contribute to growth impairment. Abnormal growth has been shown to be related to severity of respiratory dysfunction and recurrence of lung infection.[152] On the other hand, Sell and Vaucher[153] noted persistent growth delay throughout early childhood, and they concluded that, more than any other factor, delay in growth was significantly related to earlier growth parameters (prior weight, length, and head circumference). The presence or absence of BPD was not important.[153] Results of another study that compared prematures with and without BPD also indicated that growth retardation may be more directly related to birthweight and gestational age than to BPD itself.[154]

Recurrent hospitalizations are particularly frequent through the second year of life and decline in frequency thereafter. Respiratory infection is by far the most frequent cause of readmission. Recurrent illness is reported in 50% to 85% of patients[155] and rehospitalizations in 50%.[156] Exacerbations of respiratory distress, often life threatening, are primarily due to lower tract infections.[157] The most frequent infection probably is due to respiratory syncytial virus, which is particularly prevalent in the wintertime.[158,159] Extended lung damage is often a result of severe acute infection, especially when ventilator support is necessary. Other causes of readmission are bronchospasm, cor pulmonale, upper airway obstruction, surgery, systemic hypertension, and family social crises.[160]

Studies that address developmental outcomes directly related to BPD are inconclusive because study cohorts are small, the design may be flawed, or nonpulmonary risk factors are not identified. Several studies have related duration of ventilation or length of hospitalization to later outcomes. Although most of these studies indicate that longer periods of hospitalization or ventilatory support are associated with more abnormal outcomes, conclusions have varied considerably. In one report, a relationship between the duration of mechanical ventilation and abnormal pulmonary function at age 6 months could not be demonstrated.[161]

Variability of conclusions from studies of the direct impact of BPD itself is evident in a controlled study of 37 preterm infants in whom developmental delays were attributed to BPD rather than to prematurity and RDS alone. The performance of preterm infants with RDS and without BPD was comparable to that of average healthy full-term infants of comparable age.[150] In another study, a developmental quotient of less than 80 was demonstrated in 8 of 10 infants during their first evaluation between the ages of 6 and 12 months; no subsequent improvement was observed.[162]

A study by Bergman and Farrell[149] involving 112 BPD survivors born between 1987 and 1991 found that all severely impaired infants had multiple perinatal and neonatal risk factors in addition to BPD. These risk factors included severe ROP, extreme prematurity, and moderate-to-severe intraventricular hemorrhage.[149]

It is virtually impossible to arrive at unequivocal conclusions regarding the impact of nonpulmonary perinatal complications on developmental outcomes of babies with BPD. Rare is the infant who has had BPD and is free of other perinatal misadventures. In many instances, findings indicate that outcome is no different for babies with BPD than for premature infants without BPD.[149] The negative impact of intraventricular hemorrhage, which was not identified with cranial ultrasound in early studies but was identified in later ones, is cited repeatedly. When one adds to these neonatal complications the profound influence of socioeconomic and environmental factors (which often are immeasurable), accurate assessment of a direct and singular influence of BPD becomes even more elusive.

The most prominent sources of parental preoccupation during the later months of management are the abnormal pulmonary consequences of BPD. Pathophysiologic pulmonary sequelae include diminished compliance and increased resistance to airflow, expiratory airflow impediments due to bronchospasm or bronchomalacia (or both), air trapping, increased work of breathing, and reactive airway disease.[163] The most frequent signs of illness as reported in the informative data of the HIFI Study Group include crepitant rales, retractions, palatal groove, wheezing, and prolonged exhalation at rest. Stridor, subglottic stenosis, cyanosis, and tracheostomy were considerably less frequent in this study.[163]

Blayney and associates[164] evaluated pulmonary function in 32 BPD patients at 7 years of age and again at 10 years of age. All were born between 1977 and 1980, and they had grown normally. These investigators demonstrated continued improvement in lung function, and they therefore speculated that among the more recent patients with BPD only a small number would experience respiratory dysfunction in adulthood. Northway et al. reported the abnormal pulmonary residua in 26 adults who were born between 1964 and 1973.[165] Some of these patients were described in the original description of BPD,[2] and most of them had some degree of pulmonary dysfunction, including airway obstruction, airway hyperreactivity, and hyperexpansion. Furthermore, they had more respiratory infections and wheezing episodes than the controls. More than half had evidence of airway obstruction. A number of studies on children in school have also demonstrated persistent pulmonary dysfunction.[166–168]

The "New BPD"

In recent years, milder clinical disease ("new BPD") has emerged, presumably as a beneficial consequence of improved early management.[129,169] Early respiratory difficulties, range from total absence of distress at birth and up to 7-10 days later, to infants who need only hood oxygen, and yet others who require mechanical ventilatory support for short periods of time.[170] From these varied early postnatal beginnings, the subsequent clinical course may involve a few days or weeks of required oxygen supplementation. During the course of this milder BPD, breathing is moderately labored, characterized by chest retractions, rapid rates, crackling rales, and a mild but distinctly abnormal chest radiograph that is typically hazy throughout both lungs, associated with variable degrees of diffuse hyperinflation. Blood gases are moderately abnormal, but similar to the more severe classic disease. Episodes of hypoxemia and hypercarbia are common. Wheezing and acute episodes of pulmonary edema are recurrent, but neither so severe nor as frequent as in the more destructive versions of BPD. Some infants do not survive because of severe hypoalveolarization and relentless progression to extensive fibrosis. Cardiovascular complications (cor pulmonale, hypertrophy of vessel walls and partial occlusion) are rare. The milder, new expression of BPD also involves feeding difficulties and growth retardation, which are not as profound as in the more severe counterpart of the disease. In the presence of acute infection, respiratory dysfunction worsens considerably. Overall, improvement in respiratory function is gradual over a period of 3 years.[171]

Radiologic Characteristics

The radiologic and morphologic abnormalities of BPD are fairly well correlated in several reports, particularly BPD in the advanced stages.[2,11,172–174] The radiologic appearance of mild BPD (stage I) is identical to that of RDS: diffuse reticulogranularity and air bronchograms. The severity of these features is not related to the severity of subsequent changes of BPD.

Moderate BPD (stage II) is sometimes characterized by diffuse, virtually homogeneous opacification of the lungs that obscures cardiac margins. The early radiographic changes seen in mild disease often are replaced by coarse, irregularly shaped densities that are confluent and occasionally contain very small vacuolar radiolucencies (Fig. 21-1). The areas of density apparently are caused by interstitial and septal edema and by atelectasis due to the obstruction of small bronchioles with luminal debris. The small vacuolar radiolucencies represent early foci of emphysema.

In the severe form of BPD (stage III), the lucent vacuoles have expanded and are identifiable as air cysts among dense patches, which themselves have been smaller than previously described (Fig. 21-2). The cysts are evidence of progressive multifocal emphysema. The dense patches, compressed by expanding air cysts, are largely indicative of alveolar collapse, edema and fibrosis of the interstitium, and distention of lymphatics.

In advanced disease (stage IV), the lungs appear bubbly on radiography as air cysts continue to enlarge. Opacities are further reduced in size to strands, streaks, and small patches as cysts expand. Overall, the lungs are extensively hyperinflated and emphysema has progressed considerably (Fig. 21-3). The presence of cardiomegaly usually portends right-sided heart failure.

Edwards et al.[172,175] have aptly indicated that this classic progression through the radiographic stages first described by Northway et al. has largely disappeared. Thus, the dense opacification that was described for stage II is now uncommon; the bubbled pattern that characterized stage III is likewise infrequent. The appearance of stage IV is less dramatic. Hyperexpansion is less severe and the typical streaky opacities between large areas or radiolucency are not so pronounced; rather, the streaks are somewhat delicate and their dispersion throughout hyperexpanded lungs is more uniform. These subtle radiologic abnormalities are nevertheless associated with a persistent need for O$_2$ therapy for several weeks, whether by hood or ventilator. The chest radiograph often is optimistic compared to the actual severity of pulmonary pathology. In more than half of published cases, x-ray appearance "lagged behind" the actual stage of pathology.[175] Despite the clinical course, the radiographic changes may remain subtle for as long as 3 weeks. Hyperexpansion is marginal; streaky densities are discernible, but their significance is equivocal. At approximately 3 to 4 weeks, the radiographic changes are more clearly indicative of BPD.

Although the milder clinical course and radiographic appearance have been noteworthy in the last 10 years, so has the increase in the number of surviving infants whose birthweights are less than 1000 g.

Management

Respiratory Support

Mechanical ventilation both induces and treats BPD. The goals in maintaining mechanical support are brevity and attenuation, each of which is ultimately influenced by the severity of disease. The shortest possible course depends on multiple factors, including nonrespiratory management.

In 1987, Avery et al.[16] reported a survey of BPD incidence among eight centers, and one of them (Columbia University) had the lowest rate. More than a decade later, Van Marter et al.[27] compared respiratory management at Columbia in New York to two hospitals in Boston. There was a significantly higher rate of BPD in Boston, which the authors ultimately attributed to their more frequent use of mechanical ventilation than in New York. Expressed more positively, the lower incidence in New York was related to the less frequent initiation of

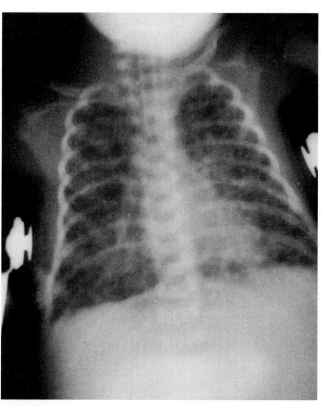

Figure 21-2. Severe (stage III) bronchopulmonary dysplasia. The small radiolucent vacuoles have expanded. They are now cysts, representing multifocal emphysema. Dense patches are collapsed alveoli, interstitial edema, and fibrosis.

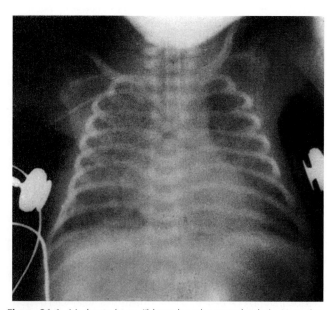

Figure 21-1. Moderate (stage II) bronchopulmonary dysplasia. Note virtually homogeneous density of both lungs that is cast by interstitial edema and atelectasis. A few small round radiolucencies are dispersed through both lungs. (From Korones SB: High-Risk Newborn Infants: The Basis for Intensive Nursing Care, 4th ed. St. Louis, C.V. Mosby, 1986, p. 262.)

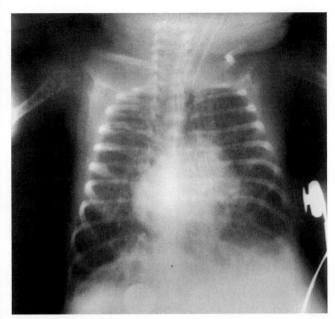

Figure 21-3. Advanced (stage IV) bronchopulmonary dysplasia. The lungs are now bubbly because air cysts continue to expand. The lungs are extensively hyperinflated. (From Korones SB: High-Risk Newborn Infants: The Basis for Intensive Nursing Care, 4th ed. St. Louis, C.V. Mosby, 1986, p. 262.)

mechanical ventilation. In recent years, mechanical ventilation has been avoided by use of nasal CPAP, even from the first minutes after birth in the smallest babies.[176] Several investigators have observed a marked diminution in BPD rates as a consequence.[177–179] Duration of ventilatory support and length of hospital stay are also diminished with preferential use of nasal CPAP. When applied post intubation it reduces the incidence of respiratory difficulties, such as apnea and respiratory acidosis.[176,177,180–182] A variety of nasal CPAP delivery modalities have been evaluated (continuous flow, variable flow, bubble CPAP, nasal prongs, nasopharyngeal tubes, face mask), but the superiority of one over the other has not been established (see Chapter 8). Nasal CPAP seems to improve a number of measured outcomes. It is apparent, however, that the avoidance of mechanical ventilation is the fundamental benefit, modality of delivery notwithstanding. Among infants for whom respiratory support was unavoidable, Van Marter et al.[27] found an elevated risk of BPD when, on the day of birth, peak inspiratory pressure (>25 cm H_2O) and FIO_2 (1.0) were high.

If mechanical support is unavoidable, respiratory settings must minimize baro-volutrauma and O_2 toxicity. PaO_2 should be maintained between 60 and 80 mm Hg; $PaCO_2$ may rise to 60 mmHg, provided pH does not fall below 7.20. A meta-analysis from the Cochrane Neonatal Review Group[183] involving two studies found no evidence supporting the use of "permissive hypercapnia" to prevent or reduce morbidity or mortality. Inspiratory times should generally range between 0.3 and 0.4 seconds; flow rates of 5 to 7 L/min are desirable. The longer the inspiratory time (beyond 0.6 seconds), the greater the likelihood of air leak and cardiovascular dysfunction, particularly at high peak pressures. However, longer inspiratory times of 0.5 to 0.6 seconds have been suggested for improving alveolar ventilation.[184] PEEP is variable. It may be required at levels as high as 6 cm H_2O to minimize airway resistance and to enhance alveolar ventilation. In most instances, 4 to 5 cm H_2O is sufficient for these purposes. Inappropriately high levels of PEEP impair alveolar ventilation, diminish lung perfusion and cardiac venous return, and increase the intensity of baro-volutrauma. FIO_2 must be maintained at levels that provide optimal PaO_2. FIO_2 may vary extensively from hour to hour or from day to day. FIO_2 must provide optimal PaO_2, but excessive concentrations must be avoided because they may worsen hyperoxic lung damage.

Weaning should be accomplished with sensitive perception of respiratory needs. When peak pressures are reduced to 12 cm H_2O and FIO_2 has declined to 0.6, the respiratory rate can be reduced at a slow pace, generally in decrements of five breaths. Establishment of spontaneous breathing requires gradual diminution of dependence on mechanical support. As the rate is diminished, evaluation of spontaneous breathing (air movement) with the stethoscope is helpful for determining a baby's capacity to breathe independently. A rate of no more than 5 breaths/min should be maintained for at least 4 hours before extubation is attempted.

Evaluation of arterial blood gases by percutaneous arterial sampling is impractical because spurious results from the painful sampling procedure preclude any value in guidance. The same may be said for capillary sampling, which is equally painful and is also inaccurate in any circumstances.[185] Transcutaneous PaO_2 determination is not reliable after a few days postnatally. Oxygen saturation by pulse oximetry is the most practical method currently in use. Arterial O_2 saturations between 90% and 95% usually indicate a PaO_2 of no less than 50 mm Hg and no more than 100 mm Hg.[186,187]

After the infant is weaned from the ventilator, O_2 supplementation may be essential for weeks or months. At first, this is best provided with a hood or nasal CPAP. When FIO_2 is diminished to less than 0.3, O_2 is best administered via nasal cannula. The flow rate in fractions of liters per minute as delivered with a nasal cannula cannot be directly correlated with specific FIO_2, but estimations are possible (see Appendix 34). Adequate arterial O_2 levels should be maintained as steadily as possible so that pulmonary vasoconstriction is prevented.[137,188] Pulmonary vascular beds are exquisitely sensitive to periods of hypoxemia. The resultant vasoconstriction is relieved by an enhanced FIO_2. Frequent periods of hypoxemia or ongoing marginal oxygenation raise pulmonary artery pressure, further stressing right-sided heart function. Desaturation after oral feeding is common but is not generally appreciated.[189] Desaturation is accentuated by fast feeding and larger volumes.

Diuretics

The rationale for use of diuretics in BPD is to treat abnormal microvascular permeability and pulmonary edema.[190,191] Lung compliance is reduced, tidal volume is diminished, and airway resistance is increased.[192] Diuretics may act directly to improve lung mechanics by reabsorption of lung fluid, unrelated to diuresis, and by reabsorption of lung fluid by the reduced extracellular fluid volume that follows diuresis.

Furosemide is the most commonly used diuretic in the long-term treatment of BPD. Its short-term benefits on pulmonary function have been shown repeatedly.[55,193–197] Whereas furosemide is a diuretic that acts on the thick ascending limb of the loop of Henle, it also has independent effects on the lungs that are not related to diuretic activity. Short-term improvement in pulmonary function appears before diuresis and probably is not related to it.[197,198] Isolated reports have indicated that pulmonary function improves in response to furosemide administration even when infants are anuric.[199] The extrarenal actions of furosemide include an increase in plasma oncotic pressure, enhancement of thoracic duct lymph flow, clearance of interstitial pulmonary edema, and diminution in lung transvascular fluid movement.[200] Furosemide also lowers pulmonary vascular resistance and improves ventilation-perfusion ratios by direct action on vascular smooth muscle. It improves clinical respiratory status, often decreasing the need for ventilatory support. The diuretic effect of furosemide is attributable to blockage of sodium, potassium, and chloride transport in the thick ascending limb of Henle. The result is significant excretion of these electrolytes, as well as of calcium and magnesium.[199]

Activity of furosemide peaks in approximately 1 to 2 hours and generally ends by 6 hours after dosage. Half-life may be as long as 24 hours in infants whose gestational age is 30 weeks or younger.[200] Half-life shortens with increasing gestational age. The dosing for furosemide and other medications for the treatment of BPD is given in Table 21-5. In babies older than 3 weeks, oxygenation and lung compliance improve with acute or chronic administration. For infants who are younger than 3 weeks, the impact of furosemide is inconsistent or undetectable.[201] Careful monitoring is mandatory in BPD infants who are treated with diuretics. Electrolyte and mineral imbalances are frequent, and supplements of potassium, sodium, and chloride often are necessary. Treatment induced hypokalemia and alkalosis may occur if the dose of the diuretic is large or repeatedly given over time, if sodium and chloride intakes are inadequate, or if KCl supplement is not administered. Infants with ongoing BPD usually have a compensated respiratory acidosis because of renal retention of bicarbonate. A pH of 7.30 to 7.40 is expected in the usual course of BPD, hypercapnia notwithstanding. However, a diuretic induced primary metabolic alkalosis causes higher pH and the infant hypoventilates.

The resultant increase in $Paco_2$ compensates for the rising pH. With an apparently elevated pCO_2, an increased dose of diuretic would seem appropriate at first thought, but in fact the dose should be reduced to alleviate the primary diuretic-induced metabolic alkalosis.[191]

Furosemide may cause hypercalciuria that advances to nephrocalcinosis when calcium is deposited in renal interstitial tissue. The etiologic role of furosemide is not as clear as is generally believed. The first report of nephrocalcinosis in preterm babies in 1982 cited a major etiologic role for furosemide.[202] Since then, the reported incidence in all prematures has varied from 20% to 64%.[203] Karlowicz et al.[204] emphasized family history of kidney stones and white race as the most important determinants of nephrocalcinosis. Jacinto et al.[205] reported overall incidence of 64%. Most but not all of the affected infants had received furosemide. Multifactorial origin was emphasized in another study of nephrocalcinosis, which was identified in 16% of all babies less than 32 weeks of gestation. These authors cited extreme prematurity, severe respiratory disease requiring ventilation, male sex, frequency and duration of gentamicin administration, and high urinary oxalate and urate excretion as major causes. Approximately half of affected infants received furosemide.[203] In a follow-up study of nine patients, Ezzedeen et al.[206] found that at a mean age of 21.3 months, calcification improved in five patients and resolved completely in four. Pope et al.[207] reported resolution of calcification 5 to 6 months after cessation of furosemide therapy in 50% of treated infants. Jones et al.[208] studied 11 prematures with calcifications and 17 controls. Children in both groups were 4 to 5 years old. They concluded that renal calcification in the neonatal period does not seem to be a major predisposition to abnormal renal function at a later age. Ototoxicity has also been associated with long-term furosemide use. These undesirable side effects notwithstanding, the benefit of improved pulmonary function that is achieved with long-term diuretic treatment is believed to outweigh the hazards.[55]

Thiazide diuretics (chlorothiazide and hydrochlorothiazide) are used in combination with spironolactone, which is potassium sparing. Studies on the short-term effectiveness of diuretic therapy with these preparations are inconclusive,[199] but a study by Kao et al.[209] indicated long-term effectiveness of spironolactone and chlorothiazide in improving pulmonary function. In extubated O_2-dependent infants, a lower FIO_2 was possible, but the duration of dependency was unaffected.[209] A Cochrane Review indicates that only a few infants have been studied in randomized trials[192]; however, in infants older than 3 weeks who were given thiazide and spironolactone, improved lung compliance was demonstrated after 4 weeks of treatment. A single study showed significantly reduced mortality among intubated infants.

Bronchodilators

The treatment of acute and sometimes life-threatening episodes of severe bronchospasm requires a rapid response to bronchodilator therapy. Increased airway resistance is characteristic of the moderate and advanced stages of BPD. The morphologic changes responsible for airway obstruction include accumulation of debris, squamous metaplasia, and bronchial muscle hypertrophy. Control of bronchial smooth muscle tone is probably the most prominent factor in acute bronchospastic

---

TABLE 21-5. Pharmacologic Agents in Management of Bronchopulmonary Dysplasia

Drug	Dosage
Diuretics	
Furosemide (intravenous, intramuscular)	1.0–2.0 mg/kg every 12 hr × 3; then once daily or every other day
Furosemide (oral)	2.0–6.0 mg/kg every 12 hr × 3; then once daily or every other day
Chlorothiazide	10–20 mg/kg every 12 hr
Spironolactone	0.5–1.5 mg/kg every 12 hr
Bronchodilators	
Albuterol (inhaled)	0.1–0.5 mg/kg every 2–6 hr
Albuterol (oral)	0.1–0.5 mg/kg every 6–8 hr
Terbutaline (subcutaneous)	0.05 mg/kg
Theophylline (oral)	5.0–6.0 mg/kg, loading dose; 1.0–2.0 mg/kg every 8–12 hr, maintenance dose
Corticosteroids	
Dexamethasone (42-day course)	0.25–0.5 $mg \cdot kg^{-1} \cdot day^{-1}$ every 12 hr for 3 days; taper every 3 days to 0.10 $mg \cdot kg^{-1} \cdot day^{-1}$ every 12 hr on day 36; then 0.10 $mg \cdot kg^{-1} \cdot day^{-1}$ on days 38, 40, and 42

episodes. Bronchial hyperreactivity is a characteristic component of BPD. Its early appearance sometimes heralds the onset of BPD, and occasionally the hyperreactivity persists even after the infant is relatively asymptomatic.

Bronchodilator therapy is used for acute bronchospastic episodes, and in some centers ongoing medication with methylxanthines (theophylline and caffeine) is used to maintain decreased airway resistance. For acute episodes, beta-adrenergic agonist therapy is generally used. Sometimes, anticholinergic therapy is used as an adjuvant. Albuterol is a specific beta$_2$-adrenergic agent that effectively reverses acute episodes of bronchospasm and causes few cardiovascular side effects. Lung compliance increases and airway resistance decreases within minutes of inhalation treatment. The effect lasts for approximately 4 hours. Cardiovascular side effects are less frequent with albuterol than with the other beta$_2$-agonists, such as isoproterenol and metaproterenol. The side effects from the latter two preparations include tachycardia, hypertension, hyperglycemia, and tremor. Albuterol is more specifically a beta$_2$-agonist than the other preparations and is currently the bronchodilator of choice. Atropine is less effective than the beta-agonists. Side effects include tachycardia, diminished intestinal motility, tremor, and inspissation of airway secretions. Ipratropium bromide is another anticholinergic preparation that dilates airways, principally the larger ones.[199]

Theophylline and caffeine are weak bronchodilators compared with the beta$_2$-agonists. Caffeine is the weaker of the two drugs. These preparations also have diuretic and respiratory stimulation effects. Their weak bronchodilating activity has led to their infrequent use in the ongoing treatment of BPD.[199]

Corticosteroids

Prenatal use of glucocorticoids is known to diminish the incidence of RDS by 50% and the recommendation of the Consensus Conference on Antenatal Steroids remains unchanged.[210] There is a suggestion, however, that betamethasone in two doses given 12 hours apart is preferred to other preparations and other schedules.[211] If the benefit and safety of a single course of prenatal steroids are now accepted widely, the status of repeated antenatal courses of treatment is largely unsettled and is not recommended except in clinical trials.[212] The incidence of BPD has not been shown to diminish after administration of antenatal steroids.

Postnatal use of glucocorticoids was widespread for a number of years[213] until poor neurodevelopmental outcomes were reported in abstract form by Yeh et al.[214] in 1997 and published fully 1 year later.[215] Before describing the apparent positive benefits and the side effects of postnatal steroids, it would perhaps be better at the outset to cite the February 2002 negative advisory jointly issued by the American Academy of Pediatrics and the Canadian Pediatric Society.[216] The statement reviewed the "short and long term effects of systemic and inhaled corticosteroids for prevention or treatment of evolving or established chronic lung disease." Because short-term benefits are limited and long-term benefits are absent, routine use of systemic dexamethasone for these purposes was "not recommended." Use of steroids postnatally should be limited to appropriate trials. Clinical use should be limited to serious situations in which maximal respiratory support is already in

place. Parents should be fully informed regarding short and long-term effects and risks, and they should agree to the use of steroids.

Postnatal steroids have been widely used to ameliorate or prevent BPD. The injury imposed by mechanical ventilation and oxygen toxicity has been observed to diminish significantly. In 1983, Mammel et al.[217] reported more rapid ventilator weaning with steroid therapy, and those observations were confirmed in 1985 by Avery et al. Lung compliance was shown to increaese.[218] Steroid treatment suppressed inflammatory mediators, lung function improved demonstrably, and earlier extubation was achieved. Postnatally administered steroids are effective by virtue of several actions.[219,220] Steroids are powerful anti-inflammatory agents, which probably is a fundamental reason for their effectiveness. They diminish the attraction and aggregation of polymorphonuclear leukocytes in the lung,[221] and they lessen the elaboration of prostaglandins, elastase, leukotrienes, interleukins, and tumor necrosis factor. Ultimately, they diminish the permeability of the pulmonary microvasculature and therefore minimize pulmonary edema. They increase diuresis and heighten beta-adrenergic activity. They dilate airways and may enhance the synthesis of surfactant and antioxidants. At the clinical level, these responses to steroids lead to alleviation of pulmonary inflammation, edema, fibrosis, and bronchospasm. Lung compliance increases and airway resistance diminishes; as a consequence, it becomes feasible to lower inspiratory pressure and F$_{IO_2}$.

The adverse acute effects of dexamethasone are multiple, but their frequency is low.[222] Earlier reports on the incidence of severe infections have not materialized in the trials of steroids for BPD. Among the acute side effects, hypertension is quite common.[218,223,224] Treatment usually is not required, but when applied it is effective. Gastrointestinal complications include perforated gastric and duodenal ulcers and life-threatening upper gastrointestinal hemorrhage.[225,226] Hyperglycemia is relatively common.[223,227–230] Occasionally, the use of insulin may be required. Adrenal gland function is suppressed during the treatment period. The effect is apparently temporary[231,232]; adrenal responsiveness is fully restored within 4 to 5 weeks after the discontinuation of steroid therapy.[200] Obstructive hypertrophic cardiomyopathy, which is reversible, has also been reported.[233,234] In one report, the cardiac effects were transient, reaching maximum intensity by week 3 of treatment and disappearing by week 6 of treatment.[234] Thickness was increased in the interventricular septum and in the right and left ventricular free walls.

The aforementioned statement on the use of postnatal corticosteroids jointly issued by the American Academy of Pediatrics and the Canadian Pediatric Society presented a comprehensive review of pertinent literature. In the studies of infants who were treated within the first 96 postnatal hours,[235,236] steroids were given intravenously. All studies except two used dexamethasone. Short-term effects were encouraging. Steroid treatment significantly diminished the combined outcome of BPD and death to the time of discharge, but there was no effect on mortality itself. The incidence of BPD was diminished, and weaning from the ventilator was easier. Acute side effects included hypertension, hypoglycemia, gastrointestinal bleeding or perforation, and hypertrophic obstructive cardiomyopathy. Pulmonary air leak and patent ductus were decreased, and there was no increase in infection, necrotizing enterocolitis, intraventricular hemorrhage, or severe ROP. A relative risk of 1.41 for periventricular leukomalacia was calculated.

The studies of infants who were treated from 7 to 14 postnatal days[195,236,237] all used dexamethasone given intravenously for 2 to 42 days. BPD combined with death was decreased at 28 days postnatal age (PNA) and at 36 weeks PMA, but mortality itself was not diminished. BPD incidence was decreased at 28 days PNA and 36 weeks PMA. Extubation at 7 and 28 days after onset of treatment was more likely in dexamethasone-treated infants. Duration of hospitalization and need for supplemental oxygen were unchanged. Incidences of pneumothorax, severe ROP, intraventricular hemorrhage, and necrotizing enterocolitis were unaffected by dexamethasone.

In the studies of infants whose steroid therapy was initiated beyond 3 postnatal weeks,[238] dexamethasone was given intravenously or enterally for 3 days to 3 weeks. Combined outcome of BPD and death was diminished in the treated group, but survival to discharge was unchanged. Dexamethasone increased compliance and decreased the need for supplemental oxygen; thus, there was a marginally significant diminution of BPD at 36 weeks PMA. Treated infants were more at risk for hypertension but not for infection, necrotizing enterocolitis, and gastrointestinal bleeding.

Although not conclusive, there is strong evidence that long-term neurodevelopmental outcomes are more likely to be dysfunctional when postnatal steroids have been given for BPD.[239] The vast majority of studies concern dexamethasone, and there are no data suggesting that another steroid would be less troublesome. Watterberg[240] and Finer et al. [241] point to three studies[215,242,243] that have shown a significantly higher incidence of neurodevelopmental dysfunction associated with pharmacologic doses of dexamethasone given to small premature infants. A short meta-analysis of the three studies revealed increased odds ratios for the occurrence of cerebral palsy or abnormal findings on neurologic evaluation. The results suggest that for every three to four treated survivors, one child would have an abnormal neurodevelopmental outcome.[241] Mertz et al.[244] reported an increased incidence of periventricular leukomalacia among steroid-treated infants (23% vs 9% in controls). In another extensive review, O'Shea and Doyle[245] expressed similar concerns about long-term outcomes. There is an urgent need to identify a less noxious corticosteroid. Trials of hydrocortisone have been suggested.[246]

In a commentary on postnatal steroids for BPD, Barrington[247] maintains that pharmacologic doses could be abandoned without increase in either mortality or the need for home oxygen. He calculated that for every 30 infants so treated, there will be four extra infants with cerebral palsy and three extra infants with some form of neurodevelopmental dysfunction.

In the meta-analysis by Banks,[248] conclusions were similar to those of other such analyses. Forty controlled studies on dexamethasone were identified, involving more than 4000 neonates. Only 18 of them (n = 2613) were included in the meta-analysis. Treating 100 ventilated infants with dexamethasone in the first 48 postnatal hours would result in 11 fewer instances of death or BPD at 36 weeks PMA. Among those infants so treated, there would be approximately 4 with gastrointestinal hemorrhage and 18 children with cerebral palsy and abnormal neurodevelopmental outcomes.

Nutrition

With only a few points of exception, providing nutrition for a premature with BPD varies little from prematures without BPD. The points of exception include the following: (1) most infants with BPD need more calories to sustain growth compared to unaffected infants; (2) increments in calorie intake usually imply an increased fluid volume that the BPD infant may not tolerate because of a propensity to develop pulmonary edema; and (3) formulas of increased calorie density (up to 30 kcal/oz) must often be fed to satisfy the requirements of high calories and relatively low fluid volume.

An etiologic relationship between deficiencies of specific nutrients and the incidence of BPD has not been unequivocally demonstrated. Vitamin E was proposed and subsequently discarded.[249] Inositol concentrations are low in premature infants, and in one multicenter study the incidence of survival with BPD was significantly reduced.[250] Inositol is a phospholipid that enhances the synthesis of surfactant. There has been no subsequent study of this issue. The most recent and most hopeful specific nutrient deficiency is vitamin A. However, even though supplemental nutrition of enriched formulas has provided for better growth and bone mass accretion, the advantage is not sustained past 3 months of age.[251] Establishing the need for specific nutrients such as antioxidant vitamins, minerals, and perhaps vitamin A requires considerably more data than are currently available. There is good evidence that nutrition has a major impact on the extent of vulnerability in the lung to injury, but there is a paucity of data indicating that nutrition can modulate the outcome of BPD.[252] The need for overall supplementation of nutrition beyond requirements for full-term infants is apparent, but further investigation is necessary before evidence-based recommendations can be formulated.[251]

There can be no concrete recommendation for caloric provision to ensure adequate growth. We hope to achieve weight increments of 20 to 30 g daily, and we provide nutrition with this goal in mind. Maximum fluid volume is 140 to 150 mL/kg/day. Protein intake is provided at 3.2 to 3.5 g/kg/day. Prescription of the remaining nutrients is similar to feedings of premature infants who do not have BPD. We use an enriched formula (30 cal/oz, 1.0 kcal/mL) that is prepared by adding powdered formula to a liquid 24 cal/oz preparation. This preparation avoids the need to add unsaturated oils, medium-chain triglycerides, and glucose polymers to provide greater calorie density. It also provides acceptable intake of protein, calcium, and phosphorus. Osmolality is maintained at 380.[253]

Vitamin A may be effective in reducing the occurrence of BPD. The first trial,[253] reported in 1987 by Shenai et al.,[113] demonstrated reduction of BPD from 85% in controls to 45% in babies given 2000 IU intramuscularly every other day for the first 4 postnatal weeks. Criticism was directed at the unusually high (85%) incidence of BPD in the control group, but this was a claimed intention to recruit infants at the highest risk for BPD.[254] Tyson et al.[117] reported a large multicenter trial that enrolled 807 infants, 405 of whom received vitamin A (5000 IU intramuscularly, three times weekly for 4 weeks). Death or BPD was the primary outcome and was significantly reduced in the vitamin A group. The risk of CLD was slightly reduced in extremely-low-birthweight infants.

EXTRANEOUS AIR SYNDROMES (AIR LEAKS)

Extraneous air syndromes are a group of clinically recognizable disorders produced by alveolar rupture and the subsequent escape of air into tissue in which air is not normally present. Table 21-6 lists the sites in which extraneous air has been reported. All the clinical variations of air leak syndrome originate in overdistended alveoli, which ultimately rupture. Overdistention may follow initial spontaneous vigorous respirations (usually larger term babies) at birth, high pressure with mechanical ventilation (either PEEP or peak inspiratory pressure), vigorous ventilatory resuscitation, and air trapping in the presence of a ball valve mechanism. Although most of the syndromes have long been known to occur spontaneously, their incidence increased as the use of ventilatory support became widespread, particularly since the advent of PEEP ventilation.[13] The occurrence of air leaks has diminished considerably since the advent of surfactant treatment and the use of less intense pressure settings for ventilator support. Beside BPD, air leak syndromes are the most frequent life-threatening complications of ventilatory assistance. The capacity for instant recognition, evaluation, and relief of these disorders is a primary requisite for personnel who assume responsibility for sustained neonatal ventilatory support.

Incidence

Few authors have reported the combined incidence of all of the air leak syndromes. Kirkpatrick et al.[255] were one of the few teams of investigators who did so, but their numbers were small. Fifteen of their 37 infants (41%) with RDS developed one or more of the syndromes. Their case reports included pulmonary interstitial emphysema (PIE), pneumomediastinum, pneumothorax, pneumoperitoneum, and air embolus. Yu et al.[256] also reported on air leaks as a group: 11% of infants with RDS (with or without ventilatory assistance) developed pneumothorax, pneumomediastinum, or interstitial emphysema. Although Thibeault et al.[257] correctly considered interstitial emphysema, pneumomediastinum, and pneumothorax as a single pathologic continuum, they did not cite incidence. Most reports describe selected clinical syndromes to the exclusion of others. A true estimate of the frequency of air leak should include all of its manifestations.

Incidence varies according to the type and severity of disease, gestational age, mode of therapy, and expertise of personnel. Complications are most frequent during treatment for RDS. Interstitial emphysema and pneumothorax, for example, were observed more often in babies with RDS than in infants with other disorders.[257,258] Frequency is also significantly influenced by the vigor of ventilatory assistance, which itself is usually a reflection of the severity of disease and "style" of ventilator support. Berg et al.[13] observed that interstitial emphysema, pneumothorax, and pneumomediastinum occurred twice as often with the use of PEEP (39.7%) than without it (20.7%). In babies with RDS, Ogata et al.[259] noted that the frequency of pneumothorax increased as therapy became more vigorous. Only 3.5% of infants were affected when assisted ventilation was not used; 11.0% when total management consisted of CPAP; 24.0% when CPAP was used at first and IPPV with PEEP later; and 3.3% when only IPPV and PEEP were used throughout the course of treatment.

Pneumopericardium was described as a "very rare condition" in neonates by Matthieu et al.[260] in 1970. These authors could find descriptions of only seven cases. In 1974, Yeh et al.[261] found 13 cases in the English literature since 1942, yet they reported four infants they had observed within a 12-month period. In 1976, Brans et al.[262] described six babies with pneumopericardium in as short a duration as 6 months in one intensive care unit. They found 57 cases in their review of the literature. Pneumopericardium, a "very rare condition" in 1970, increased in frequency until the early 1990s when use of surfactant became widespread. Most reports allude to a relationship between the increased frequency of this syndrome and the vigor of ventilatory therapy. A similar course of events has been noted for pneumoperitoneum. The association of this finding with extraneous air in thoracic structures strongly suggests the absence of gastrointestinal perforation. It was a rare event in 1972,[263,264] but it was not unusual just a few years later.[255,265,266]

Most of the clinical trials of surfactant have demonstrated a striking reduction in the incidence of pneumothorax among treated versus control babies.[22] Extraneous air syndromes will continue to occur, however, and their incidence remains related to high ventilator pressures and severe disease.

Pathogenesis

The 1939 publication by Macklin[267] and the masterful 1944 review of Macklin and Macklin[268] are the basis for our contemporary understanding of the extraneous air syndromes. Macklin postulated that all air leaks are caused by high intra-alveolar pressure that follows inhalation, insufflation, or retention of inordinately large volumes of air. The resultant pressure gradient from affected alveoli to adjacent tissue space may be of sufficient magnitude to rupture the bases of alveoli that overlie capillaries. Air escapes through disruption within the meshes of capillaries. It enters perivascular sheaths and migrates toward the hilum. More recent observations indicate that, in addition to the phenomena observed by Macklin, a somewhat different mechanism prevails in immature, surfactant-deficient lungs.[269-271] In the immature lung of baboons, rupture occurs in the small, compliant terminal airways rather than in the noncompliant, unexpanded, more distal saccules (premature alveoli).[272] The result is the more

TABLE 21-6.   Extraneous Air Syndromes

Site of Extraneous Air	Syndrome
Pulmonary interstitium (perivascular sheaths)	Interstitial emphysema
Alveoli-trabeculae-visceral pleura	Pseudocysts
Pleural space	Pneumothorax
Mediastinum	Pneumomediastinum
Pericardial space	Pneumopericardium
Perivascular sheaths (peripheral vessels)	Perivascular emphysema
Vascular lumina (blood)	Air embolus
Subcutaneous tissue	Subcutaneous emphysema
Retroperitoneal connective tissue	Retroperitoneal emphysema
Peritoneal space	Pneumoperitoneum
Intestinal wall	Pneumatosis intestinalis
Scrotum	Pneumoscrotum

frequent occurrence of PIE that usually does not progress to pneumothorax. Often, extrusions of air occur in contiguous connective tissue and, at times, in trabeculae through which air migrates to pleura to form blebs and burst into the pleural space.

Macklin also speculated that atelectasis poses a considerable risk for rupture of the adjacent expanded alveoli because they become overdistended when, during inspiration, negative pressure is applied to a reduced number of distensible alveoli for a prolonged time interval. The result is overdistention and rupture. In a lucid discussion published in 1963, Chernick and Avery[273] applied Macklin's reasoning when they postulated the pathogenesis of spontaneous pneumothorax occurring during the first few breaths of the newborn infant. When aspirated mucus or meconium prevents expansion of a sufficient number of alveoli, overdistention of already expanded alveoli causes their spontaneous rupture soon after birth. During the first few breaths, normal infants create intrapleural pressures that are 40 to 100 cm H_2O below that of the atmosphere.[274] This negative pressure is transmitted to atelectatic areas, and thus no gradient is present between unexpanded alveoli and the pleural space. However, a gradient does exist between alveoli that are distended by atmospheric pressure and the pleural space, which is transiently at 40 to 100 cm H_2O below atmospheric pressure. When a significant portion of the neonate's lung remains unexpanded during peak inspiration, the gradient between intra-alveolar and intrapleural pressures is sustained for a longer period of time than is normal in the expanded areas. Apparently, the resultant protracted tension on alveolar walls causes spontaneous ruptures.

Air in perivascular sheaths dissects toward the hilum and invades the mediastinum and thus causes pneumomediastinum. Air bubbles may accumulate at the hilum to form large blebs that sometimes compress hilar vessels. The blebs are situated where the visceral pleura reflects onto the parietal pleura. As pressure mounts, rupture of blebs at this location releases air into the pleural space to give rise to pneumothorax. Apparently, air also passes from other points in the mediastinal wall to the pleural cavity. The pathway and mechanism of extension to the pericardial space are still conjectural. The point of invasion by air may be where the pericardium reflects onto pulmonary vessels to join the pleura.

Figure 21-4 depicts the migration of air from alveolar rupture through the lung interstitium *(A)* into the pleural *(B)* and the pericardial *(C)* cavities. (The chest films correspond to the diagrams.)

Far-flung dispersion of air was noted experimentally in cats by Macklin.[267] He described "freshlets breaking through downward" to enter the retroperitoneal space and upward into the neck, chest wall, arm, axilla, and face. Pneumoperitoneum is thought to result from the extension of mediastinal air along the great vessels and esophagus into the retroperitoneal space and from there to the peritoneal cavity after rupture through the posterior peritoneum.[263,264,267] Pneumoscrotum is sometimes associated with pneumoperitoneum. Presumably, migration of air occurred from the peritoneal cavity through the processus vaginalis into the scrotum. Air embolism occurs when extremely high pressures are used for ventilatory assistance. Air may be injected directly into the pulmonary capillaries at the time of alveolar rupture.[266] Entry into blood vessels has been demonstrated experimentally in dogs when small lacerations are made in lung parenchyma. Thus, in humans, the application of very high peak inspiratory pressure to a lung of low compliance may lacerate the parenchyma, allowing the passage of air under a high head of pressure into blood vessels.[275] Another possible pathway involves the dissection of air through the subadventitial planes of pulmonary veins, thus producing both air embolus and pneumopericardium.[276]

The appearance of extraneous air, regardless of its location, always begins with distal airway or alveolar rupture and air leak. The migration of escaped air ensues through tissue planes that offer the least resistance to extension, thus giving rise to a spectrum of clinical syndromes that range from interstitial emphysema and pneumothorax to air embolism and pneumoscrotum.

Clinical Aspects of Extraneous Air Syndromes

Of the 12 syndromes listed in Table 21-6, only pneumothorax and pneumopericardium require remedial action within minutes lest death or brain damage ensue. On rare occasions, pneumomediastinum and pneumoperitoneum require the same urgent attention. Interstitial emphysema is a serious manifestation of air leak that is associated with a high rate of mortality. Although several treatment modalities have been proposed, no consistently effective treatment is presently available. Air embolus is a fatal event for which no effective therapy exists.

Pulmonary Interstitial Emphysema

PIE is a consequence of the overdistention of distal airways, and it usually occurs in the smallest babies with the most immature lungs. Ruptured ducts provide a pathway for leakage into connective tissue sheaths that envelop the airways.[269–271] When air accumulates in sheaths, PIE is the result. An alternate description of the distribution of interstitial air was demonstrated by Boothroyd and Barson.[277] Although they could not identify sites of entry, they did demonstrate that the interstitial air largely resided in lung lymphatics. The onset of abnormal clinical signs is relatively gradual. Most infants develop PIE during administration of mechanical ventilatory support. Oxygen requirements increase, and CO_2 retention may be relentless. Death eventually results from failure to adequately ventilate the baby. The extent to which death is attributable to vascular compression, particularly at the hilum, is unknown. Noncompliant overexpanded lungs impair cardiac venous return because they increase pleural pressure, which may be a reason for the increased incidence of intraventricular hemorrhage in babies with PIE.

Approximately 50% of pneumothoraces are associated with antecedent recognizable PIE. Campbell[278] observed progression to pneumothorax in 13 of 14 infants in whom the pre-existence of PIE was unquestionable. Emery[279] noted that PIE was associated with pneumothorax in 11 of 13 necropsied infants. All of the infants studies by Campbell had RDS. All of the babies studied by Emery were born at term and were otherwise well. Mechanical ventilatory assistance was not a factor in either of these studies. In an analysis of 311 infants who received ventilatory assistance over a 12-month period, the author identified 22 infants who had PIE with and without other sites of extraneous air. The gestational age of all 22 infants was 33 weeks or less. Watts et al.[130] noticed a high incidence of PIE during the first 24 hours of life among infants who later developed BPD.

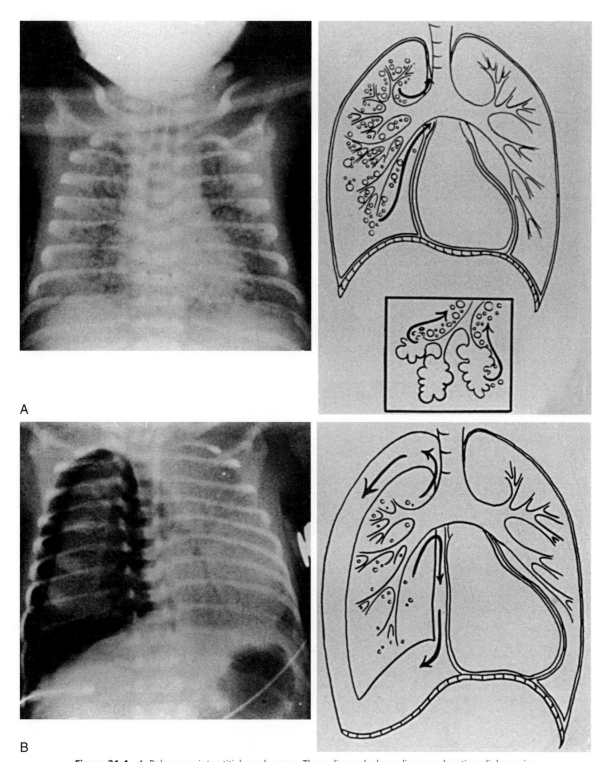

Figure 21-4. *A,* Pulmonary interstitial emphysema. The radiograph shows linear and cystic radiolucencies, which are cast by accumulation of interstitial air. The diagram depicts air leak from a ruptured alveolus *(bottom)* with escape to interstitial tissue. *B,* Pneumothorax (tension) has compressed a stiff lung, depressed the right side of the diaphragm, and displaced the heart considerably to the left. The diagram indicates a pathway of air from the interstitium into the pleural cavity.

Figure 21-4 continued on next page

PIE can only be diagnosed radiologically. Campbell[278] has clearly described the radiologic appearance. It is characterized by two basic features: radiolucencies that are linear and those that are cystlike. The linear radiolucencies vary in width; they are coarse and they do not branch. They are seen in the peripheral as well as the medial lung fields. Boothroyd and Barson[277] described the radiologic appearance of lymphatic gas as disorganized and haphazard in distribution. Accumulations were cystic and linear. The linear configurations did not branch and they extended from hilar to periphery. At autopsy, variable

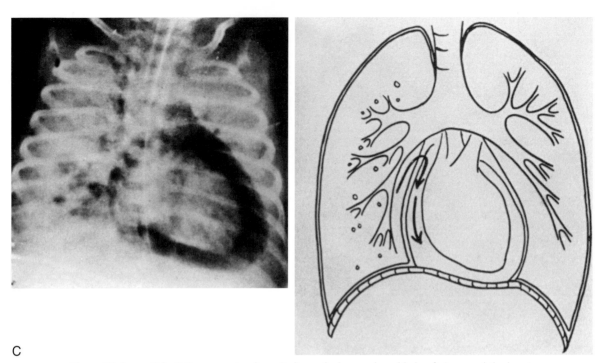

C

Figure 21-4—cont'd. *C,* Pneumopericardium. Radiograph shows a broad halo of air around the heart. Pulmonary interstitial emphysema affects the right lung. The diagram indicates the path of air from the lung interstitium to the pericardial space. (From Korones SB: High-Risk Newborn Infants: The Basis for Intensive Nursing Care, 4th ed. St. Louis, C.V. Mosby, 1986, pp. 252–253.)

distention of lymphatics was microscopically prominent. Medium-sized pulmonary arteries were frequently enveloped by markedly dilated air-filled lymphatics. Air bronchograms must be differentiated from interstitial air. The bronchial air shadows are smooth and branching. They usually are seen toward the hilar regions, particularly in the lower lobes. The cystlike radiolucencies of PIE vary in diameter from 1.0 to 4.0 mm. In some instances, they are oval or lobulated. They may be so numerous that they impart a spongy appearance. In local areas their distribution is haphazard. Figure 21-4*A* depicts a chest film that closely resembles Campbell's description. PIE may involve only one lobe, one lung, or, more usually, both lungs. It appears within 96 hours of birth in babies who are receiving ventilatory assistance. If conventional ventilator support is maintained, high-frequency (oscillatory or jet) ventilation is preferred. Attempts should be made to minimize peak inspiratory pressures, shorten inspiratory times, and reduce distending pressures. Usually the development of PIE itself imposes a need for more vigorous therapy. Intubation of the contralateral bronchus when only one lung is involved and "positional therapy" with the affected lung down have been used successfully in the management of unilateral PIE. High-frequency ventilation often alleviates PIE within 24 to 48 hours of treatment onset. An infant with PIE is described in Chapter 29, case 4.

Pneumothorax

Pneumothorax can occur spontaneously (no iatrogenic factors implicated) as a result of ventilatory assistance or, rarely, as a complication following certain procedures. The incidence of pneumothorax has declined dramatically with the use of surfactant therapy and lower ventilator pressures.

Spontaneous pneumothorax usually occurs during the first few breaths soon after birth. The vast majority of infants are asymptomatic. Radiologic surveys have demonstrated an incidence of 1.0% to 2.0% of all live births[280]; symptomatic pneumothorax, however, has been noted in only 0.05% to 0.07% of live births.[273,281–283] Most investigators have found a higher incidence of spontaneous pneumothorax in full-term infants.[273,283] Postmature infants seem to be the most vulnerable.[273,279,284]

Distress is generally evident in the delivery room or soon after arrival in the nursery. Tachypnea (to 130 breaths/min) is a universal occurrence. Malan and Heese[283] stressed the frequency and prominence of chest bulge on the involved side. Grunting, retractions, and cyanosis in room air have been noted in virtually all affected infants. As a rule, symptomatic infants have abnormal chest findings that are attributable to lung underexpansion and to displacement of the heart away from the affected hemithorax. Lubchenco[287a] was impressed with the frequency and degree of restlessness and irritability among affected neonates. Spontaneous pneumothorax is sometimes a manifestation of serious lung disease. It has long been observed in association with meconium aspiration, RDS, transient tachypnea of the newborn, pneumonia, pulmonary hypoplasia with renal anomalies, and diaphragmatic hernia. It has been encountered in infants who had RDS syndrome type II (transient tachypnea). Although spontaneous alveolar rupture is sometimes a worrisome portent of serious underlying pulmonary disease, most infants have otherwise normal lungs. Approximately 80% to 90% are mildly ill and require no therapy other than O_2 supplementation.[273]

During ventilatory assistance, when pneumothorax occurs, tension pneumothorax is common. Vigilance by expert personnel, particularly nurses, is effective for early detection; a significant number of pneumothoraces can be predicted. Early gestational age, RDS, and high ventilatory pressures are the most significant risk factors. Their presence imposes a high risk for air leak. Predictions based on chest film review are more specific. PIE is a frequent precursor. Campbell and Hoffman[258] reported 31 babies with RDS; PIE preceded pneumothorax in 15 (50%). The shortest interval between radiologic demonstration of PIE and the appearance of pneumothorax was 2 hours; the longest interval was 72 hours. Ogata et al.[259] reported virtually identical observations. Pneumomediastinum is another predictor that has long been identified as an occasional precursor of pneumothorax. Changes in oscilloscopic tracings of cardiac activity are often valuable signs. Merenstein et al.[285] identified pneumothorax before the appearance of any clinical signs if RS voltage suddenly diminished by at least 40%.

Identification and relief of pneumothorax can be accomplished within a few minutes by detection of abnormal signs. Tension pneumothorax produces abrupt duskiness or cyanosis. Ogata et al.[259] described significant declines of arterial blood pressure, heart rate, respiratory rate, and pulse pressure in 77% of their infants. They did not detect the expected abnormal chest signs. Detection of diminished breath (and heart) sounds, bulging of the affected hemithorax, and mediastinal shift to the unaffected side nevertheless are valuable early indications.

The definitive treatment of tension pneumothorax is placement of a chest tube and application of continuous suction (-10 cm H_2O), particularly if PEEP is used for ventilatory assistance. Recurrence of pneumothorax during chest drainage is frequent. Yu et al.[256] described recurrence in 9 of 14 infants. In such circumstances, the existing tube must be replaced if it is demonstrably occluded; if the tube is not blocked, a second one must be inserted. The most difficult pneumothorax that we have treated was a bilateral one that ultimately required 13 tube insertions. At one point during the course, three tubes were simultaneously operative in one of the child's pleural cavities and two in the other. At 4 years of age, this child was normal.

Pneumothorax as a result of certain procedures is rare. Leake et al.[286] reported a pneumothorax that became evident 3 hours after birth in a term infant. The mother had an amniocentesis shortly before the onset of labor and several hours before the infant's birth. They also summarized three previous reports of pneumothorax, all attributable to entry of the amniocentesis needle into the fetal chest. Anderson and Chandra[287] described three infants who developed pneumothorax following perforation of segmental bronchi by suction catheters.

Pneumopericardium

Pneumopericardium usually occurs in association with one or more of the other extraneous air syndromes. It is rare in the absence of mechanical respiratory support. In most instances, very high ventilatory pressures are used for adequate therapy. The first sign of onset is often a sudden appearance or deepening of cyanosis. Heart sounds are muffled. In the most severe cases, heart sounds are inaudible, although reduced voltage cardiac activity is evident on the oscilloscope or electrocardiograph. If sufficient air accumulates in the pericardial space, pressure within it increases and eventually stroke volume diminishes (tamponade). Arterial blood pressure falls, and in the extreme case peripheral pulses are not palpable. As hypoxia worsens, bradycardia becomes evident. Metabolic acidosis develops in response to hypoxemia and to the generally diminished tissue perfusion that results from low cardiac output due to tamponade. The most distinctive features that suggest the onset of tamponade are the abrupt appearance of cyanosis, hypotension, inaudible heart sounds associated with diminished cardiac activity visible on the electrocardiograph or the oscilloscope, and persistent pulsations of fluid in the umbilical artery catheter.[260] Radiographic diagnosis is definitive. A broad radiolucent halo completely surrounds the heart, including the inferior (diaphragmatic) surface (see Fig. 21-4C). In the lateral projection, a broad area of radiolucency separates the anterior surface of the heart from the sternum and, to a lesser extent, from the diaphragm.

Pneumopericardium varies widely in severity. I have made the diagnosis serendipitously on a routine chest film from a baby who had no abnormal cardiac signs. The pericardial air disappeared spontaneously 6 hours later (Fig. 21-5). In a review of the literature, Brans et al.[262] revealed 57 cases, to

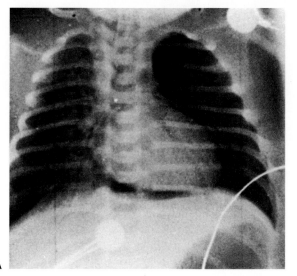
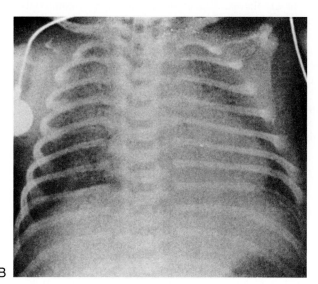

A   B

Figure 21-5. Pneumopericardium diagnosed incidentally on a routine chest film in an infant being ventilated for respiratory distress. *A,* A thin halo of air surrounds the heart and delineates the pericardium as a thin white line against air-filled lung. *B,* Spontaneous clearing of pneumopericardium 6 hours later.

which they added 6 of their own. Approximately 60% of the infants survived. Of those infants who were treated with peri- cardiocentesis, 79% survived. Conservative management was associated with 32% survival. These authors thus made a case for aggressive management with needle aspiration or catheter insertion. On the other hand, Pomerance et al.[288] and Varano and Maisels[289] opted for conservative management. The latter authors would maintain conservative therapy until cardiac tam- ponade is indicated by a decrease in aortic blood pressure.

Treatment may consist of multiple pericardial taps, as indi- cated for the accumulation of air, or involve the insertion of a pericardial tube for continuous drainage. The incidence of reac- cumulation after initial pericardiocentesis was reported to be 53% in one review.[290]

Pneumomediastinum

This is a common isolated disorder when it occurs sponta- neously in otherwise healthy infants by the same mechanisms that have been described for spontaneous pneumothorax. It also occurs spontaneously in RDS, after resuscitation at birth, and during ventilator therapy. Morrow et al.[291] found that spontaneous pneumomediastinum occurred at a rate of 25 per 10,000 live births. As observed in spontaneous pneumothorax, postmature infants were more vulnerable than others, presum- ably for the same reason: a higher incidence of meconium aspiration.

When pneumomediastinum occurs in otherwise normal infants at birth, it is generally asymptomatic. In other circum- stances, it produces mild-to-moderate abnormal clinical signs. Tachypnea, a bulging sternum, muffled heart sounds, and cyanosis occur with varying frequencies. The chest film is diag- nostic in the lateral projection.[292] Anteroposterior projections often appear spuriously normal. In the lateral view, air is seen as a radiolucent area behind the sternum or in the superior portion of the mediastinum if the infant is upright. Occasionally, the thymus is visible above the heart. In the anteroposterior view, a halo is seen around the heart; this halo does not extend to the heart's inferior (diaphragmatic) border. Sometimes the halo is so broad that it extends toward the lateral reaches of the thorax. The *spinnaker sail sign* is commonly apparent in this projection. It is produced by lifting of the thymus from the heart by the air beneath it (Fig. 21-6A and B). This sign (also called the *bat-wing* or *angel-wing* sign) should not be confused with the *sail sign,* which is a normal triangular shadow in the upper mediastinum. There is no separation of the "sail" from surrounding structures by radiolucent air. Pneumomediastinum resolves spontaneously with rare excep- tions. Careful observation is essential, but nothing more aggressive is indicated.

Pneumoperitoneum

Free air in the peritoneum usually suggests perforation of an abdominal viscus, which requires immediate laparotomy; however, in a number of reports, pneumoperitoneum was shown to follow a pulmonary air leak. Air migrates through the diaphragm[264,266,293] to the retroperitoneal space and then to the peritoneal cavity. The principal difficulty of this situation is the need to exclude the possibility of a serious surgical dis- order. The simultaneous presence of aberrant air in the chest suggests that the situation is nonsurgical. The absence of peri-

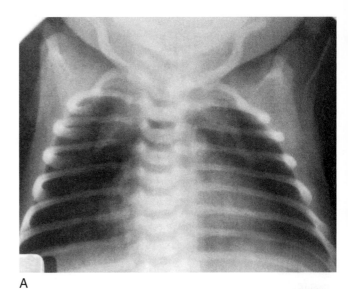

A

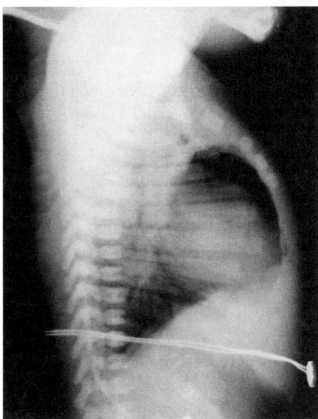

B

Figure 21-6. *A,* Anteroposterior projection of a pneumomediastinum, which has lifted both thymi lobes to produce the "spinnaker sail sign." *B,* Lateral view shows air beneath the sternum in the superior medi- astinum. (From Korones SB: High-Risk Newborn Infants: The Basis for Intensive Nursing Care, 4th ed. St. Louis, C.V. Mosby, 1986, p. 257.)

toneal fluid, normal thickness of the bowel wall, and the absence of air–fluid levels are further evidence of the nonsur- gical nature of the condition. Figure 21-7 demonstrates a curious variation of pneumoperitoneum in which air envelops the scrotum. Occasionally, massive pneumoperitoneum may compress the inferior vena cava, resulting in decreased blood return to the heart, hypotension, and metabolic acidosis.

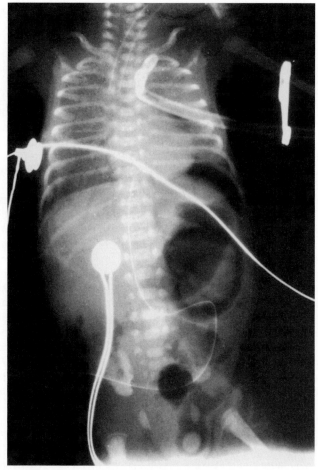

Figure 21-7. Pneumoperitoneum, pneumoscrotum. Air is evident in the peritoneal space, processus vaginalis, and the scrotum. Note also the free air beneath the left diaphragm. (From Korones SB: High-Risk Newborn Infants: The Basis for Intensive Nursing Care, 4th ed. St. Louis, C.V. Mosby, 1986, p. 260.)

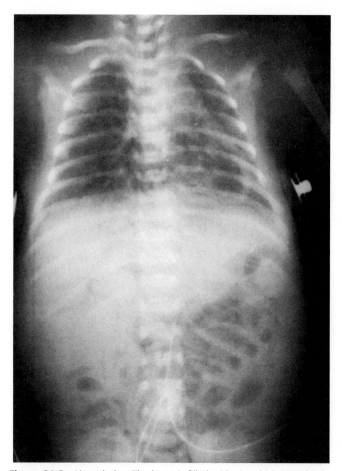

Figure 21-8. Air embolus. The heart is filled with air, which can also be seen in the portal vessels in the liver. (From Korones SB: High-Risk Newborn Infants: The Basis for Intensive Nursing Care, 4th ed. St. Louis, C.V. Mosby, 1986, p. 261.)

Air Embolus

This relatively rare condition is the most sinister of the extraneous air syndromes. It occurs when extremely high pressures are required to ventilate extremely stiff lungs. Parenchymal tears probably occur, and as a result air is injected into the pulmonary vasculature. In the infant described by Gregory and Tooley,[275] inflation pressures up to 50 cm H_2O were necessary to provide a satisfactory tidal volume. Lubens et al.[294] had to use a peak inspiratory pressure of 55 cm H_2O in the 800-g infant whom they reported. Bowen et al.[295] encountered a similar situation in the infant they studied, who developed intravascular air. Siegle et al.[296] described two infants with air embolus who were managed in their unit. Each had antecedent PIE. The clinical presentation of infants with air embolus is a catastrophic event. Sudden cyanosis and circulatory collapse become evident. The heart slows, but with each beat the air–blood mixture crackles and pops. Withdrawal of blood from the umbilical artery catheter yields alternating segments of air and blood, similar to what one would expect if a stopcock connection were loose. Radiography reveals the bizarre picture of intracardiac and intravascular air. Figure 21-8 shows air in the portal vessels as well as in the heart. No beneficial treatment for air embolism is available.

RETINOPATHY OF PREMATURITY

ROP was first described in 1942 by Terry[297] in five premature infants, each of whom had a "grayish-white, opaque membrane behind each crystalline lens." The disorder was then named *retrolental fibroplasia*. Although Terry first described the disease, it was Clifford, a Boston pediatrician, who first called attention to it. Clifford recognized unanticipated blindness on routine examination of a 4-month-old infant during a house call in the Roxbury section of Boston.[298]

Over the next decade, a long list of postulated causes accumulated, but later (between 1952 and 1955), three controlled studies demonstrated that excessive use of O_2 was associated with the development of ROP.[299-301] As a result, the routine administration of O_2 to premature infants was no longer considered tenable; it was restricted pervasively. It should be realized that these studies addressed restrictions of FIO_2; blood gas determinations were not feasible at the time. The epidemic of blindness that had transpired during the 1940s and the early 1950s receded following the restriction of O_2 use, but in the early 1960s, a newly increased mortality and a heightened incidence of cerebral palsy were thought to be a function of O_2 restriction.[302,303] There followed an era of regulated O_2 administration that could now be based on blood gas determinations

(PaO$_2$); this technique was substantially replaced with the advent of transcutaneous O$_2$ monitoring. More recently, determination of O$_2$ saturation with the use of pulse oximetry became the modality of choice. Although O$_2$ concentration was monitored assiduously with advanced technology, in 1981 Phelps[304] reported that there nevertheless was an apparent resurgence in the incidence of ROP. A "new epidemic" had materialized, and it was attributed to a remarkable increase in the survival of very small infants (<1000 g). Although today the survival of the smallest babies has been enhanced and despite careful monitoring of blood O$_2$ levels, the incidence of ROP has increased significantly.[304,305] It became apparent that O$_2$ was not the sole cause of ROP, as had been widely believed.[1,306]

Etiology

Controlled clinical trials in the early 1950s demonstrated that supplemental O$_2$ administration was a causative factor. In one cooperative study, Kinsey and Hemphill[299] reported an incidence of 71% for active ROP with the liberal use of O$_2$ versus an incidence of 33% with the curtailed use of O$_2$ in a large group of matched infants. Other studies came to the same conclusion.[300,301] However, cases had previously been reported in term infants,[307] in premature infants never exposed to O$_2$,[307] in infants with cyanotic congenital heart disease,[308] and in term infants who received exchange transfusions.[309] The cause is currently considered multifactorial.[310]

In a kitten model an angiogenic growth factor [vascular endothelial growth factor (VEGF)] has been isolated in greater concentrations from the avascular retina than from the immediately posterior vascular retina. It is proposed that, when stimulated (as by hypoxia), growth factor increases and angiogenesis is more prolific. The growth factor has been identified in the eye of the human infant.[311]

The unequivocal assumption that hyperoxia in premature infants is the sole cause of ROP has been virtually discarded.[1,312] Re-examination of the original studies[147] and accumulated evidence from numerous reports since these original studies were published have produced a perspective that is possible only after years of experience have elapsed. Although the important role of O$_2$ is evident from the earlier investigations, interpretations of the data have tended to overlook the substantial number of infants who developed ROP despite the assiduous control of low ambient O$_2$ concentrations. Also overlooked were the impressive number of infants in whom no disease was present despite their exposure to high O$_2$ concentrations. Furthermore, more than 60 infants born at term are known to have developed ROP, and the majority did not receive O$_2$. In a similar context, 95 low-birthweight infants who had never received supplemental O$_2$ were reported to have retinopathy.[1] The disease has been reported in 11 anencephalic infants, 10 of whom either were stillborn or did not survive for longer than a few days.

The issue of causation is further confused by data suggesting that retinal hypoxia may cause the neovascularization that characterizes ROP. Several studies indicate that the infants who develop ROP have more complicated courses, more hypoxemic episodes, and overall lower arterial O$_2$ levels.[313–316] In 1953, Szewczyk[317] reported an extensive favorable experience with severe ROP when infants were given O$_2$ that was gradually withdrawn. Bedrossian et al.[318,319] reported fewer cases of ROP when O$_2$ was gradually withdrawn. These clinical experiences, as well as evidence from animal studies,[320] motivated a controlled clinical trial comparing the impact of maintaining O$_2$ saturations at 96% to 99% versus 89% to 94% on progression to threshold ROP in infants identified with prethreshold ROP. The study sought to determine whether the higher O$_2$ saturations would diminish progression of the disease. The rates of progression did not differ between the two groups.[321]

In summary, views on the etiologic significance of O$_2$ therapy have changed remarkably since the original studies of the 1950s established a rigid therapeutic approach that was applied for more than 2 decades. The present epidemic of blindness differs from the first one of the 1950s.[304] It affects a population of considerably smaller infants whose birthweights are less than 1000 g. In these infants particularly, an association between the use of O$_2$ and the development of retinopathy does not appear to exist. The accumulated data indicate that ROP may not be a preventable disease, especially in infants of extremely low birthweight (<1000 g). Risk factors as summarized in an informative review of studies on ROP[310] include prematurity, O$_2$ administration, vitamin A deficiency, inositol deficiency, indomethacin therapy for prevention of patent ductus arteriosus, vitamin E deficiency, exposure to light, intravenous lipid administration, apneic episodes, transfusions of adult blood, elevated or depressed PaCO$_2$, intraventricular hemorrhage, and septicemia. None of these factors has been identified as a valid cause of ROP. Newer studies examining O$_2$ saturation targets indicate that lowering the saturation targets may reduce the incidence of ROP in the most susceptible infants without increasing neurologic dysfunctional outcomes.[321]

Incidence

All large studies to date reveal that the incidence of ROP is inversely proportional to birthweight, gestational age, or both. This finding supports the evidence that disease occurs in the nonvascularized portion of the retina and that vascularization of the retina progresses linearly with increasing gestational age. Kingham[322] found a 13% incidence (107/810) of infants discharged from an intensive care nursery. He concurred that the incidence of ROP was greatest in the least mature infants. Two thirds (71/107) of all cases were infants less than 29 weeks of gestation. ROP resolved without scarring after discharge in two thirds of infants weighing less than 1000 g. Kingham found no permanent scarring in any infant weighing more than 1500 g, and spontaneous resolution occurred in 75% of all infants with evidence of ROP at discharge (Table 21-7).

Flynn[323] examined 639 infants whose birthweights were 1500 g or less and who survived at least 28 days. The infants were admitted to the intensive care unit from 1975 to 1981. Acute proliferative disease was found in 67% of infants who weighed from 600 to 999 g, 36% of infants who weighed from 1000 to 1249 g, and 13% of infants who weighed from 1250 to 1500 g. Univariate and multivariate analysis indicated that birthweight was the most powerful predictor of disease. Duration of ventilation, particularly for infants weighing more than 1000 g, also was predictive. Oxygen therapy apparently was not predictive for the smallest infants (i.e., those weighing from 600 to 999 g), but there was a stronger association between O$_2$ and ventilation therapy in infants in the higher-weight groups (i.e., those weighing >1250 g). Shohat et al.[324] reported acute disease in 52% of infants whose birthweights ranged from 501 to 1250 g and who were discharged from their intensive care unit from 1977 to 1980.

TABLE 21-7. Long-Term Outcomes of Retinopathy of Prematurity

Birthweight (g)	No. of Patients Examined	At Discharge		Long-term Outcome	
		Normal	RLF	RLF Resolved	Permanent Scarring
<1000	118	67 (57%)	51 (43%)	33 (28%)	18 (15%)
1000–1500	467	420 (90%)	47 (10%)	40 (9%)	7 (1%)

RLF, retrolental fibroplasia (retinopathy of prematurity).
From Silverman WA: Prematurity in retrolental fibroplasia. Sight Sav Rev 39:42, 1969. Reprinted with permission of Prevent Blindness America.

The CRYO-ROP Study reported that most infants less than 27 gestational weeks had ROP (>90% at ≤25 weeks). The LIGHT-ROP Study, 10 years later, reported a similar incidence.[311]

Pathology

The human retina is immune to the toxic effects of O_2 if vascularization is complete. At 12 to 16 weeks of gestation, vascularization of the retina begins.[325] Vessels grow outward from the optic disc toward the nasal and temporal periphery of the retina. As gestation advances, the amount of avascular retina decreases progressively.[326] The human retina is not completely vascularized at term, however, a fact that probably accounts for the occasional occurrence of ROP in full-term infants. Moreover, the human fetus lives in an environment of low oxygenation. Pao_2 ranges from 25 to 35 mm Hg in the umbilical vein. At birth, the retina is exposed to relative hyperoxygenation, even if no supplemental O_2 is given. Normal Pao_2 ranges from 50 to 100 mm Hg. Hyperoxygenation (i.e., $Pao_2 > 100$ mm Hg) results in constriction and then obliteration of retinal vessels with the cessation of normal peripheral growth. This usually occurs in the temporal area, which is the slowest to vascularize. Vascular growth resumes when arterial O_2 concentration returns to normal, but this growth may be erratic.[327]

The initial ophthalmologic finding is an abnormal terminal arborization of retinal vessels. Later, a ridge of neovascularization at the junction of the vascularized and nonvascularized retina is produced by the outward growth of these vessels through the inner limiting membrane of the retina into the vitreous. The creation of an arterial venous shunt accounts for the finding of dilated tortuous vessels on the retina posteriorly.

At this point, the disease may take one of two pathways. In most infants, these vascular abnormalities resolve and vision is normal or only slightly impaired. Unfortunately, a few cases progress to yield an exudative response, which, when organized, leads to the formation of membranes between the retina and vitreous that produce retinal traction and detachment. At approximately 6 months of age, cicatricial changes begin in severely affected infants. This process may be compounded by temporal traction of the new vessels as they leave the optic disc. Concurrently, fibrous tissue continues to proliferate immediately behind the lens, producing leukoria (opaque, white pupils). Partial or total retinal detachment is the endpoint of the cicatricial process, resulting in severely impaired vision or total blindness.

Classification

Retrolental fibroplasia has long been the accepted name of this ocular disease, which was first discovered in 1941 and first described in 1942. However, the name *retinopathy of prematurity* is more appropriate. Literally, retrolental fibroplasia means "scar formation behind the lens," which is the culmination of this disorder but which occurs in only a few affected infants. ROP is a more inclusive term in that it describes abnormal events in the retina during which a number of stages unfold, beginning with vascular changes, progressing to retinal edema and detachment, and culminating in fibrosis. Progression through all of these stages to scar formation occurs in a few infants. In most, the process arrests in the early stages of vascular change, before the appearance of fibroplasia.

Various classifications of the progression of ROP have been proposed. In the modified Reese classification, the disease has been divided into two phases, active and cicatricial.[328,329]

A new international classification of ROP was published in 1984.[330] It is suggested as a replacement for the part of the Reese classification that deals with the "active phase" of the disease; however, the new classification recommends retention of the section of Reese's classification dealing with the "cicatricial phase."

The new classification deals primarily with (1) the location in which disease has been identified, (2) the extent of disease in terms of the maximum fundal area involved, and (3) the staging of the disease, which is intended to indicate the degree to which the disease has advanced.

Location

Location is expressed as zone 1, 2, or 3 (Fig. 21-9).[330] Each zone is centered on the optic disc because normal retinal vascular growth progresses peripherally from the disc toward the ora serrata.

> *Zone 1:* Posterior pole or inner zone. Extends in all directions from the optic disc to a distance twice that between the disc and the macula.
> *Zone 2:* From the edge of zone 1 peripherally to a point tangent to the nasal ora serrata and an area near the temporal anatomic equator. (Landmarks of equator are obscure; therefore, precisely defined locations are difficult to identify.)
> *Zone 3:* Remaining crescent of the fundus anterior to zone 2. This zone is the last to be vascularized.

Extent of Disease

The real extent of the disease is expressed in reference to the aggregate number of clock hours occupied by ROP changes (see Fig. 21-9).

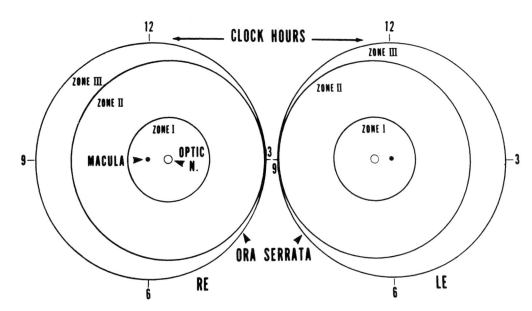

Figure 21-9. Schematic drawing of the retinas of the right eye (RE) and the left eye (LE) showing zone borders. Clock hours are used to describe the location and extent of retinopathy of prematurity. (From Garner A, Ben-Sira I, Deutman A, et al: An international classification of retinopathy of prematurity. Pediatrics 74:127, 1984. Reprinted by permission of *Pediatrics*.)

Staging of Disease: Proliferative Phase

In addition to the location and extent of the disease, the stage of advancement is also described as follows:

Stage 1: Demarcation Line

This is a flat white line within the plane of the retina that clearly delineates the vascularized posterior retina from the avascular anterior portion. Abnormal branching or arcading of vessels is recognizable immediately posterior to the demarcation line.

Stage 2: Ridge

The ridge is an expanded demarcation line that now has three dimensions because it has grown in height and width, rising above the plane of the retina. The color may be white to pink. Small tufts of new vessels may lie on the surface of the retina posterior to the ridge.

Stage 3: Ridge with Extraretinal Fibrovascular Proliferation

In addition to the structure of stage 2, extraretinal fibrovascular tissue is present. This tissue may (1) be continuous with the posterior aspect of the ridge, causing a ragged appearance; (2) be immediately posterior to the ridge but not connected to it; or (3) extend into the vitreous perpendicular to the retinal plane.

Stage 4: Retinal Detachment

Changes of stage 3 are complicated by retinal detachment that is caused by the effusion of fluid, traction, or by both. Serial examinations may be required to ascertain true detachment.

"Plus" Disease

For stages 2 and 3, add a plus sign (+) if the posterior veins are clearly enlarged and arterioles unequivocally tortuous.

Thus, stage 2 ROP with posterior vascular dilation and tortuosity would be written "stage 2+ ROP."

"Rush" Disease

This is the term used to describe severe plus disease associated with ROP in zone 1. The *rush* refers to an extremely rapid progress to retinal detachment.

"Threshold ROP"

This refers to zone 1 or 2 changes that occupy a minimum of five contiguous (uninterrupted) clock hours or an aggregate of eight clock hours of involved areas that are separated from each other.

"Prethreshold ROP"

This term refers to any ROP change that is less extensive than threshold in zone 1. In zone 2, ROP at stage 2 with plus disease or at stage 3 without plus disease is "prethreshold."

Staging of Disease: Cicatricial Phase

The published statement recommends use of the Reese classification of cicatricial disease. Table 21-8 lists the cicatricial changes.

Treatment

Cryotherapy and laser therapy are presently the only effective treatments available. In the STOP-ROP Study,[321] 82% of the treated eyes had good anatomic outcomes, that is, there was no retinal detachment, folds, or dragged discs. The recommendations of the multicenter trial reported in 1988[331] indicate that cryotherapy should be used when stage 3 is identified in more than five contiguous clock hours or when more than eight total clock hours (noncontiguous) are involved in zones 1 or 2, including the presence of plus disease.

There is no evidence that vitamin E supplementation successfully reduces the incidence of ROP.[310]

TABLE 21-8. Classification of Cicatricial Disease in Retinopathy of Prematurity

Grade	Fundus Changes
I	Small areas of retinal pigment irregularities; small scars in retinal periphery
II	Disc distortion
III	Retinal fold
IV	Incomplete retrolental mass; partial retinal detachment
V	Complete retrolental mass; total retinal detachment

Classification of Reese et al.[329] modified in Patz A: Retrolental fibroplasia. Surv Ophthalmol 14:1, 1969.

Schedule for Ophthalmologic Examination: Identification of Disease (Appendix 28)

Infants who should be examined are those whose birthweight is less than 1500 g, those who have a gestational age less than 29 weeks, or both.[332] Indirect ophthalmoscopy should be performed by an experienced ophthalmologist. The first examination should be carried out when the patient is 4 postnatal or 32 weeks PMA, and it should be repeated every 2 weeks thereafter until retinal vascularization is complete (i.e., has reached the ora serrata). The frequency of examination should be increased to weekly intervals if zone 2, stage 2, plus disease is identified or if zone 3, stage 3 disease is evident. Infants whose gestational age is 32 to 36 weeks also should be examined on this schedule if they have received supplemental O_2 for at least 6 hours.

REFERENCES

1. Lucey JF, Dangman B: A reexamination of the role of oxygen in retrolental fibroplasia. Pediatrics 73:82, 1984.
2. Northway WH Jr, Rosan RC, Porter DY: Pulmonary disease following respiratory therapy of hyaline-membrane disease. Bronchopulmonary dysplasia. N Engl J Med 276:357, 1967.
3. Bancalari EH: Neonatal chronic lung disease. In Fanaroff AA, Martin RJ (eds): Neonatal-Perinatal Medicine. Diseases of the Fetus and Infant, vol. II, 7th ed. St. Louis, Mosby, 2002, p. 1057.
4. Davis JM, Rosenfeld WN: Chronic lung disease. In Avery GB, Fletcher MA, MacDonald MG (eds): Neonatology. Pathophysiology and Management of the Newborn, 5th ed. Philadelphia, Lippincott Williams & Wilkins, 1999, p. 509.
5. Northway WH Jr: Historical perspective. Early observations and subsequent evolution of bronchopulmonary dysplasia. In Bland RD, Coalson JJ (eds): Chronic Lung Disease in Early Infancy. New York, Marcel Dekker, 2000, p. 1.
6. Northway WH Jr: An introduction to bronchopulmonary dysplasia. Clin Perinatol 19:489, 1992.
7. Northway WH Jr: Bronchopulmonary dysplasia: Then and now. Arch Dis Child 65:1076, 1990.
8. Banerjee CK, Girling DJ, Wigglesworth JS: Pulmonary fibroplasia in newborn babies treated with oxygen and artificial ventilation. Arch Dis Child 47:509, 1972.
9. Philip AGS: Oxygen plus pressure plus time: The etiology of bronchopulmonary dysplasia. Pediatrics 55:44, 1975.
10. Pusey VA, MacPherson RI, Chernick V: Pulmonary fibroplasia following prolonged artificial ventilation of newborn infants. Can Med Assoc J 100:451, 1969.
11. Edwards DK: Bronchopulmonary dysplasia today. In Milunsky A, Friedman EA, Gluck L (eds): Advances in Perinatal Medicine, vol. 3. New York, Plenum Medical Book Co., 1983, p. 117.
12. Johnson JD: Therapeutic misadventures. In Moore TD (ed): Iatrogenic Problems in Neonatal Intensive Care: Report of the Sixty-ninth Ross Conference on Pediatric Research. Columbus, OH, Ross Laboratories, 1976, p. 21.

13. Berg TJ, Pagtakhan RD, Reed MH, et al: Bronchopulmonary dysplasia and lung rupture in hyaline membrane disease: Influence of continuous distending pressure. Pediatrics 55:51, 1975.
14. Boynton BR: The epidemiology of bronchopulmonary dysplasia. In Merritt TA, Northway WH Jr, Boynton BR (eds): Bronchopulmonary Dysplasia. Boston, Blackwell Scientific Publications, 1988, pp. 19–32.
15. Farrell PM, Palta M: Bronchopulmonary dysplasia. In: Bronchopulmonary Dysplasia: Report of the 90th Ross Conference on Pediatric Research. Columbus, OH, Ross Laboratories, 1986, p. 3.
16. Avery ME, Tooley WH, Keller JB, et al: Is chronic lung disease in low birth weight infants preventable? A survey of eight centers. Pediatrics 79:26, 1987.
17. Cooke RWI: Factors associated with chronic lung disease in preterm infants. Arch Dis Child 66:776, 1991.
18. Parker RA, Lindstrom DP, Cotton RB: Improved survival accounts for most, but not all, of the increase in bronchopulmonary dysplasia. Pediatrics 90:663, 1992.
19. Bancalari E, Abdenour GE, Feller R, et al: Bronchopulmonary dysplasia: Clinical presentation. J Pediatr 95:819, 1979.
20. Shennan AT, Dunn MS, Ohlsson A, et al: Abnormal pulmonary outcomes in premature infants: Prediction from oxygen requirement in the neonatal period. Pediatrics 82:527, 1988.
21. Lemons JA, Bauer CR, Oh W, et al: Very low birth weight outcomes of the National Institute of Child Health and Human Development Neonatal Research Network, January 1995 through December 1996. Pediatrics 107:1, 2001.
22. Yost CC, Soll RF: Early versus delayed selective surfactant treatment for neonatal respiratory distress syndrome. Available at: http://www.nichd.nih.gov/cochraneneonatal/yost/yost.htm.
23. Jobe AH: Influence of surfactant replacement on development of bronchopulmonary dysplasia. In Bland RD, Coalson JJ (eds): Chronic Lung Disease in Early Infancy. New York, Marcel Dekker, 2000, p. 237.
24. Jobe AH: The new BPD: An arrest of lung development. Pediatr Res 46:641, 1999.
25. Jobe AH, Ikegami AM: Mechanisms initiating lung injury in the preterm. Early Hum Dev 53:81, 1998.
26. Yoon BH, Romero R, Kim KS, et al: A systemic fetal inflammatory response and the development of bronchopulmonary dysplasia. Am J Obstet Gynecol 181:773, 1999.
27. Van Marter LJ, Allred EN, Pagano M, et al: Do clinical markers of barotrauma and oxygen toxicity explain interhospital variation in rates of chronic lung disease? Pediatrics 105:1194, 2000.
28. Charafeddine L, D'Angio CT, Phelps DL: Atypical chronic lung disease patterns in neonates. Pediatrics 103:759, 1999.
29. Hageman JR, Adams MA, Gardner TH: Pulmonary complications of hyperventilation therapy for persistent pulmonary hypertension. Crit Care Med 13:1013, 1985.
30. Hudak BB, Egan EA: Impact of lung surfactant therapy on chronic lung diseases in premature infants. Clin Perinatol 19:591, 1992.
31. Ahlstrom H: Pulmonary mechanics in infants surviving severe neonatal respiratory insufficiency. Acta Paediatr Scand 64:69, 1975.
32. Chernick V: Epidemiology of BPD: Discussion. J Pediatr 95:855, 1979.
33. Lamarre A, Linsao L, Reilly BJ, et al: Residual pulmonary abnormalities in survivors of idiopathic respiratory distress syndrome. Am Rev Respir Dis 108:56, 1973.
34. Thibeault DW, Grossman H, Hagstrom JWC, et al: Radiologic findings in the lungs of premature infants. J Pediatr 74:1, 1969.
35. Wung J-T, Koons AH, Driscoll JM Jr, et al: Changing incidence of bronchopulmonary dysplasia. J Pediatr 95:845, 1979.
36. Romero R, Chaiworapongsa T: Preterm labor, intrauterine infection, and the fetal inflammatory response syndrome. NeoReviews 3:e73, 2002.
37. Kraybill EN, Runyan DK, Bose CL: Risk factors for chronic lung disease in infants with birth weights of 751 to 1000 grams. J Pediatr 115:115, 1989.
38. Taghizadeh A, Reynolds EOR: Pathogenesis of bronchopulmonary dysplasia following hyaline membrane disease. Am J Pathol 82:241, 1976.
39. Bonikos DS, Bensch KG, Northway WH, et al: Bronchopulmonary dysplasia: The pulmonary pathologic sequel of necrotizing bronchiolitis and pulmonary fibrosis. Hum Pathol 7:643, 1976.
40. Edwards DK, Dyer WM, Northway WH Jr: Twelve years' experience with bronchopulmonary dysplasia. Pediatrics 59:839, 1977.
41. Rhodes PG, Hall RT, Leonidas JC: Chronic pulmonary disease in neonates with assisted ventilation. Pediatrics 55:788, 1975.
42. Varsila E, Pesonen E, Andersson S: Early protein oxidation in the neonatal lung is related to development of chronic lung disease. Acta Paediatr 84:1296, 1995.

43. Frank L, Groseclose EE: Preparation for birth into an O_2-rich environment: The antioxidant enzymes in the developing rabbit lung. Pediatr Res 18:240, 1984.

44. Frank L: Antioxidants, nutrition and bronchopulmonary dysplasia. Clin Perinatol 19:541, 1992.

45. Frank L, Lewis P, Sosenko IRS: Dexamethasone stimulates fetal rat lung antioxidant enzyme activity in parallel with surfactant stimulation. Pediatrics 75:569, 1985.

46. Frank L, Sosenko IRS: Failure of premature rabbits to increase antioxidant enzymes during hyperoxic exposure: Increased susceptibility to pulmonary oxygen toxicity compared to term rabbits. Pediatr Res 29:292, 1991.

47. White CW: Pulmonary oxygen toxicity: Cellular mechanisms of oxidant injury and antioxidant defense. In Bancalari E, Stocker JT (eds): Bronchopulmonary Dysplasia. Washington, DC, Hemisphere Publishing Corporation, 1988, p. 22.

48. Contreras M, Hariharan N, Lewandoski JR, et al: Bronchoalveolar oxyradical inflammatory elements herald bronchopulmonary dysplasia. Crit Care Med 24:29, 1996.

49. Saustad OD: Chronic lung disease: The role of oxidative stress. Biol Neonate 74:21, 1998.

50. Frank L, Autor AP, Roberts RJ: Oxygen therapy and hyaline membrane disease: The effect of hyperoxia on pulmonary superoxide dismutase activity and the mediating role of plasma or serum. J Pediatr 90:105, 1977.

51. Rosenfeld W, Evans H, Concepcion L, et al: Prevention of bronchopulmonary dysplasia by administration of bovine superoxide dismutase in preterm infants with respiratory distress syndrome. J Pediatr 105:781, 1984.

52. Rosenfeld WN, Davis JM, Parton L, et al: Safety and pharmacokinetics of recombinant human superoxide dismutase administered intratracheally to premature neonates with respiratory distress syndrome. Pediatrics 97:811, 1996.

53. Davis JM, Rosenfeld WN, Parad R, et al: Improved pulmonary outcome at one year corrected age in premature neonates treated with recombinant human superoxide dismutase. Pediatr Res 47:395A, 2000.

54. Welty SE: Is there a role for antioxidant therapy in bronchopulmonary dysplasia. J Nutr 131:947S, 2001.

55. Ehrenkranz RA, Mercurio MR: Bronchopulmonary dysplasia. In Sinclair JC, Bracken MB (eds): Effective Care of the Newborn Infant. Oxford, Oxford University Press, 1992, p. 399.

56. Bonikos DS, Bensch KG: Pathogenesis of bronchopulmonary dysplasia. In Merritt TA, Northway WH Jr, Boynton BR (ed): Bronchopulmonary Dysplasia. Boston, Blackwell Scientific Publications, 1988, p. 33.

57. Frank HL, Sosenko IRS: Oxidants and antioxidants. What role do they play in chronic lung disease: In Bland RD, Coalson JJ (eds): Chronic Lung Disease in Early Infancy. New York, Marcel Dekker, 2000, p. 841.

58. Davis JM, Dickerson B, Mettay L, et al: Differential effects of oxygen and barotrauma on lung injury in the neonatal piglet. Pediatr Pulmonol 10:157, 1991.

59. Moylan FMB, Walker AM, Kramer SS, et al: Relationship of bronchopulmonary dysplasia to the occurrence of alveolar rupture during positive pressure ventilation. Crit Care Med 6:140, 1978.

60. Moylan FMB, Walker AM, Kramer SS, et al: Alveolar rupture as an independent predictor of bronchopulmonary dysplasia. Crit Care Med 6:10, 1978.

61. Rhodes PG, Graves GR, Patel DM, et al: Minimizing pneumothorax and bronchopulmonary dysplasia in ventilated infants with hyaline membrane disease. J Pediatr 102:68, 1983.

62. Boynton BR, Mannino FL, Randel RC, et al: Minimizing bronchopulmonary dysplasia in VLBW infants. J Pediatr 104:962, 1984.

63. Nillson R, Grossman G, Robertson R: Lung surfactant and the pathogenesis of neonatal bronchiolar lesions induced by artificial ventilation. Pediatr Res 12:249, 1978.

64. Poets CF, Sens B: Changes in intubation rates and outcome of very low birth weight infants: A population based study. Pediatrics 98:24, 1996.

65. deLemos RA, Coalson JJ: The contribution of experimental models to our understanding of the pathogenesis and treatment of bronchopulmonary dysplasia. Clin Perinatol 19:521, 1992.

66. Clark RH, Gerstmann DR, Jobe AH, et al: Lung injury in neonates: Causes, strategies for prevention, and long-term consequences. J Pediatr 139:478, 2001.

67. Auten RL, Vozzelli M, Clark RH: Volutrauma. What is it, and how do we avoid it? Clin Perinatol 28:505, 2001.

68. Dreyfuss D, Saumon G: Barotrauma is volutrauma, but which volume is the one responsible? [editorial]. Intensive Care Med 18:139, 1992.

69. Milner A: The importance of ventilation to effective resuscitation in the term and preterm infant. Semin Neonatol 6:219, 2001.

70. Hernandez LA, Peevy KJ, Moise AA, et al: Chest wall restriction limits high airway pressure-induced lung injury in young rabbits. J Appl Physiol 66:2364, 1989.

71. Wada K, Jobe AH, Ikegami M: Tidal volume effects on surfactant treatment responses with the initiation of ventilation in preterm lambs. J Appl Physiol 83:1054, 1997.

72. Bjorklund LJ, Ingimarsson J, Curstedt T, et al: Manual ventilation with a few large breaths at birth compromises the therapeutic effect of subsequent surfactant replacement in immature lambs. Pediatr Res 42:348, 1997.

73. Dreyfuss D, Saumon G: Ventilator induced injury: lessons from experimental studies. Am J Respir Crit Care Med 25:294, 1998.

74. Ranieri VM, Suter PM, Tortorella C, et al: Effect of mechanical ventilation on inflammatory mediators in patients with acute respiratory distress syndrome. A randomized controlled trial. JAMA 282:54, 1999.

75. Hudson LD: Progress in understanding ventilator-induced lung injury. JAMA 282:77, 1999.

76. Speer CP, Groneck P: Inflammatory mediators in neonatal lung disease. In Bland RD, Coalson JJ (eds): Chronic Lung Disease in Early Infancy. New York, Marcel Dekker, 2000, p. 147.

77. Yoon BH, Romero R, Yang SH, et al: Interleukin-6 concentrations in umbilical cord plasma are elevated in neonates with white matter lesions associated with periventricular leukomalacia. Am J Obstet Gynecol 174:1433, 1996.

78. Benirschke K: Routes and types of infection in the fetus and the newborn. Am J Dis Child 99:714, 1960.

79. Benirschke K, Driscoll SG: The Pathology of the Human Placenta. New York, Springer-Verlag, 1967.

80. Blanc WA: Pathways of fetal and early neonatal infection, viral placentitis, bacterial and fungal chorioamnionitis. J Pediatr 59:473, 1961.

81. Guinn D, Gibbs R: Infection-related preterm birth: A review of the evidence. NeoReviews 3:e86, 2002.

82. Gomez R, Romero R, Ghezzi F, et al: The fetal inflammatory response syndrome. Am J Obstet Gynecol 179:194, 1998.

83. Watterberg KL, Demers LM, Scott SM, et al: Chorioamnionitis and early lung inflammation in infants in whom bronchopulmonary dysplasia develops. Pediatrics 97:210, 1996.

84. Pacora P, Chaiworapongsa T, Maymon E, et al: Funisitis and chorionic vasculitis: The histological counterpart of the fetal inflammatory response syndrome. J Matern Fetal Neonatal Med 2002 11:18, 2002.

85. Yoon BH, Romero R, Park JS, et al: The relationship among inflammatory lesions of the umbilical cord (funisitis), umbilical cord plasma interleukins 6 concentration, amniotic fluid infection, and neonatal sepsis. Am J Obstet Gynecol 183:1124, 2000.

86. Vigneswaran R: Infection and preterm birth: Evidence of a common causal relationship with bronchopulmonary dysplasia and cerebral palsy. J Paediatr Child Health 36:293, 2000.

87. Bagchi A, Viscardi RM, Taciak V, et al: Increased activity of interleukin-6 but not tumor necrosis factor-α in lung lavage of premature infants is associated with the development of bronchopulmonary dysplasia. Pediatr Res 36:244, 1994.

88. Ghezzi F, Gomez R, Yoon BH, et al: Elevated interleukin-8 concentrations in amniotic fluid of mothers whose neonates subsequently develop bronchopulmonary dysplasia. Eur J Obstet Gynecol Reprod Biol 78:5, 1998.

89. Jonsson B, Tullus K, Brauner A, et al: Early increase of TNFα and IL-6 in tracheobronchial aspirate fluid indicator of subsequent chronic lung disease in preterm infants. Arch Dis Child 77:F198, 1997.

90. Yoon BH, Romero R, Jun JK, et al: Amniotic fluid cytokines (interleukin-6, tumor necrosis factor-α, interleukin-1β, and interleukin-8) and the risk for the development of bronchopulmonary dysplasia. Am J Obstet Gynecol 177:825, 1997.

91. Groneck P, Gotze-Speer B, Oppermann M, et al: Association of pulmonary inflammation and increased microvascular permeability during the development of bronchopulmonary dysplasia: A sequential analysis of inflammatory mediators in respiratory fluids of high-risk preterm neonates. Pediatrics 93:712, 1994.

92. Kotecha S, Wilson L, Wangoo A, et al: Increase in interleukin (IL)-1α and IL-6 in bronchoalveolar lavage fluid obtained from infants with chronic lung disease of prematurity. Pediatr Res 40:250, 1996.

93. Pierce MR, Bancalari E: The role of inflammation in the pathogenesis of bronchopulmonary dysplasia. Pediatr Pulmonol 19:371, 1995.

94. Husain AN, Siddiqui NH, Stocker JT: Pathology of arrested acinar development in postsurfactant bronchopulmonary dysplasia. Hum Pathol 29:710, 1998.

95. Ross JM, Furr PM, Taylor-Robinson D, et al: The effect of genital mycoplasmas on human fetal growth. Br J Obstet Gynaecol 1981;88:749.

96. Lamey JR, Foy HM, Kenny GE: Infection with Mycoplasma hominis and T-strains in the female genital tract. Obstet Gynecol 44:703, 1974.

97. Cassell GH, Waites KB, Gibbs RS, et al: Role of Ureaplasma urealyticum in amnionitis. Pediatr Infect Dis J 5(Suppl):S247, 1986.

98. Holtzman RB, Hageman JR, Yogev R: Role of Ureaplasma urealyticum in bronchopulmonary dysplasia. J Pediatr 114:1061, 1989.

99. Wang EEL, Cassell GH, Sanchez PJ, et al: Ureaplasma urealyticum and chronic lung disease of prematurity: Critical appraisal of the literature on causation. Clin Infect Dis 17(Suppl 1):S112, 1993.

100. Payne NR, Steinberg SS, Ackerman P, et al: New prospective studies of the association of Ureaplasma urealyticum colonization and chronic lung disease. Clin Infect Dis 17(Suppl 1):S117, 1993.

101. Crouse DT, Odrezin GT, Cutter GR, et al: Radiographic changes associated with tracheal isolation of Ureaplasma urealyticum from neonates. Clin Infect Dis 1993;17(Suppl 1):S122, 1993.

102. Cassell GH, Waites KB, Crouse DT, et al: Association of Ureaplasma urealyticum infection of the lower respiratory tract and chronic lung disease and death in very low birth weight infants. Lancet 2:240, 1988.

103. Desilva NS, Quinn PA: Phospholipase A and C activity in Ureaplasma urealyticum. J Clin Microbiol 23:354, 1986.

104. Benitz WE, Arvin AM: Infection in the pathogenesis of bronchopulmonary dysplasia. In Bland RD, Coalson JJ (eds): Chronic Lung Disease in Early Infancy. New York, Marcel Dekker, 2000, p. 163.

105. Gonzalez A, Sosenko IRS, Chandar J, et al: Influence of infection on patent ductus arteriosus and chronic lung disease in premature infants weighing 1000 grams or less. J Pediatr 128:470, 1996.

106. Frank L, Sosenko IRS: Undernutrition as a major contributing factor in the pathogenesis of bronchopulmonary dysplasia. Am Rev Respir Dis 138:725, 1988.

107. Frank L: Nutrition: Influence on lung growth, injury and repair, and development of bronchopulmonary dysplasia. In Bancalari E (ed): Bronchopulmonary Dysplasia. Washington, DC, Hemisphere Publishing Corporation, 1988, p.78.

108. Merritt TA, Boynton BR: Clinical presentation of bronchopulmonary dysplasia. In Merritt TA, Northway WH Jr, Boynton BR (eds): Bronchopulmonary Dysplasia. Boston, Blackwell Scientific Publications, 1988, pp. 179–184

109. Niermeyer S: Nutritional and metabolic problems in infants with bronchopulmonary dysplasia. In Bancalari E, Stocker TJ (eds): Bronchopulmonary Dysplasia. Washington, DC, Hemisphere Publishing Corporation, 1988, p. 313.

110. Blackfan KD, Wolbach SB: Vitamin A deficiency in infants: A clinical and pathological study. J Pediatr 3:679, 1933.

111. Hustead VA, Gutcher GR, Anderson SA, et al: Relationship of vitamin A (retinol) status to lung disease in the preterm infant. J Pediatr 105:610, 1984.

112. Shenai JP, Chytil F, Stahlman MT: Vitamin A status of neonates with bronchopulmonary dysplasia. Pediatr Res 19:185, 1985.

113. Shenai JP, Kennedy KA, Chytil F, et al: Clinical trial of vitamin A supplementation in infants susceptible to bronchopulmonary dysplasia. J Pediatr 111:269, 1987.

114. Papagaroufalis C, Cairis M, Pantazatou E, et al: A trial of vitamin A supplementation for the prevention of bronchopulmonary dysplasia (BPD) in very-low-birth-weight (VLBW) infants. Presented at the Annual Meeting of the Society for Pediatric Research in May 1988. Pediatr Res 23:518A, 1988.

115. Bental RY, Cooper PA, Sandler D, et al: The effects of vitamin A therapy on the incidence of chronic lung disease (CLD) in premature infants. Pediatr Res 27:296A, 1990.

116. Pearson E, Bose C, Snidow T, et al: Trial of vitamin A supplementation in very low birth weight infants at risk for bronchopulmonary dysplasia. J Pediatr 121:420, 1992.

117. Tyson JE, Wright LL, Oh W, et al: Vitamin A supplementation for extremely-low-birth-weight infants. N Engl J Med 340:1962, 1999.

118. Darlow BA, Graham PJ: Vitamin A supplementation for preventing morbidity and mortality in very low birthweight infants. Available at: http://www.cochranelibrary.com.

119. Brown ER, Stark A, Sosenko I, et al: Bronchopulmonary dysplasia: Possible relationship to pulmonary edema. J Pediatr 92:982, 1978.

120. Gerhardt T, Bancalari E: Lung function. In Bancalari E, Stocker JT (eds): Bronchopulmonary Dysplasia: Aspen Seminars on Pediatric Disease. Washington, DC, Hemisphere Publishing, 1988, p. 182.

121. Van Marter LJ, Leviton A, Allred EN, et al: Hydration during the first days of life and the risk of bronchopulmonary dysplasia in low birth weight infants. J Pediatr 116:942, 1990.

122. Van Marter LJ, Pagano M, Allred EN, et al: Rate of bronchopulmonary dysplasia as a function of neonatal intensive care practices. J Pediatr 120:938, 1992.

123. Bell EF, Warburton D, Stonestreet BS, et al: Effect of fluid administration on the development of symptomatic patent ductus arteriosus and congestive heart failure in premature infants. N Engl J Med 302:598, 1980.

124. Lorenz JM, Kleinman LI, Kotagal UR, et al: Water balance in very-low-birth-weight infants: Relationship to water and sodium intake and effect on outcome. J Pediatr 101:423, 1982.

125. Bell EF, Acarregui MJ: Restricted versus liberal water intake for preventing morbidity and mortality in preterm infants (Cochrane Review). Available at: http://www.cochranelibrary.com.

126. Stocker JT: Pathology of acute bronchopulmonary dysplasia. In Bancalari E (ed): Bronchopulmonary Dysplasia. Washington, DC, Hemisphere Publishing Corporation, 1988, p. 237.

127. Stocker JT: Pathology of long-standing "healed" bronchopulmonary dysplasia. In Bancalari E (ed): Bronchopulmonary Dysplasia. Washington, DC, Hemisphere Publishing Corporation, 1988, p. 279.

128. Coalson JJ: Pathology of chronic lung disease in early infancy. In Bland RD, Coalson JJ (eds): Chronic Lung Disease in Early Infancy. New York, Marcel Dekker, 2000, p. 85.

129. Jobe AH, Bancalari E: Bronchopulmonary dysplasia. Am J Respir Crit Care Med 163:1723, 2001.

130. Watts JL, Ariagno RL, Brady JP: Chronic pulmonary disease in neonates after artificial ventilation: Distribution of ventilation and pulmonary interstitial emphysema. Pediatrics 60:273, 1977.

131. Hislop AA, Haworth SG: Pulmonary vascular damage and the development of cor pulmonale following hyaline membrane disease. Pediatr Pulmonol 9:152, 1990.

132. Hislop AA, Wigglesworth JS, Desai R, et al: The effects of preterm delivery and mechanical ventilation on human lung growth. Early Hum Dev 15:147, 1987.

133. Margraf LR, Tomashefski JF, Bruce MC, et al: Morphometric analysis of the lung in bronchopulmonary dysplasia. Am Rev Respir Dis 143:391, 1991.

134. Sobonya RE, Logvinoff MM, Taussig LM, et al: Morphometric analysis of the lung in prolonged bronchopulmonary dysplasia. Pediatr Res 16:969, 1982.

135. Tay-Uyboco JS, Kwiatkowski K, Cates DB, et al: Hypoxic airway constriction in infants of very low birth weight recovering from moderate to severe bronchopulmonary dysplasia. J Pediatr 115:456, 1989.

136. Rendas A, Brown ER, Avery ME: Prematurity, hypoplasia of the pulmonary vascular bed, and hypertension: Fatal outcome in a ten month old infant. Am Rev Respir Dis 121:873, 1980.

137. Abman SH, Wolfe RR, Accurso FJ, et al: Pulmonary vascular response to oxygen in infants with severe bronchopulmonary dysplasia. Pediatrics 75:80, 1985.

138. Halliday HL, Dumpit FM, Brady JP: Effects of inspired oxygen on echocardiographic assessment of pulmonary vascular resistance and myocardial contractility in bronchopulmonary dysplasia. Pediatrics 65:536, 1980.

139. Abman SH: Pulmonary hypertension in infants with bronchopulmonary dysplasia: Clinical aspects. In Bancalari E, Stocker JT (eds): Bronchopulmonary Dysplasia. Washington, DC, Hemisphere Publishing Corporation, 1988, p. 220.

140. Goodman G, Perkin RM, Anas NG: Pulmonary hypertension in infants with bronchopulmonary dysplasia. J Pediatr 112:67, 1988.

141. Sherman FS: Cor pulmonale. In Merritt TA, Northway WH Jr, Boynton BR (eds): Bronchopulmonary Dysplasia. Boston, Blackwell Scientific Publications, 1988, p. 251.

142. Weinstein MR, Oh W: Oxygen consumption in infants with bronchopulmonary dysplasia. J Pediatr 99:958, 1981.

143. Kurzner SI, Garg M, Bautista DB, et al: Growth failure in infants with bronchopulmonary dysplasia: Nutrition and elevated resting metabolic expenditure. Pediatrics 81:379, 1988.

144. Johnson JD, Malachowski NC, Grobstein R, et al: Prognosis of children surviving with the aid of mechanical ventilation in the newborn period. J Pediatr 84:272, 1974.

145. Anderson AH, Warady BA, Daily DK, et al: Systemic hypertension in infants with severe bronchopulmonary dysplasia: Associated clinical factors. Am J Perinatol 10:190, 1993.

146. Alagappan A, Malloy MH: Systemic hypertension in very low-birth weight infants with bronchopulmonary dysplasia: Incidence and risk factors. Am J Perinatol 15:3, 1998.

147. Abman SH, Warady BA, Lum GM, et al: Systemic hypertension in infants with bronchopulmonary dysplasia. J Pediatr 104:928, 1984.

148. Johnson V: Editorial: Systemic hypertension in infants with severe bronchopulmonary dysplasia. Am J Perinatol 10:260, 1993.
149. Bergman J, Farrell EE: Neurodevelopmental outcome in infants with bronchopulmonary dysplasia. Clin Perinatol 19:673, 1992.
150. Meisels SJ, Plunkett JW, Roloff DW, et al: Growth and development of preterm infants with respiratory distress syndrome and bronchopulmonary dysplasia. Pediatrics 77:345, 1986.
151. Eichenwald EC, Stark AR: Pulmonary function in BPD and its aftermath. In Bland RD, Coalson JJ (eds): Chronic Lung Disease in Early Infancy. New York, Marcel Dekker, 2000, p. 297.
152. Cunningham CK, McMillan JA, Gross SJ: Rehospitalization for respiratory illness in infants of less than 32 weeks' gestation. Pediatrics 88:527, 1991.
153. Sell EJ, Vaucher YE: Growth and neurodevelopmental outcome of infants who had bronchopulmonary dysplasia. In Merritt TA, Northway WH Jr, Boynton BR (eds): Bronchopulmonary Dysplasia. Boston, Blackwell Scientific Publications, 1988, p. 403.
154. Vrlenich LA, Bozynski MEA, Shyr Y, et al: The effect of bronchopulmonary dysplasia on growth at school age. Pediatrics 95:855, 1995.
155. Brown ER: Bronchopulmonary dysplasia. In Rubin IL, Crocker AC (eds): Developmental Disabilities: Delivery of Medical Care for Children and Adults. Philadelphia, Lea & Febiger, 1989, p. 223.
156. Koops BL, Abram SH, Accurso FJ: Outpatient management and follow-up of bronchopulmonary dysplasia. Clin Perinatol 11:101, 1984.
157. Kinney JS, Robertsen CM, Johnson KM, et al: Seasonal respiratory viral infections: Impact on infants with chronic lung disease following discharge from the neonatal intensive care unit. Arch Pediatr Adolesc Med 149:81, 1995.
158. Groothuis JR, Gutierrez KM, Lauer BA: Respiratory syncytial virus infection in children with bronchopulmonary dysplasia. Pediatrics 82:199, 1988.
159. Groothuis JR, Simoes EA, Hemming VG: Respiratory syncytial virus (RSV) infection in preterm infants and the protective effects of RSV immune globulin (RSVIG). Respiratory Syncytial Virus Immune Globulin Study Group. Pediatrics 95:463, 1995.
160. Koops BL, Lam C: Outcome in bronchopulmonary dysplasia: Mortality risks and prognosis for growth, neurological integrity, and developmental performance. In Bancalari E, Stocker JT (eds): Bronchopulmonary Dysplasia. Washington, DC, Hemisphere Publishing Corporation, 1988, p. 403.
161. Yuksel B, Greenough A, Green S: Lung function abnormalities at 6 months of age after neonatal intensive care. Arch Dis Child 66:472, 1991.
162. Mayes L, Perkett E, Stahlman MT: Severe bronchopulmonary dysplasia: A retrospective review. Acta Pediatr Scand 72:225, 1983.
163. Bhutani VK, Abbasi S: Long-term pulmonary consequences in survivors with bronchopulmonary dysplasia. Clin Perinatol 19:649, 1992.
164. Blayney M, Kerem E, Whyte H, et al: Bronchopulmonary dysplasia: Improvement in lung function between 7 and 10 years of age. J Pediatr 118:201, 1991.
165. Northway WH Jr, Moss RB, Carlisle KB, et al: Late pulmonary sequelae of bronchopulmonary dysplasia. N Engl J Med 323:1793, 1990.
166. Andreasson B, Lindroth M, Mortensson W, et al: Lung function eight years after neonatal ventilation. Arch Dis Child 64:108, 1989.
167. Bader D, Ramos AD, Lew CD, et al: Childhood sequelae of infant lung disease: Exercise and pulmonary function abnormalities after bronchopulmonary dysplasia. J Pediatr 110:693, 1987.
168. Smyth JA, Tabachnik E, Duncan WJ, et al: Pulmonary function and bronchial hyperreactivity in long-term survivors of bronchopulmonary dysplasia. Pediatrics 68:336, 1981.
169. Bancalari E, Gonzalez A: Clinical course and lung function abnormalities during development of neonatal chronic lung disease. In Bland RD, Coalson JJ (eds): Chronic Lung Disease in Early Infancy. New York, Marcel Dekker, 2000, p. 41.
170. Rojas MA, Gonzalez A, Bancalari E, et al: Changing trends in the epidemiology and pathogenesis of neonatal chronic lung disease. J Pediatr 126:605, 1995.
171. Gerhardt T, Henre D, Feller R, et al: Serial determination of pulmonary function in infants with chronic lung disease. J Pediatr 110:448, 1987.
172. Edwards DK III: The radiology of bronchopulmonary dysplasia and its complications. In Merritt TA, Northway WH Jr, Boynton BR (eds): Bronchopulmonary Dysplasia. Boston, Blackwell Scientific Publications, 1988, p. 185.
173. Foley LC: Serial radiological findings of bronchopulmonary dysplasia. In Bancalari E, Stocker JT (eds): Bronchopulmonary Dysplasia. Washington, DC, Hemisphere Publishing Corporation, 1988, p. 192.
174. Tsai SH, Anderson WR, Strickland MB, et al: Bronchopulmonary dysplasia associated with oxygen therapy in infants with respiratory distress syndrome. Radiology 105:107, 1972.
175. Edwards DK, Northway WH Jr: Radiographic features of BPD and potential application of new imaging techniques. In Bland RD, Coalson JJ (eds): Chronic Lung Disease in Early Infancy. New York, Marcel Dekker, 2000, p. 65.
176. Aly HZ: Nasal prongs continuous positive airway pressure: A simple yet powerful tool. Pediatrics 108:759, 2001.
177. Davis PG, Henderson-Smart DJ: Nasal continuous positive airways pressure immediately after extubation for preventing morbidity in preterm infants. Available at: http://www.cochranelibrary.com.
178. De Klerk AM, De Klerk RK: Use of continuous positive airway pressure in preterm infants: Comments and experience from New Zealand. Pediatrics 108:761, 2001.
179. Lindner W, Vobeck S, Hummler H, et al: Delivery room management of extremely low birth weight infants: Spontaneous breathing or intubation? Pediatrics103:961, 1999.
180. Davis PG, Henderson-Smart DJ: Post-extubation prophylactic nasal continuous positive airway pressure in preterm infants: Systematic review and meta-analysis. J Paediatr Child Health 35:367, 1999.
181. Hammer J: Nasal CPAP in preterm infants—Does it work and how? Intensive Care Med 27:1689, 2001.
182. Higgins RD, Richter SE, Davis JM: Nasal continuous positive airway pressure facilitates extubation of very low birth weight neonates. Pediatrics 88:999, 1991.
183. Woodgate PG, Davies MW: Permissive hypercapnia for the prevention of morbidity and mortality in mechanically ventilated newborn infants. Available at: http://www.cochranelibrary.com.
184. Goldman SL, McCanre EM, Lloyd BW, et al: Inspiratory time and pulmonary function in mechanically ventilated babies with chronic lung disease. Pediatr Pulmonol 11:198, 1991.
185. Courtney SE, Weber KR, Breakie LA, et al: Capillary blood gases in the neonate. A reassessment and review of the literature. Am J Dis Child 144:168, 1990.
186. Ramanathan R, Durand M, Larrazalol C: Pulse oximetry in very low birth weight infants with acute and chronic lung disease. Pediatrics 79:612, 1987.
187. Solimano AJ, Smyth JA, Mann TK, et al: Pulse oximetry advantages in infants with bronchopulmonary dysplasia. Pediatrics 78:844, 1986.
188. Palmisano JM, Martin JM, Krauzowicz BA, et al: Effects of supplemental oxygen administration in an infant with pulmonary artery hypertension. Heart Lung 19:627, 1990.
189. Singer L, Martin RJ, Hawkins SW, et al: Oxygen desaturation complicates feeding in infants with bronchopulmonary dysplasia after discharge. Pediatrics 90:380, 1992.
190. Brion LP, Yong SC, Perez IA, et al: Diuretics and chronic lung disease of prematurity. J Perinatol 21:269, 2001.
191. Hazinski TA: Drug treatment for established BPD. In Bland RD, Coalson JJ (eds): Chronic Lung Disease in Early Infancy. New York, Marcel Dekker, 2000, p. 257.
192. Brion LP, Primhak RA, Ambrosio-Perez I: Diuretics acting on the distal renal tubule for preterm infants with (or developing) chronic lung disease. Available at: http://www.nichd.nih.gov/cochrane/brion5/brion.htm.
193. Engelhardt B, Elliott S, Hazinski TA: Short- and long-term effects of furosemide on lung function in infants with bronchopulmonary dysplasia. J Pediatr 109:1034, 1986.
194. Kao LC, Warburton D, Sargent CW, et al: Furosemide acutely decreases airways resistance in chronic bronchopulmonary dysplasia. J Pediatr 103:624, 1983.
195. Mammel MC, Fiterman C, Coleman M, et al: Short-term dexamethasone therapy for bronchopulmonary dysplasia: Acute effects and one-year follow up. Dev Pharmacol Ther 10:1, 1987.
196. Najak ZD, Harris EM, Lazzara A, et al: pulmonary effects of furosemide in preterm infants with lung disease. J Pediatr 102:758, 1983.
197. Rush MG, Engelhardt B, Parker RA, et al: Double-blind, placebo-controlled trial of alternate-day furosemide therapy in infants with chronic bronchopulmonary dysplasia. J Pediatr 117:112, 1990.
198. Barrington KJ, Finer NN: Treatment of bronchopulmonary dysplasia. A review. Clin Perinatol 25:177, 1998.
199. Rush MG, Hazinski TA: Current therapy of bronchopulmonary dysplasia. Clin Perinatol 19:563, 1992.
200. Davis JM, Sinkin RA, Aranda JV: Drug therapy for bronchopulmonary dysplasia. Pediatr Pulmonol 8:117, 1990.

201. Brion LP, Primhak RA: Intravenous or enteral loop diuretics in preterm infants with (or developing) chronic lung disease. Available at: http://www.nichd.nih.gov/cochrane/brion2/brion.htm.

202. Hufnagle KG, Khan SN, Penn D, et al: Renal calcifications: a complication of long-term furosemide therapy in preterm infants. Pediatrics 70:360, 1982.

203. Narendra A, White MP, Rolton HA, et al: Nephrocalcinosis in preterm babies. Arch Dis Child Fetal Neonatal Ed 85:F207, 2001.

204. Karlowicz MG, Katz ME, Adelman RD, et al: Nephrocalcinosis in very low birth weight neonates: Family history of kidney stones and ethnicity as independent risk factors. J Pediatr 122:635, 1993.

205. Jacinto JS, Modanlou HD, Crade M, et al: Renal calcification incidence in very low birth weight infants. Pediatrics 81:31, 1988.

206. Ezzedeen F, Adelman RD, Ahlfors CE: Renal calcification in preterm infants: Pathophysiology and long-term sequelae. J Pediatr 113:532, 1988.

207. Pope JC, Trusler LA, Klein AM, et al: The natural history of nephrocalcinosis in premature infants treated with loop diuretics. J Urol 156:709, 1996.

208. Jones CA, King S, Shaw NJ, et al: Renal calcification in preterm infants: Follow up at 4-5 years. Arch Dis Child 76:F185, 1997.

209. Kao LC, Durand DJ, McCrea RC: Randomized trial of long-term diuretic therapy for infants with oxygen-dependent bronchopulmonary dysplasia. J Pediatr 124:772, 1994.

210. Crowley P: Antenatal corticosteroid therapy: A meta-analysis of the randomized trials—1972–1994. Am J Obstet Gynecol 173:322, 1995.

211. Baud O, Foix-L'Helias L, Kaminski M, et al: Antenatal glucocorticoid treatment and cystic periventricular leukomalacia in very premature infants. N Engl J Med 341:1190, 1999.

212. NIH Consensus Statement Online 2000: Antenatal corticosteroids revisited: repeat courses 17:1, 2000.

213. Yeh TF, Torre JA, Rastogi A, et al: Early postnatal dexamethasone therapy in premature infants with severe respiratory distress syndrome: A double-blind controlled study. J Pediatr 117:273, 1990.

214. Yeh TF, Lin YJ, Lin CH, et al: Early postnatal (<12 hrs) dexamethasone (D) therapy for prevention of BPD in preterm infants with RDS: a two year follow-up study. Pediatr Res 41:188A, 1997.

215. Yeh TF, Lin YJ, Huang CC, et al: Early dexamethasone therapy in preterm infants: A follow-up study. Pediatrics 101:1, 1998. Available at: http://www.pediatrics.org/cgi/content/full/101/5/e7.

216. American Academy of Pediatrics Committee on Fetus and Newborn, Canadian Paediatric Society Fetus and Newborn Committee: Postnatal corticosteroids to treat or prevent chronic lung disease in preterm infants. Pediatrics 109:330, 2002.

217. Mammel MC, Green TP, Johnson DE, et al: Controlled trial of dexamethasone therapy in infant with bronchopulmonary dysplasia. Lancet 1:1356, 1983.

218. Avery GB, Fletcher AB, Kaplan M, et al: Controlled trial of dexamethasone in respirator-dependent infants with bronchopulmonary dysplasia. Pediatrics 75:106, 1985.

219. Bancalari E: Corticosteroids and neonatal chronic lung disease. Eur J Pediatr 157:S31, 1998.

220. Jobe AH: Glucocorticoids, inflammation and the perinatal lung. Available at: http://www.ideallibrary.com.

221. Murch SH, MacDonald TT, Wood CBS, et al: Tumour necrosis in the bronchoalveolar secretions of infants with the respiratory distress syndrome and the effect of dexamethasone treatment. Thorax 47:44, 1992.

222. Ng PC: The effectiveness and side effects of dexamethasone in preterm infants with bronchopulmonary dysplasia. Arch Dis Child 68:330, 1993.

223. Ariagno RL, Sweeney TJ, Baldwin RB, et al: Dexamethasone effects on lung function in 3 week-old ventilator dependent preterm infants. Am Rev Respir Dis 135:A125, 1987.

224. Cummings JJ, D'Eugenio DB, Gross SJ: A controlled trial of dexamethasone in preterm infants at high risk for bronchopulmonary dysplasia. N Engl J Med 320:1505, 1989.

225. Ng PC, Brownlee KG, Dear PRF: Gastroduodenal perforation in preterm babies treated with dexamethasone for bronchopulmonary dysplasia. Arch Dis Child 66:1164, 1991.

226. O'Neal EA, Chwals WJ, O'Shea MD, et al: Dexamethasone treatment during ventilator dependency: Possible life threatening gastrointestinal complications. Arch Dis Child 67:10, 1992.

227. Collaborative Dexamethasone Trial Group: Dexamethasone therapy in neonatal chronic lung disease: An international placebo-controlled trial. Pediatrics 88:421, 1991.

228. Harkavy KL, Scanlon JW, Chowdhry PK, et al: Dexamethasone therapy for chronic lung disease in ventilator dependent infants: a controlled trial. J Pediatr 115:979, 1989.

229. Kazzi NJ, Brans YW, Poland RL: Dexamethasone effects on the hospital course of infants with bronchopulmonary dysplasia who are dependent on artificial ventilation. Pediatrics 86:722, 1990.

230. Ohlsson A, Calvert S, Hosking M, et al: Randomised controlled trial of dexamethasone treatment in very low birthweight infants with ventilatory dependent chronic lung disease. Pediatr Res 25:225A, 1989.

231. Alkalay AL, Pomerance JJ, Puri AR, et al: Hypothalamic-pituitary-adrenal axis function in very low birth weight infants treated with dexamethasone. Pediatrics 86:204, 1990.

232. Rizvi ZB, Aniol HS, Myers TF, et al: Effects of dexamethasone on the hypothalamic-pituitary-adrenal axis in preterm infants. J Pediatr 120:961, 1992.

233. Ohning BL, Fyfe DA, Riedel PA: Reversible obstructive hypertrophic cardiomyopathy after dexamethasone therapy for bronchopulmonary dysplasia. Am Heart J 125:253, 1993.

234. Werner JC, Sicard RE, Hansen TWR, et al: Hypertrophic cardiomyopathy associated with dexamethasone therapy for bronchopulmonary dysplasia. J Pediatr 120:286, 1992.

235. Halliday HL, Ehrenkranz RA: Early postnatal (<96 hours) corticosteroids for preventing chronic lung disease in preterm infants (Cochrane Review). Cochrane Database Syst Rev 1:CD001146, 2001.

236. Shah V, Ohlsson A: Postnatal dexamethasone in the prevention of chronic lung disease. In David TJ (ed): Recent Advances in Paediatrics 19. London, United Kingdom: Churchill Livingstone, 2001, p. 77.

237. Halliday HL, Ehrenkranz RA: Moderately early (7–14 days) postnatal corticosteroids for preventing chronic lung disease in preterm infants (Cochrane Review). Cochrane Database Syst Rev 1:CD001144, 2001.

238. Halliday HL, Ehrenkranz RA: Delayed (>3 weeks) postnatal corticosteroids for chronic lung disease in preterm infants (Cochrane Review). Cochrane Database Syst Rev 2:CD001145, 2001.

239. Halliday H: Clinical trials of postnatal corticosteroids: Inhaled and systemic. Biol Neonate 76:29, 1999.

240. Watterberg K: Postnatal steroids for bronchopulmonary dysplasia: Where do we go from here? Neonatal Respir Dis 11: 2001, pp. 1–8.

241. Finer NN, Craft A, Vaucher YE, et al: Postnatal steroids: Short-term gain, long-term pain? J Pediatr 137:9, 2000.

242. O'Shea TM, Kothadia J, Klinepeter KL, et al: A randomized placebo-controlled trial of a 42-day tapering course of dexamethasone to reduce the duration of ventilator dependency in very low birth weight infants: Outcome of study participants at 1-year adjusted age. Pediatrics 104:15, 1999.

243. Shinwell ES, Karplus M, Reich D, et al: Early postnatal dexamethasone treatment and increased incidence of cerebral palsy. Arch Dis Child Fetal Neonatal Ed 83:F177, 2000.

244. Mertz U, Peschgens T, Kusenbach G, et al: Early versus late dexamethasone treatment in preterm infants at risk for chronic lung disease: A randomized pilot study. Eur J Pediatr 158:318, 1999.

245. O'Shea TM, Doyle LW: Perinatal glucocorticoid therapy and neurodevelopmental outcome: An epidemiologic perspective. Available at: http://www.ideallibrary.com.

246. Thebaud B, Lacaze-Masmonteil T, Watterberg K: Postnatal glucocorticoids in very preterm infants. "The good, the bad, and the ugly"? Pediatrics 107:413, 2001.

247. Barrington KJ: Postnatal steroids and neurodevelopmental outcomes: A problem in the making. Pediatrics 107:1425, 2001.

248. Banks BA: Postnatal dexamethasone for bronchopulmonary dysplasia: A systematic review and meta-analysis of 20 years of clinical trials. NeoReviews 3:e24, 2002.

249. Ehrenkranz RA, Ablow RC, Warshaw JB: Effect of vitamin E on the development of oxygen-induced lung injury in neonates. Ann NY Acad Sci 393:452, 1982.

250. Hallman M, Bry K, Hoppu K, et al: Inositol supplementation in premature infants with respiratory distress syndrome. N Engl J Med 326:1233, 1992.

251. Atkinson SA: Special nutritional needs of infants for prevention of and recovery from bronchopulmonary dysplasia. J Nutr 131:942S, 2001.

252. Sosenko IRS, Kinter MT, Roberts RJ: Nutritional issues in chronic lung disease of premature infants. In Bland RD, Coalson JJ (eds): Chronic Lung Disease in Early Infancy. New York, Marcel Dekker, 2000, p. 285.

253. Citrino C: Nutrition in the Newborn Center. Memphis, TN, The University of Tennessee, 2001.

254. Hazinski TA: Vitamin A treatment for the infant at risk for bronchopulmonary dysplasia. NeoReviews 1:e11, 2000.

255. Kirkpatrick BV, Felman AH, Eitzman DV: Complications of ventilator therapy in respiratory distress syndrome. Am J Dis Child 128:496, 1974.

256. Yu VYH, Liew SW, Roberton NRC: Pneumothorax in the newborn: Changing pattern. Arch Dis Child 50:449, 1975.

257. Thibeault DW, Lachman RS, Laul VR, et al: Pulmonary interstitial emphysema, pneumomediastinum, and pneumothorax: Occurrence in the newborn infant. Am J Dis Child 126:611, 1973.

258. Campbell RE, Hoffman RR Jr: Predictability of pneumothorax in hyaline membrane disease. Am J Roentgenol Radium Ther Nucl Med 120:274, 1974.

259. Ogata ES, Gregory GA, Kitterman JA, et al: Pneumothorax in the respiratory distress syndrome: Incidence and effect on vital signs, blood gases and pH. Pediatrics 58:177, 1976.

260. Matthieu JM, Nussle D, Torrado A, et al: Pneumopericardium in the newborn. Pediatrics 46:117, 1970.

261. Yeh TF, Vidyasagar D, Pildes RS: Neonatal pneumopericardium. Pediatrics 54:429, 1974.

262. Brans YW, Pitts M, Cassady G: Neonatal pericardium. Am J Dis Child 130:393, 1976.

263. Aranda JV, Stern L, Dunbar JS: Pneumothorax with pneumoperitoneum in a newborn infant. Am J Dis Child 123:163, 1972.

264. Donahoe PK, Stewart DR, Osmond JD III, et al: Pneumoperitoneum secondary to pulmonary air leak. J Pediatr 81:797, 1972.

265. Campbell RE, Boggs TR Jr, Kirkpatrick JA Jr: Early neonatal pneumoperitoneum from progressive massive tension pneumomediastinum. Radiology 114:121, 1975.

266. Leonidas JC, Hall RT, Rhodes PG: Pneumoperitoneum in ventilated newborns: A medical or surgical problem? Am J Dis Child 128:677, 1974.

267. Macklin CC: Transport of air along sheaths of pulmonic blood vessels from alveoli to mediastinum: Clinical implications. Arch Intern Med 64:913, 1939.

268. Macklin MT, Macklin CC: Malignant interstitial emphysema of the lungs and mediastinum as an important occult complication in many respiratory diseases and other conditions: An interpretation of the clinical literature in the light of laboratory equipment. Medicine 23:281, 1944.

269. deLemos RA, Guajardo A, Null DM Jr: Mechanisms and role of barotrauma in neonatal lung injury. In Bancalari E, Stocker JT (eds): Bronchopulmonary Dysplasia. Washington, DC, Hemisphere Publishing Corporation, 1988, p. 49.

270. Halliday HL: Other acute lung disorders. In Sinclair JC, Bracken MB (eds): Effective Care of the Newborn Infant. Oxford, Oxford University Press, 1992, p. 359.

271. Thibeault DW, Lang MJ: Mechanisms and pathobiologic effects of barotrauma. In Merritt TA, Northway WH Jr, Boynton BR (eds): Bronchopulmonary Dysplasia. Boston, Blackwell Scientific Publications, 1988, p. 79.

272. Ackerman NB Jr., Coalson JJ, Kuehl TJ, et al: Pulmonary interstitial emphysema in the premature baboon with hyaline membrane disease. Crit Care Med 12:512, 1984.

273. Chernick V, Avery ME: Spontaneous alveolar rupture at birth. Pediatrics 32:816, 1963.

274. Karlberg PJE: Breathing and its control in premature infants. In Lanman JT (ed): Physiology of Prematurity: Transactions of the Second Conference, 1957. New York, Josiah Macy Jr Foundation, 1958.

275. Gregory GA, Tooley WH: Gas embolism in hyaline-membrane disease. N Engl J Med 282:1141, 1970.

276. Grosfield JL, Boger O, Clotworthy WH: Hemodynamic and manometric observations in experimental air block syndrome. J Pediatr Surg 6:339, 1971.

277. Boothroyd AE, Barson AJ: Pulmonary interstitial emphysema—A radiological and pathological correlation. Pediatr Radiol 18:194, 1988.

278. Campbell RE: Intrapulmonary interstitial emphysema: A complication of hyaline membrane disease. Am J Roentgenol Radium Ther Nucl Med 110:449, 1970.

279. Emery JL: Interstitial emphysema, pneumothorax and "air-block" in the newborn. Lancet 1:405, 1956.

280. Davis CH, Stevens GW: Value of routine radiographic examinations of the newborn, based on a study of 702 consecutive babies. Am J Obstet Gynecol 20:73, 1930.

281. Harris LE, Steinberg AG: Abnormalities observed during the first six days of life in 8716 live-born infants. Pediatrics 14:314, 1954.

282. Howie VM, Weed AS: Spontaneous pneumothorax in the first ten days of life. J Pediatr 50:6, 1957.

283. Malan AF, Heese H de V: Spontaneous pneumothorax in the newborn. Acta Paediatr Scand 55:224, 1966.

284. Peterson HG, Pendleton ME: Contrasting roentgenographic patterns of the hyaline membrane and fetal aspiration syndromes. Am J Roentgenol Radium Ther Nucl Med 74:800, 1955.

285. Merenstein GB, Dougherty K, Lewis A: Early detection of pneumothorax by oscilloscope monitor in the newborn infant. J Pediatr 80:98, 1972.

286. Leake RD, Hobel CJ, Lachman RS: Neonatal pneumothorax and subcutaneous emphysema secondary to diagnostic amniocentesis. Obstet Gynecol 43:884, 1974.

287. Anderson KD, Chandra R: Pneumothorax secondary to perforation of sequential bronchi by suction catheters. Pediatr Surg 11:687, 1976.

287a. Lubchenco LO: Recognition of spontaneous pneumothorax in premature infants. Pediatrics 24:996, 1959.

288. Pomerance JJ, Weller MH, Richardson CJ, et al: Pneumopericardium complicating respiratory distress syndrome: Role of conservative management. J Pediatr 84:883, 1974.

289. Varano LA, Maisels MJ: Pneumopericardium in the newborn: Diagnosis and pathogenesis. Pediatrics 53:941, 1975.

290. Reppert SM, Ment LR, Todres ID: The treatment of pneumopericardium in the newborn infant. J Pediatr 90:115, 1977.

291. Morrow G III, Hope JW, Boggs TR Jr: Pneumomediastinum: A silent lesion in the newborn. J Pediatr 70:554, 1967.

292. O'Gorman LD, Cottingham RA, Sargent EN, et al: Mediastinal emphysema in the newborn: A review and description of the new extrapleural gas sign. Dis Chest 53:301, 1968.

293. Lee SB, Kuhn JP: Pneumatosis intestinalis following pneumomediastinum in a newborn infant. J Pediatr 79:813, 1971.

294. Lubens P, Jubelirer D, Steichen JJ: Massive intravascular air accumulation in a neonate. J Pediatr 88:1020, 1976.

295. Bowen FW Jr, Chandra R, Avery BG: Pulmonary interstitial emphysema with gas embolism in hyaline membrane disease. Am J Dis Child 126:117, 1973.

296. Siegle RL, Eyal FC, Rabinowitz JG: Air embolus following pulmonary interstitial emphysema in hyaline membrane disease. Clin Radiol 27:77, 1976.

297. Terry TL: Extreme prematurity in fibroblastic overgrowth of persistent vascular sheath behind each crystalline lens. Preliminary report. Am J Ophthalmol 25:203, 1942.

298. Silverman WA: Retrolental Fibroplasia: A Modern Parable. New York, Grune and Stratton, 1980.

299. Kinsey VE, Hemphill FM: Etiology of retrolental fibroplasia and preliminary report of cooperative study of retrolental fibroplasia. Trans Am Acad Ophthalmol Otolaryngol 59:15, 1955.

300. Lanman JT, Guy LP, Dancis J: Retrolental fibroplasia and oxygen therapy. JAMA 155:223, 1954.

301. Patz A, Hoeck LE, De La Cruz E: Studies on the effect of high oxygen administration in retrolental fibroplasia: Nursery observations. Am J Ophthalmol 35:1248, 1952.

302. Avery ME, Oppenheimer EH: Recent increase in mortality from hyaline membrane disease. J Pediatr 57:553, 1960.

303. McDonald AD: Cerebral palsy in children of very low birth weight. Arch Dis Child 38:579, 1963.

304. Phelps DL: Retinopathy of prematurity: An estimate of vision loss in the United States—1979. Pediatrics 67:924, 1981.

305. Bancalari E, Flynn J, Goldbert RN, et al: Influence of transcutaneous monitoring on the incidence of retinopathy of prematurity. Pediatrics 79:663, 1987.

306. James LS, Lanman JT: History of oxygen therapy and retrolental fibroplasia. Pediatrics 57(Suppl):591, 1976.

307. Brockhurst RJ, Christi MJ: Cicatricial retrolental fibroplasia: Its occurrence without oxygen administration and in full term infants. Graefes Arch Clin Exp Ophthalmol 195:113, 1975.

308. Klina R, Hodson WA, Morgan BC: Retrolental fibroplasia in a cyanotic infant. Pediatrics 50:765, 1972.

309. Stockman JA III, Oski FA: Physiological anaemia of infancy and the anaemia of prematurity. In Gladner BE (ed): Clinics in Haematology, vol. 1. Philadelphia, WB Saunders, 1978, p. 12.

310. Watts JL: Retinopathy of prematurity. In Sinclair JC, Bracken MB (eds): Effective Care of the Newborn Infant. Oxford, Oxford University Press, 1992, p. 617.

311. Phelps DL: Retinopathy of prematurity: History, classification, and pathophysiology. NeoReviews 2:e153, 2001.

312. Silverman WA: Retinopathy of prematurity: Oxygen dogma challenged. Arch Dis Child 57:731, 1982.

313. Katzman G, Satish M, Krishnan V, et al: Comparative analysis of lower and higher stage retrolental fibroplasia. Pediatr Res 16:294A, 1982.

314. Katzman G, Satish M: Letter to the editor: Hypoxemia and retinopathy of prematurity. Pediatrics 80:972, 1987.
315. Kinsey VE, Arnold AJ, Kalina RE, et al: Pao$_2$ levels and retrolental fibroplasia: A report of the cooperative study. Pediatrics 60:655, 1977.
316. Satish M, Katzman G, Krishnan V, et al: Association of physiologic state and therapeutic modalities other than oxygen. Pediatr Res 15:679A, 1981.
317. Szewczyk TS: Retrolental fibroplasia and related ocular diseases: Classification, etiology and prophylaxis. Am J Ophthalmol 36:1333, 1953.
318. Bedrossian RH, Carmichael P, Ritter J: Effect of oxygen weaning on retrolental fibroplasia. Am J Ophthalmol 53:514, 1955.
319. Bedrossian RH, Carmichael P, Ritter J: Retinopathy of prematurity (retrolental fibroplasia) and oxygen: Part I. Clinical study: Part II. Further observations on the disease. Am J Ophthalmol 37:78, 1954.
320. Phelps DL: Reduced severity of oxygen-induced retinopathy in kittens recovered in 28% oxygen. Pediatr Res 24:106, 1988.
321. The STOP-ROP Multicenter Study Group: Supplemental therapeutic oxygen for pre-threshold retinopathy of prematurity (STOP-ROP), a randomized, controlled trial. I: Primary outcomes. Pediatrics 105:295, 2000.
322. Kingham JD: Reticular dystrophy of the retinal pigment epithelium. A clinical and electrophysiologic study of three generations. Arch Ophthalmol 96:1177, 1978.
323. Flynn JT: Acute proliferative retrolental fibroplasia: Multivariate risk analysis. Trans Am Ophthalmol Soc 81:549, 1983.
324. Shohat M, Reisner SH, Krikler R, et al: Retinopathy of prematurity: Incidence and risk factors. Pediatrics 72:159, 1983.
325. Reese AB, Blodi FC: The pathology of early retrolental fibroplasia with an analysis of the histologic findings in the eyes of newborn and stillborn infants. Am J Ophthalmol 35:1490, 1952.
326. Fos RY, Kopelow SM: Development of the retinal vasculature in perinatal infants. Surv Ophthalmol 18:117, 1973.
327. Ashton N: Oxygen and growth of retinal vessels. In Kimura SJ, Caygill WM (eds): Vascular Complications of Diabetes Mellitus. St. Louis, CV Mosby, 1967, p. 3.
328. Patz A: Retrolental fibroplasia. Surv Ophthalmol 14:1, 1969.
329. Reese AB, Owens WC, King M: Classification of retrolental fibroplasia. Am J Ophthalmol 36:1333, 1953.
330. Garner A, Ben-Sira I, Deutman A, et al: An international classification of retinopathy of prematurity. Pediatrics 74:127, 1984.
331. Cryotherapy for Retinopathy of Prematurity Group: Multicenter trial of cryotherapy for retinopathy of prematurity. Pediatrics 81:697, 1988.
332. American Academy of Pediatrics Section on Ophthalmology, American Association for Pediatric Ophthalmology and Strabismus, and the American Academy of Ophthalmology: Screening examination of premature infants for retinopathy of prematurity. Pediatrics 108:809, 2001.

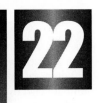

22 SURGICAL MANAGEMENT OF THE AIRWAY

MOHAMMAD A. EMRAN, MD
MARK E. GERBER, MD
ROBERT ARENSMAN, MD

Improved survival of low-birthweight infants, better and earlier detection of disease processes, better intensive care unit (ICU) support, and evolving experience mean pediatric surgeons and otolaryngologists become involved in the care of an increasing number of children with congenital or acquired airway problems. As our ability to detect abnormalities and to intubate, ventilate, and save children who would have been victims of neonatal asphyxia or respiratory distress improves, the role of the pediatric surgeon as part of the neonatal management team expands.

The surgeon assumes many roles in the management of the neonatal airway. First, the surgeon/endoscopist acts as ongoing consultant for neonates undergoing medical treatment after intubation of their airways. This includes continued endoscopic surveillance of the airway after intubation. Second, the surgeon/endoscopist functions as a primary diagnostician for infants who manifest signs of congenital upper airway obstruction and occasionally acquired upper airway obstruction. Finally, the surgeon/endoscopist may play a primary role in therapy for these patients and in providing a secure airway.

THE PEDIATRIC SURGEON AS CONSULTANT

The increased frequency of long-term intubation of neonates and the survival of some patients with severe respiratory difficulties are associated with increased airway complications. The pediatric surgeon/endoscopist has an important role in the evaluation of the airways of these patients. Other indications for neonatal endoscopy include evaluation of stridor (discussed later), persistent atelectasis, evaluation of endotracheal tube position or patency, and as an aid to difficult intubations.

Anatomic Considerations

The air passages of a neonate obviously are smaller than those of an adult or a large child, and this increases their vulnerability to obstruction.[1] The mucosa is softer, looser, and more fragile. The location of the epiglottis and larynx of a neonates airway is more cephalad and anterior than that of an adult. Of note, the cricoid cartilage is the narrowest point in an infant's upper airway. This feature not only makes the use of a cuffed endotracheal tube unnecessary in this population, but it also increases the risk of the subglottic pressure complications from prolonged intubation. Furthermore, at an infant's carina, the mainstem bronchi angulate symmetrically, unlike an adult's carina. This mandates that care be taken to listen to the chest bilaterally following intubation, because mainstem bronchus intubation is possible bilaterally.

Pathophysiology of Acquired Tracheal Stenosis

Subglottic edema can result from mechanical irritation due to the presence of an endotracheal tube. Because the cricoid cartilage is a complete ring, mucosal edema at this level of the airway can result in acute inflammation leading to mucosal ulceration, submucosal inflammation, and chondritis. The body's reparative response to these changes is fibrosis and scarring that, if severe, results in laryngotracheal stenosis.

Preventative Measures

In order to minimize this cycle of destruction, an endotracheal tube is chosen for appropriate size, and fixation is secure enough to minimize lateral or horizontal motion and prevent accidental extubation. Prolonged intubation may require nasotracheal intubation and fixation to decrease these movement problems (see Chapter 6).

NEONATAL LARYNGOSCOPY AND BRONCHOSCOPY

Flexible Endoscopy

Excellent flexible and rigid endoscopes are available for examination of the neonatal airway. In addition, ultrathin flexible bronchoscopes that are now available allow examination of the tracheobronchial tree through endotracheal tubes. These scopes are available in diameters ranging from 1.3 to 2.7 mm[2–4] and presumably allow bronchoscopic examination without interrupting positive-pressure ventilation when a swivel Y-adapter (Vigo, France) is used between the endotracheal tube and the ventilator. They are easy to maneuver and make examination in the neonatal ICU possible. Serious complications, such as perforation, are unlikely. However, the majority of these scopes do not provide capabilities for lavage or suction, and resolution is limited by current fiberoptic technology. Olympus scopes as small as 2.2-mm intraluminal size retain good maneuverability and allow some use of instruments.[5]

With the ultrathin flexible endoscopes an endotracheal tube is placed over the scope under direct vision. This is particularly useful in neonates with congenital airway obstruction or craniofacial anomalies. In these neonates, visualization of the airway with traditional laryngoscopy can be impossible.[6] The flexible endoscopes rapidly provide information about endotracheal tube position and patency. Awake flexible laryngoscopy prevents the complications of general anesthetic.[7] For major diagnostic and all therapeutic procedures, however, rigid bronchoscopy performed by an experienced pediatric bronchoscopist provides the maximum yield. Performed with appropriate anesthesia, lighting, and suction, it is associated with minimal morbidity and mortality.

Rigid Endoscopy

Rigid scopes such as the Storz, equipped with Hopkins pediatric telescopes, are available in sizes ranging from 2.5 to 5.0 mm, with telescopes available in sizes ranging from 1.9 to 4.0 mm. Larger telescopes increase resolution but at the cost of increased airway resistance as measured by peak airway pressure.[8] These scopes provide superb illumination and magnification for inspection, as well as an adequate lumen through which to insert tubes or instruments (Fig. 22-1). A technique of using the Hopkins telescope without the sheath by inserting it directly through an endotracheal tube via a Y-adapter has been described and allows continuation of endotracheal intubation and positive-pressure ventilation throughout the procedure.[9] In addition, the rigid scopes have a portal for aspiration, biopsy, and lavage that is not present on smaller flexible scopes and is useful in therapeutic procedures.[10]

When the patient's condition precludes movement to the operating room (OR), both flexible and rigid scopes are easily used in the neonatal ICU. Consequently, no infant should be denied an endoscopic examination when diagnostic or therapeutic benefits are likely. Use of photography or video cameras are useful because they provide a media for documenting findings, communicating with parents and colleagues, and teaching. In addition, video images provide more information because their dynamic nature can document transient phenomena.[5]

Evaluation of Intubation

Because most patients admitted to our neonatal ICU for intubation and ventilatory support are treated medically, the role of the pediatric surgeon/endoscopist is primarily one of consultation. Improved techniques for endotracheal and nasotracheal intubation and the development of better pediatric ventilators make it possible to maintain most children safely on respiratory support for 6 to 8 weeks with minimal concern for permanent pressure damage to the airway. After 6 to 8 weeks of endotracheal intubation, one should consider bronchoscopic evaluation (Fig. 22-1) to determine if damage has occurred and if continued intubation is appropriate management (see section on Tracheostomy).

Other Indications for Laryngoscopy and Bronchoscopy

Other indications for diagnostic bronchoscopy are listed in Table 22-1. Many of the conditions that contribute to neonatal stridor are diagnosed using bronchoscopy. Diagnosis by bronchoscopy is associated with little risk of complication compared to therapeutic bronchoscopy, which carries a greater complication risk.[11] For this reason, consideration should be given to performing operative/therapeutic bronchoscopy in the OR.

One problem occasionally encountered during bronchoscopy is decreased oxygen saturation. This is the result of partial airway obstruction by the bronchoscope. Fear of hypoxia should not be a factor in preventing bronchoscopy in an infant who truly needs it. Intratracheal oxygen administration can be done through the aspiration/suction port of the bronchoscope to prevent or limit this hypoxia.[12] If a suction port is not available, then caution is taken not to be overzealous in continuing the procedure in the presence of desaturation. Other diagnostic modalities including computed tomography (CT), magnetic resonance imaging, and angiography are used in determining upper airway obstructive pathology, and they are discussed as they pertain to use in diagnosing specific conditions.

TABLE 22-1.   Indications for Neonatal Bronchoscopy

Prolonged intubation (>6–8 weeks)
Repetitive failure of extubations
Inability to aerate all lobes of the lung (persistent atelectasis)
Clinical need for cultures or bronchial washings
Suspicion of necrotizing tracheobronchitis
Evaluation of stridor

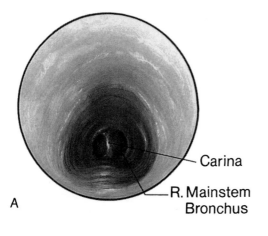
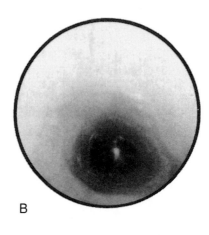

Carina

R. Mainstem
Bronchus

A

B

Figure 22-1. Normal trachea as seen through a Storz bronchoscope with a 0-degree Hopkins telescope. *A,* Artist's drawing. *B,* Photograph.

TRACHEOSTOMY

Although physicians at some centers continue endotracheal intubation if no damage is encountered on evaluation of the airway, many clinicians proceed with neonatal tracheostomy after prolonged periods of continuous ventilation. Tracheostomy is also seriously considered for infants who manifest central nervous system failure, severe bronchopulmonary dysplasia, or complex cardiovascular disease or in whom an endotracheal tube is inadequate for maintaining pulmonary toilet.

The specific technique of neonatal tracheostomy varies little from a well-performed tracheostomy at any age. Except in dire emergency, when transtracheal needle ventilation may be required, neonatal tracheostomy is performed under OR conditions, and the infant is intubated before the surgical procedure begins.

Procedure

After the landmarks of the anterior triangle of the neck are well established, a transverse or midline skin incision can be made (Fig. 22-2). Although transverse skin incisions are more cosmetic early on, the choice of skin incision appears to make little difference in the overall outcome and reflects the preference of the operating surgeon. Once the skin and subcutaneous tissues are open, midline dissection is mandatory to prevent damage to vascular or neural structures. Occasionally excision of subcutaneous fat may be necessary for proper visualization and positioning of the tracheostomy. Division of the thyroid isthmus is occasionally necessary and is easily performed with electrocautery. The cut ends may be oversewn as necessary for hemostasis. Either a simple transverse[13] or vertical H-type tracheal incision is performed in neonatal cases (Fig. 22-3). Stay sutures are placed through the cartilage of the tracheostomy site at the time the initial incision into the trachea is made so that reintubation in the early postoperative period (should it become necessary) can be achieved quickly, easily, and with minimal trauma to the neck tissues (Fig. 22-4). At no time are cartilaginous rings removed because this almost inevitably results in stricture if decannulation is successful in the future.[14–18] Today, some centers mature the stoma by suturing the skin to the tracheal wall to further facilitate replacement of the tracheostomy tube in the event of decannulation.

Because a neonatal tracheostomy is performed over an endotracheal tube if possible, the endotracheal tube is removed under direct vision as the tracheostomy tube is inserted (Fig. 22-5). This guarantees control of the neonatal airway throughout the entire procedure. Final fixation of the tube is critical, because dislodgment in the postoperative period is fatal if personnel are unable to reinsert the tube immediately. Consequently, the tube is properly secured using cloth ties tightened snugly enough to allow only two fingers to pass between the ties and the cervical skin (Fig. 22-6). Foam padding beneath the ties is used to prevent skin erosion. Suturing of the tracheostomy tube to the skin is unnecessary in children if the stoma is matured and the tube is secured as described. However, a mature stoma may increase the need for tracheocutaneous closure when the tracheostomy is no longer required. Prior to leaving the OR, the position of the tracheostomy is confirmed using flexible endoscopy.

ANTERIOR CRICOID SPLIT PROCEDURE

The improved survival of premature infants after prolonged intubation has made pressure complications increasingly

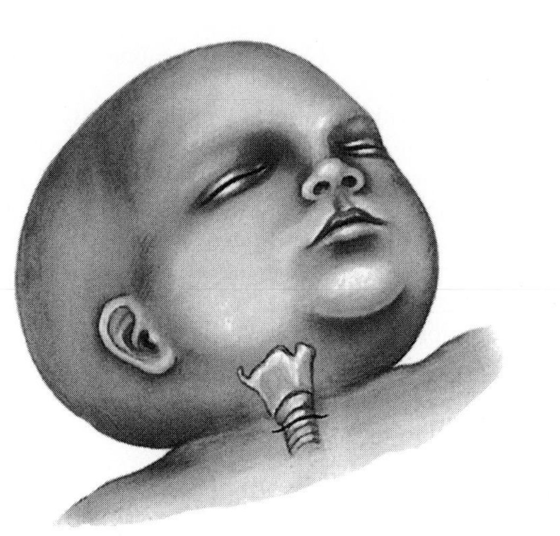

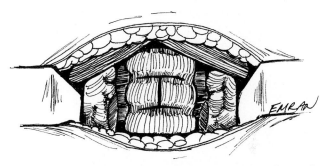

Figure 22-3. Platysma and strap muscles retracted laterally to allow midline dissection to the trachea. The thyroid isthmus is retracted or cut as necessary. An H-type tracheal incision is made at the second or third tracheal ring.

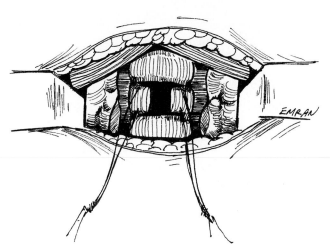

Figure 22-4. The tracheal opening is dilated. Retention sutures are sewn through the cartilages to aid postoperative reinsertion if necessary. No tracheal cartilage is removed at any time.

Figure 22-2. Transverse skin incision over tracheal rings (1 to 3).

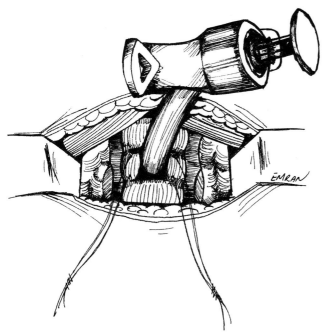

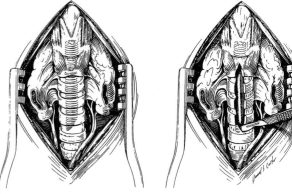

Figure 22-7. Anterior cricoid split procedure. After exposure of the anterior surface of the cricoid cartilage and upper two tracheal rings, a vertical incision is made through the cricoid and tracheal rings. Exposure of the endotracheal tube along the length of the split indicates completion of the procedure. (From Drake AF, Babyak JW, Niparko JK, et al: The anterior cricoid split: Clinical experience with extended indications. Arch Otolaryngol Head Neck Surg 114:1405, 1988. Copyright 1988, American Medical Association.)

Figure 22-5. Tracheostomy tube is inserted following slow withdrawal of the endotracheal tube under direct vision.

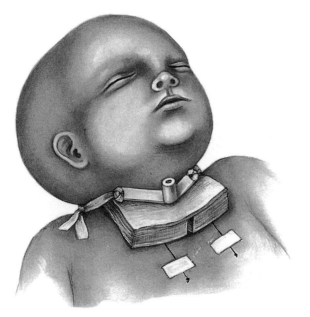

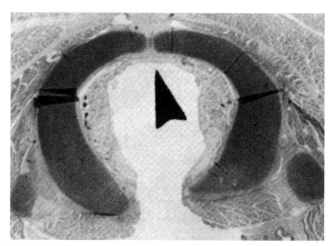

Figure 22-8. Cross-sectional specimen obtained at autopsy from a patient who had previously undergone an anterior cricoid split. The *arrow* indicates the site of the cricoid split (the posterior opening was created by the pathologist during autopsy). (From Cotton RT, Seid AB: Management of the extubation problem in the premature child: Anterior cricoid split as an alternative to tracheostomy. Ann Otol Rhinol Laryngol 89:510, 1980.)

Figure 22-6. Completed tracheostomy with dressing and tapes in place.

common. As an alternative to tracheostomy in neonates with early stages of subglottic stenosis, Cotton and Seid[19] recommend an anterior cricoid split procedure performed over an endotracheal tube. This procedure involves a transverse skin incision and a longitudinal incision through the lower aspect of the thyroid cartilage (below the vocal cords), the cricoid cartilage, and the upper two tracheal rings, as well as underlying mucosa (Fig. 22-7). The soft tissues of the neck are reapproximated over the defect via a single-layer (skin) closure. The patient remains intubated for a period of 7 to 21 days, during which time the mucosa heals by fibrosis, and tracheal stability

is re-established (Fig. 22-8). After healing has occurred, the infant is extubated.

Experience with this technique, originally described in 1980, demonstrates the procedure is a reasonable alternative in carefully selected patients, resulting in successful extubations in approximately 58% to 100% of patients.[20–27] However, when reintubation and positive-pressure ventilation become necessary in infants who have recently undergone this procedure, complications such as aerocele and persistent fistula at the site of the anterior cricoid split have been reported.[20,28] Thus, careful selection of patients for this procedure is essential, and tracheostomy remains the mainstay of initial treatment for the majority of neonates with pressure complications secondary to prolonged intubation. To decrease postoperative endotracheal tube stenting, some authors suggest stenting open the cricoid cartilage. This can be done using autologous thyroid alar cartilage, costal cartilage, or hyoid cartilage.[25,26]

TRACHEOSTOMY TUBES

The choice of an appropriate tracheostomy tube is as important as the correct technique of tracheostomy placement. Several manufacturers produce soft tubes for the pediatric and neonatal airway. These include the Shiley,[29] Bivona, and Portex. These tubes remain soft at body temperature and conform well to individual anatomy, thus reducing trauma and risk of subsequent stricture formation. In addition, the softer tubes are more comfortable for the patient and reduce the chances of cervical skin irritation or abrasions.

If a patient undergoing tracheostomy has an endotracheal tube in place, the size of the endotracheal tube can be used to guide the selection of a tracheostomy tube of appropriate size. A reasonably reliable rule is that the tracheostomy tube can be 0.5 mm larger than the correct endotracheal or nasotracheal tube. Choices of tracheostomy tubes designed to fit variations in neonatal airway include Shiley 3.0neo, 3.5neo, 4.0neo; and Portex FG 14, 15, 18, and 21. A postoperative chest radiograph indicates the tube position and eliminates the possibility of pneumothorax.

Once the stoma has stabilized, weekly changing of the tube is adequate. An alternate tube and a tube one size smaller are kept available in case a sudden replacement of the tube becomes necessary. Suctioning is performed as necessary to keep the airway clear of secretions. The details of suctioning are similar to those for endotracheal tubes (see Chapter 6).

MODALITIES FOR OXYGENATION UNTIL AIRWAY ESTABLISHMENT

Ex Utero Intrapartum Treatment Procedure

The ex utero intrapartum treatment (EXIT) procedure is a newer modality that was developed to cope with the problem of prenatal diagnosis of complicated airway problems.[30–37] It allows maintenance of the infant on placental circulation, thus maintaining oxygenation until airway access is secured. This is important when anatomy is abnormal or, in the case of cervical tumors or masses, grossly distorted, making intubation and tracheostomy difficult or impossible.

Extracorporeal Membrane Oxygenation

If intrapartum treatment is not possible and a bridge is needed until the airway can be secured, extracorporeal membrane oxygenation (ECMO) can be used to maintain oxygenation. The anatomic considerations that make airway access and tracheostomy difficult may also make vascular access in the neck challenging. In these situations, although not usually recommended, femoral access is used.

DIFFERENTIAL DIAGNOSIS OF NEONATAL UPPER AIRWAY OBSTRUCTION

Because the neonatal airway is small and can easily reach the point of critical narrowing,[38,39] the presence of stridor signals the need for rapid diagnosis and possible intervention.

TABLE 22-2. Differential Diagnosis of Neonatal Stridor (Anatomic Approach)

Nasopharynx Choanal atresia	**Larynx** Laryngeal atresia Laryngeal web Vocal cord paralysis
Tongue Idiopathic Beckwith-Wiedemann syndrome Metabolic disorders 　Hypothyroidism/ 　　lingual thyroid 　Glycogen storage disease Down syndrome	Laryngomalacia Subglottic stenosis 　Congenital/traumatic Laryngocele Laryngeal cleft Subglottic hemangioma
Oropharynx (micrognathia and glossoptosis) Pierre Robin sequence Treacher Collins syndrome Hallermann-Streiff syndrome Möbius' syndrome Freeman-Sheldon syndrome Nager syndrome	**Trachea** Intrinsic compression 　Tracheomalacia 　Tracheal stenosis 　Necrotizing tracheobronchitis Extrinsic compression 　Cystic hygroma 　Vascular rings

Neonatal stridor is easily managed medically in some cases but may represent impending fatal obstruction in others; therefore, an organized and rapid approach to diagnosis is essential.

A reasonable list of differential diagnoses for neonatal upper airway obstruction is formulated by approaching the subject anatomically, beginning in the nasopharynx and oropharynx and progressing down through the respiratory tract (Table 22-2 and Fig. 22-9).

NASOPHARYNGEAL OBSTRUCTION

Choanal Atresia

Choanal atresia[40] is a rare anomaly, with a reported incidence of 1 in 8000 births. It involves occlusion of the posterior nares by a septum with membranous (10%) or bony (90%) constitution (Fig. 22-10). The lesion may be asymptomatic if it is unilateral but may cause total airway obstruction if it is bilateral because most neonates are preferential nasal breathers. The symptoms are most evident when the patient is at rest because when infants are agitated and crying, they are able to breathe via the oropharynx. Associated anomalies include esophageal atresia, congenital cardiac lesions, colobomata, and Treacher Collins syndrome. Failure to pass a catheter through the nostril into the oropharynx suggests the diagnosis, which can be confirmed with CT scan. Acute management of a neonate with bilateral choanal atresia may require placement of an oropharyngeal airway or endotracheal intubation. Definitive surgical repair involves opening the atretic choanal plates.

OROPHARYNGEAL OBSTRUCTION

Macroglossia

The tongue is often a site of obstruction causing stertor in a neonatal patient, particularly if the tongue is disproportioately

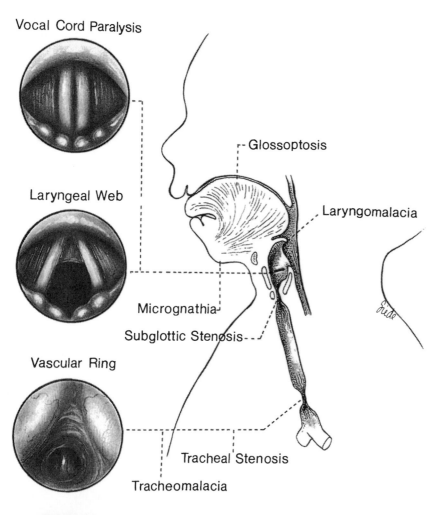

Vocal Cord Paralysis

Laryngeal Web

Vascular Ring

Glossoptosis

Laryngomalacia

Micrognathia

Subglottic Stenosis

Tracheal Stenosis

Tracheomalacia

Figure 22-9. Composite diagram of some of the lesions that result in neonatal stridor (proceeding downward through the respiratory passages).

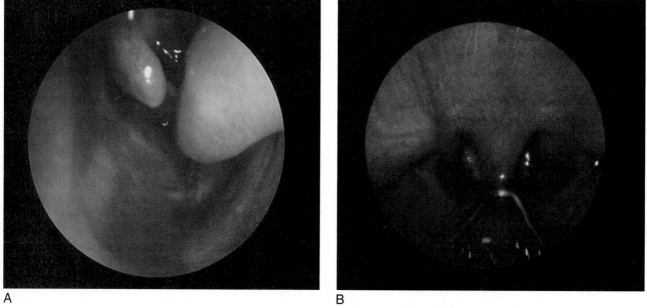

A   B

Figure 22-10. Choanal atresia. *A,* Endoscopic view. *B,* Nasopharyngeal view.

larger than the infant's oropharynx. Physical examination confirms the diagnosis. Insertion of an oral airway and prone or side positioning usually are successful for acute management of this type of airway obstruction. Several defined syndromes include macroglossia as a component.

Beckwith-Wiedemann Syndrome

Severe hypoglycemia, in many cases secondary to hyperinsulinemia, initially brought these examples of infantile gigantism to note.[41–43] Other manifestations of this syndrome include macroglossia secondary to muscular hypertrophy, visceromegaly, microcephaly, and a series of umbilical abnormalities ranging from congenital umbilical hernia to omphalocele. Affected infants may demonstrate a facial nevus flammeus, renal medullary dysplasia, and a characteristic pit on the tragus of the ear. They usually are large at term and weigh 3.5 to 5.5 kg at birth.

Lingual Thyroid

This rare condition can cause oropharyngeal obstruction.[44-46] Stertor in the presence of hypothyroidism, detected by persistent elevation of thyroid stimulating hormone on routine neonatal screening, raises the suspicion for lingual thyroid, although other lesions are more commonly responsible. This condition occurs in just over 1 in 10,000 births.

Laryngoscopy is performed to confirm a mass. This is further characterized by CT scan and thyroid scintography to aid in diagnosis. Of note, the thyroid may continue to hypertrophy during early infancy and childhood, and the respiratory complications associated with hypothyroidism, such as respiratory depression, may not occur until later.

Metabolic Disorders

Several neonatal metabolic disorders may cause macroglossia and result in congenital stridor, the best known of which are hypothyroidism and glycogen storage disease. The physical findings of macroglossia and a very high oral obstruction generally suggest the diagnosis of the underlying condition. The stridor experienced by these children usually is mild, can be managed adequately with an oropharyngeal airway, and disappears shortly after birth as a child adjusts. The diagnostic workup in these patients should be directed to the underlying metabolic disorder. Little additional diagnostic work is needed for the tracheobronchial tree.

Down Syndrome (Trisomy 21)

Affected children are easily identified by their constellation of abnormalities. Their relative macroglossia may result in a mild congenital stridor. Because Stewart[47] has reported an association between Down syndrome and congenital subglottic stenosis, endoscopy may be necessary to establish the definitive cause of the stridor.

Craniofacial Dysmorphology Syndromes

Craniofacial dysmorphology syndromes range from unusual to extremely rare. All have in common an obstruction located in the oropharynx resulting from micrognathia with glossoptosis. The upper airway obstruction varies from mild to severe, and it is important to identify the underlying problem, which usually is hereditary. One of the features of micrognathia is the associated decrease in the size of the upper airways as measured by radiography resulting in greater risk for obstruction, dysphagia, and apneic episodes in affected infants.[48]

Pierre Robin Sequence

This sequence is the most common dysmorphic syndrome with micrognathia and glossoptosis.[49-54] Approximately half of the patients also have cleft palates, perhaps attributable to protrusion of the tongue between the posterior palatine plates during embryologic development resulting in failure of normal midline fusion. The tongue often prolapses posteriorly, causing intermittent partial obstruction of the upper airway. During inspiration, negative pressure in the pharynx further retrodisplaces the tongue and may increase the degree of pharyngeal obstruction. The airway obstruction usually is resolved with insertion of an oropharyngeal airway. The child also tends to breathe more comfortably in a prone position. A child is fed by using special nipples or gavage if he or she has an associated cleft palate.

Tracheostomies are rarely necessary in these cases but seem to be preferable to surgical procedures such as glossopexy or creation of a lingual flap. These procedures usually are used in children who do not respond to conservative management. Additional surgical interventions include mandibular distraction and floor of mouth release.

Some clinicians have voiced the opinion that this syndrome really represents an etiologically heterogeneous group of anomalies resulting in micrognathia, glossoptosis, and cleft palate. This view has important implications in terms of the need for individualized treatment, depending on the particular constellation of abnormalities found in a particular patient and the causes of these abnormalities.

Treacher Collins Syndrome

Also known as mandibulofacial dysostosis, this syndrome includes an extremely variable and diffuse group of craniofacial anomalies.[55-57] Patients may manifest downward sloping palpebral fissures, colobomata of the lower lids, sunken cheekbones, and blind fistulae on an angle between the mouth and ears (Fig. 22-11). Pinnae may be deformed, deafness is common, and micrognathia is seen as well (usually less severe than that seen in Pierre Robin syndrome). The presumed genetic defect is autosomal dominant with variable penetrance.

The hypopharynx is the location of the obstruction in these children (as in children with the Pierre Robin syndrome), owing to the disproportionate relationship between the small jaw and the large tongue. These children are most often managed medically, and tracheostomy is seldom necessary.

Hallermann-Streiff Syndrome

This syndrome consists of microphthalmia, cataracts, blue sclerae, and nystagmus.[58,59] Associated anomalies include a pinched nose, micrognathia, and hypertrichosis of the scalp, eyebrows, and eyelashes (Fig. 22-12). Transmission is presumed to be autosomal dominant, although most cases are thought to represent new mutations. Congenital stridor in these infants arises from micrognathia with relative glossoptosis, and treatment is similar to that outlined for Pierre Robin or Treacher Collins syndrome.

Möbius' Syndrome

Infants with Möbius' syndrome have characteristic absences or maldevelopment of various cranial nerve nuclei.[60-64] The seventh (facial) nerve is most commonly involved, but all cranial nerves may be affected to various extents. Common physical findings include facial paralysis, ptosis, ophthalmoplegia, clubbed feet, and syndactyly. The presumed mode of transmission is an autosomal dominant defect.

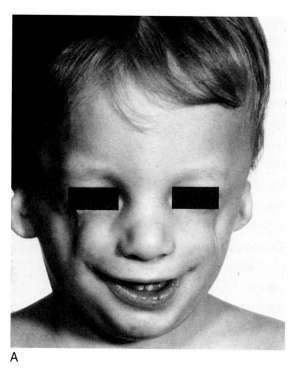
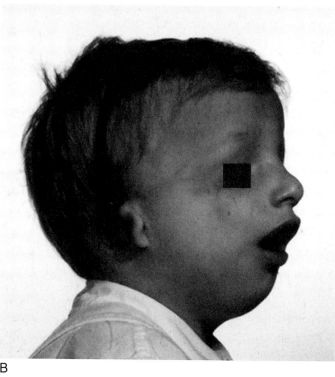

A   B

Figure 22-11. Example of a child with Treacher Collins syndrome demonstrating sunken cheek bones, downward sloping palpebral fissures, and micrognathia.

The facial immobility secondary to seventh nerve involvement causes upper airway obstruction and difficulties in chewing and swallowing. Rarely placement of a tracheostomy may be required in severe cases. Many children, however, can be successfully treated by instruction in very careful feeding techniques. Infants with associated central neurologic defects and increased risk of aspiration may benefit from fundoplication or, more radically, tracheal diversion.

Freeman-Sheldon Syndrome

Infants with this abnormality often are called "whistling faced" children.[65,66] They have hypoplastic alae nasi, clubbed feet, finger contractures, ulnar deviation of the hands, microstomia, and masklike whistling faces. Their eyes are deep set, with blepharophimosis, ptosis, and strabismus. Presumed transmission is autosomal dominant.

The noisy breathing in these children results from air forced through a narrow nasal passage. Although the sound may be alarming to family and nursing personnel, it usually does not require immediate intervention and improves as the infant grows. Upper airway endoscopic examination in these infants can be difficult or impossible. Preparations for emergent tracheostomy should be made in the child with impending respiratory failure in case of an inability to intubate.

Nager Syndrome

Nager syndrome is a rare acrofacial dysostosis that presents with upper limb malformation, mandibular and malar hypoplasia, downward slanting palpebral fissures, absent eyelashes in the medial third of the lower lids, dysplastic ears with conduc-

tive deafness, and variable degrees of palatal clefting.[67–72] Chromosome 9 abnormalities are suspected in the development of this syndrome. Airway obstruction in these patients is related to mandibular hypoplasia and tongue displacement posteriorly. Acute management often requires early tracheostomy and subsequent mandibular distraction to establish an airway and correct the defect.

LARYNGEAL ANOMALIES

An infant's larynx is the next site of possible obstruction, and laryngeal anomalies account for the majority of stridor in newborns.[73]

Laryngeal Atresia

The most extreme form of obstruction at this level, laryngeal atresia results in a desperate emergency during the first few moments of life (Fig. 22-13).[74,75] This lesion was originally described in 1826, but only 51 cases have been reported in the subsequent 160 years. Of children thus affected, few have survived. The low survival rate is attributable to the fact that the surgical intervention must occur within 2 to 5 minutes of birth.

The most dramatic physical finding is that the child is aphonic, with the absence of any cry or gasp at birth. If the lesion is immediately recognized on direct laryngoscopy, an emergency tracheostomy is performed. Diagnosis of laryngeal atresia has now been reported prenatally, and in the future clinicians may be able to prepare for emergent airway management at birth, resulting in improved survival.

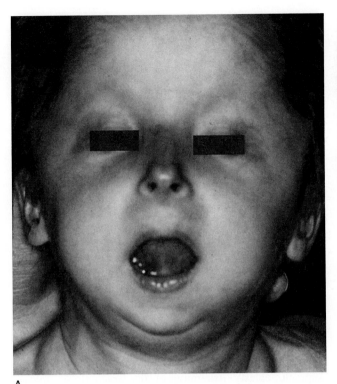
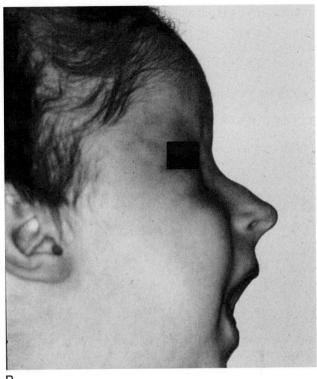

A   B

Figure 22-12. Example of an infant with Hallermann-Streiff syndrome demonstrating microphthalmia, pinched nose, micrognathia, and hypertrichosis of scalp.

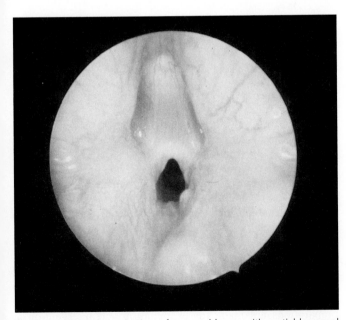

Figure 22-13. Endoscopic view of neonatal larynx with partial laryngeal atresia and a laryngeal web partially obstructing the laryngeal orifice.

Laryngeal Web

Laryngeal web accounts for approximately 5% of laryngeal anomalies (Fig. 22-13).[76–78] These lesions arise about the 10th week of intrauterine life and probably represent an arrest of the development of the larynx in the area near the vocal cords. Seventy-five percent of these lesions occur at the level of the cords; the rest are subglottic or supraglottic in about equal numbers. The web generally occurs anteriorly, and the lesions present with hoarseness/abnormal cry if they extend less than halfway back along the cords. Because the glottic area is triangular, these anteriorly placed webs reduce the glottic area by only 15% to 20% and are not sufficient to cause stridor.

If the web extends posteriorly, the symptoms may be marked. The stridor is primarily inspiratory but often has an expiratory component. The affected infant's cry is hoarse and weak. The child is rarely aphonic and often is dyspneic at rest. In addition to the stridor and voice changes, recurrent croup, recurrent tracheobronchitis, and recurrent pneumonias, although not specific to this condition, all point to chronic airway obstruction.

Laryngoscopy and bronchoscopy are performed as soon as possible. If a thin transparent web is encountered at the level of the cords, it is divided endoscopically, completely correcting the problem. Bronchoscopy is completed to rule out the possibility of associated anomalies beneath the area of the web.

If the web is thick and fibrous, no attempt is made to force the bronchoscope through the area. This kind of web often has glottic and subglottic involvement. If aeration of the child is satisfactory despite the stridor, as evidenced by arterial blood gas determinations, simple observation is sufficient management until he or she is able to undergo surgical repair. This is usually deferred until the child is 18 months to 2 years old. These extensive webs require an external approach to treat the subglottic component with possible resection or expansion with cartilage grafting. Tracheostomy serves to bypass the obstruction and to maintain the airway following surgery and is the treatment of choice if the child is dyspneic and unable to tolerate the web during infancy.

Congenital Vocal Cord Paralysis

Congenital vocal cord paralysis is the second most common cause of neonatal stridor.[73,79] In the past, birth trauma was frequently implicated in the etiology of the paralysis but now appears to be a declining cause. Intracranial lesions and the possibility of congenital cardiac lesions, especially one paralyzing the recurrent laryngeal nerve, are considered.

Fortunately, the paralysis is unilateral in 70% to 80% of cases. Some studies report that both sides are equally involved,[29] but left-sided paralysis is significant because of its association with underlying congenital cardiac anomalies. The cry of affected infants is hoarse and weak. Children with bilateral vocal cord paralysis usually have a strong cry, but the biphasic stridor is severe, especially when the children are agitated. Marked suprasternal and intercostal retractions may be present in these children.

Diagnosis is rapidly made by laryngoscopy, and treatment depends on the severity of the problem. In a unilateral paralysis with minimal or no dyspnea, simple observation is appropriate. Bilateral paralysis, generally associated with severe symptoms, necessitates tracheostomy for prevention of impending total obstruction. Once the airway is adequately secured, the cause of paralysis is explored. If the causal lesion is identified and corrected, the stridor may improve. If no lesion can be found or if it cannot safely be corrected, later fixation of the arytenoids with the vocal cords in abduction may result in satisfactory control of the stridor and decannulation of the child.

Laryngocele

This lesion is a cystic mass that arises from the laryngeal ventricle and causes external airway compression.[80] Plain x-ray, CT scan, or ultrasound that demonstrate an air- and fluid-filled mass makes the diagnosis. Treatment involves endoscopy and external excision of the mass. Tracheostomy is reserved for complicated cases only.

Laryngomalacia

According to some studies, laryngomalacia is the most common cause of neonatal stridor, accounting for 60% to 75% of cases of stridor in newborns.[73] The pathophysiology of this condition involves an immature floppy glottis that is sucked downward into the larynx at each inspiration (Fig. 22-14), producing an inspiratory stridor of varying severity. This stridor often changes with position, improving when the patient is prone and increasing in severity when the patient is supine.

Laryngomalacia occurs with a 2:1 male-to-female predominance and usually is present at birth. In 25% of cases, however, the first symptoms appear during the first or second week of life. Many of these children are reported to be micrognathic, and some may be mistakenly diagnosed with Pierre Robin syndrome.

Diagnosis is made easily by flexible awake laryngoscopy that shows a soft enfolded epiglottis. The larynx is often difficult to expose and is found high under the tongue. There is a 10% to 15% incidence of associated tracheobronchial anomalies. When symptoms are severe enough to consider surgical intervention, bronchoscopy should be performed.

The prognosis for this condition is excellent, and only on extremely rare occasions are symptoms severe enough to

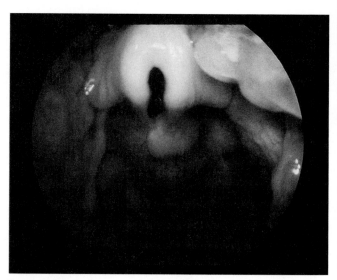

Figure 22-14. Endoscopic view of immature floppy glottis characteristic of laryngomalacia. Dynamic examination demonstrates downward displacement of glottis into larynx with inspiration.

justify surgical intervention. Maturation of the epiglottis by age 18 to 24 months results in resolution of stridor. When indicated, supraglottoplasty (trimming of the aryepiglottic folds and cuneiform cartilages) is almost universally successful in alleviating the symptoms of upper airway obstruction. Tracheostomy is only rarely required.

Congenital Subglottic Stenosis

The overall incidence of congenital subglottic stenosis is unknown, because many such cases remain unrecognized, although 39% of all subglottic lesions are estimated to be congenital.[38,47,81–83] The proposed cause is arrested development of the conus elasticus or the cricoid.

If present, stridor usually is inspiratory, progressing to biphasic with increasing severity of stenosis. It may not present until the first or second month of life. When mild, the presenting symptoms usually are initiated by an upper respiratory tract infection. Affected children often are treated for recurrent pneumonias or chronic laryngotracheobronchitis (croup). Some are not discovered until a severe episode of croup results in emergency tracheostomy or intubation. Stenosis can be identified in the early neonatal period and can be suspected by prenatal ultrasound revealing associated findings such as fetal ascites, echogenic enlarged lungs, and a dilated fluid-filled trachea.

With a prenatal diagnosis of upper airway obstruction, preparations are made for examination and intervention at the time of delivery. The diagnosis is confirmed by laryngoscopy. Bronchoscopy rules out associated defects that may be present. The mild forms (usually <50% stenosis) of this lesion usually are observed without therapy. In children with severe stenosis and marked symptoms, surgical intervention may be necessary in more than half the cases. Surgical options, which include tracheostomy and endoscopic dilation with or without laser partial excision, result in considerable improvement. When used, dilation must be gentle to prevent further damage or fibrosis of the subglottic region. For more severe degrees of stenosis, open surgical intervention becomes necessary. The outcome in this congenital group of subglottic stenosis is good, with 82% of patients in one large series successfully decannulated after one procedure. The overall outcome varies with the severity of the stenosis.

Acquired Subglottic Stenosis

Acquired subglottic stenosis, most often caused by prolonged endotracheal intubation, is explained by the sequence of events noted in the section on Pathophysiology. In its mildest form, the stenosis consists of laryngeal edema and has been reported in 30% of infants immediately after extubation. Stridor in these patients is inspiratory and presents with the first breaths after tube removal. This stridor usually resolves within 72 hours. During this 3-day period, appropriate treatment includes head elevation, humidified air, racemic epinephrine, and occasionally systemic steroids (although the efficacy of steroids have never been demonstrated conclusively by experimental study).

In its most severe form, acquired subglottic stenosis is a dense scar of well-organized fibrous tissue. Initial treatment may include graded gentle dilation with or without intralesional steroids and/or laser wedge excision. As many as half of the stenotic scars will improve and often stabilize with endoscopic management. More severe lesions or those that fail to achieve significant improvement with endoscopic management require an open approach with expansion of the stenosis, stabilization with cartilage grafts, or resection of the stenotic segment with tracheal anastomosis. These procedures can be done to avoid tracheostomy or as a staged procedure after tracheostomy is in place.

Laryngeal Cleft

Although laryngeal clefts were once considered extremely rare lesions, they have frequently been reported during the past 45 years.[80,84–87] This is probably the result of enhanced endoscopy techniques and improved ability to make the diagnosis in the antemortem period. The lesion seems to result from a failure of dorsal fusion during the chondrification of the cricoid cartilage. A midline cleft remains posteriorly and extends down between the arytenoids to various extents into the upper portion of the esophagus and trachea. Affected children often are stridorous at birth, and many have died in the past because of inadequate resuscitation. In addition to respiratory difficulties, these children aspirate and develop severe pneumonitis if they are fed without regard for the clefts. Consequently, they require recognition, stabilization, and intubation, depending upon severity. A feeding gastrostomy and fundoplication often are necessary until definitive repair is performed. Once extubation is accomplished, it is important to observe the child closely to ensure that upper airway secretions do not continuously pass into the lungs. If this proves to be a severe and ongoing problem that precipitates recurrent pneumonia and respiratory distress, it may be necessary to place a tracheostomy until surgical closure of the cleft can be achieved. During the stabilization period, evaluation for other anomalies is undertaken. Subsequently a one- to three-layered closure can be performed. Surveillance following repair is directed at preventing recurrent obstruction from granulation tissue.

Subglottic Hemangioma

Hemangiomas may be another cause of congenital subglottic obstruction.[16,39,88] The onset of symptoms is variable, as are the growth and development of these lesions. The lesions initially are small and then undergo a period of precipitous growth, followed by a long plateau and slow involution. If the lesion has grown during embryonic life, the affected child may display both inspiratory and expiratory stridor at birth. However, in most children the lesions develop shortly after birth, and several months elapse before symptoms develop. Hemangiomas on other areas of the body suggest the possibility of subglottic hemangioma. Definitive diagnosis is made by laryngoscopic and bronchoscopic examination. A bronchoscopic finding of a red or purple compressible mass just beneath the cords is generally considered sufficient to confirm the diagnosis. When such findings are seen, most pediatric surgeons believe that biopsy is contraindicated because of the risk of significant hemorrhage. Once the diagnosis is established, appropriate therapy is chosen according to the severity of symptoms. If the child is stable and has normal blood gas values at rest, observation is sufficient. If the obstruction is of sufficiently high grade to result in dyspnea, severe stridor, and possibly abnormal blood gas values, surgical intervention is considered.

Surgical options for management include (1) intralesional steroids and intubation; (2) laser partial excision; (3) open surgical excision; and (4) tracheotomy. Adjuvant measures when using options 1 and 2 include systemic steroids and α-interferon. Radiation is not used in the treatment of these children today because of the risk of thyroid malignancy. Dramatic regression of the hemangioma and prompt correction of the rare associated thrombocytopenia with the use of these agents has been reported.[87] Newer antiangiogenic agents may prove of value in treating large hemangiomas in the future, with expected decreased impingement on the airway. These medical treatments may eliminate the future need for surgical intervention beyond temporary intubation or tracheostomy in severe cases of airway obstruction.

Subglottic cysts

Subglottic cysts are not generally congenital in origin but tend to arise in neonates who have been intubated for 7 days or more but can be seen in neonates intubated for briefer periods as well.[89] Symptoms such as stridor, hoarseness, and obstructive apnea are described in patients who were low-birthweight infants. Isolated or multiple cysts usually occur in the lateral or posterior cricoid area and are identified by laryngoscopy.

Congenital cysts

Congenital cysts are another rare cause of upper airway obstruction, occurring in nearly 2 of 100,000 births.[90,91] As with the obstruction caused by the acquired form of subglottic cysts, the key to management is early detection to prevent morbidity and mortality. The management of subglottic cysts depends on the size and severity of symptoms. The natural history of the cysts is one of spontaneous resolution usually by age 1 year. Cysts causing a great deal of airway obstruction may require surgical drainage that may be preferred for early resolution of symptoms.

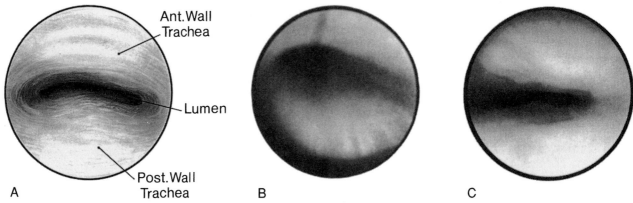

Figure 22-15. Tracheomalacia showing collapse of the trachea on expiration. The lumen is almost obliterated as the anterior wall approaches the posterior wall. *A*, Artist's drawing. *B–C*, Photographs.

TRACHEAL ANOMALIES

Internal Tracheal Lesions

Tracheomalacia

Tracheomalacia results from a failure of the cartilaginous rings to fully support the round shape of the normal trachea.[10] The cartilages are hypoplastic with an increased posterior membrane-to-cartilage ratio of 4.5:1 (normal 2:1). This allows the trachea to collapse, especially during expiration (Fig. 22-15). This condition is seen as the defect in approximately 30% of children undergoing bronchoscopic evaluation for respiratory distress, but it is only incidentally responsible for the stridor in a moderate number of the children. Stridor associated with tracheomalacia can be biphasic. If the malacia is intrathoracic, it will be predominately expiratory stridor, whereas extrathoracic malacia results in inspiratory stridor. Other signs and symptoms include prolonged expiration, cyanosis, brassy cough, apnea, feeding difficulties, retained secretions, and recurrent pneumonia. The condition is diffuse and usually occurs throughout the length of the trachea. Many of these children have associated cardiac anomalies.

Diagnosis is most simply made by rigid or flexible bronchoscopy. After the scope is passed through the vocal cords, the trachea assumes a transverse or ovoid appearance that is accentuated as expiration takes place. It frequently is difficult to see the carina as the scope advances through the trachea because of the collapse of the anterior wall. Despite rather marked findings in some children, this lesion rarely (if ever) necessitates any treatment. It can be expected to resolve spontaneously with growth and maturation. Of note, rigid bronchoscopy may be performed with the telescope only because the bronchoscope itself may stent the trachea open, which interferes with accurate diagnosis. Dynamic endoscopy with spontaneous respirations during the anesthetic maximizes the ability of endoscopist to make an accurate diagnosis.

Tracheal Stenosis

Congenital tracheal stenosis is a narrowing of the trachea secondary to complete or nearly complete cartilaginous rings.[92–95] It can involve either a short stenotic segment in an otherwise normal trachea or the entire trachea with a cylindrical tapering from the subglottic region (Fig. 22-16). Either

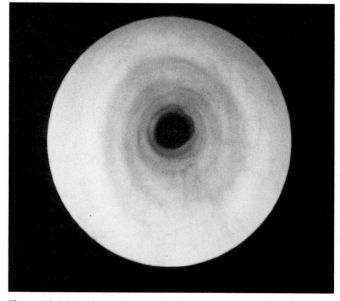

Figure 22-16. Endoscopic view of tracheal stenosis as a result of complete tracheal rings tapering to a narrow lumen.

form may demonstrate a fixed obstruction that results in inspiratory and expiratory stridor. Some of the other tracheal cartilages often are absent when this occurs, and instability of the tracheal lumen is not uncommon.

Depending on the severity of the stenosis and its length, affected children may have severe respiratory distress with cyanosis. Respiratory sounds may be weak or stridorous. Wheezing, recurrent pneumonias, and even sudden acute obstruction and respiratory arrest are possible. Lateral radiographs or xerograms of the neck and chest may show a stenotic lesion; otherwise, bronchoscopy is the best study to confirm the diagnosis.

Surgical treatment of these lesions depends on the severity of symptoms but usually is indicated because airway obstruction generally is prominent in these children. If the stenosis represents a short segment, resection and primary anastomosis can be achieved if the length of involved trachea is less than 50%. If this cannot be accomplished, the possibility of success with dilation over a long-term period is possible but dangerous because the lower airway is not adequately controlled. Tracheoplasty with a pericardial flap, cartilage grafting, slide tracheoplasty, and tracheal autograft are all surgical options.

Evaluation for other anomalies (especially heart and vascular) is performed because they are common. Complete rings have as high as a 20% to 30% association with pulmonary artery sling. Mortality can be predicted by categorizing tracheal stenosis based on severity of stenosis and presence of other anomalies. Class I patients have limited stenosis and no associated anomalies and carry a mortality of 8%. Class II patients have associated anomalies but are free from heart or lung disease and thus carry a mortality of 45%. Class III patients have significant stenosis in conjunction with heart or lung disease and have a mortality risk of 79%.

Necrotizing Tracheobronchitis

Necrotizing tracheobronchitis is a destructive process of the airway that results in sloughing of the tracheal mucosa.[96–100] The cause is unknown because cultures have consistently failed to reveal a bacterial or fungal infection. Children afflicted were generally stressed, asphyxiated, or experiencing respiratory distress and thus were all intubated and ventilated. High-frequency ventilators were initially suspected to have an association, but it has been seen in both conventional and high-frequency oscillator ventilation modalities.

Clinical presentation involves deterioration of respiratory status. Affected children generally manifest sudden carbon dioxide retention with a lack of chest wall movement that fails to respond to change in ventilator settings, change of endotracheal tubes, or intratracheal suctioning. Mortality is high unless suspicion of the lesion leads to bronchoscopy and mechanical clearing of the airway. Moreover, even if a child is able to recover from an acute episode, recurrent necrotizing tracheobronchitis or chronic strictures may result.

Total Tracheal Thrombosis

This is an anticoagulant-associated phenomenon that has been reported in patients on ECMO.[101] Airway obstruction occurs secondary to a thrombus in the airway and is managed by repeated bronchoscopy with pulmonary toilet and with meticulous attention to anticoagulation, using the least amount deemed safe.

External Tracheal Lesions

Cystic Hygroma

Cystic hygromas of sufficient size and extension that result in compression of the trachea and thus stridor have been reported.[39,75] When these lesions are severe enough to result in stridor, they almost always produce respiratory distress and require surgical intervention. The goal of the initial treatment is to relieve the compression, often by simple aspiration of fluid from the cyst. This is followed by bronchoscopy to rule out the possibility of an associated laryngotracheal anomaly and by surgical extirpation of the lesion. This is a benign lesion, and critical structures of the neck are spared if at all possible.

Vascular Rings

Vascular rings arise from anomalous formation of the great vessels that cross over or encircle the trachea and esophagus.[102–110] The variety of anomalies is extensive, but the

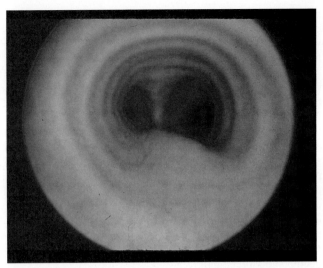

Figure 22-17. Endoscopic view of anomalous right subclavian artery with impingement on the tracheal membrane.

few categories that commonly occur and lead to problems can be classified under several headings. The structures usually responsible for stridor are the double aortic arch and the right aortic arch with left ductus arteriosus or ligamentum arteriosum. More rarely, an anomalous right subclavian artery (Fig. 22-17), anomalous left pulmonary artery sling, innominate artery, or anomalous left common carotid artery give rise to symptoms. For technical accuracy, only a few of these conditions are considered true vascular rings, that is, complete encirclement of the trachea and esophagus by vascular structures. Specifically, these lesions include the double aortic arch and the right aortic arch with left ductus. The others are more correctly referred to as *slings*, because they pass around the trachea or esophagus and compress it but do not completely encircle it.

Stridor in affected neonates usually is present from birth or appears within 1 to 2 months. With the fixed nature of the obstruction, stridor is both inspiratory and expiratory. Afflicted children have a brassy barking cough. If the compression of the vascular anomaly affects the esophagus, as it does in only a few cases, the children have associated problems with deglutition, such as regurgitation, vomiting, and aspiration.

Evaluation of these patients begins with a barium swallow that usually shows a single or double oblique indentation on the esophagus. Subsequent bronchoscopy often reveals the pulsatile compressing mass passing over the anterior portion of the trachea on either the right or left side. Depending on the location of the mass, a presumptive diagnosis can be made. Also, one can occasionally compress the pulsatile area to check for disappearance of pulses to suggest which of the vascular anomalies is present. Currently magnetic resonance angiography and CT with dye contrast make the diagnosis and contribute substantial information about the anatomy of the lesion. Today angiography is used only rarely to diagnose these anomalies.

Treatment of these lesions is surgical division of the ring when one is present. In cases of double aortic arch or right aortic arch with left ductus arteriosus, division of the ring at its narrowest portion and/or ductal ligation and division result in considerable improvement. In the case of sling lesions, the offending vessel is divided (as in treatment of the anomalous right subclavian artery). Rarely the vessel can be transposed and reanastomosed. If transection alone does not relieve the obstruction, dissection of the trachea and esophagus with vessel suspension to the anterior chest wall has been performed, with considerable improvement of symptoms.

All of these operations are performed through a standard left thoracotomy, and results have been acceptable in several large review series. The anomalous left pulmonary artery sling fortunately is one of the more rare vascular slings and continues to be the most difficult to handle surgically. This lesion usually is approached through a median sternotomy, although some surgeons have performed it through a left thoracotomy. The left pulmonary artery must be transected, moved from behind the trachea, and reanastomosed anteriorly. This results in a considerably more hazardous surgical undertaking and consequently a greater surgical mortality rate. The increased incidence of major anomalies in the tracheobronchial tree or cardiovascular system also makes this vascular malformation more difficult to handle and more lethal.

Families must be warned before surgery that a residual tracheomalacia persists and that symptoms usually abate within 6 months to 2 years after surgery. The deglutition problems improve rapidly; the stridor does not resolve as quickly because the tracheal cartilages are persistently deformed and gradual enlargement of the tracheal lumen must occur before the airway noise disappears.

Congenital Cervical Teratoma

This rare, predominantly benign neoplastic entity is now often diagnosed prenatally with ultrasound demonstrating a mass with mixed echogenicity and variable consistency. Careful planning is required for surgical management but requires immediate control of the airway, with provision made for bronchoscopy and tracheostomy should they become necessary. Maintaining the neonate on maternal circulation during cesarean section gives additional time until the airway can be secured. Tracheostomy and surgery can be troublesome because of the distortion of anatomic landmarks by the mass.

SUMMARY

By organizing the approach to neonatal airway obstruction, quick identification of etiology and ultimately of therapy can be achieved. Many of these therapies and etiologies for the conditions continue to with improved prenatal diagnosis, as better tools for evaluating the neonatal airway become available and as we become more facile in the techniques of airway management in these complicated patients.

REFERENCES

1. Barkin RM: Pediatric airway management. Emerg Med Clin North Am 6:687, 1988.
2. Finer NN, Etches PC: Fiberoptic bronchoscopy in the neonate. Pediatr Pulmonol 7:116, 1989.
3. Deres M, Kosack K, Waldschmidt J, et al: Airway anomalies in newborn infants: Detection by tracheoscopy via endotracheal tube. Biol Neonate 58:50, 1990.
4. De Blic J, Delacourt C, Scheinman P: Ultrathin flexible bronchoscopy in neonatal intensive care units. Arch Dis Child 66:1383, 1991.
5. Perez CR, Wood RE: Update on pediatric flexible bronchoscopy. Pediatr Clin North Am 41:385–400, 1994.
6. Finer NN, Muzyka D: Flexible endoscopic intubation of the neonate. Pediatr Pulmonol 12:48, 1992.
7. Berkowitz RG: Neonatal upper airway assessment by awake flexible laryngoscopy. Ann Otol Rhinol Laryngol 107:75–80, 1998.
8. Marzo SJ, Hotaling AJ: Trade-off between airway resistance and optical resolution in pediatric rigid bronchoscopy. Ann Otol Rhinol Laryngol 104(4 Pt 1):282–287, 1995.
9. Yahagi N, Kumon K, Sugimoto H, et al: A use of telescope of rigid type bronchoscope through endotracheal tube in infants [letter]. Anesth Analg 76:207, 1993.
10. Mair EA, Parsons DS: Pediatric tracheobronchomalacia and major airway collapse. Ann Otol Rhinol Laryngol 101:300–309, 1992.
11. Lindahl H, Rintala R, Malinen L, et al: Bronchoscopy during the first month of life. J Pediatr Surg 27:548–550, 1992.
12. Soong WJ, Hwang B: Intratracheal oxygen administration during bronchoscopy in newborns: Comparison between two different weight groups of infants. Zhonghua Yi Xue Za Zhi (Taipei) 63:696–703, 2000.
13. Mendez-Picou G, Ehrlich FE, Salzberz AM: The effect of tracheostomy incisions on tracheal growth. J Pediatr Surg 11:681, 1976.
14. Perrotta RJ, Schley WS: Pediatric tracheostomy: A five-year comparison study. Arch Otolaryngol 104:318, 1978.
15. Gibson R, Byrne JET: Tracheostomy in neonates. Laryngoscope 82:643, 1972.
16. Palva A, Jokinen K, Nemela T: Tracheostomy in children. Arch Otolaryngol 101:536, 1975.
17. Lynn HB, Van Heerden JA: Tracheostomy in infants. Surg Clin North Am 53:945, 1973.
18. Bardin J, Boyd AD, Hirose H, et al: Tracheal healing following tracheostomy. Surg Forum 25:210, 1974.
19. Cotton RT, Seid AB: Management of the extubation problem in the premature child: Anterior cricoid split as an alternative to tracheostomy. Ann Otol 89:508, 1980.
20. Drake AF, Babyak JW, Niparko JK, et al: The anterior cricoid split: Clinical experience with extended indications. Arch Otolaryngol Head Neck Surg 114:1404, 1988.
21. Palasti S, Respler DS, Fieldman RJ, et al: Anterior cricoid split for subglottic stenosis: Experience at the Children's Hospital of New Jersey. Laryngoscope 102:997, 1992.
22. Michna BA, Krummel TM, Tracy T Jr, et al: Cricoid split for subglottic stenosis in infancy. Ann Thorac Surg 45:541, 1988.
23. Seid AB, Canty TG: The anterior cricoid split procedure for the management of subglottic stenosis in infants and children. J Pediatr Surg 20:388, 1985.
24. Frankel LR, Anas NG, Perkin RM, et al: Use of the anterior cricoid split operation in infants with acquired subglottic stenosis. Crit Care Med 12:395, 1984.
25. Richardson MA, Inglis AF Jr: A comparison of anterior cricoid split with and without costal cartilage graft for acquired subglottic stenosis. Int J Pediatr Otorhinolaryngol 22:187–193, 1991.
26. McGuirt WF Jr, Little JP, Healy GB: Anterior cricoid split. Use of hyoid as autologous grafting material. Arch Otolaryngol Head Neck Surg 123:1277–1280, 1997.
27. Silver FM, Myer CM 3rd, Cotton RT: Anterior cricoid split. Update 1991. Am J Otolaryngol 12:343–346, 1991.
28. Patel H, Gregor B, Kleinhaus S: Aerocele, an unusual complication of anterior cricoid split. J Pediatr Surg 27:1512, 1992.
29. Othersen HB: Intubation injuries of the trachea in children: Management and prevention. Ann Surg 189:601, 1979.
30. Kalache KD, Masturzo B, Pierro A, et al: Prenatal evaluation of fetal neck masses in preparation for the EXIT procedure: The value of pulmonary Doppler ultrasonography (PDU). Prenat Diagn 21:308–310, 2001.
31. Bui TH, Grunewald C, Frenckner B, et al: Successful EXIT (ex utero intrapartum treatment) procedure in a fetus diagnosed prenatally with congenital high-airway obstruction syndrome due to laryngeal atresia. Eur J Pediatr Surg 10:328–333, 2000.
32. Crombleholme TM, Sylvester K, Flake AW, et al: Salvage of a fetus with congenital high airway obstruction syndrome by ex utero intrapartum treatment (EXIT) procedure. Fetal Diagn Ther 15:280–282, 2000.
33. Liechty KW, Crombleholme TM, Weiner S, et al: The ex utero intrapartum treatment procedure for a large fetal neck mass in a twin gestation. Obstet Gynecol 93(5 Pt 2):824–825, 1999.
34. Ward VM, Langford K, Morrison G: Prenatal diagnosis of airway compromise: EXIT (ex utero intra-partum treatment) and foetal airway surgery. Int J Pediatr Otorhinolaryngol 53:137–141, 2000.

35. Larsen ME, Larsen JW, Hamersley SL, et al: Successful management of fetal cervical teratoma using the EXIT procedure. J Matern Fetal Med 8:295–297, 1999.
36. Shih GH, Boyd GL, Vincent RD Jr, et al: The EXIT procedure facilitates delivery of an infant with a pretracheal teratoma. Anesthesiology 89:1573–1575, 1998.
37. DeCou JM, Jones DC, Jacobs HD, et al: Successful ex utero intrapartum treatment (EXIT) procedure for congenital high airway obstruction syndrome (CHAOS) owing to laryngeal atresia. J Pediatr Surg 33:1563–1565, 1998.
38. Birrell JF: Pediatric Otolaryngology. Chicago, Year Book Medical Publishers, 1978, pp. 151, 158.
39. Maze A, Bloch E: Stridor in pediatric patients. Anesthesiology 50:132, 1979.
40. Coates H: Nasal obstruction in the neonate and infant. Clin Pediatr 31:25, 1992.
41. Wiedemann HR: Complexe malformatif familial avec hernie ombilicale et macroglossi-un "syndrome nouveau"? J Genet Hum 13:223, 1964.
42. Wiedemann HR, Spranger J, Mogharei M, et al: Uber das Syndrom Exomphalos-Macroglossie-Gigantismus, uber generalisierte Muskelhypertrophie, progressive Lipo dystrophie und Miescher-Symdrom im Sinne diencephaler Syndrom. Z Kinderheilkunde 102:1, 1968.
43. Beckwith JB: Macroglossia, omphalocele, adrenal cytomegaly, gigantism, and hyperplastic visceromegaly. In Bergsma DS (ed): The First Conference on the Clinical Delineation of Birth Defects II(5). Malformation Syndromes. New York, The National Foundation, March of Dimes, 1969, p. 188.
44. Chan FL, Low LC, Yeung HW, et al: Case report: Lingual thyroid, a cause of neonatal stridor. Br J Radiol 66:462–464, 1993.
45. Maddern BR, Werkhaven J, McBride T: Lingual thyroid in a young infant presenting as airway obstruction: Report of a case. Int J Pediatr Otorhinolaryngol 16:77–82, 1988.
46. New England Congenital Hypothyroidism Collaborative: Characteristics of infantile hypothyroidism discovered on neonatal screening. J Pediatr 104:539–544, 1984.
47. Stewart DJ: Congenital abnormalities as a possible factor in the aetiology of post intubation subglottic stenosis. Anaesth Soc J 17:338, 1970.
48. Gunn TR, Tonkin SL, Hadden W, et al: Neonatal micrognathia is associated with small upper airways on radiographic measurement. Acta Paediatr 89:82–87, 2000.
49. Robin P: La chute de la base de la langue. Bull Acad Med (Paris) 89:37, 1923.
50. Robin P: Glossoptosis due to atresia and hypertrophy of the mandible. Am J Dis Child 48:541, 1934.
51. Dennison WM: The Pierre Robin syndrome. Pediatrics 36:336, 1965.
52. Shprintzen RJ: Pierre Robin, micrognathia, and airway obstruction: The dependency of treatment on accurate diagnosis. Int Anesthesiol Clin 26:64, 1988.
53. Shprintzen RJ, Singer L: Upper airway obstruction and the Robin sequence. Int Anesthesiol Clin 30:109, 1992.
54. Bath AP, Bull PD: Management of upper airway obstruction in Pierre Robin sequence. J Laryngol Otol 111:1155–1157, 1997.
55. Thompson A: Notice of several cases of malformation of the external ear, together with experiments on the state of hearing in such persons. J Med Sci 7:420, 1846.
56. Treacher Collins E: Case with symmetrical congenital notches in the outer part of each lower lid and defective development of the malar bones. Trans Ophthalmol Soc U K 20:190, 1900.
57. Franceschetti A, Klein D: The Mandibulo-facial Dysostosis: A New Hereditary Syndrome. Copenhagen, E. Muksgaard, 1949.
58. Audry C: Variete d'alopecie congenitale: Alopecie suturale. Ann Dermatol Syphiligr (Paris) (ser 3) 4:899, 1893.
59. Francois J: A new syndrome: Dyscephalis with bird face and dental anomalies, nanism, hypotrichosis, cutaneous atrophy, microphthalmia and congenital cataracts. Arch Ophthalmol 60:842, 1958.
60. Mobius PJ: Ueber angeborene doppel seitige Abduceus-Facialis-Lahmung. Munch Med Wochenschr 35:91, 1888.
61. Evans PR: Nuclear agenesis: Mobius' syndrome: The congenital facial diplegia syndrome. Arch Dis Child 30:237, 1955.
62. Henderson JL: Congenital facial diplegia syndrome: Clinical features, pathology and aetiology, a review of 61 cases. Brain 62:381, 1939.
63. Lindeman RC. Diverting the paralyzed larynx: A reversible procedure for intractable aspiration. Laryngoscope 85:157–180, 1975.
64. Cohen SR, Thompson JW: Variants of Mobius' syndrome and central neurologic impairment. Lindeman procedure in children. Ann Otol Rhinol Laryngol 96(1 Pt 1):93–100, 1987.
65. Freeman EA, Sheldon, JH: Cranio-carpo-tarsal dystrophy: An undescribed congenital malformation. Arch Dis Child 13:277, 1938.
66. Robinson PJ: Freeman Sheldon syndrome: Severe upper airway obstruction requiring neonatal tracheostomy. Pediatr Pulmonol 23:457–459, 1997.
67. Denny AD, Talisman R, Hanson PR, et al: Mandibular distraction osteogenesis in very young patients to correct airway obstruction. Plast Reconstr Surg 108:302–311, 2001.
68. Wang RY, Earl DL, Ruder RO, et al: Syndromic ear anomalies and renal ultrasounds. Pediatrics 108:E32, 2001.
69. Opitz C, Stoll C, Ring P: Nager syndrome. Problems and possibilities of therapy. J Orofac Orthop 61:226–236, 2000.
70. Vargervik K: Mandibular malformations: Growth characteristics and management in hemifacial microsomia and Nager syndrome. Acta Odontol Scand 56:331–338, 1998.
71. Friedman RA, Wood E, Pransky SM, et al: Nager acrofacial dysostosis: Management of a difficult airway. Int J Pediatr Otorhinolaryngol 35:69–72, 1996.
72. Zori RT, Gray BA, Bent-Williams A, et al: Preaxial acrofacial dysostosis (Nager syndrome) associated with an inherited and apparently balanced X;9 translocation: Prenatal and postnatal late replication studies. Am J Med Genet 46:379–383, 1993.
73. Hoka S, Sato M, Yoshitake J, et al: Management of a newborn infant with congenital laryngeal atresia. Anesth Analg 69:535, 1989.
74. Dolkart LA, Reimers FT, Wertheimer IS, et al: Prenatal diagnosis of laryngeal atresia. J Ultrasound Med 11:496, 1992.
75. Holinger PH, Brown WI: Congenital webs, cysts, laryngoceles, and other anomalies of the larynx. Ann Otol Rhinol Laryngol 76:744, 1967.
76. Cavanagh F: Stridor in children: Congenital laryngeal web. Proc R Soc Med 58:273, 1965.
77. Pennington CL: The treatment of anterior glottic webs: A reevaluation of Haslinger's technique. Laryngoscope 78:728, 1968.
78. Cohen SR: Congenital glottic webs in children. A retrospective review of 51 patients. Ann Otol Rhinol Laryngol Suppl 121:2–16, 1985.
79. Simon NP: Evaluation and management of stridor in the newborn. Clin Pediatr 30:211, 1991.
80. Chu L, Gussack GS, Orr JB, et al: Neonatal laryngoceles. A cause for airway obstruction. Arch Otolaryngol Head Neck Surg 120:454–458, 1994.
81. Richards DS, Yancey MK, Duff P, et al: The perinatal management of severe laryngeal stenosis. Obstet Gynecol 80(3 Pt 2):537–540, 1992.
82. Fearon B, Ellis D: The management of long term airway problems in infants and children. Ann Otol Rhinol Laryngol 80:669, 1971.
83. Narcy P, Contencin P, Fligny I, et al: Surgical treatment for laryngotracheal stenosis in the pediatric patient. Arch Otolaryngol Head Neck Surg 116:1047, 1990.
84. Cameron AH, Williams TC: Cleft larynx: A cause of laryngeal obstruction and incompetence. J Laryngol Otol 76:381, 1962.
85. Myer CM 3rd, Cotton RT, Holmes DK, et al: Laryngeal and laryngotracheoesophageal clefts: Role of early surgical repair. Ann Otol Rhinol Laryngol 99(2 Pt 1):98–104, 1990.
86. Holinger LD, Tansek KM, Tucker GF Jr: Cleft larynx with airway obstruction. Ann Otol Rhinol Laryngol 94(6 Pt 1):622–626, 1985.
87. Bennett EJ, Tsuchiya T, Stephen CR: Stridor and upper airway obstruction in infants. Anesth Analg (Cleve) 48:76, 1969.
88. Cohen SR: Unusual lesions of the larynx, trachea, and bronchial tree. Ann Otol Rhinol Laryngol 78:476, 1969.
89. Downing GJ, Hayen LK, Kilbride HW: Acquired subglottic cysts in the low-birth-weight infant. Characteristics, treatment, and outcome. Am J Dis Child 147:971–974, 1993.
90. Pak MW, Woo JK, van Hasselt CA: Congenital laryngeal cysts: Current approach to management. J Laryngol Otol 110:854–856, 1996.
91. Booth JB, Birck HG: Operative treatment and postoperative management of saccular cyst and laryngocele. Arch Otolaryngol 107:500–502, 1981.
92. Richardson MA, Cotton RT: Anatomic abnormalities of the pediatric airway. Pediatr Clin North Am 31:821–834, 1984.
93. Loeff DS, Filler RM: Congenital tracheal stenosis: A review of 22 patients from 1965–87. J Pediatr Surg 23:744–748, 1988.
94. Wolman IJ: Congenital stenosis of the trachea. Am J Dis Child 61:1263, 1941.
95. Hoffer ME, Tom LW, Wetmore RF, et al: Congenital tracheal stenosis. The otolaryngologist's perspective. Arch Otolaryngol Head Neck Surg 120:449–453, 1994.
96. Metlay LA, MacPherson TA, Doshi N, et al: A new iatrogenous lesion in newborns requiring assisted ventilation [letter]. N Engl J Med 309:111, 1983.

97. Tolkin J, Kirpalani H, Fitzhardinge P, et al: Necrotizing tracheobronchitis: A new complication of neonatal mechanical ventilation [abstract]. Pediatr Res 18:391A, 1984.

98. Kirpalani H, Higa T, Perlman M, et al: Diagnosis and therapy of necrotizing tracheobronchitis in ventilated neonates. Crit Care Med 13:792–797, 1985.

99. Pietsch JB, Hagaraj HS, Groff DB, et al: Necrotizing tracheobronchitis: A new indication for emergency bronchoscopy in the neonate. J Pediatr Surg 20:391, 1985.

100. Rubin SZ, Trevenen CL, Mitchell I: Diffuse necrotizing tracheobronchitis: An acute and chronic disease. J Pediatr Surg 23:476, 1988.

101. Duff B, Gruber B: Total tracheobronchial thrombosis due to extracorporeal membrane oxygenation. Ann Otol Rhinol Laryngol 105:259–261, 1996.

102. Dunbar JS: Upper respiratory obstruction in infants and children: The Caldwell lecture (1969). Am J Roentgenol Radium Ther Nucl Med 109:227, 1970.

103. Fearon B, Shortreed R: Tracheobronchial compression by congenital cardiovascular anomalies in children: Syndrome of apnea. Ann Otol Rhinol Laryngol 72:949, 1963.

104. Gustafson LM, Liu JH, Link DT, et al: Spiral CT versus MRI in neonatal airway evaluation. Int J Pediatr Otorhinolaryngol 52:197–201, 2000.

105. Nidaidoh H, Riker WL, Idriss FS: Surgical management of "vascular rings." Arch Surg 105:327, 1972.

106. Gross RE: Surgical relief for tracheal obstruction from a vascular ring. N Engl J Med 233:586, 1945.

107. Arciniegas E, Hakimi M, Hertzler JH, et al: Surgical management of congenital vascular rings. J Thorac Cardiovasc Surg 77:721, 1979.

108. Richardson JV, Doty DB, Rossi NP, et al: Operation for aortic arch anomalies. Ann Thorac Surg 31:426, 1981.

109. Backer CL, Ilbawi MN, Idriss FS, et al: Vascular anomalies causing tracheoesophageal compression: Review of experience in children. J Thorac Cardiovasc Surg 97:725, 1989.

110. Sade RM, Rosenthal A, Fellows K: Pulmonary artery sling. J Thorac Cardiovasc Surg 69:333, 1975.

CARDIOVASCULAR ASPECTS

VICTOR W. LUCAS, Jr, MD
HARLEY G. GINSBERG, MD

Optimal management of the mechanically ventilated infant requires a thorough understanding of the fetal and neonatal cardiovascular systems and of pulmonary development and pathophysiology. The lungs and heart function essentially as a unit and frequently are simultaneously and interdependently involved in disease states, especially in the newborn. Moreover, the unique flow and pressure characteristics of the transitional circulation present at birth often complicate a primary pulmonary disorder. For example, the preterm infant with respiratory distress syndrome (RDS) often develops congestive heart failure (CHF) related to a patent ductus arteriosus (PDA).[1] To evaluate and treat these complex conditions, the clinician must be able to separate the contributions of each system to the disease process. In addition, the common findings of cyanosis and respiratory distress in the term or near-term infant may be ascribed to either the cardiovascular or the pulmonary system; thus, their presence often makes precise diagnosis unclear and difficult. Knowledge of symptom complexes and their presentations, in combination with the aid of a few simple laboratory studies, enables the primary physician to consider the differential diagnosis and begin appropriate treatment.

This chapter examines the differential diagnoses of cardiac disease in the critically ill neonate, the fetal circulation, and the changes in the cardiopulmonary circulation that occur at birth and shortly thereafter. Specific conditions reviewed are persistent pulmonary hypertension of the newborn (PPHN), PDA in the preterm neonate, and medical therapy of the neonate with CHF. A detailed discussion of the postoperative management of neonates with congenital heart disease and its implications for mechanically ventilated newborns follows.

RECOGNITION AND MANAGEMENT OF THE NEONATE WITH SUSPECTED HEART DISEASE

Primary cardiac disease and the cardiovascular aspects and complications of pulmonary disease are common problems in all neonatal intensive care units. In the early neonatal period, deaths due to cardiovascular disease are surpassed in number only by those associated with prematurity. In a review of 510 consecutive neonatal interhospital transfers compiled by Merenstein and Way,[2] 39 transfers (7%) were primarily for cardiac disease. This figure did not include infants who were transferred for other reasons but had associated or secondary cardiac disease, such as RDS with a PDA or perinatal asphyxia

with ventricular dysfunction. Although many neonates with congenital heart disease are diagnosed by fetal echocardiography before birth, most infants with structural heart lesions are not discovered until after delivery. Table 23-1 lists the most common congenital heart defects based on age of presentation in the neonatal period.

The neonate with suspected heart disease may be evaluated in the modern neonatal intensive care unit in a more sophisticated and expeditious manner than was possible only a few years ago, and a definitive diagnosis can be made relatively accurately with minimally invasive techniques. Careful consideration and anticipation of the most likely diagnosis greatly improve the quality of an infant's initial care and have a positive influence on the eventual outcome.

Occasionally, the pediatrician or neonatologist may have difficulty in ascribing abnormal cardiopulmonary findings in a newborn to primary cardiac or respiratory origins. This may delay referral to a pediatric cardiologist or performance of definitive diagnostic evaluation (echocardiogram). Some clues to a cardiac diagnosis are as follows:

TABLE 23-1. Frequency Distribution of Congenital Heart Defects Based on Age at Diagnosis

Diagnosis	Percentage of Patients
Age on Admission: 0–6 days (N = 537)	
D-Transposition of the great arteries	19
Hypoplastic left heart syndrome	14
Tetralogy of Fallot	8
Coarctation of the aorta	7
Ventricular septal defect	3
Other	49
Age on Admission: 7–13 days (N = 195)	
Coarctation of the aorta	16
Ventricular septal defect	14
Hypoplastic left heart syndrome	8
D-Transposition of the great arteries	7
Tetralogy of Fallot	7
Other	48
Age on Admission: 14–28 days (N = 177)	
Ventricular septal defect	16
Coarctation of the aorta	12
Tetralogy of Fallot	7
D-Transposition of the great arteries	7
Patent ductus arteriosus	5
Others	53

Adapted from Flanagan MF, Fyler DC: Cardiac disease. In Avery GB, Fletcher MA, MacDonald M (eds): Neonatology: Pathophysiology and Management of the Newborn. Philadelphia, JB Lippincott, 1994, p. 524, with permission.

1. Heart rate increases before respiratory rate. In respiratory disease the opposite occurs.
2. Symptoms are delayed until 3 to 5 days after birth. Generally symptoms of respiratory disease occur at birth or within 1 to 2 days.
3. An electrocardiogram (ECG) demonstrates increased P-wave amplitude and/or left ventricular hypertrophy. The ECG of a normal neonatal heart reveals right ventricular hypertrophy. These abnormal findings suggest a large right atrium of tricuspid atresia or pulmonary atresia.
4. The chest x-ray film shows decreased pulmonary blood flow or the lung fields are normal or very dark. Respiratory diseases should reveal atelectasis, infiltrates, or air leaks on chest x-ray film.
5. Increasing the inspired oxygen concentration does not significantly improve the PaO_2. In respiratory disease, unless there is significant pulmonary hypertension, the PaO_2 should rise with increasing oxygen concentration.

Differential Diagnosis of Cardiac Disease in the Neonate

The newborn infant is referred for evaluation of suspected heart disease generally because of the appearance of one ore more of the following findings: heart murmur, abnormal heart rate or rhythm, CHF, cyanosis, or respiratory distress, or a combination of any of these conditions.[3]

Heart Murmur

Cardiac murmurs resulting from semilunar valve stenosis (aortic and pulmonary valves) and atrioventricular valve regurgitation (mitral and tricuspid valves) usually can be detected with the use of a stethoscope shortly after birth. The murmur associated with peripheral pulmonary artery stenosis is frequently noted quite early as well. Those defects whose murmurs depend on the pressure and resistance changes related to the transition from fetal to postnatal circulation are likely to appear somewhat later (at 1 to 2 days of life); the PDA and the small ventricular septal defect typify this category. Many serious defects (e.g., dextro-transposition, univentricular hearts) may present without murmurs in the neonatal period. Therefore, the initial absence of significant auscultatory findings in no way excludes cardiac disease.

Rhythm Disturbances

The two most common arrhythmias encountered in the newborn period are supraventricular tachycardia and congenital complete atrioventricular block, with or without underlying associated structural cardiac malformations.[4] Other less important rhythm disturbances (e.g., premature atrial beats) also are frequently seen. It is now possible in many cases to detect rhythm abnormalities with electronic fetal monitoring and fetal echocardiography. These modalities provide the clinician with advance warning and an opportunity for pharmacologic intervention in utero if indicated. After delivery, rhythm abnormalities are evaluated with standard ECG.

Congestive Heart Failure in the Neonate

CHF that is present at birth is a serious and ominous situation. The more common left-to-right shunt lesions (atrial septal defect, ventricular septal defect, PDA) do not present with CHF because of the unique pressure and resistance characteristics of the transitional circulation.[5] Common right-to-left shunt lesions (e.g., tetralogy of Fallot) are rarely associated with CHF at any age because of the reduced pulmonary blood flow and the absence of volume overload on the heart. Those situations that do give rise to CHF at birth are more likely due to rhythm or rate abnormalities (e.g., complete heart block, supraventricular tachycardia), impaired myocardial contractility (e.g., viral myocarditis, asphyxia, anomalous coronary artery), or a metabolic disturbance (e.g., thyrotoxicosis). The possibility of a peripheral arteriovenous malformation as a cause of CHF should not be overlooked; the most common of these anomalies involves the great vein of Galen and is manifest on auscultation by a continuous murmur over the skull. Those rare structural defects that present with CHF at birth usually are related to severe atrioventricular valve regurgitation (Ebstein's anomaly, atrioventricular septal defects) or to obstruction of pulmonary venous return (total anomalous pulmonary venous return). Critical aortic stenosis occasionally may present with CHF, but the typical murmur may not be present until appropriate measures are taken in order to improve ventricular function and, thus, cardiac output.[6]

Clinical Approach to the Infant with Suspected Heart Disease

The appropriate differential diagnosis of congenital heart disease is derived from consideration of the information in the history, the findings on clinical evaluation, and the results of the following simple laboratory studies:

1. Chest radiography
2. Electrocardiography
3. Doppler echocardiography
4. Arterial blood gas analysis (to include evaluation of simultaneous preductal and postductal samples)
5. Blood chemistry analysis (to include determination of electrolytes, glucose, and blood urea nitrogen)
6. Complete blood count

Maternal history may provide clues to diagnosis. For example, infants of diabetic mothers have a greater incidence of transposition of the great arteries and hypoplastic left heart syndrome.[7] All infants of diabetic mothers should be screened for low blood sugar levels because the cardiomyopathy associated with hypoglycemia may mimic congenital heart disease.

Clinical findings. Observation of the respiratory pattern may be useful in assessing the newborn with suspected heart disease. The normal respiratory rate for term newborns 2 hours after birth is less than 45 breaths/min. Table 23-2 lists some general guidelines for evaluating respiratory patterns with respect to specific disease states.

Observation of an infant's overall activity may provide pertinent information. Cyanosis and respiratory distress in a lethargic, nonresponsive infant suggest a central nervous system problem (e.g., intracranial hemorrhage), shock, or an overwhelming infection (e.g., sepsis, meningitis), rather than primary cardiac disease.

Palpation of the precordial area for assessment of cardiac activity and auscultation of the heart and lungs for detection of murmurs and abnormal respiratory sounds should be components of the initial physical examination. Cardiac examination

TABLE 23-2.   Respiratory Patterns and Specific Disease Processes

Condition	Respiration Rate	Cyanosis	Depth of Respiratory (Tidal Volume)	Intercostal Retractions	Periodic Breathing or Apnea	Grunting or Flaring of Alae Nasae
Primary pulmonary condition	+	+/−	−	+	+/−	+
Left-sided heart failure or pulmonary overcirculation	+	+/−	−	+	−	+
CHD with significant R → L shunt	+/−	++	+	+	−	−
RDS	++	+	−	++	+/−	++
Central nervous system disease	+/−	+	−	+/−	++	+/−
Pneumonia (sepsis)	+	+/−	+/−	+	+	+
Heart failure with pneumonia	++	+/−	+/−	+/−	+/−	+

CHD, congenital heart disease; R → L, right-to-left; RDS, respiratory distress syndrome.

should include careful scrutiny of the brachial and femoral pulses. Diminution or absence of the femoral pulses strongly suggests coarctation of the aorta, whereas full or bounding pulses are associated with PDA or some other aortic runoff lesion.[8]

Cyanosis

Cyanosis is simply defined as a dusky bluish color of the skin and mucous membranes. Clinically, two types of cyanosis can be identified: peripheral and central. *Peripheral cyanosis* exists when systemic arterial oxygen (O_2) saturation is normal but extraction of O_2 at the tissue level is increased. Clinically, duskiness or frank blueness of the nailbeds and peripheral extremities is seen, but the mucous membranes and tongue are pink. Peripheral cyanosis is not generally associated with significant underlying pathologic processes and usually is due to autonomic alterations in the distribution of blood flow to the skin.[9]

In contrast, *central cyanosis* exists when a pathologic process results in inadequate oxygenation of arterial blood or an admixture of venous with arterial blood. It is characterized clinically by blueness of the mucous membranes and tongue, as well as of the peripheral extremities and nailbeds. Usually the underlying pathologic process is cardiac or pulmonary, but occasionally it is hematologic or related to the central nervous system.

A number of factors influence one's ability to recognize cyanosis clinically. From a biochemical standpoint, approximately 5 g of reduced hemoglobin must be present in the circulating blood if cyanosis is to be detected with the naked eye. The bias of the observer is an important factor; a skilled nurse who is experienced in working with newborns frequently is the first to recognize the cyanotic baby in the nursery. Determination of whether cyanosis is peripheral or central may require more careful study. Other factors influencing detection of cyanosis include the site of blood gas sampling (preductal vs postductal), hemoglobin concentration (anemia vs polycythemia), and cardiac output. Arterial O_2 tension (PaO_2) is related to the affinity of hemoglobin for the oxygen molecule and is influenced biochemically by the amount of fetal hemoglobin, pH, temperature, and other factors.

Causes of cyanosis. Although many situations produce clinical cyanosis, only five possible basic physiologic abnormalities cause arterial desaturation.[9] Occasionally, two or more mechanisms may coexist, but in most clinical situations one predominates. The five abnormalities are as follows:

1. Alveolar hypoventilation
2. Right-to-left shunt
3. Ventilation-perfusion mismatching
4. Impairment of gas diffusion
5. Decreased affinity of hemoglobin for O_2

Alveolar hypoventilation. Alveolar hypoventilation occurs when inadequate gas exchange at the alveolar level leads to an accumulation of carbon dioxide (CO_2) and a reduction of O_2 in the circulating blood. Examples of conditions that give rise to such a state include central nervous system depression (intracranial hemorrhage, drugs) and disease that involves the lungs and the respiratory passages themselves. The latter includes the following:

1. Obstructions, as in choanal atresia
2. Space-occupying lesions, as in diaphragmatic hernia
3. Decreased pulmonary parenchyma, as in hypoplastic lungs
4. Decreased pulmonary compliance, as in RDS
5. Abnormal neuromuscular control, as in spinal muscular atrophy

Right-to-left shunt. In right-to-left shunt, a portion of the pulmonary arterial blood bypasses normally ventilated alveoli. This bypass results in the admixture of desaturated blood and normally oxygenated (arterial) blood. The majority of cyanotic congenital heart defects fall into this category. The classic example is tetralogy of Fallot, in which a portion of right ventricular blood completely bypasses the lung and is ejected through the ventricular septal defect directly into the aorta. Other examples are PPHN, with atrial and ductal right-to-left shunts, and intrapulmonary arteriovenous malformations.

Ventilation-perfusion mismatching. Two situations in ventilation-perfusion mismatching may cause arterial desaturation: decreased alveolar ventilation with normal or increased perfusion, and normal alveolar ventilation with decreased perfusion. In both cases, a mismatch between ventilation and perfusion occurs. Both are associated in the neonate with aspiration syndromes and regional atelectasis.

Impairment of diffusion. Impairment of diffusion is a relatively uncommon situation in newborns but may result when the acceleration of blood flow through the lungs (as in the presence of fever, atrioventricular malformation) permits insufficient time for adequate diffusion of O_2 from the alveolus into the blood. Arterial desaturation is the consequence.

Abnormal hemoglobin molecule. Certain biochemical abnormalities of the hemoglobin molecule may prevent normal coupling with O_2 and result in arterial desaturation in the presence of a normal PaO_2. The most common cause is methemoglobinemia, which commonly results from exposure to certain oxidants (nitrites, sulfonamides) or, occasionally, from a congenital deficiency of the enzyme methemoglobin reductase. Methemoglobinemia is a rare cause of clinical cyanosis, but it should not be overlooked if the more common abnormalities have been excluded.

PERSISTENT PULMONARY HYPERTENSION OF THE NEWBORN

Initial Description

In 1969, Gersony et al.[10] described "PFC syndrome" (persistence of the fetal circulation). This term has been used synonymously with PPHN; however the latter term (PPHN) is preferred because the neonatal circulation does not include the placenta. The original report described patients with "persistent characteristics of the fetal circulation in the absence of recognizable cardiac, pulmonary, hematologic or central nervous system disease." Suprasystemic pulmonary artery pressures were documented, resulting in right-to-left shunting of blood through the ductus arteriosus, foramen ovale, or both.

Fetal Circulation

Oxygenated blood leaves the placenta via the umbilical vein with a Po_2 of 30 to 40 mm Hg. Flow continues toward the left lobe of the liver and then into the portal sinus. The ductus venosus is supplied from the sinus. After traversing the liver, blood is joined by flow from the hepatic veins and empties into the inferior vena cava. Blood from the lower portion of the body mixes in the inferior vena cava with the relatively well-oxygenated blood from the placenta. Due to specific anatomic characteristics of the right atrium (Fig. 23-1), most flow (two thirds) is directed from the inferior vena cava into the right atrium to mix with blood from SVC. This blood is pumped from the right ventricle into the pulmonary artery. The remaining third passes through the foramen ovale where it mixes with pulmonary venous blood. This blood is pumped to the left ventricle and out the ascending aorta to the upper extremities, neck, and head. Approximately 90% of the right ventricular output is directed down the ductus arteriosus. The remaining 10% of flow supplies the lungs via the pulmonary artery. Systemic vascular resistance (SVR), being approximately one tenth that of the pulmonary vascular resistance (Fig. 23-2), enhances the shunting of blood from the pulmonary vascular tree to the aorta through the ductus arteriosus. The circuit is completed when blood from the aorta traverses the umbilical arteries and reaches the placenta.

Epidemiology

The incidence of PPHN has been estimated by some authors to occur in approximately 0.1% to 0.2% of all liveborn infants.[11–13] The majority of babies with PPHN are term or post term. Prematurity, however, does not exclude the diagnosis of PPHN because many of the alleged inciting influences that may be responsible for PPHN can exist throughout any part of the latter half of gestation. No race- or gender-related predispositions have been noted.

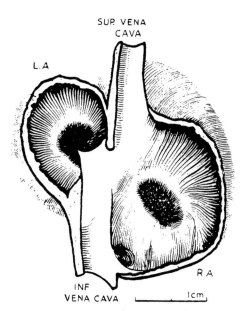

Figure 23-1. Posterior aspect of the human fetal heart at 34 weeks' gestation, with vena cava removed. INF, inferior; LA, left atrium; RA, right atrium; SUP, superior. (From Barclay AE: The Foetal Circulation and Cardiovascular System. Springfield, Ill., Charles C. Thomas, Publisher, 1945.)

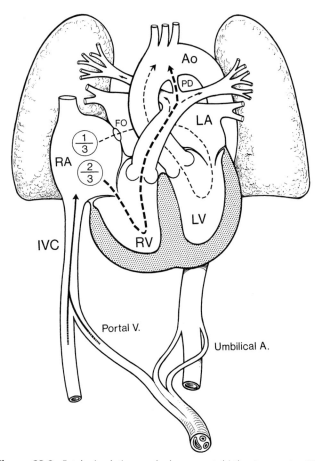

Figure 23-2. Fetal circulation and changes at birth. Ao, aorta; FO, foramen ovale; IVC, inferior vena cava; LA, left atrium; LV, left ventricle; PD, patent ductus; Portal V., portal vein; RA, right atrium; RV, right ventricle; Umbilical A., umbilical artery.

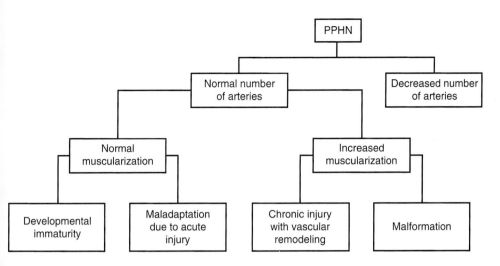

Figure 23-3. Persistent pulmonary hypertension of the newborn (PPHN) may arise from a number of different underlying pathologic states. (From Walsh-Sukys M: Persistent pulmonary hypertension of the newborn. Clin Perinatol 20:129, 1993.)

Cardiorespiratory Changes at Birth

A critical sequence of events must occur immediately after birth if an infant is to achieve adequate oxygenation and ventilation necessary for extrauterine survival. Once clamping of the umbilical cord occurs, the placental flow ceases and SVR increases. Gas exchange for the infant must then be transferred from the placenta to the lung. Pulmonary vascular bed resistance (PVR) decreases as the first breath is taken. Alveoli, which were fluid filled during fetal life, are now distended with gas, and their surface tension falls. Oxygenation is believed to play a significant role in the reduction of pulmonary vascular resistance.[14,15] Other factors contributing to decreasing pulmonary vascular resistance include lung expansion and absorption of fetal lung fluid. Vasoactive substances such as adenosine, bradykinin, prostacyclin, and endogenous nitric oxide (NO) are released and augment the decrease in pulmonary vascular resistance.

With the increase in SVR and the decrease in PVR, blood flow through the ductus arteriosus becomes left to right. The increase in the circulation to the lungs results in an increase in blood return to the left atrium and leads to functional closure of the foramen ovale. In the healthy newborn, the ductus arteriosus is believed to close over the first 24 hours of life. In certain conditions, such as hypoxia, acidosis, or sepsis, the ductus may reopen.[16]

During uterine life, the pulmonary artery and its main branches are similar to the ductus arteriosus and aorta with respect to histology of their muscular walls. The medial component or layer is smooth muscle. During the final trimester, progressive development of this layer occurs. Hypertrophy of this muscle layer may result from fetal hypoxia,[17] exposure to prostaglandin synthetase inhibitors,[18] and systemic hypertension.

Shortly after birth, a decrease in pulmonary vascular resistance is essential for survival and is accomplished by an increase in the lumen size with a decrease in arteriolar wall muscle thickness. With the first breath, alveoli are distended with gas, and capillaries are stretched proximal to these alveolar sacs. Although most of the PVR decline is accomplished in the first day, it may not be complete for 1 to 2 weeks.[19] The pulmonary circuit appears to be very sensitive to noxious stimuli, and although smooth muscle hypertrophy may take days, smooth muscle spasm can occur rapidly. Although the insulting

agent may be removed, the vasoconstrictive response may take time to "undo." Failure of the pulmonary vascular resistance to decrease and remain low results in PPHN.

PPHN is perhaps best considered the end product of a multifactorial chain of events. Walsh-Sukys[19] presented a modification of the scheme proposed by Geggel and Reid in 1984 (Fig. 23-3). Inciting stimuli include disorders of cardiac or respiratory origin such as sepsis, pneumonia, meconium aspiration pneumonitis, asphyxia, RDS, congenital diaphragmatic hernia, primary pulmonary hypoplasia, and pulmonary hypoplasia from the oligohydramnios sequence. Occasionally PPHN is idiopathic. Although infants with pulmonary hypoplasia and congenital diaphragmatic hernia may have PPHN as a result of an underlying pulmonary blood flow restriction, it is believed that PPHN in most patients is precipitated by chronic in utero hypoxia or maladaptation to the extrauterine environment.

Vasoactive substances have been shown to be capable of local blood flow regulation. Arachidonic acid is metabolized to several vasoactive agents, such as prostaglandins, thromboxanes, and leukotrienes. Bradykinin and endothelium-derived relaxing factor (EDRF) are known vasodilators as well. Some of the vasoactive substances may be intermediaries with regard to direct actions on the endothelial lining. EDRF is now believed to be a gas, NO.[20] NO has been shown to be a potent and selective pulmonary vasodilator, both in the laboratory and clinically.[21–25] NO is released from endothelial cells, vascular smooth muscle, macrophages, and platelets. It is bound tightly to hemoglobin and is rapidly oxidized, with a half-life measured in seconds. Inhaled NO (iNO) has recently become available as another mode of therapy in the treatment of PPHN in term and near-term infants. Preterm newborns with PPHN must qualify through specific research protocols to be eligible for iNO therapy. This agent is discussed later in this chapter and in Chapter 14. Active research in the uses of this agent is currently underway.

Diagnosis

Hypoxemia in a newborn out of proportion to the degree of parenchymal lung disease should prompt the clinician to consider the diagnosis of PPHN. Demonstration of right-to-left shunting through the ductus arteriosus or across the foramen ovale in light of normal cardiac examination findings should confirm this diagnosis. The most reliable and readily available method for determining PPHN may vary based on the clinical setting.

Diagnosis of PPHN may be established using a combination of the following techniques.

Physical Examination

In primary PPHN (without underlying pulmonary disease), an infant's color may appear intermittently normal or cyanotic due to the amount of shunting and the resultant systemic PaO_2. Auscultation of the thorax should reveal equal breath sounds bilaterally. The cardiac examination may reveal a single loud S_2. The physiologic "splitting" of the S_2 should return as the pulmonary hypertension subsides.

Hyperoxia Test

This test is frequently used to distinguish structural cardiac deformities from pulmonary disease. The patient is administered 100% O_2 for 5 to 10 minutes; the arterial PO_2 is then compared with the PaO_2 obtained previously. An increase in PaO_2 to greater than 150 mm Hg excludes most types of cyanotic heart defects and suggests a diagnosis of parenchymal lung disease. However, should the PaO_2 not increase, neither cyanotic heart disease nor PPHN can be eliminated from the differential diagnosis.[26] Interpretation of the hyperoxia text is given in Table 23-3.

Preductal and Postductal PaO_2

Based on the degree and location of right-to-left shunting, various levels of oxygenation are observed from preductal sites (right radial or right temporal arteries) and postductal sites (umbilical artery or lower extremity). A preductal PaO_2 of 20 mm Hg or higher compared with postductal PaO_2 is considered significant. The absence of this gradient does not exclude

PPHN because shunting at the atrial level creates no appreciable difference in preductal and postductal measurements. Detectable gradients only occur if shunting occurs from right to left across the ductus arteriosus.

Echocardiography

Two-dimensional echocardiography with color flow Doppler imaging capability is a noninvasive technique that provides very specific information about the structural integrity of the heart and about any shunting of blood flow. It can define the direction and level of shunting (ductal or atrial), along with the resultant cardiac effects such as tricuspid or pulmonic valve regurgitation. Serial two-dimensional echocardiography is beneficial in determining volume status, pump function, and cardiac response to inotropic agents.

Hyperoxia-Hyperventilation Test

In an intubated infant, the concentration of inspired O_2 is maximized and hyperventilation is begun. A ventilatory rate of greater than 100 breaths/min is established for 5 to 10 minutes, and a "critical" PaO_2 is sought. With a $PaCO_2$ that is usually less than 30 mm Hg (and not infrequently less than 20 mm Hg), a rapid improvement in systemic oxygenation associated with a decrease in pulmonary artery pressure may be seen, supporting a diagnosis of PPHN.

Cardiac Catheterization

Cardiac catheterization is reserved for a very select few infants whose diagnosis may be in doubt despite the application of the diagnostic methods listed previously. Cardiac catheterization and angiocardiography may be helpful in the evaluation of the patient who is suspected of having total anomalous pulmonary venous return with obstruction that cannot be

TABLE 23-3. Interpretation of the Hyperoxia Test

	$FiO_2 = 0.21$		$FiO_2 = 1$	
	PaO_2 (% saturation)		PaO_2 (% saturation)	$PaCO_2$
Normal	70 (95)		>300 (100)	35
Pulmonary disease	50 (85)		>150 (100)	50
Neurologic disease	50 (85)		>150 (100)	50
Methemoglobinemia	70 (95)		>200 (100)	35
Cardiac disease				
Parallel circulation*	<40 (<75)		<50 (<85)	35
Mixing with restricted PBF†	<40 (<75)		<50 (<85)	35
Mixing without restricted PBF‡	40–60 (75–93)		<150 (<100)	35
	Preductal	**Postductal**		
Differential cyanosis§	70 (95)	<40 (<75)	Variable	35–50
Reverse differential cyanosis‖	<40 (<75)	>50 (>90)	Variable	35–50

* D-transposition of the great arteries with intact ventricular septum or D-transposition of the great arteries with ventricular septal defect.
† Tricuspid atresia with pulmonary stenosis or atresia, pulmonary atresia or critical pulmonary stenosis with intact ventricular septum, or tetralogy of Fallot.
‡ Truncus arteriosus, total anomalous pulmonary venous return, single ventricle, or hypoplastic left heart syndrome.
§ Persistent pulmonary hypertension of the newborn or left ventricular outflow tract obstruction (aortic arch hypoplasia, interrupted aortic arch, critical coarctation, and critical aortic stenosis).
‖ D-transposition of the great arteries with coarctation of the aorta or interrupted aortic arch, or D-transposition of the great arteries and pulmonary hypertension.
PBF, pulmonary blood flow
Adapted from Barone MA (ed): The Harriet Lane Handbook, 14th ed. St. Louis, Mosby–Year Book, 1996; p. 155, with permission.

excluded by two-dimensional echocardiography. If possible, a Swan-Ganz catheter should be positioned in the pulmonary artery because it will be useful in guiding pharmacologic and ventilator therapy. Catheterization is only used sparingly because of the delicate nature of these patients and their intolerance to manipulation.

With no single best test for the diagnosis of PPHN, it is not surprising that more than one formula can be used for assessment of the severity of disease. Presently, the two formulas most frequently used are for the determination of the alveolar-arterial O_2 gradient ($PaO_2 - PaO_2$) and for the calculation of the O_2 index. For an in-depth discussion of these formulas, please refer to Chapter 16 on extracorporeal membrane oxygenation (ECMO). Of the two formulas, we currently find the one for O_2 index to be more useful because the O_2 index reflects the barotrauma that the patient is experiencing.

Treatment

Ideally, the treatment for PPHN should be effective and leave the patient with no long-term sequelae. Unfortunately, none of the currently available therapies can boast of this outcome with any certainty. Prompt diagnosis and referral to a tertiary medical center when appropriate should limit the mortality and, it is hoped, the morbidity associated with PPHN. Therapy, whether pharmacologic or ventilatory, should be directed toward the reduction of pulmonary artery pressure. A useful protocol for the management of neonates with PPHN is shown in Figure 23-4 (modification of a proposal by Walsh-Sukys[19]).

Ventilation Therapy

Two distinctly different modes of ventilation have been suggested for use in the treatment of PPHN. The management goals of these different techniques are summarized in Table 23-4.[19]

Hyperventilation. After the sensitivity of the pulmonary vascular bed was documented in infants, trials to achieve alkalosis by decreasing the arterial CO_2 tension ($PaCO_2$) were performed and revealed an improvement in oxygenation as well as a decrease in the pulmonary artery pressure. Hyperventilation has since become a popular mode of therapy, especially as the sophistication and reliability of neonatal ventilators has improved. With improved exhalation mechanics,

inadvertent positive end-expiratory pressure (PEEP) is reduced, and the mean airway pressure needed to achieve "critical" PaO_2 is decreased. In some infants, the "critical" $PaCO_2$ may be reached at less than 20 mm Hg (usually with subsequent pH >7.5). Frequently, in order to achieve these pH values and depressed $PaCO_2$ levels, high-frequency or oscillatory ventilation is required. Unfortunately, successful hyperventilation does not mean successful neurodevelopmental outcome. In animal models, decreased O_2 consumption and cerebral blood flow resulted from hyperventilation when $PaCO_2$ was maintained at 20 mm Hg or less.[27,28] Hyperventilation and subsequent reduction in cerebral blood flow may exacerbate cerebral ischemia in patients who have already experienced some degree of hypoxemia. Severe hypocarbia may be partly responsible for some aspects of the abnormal developmental

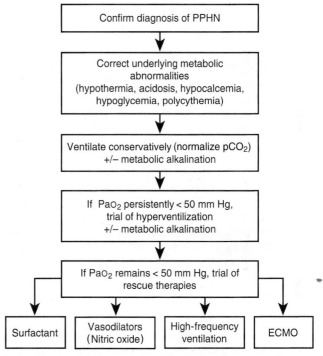

Figure 23-4. Proposed care protocol for the ventilatory management of neonates with persistent pulmonary hypertension of the newborn (PPHN). ECMO, extracorporeal membrane oxygenation. (Modified from Walsh-Sukys M: Persistent pulmonary hypertension of the newborn. Clin Perinatol 20:136, 1993.)

TABLE 23-4. Management Goals in an Aggressive Hyperventilation Approach and a More Conservative Ventilator Approach in Persistent Pulmonary Hypertension of the Newborn

	Hyperventilation*	Conservative Ventilation†
Target pH	≥7.5	≥7.25
Target $PaCO_2$ (mm Hg)	20–25	40–60
Target PaO_2 (mm Hg)	80–100	50–70
Rates (breaths/min)	Up to 100	Matched to patient's rate
Peak inspiratory pressure (cm H_2O)	High (may be >35 cm H_2O)	Minimum needed to produce chest rise
Inspiratory time (sec)	Short (0.2–0.3 sec)	Long (~0.6 sec)

* Data from Fox W, Duara S: Persistent pulmonary hypertension of the neonate: Diagnosis and clinical management. J Pediatr 103:505, 1983.
† Data from Wung JT, James LS, Kilchevsky E, et al: Management of infants with severe respiratory failure and PFC without hyperventilation. Pediatrics 76:488, 1985.

outcome seen in hyperventilated infants. In one study, over half of a group of patients who underwent hyperventilation as treatment for PPHN had audiologic abnormalities.[29] Hyperventilation, therefore, should be reserved for patients who have failed to respond to conventional ventilation therapy.

Conventional ventilation. In at least one institution, attempts at a more conventional ventilator treatment of PPHN have proved successful.[30] Accepting a $Paco_2$ of 50 to 70 mm Hg and a Pao_2 of 40 to 60 mm Hg, investigators were able to oxygenate and ventilate infants adequately and did not observe any of the long-term sequelae that were seen with hyperventilation.

In 1989, similar results were reported by Dworetz et al.[31] with their use of conventional ventilation for treatment of infants with PPHN. Although no prospective, large-scale, controlled trials comparing hyperventilation with conventional ventilation have been performed, the limited successes of both methods have presented neonatologists with the option best suited to the patient.

Metabolic Alkalization

Rather than create alkalosis with hyperventilation, clinicians have used sodium bicarbonate or tromethamine (THAM) infusions to elevate the pH of PPHN patients. This therapy has been used in lambs,[32] but no randomized controlled trial in human newborns has been performed. If this mode of treatment is selected, the practitioner should be aware of potential metabolic derangements. Hypernatremia may result from sodium bicarbonate infusions that may increase total body water and produce (or exacerbate) pulmonary edema. Tromethamine can cause hypoglycemia, hypocalcemia, hyperkalemia (especially when urine output is diminished), and respiratory depression. Skin sloughing has been reported if tromethamine extravasation occurs. Often this method is used in conjunction with mild-to-moderate hyperventilation so that pH can be raised without driving $Paco_2$ to extremely low levels.

It was demonstrated in the NICHD observational study that the alkalosis produced from hyperventilation did not equate with one created by an infusion of alkali.[33] The reader should remember that an infusion of alkali results in an increase in the production of carbon dioxide. Excretion of CO_2 occurs primarily from the lungs; therefore, increased ventilator support may be necessary when an alkali infusion is elected.

Vasodilator Therapy

Various drugs have been tried, including tolazoline, isoproterenol, chlorpromazine, prostacyclin, and iNO (see Chapter 14). The success rate has varied, but the combination of sedation, blood pressure support, mild alkalosis, NO, and careful ventilatory management has reduced our need for ECMO by more than 50%. Tolazoline hydrochloride, an alpha-adrenergic blocking agent that affects vascular smooth muscle, causing vasodilation, increased cardiac output, and decreased pulmonary *and* systemic blood pressure, has recently been removed from the market and can no longer be recommended.

Prostacyclin (PGI_2), an extremely potent vasodilator, has been used in a very limited capacity for patients with PPHN. Expansion of the lungs at birth and shortly thereafter results in PGI_2 production. Prostacyclin has been demonstrated to decrease pulmonary vascular resistance by causing vasodila-

tion of both the pulmonary arteries and veins.[34] As with tolazoline, if PGI_2 therapy is undertaken, all preparations to treat acute systemic hypotension should be made.

Nitric Oxide

iNO is the latest addition to the therapies offered for treatment of PPHN. iNO, whether in its free state or as a portion of a nitrosocompound, was thought to be the agent previously referred to as *endothelium-derived relaxing factor* (EDRF). This gas has been proven to be both a selective and potent pulmonary vasodilator.[21-25] In 1980, Furchgott and Zawadski[35] demonstrated that EDRF was required for relaxation of blood vessel tone in response to pharmacologic stimuli. Ignarro et al.[36] identified EDRF as NO. Since then, other stimuli, including sheer stress and increased oxygenation, have been shown to liberate NO and result in sustained vasodilation. NO has a very short half-life and diffuses into the vascular smooth muscle, increasing the level of cyclic guanosine monophosphate (Fig. 23-5). Hemoglobin binds NO tightly after being generated by pulmonary endothelial cells and is rapidly oxidized and inactivated. The rapidity with which this occurs results in local activity without systemic effects when NO is utilized as inhalation therapy. The utilization of NO in the treatment of neonatal PPHN came only after it had been used in animal models and in therapy of adults.[37] Unlike with other vasodilator agents, the administration of iNO is not accompanied by a decrease in systemic blood pressure. Initiation of therapy frequently begins using 20 to 40 parts per million (ppm) of iNO, with dosing adjustments as clinically warranted. The gas has been shown to be effective when used in amounts as little as 5 ppm. The response to iNO may be at least partially related to the cause of the PPHN, as well as to the time that has elapsed before the initiation of therapy.

In August 2000, the American Academy of Pediatrics (AAP) Committee on Fetus and Newborn issued its recommendations for the use of iNO.[38] The Academy suggested the initiation of iNO in centers capable of providing "multisystem support, generally including on-site extracorporeal membrane oxygenation (ECMO)." However, if iNO is offered at a center without ECMO availability, prospective establishment of a mechanism of transfer to an ECMO center must be in place. Additionally, it is essential that the transfer of patients be accomplished without interruption of iNO therapy.

Research in the use of NO in premature infants with respiratory failure has begun. Complications of NO inhalation include methemoglobinemia (rare with the use of low concentrations) and lung toxicity. Further discussion of NO use is found in Chapter 14.

Extracorporeal Membrane Oxygenation

ECMO remains the "safety net" for infants with refractory PPHN and is discussed in detail in Chapter 16.

Summary

The causes of PPHN are almost as numerous as the methods for its treatment. Early recognition and definitive echocardiographic diagnosis should afford the clinician the opportunity to provide as rapid and aggressive therapy as is warranted. Ongoing research for a "kinder, gentler" means of treating very

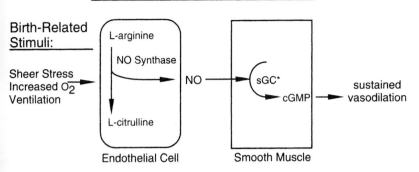

Regulation of EDRF/NO at Birth

Birth-Related Stimuli:

Sheer Stress
Increased O$_2$
Ventilation

L-arginine
NO Synthase
L-citrulline
Endothelial Cell

NO

sGC*
cGMP
Smooth Muscle

sustained vasodilation

*Soluble guanylate cyclase

Figure 23-5. Schematic representation illustrating the effects of birth-related stimuli on the pulmonary vascular endothelial cell production of nitric oxide (NO). Shear stress, increased O$_2$, and ventilation stimulate NO generation by type III NO synthase from its substrate L-arginine. NO diffuses to vascular smooth muscle, stimulating cyclic guanosine monophosphate (cGMP) production and causing vasodilation. (From Abman S, Kinsella J: Nitric oxide in the pathophysiology and treatment of neonatal pulmonary hypertension. Tufts University School of Medicine and Floating Hospital for Children Reports on: Neonatal Respiratory Diseases, 4:2, 1994.)

ill neonates with PPHN should be supported, and the use of ECMO should be limited to those patients who meet strict criteria. Neurodevelopmental follow-up should not be overlooked in determining the success of therapy.

PATENT DUCTUS ARTERIOSUS COMPLICATING RESPIRATORY DISTRESS SYNDROME

Incidence

The incidence of PDA in a full-term infant is about 1 in 2,000 live births,[39] making it a relatively common form of congenital heart disease. Siassi et al.[1] found the ductus arterious patency rate in premature infants to be significantly greater and to increase with decreasing gestational age (Table 23-5). Clearly, the incidence of patency is related to fetal maturity, but the problem of determining whether the PDA is "significant"— that is, whether it contributes to respiratory morbidity—sometimes is difficult. Several investigators have found that infants of less than 30 weeks' gestation with severe RDS who required assisted ventilation are extremely likely to have symptomatic PDA. The incidence in this subgroup approaches 75% to 80%.[40] Moreover, some trials of the use of exogenous surfactant in premature infants with RDS have demonstrated an increased incidence of symptomatic PDA after surfactant therapy.[41,42] Mouzinho et al.,[43] however, found a much lower incidence of symptomatic PDA in infants weighing less than 1500 g and of less than 34 weeks of gestation. During the period from 1987 to 1989, while practicing conservative fluid management (designed to achieve the loss of 12% to 14% of body weight during the first week of life), they found a 19% incidence of symptomatic PDA in very-low-birthweight infants and that this rate was inversely proportional to gestational age (Fig. 23-6). It appears that the incidence of symptomatic PDA may depend on a number of factors, including the severity of RDS, use of surfactant, diagnostic criteria, population selection, and use of fluid therapy and volume expanders.

Hemodynamics and Pathophysiology

The ductus arteriosus is an integral component of the fetal circulation whose direction of blood flow is from the main pulmonary artery to the descending aorta. Flow into the distal

TABLE 23-5. Incidence of Patent Ductus Arteriosus Related to Gestational Age

Gestational Age (wk)	Ductus Patency Rate (%)
28–30	70–80
31–32	40–45
34–36	21

From Slassi B, Blanco C, Cabal LA, et al: Incidence and clinical features patent ductus arteriosus in low birth weight infants: A prospective analysis of 1 consecutively born infants. Pediatrics 57:347, 1976. Reproduced by permisson of *Pediatrics*.

pulmonary arteries is limited in fetal life by a very high vascular resistance due principally to unexpanded lung tissue and, in part, to a well-developed medial muscular layer in the pulmonary arterioles. The muscularity of this medial layer is inversely proportional to the degree of fetal maturity, normally increasing to a peak at about 38 weeks' gestation. Thus, the less mature the pulmonary vascular tree, the less the resistance to blood flow through it. This maturational process becomes functionally significant when the ductus arteriosus remains patent after birth, because the magnitude of flow through the pulmonary bed is determined by the size of the ductus and by the resistance in the pulmonary bed. Shunting through the PDA results in an increase in pulmonary venous return and dilation of the left side of the heart. Increasing left ventricular end-diastolic pressure gives rise to left atrial and pulmonary venous hypertension (left-sided heart failure). This hypertension leads to transudation of fluid into the pulmonary alveoli (pulmonary edema), which in turn may result in hypoxia, pulmonary arteriolar constriction, pulmonary hypertension, and right-sided heart failure.[44]

Diagnosis

Clinical

Commonly, in a premature infant with RDS, a cardiac murmur is noted on or before the fourth day of life. The murmur may be systolic or continuous, depending on the pressure relationships between the aorta and the pulmonary artery. The murmur typically is located at the base of the heart in the second and third left intercostal spaces and may be transmitted to the back. If the left-to-right shunt is large, a mitral diastolic flow murmur is sometimes detected at the cardiac apex. The

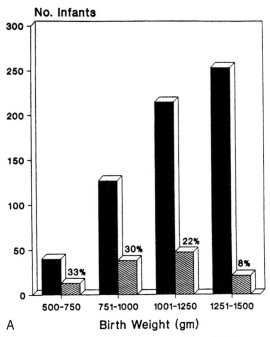

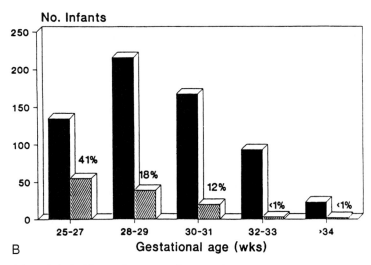

A   **Birth Weight (gm)**

B   **Gestational age (wks)**

Figure 23-6. *A,* Relationship between birthweight and the incidence of symptomatic patent ductus arteriosus (PDA) in infants surviving for longer than 72 hours. *Solid bars* represent the total number of infants studied; *cross-hatched bars* infants with symptomatic PDA. *B,* Relationship between gestational age and the incidence of symptomatic PDA in infants surviving for longer than 72 hours. *Solid bars* represent the total number of infants studied; *cross-hatched bars* infants with symptomatic PDA. (From Mouzinho AI, Rosenfeld CR, Risser R: Symptomatic patent ductus arteriosus in very-low-birth-weight infants: 1987–1989. Early Hum Dev 27:65, 1991.)

National Collaborative Study on PDA in premature infants reported that 30% of the 342 infants studied had a continuous murmur on the day of diagnosis, 59% had a systolic murmur, and 11% had no murmur.[44] The last of these represent the so-called *silent ductus* group.

Other clinical findings from the collaborative study included hyperactive precordium (47%), bounding pulses (50%), tachycardia of greater than 170 beats/min (11%), tachypnea greater than 70 breaths/min (15%), and hepatomegaly (5%).

Echocardiography

Echocardiography is the most reliable noninvasive tool for diagnosing PDA in the neonate and is now available in virtually all centers that provide care for high-risk newborns. Standard two-dimensional imaging is used for the definition of cardiac anatomy and function. High-frequency transducers make precise measurements of the ductus size routine. Doppler interrogation and color flow imaging are useful measures of the ductus shunt magnitude and of pulmonary artery pressures and have rendered obsolete the cumbersome measurements and ratios formerly obtained from M-mode studies. The development of real-time tele-echocardiography has allowed for the application of expert pediatric echocardiography (with the pediatric cardiologist's technical guidance) for prompt diagnosis and follow-up in centers without on-site cardiologists.

Medical Management

Fluid Restriction

Left-to-right shunting through a PDA imposes a volume overload on the left ventricle that is commensurate with the magnitude of the shunt. This situation may be inadvertently worsened because premature infants need relatively large volumes of fluid for the replacement of loss due to radiation or for weight maintenance or gain. Therefore, fluid restriction to 100 to 140 mL/kg/day is indicated for reduction of intravascular volume and left ventricular end-diastolic pressure. The effect of fluid restriction is lowering of pulmonary venous pressure, which increases lung compliance and promotes weaning from ventilatory support.[45] Because anemia can contribute to CHF, reduction of the workload of the heart can be achieved by maintaining the hematocrit at greater than 35%.

Digoxin

The use of digoxin in the management of CHF in the premature infant is not as effective as in the older patient, possibly because of the greater amounts of water and connective tissue in the premature myocardium.[46] Immaturity of the kidneys and liver in the preterm infant may also contribute to digoxin toxicity by prolonging its half-life. Care should be taken to adjust the dose of digoxin relative to both weight and maturity (Table 23-6). The use of digoxin in neonates for treatment of CHF secondary to PDA probably is less useful than therapy directed at ductus closure (indomethacin or ligation).

Indomethacin

Demonstration of the effects of indomethacin on ductal tissue[47] and the results of subsequent studies on the drug in clinical trials[48,49] have provided the basis for its current widespread use. A national collaborative study that included 13 medical centers and a combined patient population of

TABLE 23-6. Neonatal Digoxin Inotropic Therapy

	Weight (g)	Oral Total Digitalizing Dose (TDD)
A. Age		
Premature	500–1000	20 μg/kg or 0.02 mg/kg
	1000–1500	20–30 μg/kg or 0.02–0.03 mg/kg
	1500–2000	30 μg/kg or 0.03 mg/kg
	2000–2500	30–40 μg/kg or 0.03–0.04 mg/kg
Full-term to 1 mo	>2500	40 μg/kg or 0.04 mg/kg

1. IV dose is 75% of calculated oral TDD.
2. Acute digitalization: ⅓, ⅓, ⅓ or ½, ¼, ¼ of TDD every 8 hr.
3. Maintenance dose is ⅛ of TDD every 12 hr and is begun 12 hr after last digitalizing dose.
4. Slow digitalization: begin maintenance dose; digitalization will be complete in approximately 5 days.

B. Toxicity
1. A-V block is common (PR interval prolongation to upper limits of normal indicates digoxin effect, not toxicity).
2. Nausea, vomiting.
3. Ventricular ectopy is uncommon.
4. Toxicity suspected: withhold drug, check trough digoxin level; correct hypokalemia unless high grade A-V block is present.

A-V, atrioventricular; IV, intravenous.

TABLE 23-7. Indomethacin Treatment of Patent Ductus Arteriosus: Effect on Morbidities

	Prophylactic (0–3 days)	Early (3–10 days)	Late (>10 days)
Pulmonary hemorrhage	↓	—	—
Intraventricular hemorrhage	↓	—	—
Necrotizing enterocolitis	—	↓	↓
Respiratory distress syndrome	—	?	—
Bronchopulmonary dysplasia	—	↓	↓
Need for surgical ligation	↓	↓	↓

421 infants evaluated the efficacy of indomethacin in the management of PDA.[50] The results of this large, well-controlled study suggest that indomethacin is highly effective in closing a PDA in preterm infants. Other independent studies have supported the findings of the collaborative study.[51–53] Occasionally the ductus is initially constricted by indomethacin but subsequently reopens, necessitating repeated dosing or, occasionally, surgical closure.[54]

The administration of indomethacin has been reported to affect organ systems other than the ductus arteriosus. Because of alterations in ductal flow, there may be effects on the lungs (hemorrhage, bronchopulmonary dysplasia), the intestines (necrotizing enterocolitis), or the brain (intraventricular hemorrhage). The age of the infant when indomethacin is administered is important in determining which organ systems are affected. Table 23-7 lists the effects of indomethacin treatment on morbidities when it is given prophylactically (0 to days), early (3 to 10 days), or late (>10 days).

Dosage. The national collaborative study on PDA in premature infants used the following dosage schedule for indomethacin: 0.2 mg/kg as the initial dose, followed by 0.1 mg/kg for the second and third doses if the infant is younger than 48 hours of age. If the infant is between 2 and 7 days of age, 0.2 mg/kg is given for the second and third doses; if the infant is older than 7 days of age, 0.25 mg/kg is given for subsequent doses (Table 23-8). The time interval between doses is 12 hours. In the collaborative

TABLE 23-8. Dosage Schedule for Indomethacin (Intravenous)

Age	First Dose	Second Dose	Third Dose
<48 hr	0.2 mg/kg	0.1 mg/kg	0.1 mg/kg
2–7 days	0.2 mg/kg	0.2 mg/kg	0.2 mg/kg
≥8 days	0.2 mg/kg	0.25 mg/kg	0.25 mg/kg

From Gersony WM, Peckham GJ, Ellison RC, et al: Effects of indomethacin in preterm infants with patent ductus arteriosus: Results of a national collaborative study. J Pediatr 102:895, 1983.

study, indomethacin was administered intravenously; pharmacologic studies have shown little difference in the half-life of indomethacin whether the preparations were given orally or parenterally in infants of 32 weeks' gestation or greater. Less mature infants (less than 32 weeks' gestation) tend to metabolize the drug more slowly; thus, its half-life is prolonged.[55]

Contraindications. Because indomethacin is protein bound and competes for binding sights, it tends to depress renal function and interferes with platelet adhesiveness[56]; thus, it must be used with certain precautions. Contraindications are listed in Table 23-9. The use of furosemide for maintenance of adequate urine output during administration of indomethacin has been advocated, but its use is controversial.[57]

TABLE 23-9.   Contraindications to Use of Indomethacin

1. Blood urea nitrogen >30 mg/dL
2. Serum creatinine >1.8 mg/dL
3. Total urine output <0.6 mL/kg/hr over preceding 8 hr
4. Platelet count <60,000 mm³
5. Stool Hematest >3 + (or "moderate to large")
6. Evidence of bleeding diathesis
7. Clinical or radiographic evidence of necrotizing enterocolitis
8. Lack of parental consent

Surgical Patent Ductus Arteriosus Closure

Surgical closure of the PDA is now generally reserved for infants in whom standard medical management, including indomethacin, has failed (i.e., the ductus arteriosus is still patent after administration of three doses) or in whom contraindications to the use of indomethacin (see Table 23-9) are present. Preoperative evaluation to exclude important cardiac defects and define the aortic arch sidedness is warranted. The actual procedure, although technically straightforward and of relatively low risk,[58] is best carried out by an experienced surgeon who is well acquainted with exigencies of neonatal surgery.

Complications following PDA surgery in major medical centers are infrequent, and patients usually can be weaned promptly (within 48 hours) from ventilatory support if the PDA was the major contributor to ventilator dependency.[59] Most problems in the postoperative period arise from respiratory acidosis, hypothermia, or accidental ligation of a structure other than the PDA.[60] If surgical ligation has been delayed for several days to several weeks, weaning from the ventilator may be difficult because of chronic lung disease (bronchopulmonary dysplasia). Persistent patency of the ductus or late recanalization occasionally occurs even with ductus division. Hemodynamically significant shunts are uncommon, but, as the risks for infective endovasculitis may remain, determination of complete closure by postoperative echocardiogram is useful.

Transcatheter Management

Implanted endovascular prostheses (coils, wound nitinol devices, umbrellas) account for most patent ductus closures outside of the neonatal age group. Size constraints in the neonate, such as access vessel damage and the creation of pulmonary artery or aortic obstruction, have precluded routine application in newborns to date. Several devices in development hold promise as a therapeutic option for the future.[61]

PERIOPERATIVE MANAGEMENT OF COMPLEX NEONATAL HEART DISEASE

Advances in surgical and catheter techniques and in the perioperative management of infants with complex congenital heart defects have shifted the focus of surgical treatment toward earlier complete repair and away from palliative surgical procedures or delayed primary repair. Additionally, previously fatal lesions such as hypoplastic left heart syndrome are treated routinely with excellent results. This simply means that an increasing number of neonates are undergoing complex cardiac procedures. Successful outcome depends to a great extent on perfect preoperative stabilization and meticulous postoperative care. A coordinated multidisciplinary approach involving the cardiovascular surgeon, pediatric cardiologist, neonatologist, pediatric intensivist, intensive care nurses, respiratory therapists, and a host of ancillary personnel is essential.

Monitoring

Cardiac patients admitted to the neonatal intensive care unit setting require careful and accurate monitoring of all systems. This surveillance includes use of the standard electronic cardiorespiratory monitor that is capable of analog and digital display of heart rate (ECG), blood pressure, arterial pressure tracing, other atrial and venous waveforms (right atrial, left atrial), central venous pressures, and respiratory rate. Patients have a central arterial line so that reliable direct arterial pressure and blood gas monitoring can be performed. A transcutaneous pulse oximeter is used for continuous digital display of oxygen saturation and heart rate. Online measurement of end-tidal CO_2 and indwelling catheter measurement of oxygen saturation and blood gas data may limit the need for blood sampling.

Other aspects of monitoring include careful measurement of mediastinal and pleural tube output, urinary output, and nasogastric tube drainage. It is our usual practice to monitor serum electrolytes, blood urea nitrogen, creatinine, glucose, and calcium levels, as well as coagulation parameters (prothrombin time, partial thromboplastin time, international normalized ratio, and platelet count) preoperatively, every 6 hours on the first postoperative day, and less frequently thereafter if the patient's condition is stabilized. A chest radiograph is obtained on postoperative readmission to the intensive care unit so that the position of the endotracheal tube, intravascular catheters, and chest drainage tubes can be ascertained. In addition, serial chest radiographs are used for assessment and follow-up of conditions such as pulmonary air leaks (pneumothorax), atelectasis, and pleural effusions.[62]

Initial Ventilator Management

In the absence of coexisting lung disease, a volume preset ventilator usually is preferred. A fixed predetermined tidal volume (usually about 6 to 10 mL/kg of body weight at the outset) is delivered to the patient. Because an air leak from the trachea upon tidal volume delivery is common, notation of the returned tidal volume is most helpful in guiding changes to preset tidal volume. The rate of ventilation is initially based on what is judged appropriate for the patient's age and size. Further adjustments may be necessary after careful inspection of chest motion, auscultation, and examination of arterial blood gas values and end-tidal CO_2 monitors. Respiratory acidosis can be corrected with increases in either tidal volume or ventilatory rate (i.e., minute ventilation). Metabolic acidosis, on the other hand, usually is indicative of inadequate systemic oxygen delivery.[63]

In addition to the application of standard tidal volume and ventilatory rate settings, it usually is necessary to use continuous positive airway pressure (CPAP) or PEEP to avoid atelectasis or small airway collapse.[64,65] However, it must be remembered that both CPAP and PEEP can have an adverse effect on a patient's hemodynamic status by hindering systemic venous return and thus decreasing cardiac output.[66] In addition, the risk of pulmonary barotrauma (pneumothorax, interstitial emphysema) is increased when CPAP or PEEP levels greater than 6 to 8 cm H_2O are used.

Ventilator Strategies to Modulate Cardiac Shunting

A thorough understanding of the patient's underlying cardiac disease is requisite to planned ventilator management. For example, in the case of hypoplastic left heart syndrome, supplemental oxygen and even mild hyperventilation may decrease pulmonary vascular resistance (increase pulmonary blood flow) and thereby dramatically decrease systemic blood flow. Effective strategies to maintain or increase pulmonary vascular resistance in this setting include low tidal volume, low rate ventilation, and use of nitrogen to decrease the FIO_2 to 0.17 to 0.19 (target $PaCO_2$ 45 to 50 torr, transcutaneous saturations 80% to 85%). Alternatively, conventional ventilator settings can be used with room air plus carbon dioxide (CO_2) added to the inhalation circuit (target $PaCO_2$ 45 to 55 torr). Atelectasis is thereby avoided, but sedation or paralysis often is necessary to suppress the effects of increased respiratory drive.

Rarely, idiopathic elevation of pulmonary vascular resistance (PPHN) adversely affects the neonate with unoperated congenital heart disease. This is seen most frequently with complete transposition of the great arteries and complete atrioventricular canal defect (endocardial cushion defect) and may be associated with gestational maternal glucose intolerance. Ventilator strategies are as for PPHN alone, but the target PaO_2 and transcutaneous saturation values obviously must be individualized.

The mechanically ventilated postoperative cardiac patient usually requires an initial fraction of inspired oxygen of 0.6 to 0.8, principally due to the effects of anesthetic agents, neuromuscular blocking agents, chest wall trauma, and cardiopulmonary bypass. NO often is used to control pulmonary vascular resistance and to limit ventilation-perfusion mismatching (see Chapter 14). It should be noted that patients who have not undergone complete repair may have residual obligatory intracardiac shunting, which prevents them from attaining a normal PaO_2; this fact should be taken into account when parameters are established for weaning from the ventilator. As mentioned earlier, the highest possible PaO_2 is sometimes not a proper goal. In general, patients who have undergone complete repair can be expected to achieve a PaO_2 of 80 to 120 mmHg; patients with residual right-to-left shunts may not be able to generate PaO_2 values greater than 40 to 50 mm Hg even if they receive 100% oxygen. Understanding the surgery performed and postoperative hemodynamics can help limit excess oxygen administration and resultant toxicity.

Weaning and Extubation

A systematic approach is necessary for optimal weaning from the ventilator and for extubation. Initial efforts should be directed toward lowering high PEEP or CPAP levels in 1 to 2 cm H_2O decrements until a level of 5 cm H_2O or less is obtained. Thereafter, lowering of the FIO_2 is carried out, generally in decrements of 5% to 10% to as low as 40% FIO_2. At the same time, weaning of the respiratory rate can be accomplished by closely following the arterial pH and $PaCO_2$. The weaning process continues until the patient is breathing without mechanical assistance on physiologic CPAP (e.g., 5 cm H_2O or less) with an acceptable PaO_2 on an FIO_2 of 40% or less.[63] The entire weaning process may take from 24 to 48 hours in infants who have undergone cardiopulmonary bypass for correction of complex defects (arterial switch, tetralogy of Fallot); even longer periods of ventilatory support may be required and are not unusual. If NO is given for more than a few days, weaning below levels of 5 ppm should be done very carefully. Pulmonary artery pressure monitoring by indwelling catheter or by echocardiography is helpful to avoid acutely increased pulmonary vascular resistance from suppression of constitutive NO production ("rebound pulmonary hypertension"). Infants who undergo repair of simpler defects may often be extubated safely as early as 6 to 12 hours postoperatively.

When the decision to extubate has been made, the endotracheal tube and pharynx should be thoroughly suctioned and the nasogastric tube aspirated. The endotracheal tube is then removed and the patient placed under an oxygen hood, with the FIO_2 10% to 15% higher than that used just before extubation. A chest radiograph and arterial blood gas values are obtained within 20 to 30 minutes following extubation.

After extubation, it is our practice to administer racemic epinephrine and dexamethasone (0.1 to 0.3 mL in 2 to 3 mL normal saline) every hour for three doses. This is done so that stridor from laryngeal and subglottic edema can be prevented. Occasionally, it is necessary to give dexamethasone systemically for treatment of airway edema, especially when there has been a prolonged ventilatory course, multiple reintubations, or when significant airway obstruction is anticipated following extubation. The dose of dexamethasone is 0.5 mg/kg intravenously, and therapy is most effective when it is initiated 6 to 12 hours before extubation and is continued for 4 to 6 doses at 6-hour intervals. Routine chest physiotherapy should begin following extubation at intervals of 2 to 4 hours; this should include albuterol nebulizations every 3 to 4 hours or otherwise as required. Levalbuterol may be useful to limit undesired tachycardia that occasionally results from albuterol inhalation. Blood gas determinations should be carried out routinely at least 24 hours after extubation or as long as the patient requires supplemental oxygen.

Management of the Cardiovascular System

The primary determinant of postoperative survival is cardiac output; thus, all efforts should be directed toward ensuring that cardiac output remains adequate.[67] Cardiac output is estimated by physical examination and by measuring acid–base status and urine output. Echocardiographic measures of contractility and cardiac output are semiquantitative.[68,69] The thermodilution technique requires placement of a Swan-Ganz thermistor catheter in the pulmonary artery and has technical limitations in small infants.[68–70] Continuous monitoring of mixed venous and aortic saturations provides an excellent measure of cardiac output (arterial-venous oxygen difference) but requires an indwelling venous catheter.

The Fick equation states that cardiac output is proportional to the ventricular stroke volume multiplied by the heart rate (cardiac output = stroke volume × heart rate). Factors that influence stroke volume are ventricular preload, afterload, and myocardial contractility. Preload is reflected in the filling

TABLE 23-10.   Inotropic Agents

Agent	Dose	Comments
Dobutamine	2–10 μg/kg/min IV (40 μg/kg min maximum)	Positive inotropic with minimal chronotropic effect
Dopamine	5–10 μg/kg/min IV (50 μg/kg/min maximum)	Selective dilataton of renal bed, but alpha effect with higher doses; may increase pulmonary vascular resistance
Epinephrine	0.05–1.0 μg/kg/min IV	Positive inotropic and chronotropic effect; may cause renal ischemia; tachydysrhythmias
Isoproterenol	0.05–1.0 μg/kg/min IV	Strong inotropric and chronotropic effect; pulmonary vasodilation; systemic vasodilation may "steal" renal blood flow; tachydysrhythmias
Milrinone	0.25–0.75 μg/kg/min	Vasodilator with positive inotropic effects
Norepinephrine	0.05–1.0 μg/kg/min IV	Intense vasoconstriction

(venous) pressures of the heart and is essential to cardiac output because of the relationships expressed in the Frank-Starling mechanism (e.g., that contraction force depends on the length of muscle fibers). Preload is monitored clinically via central venous and atrial lines. It can be augmented with the infusion of 10-mL/kg aliquots of colloid (packed red blood cells, fresh-frozen plasma) or crystalloid solutions so that atrial pressures are maintained in the range from 10 to 14 mmHg.

In contrast, afterload is related to the vascular resistance or the tone of the vascular bed against which the ventricle is pumping. Most patients who have undergone open heart surgery (cardiopulmonary bypass, ventriculotomy) have both high afterload and some degree of impairment of myocardial contractility; consequently, the increase in afterload significantly reduces stroke volume, resulting in a decrease in cardiac output. Reduction in ventricular afterload involves the manipulation of vascular resistance in a number of ways. Pulmonary vascular resistance can be lowered with ventilator-induced respiratory alkalosis. Hypoxia is corrected with oxygen administration. Pharmacologic agents, such as NO, prostaglandins, milrinone, and isoproterenol, are used in various combinations to reduce pulmonary vascular resistance.

Dilation of the peripheral vascular bed can reduce systemic vascular resistance (left ventricular afterload). This usually is achieved with the use of a vasodilator such as milrinone alone or in combination with multiple inotropes. Other smooth muscle relaxants such as nitroglycerin and the alpha-blockers (e.g., phentolamine and prazosin) occasionally are used.[71–73]

Myocardial contractility is the third determinant of cardiac output. Some degree of myocardial dysfunction is almost always seen following correction of complex cardiac defects. It can be attributed to cardiopulmonary bypass, as noted earlier, to direct injury to the myocardium (ventriculotomy, resection of hypertrophic muscle), to the effects of chronic volume overload, and to a number of other factors.[74] Contractility is assessed with echocardiography, and serial follow-up studies are valuable for documenting the efficacy of treatment.

The most commonly used inotropic agents are listed in Table 23-10. These agents are discussed more extensively in Chapter 19. In addition, digoxin has been used in the past both acutely and chronically to improve myocardial contractility and control the symptoms of CHF. Table 23-6 outlines the recommendations for digoxin administration in neonatal patients.

The final determinant of cardiac output, especially in the young infant, is heart rate. Most of the inotropic drugs already discussed earlier have a chronotropic effect, particularly isoproterenol and epinephrine. Inotropic agents are frequently used in combination when a single drug does not sufficiently improve cardiac output (see Chapter 19). An inotropic drug can also be used in combination with an afterload-reducing agent (e.g., sodium nitroprusside) when increased myocardial contractility and afterload reduction are deemed necessary. Milrinone has been found to provide both inotropic support and afterload reduction. Adequate preload is essential for the successful activity of all inotropic agents and afterload-reducing agents.

Other Considerations

Although the respiratory and cardiovascular systems justifiably occupy the central position in postoperative management, it is important that the clinician not underestimate the importance of other body systems and their roles in eventual outcome.

Fluids, Electrolytes, and Nutrition

Cardiopulmonary bypass is commonly accompanied by sodium and fluid retention, along with potassium loss.[75] This effect is thought to be due to the activation of the renin-angiotensin system and of antidiuretic hormone secretion. Patients frequently are hyperglycemic in the early postoperative period, probably as a result of the stress of surgery. The initial intravenous fluids of choice are 10% dextrose in 25% normal saline in the neonate and 5% dextrose in 25% normal saline in the older child; potassium (usually, 2 mEq per 100 mL fluid) is added only after adequate renal function has been ascertained. Total fluid administration should be about two-thirds maintenance in the first 24 hours (1000 to 1200 mL/m²) and then gradually increased over the next 48 to 72 hours until full maintenance (1500 to 1800 mL/m²) is reached. If the patient has continuing fluid losses during this period or requires additional volume for preload augmentation, boluses of the appropriate fluid are given.[63] Appendix 23 lists maintenance requirements for fluids, electrolytes, and glucose. Laboratory studies monitored during the postoperative period should include frequent determinations of these parameters.

The patient undergoing cardiac surgery generally has a paralytic ileus for the first 12 to 24 hours postoperatively. This precludes enteral feeding and necessitates nasogastric drainage.

TABLE 23-11. Nutritional Care in Congestive Heart Failure

1. Calories: A. Start with 130–140 cal/kg/day and increase up to 150–170 cal/kg/day if poor weight gain or weight gain is edema fluid.
   B. Increase caloric content of standard formula (20 cal/oz) up to 24–32 cal/oz. Begin with dextrose polymer (Polycose): has 2 cal/mL, requires minimal degradation, and has only ⅙ osmotic load of free dextrose. Use medium-chain triglyceride oil (8.3 cal/mL) to obtain 32 cal/oz if Polycose causes diarrhea or if 28 cal/oz formula is ineffective.
2. Na⁺ content: Provide 2–3 mEq/kg/day for growth requirements in a low-solute formula of 7–12 mEq/L.
3. Consider nasogastric feeding if patient has anorexia or increased respiratory effort.

TABLE 23-12. Postoperative Bleeding

Coagulopathy	Prothrombin Time	Partial Thromboplastin Time	Platelets or Others	Therapy
Dilution of coagulation factors	↑ ↑	↑ ↑	↑ ↑ Thrombin time	10–15 mL/kg of FFP
Disseminated intravascular coagulation	↑ – ↑ ↑ ↑	↑ – ↑ ↑ ↑	↓ Platelets ↓ Fibrinogen ↑ Fibrin split products	FFP 10–15 mL/kg Platelets 1 unit/5 kg Vitamin K 1–5 mg IV
Heparin excess	↑	↑ ↑ ↑		1 mg/kg IV protamine sulfate; causes hypotension
Increased fibrinolysis	WNL	WNL	Platelets WNL ↑ Euglobulin lysis time	Epsilon aminocaproic acid 200 mg/kg IV, then 150 mg/kg 2 hr for 12 hr
Thrombocytopenia or platelet dysfunctions	WNL	WNL	↓ Platelet count	Platelets 1 unit/5 kg
Surgical bleeding	WNL	WNL	Normal clotting with chest drainage >3 mL/kg/hr for 3 hr or >5 mL/kg any 1 hr	Re-exploration

↑, mildly increased; ↑ ↑, moderately increased; ↑ ↑ ↑, markedly increased; FFP, fresh-frozen plasma; WNL, within normal limits.

Once bowel sounds are heard, feedings via nasogastric or transpyloric tube may be started, even if the patient is still intubated. Peripheral intravenous alimentation can be started if adequate caloric support cannot be attained with enteral feedings alone, particularly if a prolonged ventilator course is anticipated. Table 23-11 outlines the recommendations for the nutritional support of infants and young children with increased caloric requirements associated with congenital heart disease. A more complete discussion of nutritional support can be found in Chapter 24.

Hematologic Problems

Blood loss following cardiac surgery is inevitable, but excessive loss, defined as chest tube or mediastinal sump output of greater than 5 mL/kg/hour, is a serious situation, and the cause must be quickly determined. Table 23-12 outlines a systematic approach to postoperative bleeding.

Infection

Chronic malnutrition associated with congenital heart disease, the presence of arterial and venous lines, chest tubes, urinary catheters, and pacing wires all predispose the patient to the possibility of infection in the postoperative setting. It has also been determined that cardiopulmonary bypass is associated with a decrease in T- and B-lymphocyte count, and this decrease further impairs the patient's ability to combat infection.[76,77] Consequently, prophylactic antibiotic coverage is routinely given. Currently, cefazolin is administered intravenously in the operating room just before surgery is begun,

and it is continued every 6 hours for a total of eight doses or until all chest tubes and intravascular monitoring lines are removed.

Low-grade fever is extremely common in the first few postoperative days and may be related to the release of pyrogenic substances triggered by cardiopulmonary bypass. Extreme elevations of temperature, especially if associated with leukocytosis, lethargy, hypoglycemia, or decreased peripheral perfusion, point to serious infection and must be approached accordingly. Appropriate workup includes blood and urine cultures, chest radiography, and a careful physical examination that attempts to reveal the site of the infection. Broad-spectrum antibiotic coverage should be considered if evidence of infection persists.

REFERENCES

1. Siassi B, Blanco C, Cabal LA, et al: Incidence and clinical features of patent ductus arteriosus in low birth weight infants: A prospective analysis of 150 consecutively born infants. Pediatrics 57:347, 1976.
2. Merenstein GB, Way GL: Neonatal air transport and congenital heart disease. Newborn Air Transport: Mead, Johnson Conference, 1978.
3. Rowe RD, Freedom RM, Menrizi A, et al: The Neonate with Congenital Heart Disease, 2nd ed. Philadelphia, WB Saunders, 1981, p. 139.
4. Moss JA, Adams FH, Emmanouilides GC: Heart Disease in Infants, Children, and Adolescents, 2nd ed. Baltimore, Williams & Wilkins, 1977, p. 626.
5. Levin DL, Hyman AI, Heymann MA, et al: Fetal hypertension and the development of increased pulmonary vascular smooth muscle: A possible mechanism for persistent pulmonary hypertension in the newborn infant. J Pediatr 92:265, 1978.
6. Rowe RD, Freedom RM, Menrizi A, et al: The Neonate with Congenital Heart Disease, 2nd ed. Philadelphia, WB Saunders, 1981, p. 143.
7. Nadas AS, Flyer DC: Pediatric Cardiology, 3rd ed. Philadelphia, WB Saunders, 1772, p. 5.

8. Cole RB, Paul MH: Cyanotic heart disease guide to emergency management for the primary physician (part 1). Hospital Medicine, August 1979.

9. Kitterman JA: Cyanosis in the newborn infant. Pediatr Rev 4:13, 1982.

10. Gersony WM, Due GV, Sinclair JC: "PFC" syndrome (persistence of fetal circulation). Circulation 40(Suppl 3):3, 1969.

11. Goetzman BW, Riemenschneider TA: Persistence of the fetal circulation. Pediatr Rev 2:37, 1980.

12. Hageman JR, Adams A, Gardner TH: Persistent pulmonary hypertension of the newborn: Trends in incidence, diagnosis and management. Am J Dis Child 138:592, 1984.

13. John E, Roberts V, Burnard E: Persistent pulmonary hypertension of the newborn treated with hyperventilation: Clinical features and outcome. Aust Paediatr J 24:357,1988.

14. Heyman MA, Rudolph AM, Nies AS, et al: Bradykinin production associated with oxygenation in the fetal lamb. Circ Res 25:521, 1969.

15. Teitel DF, Iwamote HS, Rudolph AM: Changes in the pulmonary circulation during birth-related events. Pediatr Res 27:372, 1990.

16. Moss AJ, Adams FH, Emmanouilides GC: Heart Disease in Infants, Children and Adolescents, 3rd ed. Baltimore, Williams & Wilkins, 1983, p. 11.

17. Gersony WM, Morishima HO, Daniel SS, et al: The hemodynamic effects of intrauterine hypoxia: An experimental model in newborn lambs. J Pediatr 89:631, 1976.

18. Heymann MA, Rudolph AM: Effects of acetylsalicylic acid on the ductus arteriosus and circulation of fetal lambs in utero. Circ Res 38:418, 1976.

19. Walsh-Sukys M: Persistent pulmonary hypertension of the newborn. Clin Perinatol 20:127, 1993.

20. Moncada S, Palmer RMJ, Higgs E: Nitric oxide: Physiology, pathophysiology, and pharmacology. Pharmacol Rev 43:109, 1991.

21. Kinsella JP, McQueston JA, Rosenberg AA, et al: Hemodynamic effects of exogenous NO in ovine transitional circulation. Am J Physiol 263:H875, 1992.

22. Roberts JD, Chen TY, Kawai N, et al: Inhaled NO reverses pulmonary vasoconstriction in the hypoxic and acidotic newborn lamb. Circ Res 72:246, 1993.

23. Kinsella JP, Neish SR, Shaffer E, et al: Low dose inhalation NO therapy in PPHN. Lancet 340:819, 1992.

24. Roberts JD, Polaner DM, Lang P, et al: Inhaled NO in PPHN. Lancet 340:818, 1992.

25. Kinsella JP, Neish SR, Ivy DD, et al: Clinical responses to prolonged treatment of PPHN with low doses of inhaled NO. J Pediatr 123:103, 1993.

26. Fox WW, Duara S: Persistent pulmonary hypertension in the neonate: Diagnosis and management. J Pediatr 103:505, 1983.

27. Hansen NB, Nowicki PT, Miller RR, et al: Alterations in cerebral blood flow and oxygen consumption during prolonged hypocarbia. Pediatr Res 20:147, 1986.

28. Reuter JH, Disney TA: Regional cerebral blood flow and cerebral metabolic rate of oxygen during hyperventilation in the newborn dog. Pediatr Res 20:1102, 1986.

29. Hendricks-Munoz KD, Walton JP: Hearing loss in infants with persistent fetal circulation. Pediatrics 81:650, 1988.

30. Wung JT, James LS, Kilchevsky E, et al: Management of infants with severe respiratory failure and PFC without hyperventilation. Pediatrics 76:488, 1985.

31. Dworetz AR, Moya FR, Sabo B, et al: Survival of infants with persistent pulmonary hypertension without extracorporeal membrane oxygenation. Pediatrics 84:1, 1989.

32. Lyrene RK, Welch KA, Godoy G, et al: Alkalosis attenuates hypoxic pulmonary vasoconstriction in neonatal lambs. Pediatr Res 19:1268, 1985.

33. Walsh-Sukys MC, Tyson JE, Wright LL, et al: Persistent pulmonary hypertension of the newborn in the era before nitric oxide: practice variation and outcome. Pediatrics 105(1 Pt 1):14, 2000.

34. Cassin S, Winikor I, Tod M, et al: Effects of prostacyclin on the fetal pulmonary circulation. Pediatr Pharmacol 1:197, 1981.

35. Furchgott RF, Zawadski JW: The obligatory role of endothelial cells in the relaxation of arterial smooth muscle by acetylcholine. Nature 288:373, 1908.

36. Ignarro LJ, Buga GM, Wood KS, et al: Endothelium-derived relaxing factor produced and released from artery and vein is nitric oxide. Proc Natl Acad Sci USA 84:9265, 1987.

37. Pepke-Zaba J, Higenbottam TW, Dinh-Xuan AT, et al: Inhaled nitric oxide as a cause of selective pulmonary vasodilatation in pulmonary hypertension. Lancet 338:1173, 1991.

38. American Academy of Pediatrics Committee on Fetus and Newborn. Use of inhaled nitric oxide. Pediatrics 106(2 Pt 1):344, 2000.

39. Mitchell SC, Korones SB, Berendes HW: Congenital heart disease in 56,109 births: Incidence and natural history. Circulation 43:323, 1971.

40. Dudell G, Gersony M: Patent ductus arteriosus in neonates with severe respiratory disease. J Pediatr 104:915, 1984.

41. Taeusch HW, Keough KM, Williams M, et al: Characterization of bovine surfactant for infants with respiratory distress syndrome. Pediatrics 77:572, 1986.

42. Raju TN, Vidyasogar D, Bath R, et al: Double blind controlled trial of single-dose treatment with bovine surfactant in severe hyaline membrane disease. Lancet 1:651, 1987.

43. Mouzinho AI, Rosenfeld CR, Risser R: Symptomatic patent ductus arteriosus in very-low-birth-weight infants: 1987–1989. Early Hum Dev 27:65, 1991.

44. Ellison RC, Peckham GJ, Lang P, et al: Evaluation of the preterm infant for patent ductus arteriosus. Pediatrics 71:364, 1983.

45. Bell EF, Warburton D, Stonestreet BS, et al: Effect of fluid administration on the development of symptomatic patent ductus arteriosus and congestive heart failure in premature infants. N Engl J Med 302:598, 1980.

46. Hoffman JE: Factors affecting shunting and the development of heart failure. Persistent patency of the ductus arteriosus in premature infants. 75th Ross Conference on Pediatric Research, Columbus, Ohio, 1978.

47. Coceani F, Olley PM, Bodoch E: Lamb ductus arteriosus: Effect of prostaglandin E_2. Prostaglandin 9:299, 1975.

48. Friedman WF, Herschklau MJ, Printz MP: Pharmacologic closure of the patent ductus arteriosus in the premature infant. N Engl J Med 95:526, 1976.

49. Heymann MA, Rudolph AM, Silverman NA: Closure of the ductus arteriosus in premature infants by inhibition of prostaglandin synthesis. N Engl J Med 295:530, 1976.

50. Gersony WM, Peckham GJ, Ellison RC, et al: Effects of indomethacin in preterm infants with patent ductus arteriosus: Results of a national collaborative study. J Pediatr 102:895, 1983.

51. Brash AR, Hickey DE, Graham TP, et al: Pharmacokinetics of indomethacin in the neonate: Relation of plasma indomethacin levels to response of the ductus arteriosus. N Engl J Med 305:67, 1981.

52. Halliday HL, Hirata T, Brady JP: Indomethacin therapy for large patent ductus arteriosus in the low birth weight infant: Results and complications. Pediatrics 64:154, 1979.

53. Merritt TA, Harris JP, Ronghman K, et al: Early closure of patent ductus arteriosus in very low birth weight infants: A controlled trial. J Pediatr 99:281, 1981.

54. Ramsey JM, Murphy DJ, Vick GW, et al: Response of the patent ductus arteriosus to indomethacin treatment. Am J Dis Child 141:294, 1987.

55. Clyman RI, Heymann NA: Pharmacology of the ductus arteriosus. Pediatr Clin North Am 28:77, 1981.

56. Friedman Z, Whitman V, Maisels MJ, et al: Indomethacin disposition and indomethacin induced platelet dysfunction in premature infants. J Clin Pharmacol 18:272, 1978.

57. Yeh TF, Wilks A, Singh J, et al: Furosemide prevents the renal side effects of indomethacin therapy in preterm infants with patent ductus arteriosus. J Pediatr 101:433, 1982.

58. Eggert LD, Jung AJ, McGough EC, et al: Surgical treatment of patent ductus arteriosus in preterm infants: Four years experience with ligation in the newborn intensive care unit. Pediatr Cardiol 2:15, 1982.

59. Cotton RB, Stahlman NT, Berdu HW, et al: Randomized trial of early closure of symptomatic patent ductus arteriosus in small preterm infants. J Pediatr 93:647, 1978.

60. Fleming WH, Sarafiau LB, Brigler JD, et al: Ligation of patent ductus arteriosus in premature infants: Importance of accurate anatomic definition. Pediatrics 71:373, 1983.

61. Gray DT, Fyler DC, Walker AM, et al: Clinical outcomes and costs of transcatheter as compared with surgical closure of patent ductus arteriosus. N Engl J Med 329:1517, 1993.

62. Moes CAF: Analysis of the chest in the neonate with congenital heart disease. Radiol Clin North Am 13:251, 1975.

63. Bell TJ: Postoperative care. In Garson A Jr, Bricker JT, McNamara DG (eds): Science and Practice of Pediatric Cardiology, vol. III. Philadelphia, Lea & Febiger, 1990, p. 2253.

64. McIntyre RW, Laws AK, Ramachandran PR: Positive expiratory pressure plateau: Improved gas exchange during mechanical ventilation. Can Anaesth Soc J 16:477, 1969.

65. Kumar A, Falke KJ, Gelfin B, et al: Continuous positive-pressure ventilation in acute respiratory failure: Effects on hemodynamics and lung function. N Engl J Med 283:1430, 1970.

66. Cournand A, Mottey HL, Werko L, et al: Physiological studies of the effects of intermittent positive pressure breathing on cardiac output in man. Am J Physiol 152:162, 1948.

67. Parr GVS, Blackstone EH, Kirklin JW: Cardiac performance and mortality early after intracardiac surgery in infants and children. Circulation 51:867, 1975.

68. Nishimura RA, Callahan MJ, Schaff HV, et al: Noninvasive measurement of cardiac output by continuous-wave Doppler echocardiography: Initial experience and review of the literature. Mayo Clin Proc 59:484, 1984.

69. Morrow WR, Murphy DJ Jr, Fisher DF, et al: Continuous wave Doppler cardiac output: Use in pediatric patients receiving inotropic support. Pediatr Cardiol 9:131, 1988.

70. Callaghan ML, Weintraub WH, Coran AH: Assessment of thermodilution cardiac output in small objects. J Pediatr Surg 11:629, 1976.

71. Dillon TR, Janos GG, Meyer RA, et al: Vasodilator therapy for congestive heart failure. J Pediatr 96:623, 1980.

72. Benzing G, Helmsworth JA, Schreiber JT, Kaplan S: Nitroprusside after open-heart surgery. Circulation 54:467, 1976.

73. Stinson EB, Holloway EL, Derby G, et al: Comparative hemodynamic responses to chlorpromazine, nitroprusside, nitroglycerine, and trimethaphan after open heart operations. Circulation 51(Suppl 1):126, 1975.

74. Lappav DG, Powell J, Daggett WM: Cardiac dysfunction in the perioperative period. Anesthesiology 47:117, 1977.

75. Pacifico AD, Digerness SB, Kirklin JW: Acute alterations of body composition after open intracardiac operations. Circulation 41:331, 1970.

76. Salo M: Effect of anaesthesia and open heart surgery on lymphocyte responses to phytohaemagglutinin and concanavalin A. Acta Anaesthesiol Scand 22:471, 1978.

77. Ryhanden P, Herva E, Hollmen A, et al: Changes in peripheral blood leukocyte counts, lymphocyte subpopulations and in vitro transformation after heart valve replacement: Effect of oxygenator type and postoperative parenteral nutrition. J Thorac Cardiovasc Surg 77:259, 1979.

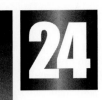

NUTRITIONAL SUPPORT

EDWARD F. BELL, MD

Advances in newborn respiratory care, in order to be fully realized, must be matched by progress in the nutritional support of premature and critically ill infants. In the early years of neonatal intensive care, efforts were focused on the problems that immediately threatened the survival of infants, and the issue of nutrition was not addressed until survival was assured. Most premature or critically ill infants received little or no nutrient intake until they were fed orally, beginning several days after birth if they survived until then. During the past several decades, advances in nutritional care have quietly accompanied and in part enabled the more highly acclaimed advances in newborn respiratory care.

In the 1950s and early 1960s, even healthy premature infants were routinely starved and thirsted for several days after birth.[1] Subsequently, earlier enteral feeding was shown to reduce the incidence of hypoglycemia and hyperbilirubinemia.[2,3] In addition, early administration of intravenous glucose was found to decrease catabolism[4] and reduce mortality in premature infants.[5,6] Improved nutritional products and increased sophistication in the use of a variety of feeding techniques today offer greater flexibility in the feeding of critically ill infants who formerly could not be fed until they were able to tolerate oral or gavage feedings.

Not only is nutritional support key to the survival of premature and critically ill infants, but their brain growth and neurodevelopmental outcome also hinge on the quantity and quality of nutrition provided during their critical early postnatal weeks. The period of maximum brain growth in the human extends from the third trimester of pregnancy through the first 18 months of postnatal life.[7] Much of this rapid growth occurs postnatally, even in full-term infants. Considerable evidence indicates that the human brain is vulnerable to the effects of nutritional deprivation during the postnatal portion of this brain growth spurt.[8–13] Undernutrition in early infancy may lead to long-term deficits in intellectual[10,11] and motor[12,13] function. For infants who require assisted ventilation, the harmful effects of malnutrition on lung development,[14,15] respiratory muscle function,[16] and lung mechanics[17] are also of great importance. Moreover, undernourished infants probably are more susceptible to bronchopulmonary dysplasia.[18–20]

Progress has been made in recent years toward defining the goals of nutritional support and the requirements of many nutrients for premature and critically ill infants, yet the requirements for many nutrients are not well defined. The determination of nutrient requirements depends on the goals set forth for the rate and composition of weight gain. The most widely accepted standard for comparison is the growth of the fetus of corresponding postmenstrual age. Despite much debate about the appropriateness and feasibility of matching fetal growth in the neonatal intensive care unit, many of the current ideas about nutritional requirements of premature infants are based on the fetal growth standard.

The infant who is ill enough to require assisted ventilation presents special problems in nutritional management. Because he or she cannot safely suck and swallow liquid feedings, a method of feeding must be used that bypasses the mouth and pharynx. The infant may have increased metabolic demands due to the severity of illness. He or she may have changes in water balance caused by both the illness and the treatment, such as assisted ventilation. The infant is more susceptible to most of the complications of feeding by various means, partly because the process of feeding may alter his or her cardiorespiratory mechanics, which are already in a tenuous state of balance.

The purpose of this chapter is to review what is known about the nutritional needs of the infant who requires assisted ventilation and how these needs can best be met. Although exact goals of nutritional therapy are hard to delineate, it should be possible, in infants who need ventilatory assistance, not only to prevent catabolism and exhaustion of endogenous energy resources but also to produce growth in lean body mass without impairing oxygen delivery to vital tissues.

NUTRITIONAL REQUIREMENTS

Water Requirement

Body Water Distribution in the Fetus and Newborn

During the third month of gestation, it is estimated that water constitutes 94% of the fetal weight. The total body water (TBW) decreases to approximately 86% by 24 weeks gestation and to about 78% by term (Fig. 24-1).[21–23] The extracellular water (ECW) and intracellular water (ICW) also change characteristically with growth. The ECW decreases from 59% of body weight at 24 weeks of gestation to about 44% at term, and the ICW increases from 27% at 24 weeks to 34% at term. The weight loss seen in the first few days of life is at least partly due to contraction of the ECW[22–27] associated with improvement of renal function.[28,29] When daily changes in body weight are used as an indicator of water balance during the first few days of life, allowance for some weight loss (5% to 15%) should be made because of these physiologic changes.

The maintenance water requirement can be accounted for by insensible water loss, renal water excretion, and stool water. In addition, water is required for growth and is produced in small amounts as a byproduct of cellular metabolism.

Insensible Water Loss

Insensible water loss (IWL) to the environment is an important factor in heat and water balance, especially in premature infants. As much as 30% of the IWL is lost through the respiratory tract as moisture in expired gas.[30,31] The balance is lost through the skin. Factors that are known to influence the rate of IWL are listed in Table 24-1.

Gestational age and body weight are both correlated inversely with IWL.[32–35] The smaller, less mature infant loses more water per kilogram because of his or her greater surface-area-to-body-weight ratio, thinner and more permeable skin, larger body water, and higher respiratory rate.

Respiratory distress may be associated with an increase in respiratory IWL. For an infant breathing spontaneously, the IWL increases with a rise in minute ventilation (respiratory rate multiplied by tidal volume).[36] The same should also be true for an infant who is being mechanically ventilated unless the gas mixture delivered by the ventilator is fully saturated.

In addition to ventilator rate, the respiratory IWL also depends on the humidity (or water vapor pressure) gradient between the patient's upper airway and the gas mixture he or she is breathing, either in a head box or incubator, or in the ventilator circuit if he or she is being assisted through nasal prongs or an endotracheal tube. Warming and humidification are desirable to prevent injury to the respiratory mucosa and to prevent blockage of an artificial airway by viscous secretions. If the temperature and water content of the inspired and expired gas are the same, the respiratory IWL will be entirely eliminated.[37] Ambient humidity also affects cutaneous evaporative water loss, but to a lesser degree than its effect on respiratory loss.[30,31,38] Hey and Katz[30] found that a threefold rise in ambient vapor pressure was accompanied by a 55% reduction in respiratory water loss and an 18% reduction in cutaneous evaporative loss.

An increase in ambient temperature above the neutral thermal zone will increase IWL as much as threefold or fourfold.[30,39,40] Similarly, elevated body temperature, whether due to fever or environmental hyperthermia, is associated with a large increase in IWL.[30,41]

Physical activity level has been shown to influence IWL.[30,41,42] The IWL in the awake, moving infant averages 37% to 70% greater than in the basal sleeping state. Crying increases the IWL to two or more times the basal state.[42]

The use of a radiant warmer increases IWL by about 50%.[33,43–47] Overhead phototherapy has been shown to increase IWL by 20% to 50%,[33,48,49] and the use of phototherapy and a radiant warmer together increases IWL more than either used alone.[45,50] The impact on IWL of fiberoptic phototherapy is not known but probably is negligible unless the blanket produces a warmer or moister microenvironment around the infant. Investigators using direct measurements of transepidermal and respiratory water loss have obtained conflicting results regarding the effect of overhead phototherapy on IWL. One group[49] measured an increase in transepidermal water loss with phototherapy, but another did not.[51]

Several devices have been shown to decrease IWL. The use of Plexiglas (rigid acrylic) heat shields for premature infants in single-walled incubators has been shown to reduce IWL by 10%

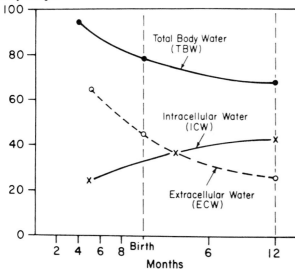

Figure 24-1. Changes in body water of the fetus and infant. (Based on data from Friis-Hansen B: Changes in body water compartments during growth. Acta Paediatr Suppl 110:1, 1957.)

TABLE 24-1.   Factors That Influence Insensible Water Loss of Infants

Factor	Change in Insensible Water Loss (per kg)
Level of maturity[32–35]	Inversely proportional to gestational age and birthweight
Respiratory distress (hyperpnea)[36]	Rises with increasing minute ventilation
High inspired or ambient humidity[30,31,38]	Respiratory insensible water loss reduced more than cutaneous
Ambient temperature above the neutral thermal zone[30,39,40]	Increase proportional to temperature
Elevated body temperature[30,41]	Increase proportional to temperature
Physical activity and crying[30,41,42]	Up to 70% increase
Radiant warmer[33,43–47]	50% increase over incubator
Phototherapy[33,45,48–50]	20%–50% increase
Plastic heat shield[32,46,52]	10%–25% reduction (in single-walled incubator)
Transparent thermal blanket[52–54] or chamber[54,55]	70% reduction in single-walled incubator,[53] 30%–50% reduction under radiant warmer[52,54,55]
Semipermeable membrane[56–58]	50% reduction
Topical agents[59,60]	50% reduction

to 25%.[32,46] The effect was more clearly evident among infants who weighed less than 1250 g[32] and is most effective if the ends of the heat shield are at least partially closed to reduce air movement near the skin. Plexiglas heat shields do not seem to be effective for infants under radiant warmers[46,52] because Plexiglas blocks the infrared energy emitted by the radiant heaters and interferes with the feedback loop that controls the heater output. A transparent thermal blanket reduced IWL by a mean of 70% in premature infants in incubators.[53] Similar blankets or chambers of thin saran[52,54] or polyvinyl chloride[55] also reduce IWL of infants under radiant warmers. Finally, both semipermeable membranes[56–58] and topical agents[59,60] have been shown to be capable of reducing IWL of premature infants by about 50%.

Renal Water Excretion

The amount of water required for urine output depends on the renal solute load and the renal concentrating ability. The full-term newborn can produce urine as dilute as 50 mOsm/L and can concentrate to around 800 mOsm/L.[61,62] The premature kidney is limited to a narrower range of osmolarity, although it has some capacity to increase free water clearance and urine volume in response to a fluid challenge.[63]

The renal solute load comes from two sources: *exogenous* (primarily electrolytes and metabolic products of nutrients) and *endogenous* (products of catabolism or changes in body composition). The commonly used commercial formulas provide a potential (exogenous) renal solute load of 18 to 24 mOsm per 100 kcal (22 to 30 mOsm/kg/day at energy intake of 125 kcal/kg/day). An intravenous infusion providing 3 mmol of NaCl and 2 mmol of KCl per kilogram per day would provide a potential renal solute load of 10 mOsm/kg/day.[64,65] The addition of 1 g of amino acids per kilogram per day would raise the potential solute load to about 16 mOsm/kg/day. If this exogenous solute were all to be excreted in the urine, that is, 10 to 30 mOsm/kg/day, a urine volume of 50 to 80 mL/kg/day would maintain the urine concentration between 125 and 600 mOsm/L. These concentrations are within the capacity of the newborn kidney, even for premature infants. In practice, the amount of solute excreted by the kidney is larger than the exogenous or potential solute load if the infant is in a catabolic state. In such cases the exogenous solute intake usually is low so that the actual solute excretion is still generally less than 30 mOsm/kg/day. On the other hand, growing infants deposit some of the exogenous solute in the body (approximately 1 mOsm per gram of weight gain[64,65]) so that the actual solute load is less than the potential. An infant receiving premature formula at 125 kcal/kg/day (30 mOsm/kg/day) and gaining 15 g/kg/day would excrete about 15 mOsm/kg/day.

The critically ill infant who requires assisted ventilation may have special problems with renal handling of water. Hypoxia or hypotension during the course of the illness may compromise kidney function by causing tubular or cortical necrosis. During the anuric or oliguric phase of acute tubular necrosis, the renal water excretion is markedly reduced and its allowance in the maintenance water calculation should be reduced accordingly. In the diuretic phase, water excretion through the kidney is markedly increased.

The renal function of infants with respiratory distress syndrome (RDS) is similar to that of infants of the same gestational age without respiratory disease so long as normal blood gases and acid-base status can be maintained.[66–68] However, if infants with RDS become hypoxic and acidotic they may have reduced renal blood flow and glomerular filtration, and a reduced threshold for renal bicarbonate excretion.[67–70] All premature infants, including those with RDS, have an increase in urine volume on the second or third day of life,[71–73] which is accompanied by a rise in plasma atrial natriuretic peptide[74–78] and contraction of the ECW compartment.[78] These changes were often temporally associated with improvement in respiratory function in the presurfactant era.

In addition to changes in renal function that may occur with pulmonary compromise from severe RDS, positive-pressure ventilation may cause water retention through effects on renal function. Continuous positive airway pressure can decrease glomerular filtration rate, sodium excretion, and free water clearance without altering renal perfusion pressure.[79] Intermittent positive-pressure ventilation impairs water and sodium excretion by several mechanisms, including increased aldosterone secretion[80] and increased production of antidiuretic hormone.[81] The underlying pulmonary disease may also cause elevated secretion of antidiuretic hormone.[82–85] Finally, it is possible for excessive airway pressures during assisted ventilation to impair glomerular filtration and solute excretion by compromising aortic pressure and renal perfusion.[86,87]

Stool Water Loss

Stool water loss usually is estimated to be about 5 mL/kg/day.[88,89] Diarrhea increases the stool water loss by an amount that can be determined by changes in body weight. Phototherapy also increases stool water loss. Jaundiced full-term infants under phototherapy lost 19 mL/kg/day in the stool, compared with losses of 7 mL/kg/day in jaundiced control infants without phototherapy.[48]

Water for Growth

The water required for growth depends on the growth rate desired, the water content of the new tissues, and any concurrent changes in body water composition. Water for growth need not be provided until after the initial period of "physiologic" weight loss, during which appropriate negative water balance is probably desirable. The water retained in new tissues during growth should be 0.5 to 0.8 L per kilogram of weight gain[90]; the higher figure applies to the least mature infants. Table 24-2 summarizes average water requirements week by week for infants with birthweight between 500 and 2000 g.[91]

Water of Oxidation

The water produced as a byproduct of metabolism is a hidden source of water intake. This "water of oxidation," subtracted from required intake in Table 24-2, consists of 0.43 mL per gram of protein oxidized, 1.07 mL per gram of fat, and 0.60 mL per gram of carbohydrate.[92] Assuming a pattern of substrate utilization similar to the subjects of Reichman et al.,[93] formula-fed premature infants should be expected to produce about 0.14 mL of water per kilocalorie expended, or between 5 and 10 mL/kg/day. This metabolic water is roughly equal to the stool water loss plus the water retained for growth. This simplification allows consideration of water requirements only in terms of insensible and urine losses.

TABLE 24-2.   Estimated Water Requirement of Low Birthweight Infants (mL/kg/day)

| Week | Component | Birthweight Range (g) | | | | | |
		501–750	751–1000	1001–1250	1251–1500	1501–1750	1751–2000
1	IWL	100	65	55	40	20	15
	Urine	70	70	70	70	70	70
	Stool	5	5	5	5	5	5
	Growth	0	0	0	0	5	5
	Oxidation	-5	-5	-5	-5	-10	-10
	Total	170	135	125	110	90	85
2	IWL	80	60	50	40	30	20
	Urine	70	70	70	70	70	70
	Stool	5	5	5	5	5	5
	Growth	0	0	5	5	10	10
	Oxidation	-5	-5	-10	-10	-10	-10
	Total	150	130	120	110	105	95
3	IWL	70	50	40	35	30	25
	Urine	70	70	70	70	70	70
	Stool	5	5	5	5	5	5
	Growth	5	5	10	10	10	10
	Oxidation	-10	-10	-10	-10	-10	-10
	Total	140	120	115	110	105	100
4	IWL	60	45	40	35	30	25
	Urine	70	70	70	70	70	70
	Stool	5	5	5	5	5	5
	Growth	10	10	10	10	10	10
	Oxidation	-10	-10	-10	-10	-10	-10
	Total	135	120	115	110	105	100

Days 3–7: Less water is given during the first 2 days to allow for "physiologic" negative water balance.
Insensible water loss (IWL) for infants above 750 g adapted from Wu PYK, Hodgman JE: Insensible water loss in preterm infants: Changes with postnatal development and non-ionizing radiant energy. Pediatrics 52:704, 1974. Increase by 40%–50% if phototherapy or radiant warmer used.
Sufficient urine to maintain concentration of 100 to 500 mOsm/L with solute excretion of 7 to 35 mOsm/kg/day.
Assuming gain of 0, 7.5, or 15 g/kg/day with 67% of gain as water.
Water of oxidation calculated as 0.14 mL/kcal expended,[92] assuming energy expenditure of 35 to 70 kcal/kg/day.
Adapted from Bell EF, Oh W: Fluid and electrolyte balance in very low birth weight infants. Clin Perinatol 6:139, 1979.

The numbers in Table 24-2 merely indicate average requirements. The amounts listed here are sufficient for most but not all low-birthweight infants. These figures are intended only as an illustration of the components of water balance and as a rough guide to help in the initial prescription of water intake. Intake must be adjusted subsequently based on such data as body weight, serum sodium concentration, and urine volume.

Energy Requirement

The energy intake required for normal growth is difficult to determine and can only be approached in the setting of a balanced diet with adequate amounts of protein and other nutrients. Previous authors[93-100] have observed that healthy premature infants gain weight at rates similar to the fetus of corresponding postmenstrual age with energy intakes as low as 106 kcal/kg/day[98] and as high as 181 kcal/kg/day[94] (Table 24-3). Within this range there appears to be no clear relation between energy intake and weight gain. It appears that an intake of 110 kcal/kg/day from high-quality infant formula or human milk is generally sufficient to support normal growth and metabolism of healthy premature infants, provided protein intake is adequate. Moreover, it seems that infants receiving high energy intakes become fatter without accelerating their gain in fat-free mass.[93,94] The energy from the diet that is not lost in the stool or urine is either expended for metabolism or stored in the body for growth. The components that comprise total energy expenditure are the minimal or resting

energy expenditure (about 40 kcal/kg/day for young premature infants), energy expended for activity, cold-induced energy expenditure, diet-induced or postprandial energy expenditure (also called the *specific dynamic action*), and energy expended for synthesis of new tissues. Some consider the last two categories to be synonymous or at least overlapping.

The total daily energy expenditure per kilogram body weight is lowest in the smallest infants and increases slightly with postnatal age in both premature and term infants.[88,101] After the first week it averages about 60 kcal/kg/day. The energy excreted in the stool and urine is about 10% of the intake. The energy stored for growth depends on the rate of gain and the composition of new tissues.

Table 24-4 lists the components used to derive the estimated requirement of 110 kcal/kg/day for healthy, growing premature infants who are enterally fed. The energy required to maintain an intravenously fed infant in a nongrowing state is considerably less, about 50 kcal/kg/day (Table 24-4). Positive nitrogen balance has been reported with intravenous feedings delivering as little as 60 kcal/kg/day,[102] but consistent growth generally requires 70 kcal/kg/day or more.

Information about the energy expenditure of infants who require assisted ventilation has until recently been limited by the technical difficulties of measuring whole-body oxygen consumption and carbon dioxide production in intubated infants. Richardson et al.[103] performed brief measurements of oxygen consumption (which is directly proportional to energy expenditure) in infants with RDS who required assisted ventilation. They found the oxygen consumption to be slightly

TABLE 24-3. Energy Intake and Weight Gain of Premature Infants

Authors	Diet	Gross Energy Intake (kcal/kg/day)	Weight Gain (g/kg/day)
Brooke et al.[94]	Formula	181	14
Reichman et al.[93]	Formula	149	17
Chessex et al.[95]	Human milk	111	15
Whyte et al.[96]	Human milk	127	15
Whyte et al.[96]	Formula	126	17
Sauer et al.[97]	Formula	130	17
Putet et al.[98]	Human milk	106	15
Putet et al.[98]	Formula	128	21
Catzeflis et al.[99]	Human milk	115	13
Catzeflis et al.[99]	Formula	113	16
Kashyap et al.[100]	Formula	130	22
Kashyap et al.[100]	Formula	155	23

TABLE 24-4. Estimated Energy Requirement of Premature Infants

	Energy Expenditure or Loss (kcal/kg/day)	
	Growing, Enterally Fed Infant*	Nongrowing, Parenterally Fed Infant
Resting energy expenditure	40	40
Activity	5	0
Cold stress	5	5
Postprandial or synthetic energy	10	0
Stool and urine energy loss	10	5
Energy for growth	40	0
Total energy requirement	110	50

Adapted from Sinclair JC, Driscoll JM Jr, Heird WC, et al: Supportive management of the sick neonate. Parenteral calories, water, and electrolytes. Pediatr Clin North Am 17:863, 1970.

higher than expected, especially during the first 24 hours of life. Billeaud et al.[104] measured oxygen consumption in mechanically ventilated premature infants with early or impending bronchopulmonary dysplasia. The oxygen consumption increased with increasing severity of lung disease, as determined by airway pressure and inspired oxygen requirement. Schulze et al.[105] measured the oxygen consumption of the lungs in premature infants with RDS who were mechanically ventilated. They found the pulmonary oxygen consumption to be 25% of the whole-body oxygen consumption and postulated that oxygen consumed by the lungs as a result of their extra work accounts for the elevated energy expenditure of infants with lung disease. Field et al.[106] found that adults with cardiorespiratory disease had a 21% reduction in oxygen consumption when they were mechanically ventilated. They attributed this difference to the work of breathing, which was about 10 times normal.

Several groups of investigators have found higher than expected rates of oxygen consumption in spontaneously breathing infants with bronchopulmonary dysplasia (BPD).[107–111] The significance of these results has been questioned in view of the methodologic difficulties presented in measuring oxygen consumption in infants who are breathing oxygen-enriched air[112]; however, the finding of increased energy expenditure in infants with BPD has been confirmed using doubly labeled water,[111] a method that should not be influenced by inspired oxygen concentration. In summary, it appears that infants ill enough to require assisted ventilation will have some increase in energy expenditure and energy requirement related to the increased work of breathing; however, this increase may be limited by use of appropriate ventilatory support.

An energy intake of 70 to 80 kcal/kg daily is sufficient to prevent starvation and promote growth in the first week of life of premature infants who are receiving the bulk of their feeding parenterally. As they become older it should be possible to increase the energy intake to 110 kcal/kg/day or more, allowing for stool losses as the proportion of energy delivered enterally increases. Finally, each infant is different, and some will require a much greater energy intake to establish growth. The ultimate tests of sufficiency of energy intake are the rate and quality of growth.

Protein Requirement

The protein requirement of newborn infants has not been firmly established. Estimates of the protein requirement of premature infants based on the rate of fetal accretion of protein are between 3.0 and 4.0 g/kg/day[113,114] (Table 24-5). These estimates are supported by experimental studies of protein turnover, nitrogen balance, and growth of premature infants. Even infants who are growing rapidly do not tolerate enteral protein intakes above 5.0 g/kg/day. Such intakes have been associated with azotemia, metabolic acidosis, fever, lethargy, diarrhea, and poor neurodevelopmental outcome.

Infants fed parenterally probably require less protein, approximately 2.5 to 3.5 g of amino acids per kilogram per day if they are growing well.[115,116] Even less should be given if an infant is critically ill and not expected to grow at the

TABLE 24-5. Advisable Daily Energy, Protein, and Nutrient Intakes for Premature Infants

Nutrient	Advisable Intake (per kg/day)	
	700–1000 g Infant	1001–1500 g Infant
Energy (kcal)	110	110
Protein (g)	4.0	3.6
Sodium (mmol)	3.6	3.0
Potassium (mmol)	2.5	2.2
Chloride (mmol)	3.2	2.6
Calcium (mg)	192	169
Phosphorus (mg)	132	118
Magnesium (mg)	7.3	6.5
Iron (mg)	2.6	2.4
Zinc (mg)	1.6	1.4
Copper (mg)	0.2	0.2

Adapted from Ziegler EE: Feeding the low birth weight infant. In Gellis SS, Kagan BM (eds): Current Pediatric Therapy, 13th ed. Philadelphia, WB Saunders, 1990, p. 713.

corresponding intrauterine rate. However, even very young premature infants who require assisted ventilation have been shown to benefit from modest amounts of intravenous amino acids (1.5 g/kg/day) begun in the first days of life.[117]

The quality of dietary protein is important. Evidence suggests that small premature infants may depend on exogenous sources of cysteine[117,118] and taurine.[119]

Fat Requirement

Linoleic acid is an essential fatty acid; it cannot be synthesized in vivo. Evidence suggests that infants also require a very small amount of linolenic acid to allow normal development of retinal and brain function.[120–122] Each of these fatty acids serves as a precursor for longer chain derivatives. Dietary essential fatty acid deficiency in infants causes dermatitis, increased susceptibility to infection, and impaired growth.[123] The requirement for essential fatty acids can be met by providing 1% of the dietary energy in the form of linoleic and linolenic acids.[124] To provide a margin of safety, the intake recommended by the Committee on Nutrition of the American Academy of Pediatrics[125] is 3% of the energy intake as essential fatty acids.

Certain biologically important long-chain polyunsaturated fatty acids, such as docosahexaenoic acid (DHA) and arachidonic acid (AA), are found in human milk but until recently were not present in commercial formulas. It has been shown that both term and premature infants have the capacity to synthesize DHA and AA.[126,127] Early studies did not show any clear long-term benefit from adding DHA and AA to infant formulas but found no evidence of toxicity from this practice.[128–130] More recently, however, formulas supplemented with DHA and AA have been shown to enhance visual and motor development in premature infants,[131] but these formulas offered no demonstrable advantage to healthy term infants.[132]

Recommendations for total lipid intake are not well established. Human milk and most commercial formulas derive 40% to 50% of their energy content from fat. The usual diet of an infant consuming human milk or infant formula contains 3.3 to 6 g of fat per 100 kcal (30% to 54% of energy). Restriction of dietary fat intake is not recommended in the first 2 years of life.

Premature infants do not absorb fat as well as term infants. The rate of bile salt synthesis, the bile salt pool, and the intraluminal concentration of bile salts are all decreased in premature infants.[133] In addition, the activity of pancreatic lipase is lower than at term.[134] The deficiencies of pancreatic lipase and bile salt activity are partly overcome by intragastric fat digestion by lingual lipase.[135] Human milk fat and vegetable fats are more easily absorbed than saturated animal fats.

Triglycerides of short-chain and medium-chain fatty acids are directly absorbed into the portal blood independent of bile salt and lipase activities. Medium-chain triglycerides (MCT) often are used as energy supplements and have been incorporated into formulas in various concentrations to enhance fat digestion. Premature infants fed formulas containing MCT show improved absorption of fat, calcium, and magnesium.[136–140] Some investigators have found enhanced nitrogen retention[136,137] or weight gain[136] in infants fed MCT, but others have not.[138,139,141] As a result of these benefits, commercial formulas designed for premature infants generally contain MCT as one of the major fat sources.

Carbohydrate Requirement

It is not possible to define an absolute requirement for carbohydrate in newborn infants. In addition to their role in preventing hypoglycemia, carbohydrates are important as metabolic fuel. Approximately half of the infant's energy needs are normally provided by combustion of carbohydrates. Moreover, brain metabolism depends on glucose as an energy source. In the premature infant, this glucose is largely derived from exogenous carbohydrate sources because of the inefficient mechanisms of gluconeogenesis; however, there is evidence that the newborn brain may utilize ketone bodies as an additional energy source.[142]

The usual dietary regimens provide roughly half of the total energy intake as carbohydrate. Fomon et al.[143] have shown that varying the portion of energy derived from carbohydrate from 34% to 62% produced no difference in linear or weight growth of term infants; 9% of the energy was derived from protein in both groups and the balance from fat.

For the infant who can be fed enterally, the type of carbohydrate to be given depends on the functional maturity of the gastrointestinal tract. The activities of most disaccharidases are adequate for digestion by 24 to 28 weeks of gestation, although the activity of lactase lags behind the others and does not fully develop until close to term.[144] Intestinal lactase activity increases to adequate functional levels within a few days after the initiation of enteral feedings, even in infants born as early as 28 weeks.[145] Activity of pancreatic amylase remains low until after term.[135,144,146] Salivary amylase activity is present even in very premature infants,[147] however, and this enzyme is thought to play a role in the initial digestion of glucose polymers,[148] a carbohydrate source often used in formulas for premature infants. Glucose transport in the intestine is limited at birth[144] and may be the rate-limiting step in carbohydrate absorption. In spite of the late gestational rise in lactase activity and the decreased capacity for intestinal glucose transport, both term and premature infants seem to tolerate the carbohydrates in human milk and commercial formulas quite well. Normal absorption and growth have been documented with formulas containing lactose, sucrose, and glucose, alone or in combination.

Mineral Requirements

Several methods have been used to estimate the infant's requirements for electrolytes and minerals. One approach is to compare the body composition of premature and term infants at birth and thus to derive the amount of a particular substance that would have accrued had the premature infant remained in utero.[149] To this amount required for the formation of new tissues can be added estimates of the amount lost through the skin, urine, and stool. This method is called the *factorial approach.* Because of the uncertainty of the derivation, the estimated requirements are increased by 10% to produce recommended or advisable intakes of nutrients (see Table 24-5).[113] An indirect approach, such as the factorial approach, must be used because nutrient requirements cannot be experimentally determined without producing deficiencies.

The requirements of sodium, potassium, and chloride derived from such calculations are similar, about 2 to 3 mmol/kg/day for the premature infant[149] and slightly less for the term infant. The recommended intakes for premature infants are 2 to 4 mmol/kg/day[113,125,150] (see Table 24-5). Very-low-birthweight infants may require additional sodium intake due to increased urinary excretion, particularly during the period of active growth.[125]

The term newborn retains an average of 30 to 40 mg of calcium per kilogram daily.[151] The recommended intake depends on the route of administration and, if given enterally, on the absorption rate. The fraction of calcium absorbed depends on the type of milk or formula, the gestational age, and the postnatal age.[151] The calcium requirement for premature infants is higher. Ziegler[113] has estimated that an enteral calcium intake of 160 to 190 mg/kg/day is necessary for small premature infants to achieve the intrauterine rate of calcium retention (see Table 24-5). The recommended intake of phosphorus is 120 to 130 mg/kg/day.[113] Poor bone mineralization (osteopenia) has been described in actively growing very-low-birthweight infants receiving inadequate intakes of calcium and phosphorus and can be prevented by oral administration of calcium in a dose of 150 to 225 mg/kg/day[152-154] with adequate phosphorus. Unsupplemented human milk does not provide adequate calcium and phosphorus intake for premature infants, but addition of a powdered mixture containing protein, lactose, minerals, and vitamins can compensate for this deficiency.[155,156] For infants fed intravenously, absorption is not a consideration, and lower intakes of calcium and phosphorus are adequate. Recommended intravenous intakes of calcium range from 60 to 90 mg/kg/day and of phosphorus 47 to 70 mg/kg/day.[157,158]

The recommended enteral intake of magnesium is 6 to 15 mg/kg/day[113,158] (see Table 24-5). Intravenous intake of 4 to 8 mg/kg/day is recommended for infants receiving total parenteral nutrition for prolonged periods.[157,158]

Iron at an intake of 2 to 3 mg/kg/day is recommended for both term and premature infants who are enterally fed.[113,125,159] During the acute care of infants requiring assisted ventilation, before enteral feeding is established, iron will most commonly be provided in the form of blood transfusions given to prevent significant anemia. Infants fed human milk should be given daily supplements of iron once an enteral intake of 100 mL/kg/day is established. Formula-fed infants should receive only iron-fortified formula, beginning with the first formula feedings. There is no need to delay the start of iron supplementation until an arbitrary age.[159-161] The advis-

TABLE 24-6. Advisable Daily Enteral Intakes of Vitamins and Trace Substances for Growing Premature Infants (per kg per day)

Vitamin A	700–1500 IU
Vitamin D	150–400 IU
Vitamin E	6–12 IU
Vitamin K	8–10 µg
Vitamin C	18–24 mg
Thiamin	0.2 mg
Riboflavin	0.3 mg
Niacin	4–5 mg
Vitamin B_6	0.2 mg
Vitamin B_{12}	0.3 µg
Folic acid	25–50 µg
Pantothenic acid	1.2–1.7 mg
Biotin	4–6 µg
Taurine	4.5–9.0 mg
Carnitine	3 mg
Inositol	32–81 mg
Choline	14–28 mg
Zinc	1 mg
Copper	0.12–0.15 mg
Selenium	1.3–3.0 µg
Manganese	7.5 µg
Iodine	30–60 µg
Chromium	0.1–0.5 µg
Molybdenum	0.3 µg

Adapted from Tsang RC, Lucas A, Uauy R, et al. (eds): Nutritional Needs of the Preterm Infant: Scientific Basis and Guidelines. Baltimore, Williams & Wilkins, 1993, p. 288.

able intakes of zinc and copper are 1.0 to 1.5 and 0.1 to 0.2 mg/kg/day, respectively[113,158] (Tables 24-5 and 24-6). Other minerals such as selenium, manganese, iodine, chromium, and molybdenum also are required in trace amounts,[150,158] as are taurine, carnitine, inositol, and choline, at least under certain conditions (Table 24-6).[158]

Vitamin Requirements

Table 24-6 lists the recommended intakes of vitamins for premature infants.[158] Vitamin E is the major natural antioxidant in the body. It protects lipid-containing cell membranes against oxidative injury and is thought to play a role in preventing neonatal oxygen toxicity.[162] The recommended enteral vitamin E intake, 6 to 12 IU/kg/day, is sufficient to compensate for variation in absorption and distribution and in the intake of other nutrients, such as iron and polyunsaturated fatty acids (PUFA), which are known to influence vitamin E intake. This level of intake is also low enough to prevent the possible toxicities associated with excessive intakes of vitamin E.[163]

The amount of vitamin E required to prevent lipid peroxidation in vulnerable tissues depends on the PUFA content of the tissues and diet.[162] Tissues containing higher levels of PUFA are more susceptible to lipid peroxidation. In addition to the recommended vitamin E intake of 6 to 12 IU/kg/day, it is advisable to keep the dietary ratio of vitamin E to PUFA at or above the level of 0.6 mg of d-alpha -tocopherol (0.9 IU) per gram of PUFA.[150,162,164] In the 1960s, premature infants fed formulas that were high in PUFA and relatively low in vitamin E sometimes developed hemolytic anemia as a result of vitamin E deficiency,[165,166] particularly if they also received large doses of iron. Most human milk samples and current infant formulas have vitamin-E-to-PUFA ratios above

0.6 mg/g.[162,167] Consequently, normal premature infants who are well enough to tolerate enteral feedings are not at risk for vitamin E deficiency. Although unproved, there may be a role for vitamin E supplementation at birth in high-risk infants requiring assisted ventilation; a single enteral dose of 20 to 30 IU/kg[168] may help to correct the relative deficiency present in the first days of life[169] as a result of low vitamin E stores, increased vitamin E utilization to quench free radicals produced by oxidative reactions, and delayed supply of vitamin E from nutritional sources.

Infants with fat malabsorption because of cholestatic liver disease or short bowel syndrome are at risk for developing vitamin E deficiency after birth. Infants who require total parenteral nutrition also may be at risk for vitamin E deficiency, particularly those who receive very little vitamin E but large amounts of PUFA in the form of lipid emulsion.[170] The vitamin E contained in parenteral multivitamin preparations is in the form of d,l-alpha -tocopheryl acetate, which is slowly hydrolyzed and relatively ineffective as an antioxidant when given by injection.[171,172] Nevertheless, small intravenous doses of vitamin E (3 IU/kg/day as alpha -tocopheryl acetate in a multivitamin preparation) seem to be sufficient to prevent vitamin E deficiency in infants receiving total parenteral nutrition[173,174] while preventing potentially toxic plasma levels of vitamin E.[163]

Despite an early study[175] showing a protective effect of intramuscular supplements of vitamin E against BPD in premature infants with RDS, subsequent studies in populations with adequate vitamin E nutrition found no effect of supplemental vitamin E on the incidence of BPD.[176–179] Several studies have shown that the incidence or severity of retinopathy of prematurity (ROP) can be reduced by administration of high-dose vitamin E supplements to premature infants.[177,178,180,181] Other trials have failed to show any such benefit.[182,183] In view of these conflicting results and the possibility of serious toxicity from large doses of vitamin E,[163] routine administration of high-dose vitamin E supplements is not recommended for prophylaxis against ROP.[184] Vitamin E supplements in the first few days of life have also been proposed to reduce the risks of periventricular and intraventricular hemorrhage in premature infants,[168,185] although the available data are not yet sufficient to allow a recommendation for dosing of vitamin E for this purpose.

Vitamin A is essential for growth and differentiation of epithelial tissues, including those in the lung. Premature infants have low stores of vitamin A at birth, and infants with lung disease have lower plasma vitamin A levels than those without lung disease.[186] A systematic review of clinical trials of vitamin A supplementation to premature infants showed that vitamin A supplementation reduced by 15% (relative risk 0.85) the likelihood that infants would require supplemental oxygen at 36 weeks postmenstrual age.[187] This calculation was based on a single large study that was the only one to report this outcome.[188] In the systematic review, mortality and other morbidities were not significantly reduced by vitamin A.[187] Because of concerns about absorption from the gastrointestinal tract, the vitamin A supplements were given by intramuscular injection in all but one of the studies included in the review. The role of vitamin A supplementation in ameliorating the severity of lung disease in premature infants is not clear. The relatively small beneficial effect must be weighed against the risks of toxicity and the need for repeated intramuscular injections.

METHODS OF FEEDING

Infants who require assisted ventilation cannot be fed orally because of the danger of pulmonary aspiration. In addition, they usually lack the strength, reflexes, and neuromuscular coordination needed to be fed orally from the breast or bottle. Alternate methods of feeding are available for these infants. Most infants can be fed small amounts of colostrum or milk by tube into the stomach as soon as the mother's milk is available. Usually, it will also be necessary to provide parenteral nutrition support.

Parenteral Feeding

Peripheral Vein Catheters

Indwelling short plastic catheters, usually 22 or 24 gauge, provide safe and convenient access to the peripheral venous circulation. Veins in the extremities are preferred over scalp veins, to prevent the parental distress caused by shaving the infant's scalp hair to expose veins. Scalp veins should be used only after extremity sites have been exhausted and, even then, only after discussing the procedure with the infant's parents. The infusion site must be carefully observed so that extravasation can be detected as soon as possible. The most common significant complication of peripheral intravenous infusions is tissue necrosis at the site of extravasation, especially if the infusate is hypertonic or acidic or contains calcium. Digital gangrene and nerve injury have been reported as complications of peripheral vein infusions. Glucose concentrations greater than 12.5% should be avoided in peripheral veins. To prevent extravasation of fluid, the catheter should be immobilized securely by adhesive tape. If the site is near a joint, the arm or leg can be splinted with a padded board.

If glucose and synthetic amino acid mixtures are the sole energy sources, it is possible to provide about 80 kcal/kg/day by peripheral venous nutrition. This figure is based on an infusion containing 12.5 g of glucose and 2.5 g of amino acid per 100 mL at a rate of 150 mL/kg/day. This level of energy intake is sufficient to provide for the maintenance energy requirement and is adequate to support growth in most infants (see Table 24-4), but it leaves the infant at risk of essential fatty acid deficiency. Intravenous lipid emulsions made from plant oils provide an important source of essential fatty acids and additional energy. The emulsion is given intravenously as a 10% or 20% solution from a separate administration set that joins the main infusate (containing glucose, amino acids, electrolytes, minerals, and vitamins) shortly before the infusion needle. Lipid emulsions provide 1.1 (10%) or 2.0 (20%) kcal/mL. Using a regimen consisting of lipid emulsion and a solution containing glucose, amino acids, electrolytes, minerals, and vitamins given by peripheral vein, it is possible to provide complete nutritional support without causing fluid overload (Table 24-7).

If lipid emulsion is infused too rapidly, serum concentrations of triglycerides and fatty acids become elevated. Small premature infants, especially those who are small for gestational age, are less tolerant of infused lipid. Hypertriglyceridemia does not generally occur if the lipid infusion rate is limited to a maximum of 0.15 g/kg/hour. In infants weighing less than 1 kg, the maximum infusion rate should be limited to 0.10 g/kg/hour.

TABLE 24-7. Energy Sources in Peripheral Venous Nutrition

	Intake (per kg/day)		
Infusate	Water (mL)	Nutrient (g)	Energy (kcal)
Dextrose (12.5 g/dL) and amino acid (2.5 g/dL) solution	135	—	—
Dextrose	—	16.9	57
Amino acids	—	3.4	13
Lipid emulsion (20%)	15	3.0	30
Total	150		100

TABLE 24-8. Effect of Nonprotein Energy Source on Gas Exchange and Ventilation in Parenterally Nourished Newborn Infants

	Low-Fat Regimen	High-Fat Regimen
Energy intake (kcal/kg/day)	75	81
Nonprotein energy source (%)		
Dextrose	85	55
Lipid emulsion	15	45
Oxygen consumption (mL/kg/min)	6.4	6.5
Carbon dioxide production (mL/kg/min)	6.9	6.2*
Respiratory quotient	1.08	0.96*
Energy expenditure (kcal/kg/day)	48	47
Ventilation (mL/kg/min)	160	142*

*Significantly lower on high-fat regimen.
From Piedboeuf B, Chessex P, Hazan J, et al: Total parenteral nutrition in the newborn infant: Energy substrates and respiratory gas exchange. J Pediatr 118:97, 1991.

Rapid infusion of lipid emulsion has been found to cause detrimental effects on pulmonary gas exchange and hemodynamics. These effects seem to occur only when the lipids are infused faster than they can be cleared from the plasma. Decreased arterial oxygen tension has been reported, but only when the lipid infusion rate exceeded 0.2 g/kg/hour.[189,190] Lipid infusions in excess of 0.2 g/kg/hour have also been found to increase pulmonary artery pressure and pulmonary-to-systemic shunting[191–193]; these effects are thought to be mediated through effects on prostanoid metabolism.[191,192,194]

The fatty acids contained in lipid emulsions have the potential to displace bilirubin from its binding sites on albumin molecules. This occurs only when the molar ratio of fatty acids to albumin exceeds 6,[195] an unlikely event with infusion rates of 0.2 g/kg/hour or less.[196]

Review of the literature suggests that adverse effects of infused lipids are more closely related to the maximum hourly infusion rate than to the total daily dose. The risks of administering lipid emulsion are minimal when the lipids are infused at rates below 0.2 g (1 mL of 20% emulsion) per kilogram per hour. In the case of critically ill infants, it should be possible to limit the rate of lipid infusion to 0.15 g/kg/hour. With this infusion rate a daily dose as high as 3.0 g/kg can be delivered, assuming 20 hours for lipid infusion with 4 hours of interruption for the infusion of medications. Because infants weighing less than 1 kg are especially intolerant of infused lipid, it is prudent to limit their infusion rate to 0.1 g/kg/hour or less. Infants who are prone to pulmonary hypertension should also be subject to limited rates of lipid infusion. With a total daily lipid dose of 2.0 g/kg (as 20% emulsion), it is possible to provide 90 kcal/kg/day with a total fluid intake of 150 mL/kg/day; with a lipid dose of 3.0 g/kg/day, 100 kcal/kg/day can be provided with a total fluid volume of 150 mL/kg/day (see Table 24-7).

Studies of respiratory gas exchange and substrate utilization in premature infants have demonstrated an important advantage to using lipid emulsion as an energy source in infants with compromised respiratory function.[197–199] Oxidation of carbohydrate produces more carbon dioxide (CO_2) per mole of oxygen consumed or per kilocalorie of energy expended than does oxidation of fat. For this reason, subjects receiving fat-free total parenteral nutrition produce more CO_2 than they would if they were receiving part of their nonprotein energy as fat. Piedboeuf et al.[198] studied 10 low-birthweight infants who were given two isocaloric intravenous nutritional regimens, low-fat (1 g/kg/day) and high-fat (3 g/kg/day), each for 5 days in a crossover design. During the low-fat (high-glucose) regimen, the infants had higher respiratory quotients and higher rates of carbon dioxide production and minute ventilation (Table 24-8). For healthy subjects without respiratory compromise, the additional CO_2 can be easily eliminated by increasing the ventilation rate. However, for subjects whose maximal unassisted ventilation is limited by disease, the extra CO_2 produced from high-glucose parenteral nutrition may require initiation of, or increase in, mechanically assisted ventilation in order to prevent an increase in arterial CO_2 tension.

Central Vein Catheters

Two types of central vein catheters are used for intravenous delivery of nutrients to newborn infants. Large-bore catheters can be inserted through a jugular vein into the superior vena cava and tunneled subcutaneously to a skin exit site on the scalp or chest. These *surgically placed central vein catheters* are used for infants who have required gastrointestinal surgery for gut malformation or necrotizing enterocolitis. Broviac and Hickman catheters are two specific types used for this purpose.

The alternative and generally preferred technique is the use of percutaneously inserted small-bore catheters, usually made of silicone elastomer (Silicone) or another nonthrombogenic material. These catheters range in caliber from 20 to 28 gauge and can be easily inserted through a slightly larger introducer needle. If carefully maintained, *percutaneous central vein catheters* may function well for weeks. They provide a safe useful technique for prolonged venous access with a much lower risk of complication than with the larger, surgically placed catheters.

Serious complications of central venous catheters include infections, which are less frequent with percutaneous central lines, and superior vena cava obstruction from thrombosis, which virtually never occurs with percutaneous central lines but is sometimes a problem with surgical central lines in small infants. With either type of central venous line, the tip of the catheter should be placed in the vena cava rather than the right atrium, to prevent cardiac thrombosis, infection, and perforation with cardiac tamponade.[200] Because of their higher complication rate, surgically placed central lines should be avoided whenever possible in newborn infants.

Umbilical Vein Catheters

During the care of an infant who is ill enough to require mechanical ventilation, umbilical vein catheters are sometimes used for monitoring central venous pressure in infants with circulatory instability or for providing temporary venous access in extremely small premature infants. Umbilical vein catheters are susceptible to the same complications as surgical central lines, that is, infection and thrombosis. The tip of the catheter should be placed in the inferior vena cava to avoid cardiac thrombosis or perforation. Once early-onset infection has been ruled out or treated and the umbilical catheter is no longer needed for venous pressure monitoring, consideration should be given to replacing the catheter with a peripheral vein catheter or a percutaneous central vein catheter. Other serious complications, including portal phlebitis and cirrhosis, have been reported with umbilical vein catheters.

Umbilical Artery Catheters

Umbilical artery catheters are frequently used to monitor arterial oxygen tension and blood pressure in critically ill newborn infants. Administration of hypertonic nutritional solutions through arterial catheters increases the already significant risk of vascular injury and thrombosis.[201,202] Parenteral nutrition solutions should not be delivered through umbilical artery catheters when alternative routes are available. When the umbilical artery must be used to deliver nutritional support, the concentrations of nutrients in the infused solution should not exceed those used in peripheral veins. Nutritional support solutions must never be infused into peripheral arterial catheters.

In summary, the relative safety of peripheral venous nutrition makes it the preferred method for parenteral feeding, although the use of percutaneous central lines offers an attractive alternative for long-term nutritional support. Hospitals caring for ventilated infants should have personnel capable of maintaining peripheral venous infusions in infants. Surgically placed central lines should be avoided whenever possible but may be needed for some infants with severe gastrointestinal dysfunction. Umbilical vein catheters can be used for short-term delivery of nutritional solutions, but longer use increases the risks of infection and thrombosis. Umbilical artery catheters should be used to deliver nutritional solutions only when other routes of administration are not available.

Enteral Feeding

Intermittent Intragastric Feeding

In addition to providing nutrients to support growth and metabolism, enteral feeding, even in very small amounts, promotes intestinal development and function. Feeding stimulates gut hormone secretion,[203,204] which promotes intestinal growth.[205,206] Enteral feeding also enhances bile flow,[207] and small amounts of feeding may help to prevent the cholestasis that often occurs with total parenteral nutrition.[208] Intermittent ("bolus") nasogastric or orogastric gavage feeding at 2- or 3-hour intervals is commonly used for feeding premature infants and other infants who are unable to be fed by nipple. Because of limitations in the mechanical and biochemical functioning of the gastrointestinal tract in infants who require assisted ventilation this method generally must be combined with intravenous nutritional support to provide sufficient intake of water, energy, and nutrients, at least initially.

Sick infants, even those requiring mechanical ventilation, usually can be fed safely by gavage, provided there is no perforation, ileus, or malformation of the gastrointestinal tract. Very small amounts of maternal colostrum or infant formula can be started within hours of birth without increasing the risk of necrotizing enterocolitis,[209-211] although feedings probably should be delayed longer in infants with significant birth asphyxia, as evinced, for example, by a very low 5-minute Apgar score. Either oral or nasal feeding tubes can be used. Nasal tubes are easier to secure and offer no disadvantage for infants who are endotracheally intubated or who are receiving nasal continuous positive airway pressure delivered by a unilateral nasal tube in the contralateral naris. Because nasal feeding tubes partially obstruct the infant's airway, they probably should not be used in infants without ventilatory support who have respiratory distress or episodic apnea.

Under certain circumstances, intermittent gavage feedings can lead to decreased arterial oxygen tension in premature and term infants, especially those with respiratory disease.[212-214] This effect is mediated by a fall in tidal volume and functional residual capacity and occurs only with feedings of 2.5 mL/kg or larger.[212] How significantly these changes in lung volume contribute to the risks of hypoxia and aspiration with feeding is not known, but the potentially hazardous relationships exist and should be kept in mind when feeding sick infants who require assisted ventilation.

Nonnutritive sucking of a pacifier during gavage feedings has been tested as a way of compensating for the lack of oral stimulation in tube-fed infants. Results of clinical studies of nonnutritive sucking have been generally inconclusive, suggesting no effect on growth or gastrointestinal function but a slight shortening of hospital stay.[215-218] This latter effect presumably indicates accelerated learning of nipple feeding as a result of the "training" effect of nonnutritive sucking.

Continuous Intragastric Feeding

An alternative method of intragastric feeding is to infuse the milk or formula continuously through an indwelling nasogastric or orogastric tube at a constant rate controlled by an infusion pump. This method offers the theoretical advantages of allowing greater volumes to be absorbed without taxing the limited gastric capacity of smaller prematures and of avoiding the volume-related postfeeding hypoxia associated with intermittent gavage.[212] Unpredictable nutrient delivery is a potential problem with continuous feeding. Human milk fat may separate from the nonfat milk and be left in the tubing or syringe.[219] This problem can be averted by positioning the infusion pump so that the opening of the syringe if pointed upward, assuring that the fat is delivered if it separates. Erratic delivery of human milk fortifier is also a potential problem.[220] Analysis of the clinical trials addressing the issue of intermittent versus continuous intragastric feeding led to the conclusion that infants fed continuously took longer to reach fully enteral feedings, but there was no difference in growth or time to discharge.[221]

Transpyloric Feeding

Intermittent nasojejunal or nasoduodenal feedings have been used successfully to feed critically ill infants. Transpyloric feeding is technically more difficult and generally offers no advantage over intragastric feeding. Systematic review of randomized trials comparing transpyloric with intragastric feeding suggests no advantage and perhaps increased risk of mortality with transpyloric feeding.[218,222] This technique, therefore, is not recommended as a routine feeding method for ventilated infants.

Human Milk for Premature and Critically Ill Infants

The advantages of human milk are by now well known to those who care for critically ill infants. The most compelling medical advantage of human milk is its protective effect against necrotizing enterocolitis in premature infants.[223] Premature infants who receive only human milk are 83% less likely to develop necrotizing enterocolitis than are their formula-fed counterparts.[223] It is important for hospitals that care for ventilated infants to provide good lactation support services. These services should include parent education and information, electric breast pumps, convenient pumping and storage facilities, and the services of trained lactation specialists. Mothers of infants who require intensive care, including assisted ventilation, should be strongly encouraged to provide their milk for their infants, even if they had planned to feed formula at home after the infant is discharged. Most mothers will agree to do this if the benefits to their infants are explained.

Combined Enteral and Parenteral Feeding

Most critically ill infants can be fed adequately and safely by some combination of the methods described. The tolerance of each infant to a particular method of feeding cannot be predicted. Infants who require mechanical ventilation cannot be fed by nipple, but they can be fed adequately with peripheral venous nutrition supplemented as tolerated with orogastric or nasogastric gavage feedings, either intermittent or continuous (Table 24-9). The advantage of even small amounts of enteral feeding for promoting gut hormone secretion and intestinal growth warrants an early attempt at enteral feeding in nearly all infants.

PRACTICAL RECOMMENDATIONS

Parenteral Feeding and Fluid and Electrolyte Management

Infants who are ill enough to require assisted ventilation should begin to receive intravenous fluids within the first hour after birth. The initial infusion should consist of 5% or 10% dextrose in water or in 0.2N saline at a rate of approximately 70% to 80% of the estimated water requirement (see Table 24-2). For example, an infant weighing 1100 g at birth should receive about 90 mL/kg, or 100 mL during the first 24 hours. This relative restriction of water intake during the first day or two of life allows for a physiologic state of negative water balance that accompanies the mobilization of ECW.[22–27] Exactly how much postnatal weight loss is desirable is not known, but the amount of fluid given should be sufficient to prevent hypernatremia and clinical signs of dehydration. In most instances, allowance for 5% to 15% weight loss in the first week of life is appropriate.

Ten percent glucose in the amount suggested previously will prevent hypoglycemia in most infants, except some who are hyperinsulinemic. Occasionally, 10% glucose in these volumes may induce hyperglycemia in very-low-birthweight infants. Thus, in infants weighing less than 1 kg at birth, 5% glucose in water should be chosen as the initial infusate (or the average if more than one solution is infused).

If sodium is not contained in the initial infusate, it is added by the second day to deliver 2.5 to 3.5 mmol/kg/day, provided

TABLE 24-9. Comparison of Feeding Methods for Ventilator-dependent Infants

Method	Advantages	Risks and Disadvantages
Peripheral vein	Not dependent on gastrointestinal function No danger of aspiration Low infection risk	Repeated infant thermal and physiologic stress Personnel effort to start and maintain infusion Risk of tissue injury with extravasation
Central vein Surgical	Higher concentrations of infused glucose Possible when other methods fail Not dependent on gastrointestinal function No danger of aspiration Low risk of necrotizing enterocolitis Less handling and cold stress	General anesthesia Vena cava thrombosis Infection Perforation of vessel or heart
Percutaneous	Same as above No need for general anesthesia Lower risk of thrombosis	Infection Perforation of vessel or heart
Intermittent intragastric	Promotes intestinal growth Promotes gut hormone secretion Promotes bile flow Reliable nutrient delivery	Bypasses salivary and lingual enzymes
Continuous intragastric	Larger volumes may be tolerated	Bypasses salivary and lingual enzymes Feeding components may separate in tubing
Transpyloric feeding	Does not rely on gastric emptying	More difficult tube placement Decreased fat absorption Possible increased mortality

the serum sodium concentration is not elevated. The practice of initially withholding sodium from premature infants in the first 24 hours of life is based on the idea that exogenous sodium may inhibit the contraction of the ECW compartment. This practice is also supported by several clinical studies.[224,225] The sodium usually is given as sodium chloride. If metabolic acidosis is present, some or all of the maintenance sodium may be given as sodium bicarbonate or sodium acetate.[226] Potassium chloride is also added to the infusion on day 2, to give 2 to 2.5 mmol/kg/day, provided the serum potassium concentration is normal and urination is well established. On the second or third day of life, the infusion rate usually is increased to deliver maintenance volumes (see Table 24-2). Careful limitation of fluid intake to these amounts has been shown to reduce the risks of patent ductus arteriosus and necrotizing enterocolitis in premature infants.[227]

Intravenous calcium supplementation should be started if the infant has signs that are attributed to hypocalcemia (tremulousness, seizures, apnea, cardiac arrhythmia). Calcium supplementation should also be considered if the serum ionized calcium concentration falls below 3.5 mg/dL in an infant who is receiving little or no enteral intake. Respiratory alkalosis due to hyperventilation increases the risk of hypocalcemic tetany.[228] The usual starting dose of parenteral calcium is 300 mg of calcium gluconate per kilogram per day as a 10% solution. This is equivalent to 28 mg of elemental calcium per kilogram per day. Several practical precautions should be taken during parenteral calcium therapy. (1) Calcium salts should not be infused along with sodium bicarbonate, because precipitation of calcium carbonate particles may occur. (2) Calcium should not be administered into an artery.[201] (3) If calcium is infused into a peripheral vein, the utmost care should be provided to avoid extravasation; this may cause tissue necrosis and sloughing, which can be severe in some instances.

Most infants who require assisted ventilation should be given parenteral amino acids, minerals, and vitamins beginning within 24 hours of birth. The only exception should be an infant who can safely be fed significant volumes of milk or formula soon after birth and whose feedings are likely to be advanced within several days to a volume sufficient to support growth. Intravenous amino acids should be started at a dose of 1.5 to 2.0 g/kg/day. The dose of amino acids should be increased once a day in increments of 0.5 g/kg/day until a dose of 2.5 to 3.0 g/kg/day is reached. It is customary to add minerals and vitamins to the parenteral infusate when intravenous amino acids are begun.

Lipid emulsion should normally be given as a part of any infant's parenteral nutrition regimen. There is debate about how soon after birth lipid emulsion should started, but the benefits probably outweigh any risks by the third or fourth day of life. Lipid emulsion must be started before the end of the first week to prevent essential fatty acid deficiency in infants who cannot be fed enterally. The lipid emulsion is begun at a rate of 0.5 to 1.0 g/kg/day (0.25 to 0.5 mL of 20% emulsion per kilogram per hour for 20 hours) and increased not more than once daily in increments of 0.5 g/kg/day to a maximum infusion rate that should not exceed 3 g/kg/day (0.15 g/kg/hour for 20 hours) for infants weighing more than 1 kg and 2 g/kg/day (0.10 g/kg/hour) for infants weighing less than 1 kg. When the maximum dose is reached, the serum triglyceride concentration should be checked during the infusion; if it exceeds 150 mg/dL, the infusion should be stopped for at least 4 hours and resumed at a slower rate. The infusion should also be stopped if the serum is lipemic by visual inspection. Toxicity from lipid emulsion is more closely tied to the maximum hourly infusion rate than to the total daily dose. The doses recommended here are safe if infused at a constant rate over 20 or more hours each day but would not be as safe if given more rapidly.

Enteral Feeding

Although extra caution is advised in the enteral feeding of infants who require assisted ventilation, intragastric gavage can be safely attempted in most cases. Two possible exceptions should be noted. First, infants with severe birth asphyxia probably should not be fed enterally for 5 to 7 days after birth because of their increased risk of necrotizing enterocolitis. Second, infants who are improving and seem likely to be extubated within 24 hours probably should not be fed enterally. The risk of feeding, however small, might best be deferred until after extubation. Glottic closure may be impaired and the danger of aspiration increased immediately after extubation.[229]

If a ventilated infant fits neither of these relative contraindications, has passed meconium, and has a soft nondistended abdomen and audible bowel sounds, then nasogastric or orogastric gavage feeding may be attempted. Small volumes and cautious progression of feedings are advisable because aspiration would be particularly harmful in an infant who already requires mechanical ventilation. The presence of an uncuffed endotracheal tube would offer only partial protection from the hazard of aspiration.

The first feeding should consist of maternal colostrum (fresh, if possible) or infant formula (2 to 5 mL/kg). The stomach should be aspirated for residual contents 3 hours later. If the stomach is empty or nearly so, the feeding can be repeated. This process is repeated every 3 hours. The feedings can be increased once or twice daily. The gastric residual volume is recorded every 3 hours. If more than 10% of the volume of the previous feeding (or 1 mL, whichever is larger) is present, the infant should be examined and at least one feeding should be omitted. If residuals of more than 10% (or 1 mL) are repeatedly found, feedings should be stopped and the patient carefully evaluated for signs of necrotizing enterocolitis and intestinal obstruction.

If enteral feeding is successful, the rate of intravenous feeding should be reduced to keep the total fluid intake the same or allow a slight increase appropriate for advancing postnatal age (see Table 24-2). After the first week or so, fluid intake usually can be increased to 1.5 times the estimated requirement in order to allow greater energy and nutrient intake.

With the methods described earlier, it should be possible to provide adequate nutrition to all infants requiring assisted ventilation, thereby allowing each the best possible chance for recovery and normal development.

REFERENCES

1. Cone TE Jr: History of the Care and Feeding of the Premature Infant. Boston, Little, Brown and Company, 1985.
2. Smallpeice V, Davies PA: Immediate feeding of premature infants with undiluted breast-milk. Lancet 2:1349, 1964.
3. Wu PYK, Teilmann P, Gabler M, et al: "Early" versus "late" feeding of low birth weight neonates: Effect on serum bilirubin, blood sugar, and responses to glucagon and epinephrine tolerance tests. Pediatrics 39:733, 1967.

4. Auld PAM, Bhangananda P, Mehta S: The influence of an early caloric intake with I-V glucose on catabolism of premature infants. Pediatrics 37:592, 1966.

5. Usher R: Reduction of mortality from respiratory distress syndrome of prematurity with early administration of intravenous glucose and sodium bicarbonate. Pediatrics 32:966, 1963.

6. Cornblath M, Forbes AE, Pildes RS, et al: A controlled study of early fluid administration on survival of low birth weight infants. Pediatrics 38:547, 1966.

7. Dobbing J, Sands J: Quantitative growth and development of human brain. Arch Dis Child 48:757, 1973.

8. Dobbing J: Infant nutrition and later achievement. Am J Clin Nutr 41:477, 1985.

9. Dobbing J: Early nutrition and later achievement. Proc Nutr Soc 49:103, 1990.

10. Stoch MB, Smythe PM: Does undernutrition during infancy inhibit brain growth and subsequent intellectual development? Arch Dis Child 38:546, 1963.

11. Evans D, Bowie MD, Hansen JDL, et al: Intellectual development and nutrition. J Pediatr 97:358, 1980.

12. Kumar A, Ghai OP, Singh N: Delayed nerve conduction velocities in children with protein-calorie malnutrition. J Pediatr 90:149, 1977.

13. Galler JR, Ramsey F, Solimano G: A follow-up study of the effects of early malnutrition on subsequent development. II. Fine motor skills in adolescence. Pediatr Res 19:524, 1985.

14. Lechner AJ: Perinatal age determines the severity of retarded lung development induced by starvation. Am Rev Respir Dis 131:638, 1985.

15. Kalenga M, Henquin JC: Protein deprivation from the neonatal period impairs lung development in the rat. Pediatr Res 22:45, 1987.

16. Arora NS, Rochester DF: Respiratory muscle strength and maximal voluntary ventilation in undernourished patients. Am Rev Respir Dis 126:5, 1982.

17. Kalenga M, Henquin JC: Alteration of lung mechanics by protein-calorie malnutrition in weaned rats. Respir Physiol 68:29, 1987.

18. Frank L, Groseclose E: Oxygen toxicity in newborn rats: The adverse effects of undernutrition. J Appl Physiol 53:1248, 1982.

19. Deneke SM, Lynch BA, Fanburg BL: Effects of low protein diets or feed restriction on rat lung glutathione and oxygen toxicity. J Nutr 115:726, 1985.

20. Wilson DC, McClure G, Halliday HL, et al: Nutrition and bronchopulmonary dysplasia. Arch Dis Child 66:37, 1991.

21. Friis-Hansen B: Changes in body water compartments during growth. Acta Paediatr Suppl 110:1, 1957.

22. Friis-Hansen B: Body water compartments in children: Changes during growth and related changes in body composition. Pediatrics 28:169, 1961.

23. Hartnold G, Bétrémieux P, Modi N: Body water content of extremely preterm infants at birth. Arch Dis Child Fetal Neonatal Ed 83:F56, 2000.

24. Cheek DB, Maddison TG, Malinek M, et al: Further observations on the corrected bromide space of the neonate and investigation of water and electrolyte status in infants born of diabetic mothers. Pediatrics 28:861, 1961.

25. Kagan BM, Stanincova V, Felix NS, et al: Body composition of premature infants: Relation to nutrition. Am J Clin Nutr 25:1153, 1972.

26. Shaffer SG, Bradt SK, Hall RT: Postnatal changes in total body water and extracellular volume in the preterm infant with respiratory distress syndrome. J Pediatr 109:509, 1986.

27. Bauer K, Bovermann G, Roithmaier A, et al: Body composition, nutrition, and fluid balance during the first two weeks of life in preterm neonates weighing less than 1500 grams. J Pediatr 118:615, 1991.

28. Aperia A, Broberger O, Elinder G, et al: Postnatal development of renal function in pre-term and full-term infants. Acta Paediatr Scand 70:183, 1981.

29. Guignard JP: Renal function in the newborn infant. Pediatr Clin North Am 29:777, 1982.

30. Hey EN, Katz G: Evaporative water loss in the new-born baby. J Physiol (Lond) 200:605, 1969.

31. Sulyok E, Jéquier E, Prod'hom LS: Respiratory contribution to the thermal balance of the newborn infant under various ambient conditions. Pediatrics 51:641, 1973.

32. Fanaroff AA, Wald M, Gruber HS, et al: Insensible water loss in low birth weight infants. Pediatrics 50:236, 1972.

33. Wu PYK, Hodgman JE: Insensible water loss in preterm infants: Changes with postnatal development and non-ionizing radiant energy. Pediatrics 52:704, 1974.

34. Okken A, Jonxis JHP, Rispens P, et al: Insensible water loss and metabolic rate in low birthweight newborn infants. Pediatr Res 13:1072, 1979.

35. Hammarlund K, Sedin G: Transepidermal water loss in newborn infants. III. Relation to gestational age. Acta Paediatr Scand 68:795, 1979.

36. Hooper JMD, Evans IWJ, Stapleton T: Resting pulmonary water loss in the newborn infant. Pediatrics 13:206, 1954.

37. O'Brien D, Hansen JDL, Smith CA: Effect of supersaturated atmospheres on insensible water loss in the newborn infant. Pediatrics 13:126, 1954.

38. Sosulski R, Polin RA, Baumgart S: Respiratory water loss and heat balance in intubated infants receiving humidified air. J Pediatr 103:307, 1983.

39. Rutter N, Hull D: Response of term babies to a warm environment. Arch Dis Child 54:178, 1979.

40. Bell EF, Gray JC, Weinstein MR, et al: The effects of thermal environment on heat balance and insensible water loss in low-birth-weight infants. J Pediatr 96:452, 1980.

41. Hammarlund K, Nilsson GE, Öberg PÅ, et al: Transepidermal water loss in newborn infants. II. Relation to activity and body temperature. Acta Paediatr Scand 68:371, 1979.

42. Zweymüller E, Preining O: The insensible water loss of the newborn infant. Acta Paediatr Scand Suppl 205:1, 1970.

43. Williams PR, Oh W: Effects of radiant warmer on insensible water loss in newborn infants. Am J Dis Child 128:511, 1974.

44. Jones RWA, Rochefort MJ, Baum JD: Increased insensible water loss in newborn infants nursed under radiant heaters. Br Med J 2:1347, 1976.

45. Bell EF, Neidich GA, Cashore WJ, et al: Combined effect of radiant warmer and phototherapy on insensible water loss in low-birth-weight infants. J Pediatr 94:810, 1979.

46. Bell EF, Weinstein MR, Oh W: Heat balance in premature infants: Comparative effects of convectively heated incubator and radiant warmer, with and without plastic heat shield. J Pediatr 96:460, 1980.

47. Kjartansson S, Hammarlund K, Sedin G, et al: Water loss from the skin of term and preterm infants nursed under a radiant heater. Pediatr Res 37:233, 1995.

48. Oh W, Karecki H: Phototherapy and insensible water loss in the newborn infant. Am J Dis Child 124:230, 1972.

49. Grünhagen DJ, de Boer MGJ, de Beaufort AJ, et al: Transepidermal water loss during halogen spotlight phototherapy in preterm infants. Pediatr Res 51:402, 2002.

50. Engle WD, Baumgart S, Schwartz JG, et al: Insensible water loss in the critically ill neonate. Combined effect of radiant-warmer power and phototherapy. Am J Dis Child 135:516, 1981.

51. Kjartansson S, Hammarlund K, Sedin G: Insensible water loss from the skin during phototherapy in term and preterm infants. Acta Paediatr Scand 81:769, 1992.

52. Baumgart S, Fox WW, Polin RA: Physiologic implications of two different heat shields for infants under radiant warmers. J Pediatr 100:787, 1982.

53. Marks KH, Friedman Z, Maisels MJ: A simple device for reducing insensible water loss in low-birth-weight infants. Pediatrics 60:223, 1977.

54. Baumgart S, Engle WD, Fox WW, et al: Effect of heat shielding on convective and evaporative heat losses and on radiant heat transfer in the premature infant. J Pediatr 99:948, 1981.

55. Fitch CW, Korones SB: Heat shield reduces water loss. Arch Dis Child 59:886, 1984.

56. Knauth A, Gordin M, McNelis W, et al: Semipermeable polyurethane membrane as an artificial skin for the premature neonate. Pediatrics 83:945, 1989.

57. Vernon HJ, Lane AT, Wischerath LJ, et al: Semipermeable dressing and transepidermal water loss in premature infants. Pediatrics 86:357, 1990.

58. Mancini AJ, Sookdeo-Drost S, Madison KC, et al: Semipermeable dressings improve epidermal barrier function in premature infants. Pediatr Res 36:306, 1994.

59. Rutter N, Hull D: Reduction of skin water loss in the newborn. I. Effect of applying topical agents. Arch Dis Child 56:669, 1981.

60. Nopper AJ, Horii KA, Sookdeo-Drost S, et al: Topical ointment therapy benefits premature infants. J Pediatr 128:660, 1996.

61. Hansen JDL, Smith CA: Effects of withholding fluid in the immediate postnatal period. Pediatrics 12:99, 1953.

62. Calcagno PL, Rubin MI, Weintraub DH: Studies on the renal concentrating and diluting mechanisms in the premature infant. J Clin Invest 33:91, 1954.

63. Leake RS, Zakauddin S, Trygstad CW, et al: The effects of large volume intravenous fluid infusion on neonatal renal function. J Pediatr 89:968, 1976.

64. Fomon SJ, Ziegler EE: Water and renal solute load. In Fomon SJ: Nutrition of Normal Infants, St. Louis, Mosby, 1993, p. 91.

65. Saigal S, Sinclair JC: Urine solute excretion in growing low-birth-weight infants. J Pediatr 90:934, 1977.

66. Siegel SR, Fisher DA, Oh W: Renal function and serum aldosterone levels in infants with respiratory distress syndrome. J Pediatr 83:854, 1973.

67. Broberger U, Aperia A: Renal function in idiopathic respiratory distress syndrome. Acta Paediatr Scand 67:313, 1978.

68. Tulassay T, Ritvay J, Bors Z, et al: Alterations in creatinine clearance during respiratory distress syndrome. Biol Neonate 35:258, 1979.

69. Torrado A, Guignard JP, Prod'hom LS, et al: Hypoxaemia and renal function in newborns with respiratory distress syndrome (RDS). Helv Paediatr Acta 29:399, 1974.

70. Guignard JP, Torrado A, Mazouni SM, et al: Renal function in respiratory distress syndrome. J Pediatr 88:845, 1976.

71. Langman CB, Engle WD, Baumgart S, et al: The diuretic phase of respiratory distress syndrome and its relationship to oxygenation. J Pediatr 98:462, 1981.

72. Bidiwala KS, Lorenz JM, Kleinman LI: Renal function correlates of postnatal diuresis in preterm infants. Pediatrics 82:50, 1988.

73. Lorenz JM, Kleinman LI, Ahmed G, et al: Phases of fluid and electrolyte homeostasis in the extremely low birth weight infant. Pediatrics 96:484, 1995.

74. Shaffer SG, Geer PG, Goetz KL: Elevated atrial natriuretic factor in neonates with respiratory distress syndrome. J Pediatr 109:1028, 1986.

75. Liechty EA, Johnson MD, Myerburg DZ, et al: Daily sequential changes in plasma atrial natriuretic factor concentrations in mechanically ventilated low-birth-weight infants. Biol Neonate 55:244, 1989.

76. Rozycki HJ, Baumgart S: Atrial natriuretic factor and postnatal diuresis in respiratory distress syndrome. Arch Dis Child 66:43, 1991.

77. Kojima T, Hirata Y, Fukada Y, et al: Plasma atrial natriuretic peptide and spontaneous diuresis in sick neonates. Arch Dis Child 62:667, 1987.

78. Modi N, Bétrémieux P, Midgley J, et al: Postnatal weight loss and contraction of the extracellular compartment is triggered by atrial natriuretic peptide. Early Hum Dev 59:201, 2000.

79. Tulassay T, Machay T, Kiszel J, et al: Effects of continuous positive airway pressure on renal function in prematures. Biol Neonate 43:152, 1983.

80. Cox JR, Davies-Jones GAB, Leonard PJ, et al: The effect of positive pressure respiration on urinary aldosterone excretion. Clin Sci 24:1, 1963.

81. Hemmer M, Viquerat CE, Suter PM, et al: Urinary antidiuretic hormone excretion during mechanical ventilation and weaning in man. Anesthesiology 52:395, 1980.

82. Paxson CL Jr, Stoerner JW, Denson SE, et al: Syndrome of inappropriate antidiuretic hormone secretion in neonates with pneumothorax or atelectasis. J Pediatr 91:459, 1977.

83. Rivers RPA, Forsling ML, Olver RP: Inappropriate secretion of antidiuretic hormone in infants with respiratory infections. Arch Dis Child 56:358, 1981.

84. Stern P, LaRochelle FT Jr, Little GA: Vasopressin and pneumothorax in the neonate. Pediatrics 68:499, 1981.

85. Rees L, Brook CGD, Shaw JCL, et al: Hyponatraemia in the first week of life in preterm infants. Part I. Arginine vasopressin secretion. Arch Dis Child 59:414, 1984.

86. Mullins RJ, Dawe EJ, Lucas CE, et al: Mechanisms of impaired renal function with PEEP. J Surg Res 37:189, 1984.

87. Svenningsen NW, Andreasson B, Lindroth M: Diuresis and urine concentration during CPAP in newborn infants. Acta Paediatr Scand 73:727, 1984.

88. Sinclair JC, Driscoll JM Jr, Heird WC, et al: Supportive management of the sick neonate. Parenteral calories, water, and electrolytes. Pediatr Clin North Am 17:863, 1970.

89. Lemoh JN, Brooke OG: Frequency and weight of normal stools in infancy. Arch Dis Child 54:719, 1979.

90. Ziegler EE, O'Donnell AM, Nelson SE, et al: Body composition of the reference fetus. Growth 40:329, 1976.

91. Bell EF, Oh W: Fluid and electrolyte balance in very low birth weight infants. Clin Perinatol 6:139, 1979.

92. Lavietes PH: The metabolic measurement of the water exchange. J Clin Invest 14:57, 1935.

93. Reichman B, Chessex P, Putet G, et al: Diet, fat accretion, and growth in premature infants. N Engl J Med 305:1495, 1981.

94. Brooke OG, Alvear J, Arnold M: Energy retention, energy expenditure, and growth in healthy immature infants. Pediatr Res 13:215, 1979.

95. Chessex P, Reichman B, Verellen G, et al: Quality of growth in premature infants fed their own mothers' milk. J Pediatr 102:107, 1983.

96. Whyte RK, Haslam R, Vlainic C, et al: Energy balance and nitrogen balance in growing low birthweight infants fed human milk or formula. Pediatr Res 17:891, 1983.

97. Sauer PJJ, Dane HJ, Visser HKA: Longitudinal studies on metabolic rate, heat loss, and energy cost of growth in low birth weight infants. Pediatr Res 18:254, 1984.

98. Putet G, Senterre J, Rigo J, et al: Nutrient balance, energy utilization, and composition of weight gain in very-low-birth-weight infants fed pooled human milk or a preterm formula. J Pediatr 105:79, 1984.

99. Catzeflis C, Schutz Y, Micheli JL, et al: Whole body protein synthesis and energy expenditure in very low birth weight infants. Pediatr Res 19:679, 1985.

100. Kashyap S, Ohira-Kist K, Abildskov K, et al: Effects of quality of energy intake on growth and metabolic response of enterally fed low-birth-weight infants. Pediatr Res 50:390, 2001.

101. Mestyán J, Fekete M, Bata G, et al: The basal metabolic rate of premature infants. Biol Neonate 7:11, 1964.

102. Anderson TL, Muttart CR, Bieber MA, et al: A controlled trial of glucose versus glucose and amino acids in premature infants. J Pediatr 94:947, 1979.

103. Richardson P, Bose CL, Bucciarelli RL, et al: Oxygen consumption of infants with respiratory distress syndrome. Biol Neonate 46:53, 1984.

104. Billeaud C, Piedboeuf B, Chessex P: Energy expenditure and severity of respiratory disease in very low birth weight infants receiving long-term ventilatory support. J Pediatr 120:461, 1992.

105. Schulze A, Abubakar K, Gill G, et al: Pulmonary oxygen consumption: A hypothesis to explain the increase in oxygen consumption of low birth weight infants with lung disease. Intensive Care Med 27:1636, 2001.

106. Field S, Kelly SM, Macklem PT: The oxygen cost of breathing in patients with cardiorespiratory disease. Am Rev Respir Dis 126:9, 1982.

107. Weinstein MR, Oh W: Oxygen consumption in infants with bronchopulmonary dysplasia. J Pediatr 99:958, 1981.

108. Kurzner SI, Garg M, Bautista DB, et al: Growth failure in bronchopulmonary dysplasia: Elevated metabolic rates and pulmonary mechanics. J Pediatr 112:73, 1988.

109. Kao LC, Durand DJ, Nickerson BG: Improving pulmonary function does not decrease oxygen consumption in infants with bronchopulmonary dysplasia. J Pediatr 112:616, 1988.

110. Yeh TF, McClenan DA, Ayahi OA, et al: Metabolic rate and energy balance in infants with bronchopulmonary dysplasia. J Pediatr 114:448, 1989.

111. de Meer K, Westerterp KR, Houwen RHJ, et al: Total energy expenditure in infants with bronchopulmonary dysplasia is associated with respiratory status. Eur J Pediatr 156:299, 1997.

112. Kalhan SC, Denne SC: Energy consumption in infants with bronchopulmonary dysplasia. J Pediatr 116:662, 1990.

113. Ziegler EE: Feeding the low birth weight infant. In Gellis SS, Kagan BM (eds): Current Pediatric Therapy 13, Philadelphia, WB Saunders, 1990, p. 713.

114. Ziegler EE: Protein in premature feeding. Nutrition 10:69, 1994.

115. Zlotkin SH, Bryan MH, Anderson GH: Intravenous nitrogen and energy intakes required to duplicate in utero nitrogen accretion in prematurely born human infants. J Pediatr 99:115, 1981.

116. Duffy B, Gunn T, Collinge J, et al: The effect of varying protein quality and energy intake on the nitrogen metabolism of parenterally fed very low birthweight (< 1600 g) infants. Pediatr Res 15:1040, 1981.

117. Rivera A Jr, Bell EF, Bier DM: Effect of intravenous amino acids on protein metabolism of preterm infants during the first three days of life. Pediatr Res 33:106, 1993.

118. Sturman JA, Gaull G, Raiha NCR: Absence of cystathionase in human fetal liver: Is cystine essential? Science 169:74, 1970.

119. Sturman JA, Rassin DK, Gaull GE: Taurine in development. Life Sci 21:1, 1977.

120. Uauy R, Birch DG, Birch EE, et al: Effect of dietary omega-3 fatty acids on retinal function of very-low-birth-weight neonates. Pediatr Res 28:485, 1990.

121. Hoffman DR, Birch EE, Birch DG, et al: Effects of supplementation with ω3 long-chain polyunsaturated fatty acids on retinal and cortical development in premature infants. Am J Clin Nutr (Suppl) 57:807S, 1993.

122. Carlson SE, Werkman SH, Rhodes PG, et al: Visual-acuity development in healthy preterm infants: Effect of marine-oil supplementation. Am J Clin Nutr 58:35, 1993.

123. Hansen AE, Stewart RA, Hughes G, et al: The relation of linoleic acid to infant feeding. Acta Paediatr Suppl 137:1, 1962.

124. Holman RT, Caster WO, Wiese HF: The essential fatty acid requirement of infants and the assessment of their dietary intake of linoleate by serum fatty acid analysis. Am J Clin Nutr 14:70, 1964.

125. American Academy of Pediatrics Committee on Nutrition: Nutritional needs of preterm infants. In Barness LA (ed): Pediatric Nutrition Handbook, 3rd ed. Elk Grove Village, Ill., American Academy of Pediatrics, 1993, p. 64.

126. Carnielli VP, Wattimena DJL, Luijendijk IHT, et al: The very low birth weight premature infant is capable of synthesizing arachidonic and docosahexaenoic acids from linoleic and linolenic acids. Pediatr Res 40:169, 1996.

127. Sauerwald TU, Hachey DL, Jensen CL, et al: Intermediates in endogenous synthesis of C22:6ω3 and C20:4ω6 by term and preterm infants. Pediatr Res 41:183, 1997.

128. Birch DG, Birch EE, Hoffman DR, et al: Retinal development of very low birthweight infants fed diets differing in omega-3 fatty acids. Invest Ophthalmol Vis Sci 33:2365, 1992.

129. Carlson SE, Werkman SH, Rhodes PG, et al: Visual acuity development in healthy preterm infants: Effect of marine oil supplementation. Am J Clin Nutr 58:35, 1993.

130. Clandinin MT, Van Aerde JE, Parrott A, et al: Assessment of the efficacious dose of arachidonic and docosahexaenoic acids in infant formulas: Fatty acid composition of erythrocyte membrane lipids. Pediatr Res 42:819, 1997.

131. O'Connor DL, Hall R, Adamkin D, et al: Growth and development in preterm infants fed long-chain polyunsaturated fatty acids: A prospective, randomized controlled trial. Pediatrics 108:359, 2001.

132. Auestad N, Halter R, Hall RT, et al: Growth and development in term infants fed long-chain polyunsaturated fatty acids: A double-masked, randomized, parallel, prospective, multivariate study. Pediatrics 108:372, 2001.

133. Watkins JB, Szczepanik P, Gould JB, et al: Bile salt metabolism in the human premature infant. Gastroenterology 69:706, 1975.

134. Zoppi G, Andreotti G, Pajno-Ferrara F, et al: Exocrine pancreas function in premature and full term neonates. Pediatr Res 6:880, 1972.

135. Hamosh M, Scanlon JW, Ganot D, et al: Fat digestion in the newborn. Characterization of lipase in gastric aspirates of premature and term infants. J Clin Invest 67:838, 1981.

136. Roy CC, Ste-Marie M, Chartrand L, et al: Correction of the malabsorption of the preterm infant with a medium-chain triglyceride formula. J Pediatr 86:446, 1975.

137. Tantibhedhyangkul P, Hashim SA: Medium-chain triglyceride feeding in premature infants: Effects of fat and nitrogen absorption. Pediatrics 55:359, 1975.

138. Okamoto E, Muttart CR, Zucker CL, et al: Use of medium-chain triglycerides in feeding the low-birth-weight infant. Am J Dis Child 136:428, 1982.

139. Sulkers EJ, von Goudoever JB, Leunisse C, et al: Comparison of two preterm formulas with or without addition of medium-chain triglycerides (MCTs). I: Effects on nitrogen and fat balance and body composition changes. J Pediatr Gastroenterol Nutr 15:34, 1992.

140. Sulkers EJ, Lafeber HN, Degenhart HJ, et al: Comparison of two preterm formulas with or without addition of medium-chain triglycerides (MCTs). II: Effects on mineral balance. J Pediatr Gastroenterol Nutr 15:42, 1992.

141. Whyte RK, Campbell D, Stanhope R, et al: Energy balance in low birth weight infants fed formulas of high or low medium-chain triglyceride content. J Pediatr 108:964, 1986.

142. Edmond J, Auestad N, Robbins RA, et al: Ketone body metabolism in the neonate: Development and the effect of diet. Fed Proc 44:2359, 1985.

143. Fomon SJ, Thomas LN, Filer LJ Jr, et al: Influence of fat and carbohydrate content of diet on food intake and growth of male infants. Acta Paediatr Scand 65:136, 1976.

144. Mobassaleh M, Montgomery RK, Biller JA, et al: Development of carbohydrate absorption in the fetus and neonate. Pediatrics 75:160, 1985.

145. Weaver LT, Laker MF, Nelson R: Neonatal intestinal lactase activity. Arch Dis Child 61:896, 1986.

146. Auricchio S, Rudino A, Murset G: Intestinal glycosidase activities in the human embryo, fetus, and newborn. Pediatrics 35:944, 1965.

147. Sevenhuysen GP, Holodinsky C, Dawes C: Development of salivary α-amylase in infants from birth to 5 months. Am J Clin Nutr 39:584, 1984.

148. Hodge C, Lebenthal E, Lee PC, et al: Amylase in the saliva and in the gastric aspirates of premature infants: Its potential role in glucose polymer hydrolysis. Pediatr Res 17:998, 1983.

149. Ziegler EE, Biga RL, Fomon SJ: Nutritional requirements of the premature infant. In Suskind RM (ed): Textbook of Pediatric Nutrition. New York, Raven Press, 1981, p. 29.

150. American Academy of Pediatrics Committee on Nutrition: Nutritional needs of low-birth-weight infants. Pediatrics 75:976, 1985.

151. Ziegler EE, Fomon SJ: Major minerals. In Fomon SJ (ed): Infant Nutrition, 2nd ed. Philadelphia, WB Saunders, 1974, p. 267.

152. Day GM, Chance GW, Radde IC, et al: Growth and mineral metabolism in very low birth weight infants. II. Effects of calcium supplementation on growth and divalent cations. Pediatr Res 9:568, 1975.

153. Steichen JJ, Gratton TL, Tsang RC: Osteopenia of prematurity: The cause and possible treatment. J Pediatr 96:528, 1980.

154. Chan GM, Mileur L, Hansen JW: Effects of increased calcium and phosphorus formulas and human milk on bone mineralization in preterm infants. J Pediatr Gastroenterol Nutr 5:444, 1986.

155. Greer FR, McCormick A: Improved bone mineralization and growth in premature infants fed fortified own mother's milk. J Pediatr 112:961, 1988.

156. Ehrenkranz RA, Gettner PA, Nelli CM: Nutrient balance studies in premature infants fed premature formula or fortified preterm human milk. J Pediatr Gastroenterol Nutr 8:58, 1989.

157. Greene HL, Hambidge KM, Schanler R, et al: Guidelines for the use of vitamins, trace elements, calcium, magnesium, and phosphorus in infants and children receiving total parenteral nutrition: Report of the Subcommittee on Pediatric Parenteral Nutrient Requirements from the Committee on Clinical Practice Issues of The American Society for Clinical Nutrition. Am J Clin Nutr 48:1324, 1988.

158. Tsang RC, Lucas A, Uauy R, et al. (eds): Nutritional Needs of the Preterm Infant. Baltimore, Williams & Wilkins, 1993.

159. Lundström U, Siimes MA, Dallman PR: At what age does iron supplementation become necessary in low-birth-weight infants? J Pediatr 91:878, 1977.

160. Hall RT, Wheeler RE, Benson J, et al: Feeding iron-fortified premature formula during initial hospitalization to infants less than 1800 grams birth weight. Pediatrics 92:409, 1993.

161. Franz AR, Mihatsch WA, Sander S, et al: Prospective randomized trial of early versus late enteral iron supplementation in infants with a birth weight of less than 1301 grams. Pediatrics 106:700, 2000.

162. Bell EF, Filer LJ Jr: The role of vitamin E in the nutrition of premature infants. Am J Clin Nutr 34:414, 1981.

163. Bell EF: Upper limit of vitamin E in infant formulas. J Nutr 119:1829, 1989.

164. Harris PL, Embree ND: Quantitative consideration of the effect of polyunsaturated fatty acid content of the diet upon the requirements for vitamin E. Am J Clin Nutr 13:385, 1963.

165. Hassan H, Hashim SA, Van Itallie TB, et al: Syndrome in premature infants associated with low plasma vitamin E levels and high polyunsaturated fatty acid diet. Am J Clin Nutr 19:147, 1966.

166. Oski FA, Barness LA: Vitamin E deficiency: A previously unrecognized cause of hemolytic anemia in the premature infant. J Pediatr 70:211, 1967.

167. Jansson L, Åkesson B, Holmberg L: Vitamin E and fatty acid composition of human milk. Am J Clin Nutr 34:8, 1981.

168. Bell EF: Vitamin E and iron deficiency in preterm infants. In Fomon SJ, Zlotkin S (eds): Nutritional Anemias. New York, Raven Press, 1992, p. 137.

169. Kelly FJ, Rodgers W, Handel J, et al: Time course of vitamin E repletion in the premature infant. Br J Nutr 63:631, 1990.

170. Gutcher GR, Lax AA, Farrell PM: Tocopherol isomers in intravenous lipid emulsions and resultant plasma concentrations. J Parenteral Enteral Nutr 8:269, 1984.

171. Newmark HL, Pool W, Bauernfeind JC, et al: Biopharmaceutic factors in parenteral administration of vitamin E. J Pharm Sci 64:655, 1975.

172. Knight ME, Roberts RJ: Tissue vitamin E levels in newborn rabbits after pharmacologic dosing. Influence of dose, dosage form, and route of administration. Dev Pharmacol Ther 8:96, 1985.

173. Gutcher GR, Farrell PM: Early intravenous correction of vitamin E deficiency in premature infants. J Pediatr Gastroenterol Nutr 4:604, 1985.

174. Phillips B, Franck LS, Greene HL: Vitamin E levels in premature infants during and after intravenous multivitamin supplementation. Pediatrics 80:680, 1987.

175. Ehrenkranz RA, Bonta BW, Ablow RC, et al: Amelioration of bronchopulmonary dysplasia after vitamin E administration. A preliminary report. N Engl J Med 299:564, 1978.

176. Ehrenkranz RA, Ablow RC, Warshaw JB: Effect of vitamin E on the development of oxygen-induced lung injury in neonates. Ann NY Acad Sci 393:452, 1982.

177. Hittner HM, Godio LB, Rudolph AJ, et al: Retrolental fibroplasia: Efficacy of vitamin E in a double-blind clinical study of preterm infants. N Engl J Med 305:1365, 1981.

178. Finer NN, Schindler RF, Grant G, et al: Effect of intramuscular vitamin E on frequency and severity of retrolental fibroplasia. A controlled trial. Lancet 1:1087, 1982.

179. Saldanha RL, Cepeda EE, Poland RL: The effect of vitamin E prophylaxis on the incidence and severity of bronchopulmonary dysplasia. J Pediatr 101:89, 1982.

180. Owens WC, Owens EU: Retrolental fibroplasia in premature infants. II. Studies on the prophylaxis of the disease: The use of alpha tocopheryl acetate. Am J Ophthalmol 32:1631, 1949.

181. Johnson L, Schaffer D, Boggs TR Jr: The premature infant, vitamin E deficiency and retrolental fibroplasia. Am J Clin Nutr 27:1158, 1974.

182. Puklin JE, Simon RM, Ehrenkranz RA: Influence on retrolental fibroplasia of intramuscular vitamin E administration during respiratory distress syndrome. Ophthalmology 89:96, 1982.

183. Schaffer DB, Johnson L, Quinn GE, et al: Vitamin E and retinopathy of prematurity. Follow-up at one year. Ophthalmology 92:1005, 1985.

184. American Academy of Pediatrics Committee on Fetus and Newborn: Vitamin E and the prevention of retinopathy of prematurity. Pediatrics 76:315, 1985.

185. Poland RL. Vitamin E for prevention of perinatal intracranial hemorrhage. Pediatrics 85:865, 1990.

186. Shenai JP, Chytil F, Jhaveri A, et al: Vitamin A status of neonates with bronchopulmonary dysplasia. Pediatr Res 19:185, 1985.

187. Darlow BA, Graham PJ: Vitamin A supplementation for preventing morbidity and mortality in very low birthweight infants (Cochrane Review). In: Cochrane Library. Oxford, Update Software, Issue 3, 2002.

188. Tyson JE, Wright LL, Oh W, et al: Vitamin A supplementation for extremely-low-birth-weight infants. N Engl J Med 340:1962, 1999.

189. Pereira GR, Fox WW, Stanley CA, et al: Decreased oxygenation and hyperlipemia during intravenous fat infusions in premature infants. Pediatrics 66:26, 1980.

190. Järnberg PO, Lindholm M, Eklund J: Lipid infusion in critically ill patients. Acute effects on hemodynamics and pulmonary gas exchange. Crit Care Med 9:27, 1981.

191. McKeen CR, Brigham KL, Bowers RE, et al: Pulmonary vascular effects of fat emulsion infusion in unanesthetized sheep. Prevention by indomethacin. J Clin Invest 61:1291, 1978.

192. Teague WG Jr, Raj JU, Braun D, et al: Lung vascular effects of lipid infusion in awake lambs. Pediatr Res 22:714, 1987.

193. Venus B, Smith RA, Patel C, et al: Hemodynamic and gas exchange alterations during Intralipid infusion in patients with adult respiratory distress syndrome. Chest 95:1278, 1989.

194. Gurtner GH, Knoblauch A, Smith PL, et al: Oxidant- and lipid-induced pulmonary vasoconstriction mediated by arachidonic acid metabolites. J Appl Physiol 55:949, 1983.

195. Kerner JA Jr, Cassani C, Hurwitz R, et al: Monitoring intravenous fat emulsions in neonates with the fatty acid/serum albumin molar ratio. J Parenter Enteral Nutr 5:517, 1981.

196. Spear ML, Stahl GE, Paul MH, et al: The effect of 15-hour fat infusions of varying dosage on bilirubin binding to albumin. J Parenter Enteral Nutr 9:144, 1985.

197. Van Aerde JEE, Sauer PJJ, Pencharz PB, et al: Effect of replacing glucose with lipid on the energy metabolism of newborn infants. Clin Sci 76:581, 1989.

198. Piedboeuf B, Chessex P, Hazan J, et al: Total parenteral nutrition in the newborn infant: Energy substrates and respiratory gas exchange. J Pediatr 118:97, 1991.

199. Salas-Salvadó J, Molina J, Figueras J, et al: Effect of the quality of infused energy on substrate utilization in the newborn receiving total parenteral nutrition. Pediatr Res 33:112, 1993.

200. Nadroo AM, Lin JL, Green RS: Death as a complication of peripherally inserted central catheters in neonates. J Pediatr 138:599, 2001.

201. Book LS, Herbst JJ, Stewart D: Hazards of calcium gluconate therapy in the newborn infant: Intra-arterial injection producing intestinal necrosis in rabbit ileum. J Pediatr 92:793, 1978.

202. Mokrohisky ST, Levine RL, Blumhagen JD, et al: Low positioning of umbilical-artery catheters increases associated complications in newborn infants. N Engl J Med 299:561, 1978.

203. Lucas A, Bloom SR, Aynsley-Green A: Metabolic and endocrine consequences of depriving preterm infants of enteral nutrition. Acta Paediatr Scand 72:245, 1983.

204. Lucas A, Bloom SR, Aynsley-Green A: Gastrointestinal peptides and the adaptation to extrauterine nutrition. Can J Physiol Pharmacol 63:527, 1985.

205. Johnson LR: Trophic actions of gastrointestinal hormones. Gastroenterology 70:278, 1976.

206. Heird WC, Schwarz SM, Hansen IH: Colostrum-induced enteric mucosal growth in beagle puppies. Pediatr Res 18:512, 1984.

207. Austin GL, Johnson SM, Shires GT III, et al: The effect of feeding on the bile salt-independent canalicular secretion in dogs. Am J Surg 135:36, 1978.

208. Benjamin DR: Hepatobiliary dysfunction in infants and children associated with long-term total parenteral nutrition. A clinico-pathologic study. Am J Clin Pathol 76:276, 1981.

209. Ostertag SG, LaGamma EF, Reisen CE, et al: Early feeding does not affect the incidence of necrotizing enterocolitis. Pediatrics 77:275, 1986.

210. Dunn L, Hulman S, Weiner J, et al: Beneficial effects of early hypocaloric enteral feeding on neonatal gastrointestinal function: Preliminary report of a randomized trial. J Pediatr 112:622, 1988.

211. Slagle TA, Gross SJ: Effect of early low-volume enteral substrate on subsequent feeding tolerance in very low birth weight infants. J Pediatr 113:526, 1988.

212. Yu VYH: Cardiorespiratory response to feeding in newborn infants. Arch Dis Child 51:305, 1976.

213. Pitcher-Wilmott R, Shutack JG, Fox WW: Decreased lung volume after nasogastric feeding of neonates recovering from respiratory disease. J Pediatr 95:119, 1979.

214. Rosen CL, Glaze DG, Frost JD Jr: Hypoxemia associated with feeding in the preterm infant and full-term neonate. Am J Dis Child 138:623, 1984.

215. Field T, Ignatoff E, Stringer S, et al: Nonnutritive sucking during tube feedings: Effects on preterm neonates in an intensive care unit. Pediatrics 70:381, 1982.

216. Bernbaum JC, Pereira GR, Watkins JB, et al: Nonnutritive sucking during gavage feeding enhances growth and maturation in premature infants. Pediatrics 71:41, 1983.

217. Ernst JA, Rickard KA, Neal PR, et al: Lack of improved growth outcome related to nonnutritive sucking in very low birthweight premature infants fed a controlled nutrient intake: A randomized prospective study. Pediatrics 83:706, 1989.

218. Steer PA, Lucas A, Sinclair JC: Feeding the low birthweight infant. In Sinclair JC, Bracken MB (eds): Effective Care of the Newborn Infant. Oxford, Oxford University Press, 1992, p. 94.

219. Greer FR, McCormick A, Loker J: Changes in fat concentration of human milk during delivery by intermittent bolus and continuous mechanical pump infusion. J Pediatr 105:745, 1984.

220. Bhatia J, Rassin DK: Human milk supplementation: Delivery of energy, calcium, phosphorus, magnesium, copper, and zinc. Am J Dis Child 142:445, 1988.

221. Premji S, Chessell L: Continuous nasogastric milk feeding versus intermittent bolus milk feeding for premature infants less than 1500 grams (Cochrane Review). In: Cochrane Library. Oxford, Update Software, Issue 3, 2002.

222. McGuire W, McEwan P: Transpyloric versus gastric tube feeding for preterm infants (Cochrane Review). In: Cochrane Library. Oxford, Update Software, Issue 3, 2002.

223. Lucas A, Cole TJ: Breast milk and neonatal necrotising enterocolitis. Lancet 336:1519, 1990.

224. Costarino AT Jr, Gruskay JA, Corcoran L, et al: Sodium restriction versus daily maintenance replacement in very low birth weight premature infants: A randomized, blind therapeutic trial. J Pediatr 120:99, 1992.

225. Hartnoll G, Bétrémieux P, Modi N: Randomised controlled trial of postnatal sodium supplementation on body composition in 25 to 30 week gestational age infants. Arch Dis Child Fetal Neonatal Ed 82:F24, 2000.

226. Ekblad H, Kero P, Takala J, et al: Water, sodium and acid-base balance in premature infants: Therapeutical aspects. Acta Paediatr Scand 76:47, 1987.

227. Bell EF, Acarregui MJ: Restricted versus liberal water intake for preventing morbidity and mortality in preterm infants (Cochrane Review). In: Cochrane Library. Oxford, Update Software, Issue 3, 2002.

228. Watchko J, Bifano EM, Bergstrom WH: Effect of hyperventilation on total calcium, ionized calcium, and serum phosphorus in neonates. Crit Care Med 12:1055, 1984.

229. Burgess GE III, Cooper JR Jr, Marino RJ, et al: Laryngeal competence after tracheal extubation. Anesthesiology 51:73, 1979.

25 CENTRAL NERVOUS SYSTEM MORBIDITY

W. THOMAS BASS, MD
ARTHUR E. KOPELMAN, MD

As a result of advances in obstetric and neonatal care, approximately 85% of premature very-low-birthweight (VLBW) infants (<1500 g) now survive. These advances include the use of antenatal steroids and surfactant, as well as improvements in respiratory support. Regrettably, the recent improvements in survival have not been accompanied by improved overall neurologic outcome. The most important reason for the continued high rate of neurodevelopmental disability is that the greatest improvements in survival have been among extremely-low-birthweight (ELBW) infants (<1000 g), the group that, by far, has the highest incidence of brain injury.[1] Also, the continuing high rate of bronchopulmonary dysplasia (BPD) among ELBW infants, a condition that is closely associated with neurodevelopmental deficits, may contribute to their poor neurologic outcomes.[2,3]

Although it is generally accepted that brain injury occurs more frequently in smaller infants with more severe lung disease,[4,5] the exact relationships between lung disease and its treatment and brain injury are unclear. Infants treated with ventilators are at risk for various disturbances in physiology implicated in the pathogenesis of brain injury, such as abnormal blood gases, fluctuations in arterial blood pressure, changes in cerebral blood flow,[6] and extra-alveolar air leak syndromes.[7] Although the use of surfactant to prevent or treat respiratory distress syndrome (RDS) has decreased the severity of these clinical disturbances, it has not had a significant impact on the incidence or severity of brain injury in premature infants. This observation, which was a surprise and a disappointment to physicians caring for premature infants, raises the question of whether RDS may be more significant as a marker of risk for brain injury than as its cause.[8] On the other hand, complications from the use of mechanical ventilation have important effects on cardiac output, cerebral blood flow, cerebral oxygenation, and cerebral venous return that at times result in brain injury. Certain approaches to mechanical ventilation have been associated with an increased incidence of brain injury.[9] The impact of ventilator and other treatments of respiratory diseases on risks for neurologic injury are noted in this chapter whenever possible. Although considerable progress has been made in the management of neonatal respiratory diseases, there is much more to learn about the impact of our therapies on the developing nervous system and how their use may relate to the pathogenesis of neonatal brain injury. Hopefully, as more is learned, the use of *neuroprotective* strategies will become a routine part of case management in the neonatal intensive care unit.

MECHANISMS OF NEURONAL INJURY AND DEATH: NECROSIS AND APOPTOSIS

Neurons have an extremely high metabolic rate and as a result are susceptible to injury from hypoxia, ischemia, hypoglycemia, and inflammation, disturbances that occur with some frequency in preterm infants with respiratory diseases. Overwhelming insult to the neuron causes immediate mitochondrial dysfunction and energy failure. As a result, membrane pumps cannot maintain ionic homeostasis, organelles become disrupted, and plasma membrane integrity is lost. The neuron then swells and bursts, and its cytoplasm is spilled into the extracellular space. The extracellular debris induces a potent inflammatory response complete with large numbers of phagocytic cells.[10] Acute, rapid neuronal death following an overwhelming injury is termed *necrosis* and is probably the major form of cell death seen in hemorrhagic infarction (see discussion later).

A second type of cell death occurs when a less severe cellular injury leads to an inappropriate activation of delayed or programmed cell death, also termed *apoptosis*. Apoptosis is part of normal brain development as the fetal brain has about 1.5 times the adult number of neurons, and the "excess" neurons that do not make proper synaptic connections or otherwise lose trophic support undergo programmed cell death.[11] Moderate degrees of hypoxia, ischemia, hypoglycemia, or inflammation can induce apoptosis to proceed inappropriately, leading to delayed death of neurons days, weeks, or months later that normally would have survived.[12] Interestingly, unlike necrosis, apoptosis does not induce an inflammatory response. Experimental[13,14] and clinical evidence[15] suggests that apoptosis may be the primary form of cell death in periventricular leukomalacia and global white matter injury (see discussion later). Most important, because apoptosis involves delayed cell death following an injury, there is hope that pharmacologic interventions following neuronal injury may prove successful in preventing neuronal death by apoptosis. Features of the two mechanisms of cell death, necrosis and apoptosis, will be evident in the following discussions of neonatal brain injury.

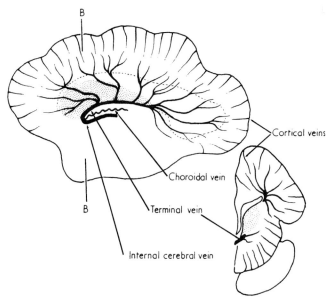

Figure 25-1. Veins related to the germinal matrix and periventricular areas at 30 weeks' gestation. (From Hambleton G, Wigglesworth JS: Origin of intraventricular hemorrhage in the preterm infant. Arch Dis Child 51:651, 1976.)

UNIQUE VULNERABILITY OF THE PRETERM BRAIN

The brain of the premature infant delivered between 24 and 32 weeks of gestation is still developing rapidly, and the unique patterns of injury seen following serious disturbances of physiology during pregnancy, labor and delivery, or early postnatal life depend upon the developmental stage at the time of the insult. The preterm infant's brain has a very high metabolic rate. The brain accounts for only 10% to 15% of body weight (as compared with 3% in the adult), but it receives 20% to 40% of the cardiac output and is responsible for 25% to 50% of oxygen and glucose consumption.[11] When caring for a fragile 24-week-gestation ELBW infant, we should appreciate that formation of the adult number of cerebral neurons, around 100 billion, is already complete, and that ongoing mitosis in the germinal matrix is now rapidly giving rise to glial cells. Unfortunately, the high metabolic rate of the preterm brain due to the active processes of rapid cell proliferation and migration, cortical organization, and myelination make it particularly vulnerable to cellular injury from ischemia, hypoxemia, hypoglycemia, and inflammation.

Because of their central importance in the pathogenesis of specific forms of brain damage in the preterm infant, four aspects of cerebral development are briefly discussed here: germinal matrix development, growth of blood vessels to support the growing cerebrum, cortical organization, and myelination.

Germinal Matrix Development

Closure of the neural tube occurs between 22 and 27 days of embryonic life.[16] The neural tube is composed of proliferating immature neuroglial cells that divide along the luminal surface of the neural tube. The postmitotic daughter cells then migrate into and populate the developing spinal cord and cerebral cortex. Cells populating the spinal cord have already completed their migration by the late second trimester. However, in the brain, periventricular masses of proliferating "germinal matrix" cells persist into the third trimester. The germinal matrix is most prominent at 24 to 28 weeks of gestation when its rich blood supply is composed of numerous poorly supported thin-walled blood vessels.[17,18] These delicate vessels are highly susceptible to disruption by disturbances in local blood pressure and flow, events that occur with some frequency if the infant is born prematurely during this period. They are the site of origin of germinal matrix and intraventricular hemorrhages.[19]

Vascular Growth to Support the Expanding Cerebral White Matter

The patterns of distribution and rates of growth of the developing venous and arterial blood supplies to the deep periventricular region of the growing cerebral white matter are relevant to the pathogenesis of the two most common major forms of severe brain injury in premature infants: periventricular hemorrhagic infarction and periventricular leukomalacia.

First, the many small medullary veins draining the periventricular white matter coalesce into the single terminal vein that courses through the germinal matrix (Fig. 25-1). Compression of this important venous confluence by a large germinal matrix or intraventricular hemorrhage, or possibly vasoconstriction of the terminal vein induced by the local release of potassium from erythrocytes in such hemorrhages, leads to *periventricular hemorrhagic infarction* (PHI), one of the major types of neonatal brain injury.[6] Localized venous congestion prevents egress of venous blood and entry of fresh oxygenated blood into the periventricular tissue, which then undergoes infarction with rupture of the distended veins converting the damaged region into a hemorrhagic infarct. This lesion is almost always unilateral or markedly asymmetric, developing ipsilateral to a pre-existing large germinal matrix or intraventricular hemorrhage.

The *arterial* blood supply of the enlarging cerebrum consists of multiple penetrating arteries from the pial surface (Fig. 25-2). The innermost region of the rapidly growing cerebrum is farthest from the in-growing penetrating arteries, so the deep periventricular white matter is most vulnerable to ischemic injury, that is, a watershed zone. In the event of significant hypotension, the immature oligodendrocytes and axons of the periventricular white matter are vulnerable to ischemic injury. This ischemic injury is termed *periventricular leukomalacia* (PVL). If the cell loss is extensive, phagocytosis of necrotic or dying tissue results in periventricular white matter cysts (cystic PVL). The penetrating arteries are even less well developed in the most immature infants, in whom cerebral perfusion is even more critically dependent upon maintenance of adequate systolic blood pressure so even relatively modest hypotension may result in diffuse leukomalacia.[20]

Cortical Organization

Cortical organizational events occur during the latter part of, and following, the stage of neuronal migration. As outlined by Volpe,[21] these organizational events involve the establishment

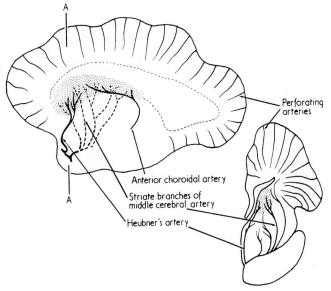

Figure 25-2. Arterial supply to the basal ganglia and periventricular areas at 30 weeks' gestation. (From Hambleton G, Wigglesworth JS: Origin of intraventricular hemorrhage in the preterm infant. Arch Dis Child 51:651, 1976.)

of transient "way station" subplate neurons, establishment of cortical plate neurons, and formation of axons, dendrites, and synaptic connections. During this time, selective elimination of "excess" neurons (apoptosis), and proliferation and differentiation of glial cells take place. These complex neuronal and neuroglial interactions can be altered by either prenatal or postnatal factors. For instance, infants who develop white matter injury, such as PVL or diffuse white matter injury, may also have a smaller volume of cortical gray matter.[22,23] This finding supports the concept that normal afferent and efferent connections are essential for normal cortical development.[24]

Myelination

Myelination of the human brain is a prolonged process that begins during the second trimester and continues for years following birth. Myelin is produced by oligodendrocytes populating the periventricular area. The progenitors of the oligodendrocyte are produced in the germinal matrix during the third trimester and postnatal period so premature infants may be delivered while oligodendrocytes are still actively proliferating and differentiating.[21] During the third trimester the oligodendrocyte enters a premyelination phase by developing linear extensions that wrap around axons. This process can be detected by magnetic resonance imaging showing an increase in the directionality of water diffusion in the periventricular region.[25] A lack of appropriate directionality of water diffusion in the periventricular region is indicative of white matter injury,[26] sometimes even when the ultrasonogram is normal.[27]

Early differentiating oligodendrocytes are especially vulnerable to many types of noxious stimuli,[28] including ischemia-reperfusion–induced free radical attack leading to cell death by apoptosis.[11,29] One possible explanation for their unusual sensitivity to free radical attack may be the high concentration of intracellular iron needed for normal differentiation; hydrogen peroxide is converted to toxic hydroxyl radicals in the presence of iron. Immature oligodendrocytes also have low levels of

catalase and glutathione peroxidase that are protective against oxidative injury.[30] Although the immature oligodendrocytes may be the primary cell lost in periventricular injury, studies suggest that astrocytes and neuronal axons are also subject to free-radical injury.[31,32] Because oligodendrocytes are responsible for myelination, it follows that deficient myelination will be a consequence of the loss of immature oligodendrocytes.

It has been shown that diffuse white matter injury may occur secondary to a perinatal inflammatory process (see section on Diffuse White Matter Injury). Although it is convenient to discuss PVL and diffuse white matter injury separately, they may represent varying degrees of severity of the same process, and in individual cases the exact etiology of the injury may not be clear. Cystic PVL may be seen on cranial ultrasound during relatively early stages of injury, but evidence of diffuse white matter injury often is not appreciated until a late ultrasound shows a diminished volume of cerebral white matter and secondary ventricular enlargement (hydrocephalus ex vacuo). Diffuse white matter injury may be a relatively common and important form of brain damage in ELBW infants that is not visualized on early cranial ultrasound.

NEUROIMAGING

Before discussing the various types of brain injury in premature infants, it is important to mention some of the strengths and limitations of the commonly used neuroimaging techniques. The preterm infant requiring a neuroimaging study often is unstable and on ventilator support. The infant's clinical condition then often dictates the choice of neuroimaging study. Computerized tomography, magnetic resonance imaging (MRI), positron emission tomography, and spectral analysis each provides different information. MRI is considered the "gold standard" to which other brain imaging techniques are compared, but it often cannot be used clinically because it requires that the critically ill infant be transported to another part of the hospital and it sometimes requires sedation. Because of its mobility, lack of ionizing radiation, and relatively low cost, cranial ultrasonography remains the most commonly used neuroimaging technique for diagnosis of brain abnormalities in the newborn.[33]

Unfortunately, lack of uniformity in describing the appearance, location, and evolution of the lesions seen on ultrasound has made it difficult to compare results of different clinical studies of neonatal brain lesions. Also, ultrasound may not detect less severe ischemic lesions, especially if they are diffuse and noncystic.[34,35] In an editorial, Paneth[36] outlined these problems and suggested a classification of brain lesions more consistent with neuropathologic findings. He proposes that abnormal findings be categorized into three groups: (1) white matter damage; (2) hemorrhage into nonparenchymal areas (i.e., ventricles); and (3) lesions in other brain locations, such as the cerebellum, basal ganglia, and brainstem. This classification properly emphasizes the almost uniform finding of cerebral white matter damage in clinically important brain injury in premature infants. In any case, one needs to pay careful attention to the diagnostic criteria used when reading or comparing studies of perinatal brain injury and outcome. Ultrasound is reasonably good at diagnosing the two major types of periventricular white matter injury, hemorrhagic infarction and leukomalacia, in the majority of patients with parenchymal lesions.[37,38]

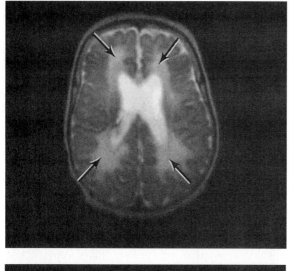

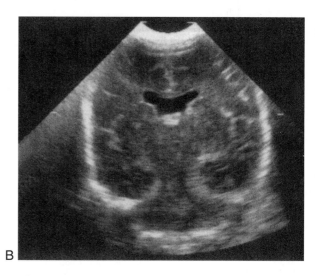

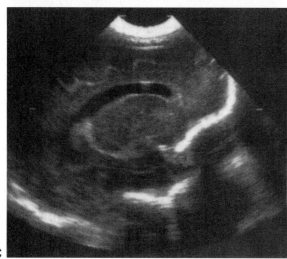

Figure 25-3. Normal echogenicity on ultrasound but diffuse excessive high signal intensity of the periventricular white matter on magnetic resonance imaging in a 530-g infant imaged at 44 weeks' postconceptual age. *A,* T2-weighted image at the midventricular level showing dilation of the lateral ventricles and high signal intensity *(arrows).* Corresponding coronal *(B)* and left *(C)* parasagittal ultrasound scans showing dilation of the ventricles and normal white matter echodensity. (From Maalouf EF, Duggan PJ, Counsell SJ, et al: Comparison of findings on cranial ultrasound and magnetic resonance imaging in preterm infants. Pediatrics 107:719, 2001.)

However, a comparison of ultrasound and MRI examinations of preterm infants showed that ultrasound accurately diagnosed germinal matrix hemorrhage, intraventricular hemorrhage, hemorrhagic parenchymal infarction, and cystic PVL, but it missed subtle diffuse white matter injury (Fig. 25-3).[39] It is likely that subtle cytotoxic edema and other subtle white matter injury predisposing to apoptosis are more easily seen with MRI, whereas hemorrhages are well visualized using ultrasound (see sections on Periventricular Leukomalacia and Diffuse White Matter Injury). As long as ultrasound remains the most common modality used clinically to look for evidence of cerebral injury in VLBW infants, we will continue to see infants in our neurodevelopmental follow-up clinics who we diagnose with cognitive, visual-spatial, and/or visual-motor deficits[40] who had a normal head ultrasound in the newborn period.

MAJOR TYPES OF BRAIN INJURY IN THE PREMATURE INFANT

Germinal Matrix Hemorrhage/Intraventricular Hemorrhage

Germinal matrix hemorrhage/intraventricular hemorrhage (GMH/IVH) is the most common type of intracranial hemor-

rhage in the premature infant seen on cranial ultrasound. Its occurrence is inversely related to birthweight and gestational age. In one large series, the incidence of GMH/IVH was 1% in infants with birthweights 1551 to 2250 g, 7% in infants 1251 to 1500 g, 16% in infants 1001 to 1250 g, 30% in infants 751 to 1000 g, and 32% in infants less than 750 g.[41] There has been a gradual reduction in the incidence of all stages of GMH/IVH over the last decade, to an incidence of approximately 20% in infants of birthweight less than 1500 g.[42]

Neuroanatomy and Pathogenesis

The pathogenesis of GMH/IVH is related to the presence of a prominent subependymal germinal matrix at the time of premature labor and birth (see discussion earlier). An elaborate capillary bed consisting of thin-walled, poorly supported vessels supplies the germinal matrix. If there are acute alterations in blood pressure and cerebral perfusion (Fig. 25-4), these tenuous capillaries are disrupted, leading to hemorrhage into the gelatinous matrix stroma.[43] With continued hemorrhage the subependymal area may become distorted, and in 80% of cases the GMH ruptures through the ependyma into the lateral ventricle.[42] The vast majority of GMH/IVH hemorrhages occur in the first few hours after birth, and 90% are detectable by ultrasound by the third postnatal day.[43] A lower incidence of GMH/IVH has been noted in female infants

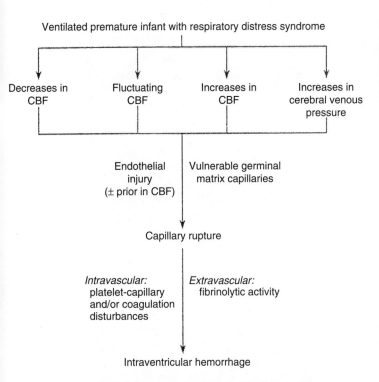

Ventilated premature infant with respiratory distress syndrome

Decreases in CBF   Fluctuating CBF   Increases in CBF   Increases in cerebral venous pressure

Endothelial injury (± prior in CBF)   Vulnerable germinal matrix capillaries

Capillary rupture

Intravascular: platelet-capillary and/or coagulation disturbances   Extravascular: fibrinolytic activity

Intraventricular hemorrhage

Figure 25-4. Interaction of major pathogenetic factors in the occurrence of germinal matrix hemorrhage/intraventricular hemorrhage in the ventilated premature infant with respiratory distress syndrome. CBF, cerebral blood flow. [From Volpe JJ: Intracranial hemorrhage: Germinal matrix-intraventricular hemorrhage of the premature infant. In Volpe JJ (ed): Neurology of the Newborn, 4th ed. Philadelphia, WB Saunders, 2001, p. 447.]

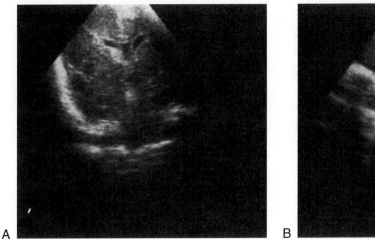
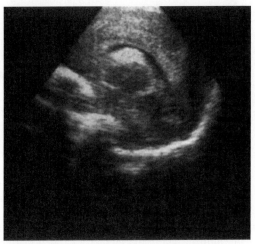

A   B

Figure 25-5. Grade I hemorrhage. Photographs from a cranial ultrasound examination with coronal (A) and parasagittal (B) views depict a right-sided grade I (germinal matrix) hemorrhage.

and in infants delivered to mothers with pregnancy-induced hypertension, and a higher incidence is seen with multiple gestation.[42,44]

Diagnosis

The most widely used classification system developed by Papile et al.[45] defines a grade I IVH as an isolated subependymal hemorrhage (Fig. 25-5), a grade II IVH by the presence of ventricular blood filling less than half of the ventricle (Fig. 25-6), and a grade III IVH as distention of the lateral ventricle, which is filled with blood (Fig. 25-7). All but the most severe forms of GMH/IVH are asymptomatic and are detected on routine cranial ultrasound studies performed on infants with risk factors such as prematurity (<32 weeks of gestation) or RDS.

Prevention

Because acute changes in blood pressure are considered important in the etiology of GMH/IVH, one would anticipate that stresses placed on the infant by an abnormal presentation, labor, or delivery would be important, but studies have not shown this consistently.[42,46] In one study, however, delivery by the vaginal route, duration of labor over 12 hours, and a trial of labor before cesarean section were associated with an increased risk of GMH/IVH.[47]

Importantly, antenatal corticosteroids have been shown to decrease the incidence of GMH/IVH by about 50%.[48–50] Although tocolytic therapy only delays delivery for a few days, its use may provide time for the obstetrician to administer a course of antenatal corticosteroids to the mother, achieving the combined benefits of reducing the incidence of GMH/IVH and

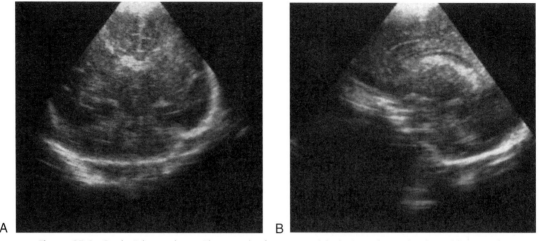

Figure 25-6. Grade II hemorrhage. Photographs from a cranial ultrasound examination with coronal (A) and sagittal (B) views depict a right-sided grade II hemorrhage (intraventricular hemorrhage without ventricular dilation).

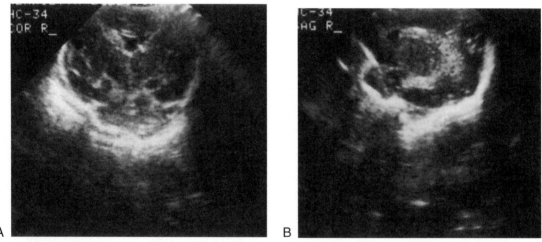

Figure 25-7. Grade III hemorrhage. Photographs from a cranial ultrasound examination with coronal (A) and sagittal (B) views depict a right-sided grade II hemorrhage (intraventricular hemorrhage with ventricular dilation).

inducing fetal lung maturity. Small studies have suggested that the use of magnesium sulfate in the mother and phenobarbital and indomethacin in the neonate significantly lowers the risk of GMH/IVH, but their use has not led to meaningful benefits and none of them has become standard care.

Air leak syndromes, such as tension pneumothorax, that compromise cardiac output and systemic blood pressure are highly associated with GMH/IVH; therefore, the use of antenatal steroids and postnatal surfactant, along with careful ventilator management to prevent these complications, is important.[7]

Several clinical studies have looked at the question of whether high-frequency ventilation (HFV) prevents GMH/IVH in preterm infants compared with conventional mechanical ventilation (CMV). A relatively large multicenter study (HIFI study) compared HFV to CMV for infants weighing 750 to 2000 g and surprisingly showed a statistically significant increase in severe intracranial hemorrhages, with 26% incidence in the HFV group compared to 18% in the CMV group ($P = 0.02$).[51] However, the study has since been criticized because the infants were not treated with surfactant and inappropriate ventilator methodology was used. The findings

nevertheless unambiguously demonstrated that clinical approaches to ventilation of VLBW infants may increase their risk for GMH/IVH. In a later study, two different approaches to administering HFV, low-pressure HFV and "optimal"-pressure HFV [defined as an increase in positive end-expiratory pressure (PEEP) $\geq$1 cm H_2O from pre-HFV baseline] were compared. A significant reduction in grade III IVH, PHI, and PVL was noted when the higher-pressure HFV was used.[52] Unfortunately, the large HIFI study continues to dominate the results of meta-analysis of all clinical trials. A meta-analysis limited to the more recent trials suggests HFV is not associated with an increase in IVH or PVL.[53] Other meta-analyses even show that the elective use of HFV reduces the rate of GMH/IVH in RDS, but they caution against its routine use until long-term neurodevelopmental outcomes demonstrate its safety.[54] To add to the uncertainty, a controlled study of VLBW infants found that early prophylactic use of HFV with a "lung volume recruitment strategy" resulted in an increased rate of severe grade III IVH or PHI compared with similar infants treated with conventional ventilation.[9] An important lesson may be that paying meticulous attention to the physiologic consequences associated with

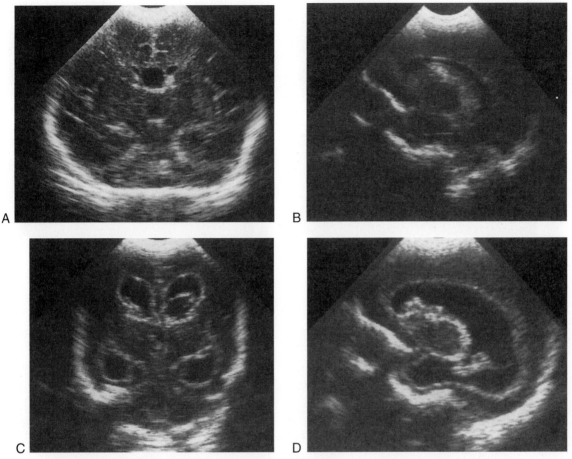

Figure 25-8. Hydrocephalus following intraventricular hemorrhage. Scans of a 4-day-old, 1200-g neonate (*A,B*) reveal bilateral subependymal hemorrhages with intraventricular extension. The ventricles are mildly dilated. Follow-up scans obtained 14 days later (*C,D*) show the development of significant ventricular dilation.

any technique of ventilator use may be as important, or even more so, than the type of ventilator used. The data available at this time do not demonstrate that use of HFV is safe for the brain of the VLBW infant, and we cannot recommend its routine use, especially because the proposed rationale for use, the prevention of chronic lung disease, has not been proven.

In most cases GMH/IVH resolves without sequelae, but occasionally a large intraventricular hemorrhage leads to posthemorrhagic hydrocephalus (Fig. 25-8) and some infants are left with neurodevelopmental deficits. The foremost clinical importance of GMH/IVH is that 15% of infants subsequently develop PHI.[33]

Periventricular Hemorrhagic Infarction

PHI refers to hemorrhagic necrosis of the periventricular white matter often associated with GMH/IVH.

Neuroanatomy and Pathogenesis

PHI is usually unilateral, or markedly asymmetric, and almost always occurs ipsilateral to a large GMH or IVH.[55] As mentioned earlier, most GMH/IVH occurs in the first 3 days of life, and the peak time of occurrence of PHI is on the fourth postnatal day. Like GMH/IVH, PHI is associated with early gestation and severe cardiopulmonary disease. PHI, once mis-

interpreted as a simple extension of IVH into the periventricular white matter, is in fact a venous infarction of the periventricular white matter.[56,57] Its location and timing are consistent with an etiologic association between IVH and PHI. GMH/IVH has been shown to obstruct the terminal vein, the common conduit through which the medullary veins drain, leading to periventricular venous infarction and hemorrhage (see earlier). This theory of pathogenesis is supported by Doppler flow studies showing decreased or absent blood flow in the terminal vein in the presence of GMH/IVH.[58] The sudden appearance and grossly hemorrhagic nature of PHI suggest that local cell death and tissue destruction occur as a result of acute ischemic necrosis.

Diagnosis

PHI usually is diagnosed by ultrasound.[37] The diagnosis of PHI requires that (1) the lesion has the appearance of a unilateral or clearly asymmetric globular or "fan-shaped" echodensity radiating from the external angle of the lateral ventricle; (2) the echodensity is located ipsilateral to a large GMH or IVH; and (3) the echodensity evolves over the next weeks into a single, large porencephalic cyst that communicates with the lateral ventricle. The early ultrasound features of PHI are shown in Figure 25-9 and its evolution into a porencephalic cyst is shown in Figure 25-10.

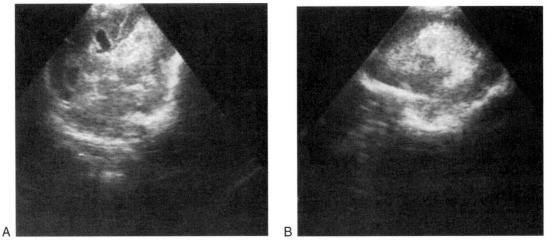

Figure 25-9. Periventricular hemorrhagic infarction. Photographs from a cranial ultrasound examination with coronal (A) and sagittal (B) views depict a left-sided intraventricular hemorrhage and periventricular white matter hemorrhage.

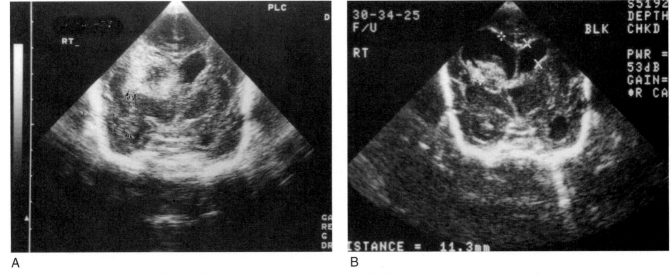

Figure 25-10. Evolution of periventricular hemorrhagic infarction. Coronal ultrasound scans of a premature infant at 4 days of age (A) and at 3 weeks of age (B). The initial right-sided intraventricular and periventricular hemorrhage has evolved into a large porencephalic cyst communicating with the right lateral ventricle. Some residual clot is seen at the base of the right lateral ventricle.

Prevention

Because PHI is a complication of GMH/IVH, its prevention is the same as for prevention of GMH/IVH, as described earlier.

Periventricular Leukomalacia

PVL is bilateral, symmetric, usually nonhemorrhagic ischemic injury of the white matter dorsal and lateral to the external angles of the lateral ventricles.[33] PVL is the most common type of cerebral injury seen on cranial ultrasound and is predictive of cerebral palsy and neurodevelopmental deficits. Both experimental and clinical studies have shed new light on potential risk factors, mechanisms of tissue injury, and potential preventive therapies.

Neuroanatomy and Pathogenesis

Coagulation necrosis with areas of liquefaction in the periventricular white matter of critically ill newborns was first described in 1962 by Banker and Larroche.[59] These investigators first noted the characteristic symmetric distribution of PVL and suggested a relationship to arterial watershed areas (border zones). Clinical circumstances associated with PVL include prematurity, postnatal survival for at least a few days, and severe cardiopulmonary disease.[60–62] The peak incidence of PVL coincides with the maximal period of myelinogenesis at 28 weeks of gestation.[63] PVL occurs in the watershed or border zones between regions supplied by the major cerebral arteries, especially near the foramina of Monro, a region located between the areas supplied by the anterior and middle cerebral arteries, and around the trigone of the lateral ventricles between the areas supplied by the middle and posterior cerebral arteries.[64]

PVL results from ischemic injury of the periventricular white matter. The brain of the very preterm infants is susceptible to ischemic injury because these infants have a pressure-passive circulation, they are prone to hypotension, and the immature oligodendrocytes populating the periventricular area are vulnerable to ischemic injury.[33] Hypocarbia also has been shown to correlate with the development of PVL (see discussion later).

Pressure-passive circulation. Total cerebral blood flow is very low in the premature infant, with measurements between 10 and 20 mL/100 g of cerebrum per minute. This is barely 20% of the blood flow to the adult cerebrum, yet normal neurologic outcome has been noted in premature infants who had measured cerebral blood flows as low as 5 mL/100 g.[65] Although both total and regional cerebral blood flow increase with postnatal age,[66–68] blood flow to the periventricular white matter remains just a fraction of that to the cerebral cortex, cerebellum, and basal ganglia.[69] Intact cerebrovascular autoregulation normally maintains constant cerebral blood flow over a range of systemic blood pressures, as cerebral arteries dilate with decreases in systemic blood pressure and constrict when systemic blood pressure rises.[33] Studies have shown that some critically ill premature infants lack this autoregulatory capability and exhibit a pressure-passive cerebral circulation.[70,71] In these infants, a decrease in systemic blood pressure is accompanied by a fall in cerebral blood flow leading to cerebral ischemia that may result in PVL. The tendency for very premature newborns to have a pressure-passive cerebral circulation may be related to an absent muscularis around the cerebral arteries and arterioles, or it may result from hypoxemia and hypercarbia associated with respiratory diseases. Ineffective cerebrovascular autoregulation has been documented by near-infrared spectroscopy in infants who subsequently developed white matter injury.[72,73]

Oligodendrocyte susceptibility. PVL primarily involves injury of the cellular elements of the developing white matter. Potential targets include radial and mature astrocytes, immature oligodendrocytes, developing axons, and vascular endothelial cells. Much of the research in this area has focused on the immature oligodendrocytes, as it has been shown that they are very sensitive not only to both free radical attack and glutamate toxicity following hypoxia/ischemia, but also to injury from proinflammatory cytokines.[30]

Studies have demonstrated the sensitivity of developing oligodendrocytes to oxygen toxicity, as seen with ischemia-reperfusion injury, and showed that addition of free radical scavengers can protect against oligodendroglial death from free radical attack.[28] The release of excessive amounts of glutamate by injured neurons may damage immature oligodendrocytes by causing glutathione depletion and further susceptibility to free radical attack.[28]

The mechanisms of cell death following ischemia-reperfusion has been a subject of great interest because this line of research may lead to the development of neuroprotective strategies. Research has shown that unlike severe ischemic insult, which rapidly results in cellular necrosis,[74] more moderate ischemic insult initiates programmed cell death by apoptosis, thus providing a window of opportunity during which to offer neuroprotective therapies[12] (see discussion of apoptosis in the section on Periventricular Leukomalacia).

Ischemia-reperfusion has been shown to injure oligodendrocytes by activating microglia and increasing proinflammatory cytokines leading to the production of reactive oxygen species.[75,76] Maternally derived proinflammatory cytokines may have similar effects. This may be important in the causation of diffuse white matter injury by proinflammatory cytokines that are produced in the inflammatory cascade resulting from low-grade perinatal infections (see discussion in section on Diffuse White Matter Injury).

Possible role of hypocarbia. Despite the very low cerebral blood flow in the premature infant, the cerebral arteries of the healthy premature infant respond normally to physiologic stimuli by vasoconstricting in response to a reduced partial pressure of carbon dioxide and vasodilating in response to reduced oxygen tension, hypercarbia, and hypoglycemia.[77]

Cerebral vasoconstriction occurring as a result of hypocarbia can lead to cerebral ischemia. In piglet studies, acute normoxemic hypocarbia with arterial carbon dioxide tensions held below 15 mm Hg was associated with a significant reduction in cerebral and total brain blood flows.[78] During hypocarbia, cerebral perfusion was reduced while blood flows to the thalamus, cerebellum, and brainstem were preserved. Hypocarbia lasting over 2 hours with $PaCO_2$ held less than 20 mm Hg resulted in reduced cerebral blood flow, oxygen delivery, oxygen extraction, and oxygen consumption.[79] This study first raised concerns that inadvertent hypocarbia, as may occur with use of high-frequency jet ventilation and other ventilator strategies, might lead to cerebral ischemia and cause PVL.

In several clinical studies, hypocarbia occurring during the first days of life in conventionally ventilated premature infants with RDS was associated with PVL.[80–83] When used during the first 72 hours of life, both patient-triggered ventilation and high-frequency jet ventilation are more frequently associated with arterial carbon dioxide tensions of less than 25 mm Hg than in similar infants treated with conventional ventilators,[84,85] and the infants who required the least ventilator support were at the greatest risk for hypocarbia on the first day. A clinical study of the association between high-frequency jet ventilation, hypocarbia, and the occurrence of cystic PVL was reported by Wiswell et al.[85] Repeated cranial ultrasonograms were obtained from a group of VLBW infants who had been treated with jet ventilation for a mean of 44 hours (range 8 to 70 hours). When they retrospectively compared the blood gas values for infants who developed cystic PVL with those who did not, they found no differences in mean $PaCO_2$, lowest $PaCO_2$, or ranges of low $PaCO_2$. However, logistic regression analysis showed that the infants who developed PVL had spent significantly more time with a $PaCO_2$ below 25 mm Hg during the first day of life.

A similar approach to analysis was used by Okumura et al.[86] to evaluate the relationship between hypocarbia and PVL. Like Wiswell et al., they studied "threshold values" for hypocarbia and calculated the area above the curve to calculate the "CO_2 index" (Fig. 25-11). They also determined the *time-averaged* values for arterial pH, respiratory rate (RR), peak inspiratory pressure (PIP), mean airway pressure (MAP), ventilator index (VI = PIP–PEEP × RR), and total respiratory rate (TRR = spontaneous respiratory rate + mechanical respiratory rate). Similar to Wiswell et al., they found that infants who subsequently developed PVL had greater time-averaged CO_2 indices, lower time-averaged $PaCO_2$, and higher time-averaged pH (on the third day of life) than infants with normal development.

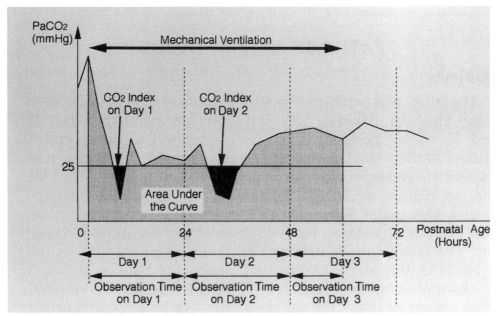

Figure 25-11. Scheme for calculation of time-averaged CO_2 index and $Paco_2$. The observation time was defined as the period when both mechanical ventilation and the arterial catheter were maintained on each day. It was sometimes shorter that 24 hours and was different among infants. The area above the curve obtained with longitudinal data for $Paco_2$ and threshold levels (= 25 mm Hg) was determined. This was calculated on each day and divided by the observation time to even the difference. The result was called the *time-averaged CO_2 index*. The area under the curve obtained with longitudinal data for $Paco_2$ was determined on each day. These data were divided by the observation time and the result was called the *time-averaged $Paco_2$*. (From Okumura A, Hayakawa F, Kato T, et al: Hypocarbia in preterm infants with periventricular leukomalacia: The relationship between hypocarbia and mechanical ventilation. Pediatrics 107:469, 2001.)

Interestingly, there were no differences in time-averaged RR, PIP, MAP, VI, or TRR between the infants who did and the infants who did not develop PVL. Thus, the ventilator settings were not higher in the infants who became hypocarbic and developed PVL than in those with normal cranial ultrasonograms, raising the question of whether infants who develop PVL have less severe lung disease (see section on Diffuse White Matter Injury).

A potential relationship between hypocarbia and neonatal brain injury is suggested by an experimental study showing that hypocarbia induces apoptosis in the hippocampus of hyperventilated hypotensive rabbits.[87] However, the possibility exists that hypocarbia in preterm infants is a marker for risk of PVL rather than its cause[86,88] (see section on Diffuse White Matter Injury).

Although the importance of low carbon dioxide tensions in causing PVL remains uncertain, this concern has led many clinicians to be increasingly vigilant to prevent hypocarbia. The safety of this approach is shown in studies of the practice of "permissive hypercarbia" during the mechanical ventilation adopted in order to minimize barotrauma in preterm infants. Less vigorous ventilation permitting higher pco_2 levels was not associated with any increase in morbidity or mortality.[89]

Diagnosis

PVL is most often diagnosed by ultrasound, although MRI has been shown to be more sensitive to subtle forms of periventricular injury. Ultrasound criteria for the diagnosis of PVL include (1) bilateral echodensities, which often develop within the first week of life at the lateral borders of the lateral ventricles; (2) minimal or no hemorrhage; and (3) evolution of the echodensities into multiple small cysts that do not communicate with the lateral ventricles (Fig. 25-12).[37] In some infants the white matter echogenicity resolves without the development of periventricular cysts. Other patients, especially ELBW infants, may show minimal or no ultrasound abnormality in the first weeks of life, only to have multiple cysts noted on a later ultrasound. Weeks later, after the cysts collapse, the ultrasound

shows a decreased white matter volume and ventriculomegaly (hydrocephalus ex vacuo) if there has been substantial white matter loss. Other infants without any abnormalities on early ultrasound will later show white matter loss and ventriculomegaly, and there is growing evidence that many of these infants have experienced diffuse white matter injury secondary to subclinical perinatal infection with increased cytokine levels, which damage the developing oligodendrocytes (see section on Diffuse White Matter Injury). Ischemia- and inflammation-induced white matter injury may coexist, and may even represent a common outcome following different types of injury. The timing and pattern of this form of brain injury is consistent with the concept of apoptosis or delayed cell death, although this has not been proven. If further research confirms that the injury results from apoptosis, it may prove possible in the future to develop therapies to prevent delayed cell death and reduce or prevent neurologic deficits.

Prevention

The list of clinical risk factors for PVL (Table 25-1) suggests several approaches to prevention.[30] Maintenance of normal cerebral perfusion by anticipating, rapidly identifying, and treating hypotension, and, conversely, avoiding cerebral vasoconstriction by carefully monitoring blood gases to prevent hypocarbia may be important measures. Research to determine whether it is possible for pharmacologic intervention to protect the immature oligodendrocytes will no doubt be a prime goal in the future. A long list of potential neuroprotectors, including free radical scavengers, glutamate receptor blockers, interventions to block the cytotoxic effects of proinflammatory cytokines, and other novel approaches, have been suggested (see section on Diffuse White Matter Injury).

Diffuse White Matter Injury

More diffuse injury of the cerebral white matter that is similar to PVL but less severe in that it does not undergo cystic change and is not seen on ultrasound during the early stage may

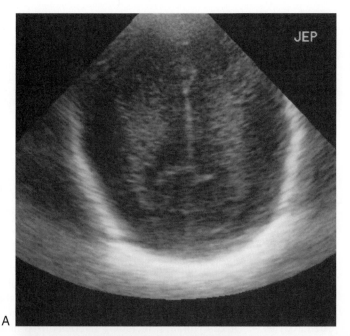

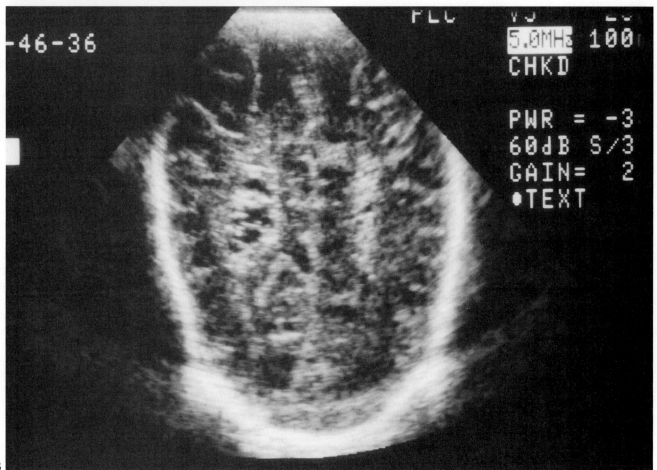

Figure 25-12. Periventricular leukomalacia. Coronal ultrasound scans of the periventricular white matter posterior to the lateral ventricles in a premature infant at 4 days of age *(A)* and 73 days of age *(B)*. The subtle bilateral periventricular echodensities noted on the initial scan have evolved into several relatively small cysts, that is, cystic periventricular leukomalacia.

be detected later by loss of white matter volume and ventriculomegaly (hydrocephalus ex vacuo). Infants with diffuse white matter injury are at high risk for neurodevelopmental delays.[35,90] The risk of neurodevelopmental problems, including cerebral palsy and delayed development, is correlated with the volume of lost brain parenchyma.

Potential mechanisms of injury to the cerebral white matter include hypoxia, ischemia, hypoglycemia, and inflammation. In recent years it has become clear that some extremely premature infants who do not experience any overt disorders of physiologic homeostasis, or show abnormalities on early head ultrasound, will show evidence of cerebral white matter

TABLE 25-1.   Possible Role of Respiratory Care in Causing Brain Injury in Extremely-Low-Birthweight Infants

Type of Lesion	Mechanism of Injury	Possible Role of Respiratory Management
GMH, IVH, PHI	Sudden fluctuations in BP and CBF	Unstable respiratory status[6] Accidental extubation Tension pneumothorax[7]
Cystic PVL	Low BP Low CBF Cerebral ischemia	Hypocarbia[85,86] Excess intrapleural pressure, with decreased cardiac filling and cardiac output (e.g., improper application of HFV)[9]
Diffuse white matter injury (noncystic)	Low-grade perinatal infection Chronic inflammation	Low-grade bronchopulmonary infection[92,102] Postnatal steroids[127,128]

BP, blood pressure; CBF, cerebral blood flow; GMH, germinal matrix hemorrhage; HFV, high-frequency ventilation; IVH, intraventricular hemorrhage; PHI, periventricular hemorrhagic infarction; PVL, periventricular leukomalacia.

damage as described on late ultrasound and may have significant motor and developmental deficits. Studies have suggested a likely role for inflammation-induced damage resulting from subclinical maternal infection as the cause of cerebral white matter injury.[91,92] This has generated considerable interest because, if verified, further research may lead to approaches to prevent this major cause of brain damage in ELBW infants. Novel approaches to alter the consequences of the inflammatory cascade have already been suggested.[93,94] Chorioamnionitis has been associated with cystic PVL and with diffuse white matter injury, suggesting that these pathologic processes may represent different levels of severity of inflammatory-mediated cerebral injury. As discussed in the section on PVL, the distinction between PVL and diffuse white matter injury often is unclear.

Equally exciting is growing evidence that perinatal infection/inflammation may play a central role in causing preterm labor, premature rupture of the membranes, and extremely preterm delivery. There also is evidence that the same perinatal inflammatory response may occur in the fetal lungs and be an important factor leading to lung injury and altered lung growth, culminating in the development of BPD. Evidence supporting these hypotheses has been reviewed. Briefly, these hypotheses are based upon studies showing that maternal bacterial vaginosis and asymptomatic chorioamnionitis (either by culture or amnionic membrane histology) are strongly associated with (1) increased levels of proinflammatory cytokines in maternal serum, amniotic fluid, cord blood, and neonatal tracheal fluid at delivery[95,96]; (2) preterm labor, premature rupture of the membranes, and ELBW delivery[97]; (3) a much higher risk for white matter injury, later cerebral palsy, and developmental delay compared with other infants of similar gestational age[92,95,98–101]; (4) less severe respiratory distress in the immediate neonatal period[99,102,103]; and (5) a higher rate of chronic lung disease.[101–103]

This construct has generated great interest as it may improve our understanding of, and provide greater insights into, possible approaches to prevention of three of the major problems in perinatal/neonatal medicine: how to prevent ELBW delivery, how to prevent chronic lung disease, and how to improve the neurologic development of ELBW infants. It also offers a possible explanation for the previously observed close association between chronic lung disease and abnormal neurologic development in ELBW infants.

Several studies suggest mechanisms by which fetal inflammatory processes may damage the cerebral white matter.

It is possible that when there is low-grade chorioamnionitis, proinflammatory cytokines released by inflammatory cells gain access to the fetal brain.[91] One such cytokine, tumor necrosis factor-α, has been shown to be highly toxic to cultured oligodendrocytes.[104] Other cytokines, including interleukin-1β and interleukin-6, are elevated in the amniotic fluid of women with chorioamnionitis and in amniotic fluid and umbilical cord blood of infants who develop PVL.[105,106] In a meta-analysis by Wu and Colford,[92] chorioamnionitis was found to be a significant risk factor for both cerebral palsy and cystic PVL. As mentioned earlier, the distinction between the forms of white matter injury is blurred, and the diagnosis made depends primarily on whether the injury is visible on early head ultrasound. Also, both perinatal infection and hypotension may occur in the same patient, further confounding attempts to distinguish between them.

Certain interesting differences exist in the epidemiology of PHI and PVL (or diffuse white matter injury). First, the incidence and severity of PHI is inversely related to gestational age and birthweight, whereas PVL tends to occur in relatively more mature preterm infants.[99,100] A possible explanation for this difference is that the period of rapid myelinogenesis begins between 28 and 32 weeks of gestation, which presumably is a vulnerable time for white matter injury.[107] Second, infants who develop PHI have a greater degree of clinical illness than those who develop PVL.[99] Infants who went on to develop PHI were found to require significantly more volume expansion and vasopressor support compared with infants who developed PVL or those with normal ultrasounds.[100] Also, indices of respiratory disease were significantly worse in the PHI group, whereas the PVL group closely mirrored the normal infants (Fig. 25-13). In the same cohort of patients, a significant association was noted between maternal chorioamnionitis and the development of PVL but not of PHI. These observations are consistent with previous observations that low-grade chorioamnionitis both enhances lung function at birth and initiates an inflammation cascade, presumably mediated by cytokines, that leads to later white matter injury (diffuse white matter injury or PVL).

An association between maternal chorioamnionitis and improved lung function at birth was first reported by Watterberg et al.[102] Subsequently, Koauge et al.[108] used a logistic regression model to show that maternal chorioamnionitis is associated with a significantly reduced risk of death in premature infants under 32 weeks of gestation. The idea of an intrauterine inflammatory process leading to initial clinical

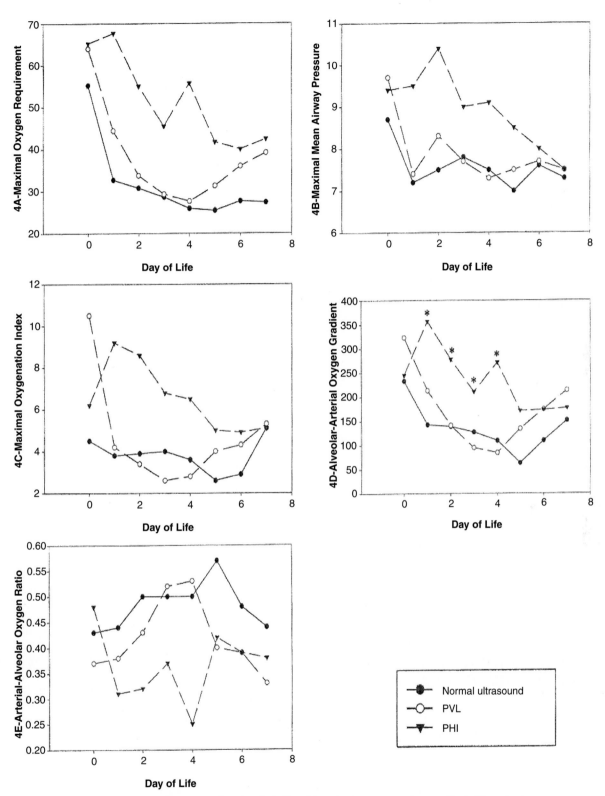

Figure 25-13. Indices of respiratory function, including *(A)* maximal oxygen requirement (Fio$_2$), *(B)* maximal mean airway pressure (MAP), *(C)* oxygenation index (OI), *(D)* alveolar-arterial oxygen gradient (AaDo$_2$), and *(E)* arterial/alveolar oxygen ratio (a/A ratio), in a cohort of premature very-low-birthweight infants. Infants with normal ultrasound scans are compared to infants who developed periventricular hemorrhagic infarction (PHI) and periventricular leukomalacia (PVL). Compared to normal infants, time-by-time analysis of variance shows significantly greater AaDo$_2$ in infants who later developed PHI (*P <0.001). Longitudinal analysis of the entire first week of life using generalized estimating equations (GEE) indicates significant differences (P <0.03) in Fio$_2$, MAP, OI, AaDo$_2$, and a/A ratio between normal and PHI infants. GEE also showed a significant difference in Fio$_2$ between infants with PHI and PVL (P <0.05). No differences were noted between the PVL group and the normal infants. (From Bass WT, Schultz SJ, Burke BL, et al: Indices of hemodynamic and respiratory functions in premature infants at risk for the development of cerebral white matter injury. J Perinatol 22:64–71, 2002.)

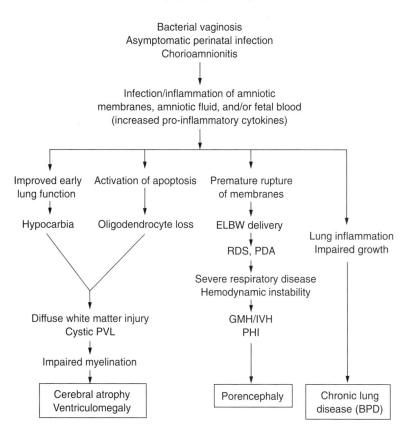

Figure 25-14. Algorithm of the potential associations of perinatal inflammation to extremely low birthweight delivery (ELBW), white matter injury, cerebral palsy, and chronic lung disease. BPD, bronchopulmonary dysplasia; GMH/IVH, germinal matrix hemorrhage/intraventricular hemorrhage; PDA, patent ductus arteriosus; PHI, periventricular hemorrhagic infarction; PVL, periventricular leukomalacia; RDS, respiratory distress syndrome.

stability and improved lung function seems counterintuitive, but studies have shown that fetal lambs exposed to endotoxin have markedly improved postnatal lung function,[109,110] an effect that is not mediated by cortisol.[111] However, other evidence suggests that, despite the improvement in early neonatal respiratory status, infants whose mothers have chorioamnionitis are at greater risk for developing chronic lung disease.[102] It is postulated that the same inflammatory process that leads to apoptosis and loss of cerebral white matter also leads to lung inflammation, altered lung growth, and chronic lung disease.[101,103] An algorithm of perinatal inflammation leading to ELBW delivery, white matter injury, cerebral palsy, and chronic lung disease is shown in Figure 25-14.

CEREBRAL INJURY ASSOCIATED WITH USE OF RESPIRATORY DRUGS

Premature infants are treated with a number of drugs intended to improve their respiratory status, including surfactants, methylxanthines, beta-mimetics, corticosteroids, sedatives, narcotic analgesics, paralytics, and diuretics. Many of these drugs are widely used despite a lack of long-term studies proving their safety for the developing central nervous system. Of particular concern to neonatologists are recent data suggesting that the use of postnatal dexamethasone in VLBW infants may result in brain damage and abnormal neurodevelopmental outcome.

Postnatal Dexamethasone

The use of postnatal dexamethasone for severe RDS evolving into BPD had gained widespread acceptance in the past decade after several randomized trials documented its usefulness in improving short-term respiratory function and achieving earlier extubation.[112–115] Recently, however, adverse effects on growth and abnormal neurodevelopmental outcome have been reported in premature infants following treatment with postnatal dexamethasone. It is unfortunate that long courses of very-high-dose dexamethasone had been used for years despite the lack of follow-up studies on the safety of such a potentially risky drug. In fact, as early as 1977, Weichsel[116] had warned about the risks of postnatal steroid use during critical periods of brain development. He cautioned that steroids given to preterm infants would likely impair brain cell division and myelination and result in long-term behavioral effects. A number of studies suggest mechanisms by which use of potent steroids in the postnatal period may adversely affect the cerebral white matter, but discussion of these mechanisms is beyond the scope of this chapter.[116–121]

Initially, short-term studies of preterm infants treated with dexamethasone suggested the possibility of neurologic problems among survivors. Poor weight gain and poor head growth were demonstrated in infants treated with dexamethasone in the first weeks of life.[122,123] These findings were particularly concerning because decreased head growth has been associated with low cognitive function.[124] As early as 1974, Fitzhardinge et al.[125] reported an increased incidence of gross neurologic and electroencephalographic abnormalities and impaired gross motor development at 1 year of age in premature infants following early steroid use.

The results of several larger long-term follow-up studies strongly suggest an association between postnatal dexamethasone use and poor neurodevelopmental outcome including cerebral palsy. Yeh et al.[126] found a higher incidence of neuromotor dysfunction and lower indices of psychomotor development at 2 years of age in prematurely born children who had been treated with dexamethasone in the newborn period. In two other studies, dexamethasone-treated infants also had a higher incidence of cerebral palsy than control infants on follow-up examination.[127,128] An increased incidence of PVL reported in two studies of dexamethasone-treated infants suggests that white matter injury from the postnatal use of dexamethasone may be responsible for the reported poor neurodevelopmental outcomes.[129,130]

Administration of much smaller doses and shorter courses of dexamethasone than were used in the past have been shown to provide short-term benefits.[131] A single dose of 0.2 mg/kg dexamethasone given within 2 hours of delivery resulted in lower ventilator settings, higher mean blood pressures, and less requirement for indomethacin for patent ductus arteriosus.[132] Others have shown similar improvements in systemic blood pressure with single-dose dexamethasone.[133] It must be remembered that these dosing schedules have not been shown to lead to long-term benefits, and their safety for neurodevelopment has not been studied.

Others have considered that steroids other than dexamethasone could provide pulmonary benefits without harming the developing brain. Methylprednisolone was shown in a small study to be as effective as dexamethasone in reducing BPD while the infants showed better weight gain, less glucose intolerance, and less PVL.[134] More recently, physiologic doses of hydrocortisone, 1 mg/kg/day for 9 days followed by 0.5 mg/kg/day for 3 days started within 48 hours of birth, were shown to improve survival without chronic lung disease. Hydrocortisone may provide a better risk-to-benefit ratio than dexamethasone,[135] but once again, while awaiting results of larger randomized clinical trials of lower doses and shorter courses of dexamethasone and/or trials of alternative steroid preparations, the clinician should carefully weigh the very real risks with the potential benefits of using postnatal corticosteroids for these patients.

Given these data, what is the place for use of postnatal steroids? In an excellent review, Finer et al.[136] state there is inadequate evidence to support the current routine use of postnatal steroids in VLBW infants and suggest that further studies of systemic or inhaled steroids must include an evaluation of neurodevelopmental outcome as a primary endpoint. Very limited steroid use may still be justified in life-threatening situations to reduce lung inflammation and improve lung function, but the clinician must balance possible benefits with proven risks of this therapy, and of course the smallest possible dose should be used. Unfortunately there are no currently established guidelines for the safe use of postnatal corticosteroids.

Antenatal Steroids

Administration of one course of antenatal steroids administered over 48 hours to women with threatened preterm labor probably is one of the most cost-effective and life-saving treatments in perinatal medicine.[137] Long-term follow up of infants whose mothers received this treatment show less RDS and air leak syndromes, a reduction in IVH, and no evidence of adverse effects.

Much of the early experimental work and the first clinical study of the effects of antenatal steroid administration on the fetus were carried out more than 3 decades ago by G.C. Liggins.[138,139] A large randomized controlled trial showed a clear reduction in RDS and neonatal death after two intramuscular injections of betamethasone administered 24 hours apart to women in preterm labor. Subsequent controlled trials, using betamethasone or dexamethasone, have supported those findings.[140,141] The Cochrane Review[141] showed there was also a significant reduction in neonatal intraventricular hemorrhage and a trend toward reduced neurodevelopmental disability among the infants.

After early follow-up studies showed that the improvements in lung function were not sustained if preterm delivery occurred more than 7 days after treatment,[139] many obstetricians began to give weekly corticosteroid courses if delivery was delayed. Because of the adverse neurologic outcomes reported following use of postnatal dexamethasone (outlined earlier), concern has been raised about possible negative consequences from repeated antenatal steroid courses. Animal studies had shown that a single dose of betamethasone given to pregnant sheep at 70% of term gestation resulted in a 10% reduction is fetal brain weight at term,[142] whereas the reduction in brain weight was 21% if four doses of betamethasone were given at weekly intervals. Other animal studies of multiple doses of maternally administered steroids showed reduced or delayed myelination,[143] a reduced number of hippocampal neurons,[144] and enhanced sensitivity to hypoxic-ischemic injury in the fetus.[145] Potential mechanisms of dexamethasone injury have been provided by experimental studies showing inhibition of neuronal growth factors and facilitation of apoptosis.[146] However, other animal studies showed potential benefits of prenatal steroid use in protecting against hypoxic-ischemic brain injury. For example, Tuor et al.[147] demonstrated reduced brain damage in rats that were pretreated with dexamethasone and then underwent unilateral carotid ligation.

Adverse neurodevelopmental effects from multiple antenatal steroid doses have not been proven in preterm infants, although the number of infants followed for the long term remains small. In a study of 200 children treated with antenatal dexamethasone, the US steroid group trial[148] found that 3.8% had a Bayley motor index below 68 compared to 6% of the control group. A larger study reported by French et al.[149] looked at 652 infants who were delivered between 20 and 32 weeks of gestation, of whom 311 had not received antenatal steroids, 123 received one course, 20 received two courses, and 23 received three or more courses of antenatal steroids. The untreated infants had a higher mortality rate, and no differences were noted in head circumference between the groups at 3 years of age. A 7.8% incidence of cerebral palsy was noted in the control group, compared with 5.1% of the infants who received one course of antenatal steroids and no infants in the groups that received multiple courses.

Three retrospective studies compared the results of cranial ultrasound examinations of infants whose mothers received and those whose mothers had not received antenatal steroids.[130,150,151] Leviton et al.[150] found the risk of developing intraventricular hemorrhage or cerebral white matter echolucencies was modestly but not significantly reduced in the steroid-treated infants. Ventriculomegaly, an important marker of white matter loss, occurred half as often in the steroid-treated infants as in those whose mothers had not received steroids. Another study also reported a 50% reduction in the incidence of PVL in preterm infants given antenatal steroids.[151] In a study by Baud et al.,[130] ultrasound examinations of premature infants not exposed to steroids were compared with those of infants exposed to antenatal betamethasone or dexamethasone. The incidence of cystic PVL was 8.4% in the untreated group, 4.4% in the betamethasone-treated group, and 11% in the dexamethasone-treated group. This study has been interpreted to suggest that antenatal betamethasone, but not dexamethasone, may be neuroprotective. It has also been suggested that dexamethasone (but not betamethasone) might be neurotoxic to the developing central nervous system whether administered prenatally or postnatally. Further studies are needed to evaluate these preliminary observations.

Because there is no current evidence from randomized trials that a single course of antenatal betamethasone increases the risk of brain injury and in fact its use has been shown to be neuroprotective, obstetricians caring for women at risk for premature delivery should routinely continue to provide this therapy.[137] The data reviewed also support the use of antenatal betamethasone rather than dexamethasone. The question of clinical benefits and risks from repeated courses is more difficult. Some of the clinical reports do not show an increased risk for the fetus' central nervous system,[152,153] but few infants have been followed for the long term. Given the adverse effects on brain development following prolonged corticosteroid exposure and especially in light of more recent studies questioning additional pulmonary benefits from multiple courses, repeated courses of corticosteroids are considered unproven and potentially harmful.[137]

Methylxanthines

Methylxanthines are a class of drugs used in virtually all premature VLBW infants despite a lack of studies demonstrating long-term safety and efficacy. Bauer et al.[154] reported increased oxygen consumption and decreased weight gain in infants receiving caffeine. The potential effects of these findings on brain development are unclear. However, increased nutritional support might be indicated in infants receiving caffeine. Of even greater concern is an animal study showing that methylxanthines may worsen brain injury following a hypoxic-ischemic event.[155] A large prospective study is underway to study the safety of caffeine use in preterm infants.

OUTCOME OF INFANTS WITH PERINATAL BRAIN INJURY

About 85% of VLBW infants now survive the neonatal period and are at risk for serious neurodevelopmental sequelae. Between 5% and 15% of survivors will have major spastic motor deficits, and as many as 25% to 50% will have less prominent motor and cognitive disabilities, including hyperactivity, attention deficit disorder, and specific learning disorders.[33] At least 50% of the tiniest surviving infants will require special education to perform at grade level or will need to be in special education classes. The difficulty in predicting future neurodevelopmental problems in individual infants is an extremely important and difficult issue as evidenced by the large number of studies published on this subject. Accurate prediction is hampered by inconsistencies between follow-up studies,[156,157] including the following: (1) individual centers usually report outcomes on a relatively small number of patients, and treatment at a center often changes over time;

(2) outcome is often reported in terms of birthweight rather than gestational age, confounding the effects of extremely premature birth and intrauterine growth restriction; and (3) reports differ in how neurologic deficits are defined.

Similar to previous experience, a study of infants with abnormalities of white matter on ultrasound confirmed that socioeconomic status was an important determinant of cognitive ability at 5 years of age.[158] Gross et al.[159] reported that family structure and stability were more important than perinatal complications in predicting academic performance at 10 years of age.

The following discussion addresses primarily the shorter-term outcomes for VLBW infants with identifiable cerebral lesions on cranial ultrasound examination. First, one must keep in mind that a birthweight less than 1500 g, even without any identifiable brain abnormality, is associated with an approximately 5% to 10% incidence of neurologic abnormality.[6] Germinal matrix bleeding (grade I IVH) and small (grade II) IVH do not lead to a significant increase in mortality or morbidity as compared with infants with normal ultrasound studies. When the amount of intraventricular blood increases and is accompanied by ventricular distension (grade III IVH), the mortality rate increases to approximately 20%, and the greater the amount of blood in the ventricles, the more likely the risk of developing posthemorrhagic hydrocephalus (PHH).[6] The 5% incidence of PHH in patients with grade I IVH increases to 55% with grade III IVH. Management of PHH is beyond the scope of this chapter, and the reader is referred to standard texts.[6]

Although abnormal neurologic outcome is sometimes seen with the more severe forms of IVH, especially with severe PHH, the highest risk for neurodevelopmental deficit exists when there is ultrasound evidence of parenchymal white matter damage, such as PHI or PVL. Although not invariably so,[160] most studies report varying degrees of spasticity and cognitive deficits among survivors with PHI or cystic PVL. Bass et al.[38] identified a cohort of 111 infants with cerebral white matter lesions and obtained 2-year follow-up data on 57 of the 76 survivors. PHI was diagnosed in 18 infants and PVL was diagnosed in 26 infants, based on previously published ultrasound criteria.[37] PHI was graded as localized (5 infants) (limited to the frontal, parietal, or occipital area) or extensive (13 infants) (involving two or more areas).[55] PVL was considered mild if there were bilateral "microcysts" smaller than 0.2 cm in dimension (12 infants), moderate if there were bilateral cysts measuring between 0.2 and 0.5 cm in diameter (6 infants), and severe if the cysts measured greater than 0.5 cm (8 infants). On follow-up, localized PHI was associated with hemiplegia in 80% of cases (one infant had no motor deficit) and an average developmental quotient of 82. Extensive PHI more often resulted in quadriplegia or mixed hemiplegia/spastic diplegia (77% of patients) and an average developmental quotient of 46. Although PHI is generally unilateral or markedly asymmetric, the frequency of extremely poor neurodevelopmental outcomes among infants with severe PHI strongly suggests the likelihood of associated cerebral white matter injury on the contralateral side that is not seen on cranial ultrasound.

The outcome of patients with PVL also was discouraging. Mild and moderate PVL were associated with spastic diplegia (in 58% and 66%, respectively) or quadriplegia (33% for both); 88% of the infants with severe PVL developed quadriplegia. The average developmental quotients for infants with mild, moderate, and severe PVL were 61, 68, and 34, respectively. The extremely poor outcomes of infants with PVL as defined in this study suggests that the appearance of cysts in the white matter, even very small ones, implies significant cerebral injury and the probable occurrence of more diffuse noncystic white matter injury that is not visualized on cranial ultrasound.

SUMMARY

The immature central nervous system is vulnerable to injury from ischemia, hypoxia, hypoglycemia, and infection/inflammation. Injury to the premature infant's brain parenchyma is seen on cranial ultrasound by either the appearance of unilateral PHI, which implies acute tissue necrosis, or by bilateral PVL, which likely represents injured areas where cells are lost by a combination of ischemic necrosis and apoptosis. Diffuse cerebral white matter injury is probably a fairly common occurrence that often is not visualized on early ultrasound but results in diffuse loss of cerebral parenchyma, so a reduction in the mass of cerebral white matter and ventriculomegaly are seen on late ultrasound. Recent evidence suggests that a cytokine-induced inflammatory process may provoke a white matter inflammatory reaction that leads to a delayed loss of oligodendrocytes by apoptosis and results in a secondary reduction in myelinated white matter tracts. The size and location of cerebral tissue loss seen on late ultrasound or other imaging study is the strongest predictor of later neurodevelopmental disability; however, socioeconomic status, parenting skills, and the home environment also play major roles in determining the child's cognitive ability.

This chapter discusses ways that respiratory support of the VLBW infant, and especially complications from that support, may result in cerebral white matter injury. Altered physiologies that may result in white matter injury include cerebral hypoperfusion and hypocarbia. Neurotoxicity from drugs commonly used to treat respiratory problems, especially postnatal dexamethasone, is discussed. Further delineation of the mechanisms of tissue injury is more than an academic exercise because a clear understanding of pathogenesis is necessary before neuroprotective strategies can be devised.

REFERENCES

1. Hack M, Friedman H, Avroy A, et al: Outcomes of extremely low birth weight infants. Pediatrics 98:931, 1996.
2. Vohr BR, Wright LL, Dusick AM, et al: Neurodevelopmental and functional outcomes of extremely low birth weight infants in the National Institute of Child Health and Human Development Neonatal Research Network, 1993–1994. Pediatrics 105:1216, 2000.
3. Perlman JM: White matter injury in the preterm infant: An important determination of abnormal neurodevelopmental outcome. Early Hum Dev 53:99, 1998.
4. Goddard-Finegold J: Periventricular, intraventricular hemorrhages in the premature newborn: Update on pathologic features, pathogenesis, and possible means of prevention. Arch Neurol 41:766, 1984.
5. Ment L: Prevention of neonatal intraventricular hemorrhage. N Engl J Med 312:1385, 1985.
6. Volpe JJ: Intracranial hemorrhage: Germinal matrix-intraventricular hemorrhage of the premature infant. In Volpe JJ (ed): Neurology of the Newborn, 4th ed. Philadelphia, WB Saunders, 2001, p. 435.
7. Mehrabani D, Gowen CW Jr, Kopelman AE: Association of pneumothorax and hypotension with intraventricular hemorrhage. Arch Dis Child 66:48, 1991.
8. Leviton A, VanMarter L, Kuban KCK: Respiratory distress syndrome and intracranial hemorrhage: Cause or association? Inferences from surfactant clinical trials. Pediatrics 84:915, 1989.
9. Moriette G, Paris-Llado J, Walti H, et al: Prospective randomized multicenter comparison of high-frequency oscillatory ventilation and conventional ventilation in preterm infants of less than 30 weeks with respiratory distress syndrome. Pediatrics 107:363, 2001.
10. Mehmet H, Edwards AD: Hypoxia, ischemia, and apoptosis. Arch Dis Child 75:F73, 1996.
11. Hutchins JB, Barger SW: Why neurons die: Cell death in the nervous system. Anat Rec 253:79, 1998.
12. Mazarakis ND, Edwards AD, Mehmet H: Apoptosis in neural development and disease. Arch Dis Child 77:F165, 1997.
13. Yoon BH, Kim CJ, Romero R, et al: Experimentally induced intrauterine infection causes fetal brain white matter lesions in rabbits. Am J Obstet Gynecol 177:797, 1997.
14. Debillion T, Gras-Leguen C, Verielle V, et al: Intrauterine infection induces programmed cell death in rabbit periventricular white matter. Pediatr Res 47:736, 2000.
15. Hargitai B, Szabo V, Hajdu A, et al: Apoptosis in various organs of preterm infants: Histopathologic study of lung, kidney, liver, and brain of ventilated infants. Pediatr Res 50:110, 2001.
16. Seller MJ: Sex, neural tube defects, and multisite closure of the human neural tube. Am J Med Genet 58:332, 1995.
17. Szymonowicz W, Schafler K Cussen LJ, et al: Ultrasound and necropsy study of periventricular haemorrhage in preterm infants. Arch Dis Child 59:637, 1984.
18. Bass WT, Singer G, Slusser J, et al: Radial glial interaction with cerebral germinal matrix capillaries in the fetal baboon. Exp Neurol 118:126, 1992.
19. Volpe JJ: Intracranial hemorrhage: Germinal matrix-intraventricular hemorrhage of the premature infant. In Volpe JJ (ed): Neurology of the Newborn, 4th ed. Philadelphia, WB Saunders, 2001, p. 429.
20. Rorke LB: Anatomic features of the developing brain implicated in pathogenesis of hypoxic-ischemic injury. Brain Pathol 2:211, 1992.
21. Volpe JJ: Neuronal proliferation, migration, organization, and myelination. In Volpe JJ (ed): Neurology of the Newborn, 4th ed. Philadelphia, WB Saunders, 2001, p. 72.
22. Marin-Padilla M: Developmental neuropathology and impact of perinatal brain damage. III. Gray matter lesions of the neocortex. J Neuropathol Exp Neurol 56:219, 1997.
23. Inder TE, Huppi PS, Warfield S, et al: Periventricular white matter injury in the premature infant is associated with a reduction in cerebral cortical gray matter volume at term. Ann Neurol 46:755, 1999.
24. Peterson BS, Vohr B, Staib LN, et al: Regional brain volume abnormalities and long-term cognitive outcome in preterm infants. JAMA 284:1939, 2000.
25. Huppi PS, Maier SE, Peled S, et al: Microstructural development of human newborn cerebral white matter assessed in vivo by diffusion tensor magnetic resonance imaging. Pediatr Res 44:584, 1998.
26. Huppi PS, Murphy B, Maier SE, et al: Microstructural brain development after perinatal cerebral white matter injury assessed by diffusion tensor magnetic resonance imaging. Pediatrics 107:455, 2001.
27. Inder T, Huppi PS, Zientara GP, et al: Early detection of periventricular leukomalacia by diffusion-weighted magnetic resonance imaging techniques. J Pediatr 134:631, 1999.
28. Back SA, Volpe JJ: Cellular and molecular pathogenesis of periventricular white matter injury. MRDD Res Rev 3:96, 1997.
29. Bass WT, Singer GA, Luizzi FJ: Transient lectin binding by white matter tract border zone microglia in the fetal rabbit. Histochem J 30:657, 1998.
30. Volpe JJ: Brain injury in the premature infant: Overview of clinical aspects, neuropathology, and pathogenesis. Semin Pediatr Neurol 5:135, 1998.
31. Dammann O, Hagberg H, Leviton A: Is periventricular leukomalacia an axonopathy as well as an oligopathy? Pediatr Res 49:453, 2001.
32. Hirayama A, Okoshi Y, Hachiya Y, et al: Early immunohistochemical detection of axonal damage and glial activation in extremely immature brain with periventricular leukomalacia. Clin Neuropathol 20:87, 2001.
33. Volpe JJ: Brain injury in the premature infant. Neuropathology, clinical aspects, pathogenesis, and prevention. Clin Perinatol 24:567, 1997.
34. Hope PL, Gould SJ, Howard S, et al: Precision of ultrasound diagnosis of pathologically verified lesions in the brains of very premature infants. Dev Med Child Neurol 30:457, 1988.
35. Kuban KC: White-matter disease in prematurity, periventricular leukomalacia, and ischemic lesions. Dev Med Child Neurol 40:571, 1998.

36. Paneth N: Classifying brain damage in preterm infants. J Pediatr 134:527, 1999.
37. Volpe JJ: Brain injury in the premature infant: Is it preventable? Pediatr Res 27:S28, 1990.
38. Bass WT, Jones MA, White LE, et al: Ultrasonographic differential diagnosis and neurodevelopmental outcome of cerebral white matter lesions in premature infants. J Perinatol 19:330, 1999.
39. Maalouf EF, Duggan PJ, Counsell SJ, et al: Comparison of findings on cranial ultrasound and magnetic resonance imaging in preterm infants. Pediatrics 107:719, 2001.
40. Jongmans M, Mercuri E, de Vries L, et al: Minor neurological signs and perceptual-motor difficulties in prematurely born children. Arch Dis Child 76:F9, 1997.
41. Sheth RD: Trends in the incidence and severity of intraventricular hemorrhage. J Child Neurol 13:261, 1998.
42. Hill A: Intraventricular hemorrhage: Emphasis on prevention. Semin Pediatr Neurol 5:152, 1998.
43. Volpe JJ: Intraventricular hemorrhage: Germinal matrix-intraventricular hemorrhage of the premature infant. In Volpe JJ (ed): Neurology of the Newborn, 4th ed. Philadelphia, WB Saunders, 2001, p. 447.
44. Shankaran S, Bauer CR, Bain R, et al: Prenatal and perinatal risk and protective factors for neonatal intracranial hemorrhage. Arch Ped Adolesc Med 150:491, 1996.
45. Papile LA, Burstein J, Burstein R, et al: Incidence and evolution of subependymal and intraventricular hemorrhage: A study of infants with birth weights less than 1,500 grams. J Pediatr 92:529, 1978.
46. Shankaran S, Cepeda E, Mauran G, et al: Antenatal phenobarbital therapy and neonatal outcome I: Effect on intracranial hemorrhage. Pediatrics 97:644, 1996.
47. Leviton A, Fenton T, Kuban KC, et al: Labor and delivery characteristics and the risk of germinal matrix hemorrhage in low birth weight infants. J Child Neurol 6:35, 1991.
48. Horbar JD: Antenatal corticosteroid treatment and neonatal outcomes for infants 501 to 1500 g in the Vermont-Oxford Trials Network. Am J Obstet Gynecol 173:275, 1995.
49. Wright LL, Verter J, Younes N, et al: Antenatal corticosteroid administration and neonatal outcome in very low birth-weight infants: The NICHD Neonatal Research Network. Am J Obstet Gynecol 173:269, 1995.
50. Leviton A, Kuban KC, Pagano M, et al: Antenatal corticosteroids appear to reduce the risk of postnatal germinal matrix hemorrhage in intubated low birthweight newborns. Pediatrics 91:1083, 1993.
51. The HIFI Study Group: High-frequency oscillatory ventilation compared with conventional mechanical ventilation in the treatment of respiratory failure in preterm infants. N Engl J Med 320:88, 1989.
52. Keszler M, Monanlou HD, Brudno DS, et al: Multicenter controlled clinical trial of high-frequency jet ventilation in preterm infants with uncomplicated respiratory distress syndrome. Pediatrics 100:593, 1997.
53. Clark RH, Dykes FD, Bachman TE, et al: Intraventricular hemorrhage and high-frequency ventilation: A meta-analysis of prospective clinical trials. Pediatrics 98(6 Pt1):1058, 1996.
54. Bhuta T, Henderson-Smart DJ: Elective high frequency jet ventilation versus conventional ventilation for respiratory distress syndrome in preterm infants. Cochrane Database Syst Rev 2:CD000328, 2000.
55. Guzzetta F, Shackelford GD, Volpe S, et al: Periventricular intraparenchymal echodensities in the premature newborn: Critical determinant of neurologic outcome. Pediatrics 78:995, 1986.
56. Takashima S, Mito T, Ando Y: Pathogenesis of periventricular white matter hemorrhages in preterm infants. Brain Dev 8:25, 1986.
57. Gould SJ, Howard S, Hope PL, et al: Periventricular intraparenchymal cerebral haemorrhage in preterm infants: The role of venous infarction. J Pathol 151:197, 1987.
58. Taylor GA: Effect of germinal matrix hemorrhage on terminal vein position and patency. Pediatr Radiol 25:S37, 1995.
59. Banker BQ, Larroche J-C: Periventricular leukomalacia of infancy. Arch Neurol 7:32, 1962.
60. Carson SC, Hertzberg BS, Bowie JD, et al: Value of sonography in the diagnosis of intracranial hemorrhage and periventricular leukomalacia: A postmortem study of 35 cases. Am J Neuroradiol 11:677, 1990.
61. de Vries LS, Wigglesworth JS, Regev R, et al: Evolution of periventricular leukomalacia during the neonatal period and infancy: Correlation of imaging and postmortem findings. Early Hum Dev 17:205, 1988.
62. Paneth N, Rudelli R, Monte W, et al: White matter necrosis in very low birth weight infants: Neuropathologic and ultrasonographic findings in infants surviving six days or longer. J Pediatr 116:975, 1990.

63. Zupan V, Gonzolez P, Tacaze-Masmonteil T, et al: Periventricular leukomalacia: Risk factors revisited. Dev Med Child Neurol 38:1061, 1996.
64. Shuman RM, Selednik LJ: Periventricular leukomalacia: A one-year autopsy study. Arch Neurol 37:231, 1980.
65. Altman DI, Powers WJ, Perlman JM, et al: Cerebral blood flow requirements for brain viability in newborn infants is lower than adults. Ann Neurol 24:218, 1988.
66. Tuor UI: Local cerebral blood flow in the newborn rabbit: An autoradiographic study of changes during development. Pediatr Res 129:517, 1991.
67. Meek JH, Tyszczuk L, Elwell CE, et al: Cerebral blood flow increases over the first three days of life in extremely preterm neonates. Arch Dis Child Fetal Neonatal Ed 78:F33, 1998.
68. Calvert SA, Ohlsson A, Hosking MC, et al: Serial measurements of cerebral blood flow velocity in preterm infants during the first 72 hours of life. Acta Paediatr Scand 77:625, 1988.
69. Borch K, Greisen G: Blood flow distribution in the normal human preterm brain. Pediatr Res 43:28, 1998.
70. Lou HC, Lassen NA, Tweed WA, et al: Pressure passive cerebral blood flow and breakdown of the blood-brain barrier in experimental fetal asphyxia. Acta Paediatr Scand 68:57, 1979.
71. Pryds O, Greisen G, Lou H, et al: Heterogeneity of cerebral vasoreactivity in preterm infants supported by mechanical ventilation. J Pediatr 115:638, 1989.
72. Watkins TW, Barbieri R, Hammer J, et al: The high pass nature of cerebral autoregulation in extremely preterm neonates and its relationship to brain injury [abstract]. Pediatr Res 49:2007, 2001.
73. Tsuji M, Saul JP, du Plessis A, et al: Cerebral intravascular oxygenation correlates with mean arterial pressure in critically ill premature infants. Pediatrics 106:625, 2000.
74. Bonofoco E, Krainc D, Ankarcrona M, et al: Apoptosis and necrosis: Two distinct events induced, respectively, by mild and intense insults with N-methyl-D-aspartate or nitric oxide/superoxide in cortical cell culture. Proc Natl Acad Sci 92:7162, 1995.
75. Fellman V, Raivio KO: Reperfusion injury as the mechanism of brain damage after perinatal asphyxia. Pediatr Res 41:599, 1997.
76. Gehrmann J, Banati RB, Wiessnert C, et al: Reactive microglia in cerebral ischaemia: An early mediator of tissue damage? Neuropathol Appl Neurobiol 21:277, 1995.
77. Pryds O: Control of cerebral circulation in the high-risk neonate. Ann Neurol 30:321, 1991.
78. Hansen NB, Brubakk AM, Bratlid D, et al: The effects of variations in $PaCO_2$ on brain blood flow and cardiac output in the newborn piglet. Pediatr Res 18:1132, 1984.
79. Hansen NB, Nowicki PT, Miller, et al: Alterations in cerebral blood flow and oxygen consumption during prolonged hypocarbia. Pediatr Res 20:147, 1986.
80. Graziani LJ, Spitzer AR, Mitchell DG, et al: Mechanical ventilation in preterm infants: Neurosonographic and developmental studies. Pediatrics 90:515, 1992.
81. Calvert SA, Hoskins EM, Fong KW, et al: Etiological factors associated with the development of periventricular leukomalacia. Acta Paediatr Scand 76:254, 1987.
82. Greison G, Munck H, Lou H: Severe hypocarbia in preterm infants and neurodevelopmental deficit. Acta Paediatr Scand 76:401, 1987.
83. Fugimoto S, Togari H, Yamaguchi N, et al: Hypocarbia and cystic periventricular leukomalacia. Arch Dis Child 71:F107, 1994.
84. Luyt K, Wright D, Baumer JH: Randomised study comparing extent of hypocarbia in preterm infants during conventional and patient triggered ventilation. Arch Dis Child Fetal Neonatal Ed 84:F14, 2001.
85. Wiswell TE, Graziani LJ, Kornhauser MS, et al: Effects of hypocarbia on the development of cystic periventricular leukomalacia in premature infants treated with high-frequency jet ventilation. Pediatrics 98:918, 1996.
86. Okumura A, Hayakawa F, Kato T, et al: Hypocarbia in preterm infants with periventricular leukomalacia: The relationship between hypocarbia and mechanical ventilation. Pediatrics 107:469, 2001.
87. Ohyu J, Endo A, Itoh M: Hypocapnia under hypotension induces apoptotic neuronal cell death in the hippocampus of newborn rabbits. Pediatr Res 48:24, 2000.
88. Dammann O, Allred EN, Kuban KCK, et al: Hypocarbia during the first 24 postnatal hours and white matter echolucencies in newborns < 28 weeks gestation. Pediatr Res 49:388, 2001.
89. Mariani G, Cifuentes J, Carlo WA: Randomized trial of permissive hypercapnia in preterm infants. Pediatrics 104:1082, 1999.

90. Leviton A, Gilles F: Ventriculomegaly, delayed myelination, white matter hypoplasia, and "periventricular" leukomalacia: Are they related? Pediatr Neurol 15:127, 1996.

91. Dammann O, Leviton A: Maternal intrauterine infection, cytokines, and brain damage in the preterm newborn. Pediatr Res 42:1, 1997.

92. Wu YW, Colford JM: Chorioamnionitis as a risk factor for cerebral palsy. A meta-analysis. JAMA 284:1417, 2000.

93. Dammann O, Leviton A: Brain damage in preterm newborns: Might enhancement of developmentally regulated endogenous protection open a door for prevention? Pediatrics 104:541, 1999.

94. Dammann O, Leviton A: Brain damage in preterm newborns: Biological response modification as a strategy to reduce disabilities. J Pediatr 136:433, 2000.

95. Dammann O, Leviton A: Infection remote from the brain, neonatal white matter damage, and cerebral palsy in the preterm infant. Semin Pediatr Neurol 5:190, 1998.

96. Hallman M: Cytokines, pulmonary surfactant and consequences of intrauterine infection. Biol Neonate 76(Suppl 1):2,1999

97. Goldenberg R, Hauth J, Andrews W: Intrauterine infection and preterm delivery. N Engl J Med 342:1500, 2000.

98. Bejar R, Wozniak P, Allard M, et al: Antenatal origin of neurologic damage in newborn infants. I. Preterm infants. Am J Obstet Gynecol 159:357, 1988.

99. Perlman JM, Risser R, Broyles RS: Bilateral cystic periventricular leukomalacia in the premature infant: Associated risk factors. Pediatrics 97:822, 1996.

100. Bass WT, Schultz SJ, Burke BL, et al: Indices of hemodynamic and respiratory function in premature infants at risk for the development of cerebral white matter injury. J Perinatol 22:64, 2002.

101. Vigneswaran R: Infection and preterm birth: Evidence of a common causal relationship with bronchopulmonary dysplasia and cerebral palsy. J Paediatr Child Health 36:293,2000.

102. Watterberg KL, Demers LM, Scott SM, et al: Chorioamnionitis and early lung inflammation in infants in whom bronchopulmonary dysplasia develops. Pediatrics 97:210, 1996.

103. Hallman M: Cytokines, pulmonary surfactant and consequences of intrauterine infection. Biol Neonate 76(Suppl 1):2, 1999.

104. Leviton A: Preterm birth and cerebral palsy: Is tumor necrosis factor the missing link? Dev Med Child Neurol 35:549, 1993.

105. Yoon BH, Romero R, Kim CJ, et al: Amniotic fluid interleukin-6: A sensitive test for antenatal diagnosis of acute inflammatory lesions of preterm placenta and prediction of perinatal morbidity. Am J Obstet Gynecol 172:960, 1995.

106. Yoon BH, Romero R, Yang SH: Interleukin-6 concentrations in umbilical cord plasma are elevated in neonates with white matter lesions associated with periventricular leukomalacia. Am J Obstet Gynecol 174:1433, 1996.

107. Gilles FH: Changes in growth and vulnerability at the end of the second trimester. In Gilles FH, Leviton A, Dooling EC, et al. (eds): The Developing Human Brain: Growth and Epidemiologic Neuropathology. Boston, Wright-PSG, 1983, p. 316.

108. Koauge S, Ohkuchi A, Minakami H, et al: Influence of chorioamnionitis on survival and morbidity in singletons live-born at < 32 weeks gestation. Acta Obstet Gynecol Scand 79:861, 2000.

109. Jobe AH, Newnham JP, Willet KE, et al: Effects of antenatal endotoxin and glucocorticoids on the lungs of preterm lambs. Am J Obstet Gynecol 182:401, 2000.

110. Willett KE, Jobe AH, Ikegami M, et al: Antenatal endotoxin and glucocorticoid effects on lung morphometry in preterm lambs. Pediatr Res 48:782, 2000.

111. Jobe AH, Newnham JP, Willett KE, et al: Endotoxin-induced lung maturation in preterm lambs is not mediated by cortisol. Am J Respir Crit Care Med 162:1656, 2000.

112. Mammel MC, Green TP, Johnson DE, et al: Controlled trial of dexamethasone therapy in infants with bronchopulmonary dysplasia. Lancet 1:1356, 1983.

113. Avery GB, Fletcher AB, Kaplan M, et al: Controlled trial of dexamethasone in respirator dependent infants with bronchopulmonary dysplasia. Pediatrics 75:106, 1985.

114. Bhuta T, Ohlsson A: Systematic review and meta-analysis of early postnatal dexamethasone for the prevention of chronic lung disease. Arch Dis Child Fetal Neonatal Ed 79:F26, 1998.

115. Halliday HL: Clinical trials of postnatal corticosteroids: Inhaled and systemic. Biol Neonate 76:29, 1999.

116. Weichsel ME: The therapeutic use of glucocorticoid hormones in the perinatal period. Potential neurological hazards. Ann Neurol 46:364, 1977.

117. Baethmann A: Steroids and brain function. In James HE, Anas NG, Perkin RM (eds): Brain Insults in Infants and Children. Orlando, Fla., Grune & Stratton, 1985, p. 4.

118. Woodbury DM: Biochemical effects of adrenocortical steroid on the central nervous system. In Lajtha A (ed): Handbook of Neurochemistry, vol. 7. New York, Plenum, 1972, pp. 255–287.

119. Murphy BP, Inder TE, Huppi PS, et al: Impaired cerebral cortical gray matter growth after treatment with dexamethasone for neonatal chronic lung disease. Pediatrics 107:217, 2001.

120. Howard H: Reductions in size and total DNA of cerebrum and cerebellum in adult mice after corticosterone treatment in infancy. Exp Neurol 22:191, 1968.

121. Tsubota S, Adachi N, Chen J, et al: Dexamethasone changes brain monoamine metabolism and aggravates ischemic neuronal damage in rats. Anesthesiology 90:515, 1999.

122. Papile LA, Tyson JE, Stoll BJ, et al: A multicenter trial of two dexamethasone regimens in ventilator-dependent premature infants. N Engl J Med 338:1112, 1998.

123. Romagnoli C, Zecca E, Vento G, et al: Effect on growth of two different dexamethasone courses for preterm infants at risk of chronic lung disease—A randomized trial. Pharmacology 59:266, 1999.

124. Stathis SL, O'Callaghan M, Harvey J, et al: Head circumference in ELBW babies is associated with learning difficulties and cognition but not ADHD in the school aged child. Dev Med Child Neurol 41:375, 1999.

125. Fitzhardinge PM, Eisen A, Lejtenyi C, et al: Sequelae of early steroid administration to the newborn infant. Pediatrics 53:877, 1974.

126. Yeh TF, Lin YJ, Huang CC, et al: Early dexamethasone therapy in preterm infants: A follow-up study. Pediatrics 101:E71, 1998.

127. O'Shea T, Kothadia J, Klinepeter K, et al: Randomized placebo-controlled trial of a 42-day tapering course of dexamethasone to reduce the duration of ventilator dependency in very low birth weight infants: Outcome of study participants at 1-year adjusted age. Pediatrics 104:15, 1999.

128. Shinwell ES, Karplus M, Reich E, et al: Early postnatal dexamethasone treatment and increased incidence of cerebral palsy. Arch Dis Child Fetal Neonatal Ed. 83:F177, 2000.

129. Merz U, Peschgens T, Kusenbach G, et al: Early versus late dexamethasone treatment in preterm infants at risk for chronic lung disease: A randomized pilot study. Eur J Pediatr 158:318, 1999.

130. Baud O, Foix-L'Helias L, Kaminski A, et al: Antenatal glucocorticoid treatment and cystic periventricular leukomalacia in very premature infants. N Engl J Med 341:1190, 1999.

131. Garland JS, Colleen PA, Pauly TH, et al: A three-day course of dexamethasone therapy to prevent chronic lung disease in ventilated neonates: A randomized trial. Pediatrics 104:91, 1999.

132. Kopelman AE, Moise AA, Holbert D, et al: A single very early dexamethasone dose improves respiratory and cardiovascular adaptation in preterm infants. J Pediatr 135:345, 1999.

133. Gaissmaier RE, Pohlandt F: Single-dose dexamethasone treatment of hypotension in preterm infants. J Pediatr 134:701, 1999.

134. Andre P, Thebaud B, Odievre MH, et al: Methylprednisolone, an alternative to dexamethasone in very premature infants at risk of chronic lung disease. Intensive Care Med 26:1496, 2000.

135. Watterberg KL, Gerdes JS, Gifford KL, et al: Prophylaxis against early adrenal insufficiency to prevent chronic lung disease in premature infants. Pediatrics 104:1258, 1999.

136. Finer NN, Craft A, Vaucher YE, et al: Postnatal steroids: Short-term gain, long-term pain? J Pediatrics 137:9, 2000.

137. Whitelaw A, Thoresen M: Antenatal steroids and the developing brain. Arch Dis Child Fetal Neonatal Ed 83:F154, 2000.

138. Liggins GC: Premature delivery of fetal lambs infused with glucocorticoids. J Endocrinol 45:515, 1969.

139. Liggins GC, Howie RN: A controlled trial of antepartum glucocorticoid treatment for the prevention of the respiratory distress syndrome in premature infants. Pediatrics 50:515, 1972.

140. Crowley P, Chalmers I, Keirse MJ: The effects of corticosteroid administration before preterm delivery: An overview of the evidence from controlled trials. Br J Obstet Gynaecol 97:11, 1990.

141. Crowley P: Prophylactic corticosteroids for preterm delivery (Cochrane review). In: The Cochrane Library. Oxford, 1999.

142. Huang WL, Beazley LD, Quinlivan JA, et al: Effect of corticosteroids on brain growth in fetal sheep. Obstet Gynaecol 94:213, 1999.

143. Quinlivan JA, Dunlop SA, Newnham JP, et al: Repeated but not single maternal administration of corticosteroid delays myelination in the brain of fetal sheep. Perinatal Neonatal Med 4:47, 1999.

144. Uno H, Lohmiller L, Thieme C, et al: Brain damage induced by prenatal exposure to dexamethasone in fetal rhesus macaques. I. Hippocampus. Dev Brain Res 53:157, 1990.

145. Tombaugh GC, Yang SH, Swanson RA, et al: Glucocorticoids exacerbate hypoxic and hypoglycaemic hippocampal injury in vitro. J Neurochem 59:137, 1992.

146. Riva Ma, Fumagalli F, Racagni G: Opposite regulation of basic fibroblast growth factor and nerve growth factor gene expression in rat cortical astrocytes following dexamethasone administration. J Neurochem 64:2516, 1995.

147. Tuor UI, Chumas PD, Del Bigio MR: Prevention of hypoxic-ischaemic damage with dexamethasone is dependent on age and not influenced by fasting. Exp Neurol 132:116, 1995.

148. US Collaborative Group on Antenatal Steroid Therapy: Effects of antenatal dexamethasone administration in the infant: Long-term follow-up. J Pediatr 104:259, 1984.

149. French NP, Hagan R, Evans SF, et al: Repeated antenatal corticosteroids: Size at birth and subsequent development. Am J Obstet Gynecol 180:114, 1999.

150. Leviton A, Dammann O, Allred EN, et al: Antenatal corticosteroids and cranial ultrasonographic abnormalities. Am J Obstet Gynecol 181:1007, 1999.

151. Canterino JC, Verma U, Visintainer PF, et al: Antenatal steroid and neonatal periventricular leukomalacia. Obstet Gynecol 97:135, 2001.

152. Smith LM, Qureshi N, Chao CR: Effects of single and multiple courses of antenatal glucocorticoids in preterm newborns less than 30 weeks' gestation. J Matern Fetal Med 9:131, 2000.

153. Goldenberg RL, Wright LL: Repeated courses of antenatal corticosteroids. Obstet Gynecol 97:316, 2001.

154. Bauer J, Maier K, Linderkamp O, et al: Effect of caffeine on oxygen consumption and metabolic rate in very low birth weight infants with idiopathic apnea. Pediatrics 107:660, 2001.

155. Schmidt B: Methylxanthine therapy in premature infants: Sound practice, disaster, or fruitless byway? J Pediatr 135:526, 1999.

156. Wood NS, Marlow N, Costeloe K, et al: Neurologic and developmental disability after extremely preterm birth. N Engl J Med 343:378, 2000.

157. Arnold CC, Kramer MS, Hobbs CA, et al: Very low birth weight: A problematic cohort for epidemiologic studies of very small or immature neonates. Am J Epidemiol 134:604, 1991.

158. Fawer CL, Besnier S, Forcada M, et al: Influence of perinatal, developmental and environmental factors on cognitive abilities of preterm children without major impairments at 5 years. Early Hum Dev 43:151, 1995.

159. Gross SJ, Mettelman BB, Dye TD, et al: Impact of family structure and stability on academic outcome in preterm children at 10 years of age. J Pediatr 138:169, 2001.

160. Shinnar S, Molteni RA, Gammon K, et al: Intraventricular hemorrhage in the premature infant. N Engl J Med 306:1464, 1982.

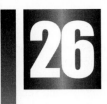

INTRAOPERATIVE MANAGEMENT

BRYAN S. KING, MD

Neonatal patients provide the anesthesiologist with some of the most complex and difficult anesthetic challenges. Over the last decade the improving survival of extremely premature infants[1] with complex medical and surgical diseases has significantly increased the challenges facing the anesthesiologist.[2,3] To confront these issues, anesthesiologists have made significant advances in their understanding of the pathophysiology of these diseases, in agents, and in techniques used for neonates requiring surgery. Despite these advances, 55% of cardiac arrests in patients younger than 18 years of age occur in the first year of life, with the vast majority of the arrests occurring secondary to a failure to ventilate the patient.[4–6]

With the introduction of inhalational anesthesia, anesthesiologists have continued to identify anesthetic risks in infants and have sought new ways to reduce these risks and provide safer anesthetics. Since the early 1950s, anesthesiologists in the United States have made significant contributions to neonatal medicine, including evaluation of the newborn's need for resuscitation (the Apgar score), the development of the first neonatal ventilator,[7] pulse oximetry, extracorporeal membrane oxygenation (ECMO), and nitric oxide (NO) therapy.[8–13] These technologic advances were coupled with clinical techniques to advance care of the most challenging and rapidly growing patient population: the premature infant.[14]

Physicians caring for neonates must recognize the special considerations and risks that their patients face when they undergo anesthesia. Knowledge of the unique physiology, anatomy, and pathology of the neonate is essential for safe intraoperative management by the anesthesiologist. In addition, an appreciation of the anesthetic techniques, pharmacologic agents, and potential intraoperative management difficulties is necessary.

Full-term newborns usually adapt rapidly to extrauterine life by converting from a fetal to a neonatal circulatory system, initiating spontaneous ventilation, maintaining adequate energy substrates, establishing renal function and fluid balance, and maintaining normal body temperature. Anesthesia and surgery exert significant stresses on the newborn during this delicate transition from intrauterine to extrauterine life. Physiologic stresses can easily cause the neonate to revert to a fetal circulation system with pulmonary hypertension, altered central control of ventilation, rapid consumption of energy substrates, decreased glomerular filtration, and thermal deregulation.

GENERAL ANESTHESIA AND THE NEONATE

A typical general anesthetic can be divided into three phases: induction, maintenance, and emergence. Induction of anesthesia begins when anesthetic agents are administered to create an adequate combination of analgesia, hypnosis, and muscle relaxation to allow for diagnostic or therapeutic interventions.[15–17] Usually a combination of intravenous and inhalational agents is used for induction according to the nature of the procedure and the coexisting medical issues. During the maintenance phase the anesthetic is designed to provide cardiorespiratory stability, hypnosis, and muscle relaxation. Emergence and recovery occur after discontinuation of the anesthetics and vary from minutes to hours according to the anesthetic used and the nature of the procedure. Induction and emergence with securing and maintaining an adequate airway are associated with the highest number of adverse events in pediatric anesthesia.[6,18,19] During all phases of the anesthetic the pediatric anesthesiologist must monitor the multisystemic impact of the anesthetic agents used and the procedures being performed on the neonate. These concerns include pain management, airway difficulties, ventilatory depression, thermal instability, rapid dehydration, and energy substrate requirements.

Inhalational anesthetics, or volatile anesthetics, are liquids that are vaporized and mixed into the patient's breathing circuit. Ether was the first volatile anesthetic administered on October 16, 1846 at Massachusetts General Hospital in Boston and was used clinically for more than 100 years. Volatile agents currently used in the United States are sevoflurane, isoflurane, desflurane, halothane, and enflurane. Cyclopropane and ether are no longer used in the United States.

Volatile anesthetics are used commonly in neonatal and pediatric anesthesia because they do not require an intravenous catheter prior to the start of a procedure. The dosing and administration are reliable and easily adjusted using modern vaporizers that deliver a precise concentration of the agent in the inspiratory gases. Clearance is primarily via exhalation with minimal amounts of metabolism depending on the agent being delivered. Volatile anesthetics are the only single agent that reliably induces the triad of analgesia, muscle relaxation, and hypnosis.

Intravenous anesthetics used frequently in neonates include propofol, thiopental, opioids, benzodiazepines, and a variety of muscle relaxants, such as succinylcholine, pancuronium, vecuronium, and cisatracurium.

Neonatal sensitivity to the cardiodepressant effects of anesthetics is demonstrated by a number of physiologic manifestations, including poor sympathetic tone, sluggish baroreceptor responses, high parasympathetic tone, and cardiac output that is determined primarily by heart rate. The volatile anesthetics are extremely vagotonic and easily potentiate an infant's high resting vagal tone to reduce heart rate[20,21] and cardiac output more rapidly than with older patients.[5,6]

NEONATAL ANESTHETIC CONCERNS

Preoperative Evaluation of the Neonate

The evaluation of the neonate begins with a prenatal history. Neonatal illness begins in utero, and a complete gestational history should be taken to identify commonly associated neonatal problems (Table 26-1). A family history of adverse reactions to anesthesia should be taken, specifically any history of prolonged paralysis (pseudocholinesterase deficiency), malignant hyperthermia, inherited defects in metabolism, and familial medical conditions, including myopathies, hemoglobinopathies, and bleeding disorders.

A history of the present illness for which the neonate requires anesthesia should consider the relevant organ systems involved. Frequently neonatal emergencies involve multiple organ systems and have a profound influence on the choice of anesthetic. When a child has one congenital malformation, the likelihood of another is increased. The anesthesiologist should have a very low threshold for ordering an echocardiogram, chest x-ray film, and abdominal ultrasound to identify congenital malformations. In utero ultrasound often may identify congenital malformations but should not be relied on to provide

postnatal diagnosis. New ultrafast magnetic resonance imaging scanners have been used to detect fetal anomalies in cases where the ultrasound has yielded equivocal results.[22]

Prior anesthetic history, drug allergy or therapy, and ventilatory management should be considered. An organized plan for intraoperative management, including premedication, if any, fasting status, drug dosages, and need for postoperative ventilation, should be developed and documented in a preanesthetic note (Table 26-2).

Baseline vital signs should be evaluated. If the child is intubated, mechanical ventilator settings are noted, especially the F_{IO_2}, rate of mechanical and spontaneous ventilation, use of continuous positive airway pressure or positive end-expiratory pressure, peak airway pressure and flows, and the ratio of inspiratory to expiratory time. Oxygen and ventilatory therapy should be maintained during transport to the operating room (OR) and during the operative procedure with an anesthesia bag or time-cycled ventilator. Baseline arterial blood or capillary gas analysis confirms the adequacy of oxygenation and ventilation. Oxygen saturation probes provide good indication of oxygenation and are essential during transport of ventilated neonates. Because even the short trip to the OR can compromise the previously stable neonate, warmed transport incubators with compressed gases are necessary for maintaining thermal stability and providing continuous ventilation.

Laboratory test data should be appropriate for the patient's history and illness and the nature of the procedure to be performed. Hematocrit, hemoglobin, and serum glucose levels should be checked prior to anesthesia. Parenteral hyperalimentation should be continued intraoperatively, with recent electrolytes checked and corrected. Urine specific gravity of 1.010 to 1.015 with urine output greater than 1 mL/kg is an indicator of adequate intravascular status (see Table 26-2).

TABLE 26-1.   Maternal History with Commonly Associated Neonatal Problems

Maternal History	Commonly Expected Problems with Neonates
Rh-ABO incompatibility	Hemolytic anemia, hyperbilirubinemia, kernicterus
Toxemia	SGA, muscle relaxant interaction with magnesium therapy
Hypertension	SGA
Drug addiction	Withdrawal, SGA
Infection	Sepsis, thrombocytopenia, viral infection
Hemorrhage	Anemia, shock
Diabetes	Hypoglycemia, birth trauma, LGA, SGA, and associated problems
Polyhydramnios	Tracheoesophageal fistula, anencephaly, multiple anomalies
Oligohydramnios	Renal hypoplasia, pulmonary hypoplasia
Cephalopelvic disproportion	Birth trauma, hyperbilirubinemia, fractures
Alcoholism	Hypoglycemia, congenital malformation, fetal alcohol syndrome, SGA

LGA, large for gestational age; SGA small for gestational age.
From Cote CJ, Todres D, Ryan JF, et al. (eds): A Practice of Anesthesia for Infants and Children, 4th ed. Philadelphia, WB Saunders, 2000.

TABLE 26-2.   Preanesthetic Checklist for Infants

- Family consent
- History and physical examination completed
  - Are additional studies needed?
  - Are appropriate laboratory results documented?
  - Is additional medical therapy indicated before surgery?
  - Correct hypovolemia
    - 10–20 mL/kg Ringers' lactate, 5% albumin, plasma, or blood
  - Correct hypoglycemia (<30 mg/dL)
    - 10% dextrose infusion, 7–11 mg/kg/min
- Preheat operating room
  - Heated humidifier
  - Radiant heater
  - Warmed prep solutions
- Anesthesia machine check
  - Appropriate endotracheal tubes, laryngoscopes, and masks
  - Suction, for oral, endotracheal, and gastric decompression
  - Backup ventilator
  - Intravenous equipment and fluids
- Medications prepared
  - Induction agents
  - Muscle relaxants
  - Analgesics
  - Atropine, epinephrine available
- Monitors
  - Temperature
  - Electrocardiograph
  - Blood pressure cuff or A-line
  - SpO_2
  - $ETCO_2$

Airway Management

Safe management of the neonatal airway is arguably the single most difficult and important task facing the anesthesia and surgical team. In 1973 Salem et al.[5] found that airway obstruction, accidental or premature tracheal extubation, and esophageal intubation were responsible for half of the cardiac arrests in their study of 73 intraoperative cardiac arrests in infants. Subsequent studies suggest that improved techniques for ventilating neonates, including the use of continuous pulse oximetry, has reduced the number of incidents involving airways but that failure to maintain an adequate airway remains a major cause of intraoperative deaths.[18,19]

The neonatal airway poses significant medical and anatomic difficulties unlike the adult airway. Induction of anesthesia results in the loss of functional residual capacity (FRC) such that lung volume falls below closing capacity of the small airways[23] and rapid arterial oxygen desaturation ensues as right-to-left intrapulmonary shunt fraction increases.[24] In the sick hypermetabolic neonate, the already diminished oxygen reserve in the lungs may be consumed even more rapidly and lead to increased risk of cardiopulmonary arrest.

The anatomy of the neonatal airway differs from that of the adult in several important ways. (1) The glottic opening is higher in the neck at the level of the third cervical vertebrae (in adults C5). (2) The more rostral position of the larynx places the epiglottis, hyoid, and tongue closer to the soft palate and roof of the mouth. The proximity of the tongue to the roof of the mouth makes visualization of the laryngeal structures more difficult and produces a more acute angulation between the plane of the tongue and the plane of the glottic opening; hence, the tongue is more likely to obstruct the view of the larynx. Straight laryngoscope blades are usually used to intubate the neonate because they more completely elevate the tongue.

Thermal Instability

Thermal instability potentially affects all neonates, whether during surgery, in the nursery, in the intensive care unit, or during transport. Intraoperative hypothermia is common in neonates, is easily overlooked, and imposes severe stresses that result in cardiac depression, hypoperfusion acidosis, and coagulopathy. Hypothermia is also associated with increased risk of infection. The etiology of neonatal temperature instability includes poor central thermoregulation, a thin insulating layer of fat, a high minute ventilation, and reduced muscle mass with poor shivering capacity. The greatest contributing factor to heat loss is the exaggerated ratio of body surface area to mass that is 2.5 or more times that of an adult.[25]

The transportation of the neonate, skin preparation, and surgical exposure lead to unavoidable heat loss. The pediatric anesthesiologist must anticipate these sources of heat loss and take steps to mitigate them, such as warming the OR well in advance of the patient's arrival, warming prep solutions, and using convective, conductive, and radiant warmers when possible.

Fluid Management

Rapid intraoperative dehydration may lead to neonatal circulatory collapse by depleting circulating fluid volume, reducing stroke volume, and promoting hypoperfusion acidosis. The newborn's large extracellular volume (40% of body weight) is rapidly reduced by fasting, insensible and operative fluid losses, gastrointestinal losses, and respiratory humidity. Renal maturation is only 80% complete by age 4 weeks and cannot provide large urine volumes during fluid overload, urine concentration during hypovolemic dehydration, or reabsorption of bicarbonate during hypoperfusion acidosis.[26,27] Thus, the neonate undergoing surgery is unable to handle a fluid overload or deficit with a strong tendency toward rapid salt and water losses promoting early dehydration and acidosis.[28] These physiologic disadvantages are even more pronounced with decreasing gestational age. Adequate fluid hydration with water and electrolytes must be provided and closely monitored during all operations on neonates.

Nutritional Imbalance

An important physiologic risk factor common to all neonates intraoperatively is a tendency toward nutritional imbalance with hypoglycemia and starvation ketosis due to low hepatic glycogen stores and stress induced metabolic workloads.[29] Unlike older children,[30] neonates are prone to hypoglycemia after relatively short periods of fasting.[31] Dextrose must be administered, along with water and electrolytes, if nutritional balance is to be maintained and if energy substrates for metabolism during fasting or surgery are to be provided. Full-term newborns require a glucose infusion of 7 to 10 mg/kg/min to maintain normoglycemia. Intraoperative infusions of glucose usually are reduced to 3 to 4 mg/kg/min because of the counterregulatory hormones released by the neuroendocrine stress response to surgery.[32,33] Attempts to completely replace large intraoperative fluid losses solely with glucose infusions may produce hyperglycemia with ketoacidosis, cardiovascular instability, and neurologic depression.

Detrimental Effects of Pain

Pain caused by surgery or injury leads to an altered physiologic condition characterized by massive sympathetic outflow mediated by the hypothalamus.[34,35] The neurohumoral response to surgery is an extreme elevation in catecholamines, insulin, growth hormone, antidiuretic hormone, beta-endorphin, aldosterone, glucagons, thyroxine, and interleukins.[36] The quantity of the stress response is related to the magnitude of the injury.[37] Higher plasma levels of the stress response markers further correlate with increased morbidity and mortality (Tables 26-3 and 26-4).[36]

The counterregulatory hormones lead to a catabolic state of increased oxygen consumption, glycogenolysis, lipolysis, and gluconeogenesis.[38] The effects seen include perioperative lactic acidemia, hypoglycemia, and negative nitrogen balance.[39] Comparable insults between infants and adults demonstrate a greater catabolic state induced in infants than in adults.[40,41] The catabolic effect of the stress response may be partly due to dysfunction of the hypothalamic-pituitary axis.[42] The resulting redistribution of proteins from skeletal muscle to provide substrate for vital organs diminishes immune function and impairs wound healing.[43,44]

Attempts to minimize the stress response have been most successful with neuraxial blockade in surgical patients.[45–47] However, this is not a safe option in septic infants in whom a concern of central nervous system (CNS) infection precludes

TABLE 26-3.   Pain and Its Effects in Neonates: Physiologic

Supporting Evidence	Fiction	Fact
Endogenous opioids (endorphins)	High plasma levels provide analgesia for several days after birth	High plasma levels indicate stress and birth asphyxia; analgesic levels in the CSF are 10,000-fold higher than observed
CV variables, $Ptco_2$, palmar sweating	Swaddling and pacifiers provide analgesia during painful procedures	$\uparrow$ HR, $\uparrow$ BP, $\downarrow$ $Paco_2$ (<50 mm Hg), and $\uparrow$ palmar sweating can be prevented with the use of local anesthetics for painful procedures
Stress hormones and their effects	Chest PT, ET suction, and intubation are performed frequently in neonates without adverse effects; light anesthetics and muscle relaxants are often administered for neonatal surgery	$\uparrow$ Plasma cortisol, epinephrine, NE, R-A-A, growth hormone, and glucagons have been measured during surgery and painful procedures; have caused hyperglycemia, ketonuria, and acidosis; can be prevented by adequate anesthesia

BP, blood pressure; CSF, cerebrospinal fluid; CV, cardiovascular; ET, endotracheal; HR, heart rate; NE, norepinephrine; PT, physiotherapy; R-A-A, rennin angiotensin aldosterone; $\uparrow$, increased; $\downarrow$, decreased.

TABLE 26-4.   Pain and Its Effects in Neonates: Anatomic

Supporting Evidence	Fiction	Fact
Nociceptive nerve endings in brain and skin	Reduced in neonates and infants	Equal to (brain) or greater than (skin) adults
Degree of peripheral nerve system myelinization and nerve conduction	Reduced myelinization indicates neurologic immaturity and inability to feel pain; neonates have slowest nerve conduction	Pain impulses are transmitted by unmyelinated C fibers and thinly myelinated A delta fibers; slower conduction speed is offset by reduced interneuron distances
Degree of central nervous system myelinization	Poor myelin insulation slows central conduction and reduces cortical pain perception	Pain tracts in spinal cord, brain stem, and thalamus are completely myelinated by 30 weeks

Data from Anand KJ, Hickey PR: Pain and its effects in the human neonate and fetus. N Engl J Med Nov 19;317:1321–1329, 1987; Lloyd-Thomas AR: Pain management in paediatric patients. Br J Anaesth 64:85–104, 1990; Anand KJ, Hickey PR: Halothane-morphine compared with high-dose sufentanil for anesthesia and postoperative analgesia in neonatal cardiac surgery. N Engl J Med 326:1–9, 1992.

transcutaneous administration of agents. Opioids and anxiolytics therefore are used liberally to attenuate the physiologic impact of pain. Clinical investigations have clearly demonstrated that these detrimental effects can be blocked and eliminated by adequate anesthesia with local anesthetics, inhaled or intravenous anesthetics, or combinations of regional and general anesthetics (Table 26-5).[48–51]

ANESTHETIC IMPLICATIONS OF PREMATURE NEONATAL PHYSIOLOGY

Marked improvements in neonatal medicine have led to improved survival of premature infants. As a result, smaller and sicker infants are coming to surgery with increasing frequency. These premature infants bring with them a variety of unique conditions with significant anesthetic consequences. The physiologic, morphologic, and technical differences between premature and term infants will be discussed using a systems approach.

Respiratory Disease of the Premature Infant

With the improvements in neonatal medicine, more premature infants now survive respiratory distress syndrome (RDS) and require surgical procedures such as ligation of the patent ductus arteriosus (PDA), ventriculoperitoneal shunting,

inguinal hernia repair, and central venous cannulation early and often during their course of treatment for RDS. Preterm infants are unable to maintain rhythmic breathing after birth and apneic episodes may be frequent. Additionally, the premature infants must work harder to breathe as a result of small airway collapse and inadequate re-expansion with each breath due to the low FRC and relative lack of surfactant.[52] The periodic breathing and increased susceptibility to the ventilatory depressant effects of anesthetics result in an increased incidence of postoperative life-threatening apnea and hypoxemia.[53,54]

The special problems that the RDS infant brings to the OR may include hypoxemia, hypercapnia, reduced pulmonary compliance, and anemia. Acquired problems may include subglottic stenosis, pulmonary O_2 toxicity, pulmonary interstitial emphysema, and bronchopulmonary dysplasia. RDS infants must be managed intraoperatively in the same manner in which they are treated in the neonatal intensive care unit, that is, with a safe airway, FIO_2 carefully titrated to a measured arterial O_2 pressure (Pao_2) of 50 to 80 mm Hg, and assisted or controlled ventilation with continuous positive end-expiratory pressure. The most reliable airway is an endotracheal tube, even for minor procedures. Mean airway pressure, peak inflating pressures, and distending pressures can be measured manometrically at the endotracheal tube so that appropriate ventilation is ensured and volutrauma[55] is prevented.[56] Hemoglobin should be restored preoperatively to at least 10 to 12 g/dL by infusion of packed red blood cells.

TABLE 26-5. Pain and Its Effects in Neonates: Behavioral

Supporting Evidence	Fiction	Fact
Simple motor responses	Neonates respond to pain with diffuse body movements, not with purposeful withdrawal of limbs	Even premature (<30 weeks gestational age) neonates have well-developed flexion responses to pinprick; such responses are often accompanied by crying grimacing, or both
Facial expressions	Facial expressions cannot be classified in neonates	In neonates, objective scores now associate distinct facial expressions with pleasure, pain, sadness, and surprise
Crying	Crying patterns cannot be correlated with initiating stimuli	Crying patterns can be classified according to the distress they indicate (pain, hunger, fear), on objective evaluation by trained observers, and on spectrographic analysis
Memory	Neonates have no memory of painful stimuli	Specific behavioral changes are present after circumcision without anesthesia and disrupt feeding schedules and parental bonding

Data from Anand KJ, Hickey PR: Pain and its effects in the human neonate and fetus. N Engl J Med 317:1321–1329, 1987; Lloyd-Thomas AR: Pain management in pediatric patients. Br J Anaesth 64:85–104, 1990; Anand KJ, Hickey PR. Halothane-morphine compared with high-dose sufentanil for anesthesia and postoperative analgesia in neonatal cardiac surgery. N Engl J Med 326:1–9, 1992.

Anemia

Despite having high initial blood volumes and hematocrits, preterm infants are susceptible to anemia caused by combinations of decreased erythropoiesis, hemolysis, vitamin E deficiency, short erythrocyte lifespan, bouts of sepsis, and frequent blood sampling for laboratory investigations.[57]

At birth, expanded blood volumes of 90 to 105 mL/kg may result from uteroplacental transfusion and delayed cord clamping.[58] High hematocrits and hemoglobin levels (16.0 to 17.0 g/dL) result from hemoconcentration within hours of birth and from the production of fetal hemoglobin (HbF) in the fetal liver and spleen (Appendix 18).[59,60] Adult hemoglobin (HbA) is also present in the fetus and neonate, but its production, which commences in fetal bone marrow at 20 weeks of gestation, lags behind that of HbF. At birth, 90% to 95% of the preterm infant's hemoglobin is HbF, compared with 65% to 85% in the full-term infant. The differences in HbF contribution to total hemoglobin at birth are important in determining red blood cell longevity, O_2-carrying capacity, and tissue oxygenation.[61]

HbA and HbF differ in structure, function, and lifespan. HbF has greater affinity for O_2 than HbA, limited ability to bind with 2,3-diphosphoglycerate (2,3-DPG), and impaired releasing capabilities (Appendix 10). These physiologic characteristics of HbF are beneficial to the fetus competing with the mother for O_2, but they are detrimental to the preterm neonate whose tissues may be starving for O_2 as a result of the stresses of RDS or surgery.[69]

Clinical investigations have demonstrated that an increase in HbA concentration by means of blood transfusion in preterm neonates with PDA may enhance ductal closure and alleviate congestive heart failure.[63,64] Possible mechanisms for transfusion-mediated ductal closure include reversal of the ratio of HbF to HbA, improvement in blood O_2 content, better tissue oxygenation, and O_2-induced ductal smooth muscle constriction.

In term infants, the hemoglobin concentration decreases rapidly and reaches a nadir of 9.0 to 11.0 g/dL (hematocrit, 30% to 33%) by 9 to 12 weeks (Appendix 18). In preterm infants, this decrease is greater and faster, reaching its nadir of 7.0 to 8.0 g/dL (hematocrit, 28% to 30%) by 4 to 8 weeks.[65,66] Anemia in the preterm infant is thus greater than in the term infant, and its severity is directly related to the degree of prematurity. Despite rapid decreases in hemoglobin levels, tissue oxygenation continues as HbA levels rise, 2,3-DPG levels increase, and the oxyhemoglobin dissociation curve moves to the right (Appendix 10).[60,67] By the third or fourth month of life, hemoglobin levels stabilize at 11 to 12 g/dL in term infants; these values are slightly lower in preterm infants.[65,66] By 1 year of age, the hemoglobin levels of term and preterm infants are comparable.[68] Hemoglobin changes during the first year of life in term and premature infants are indicated in Appendix 18.

Intracranial Hemorrhage

Intracranial hemorrhage (ICH) is a potential sequela of prematurity and low-birthweight. In addition to the cognitive impairment, neonates with ICH may require several surgeries for ventriculoperitoneal shunting as they grow older if progressive hydrocephalus develops. Premature infants are susceptible to ICH due to their immature cerebral autoregulation and fragile cerebral blood vessels.[69] Moreover, the hypertensive stress response appears to be exaggerated in premature neonates compared to older children.[70] Over the last decade a significant reduction in severity and incidence of ICH has been reported. Despite dramatic declines in ICH rates, approximately 21% of infants weighing less than 1000 g and 12% of those weighing less than 1500 g at birth are affected.[71] In the smallest preterm infants, ICH is more severe, occurs earlier, and is more often associated with a fatal outcome than in preterm infants weighing more than 700 g.[72–74] ICH in preterm infants is most commonly periventricular-intraventricular, but it may also be subdural, subarachnoid, or intracerebellar.[75]

Periventricular-intraventricular hemorrhage originates in the capillaries of the subependymal germinal matrix, which are poorly supported by connecting tissue.[72] Initial hemorrhagic lesions usually occur near the caudate nucleus in premature infants of less than 28 weeks' gestation and at the choroid plexus in preterm infants of greater than 28 weeks' gestation. Approximately 80% of cases of periventricular hemorrhage involve rupture through the ependyma and subsequent filling of the ventricular system with blood. The blood often pools in the posterior fossa, causing obliterative arachnoiditis with subsequent hydrocephalus.[75]

The pathogenesis of ICH in preterm infants appears to be related to several factors that can be differentiated as endothelial, vascular, or extravascular. The endothelial factors include immaturity and fragility of the periventricular capillary bed. Endothelial factors cannot be modified in the perioperative period, as can vascular and extravascular factors.[76] Vascular causes of ICH include impairment of cerebral autoregulation,[76] entry of a disproportionate amount of total cerebral blood flow into the periventricular circulation, fluctuation of arterial hypertension, and anatomic susceptibility to venous engorgement in the periventricular capillary bed.[72,75–77] Extravascular factors in ICH may include increased fibrinolytic activity in the periventricular region,[77] congenital or acquired hypocoagulability,[78] heparin administration,[79] and the rapid intravenous administration of colloid solutions,[80] saline, or sodium bicarbonate.[81] Such causative factors may combine in a premature infant (particularly one subjected to a perinatal asphyxial insult) to produce periventricular-intraventricular hemorrhage.

A number of commonly performed procedures have been associated with significant intracranial hypertension in preterm infants, including intratracheal suctioning,[82] awake tracheal intubation,[83] and asynchronous mechanical ventilation during spontaneous breathing.[84,85] Such procedures may predispose the preterm infant to a greater risk of ICH. Conversely, surgical closure of a PDA has not been shown to increase the risk of ICH in preterm infants.[86]

Eliminating fluctuations in blood pressure and cerebral blood flow by limiting the use of tracheal intubation, suctioning, and mechanical ventilation to anesthetized, paralyzed preterm infants has been shown to reduce intracranial pressure and possibly the risk of ICH.[87,88] Sedation with barbiturates in preterm infants with RDS has reduced the incidence of ICH in a susceptible population by eliminating stress-induced increases in arterial pressure during prolonged neonatal intensive care unit stays.[87]

Because the administration of halothane, isoflurane, fentanyl, or ketamine does not increase intracranial pressure in preterm neonates as it does in adults, premature neonates should receive an appropriate amount of anesthesia in surgery so that fluctuations in intracranial pressure are eliminated and the perianesthetic risks of ICH reduced.[85,89,90] An adequate plane of general anesthesia with combinations of titrated doses of inhaled and intravenous anesthetics and muscle relaxants can be maintained in preterm infants needing surgery. For further discussion of ICH, see Chapter 25.

Episodic Apnea

Episodic apnea occurs frequently in premature infants, usually worsens when O_2 and ventilatory therapy ceases, and can be induced by feeding or upper airway suctioning.[91] Episodic apnea can be a brief respiratory pause shorter than 15 seconds' duration (periodic breathing) or a prolonged apneic pause longer than 15 seconds' duration.[92] Apnea lasting longer than 15 seconds often is accompanied by heart rates of less than 100 beats/min for at least 5 seconds.[93] In most cases, the incidence of perioperative apnea may be inversely correlated with gestational age and weight.[92] Despite significant advances in the perioperative management of premature infants, apnea with or without bradycardia still poses one of the greatest risks following anesthesia and surgery in preterm neonates.[94] In a retrospective review of infants undergoing herniorrhaphy in the first months of life, Steward[14] was among the first to report that preterm infants were more likely to develop postoperative apnea than were full-term infants. Later, Liu et al.[53] reported a significant incidence of prolonged apnea in premature neonates younger than 41 weeks' postconceptual age. In 1987, Kurth et al.[54] reported a 37% incidence of postoperative prolonged apnea in infants of 32 to

55 weeks' postconceptual age and recommended postoperative apnea monitoring for up to 60 weeks' postconceptual age in preterm infants. This study also documented initial episodes of prolonged apnea occurring as late as 12 hours following termination of anesthesia.[54]

In 1995 Cote et al.[95] reported a meta-analysis of prospective data from eight studies of former preterm infants. Surprisingly they found no correlation of postoperative apnea with a history of necrotizing enterocolitis, neonatal apnea, RDS, bronchopulmonary dysplasia, or operative use of opioids or muscle relaxants. The analysis showed that apnea was inversely related to both gestational age and postconceptual age. The authors concluded that the risk of postoperative apnea after the infant is free of recovery room apnea is not less than 5%, with 95% statistical confidence until postconceptual age was 48 weeks with gestational age 35 weeks. The risk of postoperative apnea in the same group of infants does not fall to less than 1% with 95% statistical confidence until postconceptual age was 56 weeks with gestational age 32 weeks or postconceptual age was 54 weeks and gestational age 35 weeks.[95]

The methylxanthines, theophylline, and caffeine often are administered orally or intravenously as respiratory stimulants for the management of apnea of prematurity.[93,96–99] In 1994, Welborn et al.[100] recommended intravenous caffeine therapy 10 mg/kg after induction for preterm infants with episodic apnea, contending that it is more effective and less arrhythmogenic than theophylline therapy.[93] The pharmacologic basis for methylxanthine therapy in episodic apnea of prematurity appears to be related more to central stimulation of medullary breathing centers than to pulmonary bronchodilation and augmented diaphragmatic function.[99] Methylxanthine therapy should be continued perioperatively in preterm infants with episodic apnea, and long-acting anesthetic adjuvants, especially ketamine, barbiturates, opioids, and sedatives, should be given with caution.[92,94,96,97]

Controversy exists as to whether or not regional anesthesia reduces the risk of postoperative apnea. Some studies suggest that regional anesthesia reduces the risk of postoperative apnea, presumably by avoiding the respiratory depression caused by general anesthesia.[101–104] Regional techniques may offer an advantage, but the reports of apnea following regional anesthetics make this finding inconclusive.[101,105,106] Any sedation given, including ketamine, during a regional anesthetic leaves the infant with approximately the same risk for postoperative apnea as an infant recovering from general anesthesia.[101] Moreover, movement from an irritable infant can make the surgery more difficult, requiring sedation or conversion to a general anesthetic during the procedure (see section on Regional Anesthesia in Neonates).

At present there does not seem to be an "ideal" anesthetic that is not associated with postoperative respiratory problems. Our institution avoids elective surgery in infants less than 60 weeks' postconceptual age. The risks of postoperative apnea are discussed with the family and availability of beds and monitoring are checked prior to the onset of anesthesia. For further discussion of episodic apnea, see Chapter 3.

Retinopathy of Prematurity

Retinopathy of prematurity (ROP) is caused by intense vasoconstriction of immature retinal vessels in combination with retinal edema associated usually with exposure to a high

FIO_2 with development of high PaO_2 in retinal vessels.[107–109] Retinal hemorrhage, neovascularization, fibroproliferation, and retinal detachment with scarring may follow and result in myopia, strabismus, and, in severe cases, blindness.[110,111] Low birthweight and prematurity remain the most consistent risk factors for developing ROP.[112–115] Additional factors associated with ROP include mechanical ventilation, high FIO_2, and high PaO_2 (>70 to 90 mm Hg),[109] high O_2 saturation (>92% to 95%) in the retinal vessels, septicemia, intraventricular bleeding, and blood transfusion.[112–117]

These studies leave the anesthesiologist with the dilemma of allowing sufficient oxygenation of the vital organs while preventing the possible damaging effects of retinal hyperoxia. Because ROP appears to be multifactorial, it is unlikely that a brief episode of intraoperative hyperoxia can be entirely responsible.[118] Short-term administration of high concentrations of O_2 (for 1 to 3 minutes) before a hypoxic challenge such as tracheal intubation, extubation, or prolonged suctioning is considered acceptable and desirable and should not be avoided for fear of ROP.[119]

Although ROP usually afflicts the sickest and smallest infants, it has occurred infrequently in room air in term infants of less than 44 weeks' postconceptual age,[108,109] in cyanotic infants,[109] and even after short-term intraoperative administration of O_2 to term infants.[117,119] Because the infant's retina does not mature until 44 weeks of gestational age, it may be advisable to delay elective surgery until after that time.[120,121] If anesthesia is performed on infants younger than 44 weeks of gestation, use of pulse oximetry to maintain oxygen saturation between 93% and 95% may prevent hyperoxia.[122,123] For further discussion of ROP, see Chapter 21.

Persistent Pulmonary Hypertension of the Newborn

Large premature infants (34 to 37 weeks' gestational age), term neonates, and postmature newborns are at greater risk of persistent pulmonary hypertension of the newborn (PPHN) than the smallest premature infants. The danger of precipitating or worsening PPHN is highest in the first 3 days of life, when pulmonary artery pressures and resistances are elevated and pulmonary vascular reactivity to hypoxemia, volume fluctuations, or cardiac depression is unpredictable. Surgical interventions for situations that are not life threatening are best postponed in those infants most susceptible to PPHN until the risks of PPHN pass. For infants requiring surgery with PPHN, intraoperative NO may be helpful.[124] For further discussion of PPHN, see Chapters 23 and 24.

CONGENITAL MALFORMATIONS REQUIRING EARLY SURGICAL INTERVENTION IN NEONATES

Classification of Neonatal Surgical Emergencies

In neonates, surgical abnormalities represent a unique series of conditions seldom encountered in patients of any other age group. Careful attention to perioperative critical care and hemodynamic stabilization allows these tiny infants to undergo major corrective surgery with reduced risk. Prematurity and RDS may coexist with various congenital deformities and complicate management. Suggestions for anesthetic management of the most common surgical emergencies in newborns are presented in Table 26-6. A preanesthetic checklist is provided in Table 26-2.[125,126]

Congenital thoracic malformations requiring early surgical intervention in neonates include diaphragmatic hernia, tracheoesophageal fistula, congenital lobar emphysema (CLE), cystic adenomatoid malformation (CAM), intrathoracic masses [bronchogenic cysts (BC), pulmonary sequestration, and PDA]. Congenital malformations that cause acute abdominal emergencies requiring early surgical intervention in neonates include anterior abdominal wall defects (omphalocele, gastroschisis), small bowel obstruction (duodenal stenosis, atresia, jejunoileal atresia, malrotation, volvulus, meconium ileus), and colonic obstructions (Hirschsprung disease, meconium plug syndrome, hypoplastic left colon syndrome).

Thoracic Surgical Emergencies in Neonates

Congenital Diaphragmatic Hernia

Congenital diaphragmatic hernia (CDH) with onset of respiratory failure at birth has one of the most dramatic presentations of all thoracic surgical emergencies in neonates.[127,128] Neonates in gravest danger have large left-sided defects of the diaphragm, abnormal left lung tissue, a left hemithorax filled with intestines and abdominal viscera, and a mediastinum that is displaced into the right hemithorax and is compressing the right lung with possible right-sided pulmonary hypoplasia. Such neonates are deeply cyanotic at birth, have scaphoid abdomens, and make no respiratory effort. Neonates in less severe respiratory failure manifest varying degrees of tachypnea and cyanosis. Rarely, a neonate with CDH shows no symptoms during the first few hours or even days of life. These children with late onset of respiratory symptoms generally have small diaphragmatic defects, often on the right side, where the liver blocks significant herniation of abdominal contents into the right hemithorax. In general, neonates who develop diaphragmatic hernia after the first day of life recover quickly after surgical repairs without pulmonary hypertension or prolonged respiratory failure.[130]

Infants in acute respiratory distress from CDH at birth require prompt surgical evaluation and management. Before reduction of the hernia and repair of the hemidiaphragm, immediate management of acute respiratory failure must be undertaken and includes tracheal intubation for mechanical ventilation with rapid ventilatory rates and low peak inspired pressures. High-frequency oscillatory ventilation has been associated with a higher survival rate in neonates with CDH.[131] Ventilator-induced respiratory alkalosis with hyperoxygenation has now been shown to improve the systemic acidosis, hypoxemia, and pulmonary hypertension that characterize patients with large diaphragmatic defects. Large diaphragmatic hernias should be immediately evaluated for ECMO and NO therapy at birth when mechanical ventilation often proves to be inadequate.[132,133] Early transfer to an ECMO center should be strongly considered because respiratory demise usually is rapid. If CDH is diagnosed prenatally by ultrasound, the mother should be offered delivery in a neonatal facility that provides HFV, NO, and ECMO. The goal of preoperative mechanical hyperventilation in CDH is the control of persistent pulmonary hypertension through the

TABLE 26-6. Perioperative Management of Most Common Neonatal Emergencies

Surgical Diagnosis	Preoperative Considerations	Special Monitoring	Suggested Volatile Anesthetic	Suggested Adjuvants	Postoperative Considerations
Diaphragmatic hernia	Hypoplastic lungs, pulmonary hypertension, hypoxia, pneumothorax, gastric distention, cardiac defects, ECMO, nitric oxide	Nasogastric tube, arterial line, controlled low-pressure ventilation, Foley catheter	Sevoflurane or isoflurane, avoid N_2O	Fentanyl, morphine, muscle relaxants, epidural blockade	Anticipate postoperative intubation, nitric oxide? ECMO?
Gastroschisis	Hypovolemia, shock, hypothermia, sepsis, gastric distention	Nasogastric tube, arterial line, Foley catheter	Sevoflurane or isoflurane, avoid N_2O	Fentanyl, morphine, muscle relaxants	Tight closure with hypoventilation and caval compression, prolonged ileus, postoperative intubation
Intestinal obstruction	Hypovolemia, shock, aspiration, cystic fibrosis, Down syndrome	Nasogastric tube, large-bore IV access, Foley catheter	Sevoflurane or isoflurane, avoid N_2O	Fentanyl, morphine, muscle relaxants, epidural blockade	Ongoing third space losses, prolonged ileus, aspiration risk
Myelomeningocele	Hypothermia, sepsis, raised ICP	Careful prone positioning, precordial Doppler, line, large-bore IV evoked potentials, Foley catheter	Isoflurane or sevoflurane, N_2O/O_2	Avoid muscle relaxants, may interfere with nerve testing	Raised ICP, may need VPS, avoid prolonged sedation and hypoventilation, hypovolemia, hypothermia
Omphalocele	Hypovolemia, hypotension, hypoglycemia, hypothermia, sepsis, cardiac defects, Beckwith-Wiedemann	Radial A-line, large-bore IV access, Foley catheter	Isoflurane or sevoflurane, avoid N_2O	Fentanyl, morphine, muscle relaxants	Tight closure with hypoventilation and caval compression, prolonged ileus, postoperative intubation, hypoglycemia
Patent ductus arteriosus	Heart failure, extreme prematurity, RDS, cardiac defects	Preoperative echocardiogram, radial A-line, large-bore IV access	Avoid volatile anesthetic with severe heart failure	Fentanyl, morphine, muscle relaxants	Recurrent laryngeal nerve injury, mechanical ventilation for RDS, Cyanosis suggests ductus-dependent cardiac lesion
Pyloric stenosis	Hypokalemia, hypochloremia, metabolic alkalosis then hypoperfusion alkalosis, gastric distention, aspiration	Orogastric decompression	Sevoflurane or isoflurane	Rapid sequence intravenous induction with intubation, local infiltration of wound, narcotics usually unnecessary	Hypoglycemia, respiratory depression
Tracheoesophageal fistula	Oral secretions, aspiration, gastric distention, cardiac defects	Nasogastric tube, endotracheal tube below fistula, possible gastrostomy	Sevoflurane for inhalational induction, N_2O after fistula repair	Epidural blockade, muscle relaxants after ability to ventilate is verified	Tracheomalacia, esophageal reflux, esophageal stenosis, aspiration, pneumonitis

ECMO, extracorporeal membrane oxygenation; ICP, intracranial pressure; IV, intravenous; RDS, respiratory distress syndrome; VPS, ventriculoperitoneal shunt.
Modified after Diaz JH. Intraoperative management. In Goldsmith JP, Karotkin EH (eds): Assisted Ventilation of the Neonate, 3rd ed. Philadelphia, WB Saunders, 1991, p. 415.

achievement of the highest possible Pa_{O_2}, gradual reduction of the Pa_{CO_2} to 25 to 35 mm Hg, and maintenance of serum pH greater than 7.45 with a combination of high-frequency oscillatory ventilation, NO therapy, and alkali infusion.[134,135] No one treatment has been shown to be clearly superior to the other. ECMO usually is the ultimate treatment, but it still is associated with a high mortality.[133]

After respiratory failure has stabilized, insertion of reliable intravenous and arterial lines follows. Pulmonary hypertension with CDH causes massive right-to-left shunting of deoxygenated blood across the PDA away from the lungs and into the aorta and systemic circulation. Consequently, only the right radial artery consistently provides preductal arterial blood for gas analysis, whereas the umbilical artery provides postductal arterial blood for analysis. Many studies, however, have reported survival results and treatment protocols in CDH that are based on postductal arterial gas determinations from the umbilical artery or lower extremities.[136,137] Monitoring at both preductal and postductal arterial sites may be desirable for differential arterial blood gas comparison for detection and quantitation of pulmonary shunting after CDH repair. A combination of preductal arterial line monitoring and postductal pulse oximetry provides a less invasive but equally reliable shunt study.

Tension pneumothorax frequently complicates ventilatory management in CDH because of the high inspired pressures required for lung inflation, both of which are compressed by bowel contents (ipsilateral lung) or mediastinal structures (contralateral lung) and are often severely hypoplastic. Tension pneumothorax may occur in either side of the chest in CDH, causing loss of breath sounds on the affected side, mediastinal shifting into the opposite hemithorax, and cardiovascular collapse from insufficient venous return. Tension pneumothorax may be accompanied by tension pneumoperitoneum in neonates with CDH who are receiving mechanical ventilation with high mean airway pressures. Chest radiographs confirms tension pneumothorax, determines its site of origin, and directs immediate treatment. Placement of the properly sized thoracostomy tube (usually 10- or 12-French) is done immediately. If access to a chest tube is not readily available, then placement of an Angiocath in the second intercostal space will act as a temporizing measure.

Timing of repair is controversial. In the stable patient, repair can be done expeditiously in an elective fashion. However, in the patient with severe PPHN, repair should be delayed until the respiratory status is stable or is no longer improving. Following surgical reduction of the thoracic hernia and primary or patch repair of the hemidiaphragm, a chest tube is sometimes placed on the affected side for fluid drainage.

A nasogastric tube should be inserted as soon as possible in all neonates with CDH for decompression of the stomach, which often is distended by positive-pressure ventilation, and for reduction of the air and fluid contents of the viscera in the thoracic hernia. A Foley catheter is required in children with CDH if they are paralyzed or if the hemodynamic status warrants catheterization. Otherwise, routine use of a Foley catheter is not required as long as strict fluid balance is monitored.

Tracheoesophageal Fistula

Tracheoesophageal fistula (TEF) may present as one of four common varieties, all characterized by varying degrees of esophageal atresia and fistulous connections between the trachea and esophagus.[138,139] Neonates with TEF may have minimal symptoms or profound respiratory embarrassment. In the common forms of TEF, respiratory distress begins when orogastric secretions spill into the tracheobronchial tree, causing aspiration pneumonitis.

Once the diagnosis of TEF in a neonate has been entertained, placement of an oral sump tube in the proximal region of the esophagus prevents spillage of saliva from the obstructed esophagus into the trachea. Esophageal obstruction in TEF may be due to a blind esophageal pouch in 87% of cases or to an esophageal atresia. Because the more common varieties of TEF are not characterized by the presence of an esophagus patent to the stomach, gastric decompression usually is impossible. An emergent decompressive gastrostomy is used only in the patient with severe respiratory distress who develops abdominal distention that compromises ventilation. However, one must be ready to perform an emergency thoracotomy to ligate the fistula if, after gastric tube placement, one can no longer ventilate the baby due to preferential ventilation via the fistula. For most newborns with careful anesthesia, low peak inspiratory pressures, and proper placement of the endotracheal tube and sump tube, primary ligation of the fistula and repair of the esophageal atresia can be performed. Once the fistula is divided, further distention of the gastrointestinal tract secondary to positive-pressure ventilation does not occur. A small (6- or 8-French) nasogastric tube can be positioned carefully across the esophageal anastomosis during surgery, with the tip of the tube in the stomach for postoperative enteral feedings once bowel function returns. If, however, the nasogastric tube is accidentally withdrawn postoperatively, great care must be taken in its reinsertion because of the risk of esophageal perforation.

Immediate endotracheal intubation in neonates with TEF often is unnecessary unless the infants are very premature or have severe underlying lung disease or aspiration pneumonitis. Term neonates with excessive salivation and TEF identified shortly after birth can be easily managed preoperatively with esophageal pouch decompression, intravenous hydration, and elevation of the head of the bed. Careful attention to pouch decompression usually prevents aspiration pneumonia and allows adequate time for further diagnostic evaluation before unhurried TEF repair.

Premature neonates and infants with severe underlying lung disease or aspiration pneumonitis often require prolonged endotracheal intubation for mechanical ventilation postoperatively. Patients can be extubated as soon as clinically ready. Term neonates with stable cardiopulmonary status and no preexisting lung disease may undergo extubation at the completion of uncomplicated TEF repair. If tracheal reintubation is indicated in the postoperative period, it must be performed with extreme care with minimal bag-and-mask ventilation to avoid high airway pressures so that tracheal perforation at the suture line and/or esophageal anastomotic breakdown can be prevented.

Central venous, urinary, and intra-arterial catheters are all useful adjuncts to standard hemodynamic monitoring in unstable patients with TEF, but none of these monitors is routinely indicated in uncomplicated TEF repairs. Transcutaneous O_2 saturation monitoring is useful for confirmation of adequate tissue perfusion and oxygenation. Postoperative care and monitoring can be modified as necessary should the neonate develop postsurgical complications, hemodynamic instability, or respiratory compromise from unrecognized lung disease.

Congenital Lobar Emphysema and Cystic Adenomatoid Malformation

CLE (see also Chapter 29, Casebook 4) and congenital CAM are two uncommon neonatal thoracic emergencies characterized by lung hyperinflation that are difficult to differentiate clinically and radiographically.[140–142] In CLE, air trapping occurs within one or more lung lobes at birth, producing obstructive emphysema. Air trapping in CLE is most commonly found in the left upper lobe, followed by the right upper lobe and the right middle lobe. Cardiac anomalies are frequently seen in neonatal CLE.

CAM is also lobar in its distribution but is generally confined to one or more lower lobes. There are three types of CAM. Type I are macrocystic (>2 cm), type II are microcystic (<1 cm), and type III are large noncystic lesions that commonly cause mediastinal shift. Type I lesions may be asymptomatic; types II and III usually present in the newborn period with respiratory distress. In CAM, cystic dilation of the lower lobes with air and fluid produces lobar hyperexpansion. As a result of lobar hyperexpansion in both CLE and CAM, adjacent mediastinal structures, such as the heart and the contralateral lung, are compressed and displaced, including compromise of normal lung segments.

Prenatal ultrasound has allowed detection of these anomalies as early as 12 to 14 weeks of gestation. Some of these may spontaneously regress; however, some may continue to enlarge and lead to hydrops, severe pulmonary hypoplasia, and cardiac and caval compression resulting in fetal death. If these conditions occur, fetal intervention or delivery may be warranted.[189]

Tachypnea, tachycardia, and inadequate cardiac preload are the most common presenting features in both CLE and CAM. Tracheal intubation and mechanical ventilation often are required for immediate pulmonary stabilization in CLE and CAM. Gastric distention from air swallowing requires early nasogastric decompression. The suddenness of symptom onset in CLE or CAM often is variable. Many neonates show respiratory distress at birth; others are asymptomatic for hours, days, or even several weeks after birth. The rapidity and severity of clinical presentation in CLE or CAM determine the timing of surgical intervention.

Overzealous bag-and-mask ventilation or high-pressure mechanical ventilation may aggravate respiratory distress in CLE or CAM by increasing air trapping and mediastinal shifting or by causing tension pneumothorax. If this occurs, immediate thoracotomy with lung resection is needed.

In neonates with CLE or CAM, pulmonary resection usually is necessary. If the child is asymptomatic, the patient can be followed with elective resection at a later date if complete resolution does not occur. Although the pulmonary tissue to be resected contributes little to respiration, intra-arterial monitoring in radial or umbilical arteries is recommended during the perioperative period for frequent blood gas measurements. Because the condition of most neonates with CLE or CAM is improved dramatically by removal of the affected lobe, intra-arterial lines are generally needed for only a short time postoperatively.

Bronchogenic Cyst and Pulmonary Sequestration

Although rare, bronchiogenic cyst (BC) and pulmonary sequestration (PS) are two of the more common intrathoracic mass lesions that should be resected in neonates.[142,144,145] Although both lesions cause congenital chest masses, neonates with BC or PS are often asymptomatic at birth and are usually diagnosed on routine chest radiography during evaluation for upper respiratory infections. If the mass effect of BC or PS produces respiratory distress during the neonatal period, the mass must be of sufficient size to cause normal lung displacement and compression. A paratracheal BC may compromise tracheal air flow and cause expiratory stridor. More peripherally located pulmonary sequestrations compress branch bronchi and cause bronchomalacia, atelectasis, obstructive emphysema, and expiratory wheezing.

PS is a cystic mass of nonfunctioning lung tissue that can be intralobar or extralobar. It also has an abnormal blood supply, with all or most of its blood supply from the systemic circulation. They usually are asymptomatic and present as recurring pneumonias.

If BC and PS are symptomatic in the neonatal period, perioperative management follows that recommended for CLE and CAM. Immediate tracheal intubation is indicated for severe respiratory compromise at birth. This is seldom the case, however, and tracheal intubation is normally performed during anesthesia for thoracotomy. Normal pulmonary tissue is not usually damaged during the removal of a BC or PS; this allows tracheal extubation at the conclusion of uncomplicated surgery. Intra-arterial monitoring is useful for intraoperative blood gas monitoring but can be discontinued postoperatively and replaced with transcutaneous O_2 saturation monitoring. Thoracostomy tubes are regularly placed during chest closure for drainage of trapped intrathoracic fluids and air. Nasogastric decompression, if indicated preoperatively for gastric distention or during mechanical ventilation, can be discontinued in the postoperative period after tracheal extubation.

Patent Ductus Arteriosus

PDA is a common congenital defect in neonates, especially premature neonates. Rarely, its presence requires emergency left thoracotomy for repair unless excessive left-to-right shunting causes medically unmanageable cardiorespiratory failure. The size of the PDA and the direction and rate of its shunt flow can be determined precisely on echocardiographic examination (see also Chapter 23). When medical management of PDA with fluid restriction and intravenous indomethacin fails to close the ductus arteriosus, elective surgical closure is indicated for the management of chronic congestive heart failure. Perioperative management in PDA ligation requires insertion of an endotracheal tube if a tube is not already in place for preoperative mechanical ventilation. A dependable intravenous line is indicated for fluid therapy and transfusion, if necessary. Occasionally, the thin posterior wall of the PDA leaks or ruptures during closure. Blood loss associated with such a catastrophe is sudden and heavy, making the availability of blood products necessary prerequisites for PDA ligation. Intra-arterial pressure monitoring and a Foley catheter are indicated for monitoring of end-organ perfusion during PDA ligation.

Controversy continues about whether a thoracostomy tube is needed on the side of operation after PDA ligation. Neonates who are receiving only minimal ventilatory support preoperatively, have no evidence of pulmonary interstitial emphysema, and show no signs of thoracic bleeding or pleural air leak at the conclusion of surgery may have the hemithorax closed without tube drainage. Conversely, if chances of a pneumothorax or bleeding are reasonably high, a chest tube should be inserted during closure so that the sudden onset of hemothorax or tension pneumothorax can be prevented.

Abdominal Surgical Emergencies in Neonates

Omphalocele and Gastroschisis

Omphalocele and gastroschisis, the most common congenital defects of the anterior abdominal wall, share clinical presentations at birth. Surgical repair is more urgent in gastroschisis owing to the greater risks of sepsis and hypovolemic shock.[146] Both defects require similar medical care at birth (see Table 26-6). Early nasogastric decompression of the stomach and intestines reduces emesis and the risk of aspiration and decompresses the bowel. Immediate nasogastric decompression is especially critical in neonates with gastroschisis because this defect may cause bowel obstruction and/or vascular compromise. Neither condition is likely to cause respiratory problems immediately at birth, so many of these neonates do not require tracheal intubation and mechanical ventilation until they are anesthetized for surgery. Fluid resuscitation is begun immediately, along with broad spectrum antibiotics for the prevention of bacterial contamination of the exposed (gastroschisis) or membrane-draped (omphalocele) bowel loops. Both conditions can have profound fluid losses (more so in gastroschisis patients) and temperature instability due to exposed bowel. Maintenance of temperature by placing the bowel in a sterile plastic bag and the baby under a radiant warmer aid in the resuscitation. Surgical closure of the abdominal wall defect should follow preoperative stabilization. It may be complete primary closure, as in most patients with gastroschises and small omphaloceles, or staged reduction and secondary closure with silo placement, as in those with large omphaloceles.[147] Because neonates with omphaloceles have complete bowel coverage by chorioamnionic membranes, they may undergo unhurried elective reduction and closure of their defects unless the omphalocele ruptures. In some cases of large omphaloceles, the sac itself can be used to sequentially reduce the defect prior to closure.

Postoperatively most patients will have a Foley catheter, an endotracheal tube, and a nasogastric tube. The fluid requirements may be significant, and it is not unusual for these patients to require in excess of 250 mL/kg/day for the first few days postoperatively. Depending on whether the child was closed primarily (and the difficulty of the closure will define the postoperative course), one needs to watch for signs of abdominal compartment syndrome with careful and accurate monitoring of urine output, mean arterial pressure, and peak inspiratory pressure. Nasogastric decompression should be continued postoperatively until the bowel is functioning properly. Care should be taken to investigate fully for associated congenital anomalies, especially in a child with a large omphalocele, which frequently is accompanied by congenital cardiac defects.[148] Children with gastroschisis will tend to have greater problems with bowel function than patients with omphaloceles.

Obstructive Lesions of the Small Bowel

Obstructive lesions of the small intestines may all have a similar clinical presentation, with abdominal distention and vomiting of bile. The more common congenital causes of small bowel obstruction include duodenal obstruction (by atresia, stenosis, web, or annular pancreas),[149] midgut malrotation,[150] jejunoileal atresia,[198] and meconium ileus.[151] Lower sites of obstruction (jejunoileal atresia and meconium ileus)

are characterized by the greatest amounts of associated abdominal distention and a delayed onset of vomiting of bile. In contrast, obstruction of the upper part of the small bowel, as occurs in duodenal atresia, usually results in vomiting with the first feeding or even sooner. In addition, the abdominal contour in duodenal obstructions may appear flat because abdominal distention is limited to the stomach, which, as it distends, elevates the hemidiaphragms and not the anterior abdominal wall.

Patients with jejunoileal obstructions may feed for 1 to 3 days before emesis occurs, despite marked abdominal distention. Palpable and even visible loops of dilated bowel may be present from birth in neonates with jejunoileal small bowel obstructions.

Presurgical management of neonates with obstructions of the upper part of the small bowel includes dependable intravenous line insertion for fluid resuscitation and early gastric decompression. Nasogastric decompression prevents further emesis with hypovolemia and electrolyte imbalance, removes swallowed air from the distended stomach, and relieves the respiratory restrictions imposed by the elevation of hemidiaphragms. Further monitoring is not routinely necessary in these neonates unless sepsis or massive fluid losses have compromised hemodynamic stability.

Accurate radiographic diagnosis of the level of obstruction may follow stabilization with infusion of intravenous fluids and nasogastric decompression. Air shadows and air–fluid levels within the small bowel often are sufficient for confirmation of the radiographic diagnosis of small bowel obstructions. The double-bubble pattern of duodenal obstructions on plain abdominal radiography is quite characteristic and often eliminates the need for additional contrast (barium) studies. The multiple air–fluid levels characteristic of obstructions of the lower regions of the small bowel are not diagnostic radiographically but may be sufficient for justifying laparotomy without additional contrast studies.

Malrotation of the midgut is always a neonatal surgical emergency. Blood supply to most of the small bowel is compromised by midgut malrotation. If the bowel is not untwisted quickly, total gut infarction may occur. Marked distention is apparent on physical examination, although abdominal radiographs often show little air. Any newborn with bilious emesis has a malrotation until proven otherwise. Thus, these children all require emergent radiologic studies to confirm or rule out this diagnosis. A barium enema to document the position of the cecum is given, and a limited upper gastrointestinal series to evaluate the position of the ligament of Treitz is performed. Final confirmation of the type of midgut malrotation occurs at early laparotomy for surgical correction.

Meconium ileus, often secondary to the pancreatic insufficiency of cystic fibrosis, resembles jejunoileal atresia or malrotation in its clinical presentation. Abdominal distention is prominent, and onset of bilious emesis is often delayed beyond the first few feedings.[152] A family history of cystic fibrosis suggests the diagnosis, which requires confirmation by abdominal radiography showing a flocculent intraluminal appearance to the bowel in the right lower quadrant. An enema with diatrizoate meglumine (Gastrografin) can be both diagnostic and therapeutic in meconium ileus by demonstrating the ileal plug, softening it, and promoting its expulsion during bowel movement after the enema.[153]

Endotracheal intubation in neonates with obstructions of the upper part of the small bowel usually is indicated only during anesthesia for surgical correction by bowel resection and anastomosis. Postoperative invasive monitoring or prolonged mechanical ventilation is indicated by the neonate's clinical condition or coexisting diseases, especially RDS.

Colonic Obstruction

Clinical presentation of colonic obstruction in neonates may mimic symptoms of distal small bowel obstruction, with marked abdominal distention and copious vomiting of bile. Plain abdominal radiographs may suggest the distal location of the intestinal obstruction but cannot differentiate obstructions of the distal small bowel from those of the colon. Colonic obstruction may be confirmed by barium enema, which differentiates common colonic obstructions (Hirschsprung disease, meconium plug syndrome) from the common obstructions of the distal small bowel (meconium ileus, ileal atresia, ileocecal intussusception).

Presurgical management of neonates with congenital colonic obstructions includes insertion of dependable intravenous lines for volume and electrolyte therapy and placement of nasogastric tubes for gastric decompression and aspiration prophylaxis. Further invasive monitoring is dictated by the severity of illness (hypovolemic shock, acidosis) or by the presence of coexisting illnesses (PDA, RDS). Depending on the diagnosis and clinical condition, surgery can be done electively if decompression can be performed.

PREOPERATIVE EVALUATION

Physical Examination

As discussed previously, the preoperative examination should begin with a thorough prenatal and natal history. The anesthesiologist should also obtain a family history of myopathies and metabolic abnormalities. A family history of adverse events, such as pseudocholinesterase deficiency and malignant hyperthermia, must be determined and may warrant further testing.

The physical examination of the neonate is an "exam of opportunity"[154] that should begin with general observations of the infant's appearance. The infant should be kept in a warm environment with appropriate radiant warmers to avoid causing potentially dangerous hypothermia during the examination. The hands and stethoscope should be warmed to avoid disturbing the infant. Cyanosis, mottling, pallor, and jaundice can be readily apparent. Respiratory distress is generally one of the first signs of a sick newborn and careful attention should be paid to the infant's ventilation. Is the infant demonstrating nasal flaring, grunting, chest retractions, stridor, or wheezing? Is the abdomen scaphoid or distended? It is important to be alert to unusual features because they may indicate a specific syndrome that warrants further diagnostic procedures and interventions.

Following the general observations, one should begin with the cardiac examination, arguably the most challenging part of the physical examination. Neonatal cardiac examinations are dynamic. Closure of the ductus arteriosus and foramen ovale occurs during the first 8 hours after birth[155]; therefore, an "innocent murmur" cannot be distinguished from a pathologic murmur at birth.[156] Clues to the presence of persistent shunting may come from the presence of bounding femoral pulses, discrepancy in upper and lower extremity oxygen saturations, and

the presence of a harsh systolic murmur at the left sternal border. With left-to-right shunting the child may show signs of cardiomegaly and pulmonary edema on chest x-ray film. Blood gas measurements and echocardiogram must be performed to determine the degree and pattern of shunting in sick neonates.[157]

Evaluation of the head, neck, and upper airway for nasal patency, craniofacial deformity, and cervical range of motion to predict the quality of mask fit and the ease of tracheal intubation is essential. Existing uncuffed endotracheal tubes should be checked for appropriate size,[158] proper positioning (with auscultation and chest radiography), and, most importantly, tracheal air leak at 20 to 25 cm H_2O positive peak airway pressure.[159,160] For the neonate who has already been intubated, the size and position of the endotracheal tube should be noted and confirmed by chest x-ray film. The ventilator settings must be addressed and the ability of the ventilator located in the OR matched with the needs of the neonate. Small infants with RDS may need the ventilator from the neonatal intensive care unit to be placed in the OR to provide adequate ventilation. Moreover, the children on high frequency ventilation present a special challenge that can only be managed with a high-frequency ventilator brought into the OR.[161]

Peripheral and central lines need to be checked for patency and position, particularly umbilical lines. Fluids and hyperalimentation need to be continued without interruption to avoid overhydration or underhydration or dangerous swings in serum glucose concentrations.

Radiographic Evaluation

Preoperative chest radiography in infants requiring assisted ventilation allows the physician to confirm endotracheal tube position, evaluate heart size, and rule out pneumothorax, lobar emphysema, pulmonary interstitial disease, BC, adenomatous malformations, and pulmonary sequestration, all of which can be worsened by intraoperative administration of nitrous oxide (N_2O). Congestive heart failure, usually secondary to a PDA, necessitates preoperative evaluation (often with echocardiography) and appropriate management before elective surgery.

Ophthalmologic Evaluation

Preoperative indirect ophthalmoscopy by an experienced ophthalmologist confirms the degree of retinal maturity or severity of ROP in infants requiring long-term O_2 and ventilatory therapy for RDS.[107] As noted earlier, the clinician must take an aggressive approach to ascertain the degree of retinal maturity or the extent of existing damage before anesthetics are administered.[162]

Laboratory Evaluation

Preoperative laboratory studies in neonates should include determination of hemoglobin, hematocrit, serum glucose, and electrolytes, as well as urinalysis. Normal laboratory values are summarized in Appendices 17 to 22. Hemoglobin level should be restored to 10 to 12 g/dL with packed red blood cells if indicated (Appendix 18). Hypoglycemia should be corrected. Parenteral hyperalimentation should be continued intraoperatively so that rebound hypoglycemia is prevented.

The physical findings of dehydration (e.g., weight loss, dry mucous membranes, poor skin turgor, sunken fontanelles, sunken eyes, hypotension) should be sought, confirmed by laboratory studies, and corrected preoperatively. Urine output of 1.0 mL/kg/hour, urine specific gravity of 1.010 to 1.015, serum sodium level of 140 to 145 mEq/L, and serum potassium concentration of 4.0 to 5.5 mEq/L indicate normovolemia. All anesthetics rapidly unmask preoperative hypovolemia and, with vagal effects on heart rate, can significantly reduce cardiac output and cause electromechanical dissociation or cardiac arrest.

Fasting Status

Fasting status in newborns fed orally or by gavage should be limited to 2 hours for clear liquids and breast milk and 4 hours for formula.[163,164] All infants and, particularly, neonates with neurologic disorders such as hydrocephalus, hypoxic encephalopathy, or ICH have poor airway protective reflexes and reduced gastroesophageal sphincter tone. Regurgitation and aspiration of gastric contents are common in these infants, regardless of fasting status, and underscore the need for gastric decompression when indicated and early establishment of a tracheal airway for protection of the lungs and maintenance of ventilation. When fasting begins in premature infants or any compromised neonate, an intravenous infusion of glucose should be started so that hypoglycemia and dehydration can be prevented.

Premedication

Oral premedication in neonates is contraindicated because of the poor airway protective reflexes, reduced gastroesophageal sphincter tone, and undetermined gastric absorption. Cardiorespiratory depressants such as barbiturates, opioids, and tranquilizers can worsen common pre-existing conditions such as apnea, hypoventilation, hypoxemia, and hypotension and thus are contraindicated as premedications. Preoperative anticholinergics, such as atropine or glycopyrrolate, reduce high vagal tone, dry oral secretions, and decrease the incidence and severity of intraoperative bradycardia and hypotension from both vagal stimulation (nasogastric suctioning, endotracheal intubation) and anesthetic agents, especially halothane.[5]

The sparing of myocardial contractility by sevoflurane has made premedication with anticholinergics unnecessary in healthy infants. If needed, anticholinergics can be administered immediately before or during induction and before endotracheal intubation so that heart rate and cardiac output can be maintained. Atropine is more vagolytic and faster in onset than glycopyrrolate.[165]

Neonatal Transport

Safe transportation of the sick neonate requires that the transporting team members be knowledgeable and skilled in the needs of the critically ill neonate. The securing or maintenance of an adequate airway, preservation of temperature, and appropriate monitoring are critical. Taking the extra time to send a dedicated expert neonatal transport team to retrieve patients has been shown to result in better condition of patients upon return to the tertiary center than waiting for the arrival of patients from the referring hospital.[166] One explanation for this result may be the increased numbers of procedures, such as tracheal intubation and placement of lines,[167,168] performed by the dedicated neonatal transport team prior to transport (Fig. 26-1).

Once a neonate has arrived at a facility, transport to and from the OR should be done under the direct supervision of an anesthesiologist, certified nurse anesthetist, or both. Prior to transport, the anesthesia team should assess the patency and security of the airway. If the neonate is not intubated but is in distress, the airway should be secured prior to transportation, even for "short trips." Once the airway is satisfactory, all lines, monitoring cables, chest tubes, and urinary catheter should be sorted out and secured prior to moving the patient. Patients in a potentially unstable condition preoperatively and all postoperative patients should have a portable monitor displaying continuous electrocardiogram, pulse oximetry, automated noninvasive blood pressure, or arterial line transduction.

Transport of postoperative neonates requires that the team maintain a high level of vigilance for apnea and the need to assist ventilation. Patients may need to be intubated or

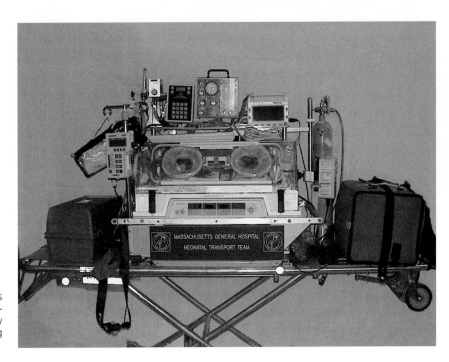

Figure 26-1. A neonatal transport isolette provides a warm stable environment with continuous monitoring. Additional equipment is available for airway management, ventilation, and fluid and drug administration.

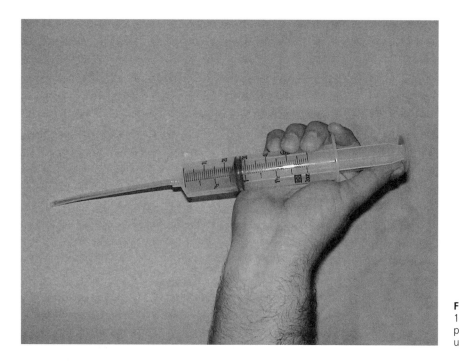

Figure 26-2. A 30-cc syringe connected to a 14-French suction catheter provides useful oropharyngeal suction when line or portable suction is unavailable.

reintubated if the airway becomes obstructed or inadequate. A tackle box with appropriately sized endotracheal tubes, laryngoscopes, masks, and drugs for resuscitation should accompany these infants. Oxygen cylinders and ventilation bags should be checked to be sure that they are full and functional. An emergency suction device can be made using a 30-cc syringe and 14-French catheter (Fig. 26-2). Some neonatal intensive care units have the capabilities, extra space, and personnel to permit certain surgical procedures (e.g., PDA ligation, gastrostomy) on site and thus avoid the potential dangers of transport.

ANESTHETIC PHARMACOLOGY

Increased infant anesthetic requirements and greater sensitivity to the cardiodepressant properties of both inhaled and intravenous anesthetics have been discussed. In addition, the limited reserves in all systems, particularly respiration, circulation, thermoregulation, and metabolism, account for the marked differences in anesthetic pharmacokinetics in neonates and adults.

Inhalation Anesthetics

Inhalational anesthetic pharmacology is unique in that uptake and clearance are primarily via the lungs. The potency of a volatile anesthetic is described by the minimum alveolar concentration (MAC) that is required to prevent nocifensive movement in response to noxious stimuli.[169] Each volatile anesthetic has a unique MAC that varies according to the age and physiologic state of the patient. The rate of uptake and distribution will correlate inversely with the solubility of the anesthetic. The blood/gas partition coefficient defines the solubility of an agent and describes how much anesthetic must be absorbed to reach anesthetic levels in the CNS where anesthetic action is thought to occur.[170,171] The differences in neonatal

TABLE 26-7. Increased Inhaled Anesthetic Requirements in Neonates Compared with Adults

Inhaled Anesthetic	Anesthetic Requirement (MAC)	
	Neonate (% Volume)	Adult (% Volume)
Halothane	1.1	0.76
Enflurane	2.0	1.70
Isoflurane	1.6	1.15
Desflurane	9.16	7.25 (18–30 years old)
		6.0 (31–65 years old)
Sevoflurane	3.3	2.69 (18–35 years old)
		1.45 (>70 years old)

MAC, minimum anesthetic concentration, which is that inspired fraction of anesthetic vapor that provides anesthesia and relaxation to 50% of a population on surgical stimulation

uptake and excretion of inhaled anesthetics are related to several factors, especially higher cardiac output, greater alveolar ventilation, and smaller FRC.[172,173]

Smoothness and rapidity of induction are essential in neonates. The neonate is more prone to laryngospasm, coughing, and rapid arterial oxygen desaturation than is the older patient.[174] An inhalational anesthetic must be nonirritating, rapid in uptake and effect, and minimal in physiologic impact.[175] For decades halothane and N_2O most closely accomplished these goals. When sevoflurane was introduced to pediatric anesthesia in the late 1980s, it rapidly became the anesthetic of choice for induction in pediatric anesthesia.[176] Most pediatric anesthesiologists now use a combination of sevoflurane and N_2O, muscle relaxants, barbiturates, and opioids for an anesthetic (Table 26-7).[177,178]

Studies have shown that full-term neonates have a lower MAC from birth to 30 days of age than older infants.[179] Infants from 30 to 180 days have a nearly 30% greater MAC than newborns or adults.[179] Preterm neonates have a lower MAC than term neonates (see Table 26-4).[180–182] The theoretical reasons for the differences in anesthetic requirements remain unclear.

Due to the higher MAC, there is a smaller margin of safety between adequate anesthesia and severe cardiorespiratory depression in infants compared to adults.[183]

The newer volatile agent sevoflurane has dramatically reduced the incidence of cardiovascular depression during general anesthesia. Prior to the introduction of sevoflurane in the 1990s, significant bradycardia may have been as high as 11% with halothane inductions. The use of sevoflurane has reduced this incidence to approximately 2%.[184]

Holzman et al.[185] compared sevoflurane and halothane using echocardiography to assess myocardial depression during anesthesia. They demonstrated that sevoflurane preserved myocardial function as measured by stress velocity index and stress-shortening index. Halothane demonstrated a reduction in contractility in this study. The application of sevoflurane in infants with cardiac disease has also demonstrated a reduction in incidence of bradycardia, desaturation, and hypotension compared to halothane.[186] The relative preservation of myocardial contractility and lack of ectopy[187] compared to halothane has further increased the attractiveness of sevoflurane over halothane.

The increased safety of sevoflurane has led to its essentially replacing halothane as the induction agent of choice for inhalational anesthesia. Following induction with sevoflurane, it is common to switch agents, discontinuing the sevoflurane and using isoflurane, enflurane, or desflurane for maintenance. The older agents have the desirable properties that they are minimally metabolized, lack the postoperative agitation associated with sevoflurane, and are less expensive.

Desflurane has several characteristics that make it desirable as a maintenance anesthetic agent. These characteristics include rapid elimination,[177] preservation of respiratory drive, reduced recovery time, and reduced incidence of postoperative apnea.[188] Desflurane is not recommended as an induction agent because of its irritating odor, and studies have demonstrated an unacceptably high level (48%) of breath holding and laryngospasm during inhalational induction.[189,190]

N_2O is no longer considered an innocuous inhaled anesthetic. N_2O dilutes the FIO_2, becomes a potent cardiovascular depressant when it is combined with narcotics, and rapidly expands air-containing cavities that are not being adequately decompressed, such as pneumothoraces, congenital lung cysts, lobar and interstitial emphysema, and obstructed stomach or bowel (see Table 26-6).[191] Compressed nitrogen or helium may serve as an O_2-diluting carrier gas in neonates for whom N_2O is contraindicated.

Intravenous Agents

Intravenous anesthetic agents can be broadly classified into three classes: the sedative-hypnotics, muscle relaxants, and opioids. Other agents include anticholinesterases, anticholinergics, and opioid antagonists (see Table 26-5). Intravenous anesthetics, such as inhalational anesthetics, have a sedative-hypnotic effect that reflects CNS concentrations of the agent. Intravenously administered agents rapidly distribute to the vessel-rich areas, such as the CNS, heart, and kidneys. Termination of effect is determined primarily by a second redistribution of the drugs to the muscle groups and less well-perfused areas of the body such as fat and bone. The pharmacokinetics for each patient vary depending on body composition, distribution of cardiac output, plasma protein level, metabolism, and excretion. The variability between patients makes it impossible to precisely anticipate the

effect of intravenous anesthetics and requires the anesthesiologist to carefully titrate the anesthetics according to each patients' response. It is well documented that the neonate is much more prone to the cardiorespiratory effects of intravenous anesthetics than the adult[192]; therefore, unit dosing of anesthetics is not only ineffective but is also unsafe.

Despite their increasing popularity and use in anesthesia for adults, most intravenous agents have not been well studied in infants. Most available pharmacokinetic information on analgesics and sedatives in immature subjects is derived from animal models.[193–195] The United States Food and Drug Administration has addressed this problem, and incentives for pharmaceutical companies to study new drugs in children are being developed.[196,197] The most frequently used intravenous sedative hypnotic agents are propofol, thiopental, and ketamine. Propofol in particular has gained favor because it has a more rapid onset and termination than thiopental or ketamine.[198–200] Propofol demonstrates less airway irritability, postoperative sedation, and nausea or vomiting.[201,202] One drawback to propofol is the pain with intravenous injection.[203] Fortunately children requiring frequent anesthetics have central venous access that circumvents the difficulties with peripheral administration. Inhalation of 50% N_2O greatly mitigates the pain due to administration of propofol.[204] An additional problem with propofol is an association with fulminant metabolic acidosis associated with long-term infusions in intensive care unit settings. This may be due to a defect in fatty acid oxidation.[205] Long-term propofol infusions once used in the intensive care setting are no longer recommended for children.[206,207]

The barbiturates thiopental and methohexital are still used frequently although they have largely been replaced by propofol. Induction with thiopental is painless and is a reasonable substitute for propofol when rapid emergence is not a consideration. The termination of effect is due to redistribution, but longer half-life in neonates may be due to a reduced clearance.[208,209] Thiopental is a myocardial depressant and vasodilator, and extreme caution is required during administration to the hypovolemic infant.[210] Methohexital administered 25 to 30 mg/kg rectally provides sedation for 60 to 80 minutes to allow brief diagnostic procedures or acts as preoperative sedation in older children.[211–214]

Ketamine, a phencyclidine derivative initially developed for veterinary use, is an intravenous anesthetic adjuvant that produces potent analgesia and sedation. Shortly after its introduction, ketamine was recommended for pediatric anesthesia because it provided greater cardiovascular stability, less respiratory depression, and better maintenance of airway protective reflexes.[215] Ketamine does provide greater cardiovascular stability in infants compromised by shock and heart failure, but it also causes prolonged sedation, an increase in oropharyngeal secretions, and more respiratory depression and airway compromise than initially considered.[215] Ketamine has proved most useful as an anesthetic in the sickest infants with cyanotic congenital heart disease who require prolonged postoperative ventilation.[215] Ketamine is not a good anesthetic choice for neonates who will be weaned from mechanical ventilation in the immediate postoperative period. When indicated, intravenous ketamine titrated to effect produces significantly shorter recovery times than large intramuscular boluses of the drug.[215]

Morphine is the most commonly used opioid in pediatric anesthesia. For infants undergoing major surgery, morphine provides long-acting reliable analgesia. It can be administered orally, intramuscularly, or intravenously. The clearance of morphine in neonates is only 9.2 mL/kg/min compared to adult clearance of 49 mL/kg/min.[216] The reduced clearance places neonates at risk for rapid accumulation and respiratory depression. In addition, the immature blood–brain barrier of a neonate in animal studies results in two to three times higher CNS concentrations of morphine in neonates than in adults.[195]

Fentanyl is a more potent, shorter-acting opioid than morphine. It is frequently used as an anesthetic adjunct to general anesthesia. It is particularly useful in cardiac anesthesia where high doses of 50 to 100 µg/kg are very effective in blocking the stress response to surgery with minimal hemodynamic consequences.[217,218] Like morphine, fentanyl has a longer half-life and diminished clearance in infants compared with older children.[219]

Remifentanil is the newest synthetic opioid. It has an extremely short half-life, does not accumulate during infusions, and is metabolized by nonspecific esterases.[220] The half-life of 3 to 5 minutes and rapid elimination may avoid the postoperative respiratory effects of other narcotics. Two main drawbacks to remifentanil are that it must be continuously administered via an intravenous line and that additional analgesics must be administered for postoperative pain control. As with other synthetic opioids, bradycardia[221] and chest wall rigidity[222] can be profound, and treatment with vagolytics and muscle relaxants should be anticipated.

In summary, all intravenous anesthetics can produce unpredictable effects in newborns and should be carefully titrated in reduced dosages at induction of anesthesia so that postoperative apnea and sedation can be avoided. The reversible agents, such as narcotics and nondepolarizing muscle relaxants, may offer more versatility and less risk of postoperative apnea than the longer-acting irreversible agents, such as barbiturates, major tranquilizers, and ketamine.

Muscle Relaxants

Neuromuscular blocking drugs (Table 26-8) now occupy a more prominent place in neonatal anesthetic management for two main reasons. First, muscle relaxants can provide optimal operating conditions and permit the reduction of doses of inhaled anesthetics, with less cardiovascular depression.[223] Second, assisted or controlled ventilation of paralyzed anesthetized infants provides improved alveolar ventilation, with less mismatching of ventilation and perfusion, than spontaneous ventilation.[29] It must be emphasized that muscle relaxants provide no analgesia or hypnosis whatsoever. They should be administered only after an adequate state of anesthesia has been obtained.

There are two types of muscle relaxants: depolarizing and nondepolarizing. The nondepolarizing muscle relaxants are further categorized into short, intermediate, and long acting. Each muscle relaxant has distinct dosage requirements, cardiovascular effects, and elimination half-lives in infants.

Succinylcholine is the only depolarizing muscle relaxants used in humans. Stead[223] suggested a reduced response to succinylcholine shortly after its introduction in the 1950s. In 1966, Nightingale et al.[224] reported that infants were more resistant to the muscle relaxant properties of succinylcholine than were adults and recommended the use of a greater dose per unit of weight. Cook et al.[225] confirmed greater infant requirements for succinylcholine on a weight-dependent basis because of the greater distribution of the drug in a larger volume of extracellular fluid in the infant compared with that in the older child and adult. Of all the muscle relaxants, succinylcholine has the most rapid onset and shortest duration. Succinylcholine, however, is plagued by several significant side effects, which include masseter spasm, arrhythmias, myoglobinemia, hyper-

TABLE 26-8.   Intravenous Anesthetic Drugs for the Neonate: Dosages and Indications

Anesthetic Agents	Premedication (mg/kg)	Induction (mg/kg)	Maintentance (µg/kg)	Intubation (mg/kg)	Reversal (mg/kg)
Anticholinergics					
Atropine	0.01–0.02				
Glycopyrrolate	0.005–0.01				
Hypnotics					
Propofol		2.5–3.0	100–150 µg/kg/min		
Thiopental		4–6			
Ketamine		0.5–2.0			
Midazolam		0.02–0.05			
Opioids					
Fentanyl		0.005–0.010	1–2 µg/kg/hr		
Morphine		0.05–0.1	10–50 µg/kg/hr		
Sufentanil		0.0001–0.0002	0.05–0.1 µg/kg/hr		
Remifentanil		0.0001	1.5–3 µg/kg/min		
Muscle Relaxants					
Succinylcholine				1–2	
Pancuronium				0.05–0.1	
Cisatracurium				0.1–0.2	
Vecuronium				0.1–0.15	
Mivacurium				0.15–0.20	
Rocuronium				0.8–1.2	
Anticholinesterases					
Neostigmine					0.05–0.08
Pyridostigmine					0.2–0.3
Narcotic Antagonists					
Naloxone					0.005–0.01

kalemia, bronchospasm, malignant hyperthermia, and cardiac arrest.[226] Because succinylcholine is the fastest acting and has the shortest duration, it is still the muscle relaxant of choice for many anesthetists in emergent situations.[227]

In contrast to succinylcholine, studies have suggested greater newborn sensitivity to the nondepolarizing muscle relaxants curare and pancuronium. Goudsouzian[228] and Cook[229] demonstrated no increased sensitivity to these agents in infants but a wide variability in response, such that some newborns are quite sensitive and others relatively resistant to muscular relaxation. The nondepolarizers should be titrated to effect (with small initial doses and reduced maintenance doses), monitored on the basis of the twitch response, and adequately antagonized at the conclusion of surgery with combinations of anticholinesterases (neostigmine, pyridostigmine) and anticholinergics (atropine, glycopyrrolate) (see Table 26-8).

The shortest-acting nondepolarizer, mivacurium, is rapidly biotransformed by plasma cholinesterases and need not be antagonized at the conclusion of surgery if normal twitch response, motor tone, and muscle movement have returned. Recovery times range from 15 to 20 minutes with mivacurium; from 40 to 60 minutes for *cis*-atracurium, vecuronium, and rocuronium; and to more than 60 minutes for pancuronium.[230] The short- and intermediate-acting nondepolarizers mivacurium, *cis*-atracurium, and vecuronium can be administered by continuous infusion during neuromuscular blockade monitoring, especially if prolonged postoperative relaxation is indicated and pancuronium and doxacurium are contraindicated by hemodynamic or renal status. Nonneuromuscular effects of muscle relaxants in infants range from histamine-mediated hypotension with succinylcholine, curare, atracurium, and mivacurium to vagolytic tachycardia with pancuronium. Variable response and resistance to antagonism are common in neonates and could indicate the need for postoperative mechanical ventilation. Hypothermia, hypocalcemia, and concomitant aminoglycoside antibiotic therapy and volatile anesthetics potentiate all nondepolarizing neuromuscular relaxants and interfere with adequate reversal.

INTRAOPERATIVE ANESTHETIC MANAGEMENT

The intraoperative anesthetic management of the neonate should provide a closely monitored continuum of analgesia, amnesia, and surgical relaxation with complete airway control, ventilatory support, and maintenance of circulation and homeostatic stability. Such a perfect anesthetic state cannot always be achieved in the high-risk infant. Frequent adjustments in levels of anesthesia and surgical muscle relaxation may be necessary.

Analgesia and amnesia can be provided with inhalation anesthetics delivered with altitude-adjusted, temperature-compensated, precision vaporizers capable of making 0.25% adjustments in inspired fractions (Fig. 26-3). Surgical relaxation can often be achieved with the use of inhaled agents alone or in combination with muscle relaxants. The exclusive use of high inspired doses of volatile anesthetics without muscle relaxants for surgical anesthesia may result in unacceptable cardiovascular depression in neonates and is not recommended. All intravenous anesthetic agents and adjuvants should be administered as accurate, incrementally titrated

dosages drawn up into clearly labeled 1-mL syringes. Drugs may be diluted with sterile saline but not mixed. A 22- to 24-gauge, nontapered Teflon intravenous catheter (not a butterfly needle) can be inserted percutaneously in most neonates, providing secure intravenous access with a reduced risk of infiltration or skin slough from subcutaneous administration of caustic anesthetic agents such as thiopental and benzodiazepines. Compared with the nursery course, the intraoperative course of newborns is one of fluctuating cardiopulmonary and volume status, temperature instability, and loss of neuromuscular irritability and tone.

Monitoring

The intra-anesthetic monitoring of the newborn must be at least as extensive as preoperative monitoring and may be more so, depending on the experience of the anesthesiologist. Minimum intra-anesthetic monitoring of neonates should include the use of a precordial or esophageal stethoscope, a temperature probe, a blood pressure cuff of appropriate size, as well as the application of an accurate, noninvasive method for determining blood pressure, continuous pulse oximetry, electrocardiography, and infrared capnometry or mass spectrometry for end-tidal CO_2 analysis (Fig. 26-4). Critically ill neonates may require additional, more invasive monitoring, such as a direct blood pressure monitoring via radial artery cannula or umbilical artery catheter. Right atrial or pulmonary artery catheters are rarely indicated in neonates (except in cardiac surgery), seldom provide reliable pressures, and often afford greater risk than benefit, even in the sickest infants.[231]

Accurate noninvasive determinations of blood pressure can be made with the use of an automated noninvasive oscillometric monitor[232,233] (Dinamap, model 847, Critikon, Inc., Tampa, FL, USA). These methods are more reliable than conventional stethoscope or oscillometric methods of blood pressure determination, but they are less accurate than intra-arterial monitoring during severe hypotension.[232,234]

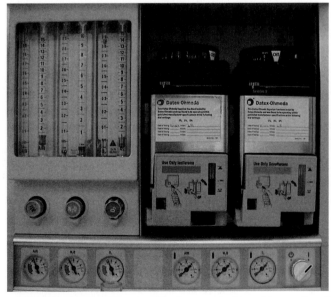

Figure 26-3. The gas delivery system of an anesthesia machine consists of the adjustable flow meters for air, nitrous oxide, and oxygen *(left)* and agent-specific vaporizers *(right)*. The pressure gauges indicate wall supply pressure and auxiliary tank pressure.

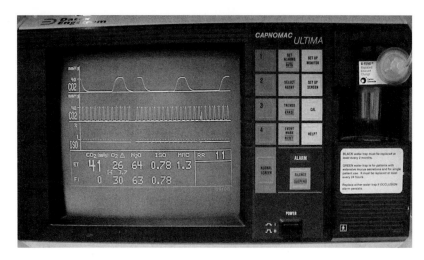

Figure 26-4. Capnography provides continues monitoring of inspiratory and expiratory concentrations of CO_2, N_2O, and the volatile agents using infrared absorption. In this example, end-tidal isoflurane (ISO) = 0.78 volume%, CO_2 = 41 mm Hg, N_2O = 64 volume%, and respiratory rate (RR) = 11 breaths/min. Oxygen cannot be detected using infrared absorption and is estimated by this particular monitor as the volume of gas not occupied by isoflurane, nitrous oxide, and carbon dioxide. For this reason a separate oxygen monitor is required on anesthesia machines.

Radiant warmers offer temperature homeostasis via servo-controlled probes that can be placed on the skin or carefully inserted into the rectum, esophagus, or nasopharynx. When using servocontrolled skin temperature probes, the clinician must take care not to cover or dislodge the probes. Tympanic membrane temperature probes may give accurate measurements that parallel brain temperature values, but they are easily dislodged and can perforate tympanic membranes.[235] Neonates with necrotizing enterocolitis or anorectal malformation are not suitable candidates for rectal temperature monitoring. With the development of servocontrolled radiant warmers designed for intraoperative use, there is a decreased need for infrared heating lamps, warming mattresses, insulating wraps, and overheated ORs, except when craniofacial surgery, in which access is limited, is performed. Heated humidification of inspired anesthetic gases should be provided during all cases lasting longer than 1 to 2 hours.[236,237]

The degree of neuromuscular block can be monitored with the use of battery-operated nerve stimulators applied to accessible peripheral nerves, such as the facial, ulnar, and posterior tibial nerves. Supplemental doses of muscle relaxants are indicated by an increase in the twitch response to electric nerve stimulation.[300]

Urine volume excretion, if monitored, should be at least 1 mL/kg/hour. Blood loss is noted and measured by calibrated suction traps and weighing of sponges. Serial determinations of arterial blood gases, glucose, electrolytes, ionized calcium, hemoglobin, and hematocrit are indicated during prolonged procedures in critically ill infants.

Intraoperative Airway Management

The technique used to manage the neonate's airway will be determined by the nature of the surgery, the medical condition of the infant, and the personal preferences of the anesthesia team. Mask ventilation is the first technique used to ventilate nearly all infants undergoing anesthesia and is taught as the most fundamental and important skill to master in pediatric anesthesia. A clear plastic mask that allows observation of the airway for secretions, vomitus, and cyanosis is recommended. The mask should fit between the chin and the bridge of the nose. Frequently the tongue will fall back during mask ventilation and obstruct the airway. Gently extending the jaw or placing on oropharyngeal airway will help to open the airway and allow adequate ventilation by mask.

The laryngeal mask airway (LMA) has been developed to allow maintenance of an open airway above the glottis without using a mask. It is relatively easy to place in the oropharynx by inexperienced personnel and has been used successfully as an alternative to mask ventilation in newborn resuscitation. The LMA is designed to be used under general anesthesia with spontaneous ventilation. The LMA works well in adult patients undergoing general anesthesia, but it difficult to use in children. In neonates it is associated with a high percentage of failure during a procedure[239,240] and suffers from malposition in nearly 50% of patients.[241,242] The high percentage of apnea in neonates undergoing general anesthesia requires intermittent ventilatory assistance that is less reliable via an LMA than an endotracheal tube. Furthermore, the LMA is unreliable when emergency medications must be administered via the respiratory mucosa. Use of the LMA has also been shown to cause increased work of breathing during anesthesia.[243] Despite the drawbacks, some clinicians prefer the LMA in healthy neonates because it is not associated with the potential complication of laryngeal edema due to instrumenting the airway.[244] Furthermore, in the child with craniofacial deformities in whom mask ventilation and direct laryngoscopy are impossible, the LMA be a life-saving device (Fig. 26-5).[245]

The neonatal glottis is funnel shaped, with the narrowest part at the level of the cricoid cartilage. Uncuffed endotracheal tubes placed below the cricoid will provide an adequate seal to allow ventilation of most neonates. Recent magnetic resonance imaging studies indicate that the cricoid cartilage is not necessarily the narrowest part of the trachea in neonates.[246] Abnormal tracheal compression or narrowing must be considered in a variety of syndromes, as well as in isolated occurrences.

For the physiologic reasons discussed, endotracheal intubation is recommended for the intraoperative airway management of neonates and for the insufflation of O_2 and anesthetic gases. Upper airway anatomy and techniques of laryngoscopy and endotracheal intubation are discussed elsewhere in this book (see Chapter 4). Some additional practical issues of airway management in neonates include quality of mask fit, selection of laryngoscope blade and endotracheal tube, awake versus anesthetized tracheal intubation, and nasotracheal versus orotracheal intubation.

An excellent mask fit for denitrogenation or bag-and-mask ventilation can often be achieved with a circular silicone Portex (Fig. 26-6).[247] A straight laryngoscope blade (Miller 0-1)

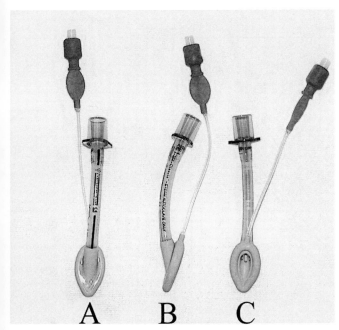

Figure 26-5. Laryngeal mask airway size 1. Dorsal view (A), lateral view (B), and ventral view (C). Once inserted into the oropharynx, the cuff is inflated and the opening seen in view C should be positioned directly over the glottic opening, with the distal tip in the upper esophageal sphincter.

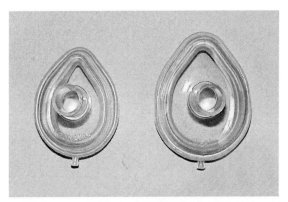

Figure 26-6. Neonatal (left) and infant (right) Portex face masks. The clear flat plastic creates a small dead space and allows observation of the lips and mouth for cyanosis and secretions during mask ventilation. A silicone bladder creates an excellent seal with the faces of most infants.

affords better glottic visibility, occupies less space in a small mouth, and can be modified to provide continuos O_2 or anesthetic insufflation (Fig. 26-7).[248,249] The appropriate sterile endotracheal tube is nontapered, made of implantation tested polyvinyl chloride, easily fits the glottis, and provides an audible tracheal air leak at a peak airway pressure of 25 cm H_2O.[159,250]

Extremely premature newborns and neonates with massive abdominal distention from intestinal obstruction, large anterior abdominal wall defects, or airway anomalies should undergo denitrogenation and awake tracheal intubation to prevent pulmonary aspiration and airway obstruction, which commonly complicate intravenous and mask inductions in such patients. In neonates requiring prolonged postoperative ventilation, a nasotracheal tube may offer greater stability than an orotracheal tube but it is more difficult to place, it often must be inserted with a Magill forceps, and it can cause epistaxis. Insufflation induction of anesthesia and muscle relaxants, if indicated, can follow establishment of a secure upper airway and auscultation of bilaterally equal breath sounds.

Intraoperative Ventilation Management

Intraoperative ventilatory management of neonates should provide insufflation of anesthetic gases, appropriate oxygenation, and adequately assisted or controlled ventilation. Spontaneous ventilation is difficult during anesthesia in neonates because of anesthetic-induced depression of alveolar ventilation and widening of the alveolar–arterial O_2 pressure gradient ($PA_{O_2} - Pa_{O_2}$).[251] Neonates in respiratory failure preoperatively need similar O_2 and ventilatory management intraoperatively, with careful titration of F_{IO_2}, monitoring of peak inspiratory pressures, and positive end-expiratory pressure, when indicated. The adequacy of oxygenation and ventilation should be continuously assessed by evaluation of color, breath sounds, chest excursion, end-tidal CO_2, and pulse oximetry. Transcutaneous oximetry provides more reliable noninvasive monitoring of oxygenation than transcutaneous O_2 tension monitoring because of frequent anesthetic-induced alterations in skin perfusion and fluctuations in skin temperature.[252] Recommended F_{IO_2} values and safe limits for arterial and tissue oxygenation in neonates have already been presented.

Apparatus for administering gas anesthesia and ventilating the neonate during surgery should have minimal dead space, impose little resistance to breathing, eliminate CO_2 adequately, and allow assisted or controlled ventilation. Anesthesia breathing circuits should be compact, lightweight, easy to clean and maintain, and allow for heated humidification of inspired gases. To meet these needs, various nonrebreathing modifications of Ayre's T-piece system[253] have been developed, including the Jackson-Rees[254] modification, the Mapleson D circuit system,[255] and the Bain[256] modification of the Mapleson C circuit (Fig. 26-8). These breathing systems require a fresh gas flow of at least twice minute ventilation to prevent rebreathing and CO_2 retention. The use of non-rebreathing circuits has been advocated in infants because they impose less resistance with no mechanical valves. In 1988 Rasch et al.[257] anesthetized infants with both open and circle systems and found no difference in PET_{CO_2}, Ptc_{CO_2}, respiratory rate, pH, or Pa_{CO_2} between the two groups. Although there was lower resistance to ventilation using the Jackson-Rees system than a circle system, both systems had lower resistances for almost all flows tested than breathing through an endotracheal tube alone. The advantages of the circle system are that it allows for low flows with conservation of anesthetic agents, heating, and humidification without an additional humidifier.

During the course of operations in the chest or upper abdomen, hand ventilation is preferred to mechanical ventilation during delicate surgical dissection intraoperatively because the former affords better appreciation of subtle changes in lung compliance and lower airway resistance and can be timed with surgical movements. The use of mechanical ventilation with a volume-cycled or, preferably, pressure-cycled ventilator and an infant circle system and soda-lime CO_2 absorption is advocated for surgical procedures lasting longer than 1 to 2 hours and for cardiothoracic surgery (Fig. 26-9).

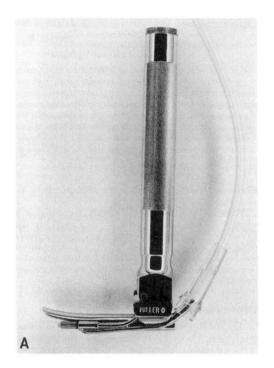

A

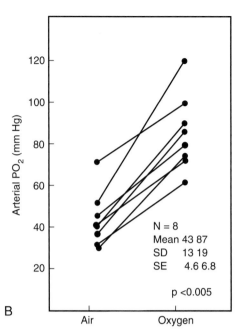

B

Figure 26-7. *A,* The "oxyscope," a modified Miller 0 laryngoscope that delivers oxygen and volatile agents at the tip of the blade during laryngoscopy. *B,* Increased Pao$_2$ levels were achieved during laryngoscopy in spontaneously ventilating infants. (From Todres ID, Crone RK: Experience with a modified laryngoscope in sick infants. Crit Care Med 9:544–545, 1981.)

(graph B labels: Arterial PO$_2$ (mm Hg); Air; Oxygen; N = 8; Mean 43 87; SD 13 19; SE 4.6 6.8; p <0.005)

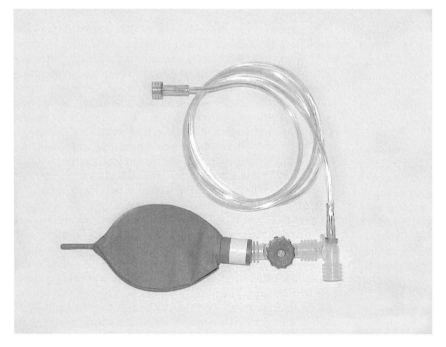

Figure 26-8. Modified Mapleson **C** circuit with a variable pressure-release valve useful for providing continuous positive airway pressure and positive-pressure ventilation during short procedures and transportation.

The Narkomed 6000 (Dragon Medical, Germany) is an anesthesia machine easily adjusted for pediatric use by application of a low-compliance pediatric circuit. The Siemens Servo 900C ventilator (Siemans Medical) has been modified for intra-anesthetic use with a soda-lime CO$_2$ absorber and allows for hand ventilation through a low-resistance infant circle-circuit.[258] Both the Narkomed 6000 and the Siemens 900C ventilators have similar performance profiles. The Narkomed 6000 has the advantage of inline vaporizers for continuous administration and monitoring of volatile anesthetics. The Narkomed 6000 is capable of ventilating patients in both tidal volume and pressure control modes with volume resolution of 1 mL and pressure resolution of 1 cm H$_2$O.[259] The intraoperative use of adult circle systems and adult ventilators for infants can be accomplished with careful attention to airway pressures but is not recommended.[260]

Intraoperative Fluid Management

Fluid management in the neonate begins with securing stable intravenous access (IV). In the healthy full-term neonate, inhalational induction usually is performed first, followed by securing an IV. Contrary to popular myth, pediatric anesthesiologists are not magicians at finding IVs in infants; the volatile anesthetics used render the infants immobile and dilate their veins. A 24-gauge IV is adequate for most minor procedures. For any operation with significant risk of blood loss, two or more IVs of 22 gauge or larger should be placed. In critically ill neonates in whom inhalational induction would not be tolerated, the IV should be established first and appropriate fluid resuscitation begun prior to the anesthetic. Intraosseous (IO) access may serve as a bridge until peripheral or central venous access can be

TABLE 26-9. Fluid Replacement for Intraoperative Third Space Losses*

Nature of Surgery	Third Space Requirements
Minimal tissue trauma	3–4 mL/kg/hr
Large areas of denuded skin	5–7 mL/kg/hr
Large area of exposed bowel	10–15 mL/kg/hr

* Estimates only and do not include replacement for preoperative deficit, blood loss, or maintenance requirements. Adapted from McCallion J, Bacsik J: Children's Hospital Department of Anesthesia Handbook, 7th ed. Boston, 2001, p. 74.

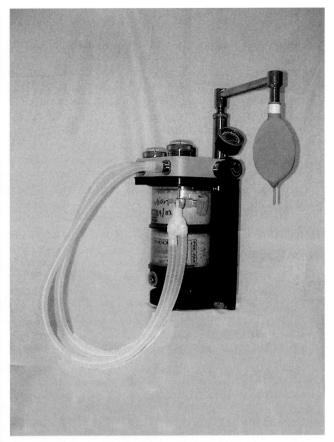

Figure 26-9. Pediatric circle system with CO_2 absorber. Anesthetic gases are adjusted and delivered into the circuit (see Fig. 26-3), and excess gases are removed via a scavenging system.

obtained.[261] Anesthetics, crystalloids, blood products, and pressors can all be administered via IO access, although with less reliability than intravenous routes.[262] IO lines may be associated with significant complications, including dislodgment, compartment syndrome, growth plate damage, and limb loss.[263,264]

Intraoperative fluid requirements can be categorized as maintenance requirement and surgical requirements. Maintenance fluid should provide adequate free water and electrolytes necessary for normal metabolism. The preoperative deficit is calculated by multiplying the hourly fluid requirements by the number of hours the neonate has been NPO (nothing by mouth). Commonly the first half of the deficit is given over the first hour of surgery and the second half is distributed over the next 2 hours, in addition to the normal hourly maintenance. Addition of glucose for short procedures usually is not necessary because the stress response raises plasma glucose levels. Neonates with long periods of fasting should have glucose added at a rate of 3 to 4 mg/kg/min with frequent blood sugar analysis.[32,265] Adequacy of fluid replacement should be continuously assessed by vital signs, peripheral perfusion, urine output, peripheral perfusion, electrolytes, and hematocrits.[266]

Surgical fluid requirements usually exceed maintenance fluid requirements considerably. Surgical trauma causes capillary leak and extravasation of isotonic fluid into the extravascular spaces, the so-called *third space*. Evaporative fluid loss from abdominal contents and respiratory mucosa should be accounted for and replaced. Finally, blood loss must be accounted for and replaced accordingly. Acute blood loss of less than 10% of estimated blood volume can be replaced with crystalloid solutions, provided the preoperative hematocrit is greater than 40% in the full-

term newborn or premature infant and greater than 30% in older infants.[267] Blood losses greater than 10% of estimated blood volume should be replaced with warmed infusions of salt-poor albumin, fresh-frozen plasma, or, preferably, packed erythrocytes, as indicated by serial hematocrits, measured bleeding, cardiovascular function, and clotting status. All banked blood should be filtered through a 40-μm mesh filter.

Prior to the onset of surgery, the maximum allowable blood loss (MABL) for a neonate should be calculated based on age, weight, current hematocrit (Hct), and minimum acceptable hematocrit.[268] Estimated blood volume (EBV) for neonates ranges from 80 to 90 mL/kg for full-term infants to 90 to 100 mL/kg for premature infants.

$$MABL = \frac{EBV \times (\text{Patient's Hct} - \text{Minimum accepted Hct})}{\text{Patient's Hct}}$$

Intraoperative urinary output, if measured, should be at least 1 to 2 mL/kg/hour, and the urine should have a specific gravity between 1.005 and 1.015. Maximum urine concentration in a premature infant is indicated by a specific gravity of 1.018 (or 800 mOsm/L), but it may be as high as 1.025 (1000 mOsm/L) in full-term infants. The specific gravity of neonatal urine may be spuriously elevated by high-molecular-weight solutes (e.g., sugars and proteins). Under normal circumstances, urinary volume is a more useful indicator of hydration in neonates than specific gravity. For major procedures, Furman et al.[269] have suggested a simple fluid replacement schedule for supplementing maintenance fluids, restoring third space losses, and replacing preoperative losses (Table 26-9).

Thermal Management

Attention to thermal management in the newborn is critical. Neonates are particularly susceptible to hypothermia in the OR, where the ambient environment tends to be kept cool and the effects of anesthesia abolish the normal thermoregulatory mechanisms. Hypothermia in the newborn results in a release of catecholamines, glucocorticoids, and thyroxine, as in the neuroendocrine stress response.[270,271] The physiologic consequences include increased oxygen consumption, increased CO_2 production, increased clotting times, left shift of the oxyhemoglobin curve, and, in extreme cases, metabolic acidosis, myocardial dysfunction, increased pulmonary artery pressures, arrhythmias, and death.

A neutral thermal environment is the range of ambient temperatures at which metabolic rate is minimal and temperature regulation is achieved by nonevaporative physical processes alone. The range of the neutral thermal environment in infants is limited. In full-term infants, increases in oxygen consumption are minimal, at skin surface to environmental temperature gradients of only 2° to 4°C. Thus, at environmental temperatures of 32° to 34°C and abdominal skin temperature of 36°C, the resting newborn infant usually is in a state of minimal increased oxygen consumption.[272,273]

Anesthesia decreases the threshold temperature to hypothermia-induced thermogenesis by 2.5°C.[274] This decreases the temperature at which an infant will passively allow its temperature to fall before initiating rewarming. Heat loss occurs through radiation, conduction, evaporation, and convection. In a thermoneutral environment, radiation is responsible for 39% of heat loss, with convection accounting for 34% of heat loss.[275] As the ambient temperature decreases in the OR, radiant heat loss alone accounts for more than 50% of heat loss, thus the emphasis on prewarming the OR prior to the arrival of the neonate.

Heat loss during anesthesia undergoes three phases described by Sessler[274]: internal redistribution of heat, thermal imbalance, and thermal steady state or rewarming. Induction of anesthesia reduces the temperature differential between the warm core and cooler extremities by vasodilation. The patient continues to redistribute heat and lower core body temperature until the difference between the skin and environment becomes thermoneutral, with heat production matching heat loss. After approximately 80 minutes,[276] a mildly hypothermic infant will begin to rewarm using nonshivering thermogenesis to return core temperature to nearly normal. Neonates are more capable of rewarming than are children or adults under anesthesia.[276]

Nonshivering thermogenesis is seen only in infants and children. During anesthesia, the hypothermic infant will increase noradrenaline levels, oxygen consumption, and CO_2 production. Nonshivering thermogenesis occurs primarily through metabolism in brown fat, but it also can occur in the skeleton, liver, brain, and white fat.[277] Brown fat is approximately 2% to 6% of the full-term infants' body weight. It is packed with mitochondria and has an abundant vascular supply. Beta-sympathetic activation leads to uncoupled oxidative phosphorylation and subsequent heat production. Beta blockade and volatile agents can inhibit nonshivering thermogenesis.[278]

Techniques to maintain the body temperature of neonates during surgery are simply the four principles of heat loss in reverse. Radiant warming is done by thoroughly preheating the OR and applying radiant lights when possible. Heating and humidifying inspired gases and warming prep solutions and irrigation fluid minimize evaporative heat loss. Placing a water-heated blanket beneath the patient accomplishes conductive warming. Convective warming is via forced warm air from a "Bair hugger."[279]

Regional Anesthesia in Neonates

Any peripheral and central nerve block performed on adults theoretically can be performed on infants.[280] The advantage to regional anesthesia is that it may not cause the respiratory and cardiovascular depression of general anesthesia and opioids. It is also superior to general anesthesia in blocking the neuroendocrine stress response and lowering postoperative pain scores.[281,282] Unlike an adult, the anesthetized infant or child cannot verbalize the CNS symptoms that are the earliest signs of local anesthetic toxicity and intravascular injection. Detection of intravascular injection therefore is much more difficult, even with the use of epinephrine-containing local

anesthetics in infants.[283] As such, most practitioners limit regional techniques to central blockade, local infiltration,[284] and inguinal and penile blocks.[285] These particular blocks are easy to perform and have low complication rates.[286] A new formulation of bupivacaine microspheres may reduce the concern of local anesthetic toxicity and dramatically prolong the duration of analgesia to 5.5 days.[287]

Central neuraxial blockade in infants consists of caudal, spinal, and continuous caudal administration of local anesthetics. Caudal anesthesia with lidocaine or bupivacaine has been used successfully to provide the sole anesthetic or a combined general-regional anesthetic for preterm and term newborns and older infants undergoing lower abdominal and lower extremity surgery (Fig. 26-10). Spinal anesthesia with lidocaine, tetracaine, or bupivacaine has been recommended as an alternative to general anesthesia in former premature infants undergoing minor surgical procedures[288-290] (Table 26-10).[290] Failure rates for spinal anesthesia in neonates may be as high as 10%.[291]

Successful regional anesthesia in neonates does not ensure cardiopulmonary stability or airway patency, and it is not recommended as the sole anesthetic for unstable neonates who may require assisted or controlled ventilation postoperatively. Regional anesthesia can be combined with general anesthesia in neonates in order to reduce inspired anesthetic fractions and provide better postoperative analgesia, especially after infraumbilical or lower extremity surgery. My preference is to combine single-dose caudal blocks with bupivacaine and general endotracheal anesthesia for preterm and full-term neonates and to reserve continuous epidural-general anesthesia for thoracic procedures.

Termination of Anesthesia

At the completion of surgery, several decisions must be made, including whether neuromuscular blockade should be reversed, when the trachea should be extubated, and the course of postoperative pulmonary management. Massive blood loss, systemic hypotension, hypothermia, or hypocalcemia are contraindications to reversal of the effects of nondepolarizing muscle relaxants. Only when the infant is conscious and vigorous can the endotracheal tube be removed. Careful reassessment of adequacy of oxygenation and ventilation then determines the proper timing of tracheal extubation. Endotracheal tubes that are to remain in place postoperatively must be re-evaluated with regard to proper placement and patency.

POSTANESTHETIC MANAGEMENT

Postoperatively, neonates must be swiftly and safely transported to postanesthetic recovery areas in warmed isolettes with continuous monitoring and portable respirators. Postanesthetic recovery areas may include adult recovery rooms, nurseries for full-term infants, and pediatric or neonatal intensive care units. Regardless of the recovery area, careful monitoring for pain, apnea, hypotension, hypothermia, and prolonged sedation must continue for a period before discharge to nonintensive care areas. Several scoring systems are available for evaluation of an infant's cardiopulmonary and neu-

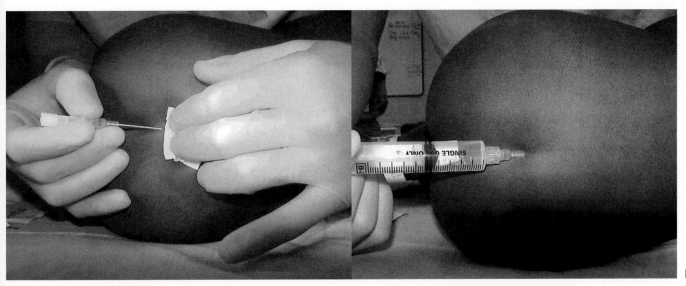

B

Figure 26-10. Placement of a caudal epidural blockade. *A,* A 20-gauge Angiocath is placed through the sacrococcygeal ligament. *B,* The stylet is removed, and local anesthetic is injected through the Angiocath.

TABLE 26-10. Anesthetics for Neonatal Neuraxial Blockade

Type of Block	Local Anesthetics	Dose	Duration of Analgesia
Spinal	Lidocaine 5%	2 mg/kg	45 min
	Bupivacaine 0.5% with epi 20 μg	0.8 mg/kg	70 min
	Tetracaine 0.5% with epi 40 μg	0.5–1.0 mg/kg	80–120 min
Single dose caudally administered	Bupivacaine 0.25%	2 mg/kg	4–6 hr
Epidural blockade	Bupivacaine 0.1%	0.1–0.2 mL/kg/hr	Days
Continuous epidural blockade	Chloroprocaine 1.5%	0.1–0.2 mL/kg/hr	Days

robehavioral well-being in postanesthetic recovery areas.[292] Premature neonates, sudden infant death syndrome survivors and their siblings, and all infants with episodic apnea must be carefully monitored for apnea for at least 12 to 24 hours postoperatively. Postoperative alveolar hypoventilation may be the result of inadvertent intraoperative hypocapnia, hypothermia, prolonged narcosis, inadequate reversal of neuromuscular blockade, or hypocalcemia. Prior to the extubation it is essential that the neonate demonstrate a consistent and stable respiratory pattern. Prolonged narcosis may require the administration of a diagnostic dose of naloxone (0.005 to 0.01 mg/kg), which results in dramatic recovery in patients in whom opioids have caused postoperative apnea. Inadequate reversal of the effects of nondepolarizing muscle relaxants can be easily excluded as a cause of postoperative hypoventilation with evaluation of twitch and post-tetanic response to electrical stimulation of a peripheral motor nerve. If hypothermia, hypocalcemia, and concomitant aminoglycoside antibiotic therapy can be excluded, a second dose of atropine and neostigmine can be administered to antagonize residual neuromuscular block (see Table 26-4). Postanesthetic cardiovascular monitoring should continue and includes electrocardiography and accurate blood pressure determination with a Dinamap oscillometric microprocessor or arterial line probe. Thermal and fluid balance must be maintained.

COMPLICATIONS OF ANESTHESIA

Recognition of anesthetic risks and careful attention to the details of airway management, ventilatory control, and vigilant monitoring prevent the most common intraoperative problems in newborns, that is, cardiovascular and respiratory accidents.[293] Several less serious complications may occur intraoperatively in neonates, including corneal abrasions, lip lacerations, intravenous line infiltrations, electrocautery or heating lamp burns, endobronchial intubation, and postextubation laryngeal edema. The clinician can prevent these complications by devoting careful attention to details such as taping the eyelids, performing gentle laryngoscopy, inspecting intravenous sites, grounding electrocautery instruments, keeping radiant heaters at least 60 cm away from the patient, and auscultating frequently for bilateral equal breath sounds.

Postextubation laryngeal edema manifesting as inspiratory stridor is unusual in newborns and most common in patients between the ages 2 and 5 years.[159] Initial management should be conservative, involving humidification, steroid administration, and use of nebulized epinephrine. No improvement or worsening of stridor are indications for endoscopic evaluation to rule out congenital anomalies, acquired subglottic stenosis, or laryngeal damage. Neonates who have required prolonged endotracheal intubation and assisted ventilation for respiratory failure are at higher risk for acquired subglottic stenosis and postextubation stridor (see Chapter 22).[294,295]

POSTOPERATIVE CRITICAL CARE MANAGEMENT OF NEONATES

The basic techniques for operative correction and postoperative management of a number of congenital malformations were discussed earlier in this chapter (see Table 26-2). Since the early 1970s, four postoperative management advances have helped to ensure good outcomes for high-risk neonates who are recovering from major surgical interventions and are still struggling to complete their difficult transition from intrauterine to extrauterine life. These advances include (1) improved antibiotic therapy; (2) fluid, electrolyte, and nutritional replacement and supportive therapy; (3) extracorporeal respiratory support with ECMO; and (4) inhaled NO therapy.

CONCLUSION

Successful intraoperative management of the neonate requires timing, teamwork, an appreciation of the involved risks, and a firm understanding of neonatal physiology. The pediatric anesthesiologist does not regard the neonate as a small adult and has developed unique skills and equipment to provide optimum intraoperative care to the high-risk infant. The neonatologist should not regard the infant's intraoperative course as an extension of a stable nursery course. Environments are constantly changing and radically different, and new problems are encountered. Much effort and extreme surveillance are required to return the neonate to a postoperative unit in homeostatic balance.

ACKNOWLEDGMENT

The author thanks Michael J. Goretsky, MD, Assistant Professor of Clinical Surgery & Pediatrics at Eastern Virginia Medical School, for his review of the section on surgical management of neonatal surgical emergencies.

REFERENCES

1. Kohelet D, Arbel E, Tavori I, et al: Survival of a 300 gram infant. Harefuah 140:1018–1020, 1118, 1119, 2001.
2. Agustines LA, Lin YG, Rumney PJ, et al: Outcomes of extremely low-birth-weight infants between 500 and 750 g. Am J Obstet Gynecol 182:1113–1116, 2000.
3. Breborowicz GH: Limits of fetal viability and its enhancement. Early Pregnancy 5:49–50, 2001.
4. Rackow H, Salinitre E, Green LT: Frequency of cardiac arrest associated with anesthesia in infants and children: Report of 66 original cases. Pediatrics 28:697, 1961.
5. Salem MR, Bennett EJ, Schwass JF, et al: Cardiac arrest related to anesthesia: Contributing factors in infants and children. JAMA 233:238, 1975.
6. Keenan RL, Boyan CP: Cardiac arrest due to anesthesia: A study of incidence and causes. JAMA 253:2373, 1985.
7. Kirby RR, Robison EJ, Schulz J, et al: Continuous flow ventilation as an alternative to assisted or controlled ventilation in infants. Anesth Analg 51:871, 1972.
8. Zapol WM, Schneider R, Snider M, et al: Partial bypass with membrane lungs for acute respiratory failure. Int Anesthesiol Clin 14:119–133, 1976.
9. Roberts JD, Polaner DM, Lang P, et al: Inhaled nitric oxide in persistent pulmonary hypertension of the newborn. Lancet 340:818–819, 1992.
10. Reid DH: A method of continuous measurement of arterial-oxygen tension. Lancet 1:1242, 1966.
11. Apgar V: The newborn (Apgar) scoring system. Reflections and advice. Pediatr Clin North Am 13:645–650, 1966.
12. Apgar V: A proposal for evaluation of the newborn infant. Anesth Analg 32:260, 1953.
13. Campbell DI, Shanks CA, Flachs J, et al: Accurate volume ventilation of neonates with maintenance of humidification. Anaesth Intensive Care 3:295–298, 1975.
14. Steward DJ: Premature infants are more prone to complications following minor surgery than are term infants. Anesthesiology 56:304, 1982.
15. Stephen CR: Elements of pediatric anesthesia. Springfield, Ill., Charles C. Thomas, 1954, p. 67.
16. Denman WT, Swanson EL, Rosow D, et al: Pediatric evaluation of the bispectral index (BIS) monitor and correlation of BIS with end-tidal sevoflurane concentration in infants and children. Anesth Analg 90:872–827, 2000.
17. Rosow C, Manberg PJ: Bispectral index monitoring. Anesthesiol Clin North America 19:947–966, xi, 2001.
18. Morray JP, Geiduschek JM, Ramamoorthy C, et al: Anesthesia-related cardiac arrest in children: Initial findings of the Pediatric Perioperative Cardiac Arrest (POCA) Registry. Anesthesiology 93:6–14, 2000.
19. Cote CJ: Anesthesia-related cardiac arrest in children. Anesthesiology 94:933; discussion 934–935, 2001.
20. Groome LJ, Loizou PC, Holland SB, et al: High vagal tone is associated with more efficient regulation of homeostasis in low-risk human fetuses. Dev Psychobiol 35:25–34, 1999.
21. Massin M, von Bernuth G: Normal ranges of heart rate variability during infancy and childhood. Pediatr Cardiol 18:297–302, 1997.
22. Wagenvoort AM, Bekker MN, Go AT, et al: Ultrafast scan magnetic resonance in prenatal diagnosis. Fetal Diagn Ther 15:364–372, 2000.
23. Damgaard-Pedersen K, Qvist T: Pediatric pulmonary CT-scanning. Anaesthesia-induced changes. Pediatr Radiol 9:145–148, 1980.
24. Serafini G, Cornara G, Cavalloro F, et al: Pulmonary atelectasis during paediatric anaesthesia: CT scan evaluation and effect of positive end-expiratory pressure (PEEP). Paediatr Anaesth 9:225–228,1999.
25. Motil KJ, Blackburn MG: Temperature regulation in the neonate. A survey of the pathophysiology of thermal dynamics and of the principles of environmental control. Clin Pediatr (Phila) 12:634–639,1973.
26. Dierdorf SF, Krishna G: Anesthetic management of neonatal surgical emergencies. Anesth Analg 60:204–215,1981.
27. Arant BS, Greifer I, Edelmann CM Jr, et al: Effect of chronic salt and water loading on the tubular defects of a child with Fanconi syndrome (cystinosis). Pediatrics 58:370–377, 1976.
28. Edelmann CM, Soriano JR, Bolchis H, et al: Renal bicarbonate resorption and hydrogen ion excretion in normal infants. J Clin Invest 46:1309, 1967.
29. Hinkle AJ, Alper MH: Anesthetic Considerations for Neonatal Surgery. ASA Refresher Courses in Anesthesiology. Philadelphia, JB Lippincott 1982, p. 123.
30. Nilsson K, Larsson LE, Andreasson S, et al: Blood-glucose concentrations during anaesthesia in children. Effects of starvation and perioperative fluid therapy. Br J Anaesth 56:375–379, 1984.
31. Halamek LP, Benaron DA, Stevenson DK: Neonatal hypoglycemia, part I: Background and definition. Clin Pediatr (Phila) 36:675–680, 1997.
32. Lilien LD, Rosenfield RL, Baccaro MM, et al: Hyperglycemia in stressed small premature neonates. J Pediatr 94:454–459,1979.
33. Srinivasan G, Jain R, Pildes RS, et al: Glucose homeostasis during anesthesia and surgery in infants. J Pediatr Surg 21:718–21, 1986.
34. Sedowofia K, Barclay C: The systemic stress response to thermal injury in children. Clin Endocrinol (Oxf) 49:335–341, 1998.
35. Anand KJ: The stress response to surgical trauma: From physiological basis to therapeutic implications. Prog Food Nutr Sci 10:67–132, 1986.
36. Hill AG, Hill GL: Metabolic response to severe injury. Br J Surg 85:884–890, 1998.
37. Smith A, Barclay C: The bigger the burn, the greater the stress. Burns 23:291–294, 1997.
38. Greisen J, Juhl CB, Grofte T: Acute pain induces insulin resistance in humans. Anesthesiology 95:578–584, 2001.
39. Bouwmeester NJ, Anand KJ: Hormonal and metabolic stress responses after major surgery in children aged 0–3 years: A double-blind, random-

ized trial comparing the effects of continuous versus intermittent morphine. Br J Anaesth 87:390–399, 2001.

40. Anand KJ, Sippell WG: Does halothane anaesthesia decrease the metabolic and endocrine stress responses of newborn infants undergoing operation? Br Med J (Clin Res Ed) 296:668–672, 1988.
41. Swedberg K, Eneroth P: Hormones regulating cardiovascular function in patients with severe congestive heart failure and their relation to mortality. CONSENSUS Trial Study Group. Circulation 82:1730–1736, 1990.
42. Wilmore DW: Metabolic response to severe surgical illness: Overview. World J Surg 24:705–711, 2000.
43. Ogawa K, Hirai M, Katsube T: Suppression of cellular immunity by surgical stress. Surgery 127:329–336, 2000.
44. Clark MA, Plank LD, Hill GL: Wound healing associated with severe surgical illness. World J Surg 24:648–654, 2000.
45. Rao MV, Chari P, Malhotra SK, et al: Role of epidural analgesia on endocrine and metabolic responses to surgery. Indian J Med Res 92:13–16, 1990.
46. Brandt MR, Fernades A: Epidural analgesia improves postoperative nitrogen balance. Br Med J 1:1106–1108, 1978.
47. Mizutani A, Hattori S, Yoshitake S: Effect of additional general anesthesia with propofol, midazolam or sevoflurane on stress hormone levels in hysterectomy patients, receiving epidural anesthesia. Acta Anaesthesiol Belg 49:133–139, 1998.
48. Anand KJ, Hickey PR: Pain and its effects in the human neonate and fetus. N Engl J Med 317:1321–1329, 1987.
49. Lloyd-Thomas AR: Pain management in paediatric patients. Br J Anaesth 64:85–104, 1990.
50. Anand KJ, Hickey PR: Halothane-morphine compared with high-dose sufentanil for anesthesia and postoperative analgesia in neonatal cardiac surgery. N Engl J Med 326:1–9, 1992.
51. Giesecke K, Hamberger B: High- and low-dose fentanyl anaesthesia: Hormonal and metabolic responses during cholecystectomy. Br J Anaesth 61:575–582, 1988.
52. Todisco T, de Benedictis FM, Iannacci L, et al: Mild prematurity and respiratory functions. Eur J Pediatr 152:55–58, 1993.
53. Liu LM, Cote CJ, Goudsouzian NG, et al: Life-threatening apnea in infants recovering from anesthesia. Anesthesiology 59:506–510, 1983.
54. Kurth CD, Spitzer AR, Broennle AM, et al: Postoperative apnea in preterm infants. Anesthesiology 66:483–488, 1987.
55. Chao DC, Scheinhorn DJ: Barotrauma vs volutrauma. Chest 109:1127–1128,1996.
56. Auten RL, Vozzelli M, Clark RH: Volutrauma. What is it, and how do we avoid it? Clin Perinatol 28:505–515, 2001.
57. Diaz JH: Anesthetic management of premature neonates, term neonates, and infants. In Diaz JH (ed): Perinatal Anesthesia and Critical Care. Philadelphia, WB Saunders, 1991, pp. 281–321.
58. Mock DM, Bell EF, Lankford GL, et al: Hematocrit correlates well with circulating red blood cell volume in very low birth weight infants. Pediatr Res 50:525–531, 2001.
59. Usher R, Lind J: Blood volume of the newborn premature infant. Acta Paediatr Scand 54:419, 1965.
60. Delivoria-Papadopoulos M, Roncevic NP, Osid IA: Postnatal changes in oxygen transport of term, premature, and sick infants: The role of red cell 2,3,-diphosphoglycerate and adult hemoglobin. Pediatr Res 5:235, 1971.
61. Oski IA: Clinical implications of the oxyhemoglobin dissociation curve in the neonatal period. Crit Care Med 7:412, 1979.
62. Goldsmith JP, Karotkin EH: Appendix 10. In Goldsmith JP, Karotkin EH (eds): Assisted Ventilation of the Neonate, 2nd ed. Philadelphia, WB Saunders, 1988, p. 437.
63. Rosenthal A: Hemodynamics in physiologic anemia of infancy. N Engl J Med 306:538, 1982.
64. Lister G, Hellenbrand WE, Kleinman CS, et al: Physiologic effects of increasing hemoglobin concentration in left-to-right shunting in infants with ventricular septal defects. N Engl J Med 306:502, 1982.
65. Glader BE: Erythrocyte disorders in infancy. In Avery ME, Taeusch HW (eds): Schaffer's Diseases of the Newborn, 5th ed. Philadelphia, WB Saunders, 1984, pp. 581–615.
66. Dallman PR: Anemia of prematurity. Annu Rev Med 32:143, 1981.
67. Oski FA: Clinical implications of the oxyhemoglobin dissociation curve in the neonatal period. Crit Care Med 7:412–418, 1979.
68. Goldsmith JP, Karotkin EH: Appendix 26. In Goldsmith JP, Karotkin EH (eds): Assisted Ventilation of the Neonate, 2nd ed. Philadelphia, WB Saunders, 1988, p. 452.
69. Papile LA, Burstein J, Burstein R, et al: Incidence and evolution of subependymal and intraventricular hemorrhage: A study of infants with birth weights less than 1,500 gm. J Pediatr 92:529–534, 1978.

70. Anand KJ: Neonatal stress responses to anesthesia and surgery. Clin Perinatol 17:207–214, 1990.
71. Sheth RD: Trends in incidence and severity of intraventricular hemorrhage. J Child Neurol 13:261–264, 1998.
72. Levene ME, Fawer CL, Lamont RF: Risk factors in the development of intraventricular haemorrhage in the preterm neonate. Arch Dis Child 57:410, 1982.
73. Ment LR, Duncan CC, Ehrenkranz RA, et al: Intraventricular hemorrhage in the preterm neonate: Timing and cerebral blood flow changes. J Pediatr 104:419, 1984.
74. Perlman JM, Volpe JJ: Intraventricular hemorrhage in extremely small premature infants. Am J Dis Child 140:1122–1124, 1986.
75. Pape KE, Wigglesworth JS: Haemorrhage, Ischemia and the Perinatal Brain. Philadelphia, JB Lippincott, 1979.
76. Lou HC, Lassen NA, Friis-Hansen B: Impaired autoregulation of cerebral blood flow in the distressed newborn infant. J Pediatr 94:118, 1979.
77. Fujimura M, Salisbury DM, Robinson RO, et al: Clinical events relating to intraventricular haemorrhage in the newborn. Arch Dis Child 54:409, 1979.
78. McDonald MM, Johnson ML, Rumack CM, et al: Role of coagulopathy in newborn intracranial hemorrhage. Pediatrics 74:26, 1984.
79. Lesko SM, Mitchell AA, Epstein MF, et al: Heparin use as a risk factor for intraventricular hemorrhage in low-birth-weight infants. N Engl J Med 314:11.56, 1986.
80. McDonald MM, Koops BL, Johnson ML, et al: Timing and antecedents of intracranial hemorrhage in the newborn. Pediatrics 74:32, 1984.
81. Wheeler AS, Sadri S, Gutsche BB, et al: Intracranial hemorrhage following intravenous administration of sodium bicarbonate or saline solution in the newborn lamb asphyxiated in utero. Anesthesiology 51:517, 1979.
82. Fanconi S, Duc G: Intracranial auctioning in sick preterm infants: Prevention of intracranial hypertension and cerebral hypoperfusion by muscle paralysis. Pediatrics 79:538, 1987.
83. Friesen RH. Honda AT, Thieme RE: Changes in anterior fontanel pressure in preterm infants during tracheal intubation. Anesth Analg 66:874, 1987.
84. Perlman JM, Goodman S, Kreusser M, et al: Reduction in intraventricular hemorrhage by elimination of fluctuating cerebral blood flow velocity in preterm infants with respiratory distress syndrome. N Engl J Med 312:1353, 1985.
85. Friesen RH, Honda AT, Thieme RE: Perianesthetic intracranial hemorrhage in preterm neonates. Anesthesiology 67:814–816, 1987.
86. Strange MJ, Myers G, Kirklin JK, et al: Surgical closure of patent ductus arteriosus does not increase the risk of intraventricular hemorrhage in the preterm infant. J Pediatr 107:602–604, 1985.
87. Donn SM, Roloff DW, Goldstein GW: Prevention of intraventricular haemorrhage in preterm infants by phenobarbitone. A controlled trial. Lancet 2:215–217, 1981.
88. Anwar M, Kadam S, Hiatt IM, et al: Phenobarbitone prophylaxis of intraventricular haemorrhage. Arch Dis Child 61:196–197, 1986.
89. Friesen RH, Thieme RE, Honda AT, et al: Changes in anterior fontanel pressure in preterm neonates receiving isoflurane, halothane, fentanyl, or ketamine. Anesth Analg 66:431–434, 1987.
90. Berry FA, Gregory GA: Do premature infants require anesthesia for surgery? Anesthesiology 67:291–293,1987.
91. Kattwinkel J: Apnea in the neonatal period. Pediatr Rev 2:115, 1980.
92. Welborn LG, Ramirez N, Oh TH, et al: Postanesthetic apnea and periodic breathing in infants. Anesthesiology 65:658, 1986.
93. Welborn LG, DeSoto H, Hannallah RS, et al: The use of caffeine in the control of postanesthetic apnea in former premature infants. Anesthesiology 68:796, 1988.
94. Gregory GA, Steward DJ: Life-threatening perioperative apnea in the "ex-preemie." Anesthesiology 59:495, 1983.
95. Cote CJ, Zaslavsky A, Downes JJ, et al: Postoperative apnea in former preterm infants after inguinal herniorrhaphy. A combined analysis. Anesthesiology 82:809–822, 1995.
96. Durand DJ, Goodman A, Ray P, et al: Theophylline treatment in the extubation of infants weighing less than 1,250 grams: A controlled trial. Pediatrics 80:684–688, 1987.
97. Aranda JV, Gorman W, Bergsteinsson H, et al: Efficacy of caffeine in treatment of apnea in the low-birth-weight infant. J Pediatr 90:467–472, 1977.
98. Aranda JV, Sitar DS, Parsons WD, et al: Pharmacokinetic aspects of theophylline in premature newborns. N Engl J Med 295:413–416, 1976.
99. Aranda JV, Turmen T: Methylxanthines in apnea of prematurity. Clin Perinatol 6:87–108, 1979.

100. Welborn LG, Greenspun JC: Anesthesia and apnea. Perioperative considerations in the former preterm infant. Pediatr Clin North Am 41:181–198, 1994.

101. Welborn LG, Rice LJ, Hannallah RS, et al: Postoperative apnea in former preterm infants: Prospective comparison of spinal and general anesthesia. Anesthesiology 72:838–842, 1990.

102. Frumiento C, Abajian JC, Vane DW: Spinal anesthesia for preterm infants undergoing inguinal hernia repair. Arch Surg 135:445–451, 2000.

103. Veverka TJ, Henry DN, Milroy MJ, et al: Spinal anesthesia reduces the hazard of apnea in high-risk infants. Am Surg 57:531–534, 1991; discussion 534–535.

104. Krane EJ, Haberkern CM, Jacobson LE: Postoperative apnea, bradycardia, and oxygen desaturation in formerly premature infants: Prospective comparison of spinal and general anesthesia. Anesth Analg 80:7–13, 1995.

105. Kunst G, Linderkamp O, Holle R, et al: The proportion of high risk preterm infants with postoperative apnea and bradycardia is the same after general and spinal anesthesia. Can J Anaesth 46:94–95, 1999.

106. Watcha MF, Thach BT, Gunter JB: Postoperative apnea after caudal anesthesia in an ex-premature infant. Anesthesiology 71:613–615, 1989.

107. Kinsey VE, Arnold HJ, Kalina RE, et al: PaO$_2$ levels and retrolental fibroplasia: A report of the cooperative study. Pediatrics 60:655–668, 1977.

108. Shohat M, Reisner SH, Krikler R, et al: Retinopathy of prematurity: Incidence and risk factors. Pediatrics 72:159–163, 1983.

109. Weiter JJ: Retrolental fibroplasia: An unsolved problem. N Engl J Med 305:1404–1406,1981.

110. O'Connor AR, Stephenson T, Johnson A, et al: Long-term ophthalmic outcome of low birth weight children with and without retinopathy of prematurity. Pediatrics 109:12–18, 2002.

111. Kaiser RS, Trese MT, Williams GA, et al: Adult retinopathy of prematurity: Outcomes of rhegmatogenous retinal detachments and retinal tears. Ophthalmology 108:1647–1653, 2001.

112. Charan R, Dogra MR, Gupta A, et al: The incidence of retinopathy of prematurity in a neonatal care unit. Indian J Ophthalmol 43:123–126, 1995.

113. Seiberth V, Linderkamp O: Risk factors in retinopathy of prematurity. A multivariate statistical analysis. Ophthalmologica 214:131–135, 2000.

114. Bassiouny MR: Risk factors associated with retinopathy of prematurity: A study from Oman. J Trop Pediatr 42:355–358, 1996.

115. Nodgaard H, Andreasen H, Hansen H, et al: Risk factors associated with retinopathy of prematurity (ROP) in northern Jutland, Denmark 1990–1993. Acta Ophthalmol Scand 74:306–310, 1996.

116. Holmstrom G, Broberger U, Thomassen P: Neonatal risk factors for retinopathy of prematurity—A population-based study. Acta Ophthalmol Scand 76:204–207, 1998.

117. Phibbs RH: Oxygen therapy: A continuing hazard to the premature infant. Anesthesiology 47:486–487, 1977.

118. Flynn JT: Oxygen and retrolental fibroplasia: Update and challenge. Anesthesiology 60:397–399, 1984.

119. Betts EK, Downes JJ, Schaffer DB, et al: Retrolental fibroplasias and oxygen administration during general anesthesia. Anesthesiology 47:518, 1977.

120. Quinn GE, Betts EK, Diamond GR, et al: Neonatal age (human) at retinal maturation. Anesthesiology 55:S326, 1981.

121. Breton ME, Quinn GE, Schueller AW: Development of electroretinogram and rod phototransduction response in human infants. Invest Ophthalmol Vis Sci 36:1588–1602, 1995.

122. Bucher HU, Fanconi S, Baeckert P, et al: Hyperoxemia in newborn infants: Detection by pulse oximetry. Pediatrics 84:226–230,1989.

123. Cote CJ, Todres D, Ryan JF, et al. (eds): A Practice of Anesthesia for Infants an Children, 4th ed. Philadelphia, WB Saunders, 2000, p. 45.

124. Morris GN, Rich GF: Inhaled nitric oxide as a selective pulmonary vasodilator in clinical anesthesia. AANA J 65:59–67, 1997.

125. Downes JJ: Anesthesia and postoperative care of the newborn. In Dannemiller FJ (ed): Society of Air Force Anesthesiologists 24th Annual Review Course Lecture Notes #105. San Antonio, Texas, United States Air Force, 1977.

126. Broennle AM: The neonate: Intraoperative management. American Society of Anesthesia Refresher Course Lectures, #126, 1977.

127. Bochdalek VA: Einige Betrachtungen uber die Enstehung des angeborenen Zwerchfellbruches: als Beitrag zur pathologischen Anatomie der Hernien. Vierteljahresschrift Prakt Heilkund 3:89, 1848.

128. Adelman S, Benson CD: Bochdalek hernias in infants: Factors determining mortality. J Pediatr Surg 11:569–573, 1976.

129. Adzick NS, Harrison MR, Glick PL: Diaphragmatic hernia in the fetus: Prenatal diagnosis and outcome in 94 cases. J Pediatr Surg 20:357–361, 1985.

130. Beresford MW, Shaw NJ: Outcome of congenital diaphragmatic hernia. Pediatr Pulmonol 30:249–256, 2000.

131. Cacciari A, Ruggeri G, Mordenti M: High-frequency oscillatory ventilation versus conventional mechanical ventilation in congenital diaphragmatic hernia. Eur J Pediatr Surg 11:3–7, 2001.

132. The Congenital Diaphragmatic Hernia Study Group: Does extracorporeal membrane oxygenation improve survival in neonates with congenital diaphragmatic hernia? J Pediatr Surg 34:720–724, 1999; discussion 724–725.

133. Lally KP: Extracorporeal membrane oxygenation in patients with congenital diaphragmatic hernia. Semin Pediatr Surg 5:249–255, 1996.

134. Fox WW, Duara S: Persistent pulmonary hypertension in the neonate: Diagnosis and management. J Pediatr 103:505–514, 1983.

135. Mok Q, Yates R, Tasker RC: Persistent pulmonary hypertension of the term neonate: A strategy for management. Eur J Pediatr 158:825–827, 1999.

136. Raphaely RC, Downes JJ Jr: Congenital diaphragmatic hernia: Prediction of survival. J Pediatr Surg 8:815–823, 1973.

137. Kaiser JR, Rosenfeld CR: A population-based study of congenital diaphragmatic hernia: Impact of associated anomalies and preoperative blood gases on survival. J Pediatr Surg 34:1196–1202, 1999.

138. Gross RE: Surgery of Infancy: Its Principles and Techniques. Philadelphia, WB Saunders, 1953, pp. 75–102.

139. Kluth D: Atlas of esophageal atresia. J Pediatr Surg 11:901–919, 1976.

140. Bolande RB, Schneider AF, Boggs JD: Infantile lobar emphysema: Etiological concept. AMA Arch Pathol 61:289, 1956.

141. Cremin BJ, Movsowitz H: Lobar emphysema in infants. Br J Radiol 44:692–696, 1971.

142. Buntain WL, Isaacs H Jr, Payne VC Jr: Lobar emphysema, cystic adenomaloid malformation, pulmonary sequestration, and bronchogenic cyst in infancy and childhood: A clinical group. J Pediatr Surg 9:85–93, 1974.

143. Adzick NS, Harrison MR, Glick PL, et al: Fetal cystic adenomatoid malformation: Prenatal diagnosis and natural history. J Pediatr Surg 20:483–488, 1985.

144. Haller JA Jr, Golladay ES, Pickard LR, et al: Surgical management of lung bud anomalies: Lobar emphysema, bronchogenic cyst, cystic adenomatoid malformation, and intralobar pulmonary sequestration. Ann Thorac Surg 28:33–43, 1979.

145. Evrard V, Ceulemans J, Coosemansw, et al: Congenital parenchymatous malformations of the lung. World J Surg 23:1123–1132, 1999.

146. Schuster SR: Omphalocoele, hernia of the umbilical cord and gastroschisis. In Ravith MM, Welch KJ, Bensen CD, et al. (eds): Pediatric Surgery, 3rd ed. Chicago, Year book Medical Publishers, 1979, pp. 778–801.

147. Allen RG, Wrenn EL Jr: Silon as a sac in the treatment of omphalocele and gastroschisis. J Pediatr Surg 4:3–8, 1969.

148. Cantrell JR, Haller JA, Ravitch MM: A syndrome of congenital defects involving the abdominal wall, sternum, diaphragm, pericardium and heart. Surg Gynecol Obstet 107:602, 1958.

149. Lynn HB: Duodenal obstruction: Atresia, stenosis, and annular pancreas. In Ravith MM, Welch KJ, Bensen CD, et al. (eds): Pediatric Surgery, 3rd ed. Chicago, Year book Medical Publishers, 1979, pp. 902–911.

150. Andrassy RJ, Mahour GH: Malrotation of the midgut in infants and children: A 25-year review. Arch Surg 116:158–160, 1981.

151. Nixon HH, Tawes R: Etiology and treatment of small intestinal atresia: Analysis of a series of 127 jejunoileal atresias and comparison with 62 duodenal atresias. Surgery 69:41–51, 1971.

152. Ziegler MM: Meconium ileus. Curr Probl Surg 31:731–777, 1994.

153. Kalayoglu M, Sieber WK, Rodnan JB, et al: Meconium ileus: A critical review of treatment and eventual prognosis. J Pediatr Surg 6:290–300, 1971.

154. Cote CJ, Todres D, Ryan JF, et al. (eds): A Practice of Anesthesia for Infants an Children, 4th ed. Philadelphia, WB Saunders, 2000, p. 39.

155. Walther FJ, Benders MJ, Leighton JO: Early changes in the neonatal circulatory transition. J Pediatr 123:625–632, 1993.

156. Arlettaz R, Archer N, Wilkinson AR: Natural history of innocent heart murmurs in newborn babies: Controlled echocardiographic study. Arch Dis Child Fetal Neonatal Ed 78:F166–F170, 1998.

157. Rein AJ, Omokhodion SI, Nir A: Significance of a cardiac murmur as the sole clinical sign in the newborn. Clin Pediatr (Phila) 39:511–520, 2000.

158. Smith RM: Anesthesia for Infants and Children, 4th ed. St. Louis, CV Mosby, 1980, p. 175.

159. Koka BV, Jeon IS, Andre JM, et al: Postintubation croup in children. Anesth Analg 56:501–505, 1977.

160. Pettignano R, Holloway SE, Hyman D, et al: Is the leak test reproducible? South Med J 93:683–685, 2000.

161. Scuderi J, Elton CB, Elton DR: A cart to provide high frequency jet ventilation during transport of neonates. Respir Care 37:129–136, 1992.

162. Teoh SL, Boo NY, Ong LC, et al: Duration of oxygen therapy and exchange transfusion as risk factors associated with retinopathy of prematurity in very low birthweight infants. Eye 9(Pt 6):733–737, 1995.

163. Ferrari LR, Rooney FM, Rockoff MA: Preoperative fasting practices in pediatrics. Anesthesiology 90:978–980, 1999.

164. Sethi AK, Chatterji C, Bhargava SK, et al: Safe pre-operative fasting times after milk or clear fluid in children. A preliminary study using real-time ultrasound. Anaesthesia 54:51–59, 1999.

165. Eger EI II: Atropine, scopolamine, and related compounds. Anesthesiology 23:356, 1965.

166. Arroe M, Steensgard J, Greisen G: Emergency transport of newborn infants—Fetch or bring? Ugeskr Laeger 163:1093–1097, 2001.

167. Leslie AJ, Stephenson TJ: Audit of neonatal intensive care transport—Closing the loop. Acta Paediatr 86:1253–1256, 1997.

168. Kronick JB, Frewen TC, Kissoon N, et al: Influence of referring physicians on interventions by a pediatric and neonatal critical care transport team. Pediatr Emerg Care 12:73–77, 1996.

169. Eger EI II, Saidman LJ, Brandstater B: Minimum alveolar anesthetic concentration: A standard of anesthetic potency. Anesthesiology 26:756–763, 1965.

170. King BS, Rampil IJ: Anesthetic depression of spinal motor neurons may contribute to lack of movement in response to noxious stimuli. Anesthesiology 81:1484–1492, 1994.

171. Antognini JF: The relationship among brain, spinal cord and anesthetic requirements. Med Hypotheses 48:83–87, 1997.

172. Eger EI 2nd, Bahlman SH, Munson ES: The effect of age on the rate of increase of alveolar anesthetic concentration. Anesthesiology 35:365–372, 1971.

173. Brandom BW, Brandom RB, Cook DR: Uptake and distribution of halothane in infants: In vivo measurements and computer simulations. Anesth Analg 62:404–410, 1983.

174. Tay CL, Tan GM, Ng SB: Critical incidents in paediatric anaesthesia: An audit of 10000 anaesthetics in Singapore. Paediatr Anaesth 11:711–718, 2001.

175. Piat V, Dubois MC, Johanet S, et al: Induction and recovery characteristics and hemodynamic responses to sevoflurane and halothane in children. Anesth Analg 79:840–844, 1994.

176. Delgado-Herrera L, Ostroff RD, Rogers SA: Sevoflurane: Approaching the ideal inhalational anesthetic: A pharmacologic, pharmacoeconomic, and clinical review. CNS Drug Rev 7:48–120, 2001.

177. O'Brien K, Robinson DN, Morton NS: Induction and emergence in infants less than 60 weeks post-conceptual age: Comparison of thiopental, halothane, sevoflurane and desflurane. Br J Anaesth 80:456–459, 1998.

178. Vivon E: Induction and maintenance of anesthesia. In Rees GT, Gray TC (eds): Paediatric Anesthesia: Trends in Current Practice. London, Butterworths, 1981, p. 101.

179. Lerman J, Robinson S, Willis MM, et al: Anesthetic requirements for halothane in young children 0–1 month and 1–6 months of age. Anesthesiology 59:421–424, 1983.

180. LeDez KM, Lerman J: The minimum alveolar concentration (MAC) of isoflurane in preterm neonates. Anesthesiology 67:301–307, 1987.

181. Taylor RH, Lerman J: Minimum alveolar concentration of desflurane and hemodynamic responses in neonates, infants, and children. Anesthesiology 75:975–979, 1991.

182. Lerman J, Sikich N, Kleinman S, et al: The pharmacology of sevoflurane in infants and children. Anesthesiology 80:814–824, 1994.

183. Cote CJ, Todres D, Ryan JF, et al. (eds): A Practice of Anesthesia for Infants an Children, 4th ed. Philadelphia, WB Saunders, 2000, p. 133.

184. Kataria B, Epstein R, Bailey A, et al: A comparison of sevoflurane to halothane in paediatric surgical patients: Results of a multicentre international study. Paediatr Anaesth 6:283–292, 1996.

185. Holzman RS, van der Velde ME, Kaus SJ, et al: Sevoflurane depresses myocardial contractility less than halothane during induction of anesthesia in children. Anesthesiology 85:1260–1267, 1996.

186. Russell IA, Miller Hance WC, Gregory G: The safety and efficacy of sevoflurane anesthesia in infants and children with congenital heart disease. Anesth Analg 92:1152–1158, 2001.

187. Krane EJ, Su JY: Comparison of the effects of halothane on newborn and adult rabbit myocardium. Anesth Analg 66:1240–1244, 1987.

188. Wolf AR, Lawson RA, Dryden CM, et al: Recovery after desflurane anaesthesia in the infant: Comparison with isoflurane. Br J Anaesth 76:362–364, 1996.

189. Taylor RH, Lerman J: Induction, maintenance and recovery characteristics of desflurane in infants and children. Can J Anaesth 39:6–13, 1992.

190. Zwass MS, Fisher DM, Welborn LG, et al: Induction and maintenance characteristics of anesthesia with desflurane and nitrous oxide in infants and children. Anesthesiology 76:373–378, 1992.

191. Brodsky JB, Cohen EN: Adverse effects of nitrous oxide. Med Toxicol 1:362–374, 1986.

192. Boutroy MJ: Drug-induced apnea. Biol Neonate 65:252–257, 1994.

193. Turner S, Longworth A, Nunn AJ, et al: Unlicensed and off label drug use in paediatric wards: Prospective study. BMJ 316:343–345, 1998.

194. Carmichael EB: The median lethal dose (Ld50) of pentothal sodium for both young and old guinea pigs and rats. Anesthesiology 8:589, 1947.

195. Kupferberg HJ, Way EL: Pharmacologic basis for the increased sensitivity of the newborn rat to meperidine and morphine. J Pharmacol Exp Ther 141:105, 1963.

196. Tauer CA: Testing drugs in pediatric populations: The FDA mandate. Account Res 7:37–58, 1999.

197. Conroy S, McIntyre J, Choonara I: Unlicensed and off label drug use in neonates. Arch Dis Child Fetal Neonatal Ed 80:F142–144, 1999; discussion F144–145.

198. Johnston R, Noseworthy T, Anderson B, et al: Propofol versus thiopental for outpatient anesthesia. Anesthesiology 67:431–433, 1987.

199. Lebovic S, Reich DL, Steinberg LG, et al: Comparison of propofol versus ketamine for anesthesia in pediatric patients undergoing cardiac catheterization. Anesth Analg 74:490–494, 1992.

200. Doze VA, Westphal LM, White PF: Comparison of propofol with methohexital for outpatient anesthesia. Anesth Analg 65:1189–1195, 1986.

201. Borgeat A: Recovery from propofol and its antiemetic effect in pediatric anesthesia. Cah Anesthesiol 41:231–234, 1993.

202. Martin TM, Nicolson SC, Bargas MS: Propofol anesthesia reduces emesis and airway obstruction in pediatric outpatients. Anesth Analg 76:144–148, 1993.

203. Valtonen M, Iisalo E, Kanto J, et al: Propofol as an induction agent in children: Pain on injection and pharmacokinetics. Acta Anaesthesiol Scand 33:152–155, 1989.

204. Author's observations.

205. Wolf A, Weir P, Segar P, et al: Impaired fatty acid oxidation in propofol infusion syndrome. Lancet 357:606–607, 2001.

206. Hanna JP, Ramundo ML: Rhabdomyolysis and hypoxia associated with prolonged propofol infusion in children. Neurology 50:301–303, 1998.

207. Hatch DJ: Propofol-infusion syndrome in children. Lancet 353:1117–1118, 1999.

208. Gaspari F, Marraro G, Penna GF, et al: Elimination kinetics of thiopentone in mothers and their newborn infants. Eur J Clin Pharmacol 28:321–325, 1985.

209. Garg DC, Goldberg RN, Woo-Ming RB: Pharmacokinetics of thiopental in the asphyxiated neonate. Dev Pharmacol Ther 11:213–218, 1988.

210. Gelissen HP, Epema AH, Henning RH: Inotropic effects of propofol, thiopental, midazolam, etomidate, and ketamine on isolated human atrial muscle. Anesthesiology 84:397–403, 1996.

211. Sedik H: Use of intravenous methohexital as a sedative in pediatric emergency departments. Arch Pediatr Adolesc Med 155:665–668, 2001.

212. Pomeranz ES, Chudnofsky CR, Deegan TJ: Rectal methohexital sedation for computed tomography imaging of stable pediatric emergency department patients. Pediatrics 105:1110–1114, 2000.

213. Alp H, Guler I, Orbak Z, et al: Efficacy and safety of rectal thiopental: Sedation for children undergoing computed tomography and magnetic resonance imaging. Pediatr Int 41:538–541, 1999.

214. Beekman RP, Hoorntje TM, Beek FJ, et al: Sedation for children undergoing magnetic resonance imaging: Efficacy and safety of rectal thiopental. Eur J Pediatr 155:820–822, 1996.

215. White PF, Way WL, Trevor AJ: Ketamine—Its pharmacology and therapeutic uses. Anesthesiology 56:119–136, 1982.

216. Lynn A, Nespeca MK, Bratton SL: Clearance of morphine in postoperative infants during intravenous infusion: The influence of age and surgery. Anesth Analg 86:958–963, 1998.

217. Duncan HP, Cloote A, Weir PM, et al: Reducing stress responses in the pre-bypass phase of open heart surgery in infants and young children: A comparison of different fentanyl doses. Br J Anaesth 84:556–564, 2000.

218. Newland MC, Leuschen P, Sarafian LB: Fentanyl intermittent bolus technique for anesthesia in infants and children undergoing cardiac surgery. J Cardiothorac Anesth 3:407–410, 1989.

219. Koehntop DE, Rodman JH, Brundage DM, et al: Pharmacokinetics of fentanyl in neonates. Anesth Analg 65:227–232, 1986.

220. Ross AK, Davis PJ, Dear Gd GL, et al: Pharmacokinetics of remifentanil in anesthetized pediatric patients undergoing elective surgery or diagnostic procedures. Anesth Analg 93:1393–1401, 2001.

221. Reid JE, Mirakhur RK: Bradycardia after administration of remifentanil. Br J Anaesth 84:422–423, 2000.

222. Breslin DS, Reid JE, Mirakhur RK, et al: Sevoflurane–nitrous oxide anaesthesia supplemented with remifentanil: Effect on recovery and cognitive function. Anaesthesia 56:114–119, 2001.

223. Stead AL: The response of the newborn to muscle relaxants. Br J Anaesth 27:124, 1955.

224. Nightingale DA, Glass AG, Bachman L: Neuromuscular blockade by succinylcholine in children. Anesthesiology 27:736, 1966.

225. Cook DR, Wingard LB, Taylor FH: Pharmacokinetics of succinylcholine in infants, children, and adults. Clin Pharmacol Ther 20:493–498, 1976.

226. Goudsouzian N: Muscle relaxants in children. In Cote CJ, Todres D, Ryan JF, et al. (eds): A Practice of Anesthesia for Infants and Children, 4th ed. Philadelphia, WB Saunders, 2000, pp. 200–202.

227. Robinson AL, Jerwood DC, Stokes MA: Routine suxamethonium in children. A regional survey of current usage. Anaesthesia 51:874–878, 1996.

228. Goudsouzian NG: Maturation of neuromuscular transmission in the infant. Br J Anaesth 52:205–214, 1980.

229. Cook DR: Muscle relaxants in infants and children. Anesth Analg 60:335–343, 1981.

230. Goudsouzian N: Muscle relaxants in children. In Cote CJ, Todres D, Ryan JF, et al. (eds): A Practice of Anesthesia for Infants and Children, 4th ed. Philadelphia, WB Saunders, 2000, pp. 200–202.

231. Morgan BC: Complications from intravascular catheters. Primum non nocere. Am J Dis Child 138:425–426, 1984.

232. Friesen RH, Lichtor JL: Indirect measurement of blood pressure in neonates and infants utilizing an automatic noninvasive oscillometric monitor. Anesth Analg 60:742–745, 1981.

233. Cullen PM, Dye J, Hughes DG: Clinical assessment of the neonatal Dinamap 847 during anesthesia in neonates and infants. J Clin Monit 3:229–234, 1987.

234. Lui K, Doyle PE, Buchanan N: Oscillometric and intra-arterial blood pressure measurements in the neonate: A comparison of methods. Aust Paediatr J 18:32–34, 1982.

235. Bissonnette B, Sessler DI, LaFlamme P: Intraoperative temperature monitoring sites in infants and children and the effect of inspired gas warming on esophageal temperature. Anesth Analg 69:192–196, 1989.

236. Chalon J, Patel C, Ali M, et al: Humidity and the anesthetized patient. Anesthesiology 50:195–198, 1979.

237. Chalon J, Loew DA, Malebranche J: Effects of dry anesthetic gases on tracheobronchial ciliated epithelium. Anesthesiology 37:338–343, 1972.

238. Cote CJ, Todres D, Ryan JF, et al. (eds): A Practice of Anesthesia for Infants and Children, 4th ed. Philadelphia, WB Saunders, 2000, pp. 196–199.

239. Harnett M, Kinirons B, Heffernan A, et al: Airway complications in infants: Comparison of laryngeal mask airway and the facemask-oral airway. Can J Anaesth 47:315–318, 2000.

240. Park C, Bahk JH, Ahn WS, et al: The laryngeal mask airway in infants and children. Can J Anaesth 48:413–417, 2001.

241. Rowbottom SJ, Simpson DL, Grubb D: The laryngeal mask airway in children. A fibreoptic assessment of positioning. Anaesthesia 46:489–491, 1991.

242. Mizushima A, Wardall GJ, Simpson DL: The laryngeal mask airway in infants. Anaesthesia 47:849–851, 1992.

243. Keidan I, Fine GF, Kagawa T, et al: Work of breathing during spontaneous ventilation in anesthetized children: A comparative study among the face mask, laryngeal mask airway and endotracheal tube. Anesth Analg 91:1381–1388, 2000.

244. Grebenik CR, Ferguson C, White A: The laryngeal mask airway in pediatric radiotherapy. Anesthesiology 72:474–477, 1990.

245. Walker RW: The laryngeal mask airway in the difficult paediatric airway: An assessment of positioning and use in fibreoptic intubation. Paediatr Anaesth 10:53–58, 2000.

246. Reed JM, O'Connor DM, Myer CM 3rd: Magnetic resonance imaging determination of tracheal orientation in normal children. Practical implications. Arch Otolaryngol Head Neck Surg 122:605–608, 1996.

247. Palme C, Nystrom B, Tunell R: An evaluation of the efficiency of face masks in the resuscitation of newborn infants. Lancet 1:207–210, 1985.

248. Todres ID, Crone RK: Experience with a modified laryngoscope in sick infants. Crit Care Med 9:544–545, 1981.

249. Diaz JH: Further modifications of the Miller blade for difficult pediatric laryngoscopy. Anesthesiology 60:612–613, 1984.

250. Litman RS, Keon TP: Postintubation croup in children. Anesthesiology 75:1122–1123, 1991.

251. Seo K, Someya G, Tanaka Y, et al: Sevoflurane and isoflurane reduce oxygen saturation in infants. Anesth Prog 47:3–7, 2000.

252. Poets CF, Southall DP: Noninvasive monitoring of oxygenation in infants and children: Practical considerations and areas of concern. Pediatrics 93:737–746, 1994.

253. Ayre P: Anaesthesia for intracranial operation. Lancet 1:561, 1937.

254. Rees GJ: Anaesthesia in the newborn. Br Med J 2:1419, 1950.

255. Mapleson WW: The elimination of rebreathing in various semiclosed anaesthetic systems. Br J Anaesth 26:323, 1954.

256. Bain JA, Spoerel WE: Flow requirements for a modified Mapleson D system during controlled ventilation. Can Anaesth Soc J 20:629, 1973.

257. Rasch DK, Bunegin L, Ledbetter J, et al: Comparison of circle absorber and Jackson-Rees systems for paediatric anaesthesia. Can J Anaesth 35:25–30, 1988.

258. Stayer SA, Bent ST, Campos CJ, et al: Comparison of NAD 6000 and servo 900C ventilators in an infant lung model. Anesth Analg 90:315–321, 2000.

259. Narkomed 6000 Operations Manual, Draeger Medical, Inc., 2001.

260. Jeffery MF: Optimal performance of the Narkomed 6000 Divan ventilator for pediatric patients: Choose the right circuit! Clinical Practice Bulletin 8, Drager Medical Inc, 2001.

261. Rosetti VA, Thompson BM, Miller J, et al: Intraosseous infusion: An alternative route of pediatric intravascular access. Ann Emerg Med 14:885–888, 1985.

262. Hodge D 3rd: Intraosseous infusions: A review. Pediatr Emerg Care 1:215–218, 1985.

263. Melker RJ, Miller G, Gearen P, et al: Complications of intraosseous infusion. Ann Emerg Med 19:731–732, 1990.

264. Moscati R, Moore GP: Compartment syndrome with resultant amputation following intraosseous infusion. Am J Emerg Med 8:470–471, 1990.

265. Welborn LG, McGill WA, Hannallah RS, et al: Perioperative blood glucose concentrations in pediatric outpatients. Anesthesiology 65:543–547, 1986.

266. Filston HC: Fluid and electrolyte management in the pediatric surgical patient. Surg Clin North Am 72:1189–1205, 1992.

267. Liu LMP: Pediatric blood and fluid therapy. ASA Refresher Course in Anesthesiology. Philadelphia, JB Lippincott, 1984, p. 112.

268. Bourke DL, Smith TC: Estimating allowable hemodilution. Anesthesiology 41:609–612, 1974.

269. Furman EB, Roman DG, Lemmer LA: Specific therapy in water, electrolyte and blood-volume replacement during pediatric surgery. Anesthesiology 42:187–193, 1975.

270. Gale CC: Neuroendocrine aspects of thermoregulation. Annu Rev Physiol 35:391–430, 1973.

271. Granberg PO: Human endocrine responses to the cold. Arctic Med Res 54:91–103, 1995.

272. Adamsons K, Gandy JM: The influence of thermal factors upon oxygen consumption of the newborn infant. J Pediatr 66:495–508, 1965.

273. Adams AK, Nelson RA, Bell EF, et al: Use of infrared thermographic calorimetry to determine energy expenditure in preterm infants. Am J Clin Nutr 71:969–977, 2000.

274. Sessler DI: Perianesthetic thermoregulation and heat balance in humans. FASEB J 7:638–644, 1993.

275. Hammarlund K, Nilsson GE, Oberg PA: Transepidermal water loss in newborn infants. V. Evaporation from the skin and heat exchange during the first hours of life. Acta Paediatr Scand 69:385–392, 1980.

276. Bissonnette B: Thermoregulation and pediatric anesthesia. Curr Opin Anesthesiol 6:537–542, 1993.

277. Dawkins MJ, Scopes JW: Non-shivering thermogenesis and brown adipose tissue in the human new-born infant. Nature 206:201–202, 1965.

278. Ohlson KB, Mohell N, Cannon B, et al: Thermogenesis in brown adipocytes is inhibited by volatile anesthetic agents. A factor contributing to hypothermia in infants? Anesthesiology 81:176–183, 1994.

279. Borms SF, Engelen SL, Himpe DG, et al: Bair hugger forced-air warming maintains normothermia more effectively than thermo-lite insulation. J Clin Anesth 6:303–307, 1994.

280. Ross AK, Eck JB, Tobias JD: Pediatric regional anesthesia: Beyond the caudal. Anesth Analg 91:16–26, 2000.

281. Solak M, Ulusoy H, Sarihan H: Effects of caudal block on cortisol and prolactin responses to postoperative pain in children. Eur J Pediatr Surg 10:219–223, 2000.

282. Grass JA: The role of epidural anesthesia and analgesia in postoperative outcome. Anesthesiol Clin North America 18:407–428, viii, 2000.

283. Moore DC, Batra MS: The components of an effective test dose prior to epidural block. Anesthesiology 55:693–696, 1981.

284. Reid MF, Harris R, Phillips PD, et al: Day-case herniotomy in children. A comparison of ilio-inguinal nerve block and wound infiltration for post-operative analgesia. Anaesthesia 42:658–661, 1987.

285. Giaufre E, Dalens B, Gombert A: Epidemiology and morbidity of regional anesthesia in children: A one-year prospective survey of the French-Language Society of Pediatric Anesthesiologists. Anesth Analg 83:904–912, 1996.

286. Shandling B, Steward DJ: Regional analgesia for postoperative pain in pediatric outpatient surgery. J Pediatr Surg 15:477–480,1980.

287. Curley J, Castillo J, Hotz J, et al: Prolonged regional nerve blockade. Injectable biodegradable bupivacaine/polyester microspheres. Anesthesiology 84:1401–1410, 1996.

288. Abajian JC, Mellish RW, Browne AF, et al: Spinal anesthesia for surgery in the high-risk infant. Anesth Analg 63:359–362, 1984.

289. Somri M, Gaitini L, Vaida S, et al: Postoperative outcome in high-risk infants undergoing herniorrhaphy: Comparison between spinal and general anaesthesia. Anaesthesia 53:762–766, 1998.

290. William JM, Stoddart PA, Williams SA, et al: Post-operative recovery after inguinal herniotomy in ex-premature infants: Comparison between sevoflurane and spinal anaesthesia. Br J Anaesth 86:366–371, 2001.

291. Kokki H, Hendolin H: Comparison of 25 G and 29 G Quincke spinal needles in paediatric day case surgery. A prospective randomized study of the puncture characteristics, success rate and postoperative complaints. Paediatr Anaesth 6:115–119, 1996.

292. Aldrete JA, Kroulik D: A postanesthetic recovery score. Anesth Analg 49:924, 1974.

293. Rackow H, Salinitre E, Green LT: Frequency of cardiac arrest associated with anesthesia in infants and children: Report of 66 original cases. Pediatrics 28:697, 1961.

294. Rivera R, Tibballs J: Complications of endotracheal intubation and mechanical ventilation in infants and children. Crit Care Med 20:193–199, 1992.

295. Jones R, Bodnar A, Roan Y, et al: Subglottic stenosis in newborn intensive care unit graduates. Am J Dis Child 135:367–368, 1981.

TRANSPORT OF VENTILATED INFANTS

GARY PETTETT, MD
GERALD B. MERENSTEIN, MD

For nearly 2 decades the neonatal mortality rate has steadily declined. Improved survival, especially among lower-birthweight infants, has been associated with the development of regional neonatal intensive care centers.[1-4]

Interhospital transport services are an integral part of regional organization. Early identification and transfer of critically ill infants to an intensive care center significantly reduces regional neonatal morbidity and mortality.[1]

The neonatal transport service functions as an extension of the newborn intensive care unit (NICU) and is designed to provide tertiary-level care throughout its referral region. In the United States, the majority of births occur in hospitals that lack the personnel, equipment, or facilities for newborn intensive care. It is estimated that 6% of all newborn infants require some form of resuscitation or transfer to a NICU.[6] The number increases dramatically as birthweight diminishes. As many as 80% of babies weighing less than 1500 g may require some form of resuscitation at birth. Despite efforts to identify high-risk pregnancies as early in gestation as possible, nearly one third of all very-low-birthweight infants continue to be delivered in community hospitals that are not equipped to manage critically ill infants.[7] Rapidly advancing labor, undiagnosed fetal disorders, and unanticipated complications, including neonatal asphyxia, continue to be significant causes of perinatal morbidity and mortality. Nearly half of those infants who require resuscitation have no evidence of fetal distress before delivery and are born to mothers who were believed to be at low risk for perinatal complications.[6,8] For infants who require transport, the care they receive in the early postnatal period can have an important influence on subsequent morbidity and mortality. Adequate resuscitation and stabilization before transfer lowers morbidity and improves the chances of survival.[9-11]

With the introduction of newer treatment modalities, advances in technology, and a more aggressive approach to perinatal care, the number of critically ill infants requiring transport has increased significantly. Better medical and surgical care has altered the perinatal management and has improved survival for many anomalies and other illnesses with high mortality rates. This increasingly complex intensive care environment requires more sophisticated transport equipment and more highly trained transport personnel to ensure a proper continuum of care.

Pulmonary disorders continue to be the most common problems encountered in the transport of critically ill infants. In 1978, Hackel[12] estimated that as many as 45% of all transported infants required some form of ventilatory assistance. Today, respiratory disease and the need for some measure of ventilatory support still account for approximately 50% of all newborn transports (Neonatal Transport Service, Children's Mercy Hospital, Kansas City, MO, USA). This chapter reviews the basic elements of support and stabilization for infants who require ventilatory assistance during transport. More detailed discussions of pathophysiology or clinical management of specific diseases can be found in other chapters of this book.

TRANSPORT TEAM

The transport team must be adequately trained and equipped to provide supportive care for a wide variety of neonatal disorders and their potential complications. Informal, poorly organized transport services are hazardous and may seriously jeopardize an infant's condition.[9] Basic prerequisites for transport personnel include proficiencies in pathophysiologic mechanisms of neonatal disease, technical skills of tertiary care, and principles of clinical management in the transport environment. Team members should be skilled in neonatal resuscitation and stabilization and should be capable of modifying treatment algorithms to fit the transport setting.

The importance of adequate training for transport personnel is well recognized.[9,10,13] Most transport services use experienced NICU nursing personnel as the nucleus of their team. NICU experience is supplemented with additional cognitive training, skills workshops, situational scenarios, and a period of closely supervised transport experience. However, NICU experience, even when supplemented with additional training, may not be sufficient to maintain expertise in the transport environment. Many of the unique challenges encountered during transport (excessive noise, vibration and rotation forces, low-level lighting, and variable ambient temperatures/humidity) are difficult to simulate during classroom training. Team members should participate in transports with sufficient regularity to maintain both their technical skills and their ability to treat patients effectively in various transport settings (e.g., ambulance, aircraft, or community hospital). High-volume transport services have the advantage of developing full-time transport teams dedicated solely to neonatal transport. Smaller services that use team members on a more infrequent basis need to invest considerably more time and effort in the maintenance of technical skills and decision-making processes. The number of personnel assigned to the transport service may need to be adjusted to ensure that each team member has sufficient opportunities to maintain his or her experience in the transport environment.

Neonatal transports are most efficient when the transport team consists of at least two individuals. At the referring hospital, one individual (transport nurse/physician) can assess a patient and complete necessary procedures (e.g., peripheral intravenous lines, Chemstrip, blood gas analysis) while the other (respiratory therapist, paramedic, emergency medical technician) tends to administrative procedures (e.g., medical records, charting) and prepares the transport incubator and monitoring systems to transport the infant. Because pulmonary disorders affect approximately half of all transported infants, neonatal respiratory therapists seem to be the most logical additions to the transport team. For infants who require ventilatory support, the respiratory therapist provides expertise in the management of both the airway and the respiratory support equipment (e.g., ventilator, oxygen [O_2] source, oxyhood). When ventilatory assistance is not necessary, the respiratory therapist has been cross-trained to assist the transport nurse with basic stabilization of the infant in preparation for transport. Whatever composition is chosen, transport participants should be cross-trained and capable of supporting all transport procedures. All transport personnel should participate in the same selection, training, and evaluation processes.

For various reasons, physicians (attending staff or neonatal fellows) and advanced practice nurses are best used only when the need for their additional expertise can be reasonably anticipated. With a well-trained, experienced transport team, fewer than 10% of all transports may require physician or nurse practitioner involvement.

EQUIPMENT

Basic support equipment and medications for interhospital transport are listed in Tables 27-1 to 27-3. Medications and consumable supplies can be carried in a well-organized transport box or lightweight backpacks (Fig. 27-1).

The safety and efficiency of neonatal transport are dependent on the availability of properly functioning equipment. One of the most important nontransport functions of team members is equipment maintenance. Equipment and supplies to be used during transport should be ready to go at all times. Consumable supplies should be checked and replenished after every transport. The incubator, monitors, and ventilatory equipment should be regularly reviewed for preventive maintenance and periodically tested for proper function. Portable battery-powered electronic devices should be plugged into power supplies for charging when not in use. The capacity of gas cylinders (air and O_2) should be checked both before and after each transport. Tanks should be labeled with their current status (full, used, empty) and replaced with new tanks if insufficient volume remains.

The transport incubator is the centerpiece of support equipment. Modular transport incubators have largely replaced the ingeniously fabricated but often cumbersome transport systems of the past. Many of the larger equipment items listed in Table 27-2 can be incorporated into the modular incubator and may be more economical to purchase as an integrated unit. Transport personnel should be thoroughly familiar with the equipment used in transport. Diagnosing and troubleshooting the most common types of malfunction should be part of their training program. Many of these devices have been incorporated into the transport environment but have not been system-

TABLE 27-1. Supplies

Feeding tubes (5, 6, 8 French)	Intravenous arm boards
Arterial catheters (3.5, 5 French)	Angiocatheters (18, 22, 24 gauge)
Three-way stopcock	Trocars (10, 12 French)
Catheter adapters (18, 20, 21)	Intravenous extension tubing, T-connectors
Scalp vein needle (21, 23, 25)	Buretrol
Plastic medicine cups	Bulb syringe
Intravenous pump tubing	Sterile gauze (roll)
Alcohol swabs	Tape measure
Cotton balls	K-Y jelly
Band-Aids	Scissors
Umbilical tape	Hemostats
Clear tape (½ inch, 1 inch)	Pencil flashlight
Alcohol	Intravenous fluids ($D_{10}W$, D_5W, NS), 500-mL resuscitation bags
Povidine-iodine solution	Tuberculin syringe with needles
Tincture of benzoin	Gauze swabs (2 × 2 inches, 4 × 4 inches)
Lancets	Thermometer
Chemstrips	Pacifier
Capillary tubes	Monitor electrodes
Umbilical catheters, single and double lumen (3.5, 5 French)	Nasal CPAP prongs (small, large)*
Butterfly needles (19, 23, 25 gauge)	Spare laryngoscope bulbs*
Alcohol and Betadine swabs	Spare laryngoscope batteries*
Meconium aspirator	Endotracheal tubes and adapters (2.5, 3.0, 3.5, 4.0 mm)*
Omphalocele bag (sterile)	Bayonette or Magill forceps*
Capillary and blood collection tubes	Thoracostomy tubes*
Stockinette caps	Heimlich valves*
Suction catheters (6, 8 French)	Y-connectors*
Sterile gloves (sizes 6–8)	5-to-1 (Christmas tree) adapter*
Syringes (1, 3, 5, 10 mL)	Oxygen tubing*
Safety pins, rubber bands	Umbilical catheter tray
	Thoracostomy tray*

* Supplies needed specifically for respiratory support.
CPAP, continuous positive airway pressure.

atically tested for either durability or reliability. Monitors with lighted display screens may be subject to distortion from motion or vibrational and rotational forces. Vital signs and other measurements reported by these instruments may be inaccurate and could require a more direct method of assessment. The use of physiologic monitoring systems during air transport may present a risk for electromagnetic interference with aircraft navigational or other flight instruments. The flight crew and transport team should be aware of the potential for electric interference and should coordinate their efforts to minimize the chance of in-flight errors. Recurrent equipment problems should be noted in transport records so that they can be addressed by the hospital biomedical maintenance staff, equipment manufacturer, or appropriate regulatory agencies.

The Bio-Med MVP-10 ventilator is the prototypic transport ventilator for infants (Fig. 27-2). This system offers the advantage of a simple integrated unit with a time-cycled, pressure-limited fluidic ventilator requiring only 3 L/min of flow to activate. The ventilator itself is small (8 × 9 × 3 inches) and lightweight (2.3 kg) and provides capability for intermittent positive-pressure ventilation, intermittent mandatory ventilation, positive end-expiratory pressure, and continuous positive airway pressure (CPAP). The MVP-10 has been incorporated into many of the most popular modular transport incubators. In this modular design, gases for the ventilator can be supplied by E cylinders of air and O_2, which are mounted directly on the transport incubator frame. One full E cylinder of O_2 lasts approx-

TABLE 27-2.   Equipment

Oxygen face mask (0, 1, 2)*	Oxygen tubing
Manual resuscitation apparatus	Pulse oximeter sensors and cable
Nebulizer*	Laryngoscope blades (no. 0,
Laryngoscope (penlight handle)	no. 1)
Oxygen cylinder wrench*	Laryngoscope bulbs
Battery-operated intravenous	Dry cell batteries (various sizes)
pump	Electrocardiogram leads
Chemical warming mattress	Oxygen–air blender*
Radiant heat shield	Oxygen monitor*
Oxygen hood*	Cardiorespiratory monitor
Infant Magill forceps	Airway pressure monitor*
Pulse oximeter	Incubator with built-in ventilator
Blood pressure monitor,	Adequate cylinders of oxygen
disposable cuffs (sizes 2–5)	and air with appropriate
Oral airways	fittings, flow and pressure
	gauges*
	Nitric oxide delivery system

* Equipment needed for ventilatory support in transport.

TABLE 27-3.   Drugs

5% Albumin
Adenosine
Calcium chloride 10%
$D_{10}W$ (250 mL)
Digoxin 100 μg/mL
Epinephrine, 1:10,000
Furosemide (Lasix), 10 mg/mL
Naloxone (Narcan), 0.02 mg/mL
Dopamine, 200-mg vial
Atropine, 0.1 mg/mL
Phenytoin (Dilantin), 250 mg/5 mL
Sodium bicarbonate 4.2%, 10 mL
Sodium chloride, 3 mEq/mL
Sodium phenobarbital, 65 mg/mL (powder)
Vitamin K (AquaMEPHYTON)
Lactated Ringer's solution, 250 mL
Water for injection
Calcium gluconate
Isotonic saline vials, 20 mL
Ampicillin
Gentamicin/cefotaxime
Dobutamine
Surfactant
Heparin flush solution
Lacri-Lube
Lidocaine 1%
Adenosine
Aminophylline
Pancuronium bromide (Pavulon)
Midazolam (Versed)
Morphine
Fentanyl
Diazepam (Valium)

imately 1 hour at a flow rate of 10 L/min. The mounted E cylinders should be used only when an infant is being transferred to or from the transport vehicle. In transport, ventilatory gases should be obtained from larger H or M cylinders, which are part of the ambulance of aircraft configuration. Table 27-4 lists the characteristics and expected life of various sizes of gas cylinders at differing flow rates. Familiarity with this information may be particularly important for longer transports or for infants who require higher concentrations of inspired O_2 (FIO_2).

In addition to the mechanical ventilator, proper equipment for manual ventilation should be available on all transports. An anesthesia bag, tubing of appropriate sizes, a pressure manometer, endotracheal adaptors, and various sizes of face masks should be part of the transport equipment inventory. For infants who require ventilatory assistance, brief periods of manual support may be necessary during initial stabilization, when moving the infant between the bed and incubator, or while ventilator adjustments are being made. As with all mechanical devices, the possibility of an unexpected ventilator failure exists. The manual ventilation apparatus should be fully assembled in the incubator for immediate use if necessary. We suggest having manual ventilatory support readily available on all transports, regardless of an infant's respiratory status, as a reasonable precaution before transport.

The inability to monitor or assess oxygenation has been a significant problem in transporting infants who require ventilatory assistance. The development of pulse oximetry as a noninvasive method for continually monitoring arterial O_2 saturation has become one of the more important technologic advances applicable to the transport environment. Pulse oximetry has been shown to be a safe, accurate, and reliable method of O_2 monitoring of infants in special care nurseries.[14] Compared with transcutaneous monitoring, pulse oximetry is a more reliable device for both unstable and chronically ill infants.[15] Pulse oximetry is also less cumbersome to apply than the heated sensor of transcutaneous monitors and requires less rigorous calibration to initiate monitoring. The incorporation of pulse oximetry into standard cardiorespiratory monitors and the availability of lightweight pulse oximetry units makes this technology readily adaptable to the transport setting.

TRANSPORT VEHICLE

The selection of the transport vehicle is based on various factors: weather conditions, terrain, distance, size of the transport team, ground traffic, and vehicle availability. The transport vehicle must be designed to allow for the continuation of patient care throughout transfer.

Appropriate adapters must be available to connect transport equipment to the ambulance/aircraft power and gas supply. Lockdown devices ensure stability of the transport incubator while the vehicle is in motion and prevent shifts should sudden decelerations or accelerations occur. For busy transport services, the use of mobile intensive care units specifically designed for pediatric or neonatal intensive care can solve most of the problems related to equipment and vehicle compatibility. Standard ambulances for transporting adult patients may not meet the special needs of neonatal transport equipment and may require prior planning or modification for additional battery power, ventilatory gases, and stabilization of the incubator. Total transport time is an important additional factor to consider in vehicle selection. The transport team should maintain a record of average vehicle-specific transport times for their most frequent referral sources and provides those estimates to the referring hospital/physician when accepting a patient for transfer. Updated estimates of anticipated arrival time can be provided as the team leaves the center or while in route (longer transports) so that the referring hospital can make appropriate plans for continuation of the infant's care.

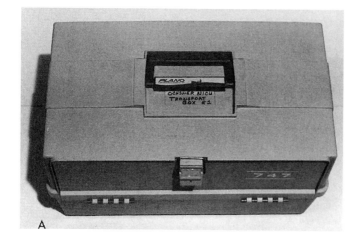

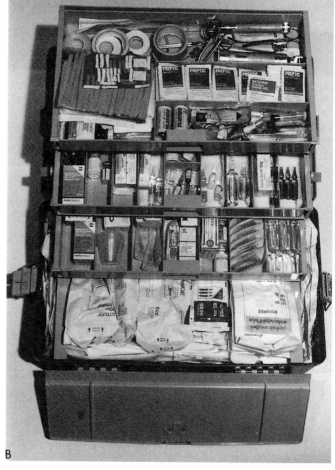

Figure 27-1. Transport box. *A,* Closed. *B,* Open.

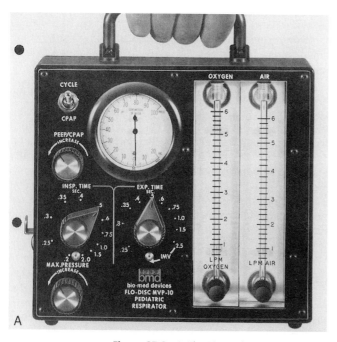

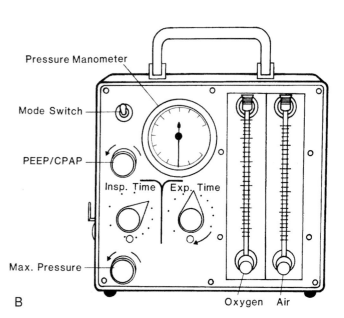

Figure 27-2. *A,* The Bio-Med MVP-10 handheld portable respirator. (Courtesy of Bio-Med Devices, Inc., Madison, CT, USA.) *B,* Diagram of front panel. PEEP/CPAP, positive end-expiratory pressure/continuous positive airway pressure.

TABLE 27-4. Characteristics of Portable Gas Cylinders

	Specifications of Oxygen Cylinders (E, M, H Type)					
	Capacity					
Cylinder Type	(cu ft)	(gal)	(L)	Height (Inches)	Diameter (Inches)	Weight of Full Tank (lb)
E	22	165	620	20	4–1/4	15
M	122	900	3450	46	7–1/8	86
H	244	1800	6900	55	9	130

	Volume and Flow Duration of Oxygen in Three Cylinder Sizes											
	Full			¾			½			¼		
Cylinder Type	E	M	H	E	M	H	E	M	H	E	M	H
Contents (cu ft)	22	107	244	16.5	80.2	193	11	53.5	122	5.5	26.8	6
Liters	622	3028	6900	466.5	2271	5175	311	1514	3450	155.5	757	172
Pressure (psi)		2000			1500			1000			500	

	Approximate Number of Hours of Flow in Three Cylinder Sizes											
	Full			¾			½			¼		
Cylinder Type	E	M	H	E	M	H	E	M	H	E	M	H
Flow Rate(L/min)												
2	5.1	25	56	3.8	18.5	42	2.5	12.5	28	1.3	6	14
4	2.5	12.6	28	1.8	10.4	21	1.2	6.3	14	0.6	3.1	7
6	1.7	8.4	18.5	1.3	6.3	13.7	0.9	4.2	9.2	0.4	2.1	4.5
8	1.2	6.3	14	0.9	4.6	10.5	0.6	3.1	7	0.3	1.5	3.5
10	1	5	11	0.7	3.7	8.2	0.5	2.5	5.5	0.2	1.2	2.7
12	0.8	4.2	9.2	0.6	3	6.7	0.4	2.1	4.5	0.2	1	2.2
15	0.6	3.4	7.2	0.4	2.5	5.5	0.3	1.7	3.5	0.1	0.8	1.7

RESUSCITATION AND STABILIZATION

Adequate resuscitation and stabilization of critically ill newborn infants has an important bearing on their survival and their ability to tolerate transport. The American Academy of Pediatrics and the American Heart Association have developed a detailed stepwise training program (Neonatal Resuscitation Program) to teach delivery room personnel basic resuscitation and stabilization of newborn infants[16] (see Chapter 4). Implementation of this or similar programs in hospitals that provide obstetric services can help ensure that proper equipment and adequately trained personnel are available at all deliveries. Members of the transport team should be proficient in resuscitation and should be capable of modifying treatment algorithms to fit the transport environment.

For high-risk infants who do not require resuscitation, efforts should be directed toward stabilizing the infant for transport. *Stabilization* is defined as the identification of those factors that, if not corrected, may lead to deterioration of the infant's condition. Important factors in the stabilization process include the following:

• Maintenance of ventilation and oxygenation
• Correction of acid–base disorders
• Treatment of pulmonary air leaks
• Cardiovascular support
• Thermal support
• Metabolic support

An unhurried assessment of each of these factors followed by appropriate corrective actions can prevent more serious intratransport problems. Stabilization of infants who require ventilatory support may include radiographic studies to assess or diagnose lung disease and to localize the placement of intravascular catheters, an endotracheal tube, or a thoracostomy drainage tube. Despite the inherent tendency to expedite the transport process, time spent stabilizing infants before leaving the referring hospital is an important investment in a safe and effective transport. No matter how small the referring unit or how limited its resources, the local environment is generally free of constraints found in transport vehicles (noise, motion, poor lighting, limited space).

Ventilation and Oxygenation

The transition from fetal to neonatal life is associated with a series of complex physiologic changes. Although respiratory gas exchange often stabilizes with the first 5 hours of life, complete cardiopulmonary adaptation may require much of the first 24 hours of postnatal life. Even at completion of these adaptive changes, newborn infants still have significant alveolar-arterial O_2 differences, which may be attributable to continuing venoarterial (fetal) shunts or perfusion of persistently atelectatic lung segments.[17] The magnitude of these ventilation-perfusion abnormalities is higher in infants born prematurely.[18]

Events that prevent or delay the completion of this transitional process may interfere with respiratory gas exchange. Clinical manifestations of impaired respiratory function include cyanosis, tachypnea, chest wall retractions, and audible expiratory grunting.

Stabilization of infants with signs of respiratory distress begins by ensuring a clear and secure airway. Fluid and particulate matter should be cleared from the mouth (first), oropharynx, and nose using either a bulb syringe or suction catheter. Infants who are born through thick, meconium-stained amniotic fluid should have their upper airway cleared on the perineum or abdomen (cesarean section) before the chest and remainder of the body are delivered.[19,20] Immediately after delivery, the vocal cords should be visualized and particulate matter cleared (suctioned) from the area just above the cords. Endotracheal intubation and suctioning of the lower airway with a meconium aspirator can remove aspirated material from below the vocal cords and prevent or diminish the severity of subsequent respiratory disease.[21] When meconium-stained fluid is found in the lower airway, repeated efforts to remove additional material must be weighed against the infant's clinical status. Repeated endotracheal suctioning should be coordinated with respiratory (oxygenation) and cardiovascular (heart rate, perfusion) support to minimize the potential hypoxic-ischemic organ damage.

Anatomic obstruction of the airway may occur in infants with micrognathia, macroglossia, and cleft palate (Pierre Robin sequence, Beckwith-Coombs syndrome) or a choanal atresia. Positioning these infants in the prone position, which allows gravitational forces to pull the chin and tongue away from the posterior oropharynx, may help keep the airway patent. If positioning is ineffective, insertion of a plastic oral airway or endotracheal tube may be necessary to keep the tongue away from the posterior pharynx and airway.[5] In rare infants with severe micrognathia, glossoptosis, and an intact palate, intubation can be exceedingly difficult, and emergency tracheotomy may be required to secure an effective airway.

Proper positioning may be important in small premature infants. Airway obstruction can occur as a result of poor tongue control and from excessive flexion or extension of the neck. Prone positioning and stabilization of the head and neck help maintain an adequate airway in spontaneously breathing premature infants who do not require intubation.

Excessive secretions may be a significant problem in infants with esophageal atresia and a blind upper pouch. An oral or nasal feeding tube should be inserted into the upper pouch and secretions cleared before the infant is moved. During transport, the tube should be connected to continuous or intermittent suction to keep the pouch and upper airway free of secretions.

Measurement of arterial blood gases [pH, arterial partial pressure of oxygen (Pao_2), partial pressure of carbon dioxide ($Paco_2$)] is the most sensitive method for assessing respiratory gas exchange and should be performed in any infant who exhibits signs of respiratory distress. If the Pao_2 is less than 60 mm Hg, supplemental O_2 should be provided. The Fio_2 can be regulated by the use of an air–O_2 blender. To prevent unnecessary heat loss and the development of thick, dry airway secretions, supplemental O_2 should be heated (to body temperature) and humidified during administration.

Cyanosis involving the trunk and mucous membranes is an indication of significant hypoxemia. Visible cyanosis occurs when desaturated hemoglobin levels reach 3 to 5 g/dL. Assuming an otherwise normal hemoglobin concentration (15 g/dL), the appearance of cyanosis corresponds with an O_2 saturation of 75% to 80% (or less) and a Pao_2 that may be as low as 30 to 50 mm Hg. Cyanotic infants should be administered O_2 in sufficient amount the relieve the cyanosis. Documentation of hypoxemia and desaturation by arterial blood gas is helpful but should not significantly delay oxygen administration.

Continuous O_2 administration should be accompanied by frequent assessment of arterial oxygenation or periodic blood gas analysis. Pulse oximetry provides a rapid, continuous, and noninvasive method of monitoring arterial oxygenation (saturation). In the absence of significant acidosis or hypercarbia, pulse oximetry may reduce the need for frequent arterial blood gas sampling. What saturation values should be accepted as normal or safe and representative of appropriate oxygenation remains uncertain.[15] Levels of O_2 saturation that may seem clinically acceptable can be associated with Pao_2 low enough to produce increased pulmonary vascular resistance. Because of high hemoglobin F levels, saturations of 85% to 90% in newborn infants correspond with Pao_2 of only 35 to 45 mm Hg. Conversely, when saturations reach 100%, reliable estimates of Pao_2 or the degree of hyperoxia are no longer possible. In preterm infants younger than 1 week of age, saturations of ≥92% were associated with Pao_2 as low as 46 mm Hg, whereas saturations of ≥97% were associated with Pao_2 as high as 122 mm Hg.[14] To restrict Pao_2 values to ≥60 mm Hg and ≤90 mm Hg, a conventionally acceptable range, saturations by pulse oximetry should be maintained between 94% and 98%, a difficult task in an NICU and perhaps even more so in a transport vehicle.

Oxygen requirements that exceed 0.60 Fio_2 to maintain a Pao_2 greater than 60 mm Hg suggest a need for more effective ventilatory support. Infants with respiratory distress syndrome (RDS) or extensive atelectasis may benefit from CPAP.[22] In larger infants (>1500 g), CPAP may be administered through nasal prongs. Smaller infants and those who do not respond to nasal CPAP may benefit from intubation and direct endotracheal CPAP. CPAP should begin at 4 to 5 cm H_2O and can be increased slowly to a maximum of 8 to 10 cm H_2O with careful monitoring of both Pao_2 and $Paco_2$ (see Chapter 8).

Although apnea is a relative contraindication to CPAP, some infants may respond to the initiation of stretch receptor reflexes in the lower airways with spontaneous respirations.[23] CPAP should be used with caution and vigilance in transported infants with significant air trapping (e.g., aspiration syndromes). Overdistention of lung segments with trapped air may increase the risk of pulmonary air leaks.

The decision to intubate an infant should be made before leaving the referring institution. Indications for endotracheal intubation include apnea, progressive respiratory failure ($Paco_2$ >60 mm Hg, Pao_2 <60 mm Hg in Fio_2 of 1.0), CPAP failure, and severe respiratory distress. Elective intubation may be considered whenever an infant's clinical condition suggests that it may be necessary before arrival at the intensive care unit. Endotracheal tubes may be inserted through either the nose or mouth. Although nasotracheal tubes tend to be more stable and inadvertent extubation is less likely, proper attention to tube position is necessary to prevent damage to the nares and turbinates.[24,25]

Differentiating severe pulmonary disease from cyanotic congenital heart disease can be difficult. A large cardiac shadow on a chest radiograph, heart murmur, profound cyanosis without significant respiratory distress, failure to respond to high ambient O_2 concentrations (hyperoxia test), and hypoxemia with a normal pH and $Paco_2$ all are suggestive of congenital heart disease. Although infants with heart disease will not likely be harmed by ventilatory support, seemingly small increases in Pao_2 may adversely affect infants with ductal-dependent cardiac lesions. When the probability of cardiac disease is high, the use of a prostaglandin E_1 infusion

(0.05 to 0.1 µg/kg/min) to maintain ductal patency may be warranted until more definitive studies can be performed.

Acid–Base Disorders

Infants who have experienced fetal or intrapartum distress frequently present with a mixed respiratory and metabolic acidosis. Early neonatal respiratory disease can aggravate this process, resulting in more severe acidosis. Alterations in acid–base balance may have profound effects on the circulation and respiratory gas exchange. Severe acidosis (pH <7.05, base deficit >15 mEq/L) and hypercapnia ($Paco_2$ >50 mm Hg) impair cardiac function and diminish pulmonary blood flow.

Correction of acid–base disorders may require the use of assisted ventilation and the administration of a buffering agent. $Paco_2$ is a function of minute ventilation. Ventilatory adjustments that increase tidal volume or respiratory rate improve carbon dioxide elimination and lower $Paco_2$. When ventilation ($Paco_2$) can be controlled, sodium bicarbonate is an effective buffering agent.[26] Sodium bicarbonate should be administered as a 0.5 mEq/mL solution and infused at a rate of approximately 1 mL/kg/min (to a maximum of 5 mEq/kg) or as a single (slow) bolus infusion of 1 to 3 mEq/kg. Rapid infusion of bicarbonate may create significant disparities in extracellular and intracellular pH and further reduce cardiac contractility.[27,28] Administration of more concentrated solutions (0.9 mEq/mL) may result in transient hypernatremia[29–31] and may increase the risk of intraventricular hemorrhage in small premature infants.[32,33] If blood gas results are available, the dose of buffer can be calculated from the following equation:

$$mEq \text{ buffer} = 0.3 \times \text{body weight (kg)} \times \text{base deficit (mEq/L)}.$$

Pulmonary Air Leak

Extravasation of air into the lung parenchyma and plural spaces is a serious and potentially life-threatening complication. Air leaks originate in overdistended segments of the lung. Rupture of small airways or respiratory saccules allows air to escape into the pulmonary interstitium. From the interstitium, air migrates along the neurovascular and peribronchial channels toward the hilum, where it can enter the mediastinum or pleural and pericardial spaces. Depending on their location, pulmonary air leaks can have a profound effect on an infant's respiration and circulation (see Chapter 21).

Pneumothorax occurs when free air accumulates between the parenchymal and parietal pleura. Clinical symptoms depend on the size of the pneumothorax and the amount of tension produced. Small, low-tension pneumothoraces may occur in as many as 15% to 20% of otherwise healthy infants with no underlying pulmonary disease. Not infrequently, many of these infants have received some form of positive-pressure ventilation during stabilization. Symptoms most often consist of mild tachypnea, which leads to discovery of a small pneumothorax on a diagnostic chest radiograph. Most of these small pneumothoraces resolve spontaneously and do not require specific treatment. Thoracentesis may damage underlying lung and aggravate the size of the pneumothorax. Oxygen supplementation occasionally may be needed to maintain O_2 saturation or Pao_2; however, there is no convincing evidence that prolonged exposure to a high Fio_2 (1.00) hastens resolution.

Larger pneumothoraces, which invariably generate a significant amount of intrapleural tension, occur in infants with underlying lung disease and are most frequent in those infants who require ventilatory assistance. Increasing pressure in the pleural space collapses the lung, depresses the hemidiaphragm on the affected side, and causes the mediastinum and great vessels to shift toward the contralateral side. High intrathoracic pressures impede venous return and interrupt respiratory gas exchange in the collapsed lung. Signs of a tension pneumothorax include sudden deterioration in an infant's condition (profound cyanosis and increased respiratory effort) and lateral shift in heart tones and the point of maximal impulse. Blood gas analysis reveals an unexplained increase in $Paco_2$ and diminished oxygenation. Restoration of adequate gas exchange requires immediate relief of intrapleural pressure. Localization of air may be determined from clinical signs (shifted heart tones), differential transillumination of the hemithoraces,[35] or radiographic examination. When none of these alternatives is readily available, thoracentesis with a butterfly or angiocatheter needle attached to an underwater seal may be diagnostic. Evacuation of a tension pneumothorax generally requires placement of a thoracostomy drainage tube. The tube should be connected to an underwater seal to prevent reaccumulation during transport. Clinical evidence of improved respiration or radiographic confirmation of resolution should be obtained before transporting the infant. Although pneumothorax might be expected to occur more frequently during air transport because of changes in barometric pressure with altitude, this hypothesis has not been confirmed.

Air that dissects into the pericardium (pneumopericardium) may produce signs of cardiac tamponade (diminished pulses, distant heart sounds, poor perfusion) and is an equally emergent condition. Pericardiocentesis is necessary to remove the air and relieve pericardial pressure. Recurrence of pneumopericardium is possible but less likely than for tension pneumothorax. Once the pressure has been relieved, careful monitoring of cardiac function is imperative.

Air that remains trapped in the pulmonary interstitium presents as pulmonary interstitial emphysema, which is diagnosed by the appearance of small linear streaks of air in the lung parenchyma on chest radiographs. Accumulation of interstitial air may lead to reduced lung compliance and poor gas exchange. Although there is no specific treatment, severe pulmonary interstitial emphysema confined to one lung may be treated by unilateral intubation of the unaffected lung. Unilateral intubation should be attempted only when absolutely necessary and under the supervision of experienced personnel.

Accumulations of mediastinal air (pneumomediastinum) may be large and occasionally difficult to differentiate from pneumothoraces. A cross-table lateral chest radiograph may be helpful in demonstrating anterior (substernal) mediastinal air. Pneumomediastinum may cause or exacerbate respiratory symptoms but does not generally lead to acute deterioration. Removal of air by transthoracic needle aspiration is rarely helpful and presents a significant risk for developing mediastinitis. A pneumomediastinum may, however, be the antecedent of a tension pneumothorax. The transport team should be aware of this potential risk and should be prepared to diagnose and relieve a pneumothorax should it occur.

Cardiovascular Support

Assessment of the circulation in infants with acute pulmonary disease can be difficult. Oxygen, carbon dioxide, and the hydrogen ion concentration all have direct effects on the cardiovascular system that may either mimic or mask vascular compromise.

Control of respiratory gas exchange and correction of acid–base disturbances are important prerequisites to determining the need for volume expansion or other cardiovascular support.

Low blood pressure, persistent metabolic acidosis, diminished urine output (<1 mL/kg/hour), cool and pale extremities, delayed cutaneous capillary refill, and tachycardia are the most frequent signs of hypovolemia. With severe acidosis, peripheral vasoconstriction may result in falsely elevated extremity blood pressures. An umbilical artery catheter attached to a pressure transducer and monitor display is more likely to reveal both low pressures and a narrowed aortic waveform indicative of low vascular volume.[36] Changes in hematocrit often do not reflect either the severity or extent of acute volume losses. A low or falling hematocrit generally appears after administration of crystalloid or colloid volume expanders and revascularization of interstitial fluid. A low central venous (right atrial) pressure[37] or central venous oxygen tension[38] measured through an umbilical venous catheter can be helpful in differentiating hypovolemic shock from that due to factors such as cardiac tamponade, pneumopericardium, pneumothorax, or an overdistended lung. Distinguishing hypovolemic shock from septic (distributive) shock can be extremely difficult. Appropriate antibiotics should be started in infants with hypotension/shock until appropriate cultures or other studies to assess the possibility of infection can be performed.

The objective in treating hypovolemia is prompt restoration of tissue perfusion and oxygenation. Volume expansion and cardiovascular support should be initiated rapidly enough to prevent secondary effects of hypoperfusion (increased capillary permeability and acute pulmonary damage). However, volume expansion that is too rapid may be equally deleterious. Rapid administration of volume expanders may not allow the peripheral vascular bed to adjust to the acutely increased vascular volume. Capillary engorgement and hemorrhage may result from the rapid expansion of vascular beds that are already maximally vasodilated. Especially vulnerable locations in small infants include the germinal matrix and periventricular area of the brain, resulting in intraventricular hemorrhage.

Whole blood is the ideal volume expander, providing both vascular volume (plasma) and red blood cells for O_2 delivery to the tissues. Repeated small infusions of blood (5 mL/kg over 5 minutes) cross-matched against the mother before delivery is the fluid of choice for newborn infants.[39] Type O Rh-negative blood traditionally has been used as the universal donor blood, but reports of occasional reactions from minor group incompatibilities warrant caution. In the absence of whole blood, packed red blood cells are a reasonable alternative. Equal volumes of packed cells and 5% albumin or normal saline provide both volume expansion and added O_2-carrying capacity. If crystalloid or colloid solutions are the only solutions available, packed red blood cells still need to be given at a later time to replace lost or diminished cell volume.

Restoration of the circulation should be monitored closely. Reperfusion of previously constricted vascular beds often leads to mobilization of lactic and pyruvic acids. Despite clinical evidence of improved perfusion, both pH and the base excess (deficit) may fall. Additional buffer base may be needed to correct the acid–base balance. Infants who continue to demonstrate poor cardiovascular function despite volume expansion and acid–base adjustment may benefit from additional pharmacologic support. Administration of dopamine at low infusion rates (3 to 5 µg/kg/min) may provide peripheral vascular support while preserving renal perfusion and minimizing inotropic activity. If low perfusion is thought to have a significant cardiogenic component, dobutamine can be administered either alone or in conjunction with dopamine to improve cardiac output and tissue perfusion and prevent renal or mesenteric vasoconstriction.

Thermal Support

The ideal thermal environment for a newborn infant is defined as the range of ambient temperatures within which metabolic rate (O_2 consumption) is at a minimum and temperature regulation is achieved by nonevaporative vasomotor processes.[40] Differences in birthweight, intrauterine growth, and postnatal age all influence the minimal metabolic rate and thermoneutral temperatures.[41] Weight-specific thermoneutral temperatures range from 32° to 34°C for 3-kg infants to 35° to 36°C for 1-kg infants (Appendix 12).

Heat production in newborn infants occurs in the metabolic activity of brown fat stores located in the neck and the interscapular and perirenal areas.[42] Heat produced in these fat stores warms the perfusing capillary blood, which disseminates the heat throughout the body. Brown fat is characterized by both a high metabolic rate and high blood flow. Hypoxemic or hypovolemic infants may be incapable of supplying sufficient O_2 or blood flow to brown fat stores to maintain core body temperature. Low-birthweight infants have diminished brown fat stores and larger surface-to-body mass ratio, which increases their risk for uncompensated heat loss.[43,44]

Controlled clinical trials have demonstrated the importance of thermal support in decreasing morbidity and mortality among small or acutely ill infants.[43–45] Conservation of body heat can be facilitated by minimizing conductive, convective, radiant, and evaporative heat loss during transport. Conductive heat can be minimized by preheating the transport incubator bed and blankets or by using a chemical heating mattress. Convective losses are diminished by avoiding direct air (ambient) currents through or around the incubator. The use of Plexiglas heat shields and double-walled incubators reduces radiant heat loss. Evaporative heat losses are minimized by keeping the skin surface dry, covering the trunk and lower body with a clear plastic blanket, and heating and humidifying inspired gases. Additional efforts to control environmental temperature may be required for transports during the winter months or when more extreme climate changes occur. The use of thermal wrapping (parka) for the incubator may reduce heat loss in cold weather.

Minimal rates of O_2 consumption and metabolic activity and normal core body temperature occur when an infant's abdominal skin temperature is kept between 36° and 36.5°C.[46] The use of incubators with a thermostatic skin sensor and servocontrolled heat source may help regulate environmental and body temperature more accurately than manual monitoring techniques. Excess heat generated from the operation of monitoring and other support equipment in modular transport incubators may also improve heat balance during transport.

Metabolic Support

Glucose is the primary metabolic substrate for both a fetus and a newborn. During the third trimester of pregnancy, a fetus converts an increasing amount of maternally supplied glucose to glycogen stores in the liver and other body organs. At birth, a healthy full-term infant uses these glycogen stores to help maintain serum glucose concentrations during the transitional period.

An infant's ability to regulate glucose during the transition to extrauterine life depends on the developmental status of glucoregulatory pathways (glycogenolysis, gluconeogenesis) and the availability of glycogen stores. Perinatal events that affect enzymatic development (prematurity), alter glycogen stores (prematurity, intrauterine growth retardation), or increase glucose use (perinatal/neonatal stress, hyperinsulinism) may impair glucose homeostasis. Insufficient glycogen stores or incompletely developed glycolytic mechanisms impair endogenous glucose production and increase the risk of hypoglycemia.[47,48]

Infants with hypoxemia may be particularly vulnerable to adverse effects of hypoglycemia. In combination, these disorders may lead to brain injury at degrees where either alone would not be likely to do so. Maintenance of glucose homeostasis is therefore of particular interest for infants with respiratory disorders or evidence of impaired oxygenation.

The definition of hypoglycemia is based largely on clinical observation. The inability to reliably correlate plasma or blood glucose levels with tissue use rates accounts for much of the uncertainty in precisely defining chemical hypoglycemia. A plasma glucose concentration of 40 mg/dL is a conservative but probably safe threshold for diagnosing hypoglycemia. The method used to measure glucose concentrations may also influence the definition of hypoglycemia. Rapid bedside techniques that use glucose oxidase-impregnated plastic strips measure whole blood glucose. Whole blood glucose concentrations may be 10% to 15% lower than that measured in plasma. Wider discrepancies can occur in infants with elevated hematocrits (polycythemia). Although these bedside tests provide a rapid and relatively simple technique for monitoring glucose levels, low (or high) glucose concentrations should be confirmed by laboratory analysis of plasma glucose.

Early intravenous support with a constant glucose infusion has been shown to prevent hypoglycemia and reduce morbidity and mortality in high-risk infants.[49] As part of the stabilization process, an intravenous line should be established and a constant intravenous infusion of glucose should be administered during transport. Glucose infusion rates of 4 to 6 mg of glucose per kilogram of body weight per minute mimic normal endogenous production rates and should be capable of maintaining a normal serum glucose level in a stabilized infant.[50] Hypoglycemic infants (plasma glucose <40 mg/dL) should receive a bolus intravenous loading dose of 2 mL/kg of $D_{10}W$, followed by a continuous glucose infusion.[51] Rapid injection of higher concentrations of glucose ($D_{25}W$, $D_{50}W$) should be avoided for two reasons. First, they have a very high osmolality, which can damage the intravenous infusion site and produce significant osmolal changes (fluid compartment shifts, intraventricular hemorrhage) in very small infants. Second, high concentrations of glucose produce wide swings in plasma glucose levels. Rapid elevation of plasma glucose may induce a compensatory insulin response, ultimately resulting in an even more profound hypoglycemia.

During transport, blood glucose levels should be monitored regularly. Infants with increased glucose use or exceptionally high insulin levels (infants of diabetic mothers) may require glucose infusion rates as high as 9 to 12 mg/kg/min or higher. Excess fluid requirements obligatory to higher glucose infusion rates may be minimized by altering the concentration of the glucose infusate. Peripheral intravenous sites generally can tolerate infusion of concentrations up to $D_{12}W$ without vascular damage or infiltration. If higher concentrations are required ($D_{15}W$, $D_{20}W$), a centrally placed umbilical catheter should be used for infusion. Profoundly hypoglycemic infants (nesidioblastosis, pancreatic islet cell adenoma) who do not respond to increasing glucose infusion rates may require the use of pharmacologic agents such as glucagon, steroids, or diazoxide. The use of these drugs in the transport setting requires consultation and careful supervision by an experienced physician in charge of the transport.

Very small infants (<1000 g) may be particularly sensitive to glucose infusions and can become severely hyperglycemic at apparently normal glucose infusion rates (4 to 6 mg/kg/min).[52] Rather than severely restricting fluid intake, a lower concentration of glucose ($D_{7.5}W$, D_5W) should be used; however, the concentration of glucose should never be lower than D_5W. These lower-glucose fluids are extremely hypotonic and may precipitate intravascular hemolysis.

The management of glucose homeostasis in the transport of acutely ill infants can be a challenging problem. Frequent monitoring and adjustment in infusion rates may be necessary to ensure maintenance of euglycemia.

NEWER TREATMENT METHODS

During the last 10 years, several advances have been made in the technology and treatment of critically ill infants. The introduction of surfactant replacement therapy for infants with RDS, development of new modes of ventilatory support [high-frequency ventilation (HFV), extracorporeal membrane oxygenation (ECMO)], the use of inhaled nitric oxide (iNO) for pulmonary hypertension, and the introduction of newer surgical approaches to previously lethal or life-threatening malformation (hypoplastic left ventricle syndrome, organ transplantation) have significantly changed the clinical management of many diseases with previously high mortality rates. As a result, neonatal transport services are transporting a greater number of more critically ill infants to regional centers for one or more of these newer treatment regimens.

Surfactant Replacement

The development of exogenous surfactant compounds for administration to infants with surfactant deficiency has had a significant impact on the morbidity and mortality of infants with RDS.[53,54] Both prophylactic administration to all low-birthweight infants in the delivery room and selective administration to infants with confirmed RDS have been used successfully in the treatment of this most common form of neonatal respiratory disease (see Chapter 20).[55,56]

Experience with surfactant replacement in the transport environment is not widely reported. Endotracheal administration is associated with certain risks of respiratory compromise (desaturation, hypoxemia, bradycardia)[57,58] and should be performed only by experienced personnel. In infants with untreated patent ductus arteriosus, increased pulmonary blood flow has been associated with the occurrence of pulmonary hemorrhage after surfactant administration.[58,59] At present, administration of exogenous surfactants in the transport setting probably should be restricted to those infants who will most likely receive immediate benefit and should be undertaken only with close supervision and adequate experience with the technique of administration. When transport time is short and the infant's disease may be relatively mild, administration of surfactant may well be delayed until arrival in the NICU. If an adverse response occurs (significant bradycardia, cyanosis), administration should be discontinued and further attempts delayed until after transport. The use of artificial surfactants for other pulmonary diseases in which endogenous surfactant consumption may occur (meconium aspiration, pneumonia, persistent pulmonary hypertension of the newborn) is still largely theoretical. Expanded use of surfactant for other respiratory disorders should await sound clinical evidence of safety and efficacy.

High-Frequency Ventilation/Extracorporeal Membrane Oxygenation

The development of techniques for HFV and cardiopulmonary bypass (ECMO) has led to a much more aggressive approach to severe neonatal lung disease. HFV has been shown to be a useful alternative to conventional ventilation in the rescue of infants from severe pulmonary air leak syndromes.[60,61] HFV may be effective in reducing the need for ECMO in infants who fail to respond to conventional ventilation.[62]

ECMO is a technique of cardiopulmonary bypass modified for longer-term use in neonates. ECMO is a highly invasive technique requiring surgical cannulation of one or more major vascular structures. Technical limitations currently restrict the use of ECMO to infants weighing more than 2000 g. Candidates for ECMO include infants who have congenital diaphragmatic hernia (CDH), meconium aspiration, persistent pulmonary hypertension, RDS, or pneumonia/sepsis and who have failed to respond to conventional methods of ventilation. Criteria for eligibility for ECMO reflect circumstances that have had a historical mortality rate in excess of 80%. With the possible exception of CDH (survival rate 60%), survival rates for ECMO are now in excess of 80% to 90% at many centers. Infants with meconium aspiration syndrome have the best survival rate at 93% to 95%.[64] Long-term morbidity has diminished with refinements in ECMO equipment and greater experience with patient management. The proportion of infants judged to be normal after ECMO treatment ranges from 64% to 86%[65] (see Chapter 16).

With the advent of ECMO, the treatment of infants with CDH has received new interest. Early antenatal identification of CDH provides an opportunity to search (by ultrasound) for additional anomalies and to look for chromosomal aberrations. Arrangements should be made to have pregnancies with known fetal CDH delivered in facilities familiar with their management and capable of providing the level of ventilatory support necessary.[66] Despite the best obstetric efforts, however, many of these infants will continue to be unanticipated problems for community hospital delivery services. In an effort to improve preoperatively the condition of infants with CDH, most centers have adopted a more aggressive approach to early neonatal management. The majority of infants with CDH are otherwise vigorous, healthy, full-term infants. Many require some form of ventilatory support at or shortly after birth. Immediate endotracheal intubation, paralysis, sedation, and insertion of a nasogastric or orogastric tube are recommended to limit the amount of air that accumulates in the herniated bowel postnatally.

Transporting critically ill infants to regional centers for HFV or ECMO has added a significantly greater dimension of complexity to neonatal transport and has raised several questions with significant ethical overtones. As the health care marketplace has become increasingly competitive, hospitals have been eager to expand their perinatal services to include various levels of neonatal intensive care. Driven largely by economic forces, many of these centers appear in hospitals where the degree of expertise in the neonatal unit exceeds that of other hospital/medical services. Infants with complex medical or surgical disorders are being delivered in these units even though referral to a regional facility eventually will be necessary to fully evaluate and treat these infants. Infants who are failing to respond to conventional ventilator treatment are often kept in local units until the need for HFV or ECMO is inevitable. Many of these critically ill infants are so unstable that even the most well-planned transport is a significant risk. Increasingly more often, our transport team spends a significant portion of their time with prolonged resuscitation of infants who are referred far too late in their disease to benefit from any form of extended therapy. These infants may well represent the most unsatisfactory aspect of neonatal care in the 1990s.

Nitric Oxide

Since the last edition of this text, iNO has been found to be an effective treatment for certain types of pulmonary hypertension in newborn infants. Portable delivery systems are commercially available and adaptable to the transport environment.

One of the more difficult issues with using iNO in the transport setting is the ability to identify those infants who are most appropriate therapeutic candidates. Until we have greater experience with iNO in transport, its use probably should be limited to those transport services whose NICUs can provide ongoing support with, and training in, iNO use (see Chapter 14).

CONCLUSION

The development of regional neonatal intensive care centers and interhospital transport services for critically ill infants have been important factors in decreasing perinatal morbidity and mortality. Rapid advances in technology, the development of newer forms of treatment, a better understanding of perinatal pathophysiology, and a more aggressive approach to perinatal care have added to the complexity and challenges of neonatal transport services. This chapter has presented an objective approach to stabilization and basic support of infants who require ventilation during neonatal transport. Successful transport is the result of careful systematic evaluation of a patient by individuals who are skilled in the care of newborn infants. No matter how complex or sophisticated our technologic support becomes, adequate stabilization of patients will always be a critical determinant of a successful outcome.

REFERENCES

1. Usher RH: The role of the neonatologist. Pediatr Clin North Am 17:199, 1970.
2. Rudolph AJ: Problems of neonatal intensive care units. In Lucey J (ed): Report of the 59th Ross Conference in Pediatric Research, Columbus, OH, Ross Laboratories, 1969, p. 15.
3. Brann AW Jr: Perinatal health care in Mississippi, 1973. In Sunshine P (ed): Regionalization of Perinatal Care. Report of the 66th Ross Conference in Pediatric Research, Columbus, OH, Ross Laboratories, 1974, p. 27.
4. Schneider JM: Developmental and educational aspects of a regionalization program. In Sunshine P (ed): Regionalization of Perinatal Care. Report of the 66th Ross Conference in Pediatric Research, Columbus, OH, Ross Laboratories, 1974, pp. 14–19.
5. Reference deleted in proofs.
6. Jain L, Vidyasagar D: Cardiopulmonary resuscitation of newborns. Pediatr Clin North Am 40:287, 1993.
7. Bose CL: Neonatal transport. In Avery GB, Fletcher MA, MacDonald MG (eds): Neonatology. Philadelphia, JB Lippincott, 1994, pp. 41–53.
8. Segal S: Transport of High Risk Newborn Infants. Canadian Pediatric Society, Ottawa, Ontario 1972.
9. Chance GW, O'Brien MJ, Swyer PR: Transportation of sick neonates, 1972: An unsatisfactory aspect of medical care. Can Med Assoc J 109:947, 1973.
10. Chance GW, Matthew JD, Cash J, et al: Neonatal transport: A controlled study of skilled assistance. J Pediatr 93:662, 1978.
11. Shenai JP, Major CW, Gaylord MS, et al: A successful decade of regionalized perinatal care in Tennessee: The neonatal experience. J Perinatol 11:137, 1991.
12. Hackel A. Ventilation. In Graven S (ed): Report of Mead Johnson Conference on Newborn Air Transport. Evanston, IL, Mead Johnson, 1978, p. 55.
13. Pettett G, Merenstein GB, Battaglia FC, et al: An analysis of air transport results in the sick newborn. I: The transport team. Pediatrics 55:774, 1975.
14. Hay WW Jr, Brockway JM, Eyzaquirre M: Neonatal pulse oximetry: Accuracy and reliability. Pediatrics 83:717, 1989.
15. Hay WW Jr, Thilo E, Curlander JB: Pulse oximetry in neonatal medicine. Clin Perinatol 18:441, 1991.
16. American Heart Association/American Academy of Pediatrics: Textbook of Neonatal Resuscitation. Dallas, Tex., American Heart Association, 1990.
17. Bolton DPG: Diffusional inhomogeneity: Gas mixing efficiency in the newborn lung. J Physiol 286:447, 1979.
18. Parks CR, Woodrum DE, Alden ER, et al: Gas exchange in the immature lung. I: Anatomical shunt in the premature infant. J Appl Physiol 36:103, 1974.
19. Carson BS, Losey RW, Bowes WA Jr, et al: Combined obstetric and pediatric approach to prevent meconium aspiration syndrome. Am J Obstet Gynecol 126:712, 1976.
20. Gregory GA, Gooding CA, Phibbs RH: Meconium aspiration in infants: A prospective study. J Pediatr 85:848, 1974.
21. Linder N, Aranda JV, Tsur M, et al: Need for endotracheal intubation and suction in meconium stained neonates. J Pediatr 112:613, 1988.
22. Gregory GA, Kitterman JA, Phibbs RH, et al: Treatment of the idiopathic respiratory distress syndrome with continuous airway pressure. N Engl J Med 284:1333, 1971.
23. Martin RJ, Nearman H, Katona P, et al: A deflation Hering-Breuer reflex in the preterm infant: A mechanism by which low continuous positive pressure (CPAP) decreases apnea. Pediatr Res 10:424A, 1976.
24. Jung AL, Thomas GK: Stricture of the nasal vestibule: A complication of nasotracheal intubation in newborn infants. J Pediatr 85:412, 1974.
25. Pettett G, Merenstein GB: Nasal erosion with nasotracheal intubation. J Pediatr 87:149, 1975.
26. Ostrea EM, Odell GB: The influence of bicarbonate administration on blood pH in a "closed system": Clinical implications. J Pediatr 80:671, 1972.
27. Graf H, Leach W, Arieff AI: Evidence for detrimental effect of bicarbonate therapy in hypoxic lactic acidosis. Science 227:754, 1985.
28. Kette F, Weil MH, Gazmuroi RJ: Buffer solutions may compromise cardiac resuscitation by reducing coronary perfusion pressure. JAMA 266:2121, 1991.
29. Baum JD, Robertson NRC: Immediate effects of alkaline infusion in infants with respiratory distress syndrome. J Pediatr 87:255, 1975.
30. Seigel SR, Phelps DL, Leake RD, et al: The effects of rapid infusion of hypertonic sodium bicarbonate in infants with respiratory distress syndrome. Pediatrics 51:651, 1973.
31. Matter JA, Neil MH, Shubin H, et al: Cardiac arrest in the critically ill, II: Hyperosmolar states following cardiac arrest. Am J Med 56:162, 1974.
32. Simmons MA, Adcock EW, Bard H, et al: Hypernatremia and intracranial hemorrhage in neonates. N Engl J Med 291:6, 1974.
33. Turbeville DF, Bowen FW, Killam AP: Intracranial hemorrhages in kittens: Hypernatremia versus hypoxia. J Pediatr 89:294, 1976.
34. Wiklund L, Oquist L, Skoog G, et al: Clinical buffering of metabolic acidosis: Problems and a solution. Resuscitation 12:279, 1985.
35. Kuhns LR, Bednared FJ, Wyman ML, et al: Diagnosis of pneumothorax or pneumomediastinum in the neonate by transillumination. Pediatrics 56:355, 1975.
36. Kitterman JA, Phibbs R, Tooley WH: Aortic blood pressure in normal newborn infants during the first 12 hours of life. Pediatrics 44:959, 1969.
37. Kitterman JA, Phibbs RH, Tooley WH: Catheterization of umbilical vessels in newborn infants. Pediatr Clin North Am 17:895, 1970.
38. Weil MH, Rackrow EC, Trevino R, et al: Difference in acid base state between venous and arterial blood during cardiopulmonary bypass resuscitation. N Engl J Med 315:153, 1986.
39. Paxton CL: Neonatal shock in the first postnatal day. Am J Dis Child 132:509, 1978.
40. Bligh J, Johnson KG: Glossary of terms for thermal physiology. J Appl Physiol 35:941, 1973.
41. Hey EN: The relationship between environmental temperature and oxygen consumption in the newborn baby. J Physiol 200:589, 1969.
42. Bruck K: Temperature regulation in the newborn infant. Biol Neonate 3:65, 1961.
43. Jolly H, Molyneux P, Newell DJ: A controlled study of the effect of temperature on premature babies. J Pediatr 60:889, 1962.
44. Miller JA Jr, Miller FS, Westin B: Hypothermia in the treatment of asphyxia neonatorum. Biol Neonate 6:148, 1964.
45. Silverman WA, Fertig JW, Berger AP: The influence of thermal environment upon the survival of newly born premature infants. Pediatrics 22:876, 1958.
46. Silverman WA, Sinclair JC, Agate EJ: The oxygen cost of minor changes in heat balance of small newborn infants. Acta Paediatr Scand 55:294, 1966.
47. Raivio KO, Hallman N: Neonatal hypoglycemia I: Occurrence of hypoglycemia in patients with various neonatal disorders. Acta Paediatr Scand 57:517, 1968.
48. Lubchenco LO, Bard H: Incidence of hypoglycemia in newborn infants classified by birth weight and gestational age. Pediatric 47:831, 1971.
49. Lubchenco LO, Delivoria-Papadopoulos M, Butterfield LJ, et al: Long term follow-up studies of prematurely born infants. I: Relationship of handicaps to nursery routines. J Pediatr 80:501, 1972.
50. King KC, Adams PAJ, Clement GA, et al: Infants of diabetic mothers: Attenuated glucose uptake without hyperinsulinemia during continuous glucose infusion. Pediatrics 44:381, 1969.
51. Lillen LO, Grajwer LA, Pildes RS: Treatment of neonatal hypoglycemia with continuous intravenous glucose infusion. J Pediatr 91:779, 1977.
52. Dweck HS, Cassidy G: Glucose intolerance in infants of very low birth weight. Pediatrics 53:189, 1974.
53. Long W, Thompson T, Sundell H, et al: Effects of two rescue doses of a synthetic surfactant on mortality rate and survival without bronchopulmonary dysplasia in 700 to 1350-gram infants with respiratory distress syndrome. J Pediatr 118:595, 1991.
54. Long W, Corbet A, Cotton R, et al: A controlled trial of synthetic surfactant in infants weighing 1250 g or more with respiratory distress syndrome. N Engl J Med 325:1696, 1991.
55. Mercier CE, Soll RF: Clinical trials of natural surfactant in respiratory distress syndrome. Clin Perinatol 20:711, 1993.
56. Corbet A: Clinical trials of synthetic surfactant in the respiratory distress syndrome of premature infants. Clin Perinatol 20:737, 1993.
57. Horbar JD, Wright LL, Soll RF, et al: A multicenter randomized trial comparing two surfactants for the treatment of neonatal respiratory distress syndrome. J Pediatr 123:757, 1993.
58. Liechty EA, Donovan E, Purohit D, et al: Reduction of neonatal mortality after multiple doses of bovine surfactant in low birthweight neonates with respiratory distress syndrome. Pediatrics 88:19, 1991.
59. Hoekstra RE, Jackson JC, Myers TF, et al: Improved neonatal survival following multiple doses of bovine surfactant in very premature neonates at risk for respiratory distress syndrome. Pediatrics 88:10, 1991.
60. Kessler M, Donn SM, Bucciarelli RL, et al: Multicenter controlled trial comparing high-frequency jet ventilation and conventional mechanical ventilation in newborn infants with pulmonary interstitial emphysema. J Pediatr 119:85, 1991.
61. Clark RH, Gerstmann DR, Null DM, et al: Pulmonary interstitial emphysema treated by high-frequency oscillatory ventilation. Crit Care Med 14:926, 1986.

62. Clark RH, Yoder BA, Sell MS: Prospective, randomized comparison of high-frequency oscillation and conventional ventilation in candidates for extracorporeal membrane oxygenation. J Pediatr 124:447, 1994.
63. Clark RH: High-frequency ventilation. J Pediatr 124:661, 1994.
64. Kanto WP Jr: A decade of experience with neonatal extracorporeal membrane oxygenation. J Pediatr 124:335, 1994.
65. Schumacher RE: Extracorporeal membrane oxygenation: will this therapy continue to be as efficacious in the future? Pediatr Clin North Am 40:1005, 1993.
66. Howell CG, Hatley RM, Boedy RF, et al: Recent experience with diaphragmatic hernia and ECMO. Ann Surg 211:793, 1990.

28 PULMONARY OUTCOME AND FOLLOW-UP

CHERYL MARCO NAULTY, MD

According to data published by the National Institute of Child Health and Human Development (NICHD) Neonatal Research Network, neonatal and infant survival rates have increased significantly in all birthweight (BW) categories over the past several decades (Fig. 28-1).[1] From 1988 to 1994, the largest increase in survival was for infants whose BW was greater than 1000 g. The most recently reported survival rates for very-low-birthweight (VLBW) infants[2] reflect these improved rates: 93% for BW 1001 to 1500 g, 85% for BW 751 to 1000 g, and 50% for BW 501 to 750 g. The incidence of major morbidities [chronic lung disease (CLD), severe intracranial hemorrhage, proven necrotizing entero-colitis (NEC)] was 12%, 44%, and 58% for the same respective BW categories. In a comparison of the change in overall major morbidity between 1988 and 1994, there was a significant decrease in all BW categories except for those infants weighing 501 to 750 g at birth. However, when evaluating outcomes of survivors only, the incidence of major morbidities decreased 17% to 41% in all BW categories (Fig. 28-1). Contributing factors to the overall decrease in mortality and morbidity were the use of exogenous surfactant, antenatal antibiotics, antenatal steroids, and more physiologically based ventilator strategies. Despite all these current therapeutic breakthroughs, however, there has not been a similar reduction over the years in the incidence of CLD and the associated childhood pulmonary morbidities.

Before addressing pulmonary outcomes and the long-term follow-up of neonatal survivors, it should be recognized that there are multiple issues that affect and influence the interpretation of outcome studies in general. At the very least, any report of the effect of a particular therapeutic strategy on a cohort of infants, at an age when full outcome measures can be assessed, may yield data on therapies that have long since changed. Hence, outcome studies are like a moving target, whose baseline is constantly changing.

In order to have the best understanding of the long-term pulmonary outcome, there should be a clear definition of the nature and severity of the neonatal pulmonary morbidity. In 1967, Northway et al.[3] first recognized that not all infants with hyaline membrane disease (HMD) recovered completely. Some went on to develop a chronic pulmonary syndrome. Northway et al. named the syndrome *bronchopulmonary dysplasia* (BPD). The definition of BPD or CLD has evolved significantly over time. The original criteria for BPD reported by Northway et al.[3] were based on an orderly progression of clinical, radiologic, and pathologic changes, beginning with severe HMD during the first week of life (stages I and II). Stages III and IV defined the

progression over the next several weeks to a severe chronic obstructive pulmonary disease, frequently complicated by cor pulmonale.[4] However, as smaller, less mature infants have survived and the approach to ventilator strategies has changed, the distinct stages as described by Northway et al. have become less clear. The radiologic abnormalities in extremely-low-birthweight infants do not seem to be similar to the original descriptions of Northway et al. In 1979, Tooley[5] introduced the current most widely used definition of CLD. He proposed that any infant who required additional oxygen at 1 month or 30 days of age with any radiologic abnormality of the lung parenchyma could be considered to have CLD or BPD. It should be recognized, however, that the length of time required for additional oxygen might be as much a function of immaturity and the policies of the particular nursery unit as reflective of the severity of the lung pathology. Most recently, Shennan et al.[6] found that, irrespective of gestational age at birth, the requirement for additional oxygen at 36 weeks of gestational age was a better predictor of abnormal long-term outcome and more likely to reflect an increased probability of abnormal pulmonary signs and symptoms in infancy.

The timing and choice of lung function measurements are important variables that influence the reporting of long-term outcome. The timing of the measurements will reflect the dominant changes occurring at the time of the testing: acute lung injury during the first 6 months and healing, remodeling, and growth in later childhood. It is not until 5 to 6 years of age that pulmonary function tests become more reliable. Total lung capacity (TLC) and vital capacity are related to overall body weight and increase with growth. Obstructive airway disease is a primary component of pulmonary dysfunction in BPD, and the best way to assess this is through forced expiratory maneuvers. With more severe disease, there is a rapid decrease in flow, expiration ends prematurely secondary to the narrowing of the small airways, and the flow–volume curve is concave following the point of maximum flow[7] (Fig. 28-2).

Further complicating the picture is the difficulty in separating out the influence of prematurity and LBW alone on pulmonary function in later childhood. Where does the role of various antenatal factors fit into the puzzle: fetal nutrition, exposure to cigarette smoke in utero, and a history of family atopy and asthma? Finally, consideration must be given to the relationship of lung functions to clinical symptoms, as well as the interaction of pulmonary dysfunction with later respiratory illnesses, and overall growth and health status and neurodevelopmental factors.

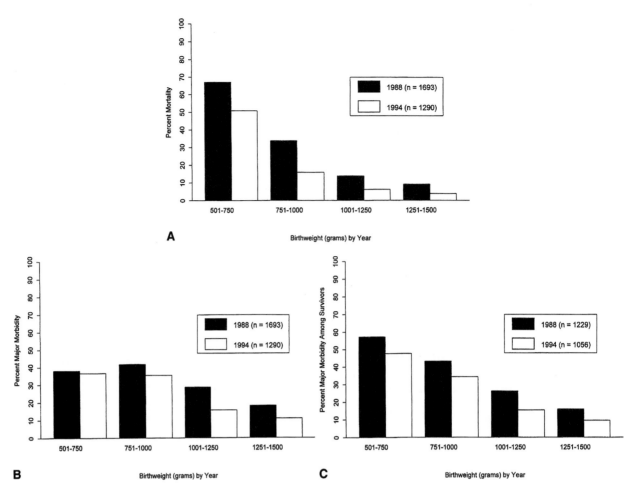

Figure 28-1. *A,* Mortality rate for very-low-birthweight (VLBW) infants cared for in National Institute of Child Health and Human Development Neonatal Research Network Centers (n = 5) in 1988 and 1994 by 250-g birthweight intervals. *B,* Major morbidity for all VLBW infants cared for in National Institute of Child Health and Human Development Neonatal Research Network Centers (n = 5) in 1988 and 1994 by 250-g birth weight intervals, including severe intracranial hemorrhage, chronic lung disease, and confirmed necrotizing enterocolitis. *C,* Major morbidity among VLBW survivors cared for in the National Institute of Child Health and Human Development Neonatal Research Network (n = 5) in 1988 and 1994 by 250-g birth weight intervals, including severe intracranial hemorrhage, chronic lung disease, and confirmed necrotizing enterocolitis. (Reprinted from Stevenson DK, Wright LL, Lemons JA, et al: Very low birth weight outcomes of the National Institute of Child Health and Human Development Neonatal Research Network, January 1993 through December 1994. Am J Obstet Gynecol 179:1635, 1998.)

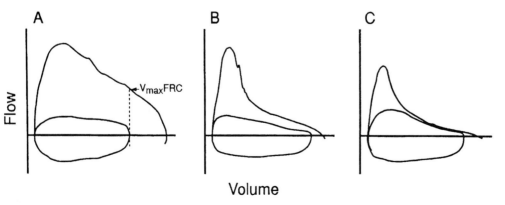

Figure 28-2. Schematic of typical partial expiratory flow–volume loops. *A,* Normal infant. *B,* Infant with mild air flow limitation (infant with history of respiratory distress syndrome). *C,* Infant with bronchopulmonary dysplasia. (Reprinted from Bhutani VK, Abbasi S: Long-term pulmonary consequences in survivors with bronchopulmonary dysplasia. Clin Perinatol 19:649, 1992.)

PULMONARY STATUS OF PREMATURELY BORN INFANTS

The literature is clearly divided on the independent correlation of BW and neonatal pulmonary disease with pulmonary abnormalities in later childhood. As early as 1928, Capper[8] commented on an increased incidence of respiratory infections in surviving premature infants. Later, a national survey of the health of a group of prematurely born and full-term infants conducted in England revealed that almost twice as many premature infants as full-term infants died or were admitted to a hospital, most frequently because of pneumonia.[9] The question is whether it is the effect of the type and severity of the neonatal lung disease, the evolving neonatal treatment and the subsequent interaction of intercurrent respiratory illness, or the child's individual constitution as reflected in BW and prematurity that puts these infants at risk for childhood pulmonary morbidities.[10]

A 1991 study published in the *British Medical Journal*[11] reported that LBW in term infants might be an independent predictor of lung function and death from chronic obstructive pulmonary disease in adult life. These data, known as the *Barker effect,* were based on a retrospective study of more than 6000 adult males, born between 1911 and 1930, with known recording of BW and childhood illness. Death from chronic obstructive airway disease in adult life was strongly associated with LBW alone.

Various studies relative to LBW and VLBW infants argue for the contribution of prematurity alone to later evidence of obstructive airways disease and hyperreactivity. Chan et al.[12] reported abnormal flow measurements and increased airway responsiveness in low-birthweight (LBW) infants compared to full-term controls at 7 years of age. The airway responsiveness was clinically significant and irrespective of neonatal respiratory illness or treatment. Similar data were reported from studies by Tammela et al.[13] and Mansell et al.[2] They reported no differences in TLC and forced vital capacity (FVC) between LBW and term infants but significantly lower flow values in LBW children at 6 to 10 years. In school-aged children, reduced lung function and respiratory symptoms, especially wheezing, were associated with LBW, regardless of respiratory complications at birth.[14,15] Every week more of gestation reduced the risk of wheezing by 10%.[15] In a very well-designed study, Galdis-Sebaldt et al.[16] found decreased forced expiratory volume in 1 second (FEV_1), air trapping, and increased airway responsiveness to methacholine in all VLBW infants with or without HMD, but not in infants with HMD whose BW was greater than 1500 g. In 1995, Rojas et al.[17] reported CLD as frequent sequela in VLBW infants with mild or no respiratory distress syndrome (RDS). In this population, the development of late episodes of patent ductus arteriosus (PDA) in association with a nosocomial infection seemed to play a role.

Equally compelling are those studies that relate HMD and mechanical ventilation in the neonatal period to later abnormal lung function. The severity of the neonatal respiratory illness, along with the occurrence of complications such as prolonged ventilation and pneumothorax, has been associated with increased respiratory morbidity and significantly lower forced expiratory flow measurements in VLBW infants without BPD at ages up to 18 years.[18-21] In most cases, however, the differences were small, there was no correlation with clinical symptoms, and the children showed improvement in lung functions with age beyond 8 years.[18,19] In a study of VLBW infants with and without BPD compared to controls at age 11 years, Kennedy et al.[22] found only a small contribution of gestational age and BW to decreased expiratory flow rates. Together BW and gestational age accounted for only 16% of the variance in FEV_1. The best predictors for abnormal lung function were days receiving supplemental oxygen and a reported family history of asthma, which together accounted for a 43.4% reduction in FEV_1. In addition, Kennedy et al.[22] reported a "dose effect" of supplemental oxygen on the subsequent FEV_1, with little effect associated with less than 20 days of O_2 but a decline of 3% in FEV_1 for every extra week of supplemental oxygen beyond 20 days. It should be noted, however, that although there were statistically significant reductions in flow values the overall lung function measurements were within the published norms for full-term children of similar age.

FOLLOW-UP OF INFANTS WITH ASSISTED VENTILATION AND BRONCHOPULMONARY DYSPLASIA

In 1990, Northway et al.[23] reported in the *New England Journal of Medicine* the follow-up to adolescence of 26 children with BPD who were born between 1964 and 1973. The majority had abnormalities in pulmonary function testing, with evidence of hyperinflation and small airway obstruction. Most of the abnormalities were mild to moderate, and only 6 of the 26 were clinically symptomatic. The chest x-ray findings were subtle, but computerized tomographic findings revealed multifocal areas of reduced lung attenuation and perfusion.[24]

These data, along with other reports of populations from the 1970s and 1980s,[25-28] found that BPD did not appear to interfere with parenchymal lung growth, as TLC and FRC increased normally with age, but BPD did result in small airway obstruction and hyperreactivity. One may conclude from these findings that infants with BPD have normal alveolar formation but also have persistent damage to their small airways.

In comparisons of large cohorts of VLBW children to healthy term infants at school age, abnormalities in lung function were present only in those with BPD.[29,30] Preterm infants without BPD, even if they had been treated with intermittent positive-pressure ventilation, showed no differences in lung function from the term infants. The abnormalities found in the children who had BPD included higher residual volumes, indicative of air trapping, and significant decreases in FVC, FEV_1, and $FEF_{25\%-75\%}$, reflecting airflow obstruction. These differences increased when BPD was defined as oxygen dependence at 35 weeks of postconceptional age (PCA). However, in most studies, although various pulmonary function measurements were significantly reduced in infants with BPD, the values were either within or close to the normal range and, therefore, not clinically significant.

In outcomes that focus on infants with more severe BPD, there is clear evidence of more significant long-term sequelae. Mallory et al.[31] looked at 11 infants with BPD and tracheostomies at up to 3 years of age and compared those ventilated for less than 5 months with those ventilated for more than 10 months. All showed an increase in FVC with age, reaching normal values by 3 years. In contrast, mean expiratory flows ($MEF_{25\%}$) were very abnormal in all patients. Those with shorter ventilatory times and less severe BPD had a gradual increase in expiratory flow rates of up to 40% of predicted by 3 years, whereas those with more severe disease had no change in flow values and remained at only 10% of predicted at 3 years of age. Jacob et al.[32] described a population with severe BPD in which all infants were on oxygen at 44 weeks PCA and all were discharged home on O_2. At 11 years of age, these children all showed significant gas trapping and hyperinflation, and mean FEV_1 was 65% of predicted compared to preterm infants without BPD. The severity of these abnormalities was inversely related to the duration of O_2 use.

EXERCISE TOLERANCE

Although many studies have found statistically significant, but not clinically relevant, abnormalities in pulmonary function measurements in children with BPD, there is some evidence suggesting that exercise tolerance in these children may not be normal. Maximum oxygen consumption and the anaerobic threshold are recognized markers of exercise performance. The failure of an adequate increase in minute ventilation during exercise to meet the high metabolic demands equals the hallmark of the cardiorespiratory response to exercise in children with BPD.[33] This certainly raises concerns about possible declining exercise capacity into adulthood.

Bader et al.[34] described 10 BPD survivors who underwent exercise testing at a mean age of 10.6 years. These patients had a decrease in arterial O_2 saturation to pre-exercise levels at maximum workload, whereas six age-matched normal controls born at term did not. No differences in maximum O_2 consumption were noted between these two groups. The pre-exercise transcutaneous carbon dioxide tension was higher and remained high at maximum workload in the BPD group compared with the control group. Later studies demonstrated BPD patients, tested up to 12 years of age, had limited ventilatory reserve, a lower anaerobic threshold, and were more likely to have O_2 desaturations during exercise.[33,35,36] Even when no significant cardiopulmonary limitations to exercise were found, those with BPD had higher respiratory rates with normal tidal volumes in response to exercise, rather than an increase in tidal volume, as occurred with control children. There may be certain qualitative adaptations to cardiopulmonary responses to exercise in children with BPD that are distinct from term infants.[37]

PATHOLOGY

The literature seems to suggest that BPD does not interfere with parenchymal lung growth,[23,25,28,38] but there is reported evidence of small airway obstruction suggestive of dysanaptic lung growth, that is, normal growth of lung volume but not of airway size.[39] A look at the pathology of those infants who die a result of their respiratory disease beyond the acute phases of BPD might provide some insight into the morphology associated with the abnormal pulmonary function findings.

In 1986, Stocker[40] described the pathology of 28 infants born between 1974 and 1984, who all had severe BPD and died at 3 to 40 months of age. The cause of death was progressive respiratory failure in 68%, and an additional 18% died of pneumonia superimposed on long-standing BPD. The original lung injury leading to BPD was characterized by necrotizing bronchiolitis, alveolar cell hyperplasia, and bronchiolar squamous

metaplasia. The main residual feature in the "healed" stage of BPD was focal alveolar septal fibrosis. The degree of fibrosis and parenchymal involvement varied considerably, with severe fibrosis in one area and normally inflated or hyperinflated lung in adjacent lobes. Stocker postulated that the variability might be related to a "protective effect" of the necrotizing bronchiolitis. The occlusion of the bronchioles by the inflammatory debris might actually shield the distal sublobule from the high oxygen tensions and ventilatory pressures. With healing, there might be absorption and recanalization, leaving a normal or less damaged parenchyma "downstream." Alternatively, the exudates might be absorbed into the alveolar wall, resulting in fibrosis, or the debris might become organized tissue, resulting in total obliteration of the alveolar space (Fig. 28-3). The morphologic features as described in this study might account for the clinical studies on infants who demonstrated increased small airway resistance, increased functional residual capacity, maldistribution of ventilation, and airway hyperreactivity.

With the continuing advancement in mechanical ventilation and the current widespread use of surfactant, the classic pathologic features of BPD are now seldom seen. The characteristic lung injury of BPD is now one of minimal-to-moderate diffuse alveolar septal fibrosis.[41] The pathologic alterations are thought to be primarily mediated by highly reactive oxygen species after respiratory therapy.[42] Husain et al.[41] found that the alveolar septal fibrosis was a mild diffuse injury that resulted in slowing of alveolar saccular and alveolar development. They reported that the ratio of the radial alveolar counts to the mean linear intercept (RAC/MLI), which reflects the comparison of the number of alveoli and their size, was significantly lower in the infants with BPD. RAC is a measure of the complexity of alveolar development, and these values were significantly decreased in BPD infants. In contrast, MLI, which is a measure of alveolar size, was significantly increased, reflecting hyperinflation of the alveoli.[41,43] This suggests that there is an "acinar arrest" during the time when normal infants have rapid alveolar development. There is a failure to increase the complexity of the acinus and a compensatory hyperexpansion of the lung with growth of the thorax. This combination of hyperinflation and decrease in alveolar number would explain the seemingly normal TLC but otherwise severe impairment in lung function. They postulate that, in the absence of necrotizing bronchiolitis, there are no "protected" acini. All acini are uniformly exposed to the ventilatory pressures and oxygen tensions, leading to this partial or complete arrest in acinar development. Further, they found that surfactant therapy did not alter this inhibited development in infants with severe BPD.[41] To add to this picture, early postnatal dexamethasone (Decadron) therapy in rats was found to inhibit outgrowth of new interalveolar septa, leading to a mature but emphysematous lung with larger and fewer air spaces.[44,45]

In conclusion, data on the influence of prematurity on long-term pulmonary function are conflicting. All infants with BPD seem to have some degree of small airway obstruction, but the abnormalities may not be clinically relevant in many cases. Good long-term studies on the combined effects of surfactant therapy, use of antenatal and postnatal steroids, and application of new modes of ventilation are yet to be done. There is some early pulmonary function data from a follow-up study at 1 year on a small number of preterm infants who were treated with surfactant replacement for RDS.[46] No significant differences in pulmonary functions were noted in early infancy. However, in late infancy the mean maximal expiratory flow in the surfac-

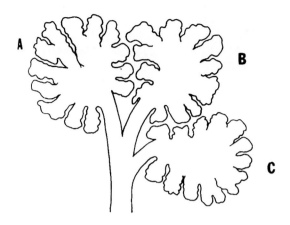

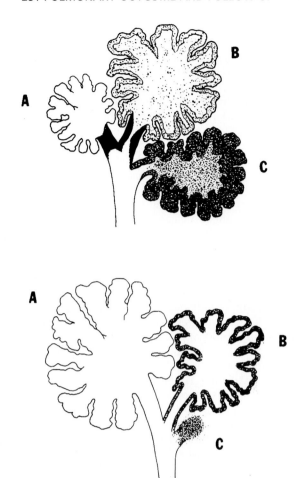

Figure 28-3. *Top left,* Schematic drawing of normally expanded and aerated pulmonary lobules. *Top right,* Acute bronchopulmonary dysplasia. *A,* Necrotizing bronchiolitis occludes the bronchiolar lumen, "protecting" the parenchyma distal to it from the high oxygen tension and pressure used in maintaining adequate oxygenation. *B,* The bronchiole is narrowed by mucosal hyperplasia and muscular hypertrophy, thereby reducing the amount of pressure and oxygen tension in the lobule distal to it. Alveolar cell hyperplasia, septal fibroplasia, and alveolar macrophage dysplasia occur to a mild-to-moderate degree. *C,* The bronchiole is widely patent, exposing the distal sublobule to the full ventilatory pressure and oxygen tension. The alveolar lumina are largely obliterated by alveolar macrophages, alveolar cell hyperplasia, and marked septal fibroplasia. *Bottom right,* Long-standing "healed" bronchopulmonary dysplasia (LSHBPD). *A,* With resolution of the necrotizing bronchiolitis that occluded the lumen of the bronchiole, the uninjured sublobule overexpands to compensate for the less expansile injured portions of lung *(B,C). B,* With resolution of the mild-to-moderate injury incurred by the parenchyma during the acute stages of bronchopulmonary dysplasia, the sublobule displays the hallmark of LSHBPD—septal fibrosis. *C,* The sublobule is virtually obliterated by organization of the severe acute bronchopulmonary dysplasia. (Reprinted from Stocker JT: Pathologic features of long-standing "healed" bronchopulmonary dysplasia: A study of 28 3- to 40-month-old infants. Hum Pathol 17:959, 1986.)

tant-treated group was significantly higher than in the placebo-treated infants. Finally, there is still the question of whether there are more subtle abnormalities that can only be discerned by challenging the capacity and endurance of lung function in children, and whether these subtleties will lead to increasing problems with age into the adult years.

FAMILY AND GENETIC FACTORS AND LATER RESPIRATORY ABNORMALITIES

In 1980, Nickerson and Taussig[47] reported an unusual incidence of a family history of asthma in ventilated RDS patients who developed BPD. They compared 21 RDS survivors without BPD with 23 with BPD and found that the BPD infants were significantly younger and smaller. In addition, 17 of the 23 infants (77%) with BPD had a family history of asthma compared with only 7 of 21 infants (33%) without BPD. Nickerson and Taussig[47] speculated that the development and/or severity of the BPD might be related to a genetic predisposition of airways to become highly reactive following exposure to one or more etiologic factors. It should be noted, however, that their incidence of a family history for asthma in 33% of the infants without BPD is high in comparison to the normal population.

The relationship between a family history of asthma and/or atopy and the development of BPD is controversial at best. To add to the confusion, various associations are made among a variety of genetic and perinatal factors and later respiratory abnormalities, including gender, ethnicity, prematurity, RDS, BPD, and familial history. Riedel[48] reported that bronchial hyperreactivity elicited by histamine inhalation had significant statistical correlation with the duration of neonatal ventilation, BW, and gestational age. Several studies showed a high prevalence of a family history of asthma or atopy among prematurely born children, who had recurrent respiratory symptoms or wheezing in early childhood.[49,50] In males from a large epidemiologic study, BW less than 1500 g, prematurity, and RDS were significant predictors of childhood asthma up to 4 years of age.[51] Von Mutius et al.[50] found that premature female infants had a higher prevalence of asthma and decreased lung function at 9 to 11 years of age, especially if they required mechanical ventilation. An ethnic influence on lung function has been described in normal, full-term children.[52] FEV_1 and FVC were found to be significantly lower in children of African and Indian origin than in those of European origin.

Bertrand et al.[53] studied the role that familial factors may play in the long-term sequelae of RDS. They looked at prematurely born infants with and without RDS and their full-term siblings as controls. An additional group of full-term children with no personal or family history of asthma or allergies was studied. They found that premature children, regardless of a previous history of RDS, and their full-term siblings had increased airway hyperreactivity. In a 1995 study, Hagen et al.[54] examined the relationship between a family history of asthma, neonatal CLD, and oxygen dependency in a group of infants of 24 to 30 weeks' gestation. They found that prematurity, and not a family history of asthma, was the dominant factor in the prevalence of CLD. However, infants with a family history of asthma were more likely to be oxygen dependent at term (odds ratio 11.0, 95% confidence interval 2.3, 53.0). They concluded that infants with CLD and a family history of asthma were more likely to develop severe CLD and experience a delay in recovery, as measured by the need for prolonged supplemental oxygen.

Hyperreactivity in both bronchial and uterine smooth muscle might account for the association between asthma and premature births.[55] Parents with a family history of asthma might be more likely to give birth to VLBW infants. Kramer et al.[56] described an association between spontaneous preterm labor and maternal asthma. In 1988, Chan et al.[57] reported that increased airway responsiveness to histamine in LBW infants and a full-term reference population was significantly related to a history of asthma in first-degree relatives (natural parents and siblings). However, they found no increase in the prevalence of maternal asthma or of airway responsiveness to histamine in the mothers, thus failing to support the hypothesis that maternal smooth muscle hyperreactivity (both uterine and airway) has a causative role in premature labor and subsequent bronchial hyperresponsiveness in their prematurely born children.

To date, available studies have not been able to conclusively associate a maternal or family history of asthma and neonatal respiratory disease in premature infants. The role of maternal bronchial hyperreactivity or asthma in the etiology of premature labor remains controversial.[58] Data do seem to support, however, a strong association between a family history of asthma and childhood asthma in VLBW infants, regardless of the development of RDS or BPD. On the other hand, BPD is associated with childhood asthma regardless of the family history. Finally, there may be a link between a family history of asthma or atopy and the severity of the CLD or the duration of oxygen dependence.

SOME CONSIDERATIONS ON THE ROLE OF AIRWAY INJURY IN THE DEVELOPMENT OF CHRONIC PULMONARY SEQUELAE

Mucosal and submucosal necrosis with inflammation have been described at the vocal cords, in the subglottic region of the larynx, and in the trachea following endotracheal intubation for assisted ventilation.[59,60] The severity of the lesion was related to the duration of intubation and to the presence of bacterial infection.[59] No lesions were seen in children who had not been intubated.

At the more extreme end of the spectrum of airway injury from endotracheal intubation is the development of subglottic stenosis.[61,62] Movement of the endotracheal tube has been judged to be a contributing causative factor, and orotracheal intubation has been associated with a higher incidence of subglottic stenosis than has nasotracheal intubation.[63,64] Following mechanical injury to the ciliated respiratory epithelium, squamous metaplasia may occur.[65] This may lead to impaired clearance of pulmonary secretions and thus to a predisposition toward pulmonary infection. In addition, the potential for premalignant change, particularly with regard to the propensity for the occurrence of neoplasia in the area of the larynx and vocal cords, needs to be evaluated on a prospective, long-term basis.

Squamous metaplasia of the respiratory epithelium occurs in vitamin A deficiency.[66] Premature infants have been reported to have levels of vitamin A that are in the deficient range.[67,68] In the study of Hustead et al.,[67] the ventilated premature infants who developed BPD had lower levels of vitamin A at birth and at age 3 weeks than those who did not have BPD. In addition, the dietary intake of vitamin A has been reported to be lower in the mothers of premature infants who developed BPD.[69] Shenai et al.[70] reported that supplementation with vitamin A resulted in an approximately 50% decrease in the incidence of BPD and a decrease in the incidence of respiratory illness. However, Pearson et al.[71] did not find a reduction in the incidence of BPD with vitamin A supplementation. Pearson et al. and Shenai et al. have speculated that this differing experience may be a result of the greater use of exogenous surfactant and postnatal steroids in the more recently studied patients of Pearson et al.

Exposure to high FIO_2 damages ciliated epithelial cells in the bronchi[72] and the trachea[73] and decreases the velocity of the tracheal clearance of mucus.[74] Free oxygen radicals, including the superoxide anion (O_2^-), accumulate, producing inhibition of cell growth and cell damage.[75] Injury to the pulmonary alveolar macrophages results in a release of chemoattractant substances that causes an outpouring of polymorphonuclear leukocytes.[76] These leukocytes contain collagenases and elastases that can cause further damage to connective tissue in the lung. The administration of liposome-encapsulated catalase to experimental animals prevented the histologic changes of chronic pulmonary O_2 toxicity.[77] The administration of superoxide dismutase to premature infants with RDS has been reported to reduce the incidence of,[78] but not totally prevent, the development of BPD.

It appears likely that the prevention of BPD will require a multifaceted approach, and attention will need to be devoted simultaneously to several factors related to their pathogenesis.

The accumulating information suggests that prematurity is such a strong determinant of these sequelae that a reduction in its incidence itself might be expected to result in a reduction in the frequency of later pulmonary sequelae.

GROWTH AND LATER RESPIRATORY ILLNESS

It has generally been accepted that growth failure is a major problem in infants with CLD. Markestad and Fitzhardinge[79] found growth retardation associated with severe and prolonged respiratory dysfunction in 26 survivors with BPD. The average height and weight at term were at or below the third percentile. Subsequent growth occurred at an accelerated rate following improvement of respiratory symptoms. Vohr et al.[80] and Meisels et al.[81] both reported that infants with BPD were at greater risk for growth retardation in the second year than those with RDS alone. This growth failure is thought to be related to increased oxygen consumption and increased respiratory energetics secondary to abnormal pulmonary mechanics.[82] Additional contributing factors are decreased caloric intake related to abnormal sucking patterns, palatal abnormalities, and iatrogenic fluid limitations.

Later studies do not necessarily support these observations. Vrlenick et al.[83] criticized prior reports based on problems with small sample size, short length of follow-up, timing of the follow-up, variable definitions of growth failure, and failure to consider confounding neonatal, neurologic, and demographic risk variables. Although their data initially supported differences in growth outcome among VLBW infants with and without BPD, no difference in any growth parameters was found when accounting for all covariates.[80,81] Likewise, Chye and Gray[84] and Davidson et al.[85] reported growth patterns of infants with BPD similar to other VLBW infants who were ventilated but did not develop BPD. All VLBW infants who were ventilated, with or without subsequent BPD, had significant growth delays in all parameters, and growth velocity at 21 months was similar in both groups.[85] BW, not respiratory status, was the best predictor for post term growth measurements at 12 and 21 months.

Is poor nutritional health related to factors other than BPD per se? Data reported by deRegnier et al.[86] indicated that growth patterns are established early. By the first 2 to 4 weeks of life, infants with BPD had lower protein and energy intakes. They took longer to achieve full enteral feedings and were lower in all growth parameters, as well as in arm muscle and fat measurements, than VLBW infants without BPD. When BPD infants were able to tolerate full enteral intake, they were able to accrete muscle and fat at a normal rate but were unable to catch up to their peers.[86] VLBW infants both with and without BPD have a bone mineral content well below that of full-term infants in the first year.[87] Singer et al.[88] assessed the feeding patterns of VLBW infants close to term gestation. The infants were more difficult to feed and spent less time sucking and more time in nonfeeding behaviors than VLBW infants without BPD, as well as healthy term infants. As a result, the BPD infants ingested lower volumes and fewer calories; however, no long-term growth data were reported.

Infants with LBW, especially those with chronic sequelae of assisted ventilation, are believed to have an increased risk of developing frequent and severe infections, especially in the lower respiratory tract. As early as 1968, Lewis[89] reported that 11 of 63 RDS survivors in London, England, required later hospital admission for bronchiolitis or bronchopneumonia. Preterm infants during the first 1 to 3 years have increased and recurrent symptoms of coughing and wheezing, an increased need for antibiotics and other medical care, and were more often hospitalized than full-term infants.[20,49,90–92] In a large series that followed RDS survivors for at least 3 years, Stahlman et al.[93] reported that 23% were found to have experienced repeated episodes of wheezing or pneumonia, or chronic respiratory symptoms. Data from a questionnaire survey of the respiratory history of 7-year-old children whose BW was less than 2000 g were compared with those from a reference group of local school children.[94] The comparison showed frequent cough was significantly more common among VLBW children who had received neonatal respiratory treatment. The prevalence of cough correlated with the neonatal O_2 score (based on the duration and the fractional inspired oxygen concentration used), but not with the use of mechanical ventilation.[53] The incidence of wheezing was not increased in this group of prematurely born children.

The rate of lower respiratory tract infections in infants with BPD has been reported to be significantly higher in comparison with that for the positive-pressure–ventilated RDS survivors without BPD.[80] Kitchen et al.[95] followed three cohorts of infants (group 1: 500–999 g BW; group 2: 1000–1500 g BW; group 3 >2500 g BW) up to 8 years of age. They found that all VLBW infants had more wheezing illnesses and more hospital admissions for respiratory problems in the first 2 years than the normal term infants. From 2 to 8 years, however, respiratory health and decreased expiratory flow measurements, indicative of obstruction, were not related to BW, but they were associated with continuing respiratory illnesses at 8 years, especially asthma and bronchiolitis.[95] Beyond 5 years of age, Korhonen et al.[91] found respiratory infections were more common only in infants who had BPD. deKleine et al.[19] associated increased treatments for pneumonia and increased hospital admissions for respiratory infections during the first 4 years with the diagnosis of BPD. After 8 years, BPD patients did not have increased respiratory symptoms over children who had HMD but no assisted ventilation, indicating improvement with age.

Furman et al.[96] reported that infants with CLD had a mean hospital stay in the first year of 153 days, the majority of which was the initial neonatal stay. However, up to 50% were rehospitalized within the first year and 37% in the second year. Cardiac and respiratory causes predominated as the primary reasons for rehospitalization, with respiratory causes representing the majority. They concluded that the duration of neonatal stay and the total duration of hospitalization in the first year were significantly associated with all measures of the severity of CLD, and the duration of hospitalization in the first year might be the more useful index of overall morbidity.[96]

In summary, the evidence indicates that later respiratory illness is more common among those who were born prematurely, appears to be increased in frequency in the children who had RDS, and is further increased in those who develop BPD. Encouragement can be taken from the fact that there seems to be improvement with age in all categories. It is particularly important that these children avoid smoking and environmental pollutants in order to minimize their risk for later impairment of pulmonary function. The impact of maternal smoking of one or more packs per day on lowering the age of onset of lower respiratory infections and on increasing the incidence of wheezing and nonwheezing illness in infancy needs to be emphasized when the parents of these children are counseled.[97]

Respiratory syncytial virus (RSV) is one of the major causes of respiratory morbidity in premature infants, especially those with CLD.[98] In general, an immunologic factor may contribute to the increased incidence of lower respiratory tract infections in prematurely born infants. Maternal immunoglobulin G is transferred to the fetus during the third trimester of pregnancy,[99,100] and serum immunoglobulin G levels at birth correlate directly with gestational age.[99,101] Hypogammaglobulinemia in infants weighing less than 1500 g at birth has been observed at 6 months of age and was associated with an increase in respiratory infections.[102] Premature infants of less than 28 weeks' gestation have been found to have significantly lower levels of specific antibodies against RSV and lower mean titers of neutralizing antibody than term infants.[103] This possibility has been suggested as an explanation for the higher incidence of RSV infection observed in prematurely born infants,[104,105] but these authors believed that the lower specific antibody levels did not entirely account for the increased incidence of infection and that other immunologic factors or structural differences must also be involved.

In the first year of life, 15% to 22% of all RVS-infected children, regardless of BW, develop lower respiratory tract infections and 0.5% to 2% of previously healthy infected children require hospitalization. The mortality rate in hospitalized infants is 0.5% to 1%. RSV infection is the major cause of hospitalization of infants with BPD during the winter months,[106] with rates ranging from 2.7% to 45%.[98,107] Meert et al.[108] found that of all infants hospitalized secondary to RSV infections, those with BPD had an increased length of stay, increased days on the ventilator and on supplemental oxygen, increased physiologic instability, and an increased rate of nosocomial infections. Infants with BPD are clearly more susceptible to more severe and prolonged illness from RSV than the healthy term population and may develop severe pulmonary compromise as a result of their infection at an older age than children without BPD.

The use of RSV immune globulin intravenous (RSV-IGIV), RespiGam (Massachusetts Public Health Biologic Laboratories and MedImmune, Inc., Gaithersburg, MD, USA), and the more recently developed intramuscular monoclonal antibody palivizumab (Synagis, MedImmune) provide an approach to the prevention or amelioration of RSV infections in high-risk infants.[109] Prophylactic use of palivizumab in a high-risk pediatric population resulted in a 55% reduction in the risk of hospitalization attributable to RSV infections. Infants and children with CLD and prematurely born infants without CLD experienced a reduced number of hospitalizations and a decrease in the severity of illness.[110] The American Academy of Pediatrics currently recommends that palivizumab or RSV-IGIV prophylaxis be considered for infants and children younger than 2 years of age with CLD, who have required medical therapy for their CLD within 6 months before the anticipated RSV season.[109] In addition, infants born at 32 weeks of gestation or earlier without CLD may be at high risk based on gestational and chronologic age at the beginning of the RSV season and should also be considered for prophylaxis.

NEURODEVELOPMENTAL OUTCOME

The impact of CLD or BPD on long-term neurodevelopmental outcome is unclear. As in most long-term outcome studies, the sample size, heterogeneity of the population, lack of controls, timing of the assessments, as well as what was measured and the variables considered, strongly influence the results. What is the effect of long-term ventilation? Is the outcome no different from the rest of the preterm population but only influenced by the degree of intraventricular hemorrhage (IVH)? How do socioeconomic and environmental factors affect the equation? Is the impact on motor developmental performance, cognitive performance, or both?

Early studies are discouraging. LBW infants with BPD did not function as well as those with RDS alone.[81] They had lower scores on both the Bayley[111] mental developmental index (MDI) and psychomotor developmental index (PDI) and a higher rate of neurologic impairment.[112] At 36 months, children with BPD and/or IVH were functioning in the subnormal range for their mental scores and in the low-average range for motor development, significantly below infants with RDS and no IVH.[113] Perlman and Volpe[114] described an extrapyramidal movement disorder that was observed in 10 premature infants with severe BPD. The natural history was partial or complete resolution or a static course. These studies, however, did not separate out the effect of BPD from other important perinatal variables, especially IVH.

Long-term follow-up studies in older children have revealed a hidden morbidity not apparent until the school-age years. Vohr et al.[115] reported lower scores in perceptual motor integration, more problems with motor coordination, and a greater need for academic support in a group of 10- to 12-year-old children who had BPD, even after eliminating those with cerebral palsy from the analysis. Others described CLD associated with long-term effects on cognitive functions related to visuomotor integration and visuospatial problem solving,[116] lower full-scale IQ and performance IQ scores,[117] and lower scores in the cognitive domains of language and memory, which persisted even after controlling for BW, gestational age, and severity of IVH.[118] Katz-Salamon et al.[119] found that CLD alone had a deleterious effect on the early developmental of certain psychomotor functions such as hand–eye coordination, but they did not have any longer-term correlations. Majnemer et al.[120] assessed outcome in VLBW infants with and without BPD at 10 years. Neurologic abnormalities, including subtle neurologic signs, cerebral palsy, microcephaly, and behavioral difficulties, were highly prevalent in the BPD group (71% compared with 19% in the control group). Severe IVH occurred with equal frequency in both groups. BPD infants were twice as likely to have difficulties in gross and/or fine motor skills and postural stability than their peers. The overall motor function correlated with the severity of the lung disease, as measured by the duration of hospitalization, duration of home oxygen therapy, and decreased lung function at school age, and not the degree of prematurity.[120]

In 1997, Singer et al.[121] reported the outcome of three groups of infants at 3 years of age: VLBW infants, with and without BPD, and full-term controls. BPD was a significant independent predictor of poorer motor outcome, associated with a 10- to 12-point decrement in the PDI scores. BPD and the neurologic risk score together accounted for 21% of the variance in the motor outcome. Minority race, lower social class, lower BW, and neurologic risk predicted poorer mental developmental outcome at 3 years. After controlling for these risks, BPD did not predict the MDI. In terms of mental outcome, children with a history of VLBW and BPD, who did not have neurologic sequelae, had similar outcomes to VLBW infants without BPD.[121]

In contrast, there are several reports of infants with CLD whose outcomes were more associated with central nervous system complications or prematurity than BPD, the duration of mechanical ventilation, or oxygen therapy.[122–124] Children who had BPD had lower mean psychometric scores compared to controls, but the differences disappeared when those with severe IVH were excluded.[122] Giacoia et al.[125] studied preterm children at 11 to 12 years of age. Although all preterm children were lower with regard to performance and full-scale IQ scores compared with the term controls, there was no difference in the proportion of children with borderline or low IQ between those with and those without BPD. In a later study, Gregoire et al.[126] compared the outcome of children with BPD based on the two different definitions: oxygen dependent at 28 days and not at 36 weeks PCA versus oxygen dependent at 36 weeks PCA. These children were compared at 18 months to other VLBW children who did not meet either definition for BPD. The children with milder BPD (oxygen dependent at 28 days and not 36 weeks PCA) were comparable to those without BPD in terms of neurodevelopmental outcome. Those with more severe BPD had a statistically significantly lower mean developmental quotient, although their scores were still within the normal range. This difference remained significant even when excluding severe IVH and periventricular leukomalacia (PVL).[126] Robertson et al.[127] also found some subtle variance in IQ and psychoeducational scores associated with more severe BPD. These data suggest that oxygen dependence at 36 weeks PCA might be a better predictor of later developmental delays.[126,127]

Overall the incidence of severe prematurity is not decreasing, and infants of less than 1000 g BW are surviving more frequently. Everyone involved with the care of high-risk neonates would like to be able to reliably predict the long-term outcome. Short-term, two-year outcomes can be predicted by the "alphabet soup of neonatal diseases": BPD, PDA, IVH, PVL, RDS, NEC.[128] The more diagnoses and the greater the severity, the more likely the surviving infant will have adverse findings on assessment at 18 to 24 months. However, the early predictors of disease severity and adverse outcomes at 18 to 24 months are not strong predictors of behavioral and school-age problems. Parental education, parental socioeconomic status, and other indicators of the environment take on more significance with age.[128,129] The strongest predictors of a good outcome are better parental education, childrearing by two parents, a stable family composition, and geographic residence at one location for greater than 10 years.[129] "Over time the neonatal risk factors become less critical as environmental influences play a synergistic relationship between biological and environmental risk factors, making preterm children especially vulnerable to non-

optimal environmental influences."[129] Furthermore, there is essentially no information on very late outcomes into adulthood and aging.

EXTRACORPOREAL MEMBRANE OXYGENATION

Medical Morbidity

The general criterion for extracorporeal membrane oxygenation (ECMO) use is a high mortality rate (>80%) related to the severity of the underlying illness. The most common diagnoses for which ECMO has been used are meconium aspiration syndrome (MAS), primary pulmonary hypertension, RDS, congenital diaphragmatic hernia (CDH), and group B streptococcus or other causes of pneumonia and sepsis. The illnesses leading to the need for ECMO treatment plus the treatment itself are all significant factors for the long-term sequelae. Underlying the diagnoses are the various physiologic problems related to the severity of the disease: hypoxia, stress, acidosis, hypotension, and the problems related to treatment prior to initiating ECMO[130] (hyperventilation-induced alkalosis, seizures, and intracranial hemorrhage). Finally, the potential complications of ECMO itself, including risks related to heparinization, equipment failure, and ligation of the carotid artery, must be factored into the equation.

Studies of the long-term outcome following ECMO often report just the ECMO population without reference to non-ECMO survivors. The outcome of ECMO survivors should really be compared to the outcome of infants with similar underlying diagnoses who were not treated with ECMO, in order to try to sort out the compounding effects of the ECMO therapy itself on the outcome.[131] Walsh-Sukys et al.[132] described their comparison of ECMO-treated children and children treated with conventional ventilation. They found an increased incidence of CLD in the children treated with conventional ventilation, but the neurodevelopmental outcomes were similar. In a later study, Rais-Bahrami et al.[133] compared the neurodevelopmental outcome at 5 years of age of survivors who were treated with ECMO and those patients they defined as near-miss ECMO. The near-miss ECMO group consisted of infants transported to their hospital because of failure to respond to medical management, with the intention of initiating ECMO, but who recovered without the use of bypass. They found similar rates of handicapping conditions in both groups as well.[133]

The major medical morbidity of ECMO survivors in the first year is related to respiratory illness.[134] Of all survivors, 62% had a history of taking, or were receiving, medications for a respiratory illness, and 25% were rehospitalized for respiratory problems during the first year. In addition, 26% had evidence of growth failure and 6% were seen for a nonstatic neurologic problem.[134] The most consistent abnormal growth parameter was microcephaly, and all children with microcephaly had associated respiratory and/or neurologic illness.[134,135] Dodge et al.,[136] however, reported an only 25% incidence of respiratory problems at 2 years, using the need for long-term respiratory medications or a tracheostomy as their criteria for respiratory morbidity. The majority of ECMO survivors have shown abnormal pulmonary mechanics at 6 months of age with increased airway resistance,[137] but lung function was slightly better compared to that of infants treated with conventional management for similar diagnoses.[138]

Certain variables during the acute course may interact with the underlying diagnosis to affect the overall outcome. Kornhauser et al.[139] found that the major risk for BPD after ECMO was the duration of mechanical ventilation. Infants at highest risk were those who had received more than 96 hours of mechanical ventilation prior to beginning ECMO. In a comparison of patients treated with ECMO and a cohort of infants treated with conventional or high-frequency ventilation, Vaucher et al.[140] demonstrated a 50% reduction in the incidence of CLD in the ECMO-treated children.

Children with RDS and MAS often have more medical complications, longer medical courses prior to being placed on ECMO, and more mechanical pulmonary complications that may all affect the overall long-term outcome.[131] CLD can result from both the pulmonary effects of meconium itself, as well as the ventilator-induced lung injury. In addition, the extrapulmonary effects of prolonged severe hypoxia, particularly on the brain, contribute to the long-term neurologic outcome. Prior to the use of ECMO for MAS, survivors were found to have a higher prevalence of asthmatic symptoms and abnormal bronchial reactivity than the general population.[141] Similarly, Swaminathan et al.[142] documented evidence of hyperinflation, increased closing volume, airway obstruction, and airway hyperreactivity. The current worldwide survival rate for more than 5000 neonates with MAS receiving ECMO support is 94%.[143] This is the highest survival rate for any neonatal condition that meets eligibility criteria for ECMO. In their follow-up study of ECMO survivors, Bernbaum et al.[144] reported a 33% incidence of BPD in ECMO-treated MAS patients at discharge, but by follow-up at 1 year the majority of patients had significant clinical improvement in respiratory status. The majority of their MAS patients also had some form of feeding dysfunction requiring supplemental tube feedings at discharge, but by 1 year of age their entire MAS population was being fed normally.[144]

The most complex group of patients to survive with ECMO support consists of those with CDH. These infants have the highest initial mortality rate, require the longest periods of ECMO and ventilatory support, and later have a high incidence of gastroesophageal reflux, feeding problems, and failure to thrive.[144–146] The overall incidence of BPD in ECMO patients at discharge was 40% in the survivors studied by Bernbaum et al.[144] However, they documented BPD in 63% of those with CDH as compared to less than half of the patients in the other diagnostic categories.[144] At follow-up at age 1 year, 50% of the CDH population continued to have requirements for supplemental oxygen, diuretics, or bronchodilators as compared to only 17% of the MAS population. Schwartz et al.[147] found evidence that pulmonary hypertension (PHT) persists or recurs well beyond the neonatal period in a significant portion of ECMO-treated children with CDH. Thirty-eight percent of the children, who were studied at a mean age of 3.8 ± 2.2 years, met echocardiographic criteria for PHT, although only a very small number had any clinical symptoms of PHT. Most of those patients with PHT had wheezing and some degree of exercise intolerance.[147]

Neurodevelopmental Outcome

The overall survival rate for infants treated with ECMO is 82%, and the vast majority of the survivors have a normal neurologic examination, fall within the normal range for developmental measures, and have intelligence scores in the average range. Bernbaum et al.[144] and Glass et al.[135] reported mean Bayley[111] scores of ECMO survivors within the normal range at 1-year follow-up. However, this masks a large minority with poor outcomes, associated either with ongoing cardiopulmonary or neurologic problems.[131] Children who are considered handicapped or who have one or more major disabilities have been reported in up to 10% to 36% of ECMO survivors.[134,136,148–150] The handicapping sequelae included spastic cerebral palsy, sensorineural hearing loss (SNHL), and cognitive deficiencies at school age. Studies reporting on later intellectual scores for ECMO survivors found that 10% to 30% of children had IQ scores greater than 1.5 to 2 SD below the mean normal range, and up to 35% of those children with seemingly normal outcomes qualified for special services at school age.[131] In follow-up studies of ECMO survivors at 5 years of age, Glass et al.[149] described a general lowering of IQ, a significant difference on multiple neuropsychological measures, and three times the incidence of behavior problems in ECMO survivors compared to normal full-term controls. This same group reported that the probability of disability at age 5 years was associated with the severity of brain lesions identified by routine cranial ultrasonography and computed tomography.[151] The severity of neonatal neuroimaging was inversely associated with decreased intellectual status, greater neuropsychological deficits across all domains, and poorer preacademic skills.

Some studies have reported a higher incidence of right-sided cerebral lesions after ECMO and attribute the lateralized brain abnormalities to the ligation of the right common carotid artery (RCCA).[152,153] However, Graziani et al.[154] did not find that post-ECMO neuroimaging or clinical evaluations indicated a selective or greater injury to the right cerebral hemisphere and believed that the long-term consequences of RCCA ligation have not been determined. Reconstruction of the RCCA immediately following decannulation has been done successfully.[155] Follow-up studies comparing patients with reconstruction to those whose RCCA was left ligated found significantly fewer brain scan abnormalities and less cerebral palsy (CP) in the reconstructed patients but similar scores on developmental and IQ testing.[156] The long-term consequences of RCCA ligation and the risks and benefits of RCCA reconstruction remain unknown.

SNHL has been identified as a significant complication in survivors of persistent PHT[157–159] and is the most common single neurosensory morbidity in ECMO survivors.[160] The incidence ranges between 3% and 21% of children.[134,149,150] Although some children may be diagnosed early with ABR screening, SNHL may present later as an isolated high frequency loss with progressive deterioration, and therefore, remain undetected for several years.[160] The exact mechanism for the SNHL remains unknown, but may be associated with various aggressive therapies commonly employed in this population prior to the initiation of ECMO. Hyperventilation has been associated with hearing loss while permissive hypercapnia might be protective.[157] Future research and a large population study are needed to determine the relationship of SNHL to the primary diagnosis and mode of treatment.

In their study published in 1996, Gringlas et al.[161] concluded that the primary diagnoses associated with the requirement for ECMO were not predictive of later developmental outcome. Nield et al.[162] reported no difference in functional status or neurologic sequelae at 3.5 years among children in different diag-

TABLE 28-1. Predictors of Neurodevelopmental Outcome at 12 to 30 Months

Outcome	Risk Factor	OR	CI	P Value
Neuromotor outcome				
Suspect or abnormal	CLD	2.60	0.97–0.99	0.005
	PPHN	4.40	1.16–16.49	0.01
	Neuroimaging abnormality*	5.10	1.55–17.09	0.01
Cerebral palsy	Neuroimaging abnormality*	10.30	1.56–67.83	0.001
	Gestational age	0.60	0.37–0.96	0.03
Developmental outcome				
MDI <84	Male gender	2.20	0.99–4.86	0.05
PDI <84	Neuroimaging abnormality*	6.30	1.72–23.32	0.006
	CLD	2.21	1.13–4.34	0.02
	Qualifying Pao$_2$	1.06	1.00–1.10	0.05
Adverse outcome†	Neuroimaging abnormality*	6.43	1.89–21.89	0.003
	CLD	2.38	1.23–4.59	0.01

* Moderate or severe.
† Neuromotor, neurosensory, or developmental.
CI, 95% Confidence interval; CLD, chronic lung disease; MDI, mental developmental index; OR, odds ratio; PDI, motor developmental index, PPHN, persistent pulmonary hypertension of the newborn.
From Vaucher YE, Dudell GG, Bejar R, et al: Predictors of early childhood outcome in candidates for extracorporeal membrane oxygenation. J Pediatr 128:115, 1996.

TABLE 28-2. Primary Diagnosis, Gestational Age, Birthweight, and Outcome in 181 Survivors of Neonatal Venoarterial (n = 152) or Venovenous (n = 29) Extracorporeal Membrane Oxygenation

	Outcomes			
	Normal		Suspect§	Abnormal‖
Neonatal Factors*	12–46 mo† (n = 96)	4.8–6 yr‡ (n = 34)	4.8–6 yr (n = 17)	16 mo–8 yr (n = 34)
Primary diagnosis				
MAS/PPHN	63	23	9	20
Diaphragmatic hernia	12	4	0	2
RDS/HMD	8	5	7	6
Sepsis/pneumonia	13	2	1	6
Gestational age, weeks (mean [SD])	39.4 (±2)	40.1 (±2)	39.6 (±2)	39.2 (±2)
Birthweight, kg (mean [SD])	3.31 (±0.6)	3.33 (±0.5)	3.20 (±0.5)	3.18 (±0.5)

* No significant differences in primary diagnosis, gestational age, or birthweight among the four groups: Chi-squared test.
† Presumed normal because of young age. No definite evidence of MR, CP, or Sensorineural hearing loss (SNHL).
‡ Wechsler Preschool and Primary Scales of Intelligence—Revised (WPPSI-R) full scale IQ ≥85; normal neurologic examination, and normal hearing thresholds for both ears at school age.
§ WPPSI-R full-scale IQ between 71 and 84, without CP and SNHL at school age.
‖ CP (n = 17); SNHL without CP or MR (n = 12); MR without CP or SNHL (n = 5).
MAS/PPHN; Meconium aspiration syndrome/persistent pulmonary hypertension of the newborn; RDS/HMD; respiratory distress syndrome/hyaline membrane disease.
From Graziani LJ, Gringlas M, Baumgart S: Cerebrovascular complications and neurodevelopmental sequelae of neonatal extracorporeal membrane oxygenation. Clin Perinatol 24:664, 1997.

nostic categories. Robertson et al.[163] noted no differences in neurodevelopmental disabilities, and mean Bayley MDI and PDI scores at 2 years of age were within the normal range for a group of ECMO-treated patients compared with infants who met ECMO criteria but were treated with conventional ventilation because of lower oxygenation indices after transfer. The risk factors for poor neurodevelopmental outcome might be related to the increased severity of the underlying illness and the various treatment modalities used prior to ECMO rather than either the specific respiratory diagnosis or the ECMO therapy itself. Hofkosh et al.[150] and Kornhauser et al.[139] both distinguished survivors with BPD as having worse developmental outcomes. These findings were further substantiated by the published results of Vaucher et al.,[140] whose data showed that infants treated with ECMO were as likely to have normal neurologic examinations as those managed with alternative treatment strategies. Major disabilities were more common in infants with CLD, and CLD increased the risk of neurodevelopmental delay at 12 to 30 months after adjusting for other variables such as respiratory diagnosis and treatment modality (Table 28-1). Kumar et al.[164] found that longer duration of ventilation and use of supplemental oxygen were significantly associated with abnormal neurodevelopmental outcome. ECMO survivors with CDH were noted to have increased neurologic sequelae and lower cognitive scores.[165,166] However, this higher incidence of neurologic sequelae in the CDH population might be due to the increased severity of illness, as reflected in lower Apgar scores, decreased initial and best Po$_2$, and the need for surgical patch closure of either the diaphragm or abdomen.[167] Graziani et al.[168] studied the outcome of

TABLE 28-3. Cerebral Palsy (n = 17) Compared with Normal School-Age Outcome (n = 34) in 51 Venoarterial ECMO Survivors: Neonatal Clinical Features

Clinical Features	Normal* (n = 34)	Cerebral Palsy† (n = 17)	P Value‡
Lowest pH Pre-ECMO	7.16±0.19	7.19±0.23	NS
Lowest Pao$_2$ Pre-ECMO	29.9±8.5	31.6±23.5	NS
Lowest Paco$_2$ Pre-ECMO	22.9±9.6	18.5±7.7	NS
Oxygenation index§	63.7±46.9	92.7±64.5	<0.02
Lowest systolic blood pressure‖	46.2±9.5	40.9±11.3	<0.01
CPR before ECMO (n[%])	0 (0)	8 (47)	<0.0001

Data represent mean ± SD, except for (CPR). Gestational age, birthweight, Apgar scores, age at start of extracorporeal membrane oxygenation (ECMO), duration of ECMO, and highest neonatal indirect bilirubin level did not differ significantly between the two groups.
* Normal neurologic examination full-scale WPPSI-R IQ scores >84, and normal bilateral hearing at age 4.8–6.0 years.
† Spastic form of CP at age 15 months to 8 years, confirmed by repeated examinations.
‡ Chi-square or Kruskal-Wallis tests of significance. NS, not significant.
§ Last oxygenation index before ECMO. Normal, n = 15; cerebral palsy, n = 6.
‖ In mm Hg, before or during ECMO.
Pao$_2$, partial pressure of oxygen; Paco$_2$, partial pressure of carbon dioxide (lowest value (mm Hg) in postductal arterial blood before ECMO).
CPR, vigorous cardiopulmonary resuscitation prior to ECMO exclusive of the immediate resuscitation at birth. Percentage calculated from the total number of survivors in each column.
From Graziani LJ, Gringlas M, Baumgart S: Cerebrovascular complications and neurodevelopmental sequelae of extracorporeal membrane oxygenation. Clin Perinatol 24: 665, 1997. Adapted from Graziani LJ, Baumgart S, Desai S, et al: Clinical antecedents of neurologic and audiologic abnormalities in survivors of neonatal ECMO. J Child Neurol 12: 415–422, 1997.

181 ECMO survivors to determine the neonatal clinical correlates of severe cardiorespiratory failure treated with ECMO and the neurodevelopmental sequelae. Their results indicated that there were no differences in outcome among the primary diagnostic groups requiring ECMO (Table 28-2). The risk for cerebral palsy was increased in infants who had hypotension (systolic blood pressure below 39 mm Hg) or required cardiopulmonary resuscitation prior to ECMO (Table 28-3). In addition, the risk for SNHL was associated with profound hypocarbia before initiation of ECMO therapy.[168]

The development of techniques for the mechanical ventilation of infants with respiratory failure should be considered one of the major advances in medical therapy in the past several decades. As improvements in assisted ventilation and other supportive technologies allow for the survival of smaller and more severely ill newborns, comprehensive long-term follow-up of these babies remains essential, both for the documentation and critical evaluation of evolving patient care and for the detection of any potentially handicapping conditions in children who have survived neonatal intensive care. The interactions between lung growth and repair of lung injury and brain growth and early brain injury in growing children remain speculative at best. The discovery of abnormal outcomes in groups of patients may lead to improvements in clinical practice. The early detection of abnormalities in an individual child permits anticipatory guidance for the family and the child, as well as the provision of appropriate early intervention services in order to minimize the impact of any impairment. Only through careful follow-up can care be improved for patients, both present and future.

REFERENCES

1. Stevenson DK, Wright LL, Lemons JA, et al: Very low birth weight outcomes of the National Institute of Child Health and Human Development Neonatal Research Network, January 1993 through December 1994. Am J Obstet Gynecol 179:1632, 1998.
2. Mansell AL, Driscoll JM, James LS: Pulmonary follow-up of moderately low birth weight infants with and without RDS. J Pediatr 110:111, 1987.
3. Northway WH, Rosan RC, Porter DY: Pulmonary disease following respiratory therapy of hyaline membrane disease: Bronchopulmonary dysplasia. N Engl J Med 276:357, 1967.
4. O'Brodovich HM, Mellins RB: Bronchopulmonary dysplasia. Am Rev Respir Dis 132:694, 1985.
5. Tooley WH: Epidemiology of bronchopulmonary dysplasia. J Pediatr 95:819, 1979.
6. Shennan AT, Dunn MS, Ohlsson A, et al: Abnormal pulmonary outcomes in premature infants: Prediction from oxygen requirement in the neonatal period. Pediatrics 82:527, 1988.
7. Bhutani VK, Abbasi S: Long-term pulmonary consequences in survivors with bronchopulmonary dysplasia. Clin Perinatol 19:649, 1992.
8. Capper A: The fate and development of the immature and of the premature child. Am J Dis Child 35:443, 1928.
9. Douglas JWB, Mogford C: Health of premature children from birth to four years. Br Med J 1:748, 1983.
10. Kennedy JD: Lung function outcome in children of premature birth. J Paediatr Child Health 35:516, 1999.
11. Barker DJP, Godfrey KM, Fall C, et al: Relation of birth weight and childhood respiratory infection to adult lung function and death from chronic obstructive airways disease. Br Med J 303:671, 1991.
12. Chan KN, Elliman A, Bryan E, et al: Clinical significance of airway responsiveness in children of low birth weight. Pediatr Pulmonol 7:251, 1989.
13. Tammela OKT, Linna OVE, Koivista ME: Long-term pulmonary sequelae in low birth weight infants with and without RDS. Acta Paediatr Scand 80:542, 1991.
14. Pelkonen AS, Hakulinen AL, Turpeinen M: Bronchial lability and responsiveness in school children born very preterm. Am J Respir Crit Care Med 156:1178, 1997.
15. Rona RJ, Gulliford MD, Chinn S: Effects of prematurity and intrauterine growth on respiratory health and lung function in childhood. BMJ 306:817, 1993.
16. Galdis-Sebaldt M, Sheller JR, Grogaard J, et al: Prematurity is associated with abnormal airway function in childhood. Pediatr Pulmonol 7:259, 1989.
17. Rojas MA, Gonzaloz A, Bancalari E, et al: Changing trends in the epidemiology and pathogenesis of neonatal chronic lung disease. J Pediatr 126:605, 1995.
18. Cano A, Payo F: Lung function and airway responsiveness in children and adolescents after hyaline membrane disease: A matched cohort study. Eur Respir J 10:880, 1997.
19. deKleine MJK, Roos CM, Voorn WJ, et al: Lung function 8–18 years after intermittent positive pressure ventilation for hyaline membrane disease. Thorax 45:941, 1990.
20. McLeod A, Ross P, Mitchell S, et al: Respiratory health in a total very low birth weight cohort and three classroom controls. Arch Dis Child 74:188, 1996.

21. Schraeder BD, Czjika C, Kalman DD, et al: Respiratory health, lung function and airway responsiveness in school-age survivors of very low birth weight. Clin Pediatr 37:237, 1998.

22. Kennedy JD, Edward LJ, Bates DJ, et al: Effects of birth weight and oxygen supplementation on lung function in late childhood in children of very low birth weight. Pediatr Pulmonol 30:32, 2000.

23. Northway WH, Moss RB, Carlisle KB, et al: Late pulmonary sequelae of bronchopulmonary dysplasia. N Engl J Med 323:1793, 1990.

24. Howling SJ, Northway WH, Hansell DM, et al: Pulmonary sequelae of bronchopulmonary dysplasia survivors: High resolution CT findings. Am J Radiol 174:1323, 2000.

25. Andreasson B, Lindroth M, Mortensson W, et al: Lung function eight years after neonatal ventilation. Arch Dis Child 64:108, 1989.

26. Blayney M, Kerern E, Whyte H, et al: BPD: Improvement in lung function between 7 and 10 years of age. J Pediatr 118:201, 1991.

27. Koumbourlis AC, Motoyama EK, Mutich RL, et al: Longitudinal follow-up of lung function from childhood to adolescence in prematurely born patients with neonatal chronic lung disease. Pediatr Pulmonol 21:28, 1996.

28. Kim TC, Wheeler W, Longmate J, et al: Longitudinal study of lung function in children following bronchopulmonary dysplasia. Am Rev Respir Dis 137:A18, 1988.

29. Doyle LW, Ford GW, Olinsky A, et al: Bronchopulmonary dysplasia and very low birth weight: Lung function at 11 years of age. J Paediatr Child Health 32:339, 1996.

30. Gross SJ, Iannuzzi DM, Kueselis DA, et al: Effect of preterm birth on pulmonary function at school age: A prospective controlled study. J Pediatr 133:188, 1998.

31. Mallory GB, Chaney H, Mutich RL, et al: Longitudinal changes in lung function during the first 3 years of premature infants with moderate to severe bronchopulmonary dysplasia. Pediatr Pulmonol 11:8, 1991.

32. Jacob SV, Coates AL, Lands LC, et al: Long-term pulmonary sequelae of severe bronchopulmonary dysplasia. J Pediatr 133:193, 1998.

33. Santuz P, Baraldi E, Zaramella P, et al: Factors limiting exercise performance in long-term survivors of BPD. Am J Respir Crit Care Med 152:1284, 1995.

34. Bader D, Ramos AD, Lew CD, et al: Childhood sequelae of infant lung disease: Exercise and pulmonary function abnormalities after bronchopulmonary dysplasia. J Pediatr 110:693, 1987.

35. Parat S, Moriette G, Delapuche M-F, et al: Long-term pulmonary functional outcome of bronchopulmonary dysplasia and premature birth. Pediatr Pulmonol 20:289, 1995.

36. Jacob SV, Lands LC, Coates AL, et al: Exercise ability in survivors of severe bronchopulmonary dysplasia. Am J Respir Crit Care Med 155:1925, 1997.

37. Pianosi PT, Fisk M: Cardiopulmonary exercise performance in prematurely born children. Pediatr Res 47:653, 2000.

38. Hakulinen AL, Jarvenpaa A-L, Turpeinew M, et al: Diffusing capacity of the lung in school-aged children born very preterm, with and without BPD. Pediatr Pulmonol 21:353, 1996.

39. Chernick V: Long-term pulmonary function studies in children with bronchopulmonary dysplasia: An everchanging saga. J Pediatr 133:171, 1998.

40. Stocker JT: Pathologic features of long-standing "healed" bronchopulmonary dysplasia: A study of 28 3- to 40 month-old infants. Hum Pathol 17:943, 1986.

41. Husain AN, Siddiqui NH, Stocker JT: Pathology of arrested acinar development in postsurfactant BPD. Hum Pathol 29:710, 1998.

42. McCarthy K, Bhogal M, Nardi M, et al: Pathogenic factors in bronchopulmonary dysplasia. Pediatr Res 18:482, 1984.

43. Margraf LR, Tomashifshi JF, Bruce MC, et al: Morphometric analysis of the lung. Am Rev Respir Dis 143:391, 1991.

44. Greenough A: Gains and losses from dexamethasone for neonatal chronic lung disease. Lancet 352:835, 1998.

45. Tschanz SA, Damke BM, Burri PH: Influence of postnatally administered glucocorticoids on rat lung growth. Biol Neonate 68:229, 1995.

46. Abbasi S, Bhutani VK, Gerdes JS: Long-term pulmonary consequences of respiratory distress syndrome in preterm infants treated with exogenous surfactant. J Pediatr 122:446, 1993.

47. Nickerson BG, Taussig LM: Family history of asthma in infants with bronchopulmonary dysplasia. Pediatrics 65:1140, 1980.

48. Riedel F: Longterm effects of artificial ventilation in neonates. Acta Paediatr Scand 76:24, 1987.

49. Giffin F, Greenough A, Yuksel B: Prediction of respiratory morbidity in the third year of life in children born prematurely. Acta Paediatr 83:157, 1994.

50. von Mutius E, Nicolai T, Martinez FD: Prematurity as a risk factor for asthma in preadolescent children. J Pediatr 123:223, 1993.

51. Schaubel D, Johansen H, Dutta M, et al: Neonatal characteristics as risk factors for preschool asthma. J Asthma 33:255, 1996.

52. Johnston IDA, Blanel JM, Andersson HR: Ethnic variation in respiratory morbidity and lung function in childhood. Thorax 42:542, 1987.

53. Bertrand J-M, Riley SP, Popkin J, et al: The long term pulmonary sequelae of prematurity: The role of familial airway hyperactivity and the respiratory distress syndrome. N Engl J Med 312:742, 1985.

54. Hagen R, Minutillo C, French N, et al: Neonatal chronic lung disease, oxygen dependency and a family history of asthma. Pediatr Pulmonol 20:277, 1995.

55. Evans M, Palta M, Sadek M, et al: Associations between a family history of asthma, bronchopulmonary dysplasia and childhood asthma in very low birth weight children. Am J Epidemiol 148:460, 1998.

56. Kramer MS, Coates AL, Niechoud M-C, et al: Maternal asthma and idiopathic preterm labor. Am J Epidemiol 142:1078, 1995.

57. Chan KN, Noble-Jamieson CM, Elliman A, et al: Airway responsiveness in low birth weight children and their mothers. Arch Dis Child 63:905, 1988.

58. Chan KN, Silverman M: Neonatal chronic lung disease and a family history of asthma. Pediatr Pulmonol 20:273, 1995.

59. Joshi VV, Mandavia SG, Stern L, et al: Acute lesions induced by endotracheal intubation. Am J Dis Child 124:646, 1972.

60. Rasche RFH, Kuhns LR: Histopathologic changes in airway mucosa of infants after endotracheal intubation. Pediatrics 50:632, 1972.

61. Hatch DJ: Prolonged nasotracheal intubation in infants and children. Lancet 1:1272, 1968.

62. Jones R, Bodnar A, Roan Y, et al: Subglottic stenosis in newborn intensive care unit graduates. Am J Dis Child 135:367, 1981.

63. Choffat JM, Goumax CF, Guex JC: Laryngotracheal damage after prolonged intubation in the newborn infant. In Stetson JB, Swyer PR (eds): Neonatal Intensive Care. St. Louis, Warren H. Green, 1975, p. 253.

64. Ratner I, Whitefield J: Acquired subglottic stenosis in the very low birth weight infant. Am J. Dis Child 137:40, 1983.

65. Symchych PS, Cadotte M: Squamous metaplasia and necrosis of the trachea complicating prolonged nasotracheal intubation of small newborn infants. J Pediatr 71:534, 1967.

66. Blackfan KD, Wolback SB: Vitamin A deficiency in infants. J Pediatr 3:679, 1983.

67. Hustead VA, Gutcher GR, Anderson SA, et al: Relationship of vitamin A (retinal) status to lung disease in the preterm infant. J Pediatr 105:610, 1984.

68. Shenai JP, Chytil F, Jhaveri A, et al: Plasma vitamin A and retinal-binding protein in premature and term neonates. J Pediatr 99:302, 1981.

69. Meehan MA, Falciglia HS, Galciglia GA, et al: Dietary intake of antioxidants during pregnancy and their relationship to bronchopulmonary dysplasia. Pediatr Res 31:316A, 1992.

70. Shenai JP, Kennedy KA, Chytil F, et al: Clinical trial of vitamin A supplementation in infants susceptible to bronchopulmonary dysplasia. J Pediatr 111:269, 1987.

71. Pearson EB, Bose CL, Snidow TM, et al: Trial of vitamin A supplementation in very low birth weight infants at risk for bronchopulmonary dysplasia. J Pediatr 121:420, 1992.

72. Lum H, Schwartz LW, Dungworth DL, et al: A comparative study of cell renewal after exposure to ozone or oxygen: Response of terminal bronchiolar epithelium in the rat. Am Rev Respir Dis 118:335, 1978.

73. Philpott DE, Harrison GA, Turbill C, et al: Ultrastructural changes in tracheal epithelial cells exposed to oxygen. Aviat Space Environ Med 48:812, 1977.

74. Sackner MA, Landa J, Hirsch J, et al: Pulmonary effects of oxygen breathing: A 6 hour study in normal men. Ann Intern Med 82:40, 1975.

75. Deneke SM, Fanburg BL: Normobaric oxygen toxicity of the lung. N Engl J Med 303:76, 1980.

76. Fox R, Hoidal J, Brown D, et al: Hyperoxia causes a preterminal influx of polymorphonuclear leukocytes into the lungs and is associated with increased lung lavage chemotaxim. Am Rev Respir Dis 121:340, 1980.

77. Thibeault DW, Rezaiekhaligh M, Mabry S, et al: Prevention of chronic pulmonary oxygen toxicity in young rats with liposome-encapsulated catalase administered intratracheally. Pediatr Pulmonol 11:318, 1991.

78. Rosenfield W, Evans H, Concepcion L, et al: Prevention of bronchopulmonary dysplasia by administration of bovine superoxide dismutase in preterm infants with respiratory distress syndrome. J Pediatr 105:781, 1984.

79. Markestad T, Fitzhardinge PM: Growth and development in children recovering from bronchopulmonary dysplasia. J Pediatr 98:597, 1981.

80. Vohr BR, Bell F, Oh W: Infants with bronchopulmonary dysplasia. Am J Dis Child 136:443, 1982.
81. Meisels SJ, Plunkett JW, Roloff DW, et al: Growth and development of preterm infants with respiratory distress syndrome and bronchopulmonary dysplasia. Pediatrics 77:345, 1986.
82. Bregman J, Farrell EE: Neurodevelopmental outcome in infants with bronchopulmonary dysplasia. Clin Perinatol 19:673, 1992.
83. Vrlenick LA, Bozynski MEA, Shyr Y, et al: The effect of bronchopulmonary dysplasia on growth at school age. Pediatrics 95:855, 1995.
84. Chye JK, Gray PH: Rehospitalization and growth of infants with bronchopulmonary dysplasia: A matched control study. J Paediatr Child Health 31:105, 1995.
85. Davidson S, Schrayer A, Wielunshy E, et al: Energy intake, growth, and development in ventilated very low birth weight infants with and without bronchopulmonary dysplasia. Am J Dis Child 144:553, 1990.
86. deRegnier RAD, Guilbert TW, Mills MM, et al: Growth failure and altered body composition are established by 1 month of age in infants with bronchopulmonary dysplasia. J Nutr 126:168, 1996.
87. Greer FR, McCormick A: Bone mineral content and growth in very low birth weight premature infants. Am J Dis Child 141:179, 1987.
88. Singer LT, Davillier M, Pruess L, et al: Feeding interactions in infants with very low birth weight and bronchopulmonary dysplasia. J Dev Behav Pediatr 17:69, 1996.
89. Lewis S: A follow-up study of the respiratory distress syndrome. Proc R Soc Med 61:771, 1968.
90. Yuksel B, Greenough A: Relationship of symptoms to lung function abnormalities in preterm infants at follow up. Pediatr Pulmonol 11:202, 1991.
91. Korhonen P, Koivisto AM, Ikonen S, et al: Very low birth weight, bronchopulmonary dysplasia and health in early childhood. Acta Paediatr 88:1385, 1999.
92. Greenough A: Measuring respiratory outcome. Semin Neonatol 5:119, 2000.
93. Stahlman M, Hedvall G, Lindstrom D, et al: Role of hyaline membrane disease in production of later childhood abnormalities. Pediatrics 69:572, 1982.
94. Chan KN, Noble-Jamieson CM, Elliman A, et al: Lung function in children of low birth weight. Arch Dis Child 64:1284, 1989.
95. Kitchen WH, Olinsky A, Doyle LW, et al: Respiratory health and lung function in 8 year old children of very low birth weight: A cohort study. Pediatrics 89:1151, 1992.
96. Furman L, Baley J, Borawski-Clarke E, et al: Hospitalization as a measure of morbidity among very low birth weight infants with chronic lung disease. J Pediatr 128:447, 1996.
97. Wright AL, Holberg C, Martinez FD, et al: Relationship of parental smoking to wheezing and non-wheezing lower respiratory tract illness in infancy. J Pediatr 118:207, 1991.
98. Carbonell-Estraney X, Quero J, Bustos G, et al: Rehospitalization because of RSV infection in premature infants < 33 weeks of gestation: A prospective study. Pediatr Infect Dis 19:592, 2000.
99. Hobbs JR, Davis JA: Serum gamma-G-globulin levels and gestational age in premature babies. Lancet 1:757, 1967.
100. Hyvarinen M, Zelzer P, Oh W, et al: Influence of gestational age on serum levels of alpha-1 fetoprotein, IgG globulin and albumin in newborn infants. J Pediatr 82:430, 1975.
101. Papadatos C, Papuevangelou G, Alexiou D, et al: Immunoglobulin levels and gestational age. Biol Neonate 14:365, 1969.
102. Ballow M, Cates KL, Rowe JC, et al: Development of the immune system in very low birth weight (less than 1500g) premature infants: concentration of plasma immunoglobulins and patterns of infection. Pediatr Res 20:899, 1986.
103. Mugruia de Suria T, Kumar ML, Wasser TE, et al: RSV-specific immunoglobulins in preterm infants. J Pediatr 122:787, 1993.
104. Abzug ML, Beam AC, Gyorkos EA, et al: Viral pneumonia in the first month of life. Pediatr Infect Dis 9:881, 1990.
105. Heilman CA: Respiratory syncytial and parainfluenza viruses. J Infect Dis 161:402, 1990.
106. Groothius JR, Gutierrez KM, Lauer BA: Respiratory syncytial virus infection in children with bronchopulmonary dysplasia. Pediatrics 82:199, 1988.
107. Baker KA, Ryan ME: RSV infection in infants and young children. Postgrad Med 106:97, 1999.
108. Meert K, Heidemann S, Lieh-Lai M, et al: Clinical characteristics of RSV infections in healthy vs previously compromised host. Pediatr Pulmonol 7:167, 1989.
109. American Academy of Pediatrics: Committee on Infectious Disease and Fetus and Newborn: Respiratory Syncytial Virus: Use of RespiGam (Palivizumab). Pediatrics 102:1121, 1998.
110. The PREVENT Study Group: Reduction of respiratory syncytial virus hospitalization among premature infants and infants with bronchopulmonary dysplasia using respiratory syncytial virus immune globulin prophylaxis. Pediatrics 99:93, 1997.
111. Bayley N: Bayley Scales of Infant Development. New York, Psychological Corp., 1969.
112. Skidmore MD, Rivers A, Hack M: Increased risk of cerebral palsy among very low birth weight infants with chronic lung disease. Dev Med Child Neurol 32:325, 1990.
113. Landry SH, Fletcher JM, Denson SE, et al: Longitudinal outcome for low birth weight infants: Effects of IVH and BPD. J Clin Exp Neuropsychol 15:205, 1993.
114. Perlman JM, Volpe JJ: Movement disorder of premature infants with severe bronchopulmonary dysplasia: A new syndrome. Pediatrics 84:215, 1989.
115. Vohr BR, Coll CG, Lobato D, et al: Neurodevelopmental and medical status of low birth weight survivors of bronchopulmonary dysplasia at 10–12 years of age. Dev Med Child Neurol 33:690, 1991.
116. O'Shea TM, Goldstein DJ, deRegnier R-A, et al: Outcome to 4–5 years of age in children recovered from neonatal chronic lung disease. Dev Med Child Neurol 38:830, 1996.
117. Hughes CA, O'Gorman LA, Skyr Y, et al: Cognitive performance at school age of very low birth weight infants with bronchopulmonary dysplasia. J Dev Behav Pediatr 20:1, 1999.
118. Farel AM, Hooper SR, Teplin SW, et al: Very low birth weight infants at 7 years: An assessment of the health and neurodevelopmental risk conveyed by chronic lung disease. J Learn Disabil 31:118, 1998.
119. Katz-Salamon M, Gerner EM, Jonsson B, et al: Early motor and mental development in very preterm infants with chronic lung disease. Arch Dis Child Fetal Neonatal Ed 83:F1, 2000.
120. Majnemer A, Riley P, Shevell M, et al: Severe bronchopulmonary dysplasia increases risk for later neurological and motor sequelae in preterm infants. Dev Med Child Neurol 42:53, 2000.
121. Singer L, Yarnashita T, Lilien L, et al: A longitudinal study of developmental outcomes of infants with bronchopulmonary dysplasia and very low birth weight. Pediatrics 100:987, 1997.
122. Gray PH, Burus YR, Mohay HA, et al: Neurodevelopmental outcome of preterm infants with bronchopulmonary dysplasia. Arch Dis Child 73:F128, 1995.
123. Luchi JM, Bennett FC, Jackson JC: Predictors of neurodevelopmental outcome following bronchopulmonary dysplasia. Am J Dis Child 145:813, 1991.
124. Teberg AJ, Pena I, Finello K, et al: Prediction of neurodevelopmental outcome in infants with and without bronchopulmonary dysplasia. Am J Med Sci 301:369, 1991.
125. Giacoia GP, Venkataraman PS, West-Wilson KI, et al: Follow-up of school-age children with bronchopulmonary dysplasia. J Pediatr 130:400, 1997.
126. Gregoire M-C, Lefebve F, Glorieux J: Health and developmental outcomes at 18 months in very preterm infants with bronchopulmonary dysplasia. Pediatrics 101:856, 1998.
127. Robertson CMT, Etches PC, Goldson E, et al: Eight-year school performance, neurodevelopmental and growth outcome of neonates with bronchopulmonary dysplasia: A comparative study. Pediatrics 89:365, 1989.
128. Jobe AH: Predictors of outcomes in preterm infants: Which ones and when? J Pediatr 138:153, 2001.
129. Gross SJ, Mittelman BB, Dye TD, et al: Impact of family structure and stability on academic outcome in preterm children at 10 years of age. J Pediatr 138:169, 2001.
130. Davis DW: Long-term follow-up of survivors of neonatal ECMO: What do we really know? Pediatr Nurs 24:343, 1998.
131. Gangarosa ME, Hynd GW, Cohen MJ: Developmental long-term follow-up of ECMO survivors. J Clin Child Psychol 23:174, 1994.
132. Walsh-Sukys MC, Bauer RE, Cornell DJ, et al: Severe respiratory failure in neonates: Mortality and morbidity rates and neurodevelopmental outcome. J Pediatr 125:104, 1994.
133. Rais-Bahrami K, Wagner AE, Coffman C, et al: Neurodevelopmental outcome in ECMO and near-miss ECMO patients at 5 years. Clin Perinatol 39:145, 2000.
134. Schumacher RE, Palmer TW, Roloff DW, et al: Follow-up of infants treated with extracorporeal membrane oxygenation for newborn respiratory failure. Pediatrics 87:451, 1991.

135. Glass P, Miller M, Short B: Morbidity for survivors of extracorporeal membrane oxygenation: Neurodevelopmental outcome at 1 year of age. Pediatrics 83:72, 1989.
136. Dodge NN, Engle WA, West KW, et al: Outcome of ECMO survivors at age 2 years: Relationship to status at 1 year. J Perinatol 16:191, 1996.
137. Garg M, Kurzner SI, Bautista DB, et al: Pulmonary sequelae at 6 months following ECMO. Chest 101:1086, 1992.
138. Beardsmore C, Dundas I, Poole K, et al: Respiratory function in survivors of the United Kingdom ECMO trial. Am J Respir Crit Care Med 161:1129, 2000.
139. Kornhauser MS, Baumgart S, Desai SA, et al: Adverse neurodevelopmental outcome after ECMO among neonates with bronchopulmonary dysplasia. J Pediatr 132:307, 1998.
140. Vaucher YE, Dudell GG, Bejar R, et al: Predictors of early childhood outcome in candidates for extracorporeal membrane oxygenation. J Pediatr 126:109, 1996.
141. MacFarlane PI, Heaf DP: Pulmonary function in children after neonatal meconium aspiration syndrome. Arch Dis Child 63:368, 1988.
142. Swaminathan S, Quinn J, Stabile M, et al: Long term pulmonary sequelae of meconium aspiration syndrome. J Pediatr 114:356, 1989.
143. Davis PJ, Shekerdemian LS: Meconium aspiration syndrome and extracorporeal membrane oxygenation. Arch Dis Child 84:F1, 2001.
144. Bernbaum J, Schwartz IP, Gerdes M, et al: Survivors of ECMO at 1 year of age: The relationship of primary diagnosis with health and neurodevelopmental sequelae. Pediatrics 96:907, 1995.
145. D'Agostino JA, Bernbaum JC, Gerdes M, et al: One year outcome of infants with congenital diaphragmatic hernia following extracorporeal membrane oxygenation. J Pediatr Surg 30:10, 1995.
146. VanMeurs KP, Robbins ST, Reed UL, et al: Congenital diaphragmatic hernia: Long-term outcome in neonates treated with extracorporeal membrane oxygenation. J Pediatr 122:893, 1993.
147. Schwartz IP, Bernbaum JC, Rychik J, et al: Pulmonary hypertension in children following extracorporeal membrane oxygenation therapy and repair of congenital diaphragmatic hernia. J Perinatol 19:220, 1999.
148. Flusser H, Dodge NN, Engle WA, et al: Neurodevelopmental outcome and respiratory morbidity for extracorporeal membrane oxygenation survivors at 1 year of age. J Perinatol 13:266, 1993.
149. Glass P, Wagner AE, Papero PH, et al: Neurodevelopmental status at age 5 years of neonates treated with ECMO. J Pediatr 127:447, 1995.
150. Hofkosh D, Thompson AE, Nozza RJ, et al: 10 years of extracorporeal membrane oxygenation: Neurodevelopmental outcome. Pediatrics 87:549, 1991.
151. Glass P, Bulas DIO, Wagner AE, et al: Severity of brain injury following neonatal extracorporeal membrane oxygenation and outcome at age 5 years. Dev Med Child Neurol 39:441, 1997.

152. Campbell LR, Bunyapur C, Holmes GL, et al: Right common carotid artery ligation in ECMO. J Pediatr 113:110, 1988.
153. Schumacher RE, Barks JDE, Johnston MV, et al: Right-sided brain lesions in infants following extracorporeal membrane oxygenation. Pediatrics 82:155, 1988.
154. Graziani LJ, Gringlas M, Baumgart S: Cerebrovascular complications and neurodevelopmental sequelae of neonatal extracorporeal membrane oxygenation. Clin Perinatol 24:655, 1997.
155. DeAngelis GA, Mitchell DG, Merton DA, et al: Right common carotid artery reconstruction in neonates after extracorporeal membrane oxygenation: Color Doppler imaging. Radiology 182:521, 1992.
156. Desai SA, Stanley C, Gringlas M, et al: Five year follow-up of neonates with reconstructed right common carotid arteries after ECMO. J Pediatr 134:428, 1999.
157. Marron MJ, Crisafi MA, Driscoll JM, et al: Hearing and neurodevelopmental outcome in survivors of persistent pulmonary hypertension. Pediatrics 90:392, 1992.
158. Naulty CM, Weiss IP, Herer GR: Progressive sensorineural hearing loss in survivors of persistent fetal circulation. Ear Hear 7:74, 1986.
159. Nield TA, Schier S, Ramos AD, et al: Unexpected hearing loss in high risk infants. Pediatrics 78:417, 1986.
160. Cheung P-Y, Robertson CMT: Sensorineural hearing loss in survivors of neonatal ECMO. Pediatr Rehabil 1:127, 1997.
161. Gringlas MB, Wiswell TE, Stanley C, et al: Primary diagnoses as predictors of long-term developmental outcome in school age survivors of extracorporeal life support (ECLS): A longitudinal study. Pediatr Res 39:266A, 1996.
162. Nield TA, Langenbacher D, Poulsen MK, et al: Neurodevelopmental outcomes at 3.5 years of age in children treated with ECMO life support: Relationship to primary diagnosis. J Pediatr 136:338, 2000.
163. Robertson CMT, Finer NN, Sauve RS, et al: Neurodevelopmental outcome after neonatal ECMO. Can Med Assoc J 152:1981, 1995.
164. Kumar P, Shanharan S, Behard MP, et al: Identifying at risk infants following neonatal extracorporeal membrane oxygenation. J Perinatol 19:367, 1999.
165. Ahmad A, Gangitano E, Odell RM, et al: Survival, intracranial lesions and neurodevelopmental outcome in infants with congenital diaphragmatic hernia with ECMO. J Perinatol 19:436, 1999.
166. Stolar CJH, Crisafi MA, Driscoll Y: Neurocognitive outcome for neonates treated with extracorporeal membrane oxygenation: Are infants with congenital diaphragmatic hernia different? J Pediatr Surg 30:366, 1995.
167. McGahren ED, Mallik K, Rodgers BM: Neurological outcome is diminished in survivors of congenital diaphragmatic hernia requiring ECMO. J Pediatr Surg 32:1216, 1997.
168. Graziani LJ, Baumgart S, Desai S, et al: Clinical antecedents of neurologic and audiologic abnormalities in survivors of neonatal extracorporeal membrane oxygenation. J Child Neurol 12:415, 1997.

VENTILATORY MANAGEMENT CASEBOOKS

JAY P. GOLDSMITH, MD

THERESA P. ROCA, MD

The topics of the following eight casebooks were originally published in the Second Edition of *Assisted Ventilation of the Neonate* (1988). They represent illustrations of common clinical problems associated with caring for infants supported by assisted ventilation devices. Over the last 15 years, the care of these infants has changed so dramatically that we have chosen to revisit each clinical topic for an update. After each clinical case, a diagnosis and discussion are presented that may refer the reader to previous chapters in the text. All casebooks represent summaries of actual patients treated in the neonatal intensive care unit (NICU) of the Ochsner Foundation Hospital in New Orleans, Louisiana. The authors are greatly indebted to the nurses, respiratory therapists, neonatal nurse practitioners, and residents who truly "cared for" these fragile infants with diligence, wisdom, and compassion.

CASE 1

History

A 920-g male infant was born to a 22-year-old primigravida at 27 weeks' gestation by vaginal delivery. Apgar scores were 1 and 3 at 1 and 5 minutes, respectively. The infant demonstrated signs of respiratory distress with tachypnea, retractions, and cyanosis, requiring intubation in the delivery room and administration of exogenous surfactant by 10 minutes of age. He was moved to the NICU where an umbilical artery catheter was inserted. After stabilization, he was placed on a pressure-limited, time-cycled ventilator with the following settings: peak inflating pressure (PIP) 22 cm H_2O, end-expiratory pressure 4 cm H_2O, rate 30 breaths/min, inspiratory time 0.35 seconds, inspiratory-to-expiratory ratio 1:3, flow 7 L/min, and fractional inspired oxygen (FIO_2) 0.60.

Initial blood gas values were adequate. Chest x-ray film (Fig. 29-1) demonstrated decreased lung volume, pulmonary fluid, and air bronchograms. At 12 hours of age a second dose of surfactant was given via the endotracheal tube. One hour later retractions were more severe and the infant became agitated and dusky. Arterial blood gas analysis revealed pH 7.18, $PaCO_2$ 58 torr, PaO_2 35 torr, base deficit −8, and bicarbonate 21 mEq/L. Breath sounds were equal but diminished bilaterally. No murmur was heard. Transillumination of the chest was negative bilaterally. A chest x-ray film was ordered (Fig. 29-2).

Denouement and Discussion

Hypoventilation Secondary to Worsening Respiratory Distress Syndrome

The chest x-ray films demonstrate progressive severe hypoaeration with decreased lung volume, air bronchograms, and a "ground glass" appearance of the lung fields. Clinically, this 27-week premature infant, appropriate for gestational age, represents typical progressive respiratory distress syndrome (RDS), which usually worsens over the first 48 to 72 hours of life.

Resuscitation was appropriate and the infant was given surfactant and placed on ventilatory support. Upon admission to the NICU, chest excursions and breath sounds were adequate. However, in a period of 12 hours the infant's lungs became more atelectatic, and hypoxemia, acidemia, and hypercapnia resulted. Clinically, the infant manifested severe retractions, agitation, and cyanosis.

The differential diagnosis at this point in management included the following: (1) patent ductus arteriosus (PDA); (2) sepsis; (3) intraventricular hemorrhage (IVH); (4) pulmonary air leak; (5) plugged endotracheal tube; and (6) hypoventilation. Although all of these diagnoses are complications of RDS, there are good clinical reasons to exclude many of the six possibilities.

PDA is unlikely to contribute to respiratory distress at this early stage of disease. The ductus is likely to be patent yet the pulmonary vascular resistance (PVR) is still high. As a result, shunting will either be right to left or bidirectional. As pulmonary resistance drops on day 2 or 3 of life, the flow will reverse (left-to-right), causing pulmonary overcirculation and increasing respiratory difficulty (see Chapter 23).

Sepsis, especially secondary to beta-hemolytic streptococci, is a possibility. Hypotension, poor perfusion, and large base deficits despite adequate oxygenation would further support a diagnosis of sepsis. Infants with sepsis may require less ventilatory support for adequate oxygenation than do cases of typical RDS. However, infants with sepsis and/or asphyxia often have a worse RDS course because these factors affect production of endogenous surfactant in the type II cell of the lung. This infant's blood and spinal fluid were cultured immediately after birth, and antibiotic treatment was initiated.

Catastrophic intracranial hemorrhage is a common problem in asphyxiated infants at this gestational age. Generally, clinical manifestations of a major hemorrhage occur at 36 to 48

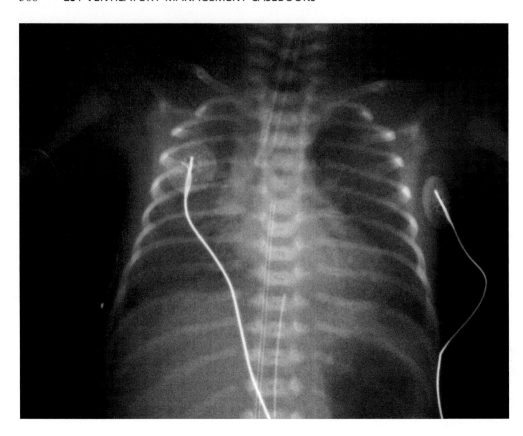

Figure 29-1. Initial chest x-ray film (anteroposterior view) taken 1 hour after birth.

hours of age and may be accompanied by hyperglycemia, hypotension, decreasing hematocrit, full fontanelle, and frequently seizures or coma.

Pulmonary air leak is a common complication of RDS requiring assisted ventilation. Bedside transillumination and the x-ray films in this case exclude the possibility, but one should remember that breath sounds radiate very well in a small chest and evaluation by stethoscope alone may be misleading. With the recent administration of the second surfactant dose, the endotracheal tube could be plugged. The tube should be suctioned or replaced, if necessary, to exclude this possibility.

Finally, this infant is suffering from simple hypoventilation. His disease has worsened because of increasing atelectasis. The ventilatory support that was adequate at birth now is inadequate despite exogenous surfactant administration, possibly secondary to the poor transition (Apgar scores 1 and 3).[1] This example highlights the need for continued and frequent reevaluation of infants on ventilatory support. Changes in disease pathology occur rapidly and require immediate attention.

Ventilatory adjustments must be made quickly to correct hypoventilation while steps are being taken to rule out other diagnostic possibilities for this infant. To correct hypoventilation when using a time-cycled, pressure-limited ventilator, the mean airway pressure ($P\overline{aw}$) should be increased. Increasing FIO_2 alone may temporarily improve oxygenation but does not improve ventilation. If the infant were on a volume ventilator, minute ventilation (i.e., tidal volume × rate/min) should be increased or the PIP inflating pressure limit should be raised.

Mean Airway Pressure

As described in Chapter 2, $P\overline{aw}$ is the average pressure delivered to the airways during a given ventilatory cycle (see Fig. 2-16). There are essentially four ways of increasing $P\overline{aw}$ if

the respiratory rate is held constant. Diagrammatically, $P\overline{aw}$ is represented by the area beneath the pressure curves of both the inspiratory and expiratory cycles and is calculated by dividing this area by its appropriate time. Calculation of $P\overline{aw}$ may be done by planimetry, a somewhat cumbersome and time-consuming task. Noninvasive devices (using a microprocessor calculation of the arithmetic mean by continuously sampling airway pressure every 10 msec) provide continuous inline determination of $P\overline{aw}$ on most modern ventilators.

Investigators in neonatal pulmonary care have advised on varied methods of ventilating neonates to achieve optimal results using conventional ventilators. Optimal ventilatory management would be indicated by the best blood gas results obtainable using the least ventilatory support (e.g., lowest PIP, lowest FIO_2, etc.) as reflected by the best survival rate and lowest rate of complications. Whereas some investigators have advocated high rate and short inspiratory time modes, others have advised the use of slow rates, low flows, and longer inspiratory times. No one method has proven efficacious for all neonatal pulmonary diseases in all stages of the disease.[2] To treat infants with RDS, other clinicians might use high-frequency ventilation as the initial therapy or as a rescue mode if the baby is inadequately managed on a conventional device.[3] Another approach might be to try nasal prong continuous positive airway pressure (CPAP) and avoid intubation and mechanical ventilation, if possible.[4] (See Chapter 8.)

Raising $P\overline{aw}$ is generally thought to improve oxygenation in babies with atelectatic disease (i.e., early-stage RDS).[5] It is generally assumed, although not proven, that the incidence of major complications (pulmonary air leak, bronchopulmonary dysplasia) is greater with increasing $P\overline{aw}$ on conventional ventilators. Our own experience demonstrates an acceptable complication rate when $P\overline{aw}$ is held at 12 cm H_2O or less. At $P\overline{aw}$ greater than 12 cm H_2O in infants weighing less than 1250 g, we consider rescue high-frequency oscillatory ventilation (HFOV)

syndrome. Danish-Swedish Multicenter Study Group. N Engl J Med 331:1051, 1994.
5. Boros SJ, Campbell K: A comparison of the effects of high frequency-low tidal volume and low frequency-high tidal volume mechanical ventilation. J Pediatr 97:108, 1980.

CASE 2

History

A 3710-g, full-term male infant was born at a community hospital to a 28-year-old gravida 4, para 2 woman. Pregnancy was reported as uncomplicated, and the fetal membranes were noted to be meconium stained at artificial rupture 5 hours prior to delivery. The infant was delivered vaginally with low forceps assistance under epidural anesthesia. Apgar scores were 3 and 6 at 1 minute and 5 minutes, respectively. The infant was meconium stained and required oxygen for 40 minutes in the delivery room. The tracheal aspirate contained no meconium, but 6 mL of meconium-stained fluid was suctioned from the stomach. The infant was given 100% oxygen by hood, but his condition deteriorated over the next several hours. Transport was requested, and at 5 hours of age the infant was intubated. During transport, he required hand ventilation to maintain adequate oxygenation. On arrival in the NICU, he was placed on a pressure-limited, time-cycled ventilator with the following settings: FIO_2 1.0, rate 60 breaths/min, PIP 30 cm H_2O, continuous distending pressure (CDP) 4 cm H_2O, inspiratory time 0.4 seconds, and flow 8 L/min. The following arterial blood gas values were obtained from analysis of a sample obtained from an umbilical artery catheter: pH 7.42, $PaCO_2$ 43 torr, PaO_2 32 torr, base excess 0, bicarbonate 21 mEq/L, and saturation 70%. The admission chest radiograph is shown in Figure 29-3. Physical examination revealed a cyanotic term infant in severe respiratory distress. The lungs were clear except for a few rales in the posterior bases. A grade 2/6 holosystolic heart murmur was heard, and the second heart sound was accentuated. The liver was palpated 1.5 cm below the right costal margin. Edema of the hands and feet was noted.

Denouement and Discussion

Persistent Pulmonary Hypertension of the Newborn

The physical examination, blood gases, and chest radiograph suggest a diagnosis of persistent pulmonary hypertension of the newborn (PPHN). Despite the history of meconium staining and the association of meconium aspiration syndrome with PPHN, the tracheal aspirate and the chest radiograph did not indicate meconium aspiration pneumonitis. In fact, the film was normal except for the streaky perihilar pattern of clearing pulmonary fluid.

Pulmonary hypertension of the newborn or persistent fetal circulation was first described in 1969 in two cyanotic term infants who did not have structural heart disease.[1] Today we know that PPHN may accompany many types of neonatal pulmonary disease, including RDS, aspiration syndromes, pneumothorax, bacterial or viral pneumonia, transient tachypnea of the newborn, wet lung syndrome, congenital diaphragmatic hernia, and perinatal asphyxia. The problem of hypoxemia due to PPHN may be more difficult to manage than the underlying disease. The most common causes of neonatal pulmonary hypertension are listed in Table 29-1.

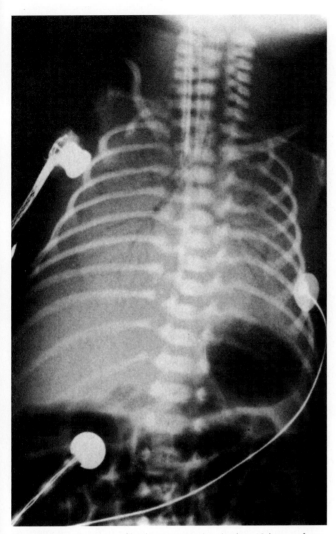

Figure 29-2. Chest x-ray film (anteroposterior view) at 12 hours of age.

to decrease the barotrauma/volutrauma of conventional devices. Additionally, infants without primary apnea appear ready for CPAP or extubation when $P\overline{aw}$ is 7 cm H_2O or less.

In this case, $P\overline{aw}$ needed to be increased to improve both oxygenation and ventilation. Whether to increase flow, inspiratory time, PIP, end-expiratory pressure, or rate in this instance is a very controversial decision. Our first choice in this instance was to increase the inspiratory time because increasing inspiratory time contributes greatly to increasing $P\overline{aw}$, allowing expansion of atelectatic alveoli at lower PIP. In this particular example, however, several settings had to be raised before the infant was adequately ventilated. By the time the baby was stabilized, the PIP was raised from 22 to 26 cm H_2O, inspiratory time from 0.35 to 0.45 seconds, and rate from 30 to 50 breaths/min.

REFERENCES

1. Kattwinkel J, Bloom BT, Delmore P, et al: High- versus low-threshold surfactant retreatment for neonatal respiratory distress syndrome. Pediatrics 106:282, 2000.
2. Mariani GL, Carlo WA: Ventilatory management in neonates: Science or art? Clin Perinatol 25:33, 1998.
3. Keszler M, Durand DJ: Neonatal high-frequency ventilation: Past, present, and future. Clin Perinatol 28:579, 2001.
4. Verder H, Robertson B, Greisen G, et al: Surfactant therapy and nasal continuous positive airway pressure for newborns with respiratory distress

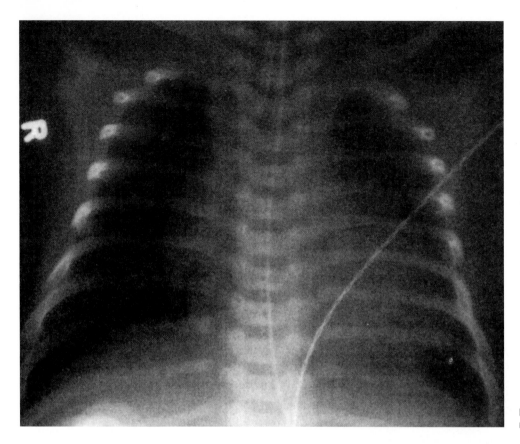

Figure 29-3. Chest x-ray film (anteroposterior view) at birth.

Pathophysiology. In the term fetus, the muscular pulmonary arterioles are constricted as 90% of the total cardiac output bypasses the lungs through intracardiac shunts at the foramen ovale and PDA. If the pulmonary vessels are abnormal or fail to dilate at birth, or if constriction occurs because of an intrapartum or postpartum event, pulmonary hypertension ensues with elevation of the right ventricular and right atrial pressures.

TABLE 29-1.   Etiologic Spectrum of Neonatal Pulmonary Hypertension

Intrauterine
UPI-SGA (chronic hypoxia)
Diaphragmatic hernia
Anencephaly
Potter syndrome
Oligohydramnios syndrome
Maternal drugs (aspirin, indomethacin)
Postmaturity

Intrapartum
Asphyxia (low Apgar score)
Aspiration (meconium/blood)
Postmaturity (UPI)

Postpartum
Primary lung disease
Metabolic disorders (hypoglycemia/hypocalcemia)
Infection (B streptococci)
Increased pulmonary blood flow
Delayed resorption of pulmonary fluid (TTN)
Hypothermia
Hyperviscosity
Intubation, CPAP
Acidosis

CPAP, continuous positive airway pressure; SGA, small for gestational age; TTN, transient tachypnea of the newborn; UPI, uteroplacental insufficiency.

Consequently, most of the right ventricular output flows through the large PDA into the lower-resistance systemic circulation. Moreover, when right atrial pressure exceeds left atrial pressure, blood return from the inferior vena cava is preferentially directed across the foramen ovale into the left atrium, thereby bypassing the lungs.

Pulmonary vasoconstriction may occur in three time periods: intrauterine, intrapartum, and postpartum. Abnormal development in utero of the pulmonary vascular bed occurs in association with congenital diaphragmatic hernia, Potter syndrome, oligohydramnios, and anencephaly. Chronic intrauterine hypoxia also may result in hypertrophy of the medial musculature of the pulmonary arterioles. Perinatal or postpartum asphyxia or other metabolic events may cause pulmonary vasospasm intrapartum or postpartum. Hypovolemia or poor myocardial function due to cardiomyopathy, hypoglycemia, hypocalcemia, or ischemia may then lead to systemic hypotension. Whereas most infants will tolerate peripartum asphyxia without evidence of serious PPHN, others are severely affected. Most neonates with PPHN are of more than 32 weeks' gestational age and have advanced development of the pulmonary arterial medial musculature. It has been shown that development of the musculature of the pulmonary arterial bed is progressive with gestational age and is appreciable after 32 weeks' gestation. Prolonged or recurrent perinatal administration of prostaglandin synthetase inhibitors (aspirin, indomethacin) to the mother also has been associated with PPHN, possibly as a result of partial constriction of the ductus arteriosus and increased pulmonary artery pressure in utero.

Diagnosis. The diagnosis of PPHN should be suspected in any hypoxic infant in whom the degree of hypoxemia is out of proportion to the severity of lung disease. The index of suspicion is high in term infants whose oxygenation fluctuates markedly with small changes in F_{IO_2}. It also is high in certain clinical settings, such as perinatal asphyxia, polycythemia, or shock; diabetic mother; or congenital diaphragmatic hernia in the term or near-term infant. Clinical manifestations of PPHN include cyanosis, a hyperactive precordium, accentuation of the second heart sound, and frequently the holosystolic murmur of tricuspid insufficiency. The infants usually are term or post-term babies with mild-to-moderate respiratory distress, and about 25% have hepatomegaly. However, increased PVR may be an important part of RDS in larger preterm infants. Arterial blood gas values or oxygen saturation values obtained simultaneously from preductal and postductal sites may show a much higher Pa_{O_2} or saturation in the preductal sample if most of the right-to-left shunting occurs across the ductus arteriosus (see Fig. 17-10). A difference of 10 torr or 5% saturation is considered diagnostic. The difference in Pa_{O_2} may not be seen in severe cases with a large right-to-left shunt across the foramen ovale and little pulmonary venous return to the heart. If the Pa_{O_2} is less than 40 torr and the infant is acidotic, there may be little difference in preductal and postductal samples.

The diagnosis of pulmonary hypertension can be confirmed by echocardiography or clinical response to certain procedures, drugs, or both (see Chapter 23). The echocardiographic findings in pulmonary hypertension include normal anatomic relationships and dilated right ventricle, right atrium, and pulmonary artery. Doppler interrogation may demonstrate right-to-left shunting across the ductus arteriosus and foramen ovale, as well as a high-velocity tricuspid regurgitant jet. An electrocardiogram may show ST-segment depression characteristic of myocardial ischemia. Chest x-ray examination is essential to assess the underlying lung or heart disease, but the findings may vary from virtually clear lungs to severe pulmonary disease.

Treatment. Treatment of PPHN includes meticulous attention to supportive measures and ventilatory management. Various therapies are aimed at dilating the pulmonary arterioles, raising systemic blood pressure, maintaining cardiac output, and preventing acidosis and hypoxia. Postnatal conditions that increase PVR, such as hypocalcemia, hypoglycemia, acidosis, hypoxia, and hyperviscosity, should be sought and treated promptly. High alveolar oxygen tension dilates the pulmonary arterial bed, thereby reducing pulmonary artery pressure. Mechanical ventilation is used to increase lung volume, and improve oxygenation (see Chapter 9). Blood pH values greater than 7.55 with Pa_{CO_2} less than 30 torr have been advised in the past to improve oxygenation, although more conservative approaches have been successful.[2] Hyperventilation can be accomplished by using very rapid respiratory rates, high PIPs, or both on time-cycled ventilators or by using high-frequency ventilation.[3] CDP is usually left at 3 cm H_2O or less on conventional devices. However, higher pressures and rates with short expiratory times on conventional ventilators may result in inadvertent positive end-expiratory pressure (PEEP), which may increase PVR. Sedation with continuously infused narcotics is used to avoid agitation that increases right-to-left shunting and to minimize pulmonary air leaks. Muscular paralysis using pancuronium bromide is infrequently used because of side effects and masking central nervous system (CNS) signs (i.e., seizures). Blood pressure is maintained by vigorous volume expansion with plasma or whole blood. If cardiac contractility is impaired, improvement may occur with correction of metabolic abnormalities or with inotropic agents.

At times, dramatic changes in oxygenation are seen with the administration of high concentrations of inspired oxygen and concomitant induction of alkalosis. We have used a combination of mild respiratory hyperventilation (P_{CO_2} 25 to 35 torr) with a regimen of sodium bicarbonate consisting of continuous intravenous infusion of 5 to 10 mEq/kg/day. However, often only gradual improvement occurs and the patient must be maintained on this regimen for several days.

Various drugs have been tried, including tolazoline, isoproterenol, chlorpromazine, prostacyclin, and inhaled nitric oxide (iNO) (see Chapters 14 and 23). The success rate has varied, but the combination of sedation, blood pressure support, mild alkalosis, nitric oxide, and careful ventilatory management has reduced the need for extracorporeal membrane oxygenation (ECMO) by more that 50%. Tolazoline hydrochloride, an alpha-adrenergic blocking agent that affects vascular smooth muscle, causing vasodilation, increasing cardiac output, and decreasing pulmonary and systemic blood pressure, has recently been removed from the market and can no longer be recommended.

When standard therapies are not effective in improving oxygenation, iNO is started at 6 to 20 ppm via the ventilator.[4] Procedures for using this drug, side effects, and weaning are described in Chapter 14. Patients who do not respond to iNO are often candidates for ECMO (see Chapter 16).[5] During treatment of PPHN, careful attention to oxygen therapy is of paramount importance. Premature or hasty reduction in the F_{IO_2} or even brief removal of the infant from oxygen for procedures such as starting an intravenous infusion, feeding, or x-ray examination has resulted in intractable hypoxemia. Similarly, infants with this disease are exquisitely sensitive to changes in ventilatory support. Very small reductions in F_{IO_2}, respiratory rate, tidal volume, or inspiratory pressure may result in a profound decrease in Pa_{O_2} due to increased vasoconstriction and exaggeration of right-to-left shunt. Therefore, any changes in ventilatory or oxygen support must be made with extreme caution. Frequent arterial blood gas sampling is essential. Simultaneous preductal and postductal oxygen saturation monitoring is extremely helpful, to compare shunting on an ongoing basis. If PPHN is reversed by oxygen therapy, hyperoxia with a Pa_{O_2} greater than 100 torr may occur. In the term infant whose retina is fully vascularized, the risk of retinopathy of prematurity from hyperoxia is minimal compared with the risk of irreversible hypoxemia. Therefore, we have tolerated mild hyperoxia (Pa_{O_2} 100 to 150 torr) until the F_{IO_2} can be reduced gradually without causing recurrence of the pulmonary hypertension.

Occasionally the diagnosis of PPHN is entertained when patients actually are underventilated on assisted ventilation. We do not start the "PPHN protocol" unless the patient has the clinical syndrome of PPHN and the Pa_{CO_2} is normal to low. The echocardiographic findings will vary according to the acid–base status of the patient at the time the study is done. A patient with hypoxemia and hypercapnia is considered underventilated until the Pa_{CO_2} is brought into the normal range.

Occasionally the management strategy for PPHN is continued for too long a period after PVR has fallen, and a large left-to-right shunt through the ductus arteriosus develops with resultant congestive heart failure. Detection of a PDA murmur is a helpful sign to start weaning from the PPHN protocol. Confirmation with an echocardiogram will assist in the weaning process.

In the present case, the diagnosis of PPHN was proved by echocardiography. Mild hyperventilation and alkalinization with bicarbonate was begun. Sedation was accomplished with a continuous infusion of fentanyl. Subsequent blood gas analysis gave the following values: pH 7.51, $PaCO_2$ 29 torr, base deficit +5, PaO_2 72 torr, and saturation 97%. Eight hours later, a right pneumothorax developed, necessitating chest tube placement. The infant deteriorated and could not be adequately oxygenated. He was switched to HFOV, and iNO 20 ppm was begun. Over the next 6 days he was gradually weaned from the iNO and assisted ventilation. At follow-up examination at 1 year of age, he was doing well and pulmonary function was normal.

REFERENCES

1. Gersony WM, Duc GV, Sinclair JC: "PFC" syndrome (persistence of the fetal circulation). Circulation 39:111, 1969.
2. Wung JT, James LS, Kilchevsky E, et al: Management of infants with severe respiratory failure and persistence of fetal circulation, without hyperventilation. Pediatrics 76:488, 1985.
3. Fox WW, Duara S: Persistent pulmonary hypertension in the neonate: Diagnosis and management. J Pediatr 103:505, 1983.
4. Roberts JD Jr, Fineman JR, Morin FC III, et al: Inhaled nitric oxide and persistent pulmonary hypertension of the newborn. The Inhaled Nitric Oxide Study Group. N Engl J Med 336:605, 1997.
5. Walsh MC, Stork EK: Persistent pulmonary hypertension of the newborn: Rational therapy based on pathophysiology. Clin Pathol 28:609, 2001.

CASE 3

History

An 832-g female was born to a 25-year-old woman at 26 to 27 weeks gestation in a local community hospital. Delivery was vaginal, presentation was vertex, and Apgar scores were 4 and 6 at 1 minute and 5 minutes, respectively. A 10% placental abruption was noted. Oxygen was administered in a hood, but progressive respiratory distress developed. Transport was arranged, and at 3 hours of age the infant was intubated by the transport team. A chest radiograph taken on arrival in the NICU revealed hypoaeration, air bronchograms, and decreased lung volume consistent with RDS. Exogenous surfactant was given via endotracheal tube. Cultures were obtained and antibiotics administered. The infant was placed on a time-cycled, pressure-limited ventilator at PIP 22 cm H_2O, rate 30 breaths/min, CDP 4 cm H_2O, FIO_2 0.80, flow 8 L/min, and inspiratory-to-expiratory ratio 1:1.5.

The patient's condition remained stable through the first 48 hours of hospitalization. She was given two additional doses of surfactant and weaned to an FIO_2 of 0.60. Intravenous fluids were restricted to 80 mL/kg/day. On the third day of life, ventilatory support was increased to PIP 26 cm H_2O and CDP 6 cm H_2O to maintain adequate blood gas values. Heart rate was 160 to 180 beats/min and blood pressure 50 to 55 mm Hg systolic/20 to 25 mm Hg diastolic. Abnormalities on physical examination were a grade 2/6 systolic heart murmur, increased pulses, and bilateral moist rales. In the next 48 hours, the patient could not be weaned from ventilatory support despite administration of furosemide (Lasix) and continued fluid restriction. All admission cultures were negative at this time. A chest radiograph was obtained (Fig. 29-4).

Denouement and Discussion

Patent Ductus Arteriosus Complicating Respiratory Distress Syndrome

The chest radiograph showed alveolar filling, pulmonary edema, and increased cardiac size consistent with a symptomatic PDA and early congestive heart failure. The echocardiogram confirmed the clinical findings. The left ventricle and left atrium were dilated, a PDA measured 3 to 4 mm in diameter, and a significant left-to-right shunt was demonstrated by color flow Doppler.

PDA is more common in premature than in term infants, and the incidence is increased if RDS is present. Siassi et al.[1] reported that PDA is present in 70% of infants born at 28 and 30 weeks' gestation, and this incidence decreases with advancing gestational age. However, with echocardiogram and color flow Doppler, left-to-right shunting through the ductus can be shown in almost every very-low-birthweight infant with RDS.

Pathophysiology. The direction and magnitude of flow through the PDA and thus the effect on ventilatory management depend on two factors: size of the PDA and relationship of pulmonary-to-systemic resistance. The factors contributing to size and patency of the ductus are unclear, but ductal maturation, reduced cholinergic innervation, and decreased responsiveness to oxygen in preterm infants may be possible factors. Several reports indicate that the in utero state of the ductus may be influenced by numerous drugs, including glucocorticoids, and that the prophylactic administration of betamethasone or dexamethasone to the mother may decrease the size and patency of the ductus.[2]

PVR is subject to many opposing factors in the premature infant with RDS. Decreased pulmonary arterial muscular tissue lowers PVR in preterm infants, but acidosis, hypercapnia, hypoxia, atelectasis, positive-pressure ventilation, and CDP all tend to increase PVR. Thus, at any given time, the preterm infant with RDS and PDA will have ductal flow dependent on the opposing forces that control PVR. Usually after surfactant administration the infant recovers from RDS at 2 to 5 days of life. As improvement occurs, PVR decreases, and a left-to-right shunt predominates, with the appearance of the characteristic murmur and increased pulse volume. The ductus usually is present earlier, but shunting may be predominantly right to left or balanced, and no significant effect is seen on the severity of the disease or ventilatory support requirements.

Diagnosis. The rapid diagnosis of a symptomatic PDA and the differentiation of pulmonary edema from primary lung disease are essential for optimal management of ventilator-dependent premature infants. Clinical examination and chest radiographs may not provide enough quantitative information for selection of appropriate therapy, especially because many PDAs are silent. Two-dimensional echocardiography and focused Doppler flow analysis have provided accurate identification of left-to-right ductal shunts and semiquantitative assessment of shunt magnitude and cardiac function. Thus, the contribution of the PDA to decreased lung compliance and increased ventilatory support requirements may be ascertained and appropriate therapy selected. Clinical and echocardiographic findings suggestive of PDA are listed in Table 29-2.

Management. Despite published strategies based on numerous studies, management of the symptomatic ductus in the ventilator-dependent preterm infant with RDS remains contro-

REFERENCES

1. Siassi B, Emmanouilides GC, Cleveland RJ, et al: Patent ductus arteriosus complicating prolonged assisted ventilation and respiratory distress syndrome. J Pediatr 74:11, 1969.
2. Abbasi S, Hirsch D, Davis J, et al: Effect of single versus multiple courses of antenatal corticosteroids on maternal and neonatal outcome. Am J Obstet Gynecol 182:1243, 2000.
3. Narayanan M, Cooper B, Weiss H, et al: Prophylactic indomethacin: Factors determining permanent ductus arteriosus closure. J Pediatr 136:330, 2000.
4. Patel J, Roberts I, Azzopardi D, et al: Randomized double-blind controlled trial comparing the effects of ibuprofen with indomethacin on cerebral hemodynamics in preterm infants with patent ductus arteriosus. Pediatr Res 47:36, 2000.
5. van Overmeire BV, Smets K, Lecoutere D, et al: A comparison of ibuprofen and indomethacin for closure of patent ductus arteriosus. N Engl J Med 343:674, 2000.

CASE 4

History

A 660-g male infant was born at a level III center after maternal/fetal transport from a community hospital due to premature rupture of membranes. The infant was born at 25 to 26 weeks gestation to a 24-year-old gravida 2, para 2 mother by vaginal delivery with vertex presentation. The neonatal team was in attendance at delivery. The infant was depressed at birth. He was intubated at 30 seconds of age and ventilated with 1.0 F_{IO_2} via resuscitation bag. Apgar scores were 2 and 5 at 1 and 5 minutes, respectively. Exogenous surfactant was given by 10 minutes of age. Attempts to place an umbilical artery catheter were unsuccessful. A radial artery blood gas at 20 minutes of age revealed pH 7.44, Pa_{CO_2} 30 torr, and Pa_{O_2} 88 torr. The infant was transferred to the NICU and placed on a pressure-limited, time-cycled ventilator at PIP 24 cm H_2O, CDP 4 cm H_2O, rate 50 breaths/min, F_{IO_2} 0.80, and inspiratory time 0.4 seconds. A radial artery catheter was placed in the right arm.

Physical examination revealed a 25 to 26 weeks gestation infant in severe respiratory distress with poor aeration in both lungs. Initial chest x-ray film obtained at 2 hours of age (Fig. 29-6) was interpreted as compatible with RDS. The infant was extremely hypotonic, and a cranial ultrasound at 5 hours of age revealed a right subependymal hemorrhage and IVH with right ventricular dilation.

Initial laboratory values were unremarkable. Over the first 12 hours of life, the infant required increasing ventilatory support to F_{IO_2} 1.0, PIP 26 cm H_2O, and breath rate 60/min. At 20 hours of age, a blood gas test revealed pH 7.04, Pa_{CO_2} 90 torr, Pa_{O_2} 45 torr, and base deficit −9.5. Physical examination revealed increased anteroposterior diameter of the chest, distant heart sounds, equal breath sounds bilaterally, and no difference between left and right hemithorax on transillumination. A chest x-ray film was ordered (Fig. 29-7).

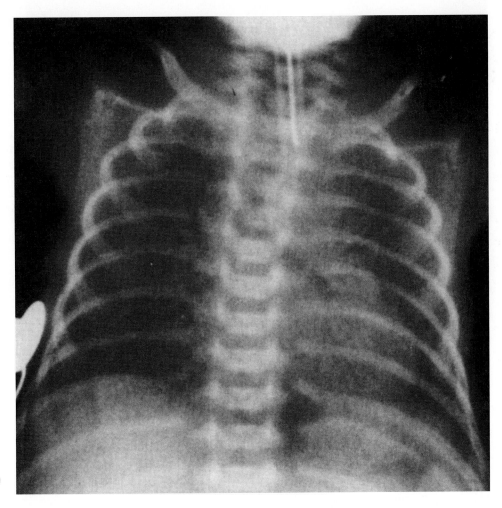

Figure 29-6. Initial chest x-ray film (anteroposterior view) at 2 hours of age.

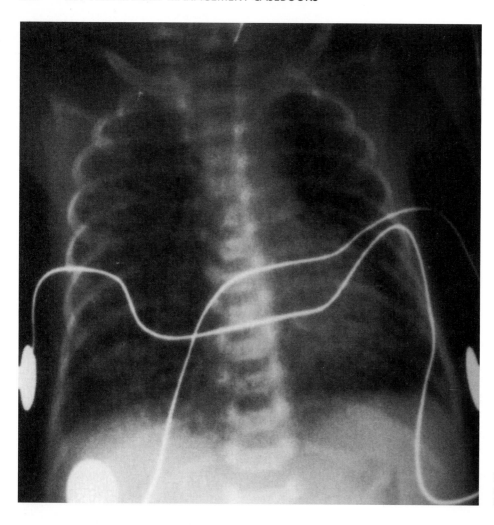

Figure 29-7. Chest x-ray film (anteroposterior view) at 20 hours of age revealing extensive pulmonary interstitial emphysema.

Denouement and Discussion

Pulmonary Interstitial Emphysema

Differential diagnosis. In premature infants with early-stage RDS, the differential diagnosis of acute onset hypercapnia includes hypoventilation, machine failure, tube blockage or malposition, or pulmonary air leak. Immediate steps should be taken to make the correct diagnosis and begin treatment. A quick observation of the infant's chest excursions and auscultation of breath sounds should determine a fairly routine algorithm (see Fig. 9-9). If air movement in the lungs is inadequate and no chest excursions are seen, the infant should be removed from the ventilator and hand ventilated with a resuscitation bag. If this produces adequate breath sounds, a machine malfunction may be the problem. If the ventilator outlet is occluded, the pressure gauge should be observed. If the gauge does not move, it may indicate one of several malfunctions: a disconnected tube, a disconnected nebulizer hood, or an internal malfunction.

If hand ventilation produces recovery (decreasing cyanosis and PaCO$_2$, increasing heart rate and blood pressure), hypoventilation is present (see Casebook 1). However, if adequate ventilation fails to improve the infant's status, usually there is a problem with the endotracheal tube or pulmonary air leak. Again, while the infant is hand ventilated, chest excursions should be observed and breath sounds auscultated. If no excursions are seen and air movement is poor, one can assume the tube is blocked or positioned in the esophagus. Use of a qualitative color-sensitive capnography device may improve recognition of

a plugged or displaced endotracheal tube.[1] If aeration is different in the left and right hemithorax, it is possible that either the tube is in a mainstem bronchus or there is a unilateral pneumothorax.

In this case, these procedures were followed and aeration was equal bilaterally. In addition, transillumination of the chest to locate a pneumothorax was negative. The chest x-ray film confirmed that the endotracheal tube was in the correct position but revealed extensive pulmonary interstitial emphysema (PIE) that was the cause of this infant's severe hypercapnia (Fig. 29-7).

Pathophysiology. PIE represents one of the many forms of barotrauma or "extraneous air syndromes" (see Chapter 21). These syndromes are a group of clinical disorders produced by pulmonary alveolar rupture and subsequent migration of air into tissue spaces where air is not normally present. Table 21-6 lists the major sites of air leak syndrome. Although many of these syndromes can occur spontaneously, the incidence is substantially increased with positive-pressure ventilation. With the advent of modern neonatal ventilators and the use of exogenous surfactant, the most severe forms of PIE are infrequently seen today, except in the most immature "micropremies."

The pathogenesis of extraneous air syndromes was first described in two reports by the Macklin and Macklin[2] in 1939 and 1944. Theoretically, all extra-alveolar air leaks are caused by high intra-alveolar pressure that follows inhalation, insufflation, or retention of excessively large volumes of air in the lung. Rupture of alveoli may follow and air escapes, entering perivascular sheaths and migrating toward the hilum. Thus, PIE is essentially characterized by air in the perivascular sheaths. This air may migrate to the pleura to form blebs. If the

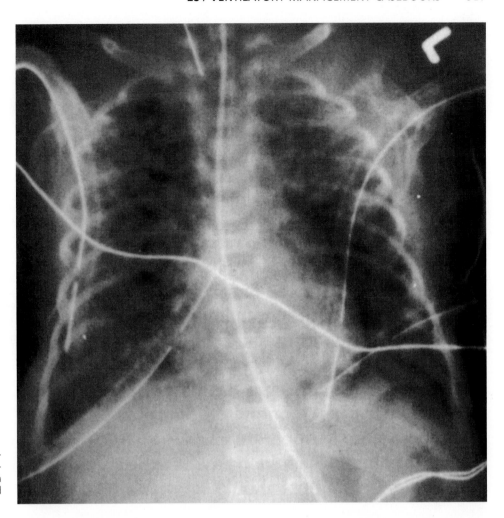

Figure 29-8. Chest x-ray film (anteroposterior view) at 3 months of age demonstrating changes of chronic lung disease, a ventricular peritoneal shunt catheter, and clips placed on the ductus arteriosus.

pleura ruptures, air is released into the intrapleural space causing a pneumothorax. However, when the pleura remains intact, the perivascular sheaths may stretch considerably as air accumulates and compresses the enveloped blood vessels. Macklin and Macklin proposed that "the most important point about pulmonic interstitial emphysema" was the "associated circulatory embarrassment."

All forms of extraneous air syndromes are preceded by migration of air through the pulmonary vascular sheaths. However, this transient passage of air usually is not clinically or radiographically evident. If air is trapped and does not escape the visceral pleura, PIE results. Although onset usually is gradual, acute PIE occasionally may develop, as in the present case. Generally, acute-onset PIE is an ominous complication of ventilatory support. Oxygen and ventilatory support requirements may be increased but often are without benefit. Increased hypercapnia and hypotension result in severe acidosis and eventual death unless intervention is successful. Death may be caused by circulatory embarrassment or impaired gas exchange resulting from air interposed between alveoli and blood vessels.

Radiographic appearance. The diagnosis of PIE is made radiographically; it is characterized by radiolucencies that are either cystlike or linear. The cystlike radiolucencies usually vary in diameter from 1.0 to 4.0 mm. Unlike air bronchograms, which are smooth and branched, linear PIE is seen in the peripheral lung fields, as well as the perihilar area. The differentiation of linear PIE from air bronchograms has obvious clinical importance.

PIE may involve one lobe, one lung, or both lungs. The severity indicated by x-ray film may range from mild to severe. When mild, only a few radiolucencies may be present in the perihilar region, having no immediate clinical significance but signaling potential future pneumothorax. Moderate-to-severe cases almost always have clinical symptomatology, including hypoxemia and hypercapnia. When unilateral, severe PIE may cause mediastinal shift to the opposite hemithorax with atelectasis of the contralateral lung. When bilateral, radiographic appearance is one of hyperexpanded lungs with a small heart and depressed diaphragms (Fig. 29-7).

Therapy. Therapy for PIE is controversial and usually inadequate in severe cases. Many extremely premature infants who suffer from significant PIE within the first 24 hours of life subsequently develop bronchopulmonary dysplasia and IVH. Frequently, the progression of PIE to pneumothorax results in the infant's dramatic improvement. On the other hand, approximately 50% of pneumothoraces are preceded by radiographically apparent PIE.

Initial treatment should be directed at ventilatory management. Attempts should be made to decrease PIP and flow rate, but disease progression usually requires even higher ventilatory support. A "low-volume" strategy using high-frequency ventilation has been advocated.[3] In our experience, the high-frequency jet ventilator used in a mode without interruption of the conventional ventilator has achieved most success. In severe cases, other therapies have been advocated. The use of 1.0 FIO_2 to allow more rapid absorption of the interstitial air has been suggested. In unilateral cases, intubation of the contralateral bronchus with resultant collapse of the affected lung has occasionally been successful.[4] Placing the infant in the lateral position with the affected side down, with no suctioning for 24 to 48 hours, has also been beneficial in some cases.[5] In extreme circumstances, visceral pleurotomy or the creation of pneumothoraces by chest tube insertion has brought symptomatic relief.

Outcome. In this case, conversion to a high-frequency oscillator was attempted without success. The infant was switched to a jet ventilator with slow improvement. Bilateral pneumothoraces developed, necessitating chest tube placement (Fig. 29-8). The infant had a prolonged course on the ventilator and developed bronchopulmonary dysplasia and grade III IVH with posthemorrhagic hydrocephalus. He required a ventricular peritoneal shunt and was discharged without supplemental oxygen at 3 months of age (Fig. 29-9).

REFERENCES

1. Roberts WA, Maniscalco WM, Cohen AR, et al: The use of capnography for recognition of esophageal intubation in the neonatal intensive care unit. Pediatr Pulmonol 19:262, 1995.
2. Macklin MT, Macklin CC: Malignant interstitial emphysema of the lungs and mediastinum as an important occult complication in many respiratory diseases and other conditions: An interpretation of the clinical literature in the light of laboratory equipment. Medicine 23:281, 1944.
3. Keszler M, Donn SM, Bucciarelli RL, et al: Multicenter controlled trial comparing high-frequency jet ventilation and conventional mechanical ventilation in newborn infants with pulmonary interstitial emphysema. J Pediatr 119:85, 1991.
4. Dickman GL, Short BL, Krauss DR: Selective bronchial intubation in the management of unilateral pulmonary interstitial emphysema. Am J Dis Child 131:365, 1977.
5. Cohen RS, Smith DW, Stevenson DK, et al: Lateral decubitus position as therapy for persistent focal pulmonary interstitial emphysema in neonates: A preliminary report. J Pediatr 104:441, 1984.

CASE 5

History

A 4670-g male infant was referred for respiratory distress to the tertiary center from a level II hospital. He had been born to a 36-year-old gravida 4, para 3 mother by cesarean section under spinal anesthesia due to cephalopelvic disproportion and nonreassuring fetal status noted by multiple variable heartbeat decelerations on electronic monitoring. Apgar scores were 1, 3, and 7 at 1, 5, and 10 minutes, respectively. The patient was intubated and hand ventilated in the delivery room. When regular spontaneous respirations were established, the infant was extubated and placed in the nursery in an oxyhood. At 90 minutes of age, the patient was reintubated for respiratory acidosis (pH 7.16). An intravenous glucose infusion was started when he developed hypoglycemia. The infant was transported to this institution on endotracheal CPAP but required intermittent mandatory ventilation (IMV) shortly after admission to the NICU.

Physical examination revealed a large-for-gestational-age infant in moderate distress. Ecchymoses were noted on the forehead; there was marked tachypnea with 1+ retractions and rales at both lung bases; duplication of the right thumb; and the liver was palpated 4 cm below the right coastal margin.

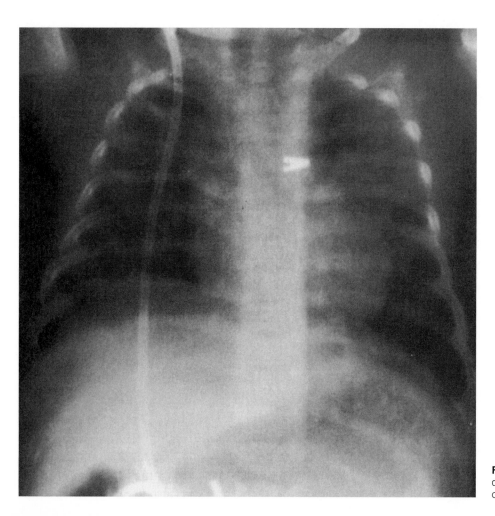

Figure 29-9. Chest x-ray at 3 months of age demonstrating ventricular peritoneal shunt catheter and silver clips on ductus arteriosus.

Neurologic examination showed a depressed infant with an incomplete Moro response, no grasp reflex, and sustained ankle and elbow clonus bilaterally.

Chest x-ray films taken on admission revealed hyperinflation with coarse infiltrates consistent with aspiration syndrome (Fig. 29-10). No meconium had been noted at delivery. The infant was placed on a time-cycled, pressure-limited ventilator. Within 24 hours, the FIO_2 was reduced from 0.75 to 0.29. An intravenous infusion of glucose 12.5% was maintained to prevent recurrent hypoglycemia. Cultures were taken and antibiotics begun. Phenobarbital was given because of perinatal asphyxia. During the first 72 hours, numerous technical problems were encountered with the endotracheal tube due to excessive mucous and tracheal secretions requiring frequent suctioning. The endotracheal tube was changed three times due to cyanosis and presumed plugging.

On the third day of life, the infant developed a holosystolic murmur, and pediatric cardiology was consulted. A two-dimensional echocardiogram revealed an endocardial cushion defect. The following day, the patient was weaned to endotracheal CPAP at +5 cm H_2O and 0.25 FIO_2. Over the next 10 days, several attempts at extubation were unsuccessful. Each attempt resulted in cyanosis, CO_2 retention, and stridor. A 3-day course of dexamethasone (Decadron) was given without success prior to the last extubation attempt. Bronchoscopy at 13 days of age revealed tracheomalacia. A chest x-ray film obtained at 16 days of age demonstrated severe bilateral hyperinflation with volume loss in the right upper lobe (Fig. 29-11). Due to continued inability to extubate the infant and known congenital heart disease, cardiac catheterization was performed at 17 days of age.

Denouement and Discussion

Extubation Failure Secondary to Congenital Vascular Ring

Weaning and extubation are important parts of neonatal ventilatory management. The patient management team (physician, nurse, respiratory therapist) must wean patients from ventilatory support as soon as possible in order to minimize complications. The longer the patient is managed with assisted ventilation, the greater the incidence of complication.

In this case, attempts to extubate the infant were unsuccessful. When this occurs, the cause must be determined so appropriate therapy can be quickly instituted and successful extubation accomplished. Table 29-3 lists the major causes of extubation failure.

Causes of extubation failure: Pulmonary. Because there are few, if any, clinically useful tests to indicate readiness for extubation, this is usually a case of trial and error. Extubation failure occurs in about one third of attempts.[1] The use of lung function studies to predict readiness for extubation is controversial.[2] Fox et al.[3] demonstrated increased pulmonary resistance in small infants who could not be extubated and suggested that immaturity and increased collapsibility of the airways might be responsible. Patients usually are weaned to low inspiratory oxygen

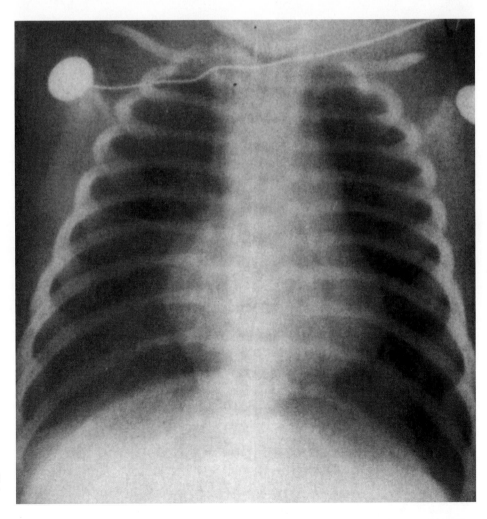

Figure 29-10. Admission chest x-ray film (anteroposterior view) demonstrating pulmonary venous and lymphatic congestion.

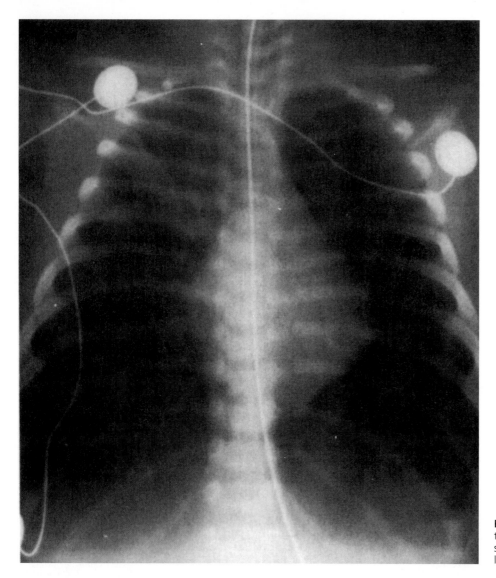

Figure 29-11. Chest x-ray film (anteroposterior view) at 16 days of age demonstrating severe bilateral hyperinflation with volume loss in the right upper lobe.

levels (<0.40 F_{IO_2}) and low ventilator settings prior to extubation attempts. A trial of endotracheal CPAP prior to extubation is usually no longer warranted.[4] Some clinicians have used $\overline{Paw}$ levels of 7 cm H_2O or less to indicate extubation readiness.

Once extubation is accomplished, the infant may develop postextubation atelectasis that may require reintubation. The right upper lobe is most frequently affected by atelectasis. Postextubation atelectasis may be minimized by nasal prong CPAP and/or chest physiotherapy. Other causes of extubation failure are pulmonary insufficiency seen in very immature infants (<1000 g) and early chronic lung disease with small airway collapse usually noted in infants who undergo assisted ventilation for more than 14 days. In both cases, the infants may require days to weeks of additional assisted ventilation before extubation is successfully accomplished.

Upper airway problems. Extubation failure may be secondary to problems encountered in the upper airway manifested chiefly by stridor. Edema secondary to traumatic, prolonged, or repeated intubations may cause severe inspiratory stridor and CO_2 retention. Tracheal secretions may be tenacious and copious and may block the upper airway and require repeated direct laryngeal suctioning. Racemic epinephrine and/or intravenous dexamethasone have been used to reduce subglottic edema after extubation. The former has been found to be

TABLE 29-3.   Major causes of Extubation Failure

I. Pulmonary
   A. Primary disease not resolved
   B. Postextubation atelectasis
   C. Pulmonary insufficiency of prematurity
   D. Bronchopulmonary dysplasia
   E. Eventration or paralysis of diaphragm
II. Upper Airway
   A. Edema and/or excess tracheal secretions
   B. Subglottic stenosis
   C. Laryngotracheomalacia
   D. Congenital vascular ring
   E. Necrotizing tracheobronchitis
III. Cardiovascular
   A. Patent ductus arteriosus
   B. Fluid overload
   C. Congenital heart disease with increased pulmonary flow
IV. Central Nervous System
   A. Apnea (extreme immaturity)
   B. Intraventricular hemorrhage
   C. Hypoxic ischemic brain damage/seizures
   D. Drugs (phenobarbital, magnesium sulfate, narcotics)
V. Miscellaneous
   A. Unrecognized diagnosis (nerve palsy, myasthenia gravis)
   B. Sepsis
   C. Metabolic abnormality

ineffective, and, despite its apparent usefulness, use of dexamethasone should be restricted because of long-term neurologic sequelae.[5] Prolonged intubation may cause trauma resulting in stenosis in the subglottic area. Subglottic stenosis has been reported to occur more frequently when infants are orally intubated because the endotracheal tube is more difficult to stabilize, resulting in increased tube movement and more frequent accidental extubations. Nasal tracheal intubation seems to be associated with less risk of subglottic stenosis. However, reviews by Spence and Barr[6] demonstrated that nasal intubations are more frequently associated with postextubation atelectasis probably secondary to decreased air flow from edema of the nasal passages. Stridor also can be due to vocal cord paralysis or congenital malformations such as laryngotracheomalacia, laryngeal web, or congenital vascular ring. Although the latter diagnosis is rare, it should be considered when the postextubation chest x-ray film demonstrates hyperinflation rather than atelectasis. "Necrotizing tracheobronchitis," an iatrogenic lesion of the tracheal-bronchial tree, can be seen after high-frequency ventilation and may prevent successful extubation.

Cardiovascular problems. In newborn disease states, the pulmonary and cardiovascular systems often are simultaneously involved and interdependent. RDS in a premature neonate may be complicated by PDA, which delays weaning and extubation until it is closed. PDA often does not appear clinically until postnatal day 3 or 4, coinciding with an improvement in pulmonary function and a decrease in PVR. Because many PDAs are silent, a clinician must suspect this diagnosis and look for other clues when the premature infant with RDS cannot be weaned from ventilatory support (see Casebook 3).

Intravenous fluid overload may delay weaning and/or extubation, leading to pulmonary edema and respiratory failure. Because almost all neonates are ventilated with some form of end-expiratory pressure, fluid overload may be masked until the end-expiratory pressure is removed. Certain types of congenital heart disease with left-to-right shunts also may delay weaning and cause extubation failure. In our experience, a ventricular septal defect coexisting with a patent ductus or an atrioventricular canal are the most common causes of the increased pulmonary blood flow that prevents successful extubation. This is more likely if the newborn is 2 to 4 weeks' postnatal age, when the PVR has decreased to normal levels.

Central nervous system problems. Successful unassisted respiratory function depends not only on adequate airway patency, pulmonary mechanics, and cardiac function, but also on CNS control of ventilation. Often the inability to wean a patient from ventilatory support is due to central causes, such as nerve immaturity or brain injury. Some authors have concluded that the administration of CNS stimulants (caffeine, theophylline) to treat these conditions decreases the time on assisted ventilation and facilitates successful extubation.

The bedside availability of cranial ultrasonography has made the diagnosis of germinal matrix and IVH relatively easy. The clinician may believe that brain hemorrhage and/or subsequent posthemorrhagic hydrocephalus may delay successful weaning from respiratory support. Attempts should be made to keep intracranial pressure normal to lessen CNS effects on respiratory drive.

Drug use or overdose may prevent successful extubation. The use of pancuronium (Pavulon) for respiratory paralysis obviously will prevent adequate ventilation unless reversed or allowed to wear off. Maternal administration of magnesium sulfate for preeclampsia may cause respiratory insufficiency in the infant requiring continued assisted ventilation. The use of phenobarbital for IVH prophylaxis has been noted to cause very high phenobarbital levels due to the unpredictable excretion of this drug by premature infants. We have seen several infants in whom extubation failed secondary to high phenobarbital levels administered at recommended dosages.

Miscellaneous causes. Patients in whom extubation fails despite resolution of their primary disorder require special attention. There may be an unrecognized coexisting condition such as phrenic nerve palsy, myasthenia gravis, or other rare disorders. Infants on ventilatory support often are victims of sepsis, and this diagnosis should be considered in any infant with unexplained deterioration or in whom extubation fails without obvious cause. A search for metabolic abnormalities also should be made under these circumstances.

Outcome. This infant had many possible reasons for extubation failure. Although his primary disorder had resolved, multiple intubations and tracheomalacia pointed to an upper airway cause. The infant had a complete atrioventricular canal with moderate left-to-right shunting documented by echocardiography. The infant also was on phenobarbital and had suffered a hypoxic insult at birth. Cardiac catheterization revealed a true vascular ring with double aortic arch in addition to the atrioventricular canal. X-ray films showed that when the endotracheal tube was below the level of the arch, the infant had a normal thoracic volume. However, when the endotracheal tube was above the level of the ring, the infant had massive air trapping and hyperinflation (Fig. 29-11). The infant underwent surgical division of the vascular ring and PDA ligation on the day 18 of life and was successfully extubated shortly thereafter. The majority of vascular rings can be identified with noninvasive techniques using echocardiography, barium esophagography, and/or magnetic resonance imaging.[7,8] Some surgeons still may prefer the anatomic detail provided by angiography.

REFERENCES

1. Kavvadin V, Greenough A, Dimitriou G: Prediction of extubation failure in preterm neonates. Eur J Pediatr 157:227, 2000.
2. Sinha SK, Donn SM: Weaning from assisted ventilation: Art or science? Arch Dis Child Fetal Neonatal Ed 83:F64, 2000.
3. Fox WW, Berman LS, Dinwiddie R, et al: Tracheal extubation of the neonate at 2 to 3 mm H$_2$O continuous positive airway pressure. Pediatrics 59:257, 1977.
4. Davis PG, Henderson-Smart DJ: Extubation from low-rate intermittent positive pressure versus extubation after a trial of endotracheal continuous positive airway pressure in intubated infants (Cochrane Review). In: The Cochrane Library, Issue 1, Oxford Update Software, 2000.
5. Halliday HL: Towards earlier neonatal extubation. Lancet 355:2091, 2000.
6. Spence K, Barr P: Nasal versus oral intubation for mechanical ventilation of newborn infants (Cochrane Review). In: The Cochrane Library, Issue 1, Oxford Update Software, 2000.
7. Azarow KS, Pearl RH, Hoffman MA, et al: Vascular ring: Does magnetic resonance imaging replace angiography? Ann Thorac Surg 53:882, 1992.
8. van Son JA, Julsrud PR, Hagler DJ, et al: Imaging strategies for vascular rings. Ann Thorac Surg 57:604, 1994.

CASE 6

History

A 3840-g male infant was born at a community hospital to a 21-year-old primigravida at 39 weeks gestation after an uncomplicated pregnancy. Membranes were artificially ruptured 8 hours before delivery. The infant was delivered vaginally with the use of low forceps while the mother was under meperidine analgesia. Apgar scores were 6 and 9 at 1 and 5 minutes, respectively. The infant was floppy and slow to respond to oxygen by mask in the delivery room. Upon admission to the nursery he was cyanotic, with a respiratory rate of 50 breaths/min. He was placed in a 0.30 FIO_2 oxyhood. Mild hypoglycemia was noted. Feedings were attempted, but the infant would not suck. The complete blood count was normal. The initial arterial blood gas measurements obtained at 18 hours of age in 0.30 FIO_2 by oxyhood were pH 7.39, $PaCO_2$ 31 torr, and PaO_2 41 torr. Because of intermittent cyanosis and progressive tachypnea despite an increase in the FIO_2, he was transported to the referral hospital at 24 hours of age. A septic workup was performed and antibiotics were administered. Peripheral arterial blood gas measurements in FIO_2 1.0 by oxyhood were pH 7.27, $PaCO_2$ 38 torr, PaO_2 56 torr, and base excess −9. He was given 10 mEq sodium bicarbonate.

Physical examination showed an intermittently cyanotic term infant who was tachypneic without grunting or retractions. The anteroposterior diameter of the chest was increased. The lungs were clear to auscultation. The cardiac examination revealed a heart rate of 124, increased P_2, and a grade 2/6 systolic murmur at the lower left sternal border. Good pulses were palpated in all extremities. The liver was not enlarged. A chest radiograph (Fig. 29-12) obtained at 24 hours of age revealed a normal cardiac silhouette plus a pattern of vascular congestion and alveolar filling consistent with retained pulmonary fluid (transient tachypnea of the newborn). Two-dimensional echocardiogram showed no structural heart defect. Tricuspid regurgitation and right-to-left shunting across the ductus arteriosus were demonstrated by Doppler interrogation. Simultaneous right radial arterial blood gas and umbilical artery catheter gas in 1.0 FIO_2 by oxyhood were obtained and provided the following values: pH 7.49, $PaCO_2$ 30 torr, and PaO_2 148 torr in the preductal sample; and pH 7.40 $PaCO_2$ 42 torr, and PaO_2 40 torr in the postductal sample. A diagnosis of pulmonary hypertension with accompanying transient tachypnea of the newborn was made. The infant was placed on HFOV at 9 Hz, $P\overline{aw}$ 15, amplitude 25, and FIO_2 100%. iNO was blended in the inspiratory circuit at 20 ppm.

Serial PaO_2 values were in the range from 40 to 60 torr, with a maximum of 66 torr. Despite alkalinization, mild hyperventilation, iNO, and dobutamine, the patient did not improve. At 3 days of age, the congestion had decreased significantly and the heart size remained normal (Fig. 29-13). At 7 days of age he developed progressive congestive heart failure that was unresponsive to therapy. A chest radiograph showed extensive alveolar filling, venous congestion, and cardiomegaly compatible with cardiogenic pulmonary edema (Fig. 29-14). The infant was transferred to our NICU for possible ECMO with iNO ongoing during transport. A repeat two-dimensional echocardiogram was performed with Doppler interrogation.

Denouement and Discussion

Total Anomalous Pulmonary Venous Connection Below the Diaphragm

The repeat echocardiogram demonstrated findings consistent with PPHN: dilated right ventricle and pulmonary arteries, moderate tricuspid regurgitation with the right ventricular pressure estimated at systemic levels, right-to-left shunting across an unrestricted foramen, and a large PDA with right-to-left shunting. Pulmonary foramen ovale were not seen draining into

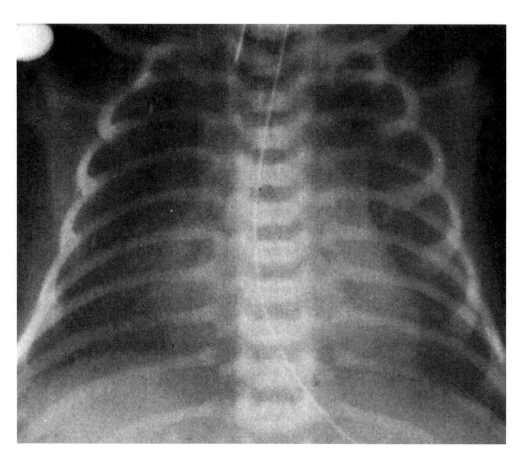

Figure 29-12. Chest x-ray film (anteroposterior view) at 24 hours of age.

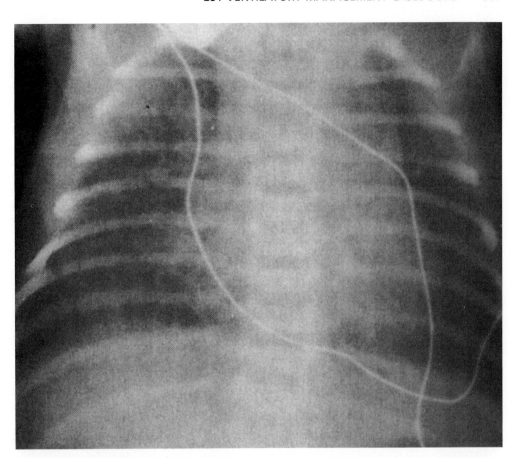

Figure 29-13. Chest x-ray film (anteroposterior view) at 3 days of age.

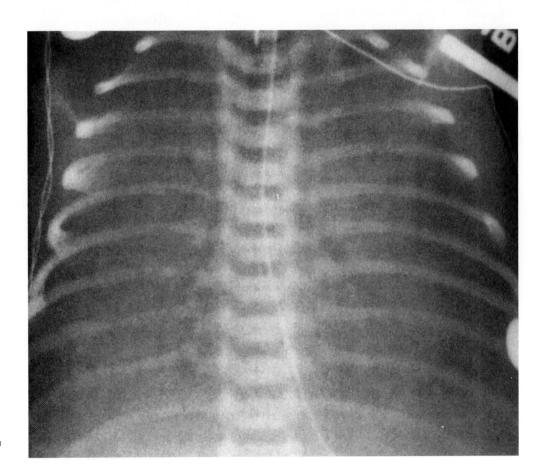

Figure 29-14. Chest x-ray film (AP view) at 7 days of age.

the left atrium. In addition, a large anomalous vertical vein was noted draining away from the heart to the liver. Color Doppler interrogation of the liver demonstrated a turbulent flow pattern suggestive of venous obstruction. The diagnosis of infradiaphragmatic total anomalous pulmonary venous connection (TAPVC) with obstruction was made. Surgical repair was performed the same day. The pulmonary hypertension persisted for several days after surgery and necessitated the use of iNO, but the patient did not require ECMO. The patient was discharged in good condition 14 days postoperatively.

TAPVC is responsible for 1% to 2% of all congenital cardiac lesions. If uncorrected, 80% of patients will die in the first year of life. The incidence in males and females is equal. TAPVC is classified by the site of the anomalous drainage: type I, supracardiac (e.g., into innominate vein, right superior vena cava); type II, cardiac (e.g., into right atrium, coronary sinus); type III, infradiaphragmatic (e.g., into the inferior vena cava, portal or hepatic veins, or ductus venosus); and type IV, mixed. Although the infradiaphragmatic type is somewhat less common, it is more likely to be obstructed and cause symptoms in the early neonatal period.[1] There is always some type of atrial communication, and the right side of the heart usually is dilated and/or hypertrophied. In the patient with pulmonary venous obstruction, the clinical features consist of cyanosis, usually no murmurs, accentuated P_2, quiet precordium, and tachypnea. Medical management of TAPVC with obstruction is generally not successful, and this diagnosis should prompt surgical repair as soon as possible.[2] ECMO may be necessary to stabilize the patient before corrective surgery.

In patients with unobstructed pulmonary venous return, the findings differ somewhat in that cyanosis usually is not as prominent. The precordium is hyperactive, the second heart sound is widely split with an accentuated P_2, and a pulmonary ejection murmur may be present with or without a tricuspid rumble. The obstructed patients are symptomatic earlier. The chest radiograph often reveals a normal-sized heart with hazy lung fields resulting from vascular congestion and pulmonary edema. Electrocardiogram usually shows right ventricular hypertrophy and right atrial enlargement. Echocardiography usually is diagnostic. Catheterization sometimes is performed when there is mixed drainage. Because the valves and ventricles usually are normal in TAPVC, surgical correction offers a good long-term prognosis.[3] However, a subset of patients have recurrent pulmonary vein stenosis that is considered lethal. Surgical repair usually consists of ligating the anomalous venous trunk distally and anastomosing it to the left atrium. Operative mortality depends upon the type of lesion and the clinical condition prior to surgery, as many patients are moribund by the time surgery is begun.

TAPVC is the cyanotic congenital heart disease that is most often misdiagnosed as PPHN (see Casebook 2) until definitive cardiac studies are performed. The major reasons for this confusion are the frequent lack of a murmur plus PaO_2 levels that may be much higher than in the other cyanotic congenital heart diseases because of better mixing of oxygenated and deoxygenated blood. Respiratory distress and other symptoms depend mainly upon degree of obstruction of the abnormal pulmonary veins, PVR, and size of the atrial communication.

In this particular patient, the initial two-dimensional echocardiogram appeared to show evidence of pulmonary veins emptying into the left atrium. With differential oxygenation of over 100 torr in preductal versus postductal blood gases and with pulmonary hypertension that responded somewhat to medical management, the attending physicians were misled until the

baby developed overt congestive failure. Lessons to be learned from this case are to assess all data as to reliability and to remember potential errors in blood gas sampling. The best explanation for the differential preductal and postductal gases would be that some room air was inadvertently mixed in the preductal sample. Note that there was a difference in both PaO_2 and $PaCO_2$. If both blood gases were technically correct, the pH and $PaCO_2$ of both samples should have been virtually identical. If one were analyzing a bubble of room air, the PO_2 would be approximately 150 torr and the PCO_2 nearly zero (see Chapter 17). Thus, in this case, room air contamination of the preductal sample would raise the PaO_2 and pH and lower the $PaCO_2$. If an umbilical venous catheter is present in the inferior vena cava, a blood gas sample from this source would demonstrate abnormally high PaO_2 because the source is near the endpoint of the pulmonary venous return. This might be an early clue to the diagnosis of TAPVC in babies presenting with signs of PPHN.

REFERENCES

1. Sano S, Brawn WJ, Mee RBB: Total anomalous pulmonary venous drainage. J Thorac Cardiovasc Surg 97:886, 1989.
2. Marino BS, Bird GL, Wernovsky G: Diagnosis and management of the newborn with suspected heart disease. Clin Perinatol 28:91, 2001.
3. Phillips SJ: Total anomalous pulmonary venous connection [letter]. Ann Thorac Surg 56:395, 1993.

CASE 7

History

A 3670-g female infant was born at 42 weeks gestation to a 32-year-old, gravida 2 mother at a level III perinatal center. The infant was born vaginally with a vertex presentation assisted by vacuum extraction under epidural anesthesia. The mother admitted she felt decreased fetal movement for several days. At delivery a tight nuchal cord was noticed and the infant was limp, with poor respiratory effort. Oxygen was administered without visible benefit, and the infant's trachea was intubated and hand ventilated. Apgar scores of 4 and 6 were assigned at 1 and 5 minutes, respectively. The infant improved and was transferred to the intensive care nursery, where arterial blood gas studies revealed pH 7.12, $PaCO_2$ 83 torr, and PaO_2 44 torr. The infant was placed on IMV via a time-cycled, pressure-limited ventilator, and an umbilical artery catheter was inserted.

Physical examination at this time revealed a post-term female infant with hyperinflation of the lungs, coarse inspiratory rales, and tachypnea. The infant had acrocyanosis and hypotonia. A chest radiograph was consistent with "aspiration syndrome." The admission white blood count was 27,200 mm/cm^3 with a differential including three metamyelocytes, eight bands, and 34 polymorphonuclear leukocytes. Platelet count was 293,000. Cultures were obtained and antibiotics were administered. The infant was placed on a PPHN protocol (see Casebook 2) with sedation, mild hyperventilation, and alkalinization. Dopamine infusion was started because of hypotension. Despite respiratory alkalosis, the patient could not be adequately oxygenated. At 24 hours of age, the infant developed bilateral pneumothoraces and was treated with chest tube drainage to suction with complete reexpansion of both lungs. Subsequently, the infant was paralyzed with pancuronium bromide with no improvement.

Multiple manipulations of the ventilator with rapid rates (100 to 150 breaths/min), reverse inspiratory-to-expiratory ratios, and hand ventilation were not successful in providing adequate oxygenation. During the last 12 hours prior to transport, the infant was almost continuously hand ventilated. The infant was then transported to this institution.

On arrival at our NICU the infant was dusky, with blood pressures of 61/31 mm Hg on dopamine. A chest radiograph (Fig. 29-15) revealed patchy areas of alveolar consolidation compatible with aspiration. Bilateral pleural catheters were in place with complete expansion of the lungs. The patient was placed on HFOV at a mean airway pressure 19 cm H_2O, amplitude 40, 9 Hz, flow 15 L/min, and FIO_2 1.0. Preductal arterial blood gases were pH 7.60, $PaCO_2$ 22 torr, HCO_3 21 mEq/L, base excess +3, and PaO_2 35 torr. Two-dimensional echocardiogram revealed a normally structured heart with dilation of the right ventricle and good ventricular function. iNO was started at 20 ppm and increased to 40 ppm without improving oxygenation. Despite HFOV, inotropic support, and iNO, the patient could not be adequately oxygenated. A conference was held with the parents.

Denouement and Discussion

Failure of Mechanical Ventilation

Despite the major advances in ventilatory technology and management of assisted ventilation made in the last 2 decades, a few patients cannot be managed with conventional or high-frequency ventilatory techniques. New protocols for treating PPHN include high-frequency ventilation, iNO, surfactant administration, and a number of pulmonary vasodilators. In recent years, various therapies have been compared, but such analysis is difficult because of the different pathophysiologies involved and lack of consensus of appropriate outcomes. A patient who survives assisted ventilation consisting of extremely high inflating pressures only to develop oxygen-dependent bronchopulmonary dysplasia and possibly succumb a year later to pneumonitis and/or cor pulmonale is not a therapeutic success. Therefore, it becomes essential in every unit to correctly predict which patients will not survive conventional and/or high-frequency ventilation and which patients will develop unacceptable complications so that appropriate interventions can be instituted as early as possible. This may require early transfer and consideration of the patient for ECMO.

Definition. Failure or potential failure of mechanical ventilation can be defined in one of four ways when patients are receiving maximal ventilatory, medical, pharmacologic, and surgical therapy: (1) death; (2) inability to adequately oxygenate the patient (unacceptably low PaO_2); (3) inability to adequately ventilate the patient (unacceptably high $PaCO_2$); and (4) potentially toxic ventilator settings or parameters predictive of poor outcome. Several groups of investigators have attempted to quantify ventilator parameters, birthweight, and/or blood gas results in order to select patients who might benefit from therapies other than conventional or high-frequency ventilation.

Neonatologists caring for infants with PPHN in a non-ECMO center face the challenge of when to refer that patient to a center with ECMO capability. PPHN can be very labile, and

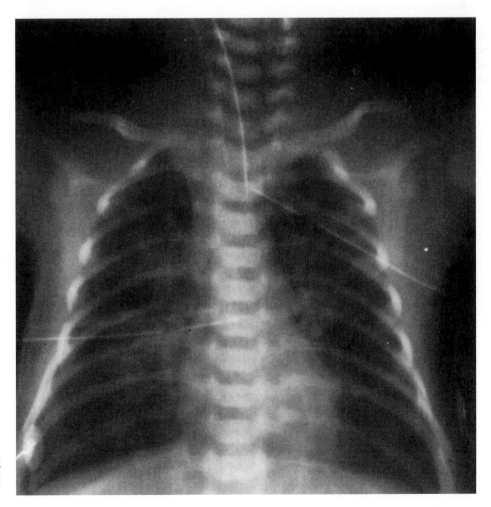

Figure 29-15. Admission chest x-ray film (anteroposterior view) demonstrating patchy alveolar consolidation with bilateral pleural catheters in place.

infants may deteriorate quickly before or during transport.[1] Predictive scoring systems have been used to identify infants who are potential candidates for ECMO.[2]

Predictive Indices

In the case presented, the patient falls into category 2, inability to adequately oxygenate despite maximal ventilatory support with adjunctive pharmacologic therapies. The patient had been given an extensive trial of conventional and high-frequency mechanical ventilation with paralysis, inotropic agents, hyperventilation, and iNO. Despite these therapies, the Pao_2 remained in an unacceptable range.

Judging the severity of PPHN allows the clinician to gauge response to various therapies, predict outcome, and direct the patient to more invasive therapies if necessary. At the present time, three techniques have been used as predictive indices.

Using postductal Pao_2, Marsh et al.[3] found that values less than 50 mm Hg in infants mechanically ventilated with 100% Fio_2 predicted a high mortality risk (sensitivity 86%, specificity 96%). Calculation of the alveolar-arterial oxygen gradient ($AaDo_2$) can also be used to judge impairment of gas exchange. Using a modified equation when the patient is breathing 100% oxygen, the calculation can be made as follows:

$$AaDo_2 = (760–47) – Paco_2 – Pao_2,$$

where 760 is atmospheric pressure at sea level and 47 is water vapor pressure. In a healthy individual breathing 100% oxygen, the oxygen gradient should be less than 200 mm Hg. Various investigators have used values ranging from 600 to 620 mm Hg for 4 to 12 hours to indicate patients with high mortality risk who are ECMO candidates. Unfortunately, the calculation must be modified when not done at sea level and can be problematic if the $Paco_2$ is driven down by hyperventilation.

The oxygen index (OI) evaluates the amount of oxygenation achieved for a given amount of mean airway pressure, thus assessing severity of disease and potential barotrauma.

$$OI = \frac{100 \times (P\overline{aw})(Fio_2)}{Pao_2}.$$

Bartlett et al.[4] reported that an OI greater than 40 in three of five blood gases taken 30 minutes apart predicted an 80% mortality risk. Most institutions use OI as an index for ECMO support, but this approach has been criticized because historical controls are used and newer therapies such as iNO have not been evaluated with this approach.

Other clinical aspects of care should alert the clinician that ECMO may be necessary. Patients with congenital diaphragmatic hernia needing ventilatory support are candidates to be managed in a center with ECMO capabilities. Likewise, patients with severe PPHN requiring high inotropic support or patients diagnosed with sepsis who have severe granulocytopenia may be ECMO candidates before they meet the ventilatory indices. Because ECMO is a highly invasive procedure, it is reserved for infants with a predicted mortality of 80% or greater. However, since the United Kingdom collaborative trial, evidence is in hand that this therapy is superior to conventional treatments for the small subset of patients who meet predictive criteria.[5]

Case Outcome

After full explanation of the invasive nature of the process and potential complications to the parents, consent was given for placement on ECMO. Cannulation of the right internal jugular vein was accomplished using veno-venous access without difficulty (see Fig. 16-3), and immediately ventilatory parameters were decreased to maintenance levels (PIP 15 cm H_2O, rate 20 breaths/min, Fio_2 0.35, flow 7 L/min) with acceptable blood gases. The patient remained on bypass with heparinization for 80 hours, at which time ECMO was discontinued. Within 48 hours after decannulation, the infant's trachea was extubated and she was weaned to room air. Studies of the CNS while the patient was on ECMO (cranial ultrasonography) and after decannulation (computed tomographic scan) showed no intracranial hemorrhage and no cortical defects. At 6-month follow-up, she was considered neurologically normal.

Summary

Each institution needs to evaluate assisted ventilation protocols continuously in order to improve outcome. Predictive indices from other centers may or may not apply in every hospital. Any patient that falls into an 80% predictive mortality group may be considered a potential candidate for more invasive interventions, provided all screening criteria are met and parents are fully informed and agree. Candidates for ECMO at our institution must meet the following criteria: (1) weight greater than 2000 g; (2) less than 7 days of assisted ventilation; (3) no evidence of intracranial hemorrhage; (4) quality of life potential; (5) parental consent; (6) reversible pulmonary disease; and (7) predicted 80% or greater mortality. Those institutions that do not have facilities such as high-frequency ventilation, iNO, or ECMO available should consider transfer of appropriate patients to centers having these facilities when predictive indices indicate that the child probably would not survive with conventional mechanical ventilation alone. Some clinicians have suggested that infants with an OI of 20 to 25 be transferred to centers with ECMO capability.[1]

REFERENCES

1. Boedy RF, Howell CG, Kanto WP Jr: Hidden mortality rate associated with extracorporeal membrane oxygenation. J Pediatr 117:462, 1990.
2. Schumacher RE, Baumgart S: Extracorporeal membrane oxygenation 2001: The odyssey continues. Clin Perinatol 28:629, 2001.
3. Marsh TD, Wilkerson SA, Cook LN: Extracorporeal membrane oxygenation selection criteria: Partial pressure of arterial oxygen versus alveolar–arterial oxygen gradient. Pediatrics 82:162, 1988.
4. Bartlett RH, Roloff DW, Cornell RG, et al: Extracorporeal circulation in neonatal respiratory failure: A prospective randomized study. Pediatrics 76:479, 1985.
5. UK collaborative randomised trial of neonatal extracorporeal membrane oxygenation. UK Collaborative ECMO Trial Group. Lancet 348:75, 1996.

CASE 8

History

A 3150-g female infant was delivered precipitously in the labor room of a community hospital to a 21-year-old gravida 3, para 1 woman. Membranes ruptured at delivery. The amniotic fluid was noted to be meconium stained. The infant cried at birth and appeared to be vigorous. Apgar scores of 7 and 9 were assigned at 1 and 5 minutes, respectively. The trachea was not intubated for meconium aspiration. Oxygen at 1.0 FIO_2 was provided by oxyhood for cyanosis, and the first arterial blood gas revealed pH 7.19, $Paco_2$ 54 torr, Pao_2 29 torr, HCO_3 20 mEq/L, and base excess −9. The infant appeared to have increasing respiratory distress, and she was intubated at approximately 20 minutes of age. Mechanical ventilation with a conventional time-cycled ventilator was begun using the following settings: PIP 20 cm H_2O, CDP +4 cm H_2O, and IMV rate 30 breaths/min. Follow-up blood gases showed pH 7.32, $Paco_2$ 41 torr, Pao_2 108 torr, and base excess −6. After a septic workup was performed and antibiotics were administered, the infant was transferred to a tertiary care hospital at 10 hours of age.

Chest radiographic examination on admission revealed bilateral alveolar filling with hyperexpansion and moderate cardiomegaly compatible with retained pulmonary fluid and/or meconium aspiration (Fig. 29-16). Through the first 13 hours of life, the infant demonstrated metabolic acidosis that required a total of 15.5 mEq of sodium bicarbonate to correct the base deficit. Meconium-stained fluid was suctioned from the trachea. When agitated, the infant's oxygen saturations fell to 50%. Pancuronium bromide was administered. The subsequent blood gases confirmed respiratory acidosis with pH 7.19, $Paco_2$ 59 torr, and Pao_2 53 torr. The PIP and rate were increased to 24

and 40, respectively, and the FIO_2 was increased to 1.0. The CDP was increased to +5 cm H_2O. Respiratory acidosis persisted until the PIP was increased to 28 cm H_2O with a rate of 50 breaths/min. With pH 7.43, $Paco_2$ 40 torr, and Pao_2 65 torr, the diagnosis of pulmonary hypertension of the newborn (PPHN) was considered, and further attempts at hyperventilation were made, resulting in an increase of the ventilatory parameters to PIP 30 cm H_2O, PEEP +6 cm H_2O, and rate 60 breaths/min. Resultant blood gases showed pH 7.57, $Paco_2$ 30 torr, and Pao_2 55 torr. Repeat chest radiographic films at 20 hours of age showed continued hyperexpansion of the lungs (Fig. 29-17). A two-dimensional echocardiogram obtained at 25 hours of age showed normal cardiac structure with no significant right-to-left shunting at the atrial or ductal level.

Denouement and Discussion

Iatrogenic Overexpansion Resulting in Poor Lung Compliance

After the diagnosis of pulmonary hypertension was ruled out, the patient was reevaluated and pancuronium bromide was discontinued. The PIP was decreased from 30 to 24 cm H_2O and PEEP was decreased from 6 to 4 cm H_2O without deterioration of the blood gases. Four hours later the infant was noted to have some spontaneous respiratory effort and the Pao_2 was

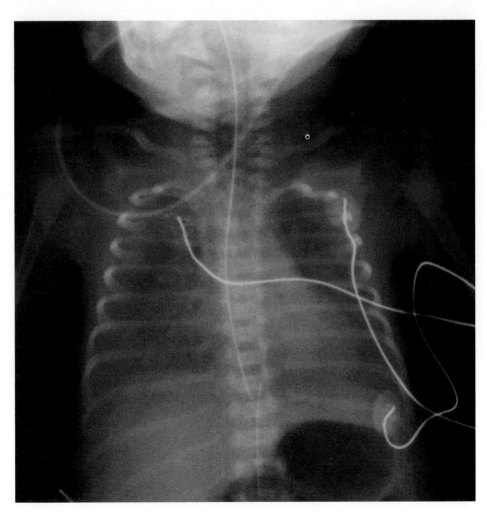

Figure 29-16. Chest x-ray film (anteroposterior view) at 11 hours of age.

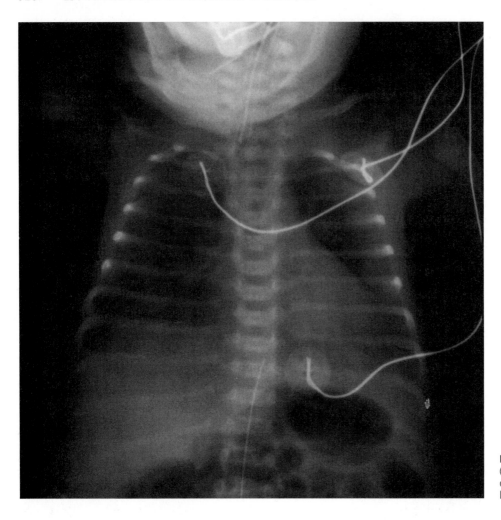

Figure 29-17. Repeat chest x-ray film (anteroposterior view) at 20 hours of age demonstrating mild hyperexpansion of the lungs.

116 torr. The PIP was further decreased to 20 cm H_2O and the infant was weaned to extubation 24 hours later.

By paralyzing this infant with pancuronium bromide, proportionately more pressure was being transmitted to the lungs, because some of the chest recoil is eliminated by muscle paralysis and relatively little pressure is required to expand the chest wall of a neonate.[1] The infant developed respiratory acidosis resulting from the sudden decrease in minute volume when her spontaneous respirations were eliminated by pancuronium bromide and not immediately compensated by an increase in the ventilator rate. Instead of simply increasing the rate, both the rate and PIP were increased, which served to increase the distention of the alveoli already compromised by air trapping caused by the mild meconium aspiration. The ventilation-perfusion abnormality was increased by these maneuvers, thus worsening blood gases and leading to an erroneous diagnosis of PPHN.

The major force contributing to lung elastic recoil in the newborn is produced by surface tension at the air–alveolar interface. In term newborns with adequate surfactant, alveoli with large radii will require little pressure to remain open or be further expanded, as shown by the Laplace relationship (pressure = 2 × surface tension/radius). As noted in Chapter 2, when alveoli are overexpanded, they are in the uppermost flat portion of their pressure–volume or compliance curve, where little extra volume is achieved despite large changes in pressure (see Fig. 2-3). Compliance describes the relationship between a given change in volume and the pressure required to produce that change. Dynamic compliance is measured in newborns at the point of no flow (i.e., end-inspiration or end-expiration). Note that in Figure 2-3 the lung compliance curve of the newborn describes an S shape overall. At the lower end of the curve (area A), little volume increase is achieved despite major pressure changes (stiff lungs). In the midportion (area B), where tidal volume breathing normally takes place, compliance is directly and linearly related to lung volume (with each unit pressure increase there is a unit increase in lung volume). The steeper this curve, the greater the compliance or elasticity of the lung. The flatter the curve, the less compliant (or more stiff) the lung. At the uppermost portion of the curve (area C), the compliance decreases as lung volume approaches total lung capacity. Moreover, ventilation of patients in the uppermost portion of the curve may result in transmission of excessive pressure to the mediastinum, thus impeding thoracic venous return, decreasing cardiac output, and reducing systemic blood pressure.

Thus, clinicians managing infants requiring assisted ventilation should attempt to ventilate these infants in the midportion of their lung compliance curve. This is not always possible considering the pathophysiology of the disease process or specialized treatment methods for specific situations.

Finding the optimal PEEP for a given patient in a specific clinical situation is often difficult. At a given compression or driving pressure (PIP–PEEP), functional residual capacity is determined by the PEEP. Ventilating infants at the optimal functional residual capacity will improve lung compliance and decrease mean airway pressure. This concept is illustrated in Figure 18-10.[2]

In this case, the patient care team believed that the large alveolar-arterial oxygen gradient observed when the infant's blood gases were relatively normal on assisted ventilation (pH 7.43, $Paco_2$ 40 torr, Pao_2 65 torr) indicated possible pulmonary hypertension and shunting at the foramen ovale and/or ductal levels. No attempt was made at that time to confirm their suspicions by simultaneous preductal and postductal sampling of blood gases, simultaneous preductal and postductal oxygen saturations, or two-dimensional echocardiography. The patient was hyperventilated for treatment of pulmonary hypertension with no improvement in the infant's condition or blood gases. Therefore, the assumption that the large alveolar-arterial oxygen gradient was caused by intracardiac shunting was incorrect, and the infant's large gradient was likely due to intrapulmonary shunt and ventilation-perfusion mismatch.

In any case of suspected pulmonary hypertension of the newborn, attempts must be made to document by two-dimensional echocardiography and/or simultaneous preductal and postductal blood gases that this condition does exist.[3] Obviously, the ventilatory treatment of pulmonary hypertension by hyperventilation is fraught with potential compli-cations, including pulmonary air leak and overdistention of alveoli. This therapy has been used less frequently by clini-cians since published reports of long-term sequelae to this technique, such as hearing loss and stroke, and the availabil-ity of iNO.[4]

This infant responded to the drop in CDP and PIP by a dra-matic improvement in blood gases when her lung compliance fell into area B of the lung compliance curve. The lesson to be learned from this case is to be aware of the adverse effects that excessive positive pressure can have on an infant with loss of elastic recoil from the chest and subsequent overdistention of alveoli already compromised by air trapping seen in aspiration syndromes.

REFERENCES

1. Bhutani VK, Abbasi S, Sivieri EM: Continuous skeletal muscle paralysis: Effect on neonatal pulmonary mechanics. Pediatrics 81:419, 1988.
2. Bhutani VK, Sivieri EM: Clinical use of pulmonary mechanics and wave-form graphics. Clin Perinatol 28:487, 2001.
3. Walsh MC, Stork EK: Persistent pulmonary hypertension of the newborn: Rational therapy based on pathophysiology. Clin Perinatol 28:609, 2001.
4. Walsh-Sukys MC, Tyson JE, Wright LL, et al: Persistent pulmonary hyper-tension of the newborn: Practice variation and outcome in the era before nitric oxide. Pediatrics 105:14, 2000.

APPENDICES

1. Modes of neonatal ventilation with advantages and disadvantages.
2. Lung volumes in the infant.
3. Changes in respiratory system dimensions with growth.
4. Effect of age on lung size.
5. Lung volume in full-term and premature newborns.
6. Allen's test.
7. Procedure for obtaining capillary blood gases.
8. A, Arterial blood gas values in normal full-term infants.
   B, Arterial blood gas values in normal premature infants.
9. Blood gas values in cord blood and in arterial blood at different ages during the neonatal period.
   A, Oxygen tension.
   B, Carbon dioxide tension.
   C, pH.
   D, Base excess.
10. Hemoglobin-oxygen dissociation curves.
11. Siggaard-Andersen alignment nomogram.
12. Neutral thermal environmental temperatures.
13. A, Maturational assessment of gestational age.
    B, Classification of newborns (both sexes) by intrauterine growth and gestational age.
14. Heart rates in premature and full-term neonates.
15. Systolic and diastolic blood pressure in newborn infants.
16. Mean blood pressure and pulse pressure in newborn infants.
17. Blood chemistries.
    A, Normal blood chemistry values, term infants.
    B, Normal blood chemistry values, low-birthweight infants, capillary blood, first day.
    C, Blood chemistry values in premature infants during the first 7 weeks of life (birthweight, 1500–1750 g).
18. Hematologic values in newborn infants.
    A, Normal hematologic values during the first 14 days of life.
    B, Changes in hemoglobin and reticulocyte count in term and preterm infants.
19. Leukocyte values and neutrophil counts in term and premature infants.
    A, Leukocyte values in term and premature infants.
    B, Total neutrophil count reference range in the first 60 hours of life.
20. Platelets.
    A, Venous platelet counts in normal low-birthweight infants.
    B, Platelet counts in full-term infants.
21. Coagulation factors and test values in term and premature infants.
22. Cerebrospinal fluid values in term and premature infants.
23. Daily maintenance fluid, mineral, and glucose requirements for term neonates.
24. Perinatal transport record.
    A, Historical data.
    B, Transport data.
25. Neonatal ICU flow sheet.
26. A, Neonatal resuscitation record.
    B, Evaluation of code performance.
27. Delivery room care of the neonate: neonatal resuscitation.
28. Clinical considerations in the use of oxygen.
29. Executive summary: final COBRA regulations.
30. OSHA Guidelines for occupational exposure.
    A, Universal precautions for use with all patients.
    B, Specific guidelines.
31. FDA Safety Alert: Hazards of heated-wire breathing circuits.
32. Effective F_{IO_2} conversion tables for infants on nasal cannula.
33. Neonatal indications and dosages for administration of selected drugs.
34. Frequently used abbreviations.

A P P E N D I X   1
MODES OF VENTILATION (WITH ADVANTAGES AND DISADVANTAGES)

Mode Classification	Principle of Operation	Advantages	Disadvantages
Time-cycled, pressure limited	PIP set during inspiration flow of gas delivered to achieve pressure desired. Flow down after PIP attained until inspiratory phase completed.		
Volume control (not actually a mode, but indicates what is constant during the ventilated breath delivery, and should be used as a prefix for each "mode", e.g., VC-SIMV)	Volume constant, pressure variable.		High PIPs with decreasing lung compliance and/or airway resistance.
Synchronized or patient-triggered ventilation (PTV)	Inspiratory phase initiated by patient's own inspiratory effort. Methods of triggering: 1. Impedance (thorax-Sechrist SAVI). 2. Motion (Infrasonic's Star-sync. 3. Pressure: senses decrease in baseline pressure with patient inspiratory effort. 4. Flow: senses decrease in baseline flow. secondary to patient's inspiratory effort. 5. Volume: triggers inspiration in response to preset volume loss.	Improves patient-ventilator synchrony. Flow triggering has become the standard on all current ventilators. Flow triggering has been shown to decrease the amount of work needed to trigger. Volume triggering's advantage over flow triggering: decreased "noise" from circuit condensate decreases potential of false triggering.	Auto-cycling if too sensitive or variable leak around ETT. Patient "locked out" if not sensitive enough. Volume triggering (Drager Babylog) has not been adequately evaluated. Disadvantage of volume triggering versus flow triggering: the delay from the signal processing may produce phase lag.
IMV	Preset mandated breaths are delivered at a set frequency independent of the patient's spontaneous breaths.		Breath stacking Potential for air leak
SIMV	A version of IMV in which the ventilator sets up a timing window around the scheduled delivery of a mandatory breath in an attempt to deliver the mandated breath in conjunction with the patient's inspiratory effort. If no effort is detected during the timing window, the ventilator will deliver the scheduled mandated breath.	Primarily used as weaning strategy due to range of ventilator breaths. Improves patient-ventilator synchrony. Prevents breath stacking and potential for air leak/gas trapping/volutrauma.	Same as for *Synchronized or patient-triggered ventilation*
Pressure Control (not actually a mode, but indicates what is constant during the ventilated breath delivery, and should be used as a prefix for each "mode," e.g., PC-SIMV + PS)	Pressure constant, volume variable: flow variable (decelerating waveform). Constant PIP (square pressure waveform).	Better gas distribution. Rapid pressurization helps overcome airway resistance.	Variable volumes in face of changing lung compliance or lung resistance with potential for hypo- or hyper-inflation.
Pressure-regulated volume control (Servo 300) (patient- or machine-triggered, pressure limited and time cycled, with tidal volume as the conditional variable used to change the pressure limit)	Variable flow rate (decelerating waveform) but targets specific tidal volume. A dual-control mode. Inspiration is pressure controlled within a breath, but the pressure	Good if you need high PIP. Combines guaranteed tidal volume with pressure-limited features. Limits PIP (within a given range), avoiding lung overinflation while maintaining the	An assist-control mode; therefore there is the potential for hyperventilation if the patient is not well-sedated or paralyzed and the patient becomes tachypneic. Not a "weaning" mode.

APPENDIX 1
MODES OF VENTILATION (WITH ADVANTAGES AND DISADVANTAGES)—CONT'D

Mode Classification	Principle of Operation	Advantages	Disadvantages
	limit is automatically adjusted up or down (based on the calculated value for respiratory system compliance derived from a "test" breath) to achieve a preset tidal volume. A form of pressure-limited, time-cycled ventilation that uses tidal volume as a feedback control for continuously adjusting the pressure limit.	advantage of volume control (delivering a consistent minute ventilation even in the face of changing lung mechanics).	
Pressure support (Pressure controlled, patient-triggered, pressure limited, patient cycled)	Spontaneous breathing mode in which a patient's inspiratory effort is assisted by the ventilator up to a preset inspiratory pressure. Inspiration is terminated when inspiratory flow reaches either a minimum level or a percentage of the initial inspiratory flow. The patient determines his or her own rate, inspiratory time, and tidal volume. A secondary safety termination typically includes time. This prevents prolonged inspiratory times in the presence of air leaks where flow criteria may not be met.	Weaning. Decreases WOB by overcoming resistance of ETT.	If used just to overcome resistance of the ETT: there is no further decrease in WOB when pressures of >10 cm H_2O are applied.
Proportional assist ventilation (PAV): Evita ventilator by Drager, whose term for this is "proportional pressure support" (pressure controlled, patient triggered, pressure limited, and flow cycled)	A spontaneous mode that is a form of pressure control in which pressure will vary continuously throughout inspiration and is proportional to the volume and flow signals (flow and volume are controlled by parameters based on patient effort; the greater the patient effort, the faster the flow, and the higher the tidal volume).	Potentially the most "comfortable" form of ventilation.	Experimental. Not approved for infant ventilation.
Volume-assured pressure support (VAPS): Bird 8400 Sti or T-Bird Vent (pressure controlled, patient or time triggered, pressure limited, and flow cycled)	A dual-control mode in which adjustments are made within the breath to achieve a target volume. Ventilation starts inspiration in pressure control. If the target volume has not been delivered by the time inspiratory flow decays to a preset inspiratory flow, the ventilator switches to volume control.	Limits PIP (within a given range), which avoids lung overdistension while maintaining the advantage of volume control (delivering a constant minute ventilation even if changes in lung mechanics occur).	
CPAP (pressure controlled, patient triggered, patient cycled, unsupported spontaneous breathing	Mode of operation (debated as to whether truly a "mode," because no tidal volume is generated by the ventilator) in which a preset pressure is maintained while the patient is allowed to breathe spontaneously. Patient determines his or her own rate and tidal volume.	Increases mean airway pressure and therefore oxygenation. Possibly decreases WOB if optimizes FRC and ventilation/perfusion matching.	

Abbreviations:
PIP = peak inspiratory pressure; IMV = intermittent mandatory ventilation; SIMV = synchronized intermittent mandatory ventilation; ETT = endotracheal tube; WOB = work of breathing

APPENDIX 2
LUNG VOLUMES IN THE INFANT

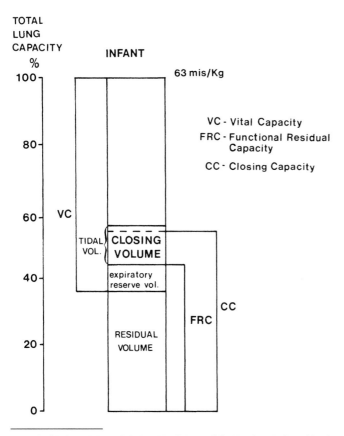

From Smith CA, Nelson NM: The Physiology of the Newborn Infant. 4th ed. Springfield, IL, Charles C Thomas, Publisher, 1976.

APPENDIX 3
CHANGES IN RESPIRATORY SYSTEM DIMENSIONS WITH GROWTH*

	Newborn to 1 Month	Infant
Chest, diameter (cm)		
Transverse	10	14
Anteroposterior	7.5	9
Trachea, length (mm)	40/57	42/67
Diameter (mm)	4	5
CSA (mm²)	26	34
Mainstem bronchi		
Diameter (mm)	4	4
CSA, right/left (mm²)	—	20/13
Bronchioles, diameter (mm)	0.3	0.4
CSA (mm²)	0.07	0.12
Terminal bronchioles		
Diameter (mm)	0.2	0.3
Internal diameter (mm)	0.1	0.12
CSA	0.03	0.07
Alveoli, diameter (mm)	0.05	0.06–0.07
Surface area (m²)	2.8	6.5
Body length (cm)	50	—
Weight (kg)	3.4	—
Surface area (m²)	0.21	0.3
Lung weight (gm)	50	70
Dead space (mL)	7–8	—

Abbreviation: CSA = cross-sectional area.
* Values from Engel S (autopsy data) and Fearon B, and Whalen JS (living subjects); (autopsy/living).
From Scarpelli EM (ed): Pulmonary Physiology of the Fetus, Newborn, and Child. Philadelphia, Lea & Febiger, 1975. Reprinted by permission.

APPENDIX 4
EFFECT OF AGE ON LUNG SIZE*

Age	No. of Cases Studied	Alveoli (× 106)	Respiratory Airways (× 106)	Air-tissue Interface (m²)	Body Surface Area (m²)	Generations of Respiratory Airways
Birth	1	24	1.5	2.8	0.21	—
3 mo	3	77	2.5	7.2	0.29	21
7 mo	1	112	3.7	8.4	0.38	—
13 mo	1	129	4.5	12.2	0.45	22
22 mo	1	160	7.1	14.2	0.50	—
4 y	1	257	7.9	22.2	0.67	—
8 y	1	280	14.0	32.0	0.92	23
Adult		296	14.0	75.0	1.90	23
Approximate fold-increase, birth to adult	—	10	10	21	9	—

* Values from Dunnill MS.
From Thibeault DW, Gregory GA (eds): Neonatal Pulmonary Care. Menlo Park, CA, Addison-Wesley Publishing Co., 1979, and Scarpelli EM (ed): Pulmonary Physiology of the Fetus, Newborn, and Child. Philadelphia, Lea & Febiger, 1975.

APPENDIX 5
LUNG VOLUME IN FULL-TERM AND PREMATURE NEWBORNS

Reference	Method	Weight (kg)	Age	Lung Volume
Berglund and Karlberg	Helium	2.0–5.0	0.5–7 d	27 mL/kg
Klaus et al.	Plethysmography	2.3–4.1	11–20 min	23 mL/kg
			30–40 min	29 mL/kg
			25–48 h	28 mL/kg
			>96 h	39 mL/kg
Nelson et al.	Plethysmography	1.3–4.0	16 h–71 d	40.6 mL/kg
	N$_2$ washout	1.3–4.0	16 h–71 d	31.3 mL/kg
Kraus and Auld	Plethysmography	>1.75	<24 h	2 mL/cm
	Helium	>1.75	<24 h	1.3 mL/cm
	Plethysmography	>1.75	3–6 d	1.8 mL/cm
	Helium	>1.75	3–6 d	1.4 mL/cm
	Plethysmography	<1.75	<24 h	1.7 mL/cm
	Helium	<1.75	<24 h	0.9 mL/cm
	Plethysmography	<1.75	12–19 d	0.9 mL/cm
	Helium	<1.75	12–19 d	0.8 mL/cm
Lacourt and Polgar	Plethysmography	0.68–2.65 (prematures)	1–72 d	30.4 mL/kg 1.12 mL/cm
	Plethysmography	1.5–3.6 (full-term)	1–18 d	32.4 mL/kg 1.72 mL/cm
Ronchetti et al.	Plethysmography	1.38–2.6	4–28 d	37.5 mL/kg
	Helium	1.38–2.6	4–28 d	29.5 mL/kg

From Thibeault DW, Gregory GA (eds): Neonatal Pulmonary Care. Menlo Park, CA, Addison-Wesley Publishing Co., 1979, and Scarpelli EM (ed.): Pulmonary Physiology of the Fetus, Newborn, and Child. Philadelphia, Lea & Feblger, 1975.

APPENDIX 6
ALLEN'S TEST

Gently squeeze the hand to partially empty it of blood. Apply pressure to both the ulnar and radial arteries. Then remove pressure from the hand and the ulnar artery. If the entire hand flushes and fills with blood, the ulnar artery can supply the hand with blood and the radial artery can be safely punctured or cannulated.

APPENDIX 7
PROCEDURE FOR OBTAINING CAPILLARY BLOOD GASES

1. Equipment needed:
   75-µL capillary tube (heparinized)
   Monocet lancet (3-mm)
   Alcohol sponge
   Metal stirrer and magnet
   Sealing wax

2. Procedure for obtaining capillary blood gases:
   Wash hands
   Warm infant's foot for 3 minutes with water at body temperature or slightly warmer. Use thermometer. Water temperature should not exceed 39° C (101–104° F).
   Cleanse heel with alcohol sponge
   Puncture with Monocet lancet
   Wipe away first drop of blood
   Collect blood in sample tube by holding tube below level of puncture and allow blood to flow freely into tube. Avoid squeezing heel to fill tube, as this introduces serum and venous blood, and renders the sample inaccurate. Avoid introducing air into the tube.
   Hold an alcohol sponge against the puncture site to stop flow
   Place metal stirrer in tube
   Slide the magnet along the tube to move the stirrer and mix the blood
   Seal the ends of the tube
   Send to the laboratory for analysis

APPENDIX 8

A, ARTERIAL BLOOD GAS VALUES IN NORMAL FULL-TERM INFANTS*

		Umbilical Vein	Umbilical Artery	5–10 min	20 min	30 min	60 min	5 h
pH	$\bar{x}$	7.320	7.242	7.207	7.263	7.297	7.332	7.339
	SD	0.055	0.059	0.051	0.040	0.044	0.031	0.028
P_{CO_2} (mm Hg)	$\bar{x}$	37.8	49.1	46.1	40.1	37.7	36.1	35.2
	SD	5.6	5.8	7.0	6.0	5.7	4.2	3.6
P_{O_2} (mm Hg)	$\bar{x}$	27.4	15.9	49.6	50.7	54.1	63.3	73.7
	SD	5.7	3.8	9.9	11.3	11.5	11.3	12.0
Standard bicarbonate	$\bar{x}$	20.0	18.7	16.7	17.5	18.2	19.2	19.4
(mEq/L)	SD	1.4	1.8	1.6	1.3	1.5	1.2	1.2

		24 h	2 d	3 d	4 d	5 d	6 d	7 d
pH	$\bar{x}$	7.369	7.365	7.364	7.370	7.371	7.369	7.371
	SD	0.032	0.028	0.027	0.027	0.031	0.023	0.026
P_{CO_2} (mm Hg)	$\bar{x}$	33.4	33.1	33.1	34.3	34.8	34.8	35.9
	SD	3.1	3.3	3.4	3.8	3.5	3.6	3.1
P_{O_2} (mm Hg)	$\bar{x}$	72.7	73.8	75.6	73.3	72.1	69.8	73.1
	SD	9.5	7.7	11.5	9.3	10.5	9.5	9.7
Standard bicarbonate	$\bar{x}$	20.2	19.8	19.7	20.4	20.6	20.6	21.8
(mEq/L)	SD	1.3	1.4	1.4	1.7	1.7	1.9	1.3

* Values from Koch and Wendel. Blood obtained through umbilical artery line. P_{O_2} and P_{CO_2} measured with Clark and Severinghaus electrodes.
From Bancalari E: Pulmonary function testing and other diagnostic laboratory procedures. In Thibeault DW, Gregory GA (eds): Neonatal Pulmonary Care. Reading, MA, Addison-Wesley Publishing Co., 1979, p 123, Table 7–4. Used by permission.

B, ARTERIAL BLOOD GAS VALUES IN NORMAL PREMATURE INFANTS*

		3–5 h	6–12 h	13–24 h	25–48 h	3–4 d	5–10 d	11–40 d
pH	$\bar{x}$	7.329	7.425	7.464	7.434	7.425	7.378	7.425
	SD	0.038	0.072	0.064	0.054	0.044	0.043	0.033
P_{CO_2} (mm Hg)	$\bar{x}$	47.3	28.2	27.2	31.3	31.7	36.4	32.9
	SD	8.5	6.9	8.4	6.7	6.7	4.2	4.0
P_{O_2} (mm Hg)	$\bar{x}$	59.5	69.7	67.0	72.5	77.8	80.3	77.8
	SD	7.7	11.8	15.2	20.9	16.4	12.0	9.6
Base excess (mEq/L)	$\bar{x}$	−3.7	−4.7	−3.0	−2.3	−2.9	−3.5	−2.1
	SD	1.5	3.1	3.3	3.0	2.3	2.3	2.2

* Values from Orzalesi et al. Mean birth weight, 1.76 kg; gestational age, 34.5 wk. Blood obtained from radial, temporal, or umbilical artery. P_{O_2} measured with Clark electrode, and P_{CO_2} calculated with use of the Siggaard-Andersen nomogram.
From Bancalari E: Pulmonary function testing and other diagnostic laboratory procedures. In Thibeault DW, Gregory GA (eds): Neonatal Pulmonary Care, Reading, MA, Addison-Wesley Publishing Co., 1979, p 123, Table 7–5. Used by permission.

APPENDIX 9
BLOOD GAS VALUES IN CORD BLOOD AND IN ARTERIAL BLOOD AT DIFFERENT AGES DURING THE NEONATAL PERIOD

A, OXYGEN TENSION

	UV	UA	5–10 min	20 min	30 min	60 min	5 h	24 h	2 d	3 d	4 d	5 d	6 d	7 d
Po$_2$ (mm Hg) $\bar{x}$	15.9	27.4	49.6	50.7	54.1	63.3	73.7	72.7	73.8	75.6	73.3	72.1	69.8	73.1
SD	3.8	5.7	9.9	11.3	11.5	11.3	12.0	9.5	7.7	11.5	9.3	10.9	9.5	9.7
Range	7	15	33	31	31	38	55	54	62	56	60	56	55	57
	23	40	75	85	85	83	106	95	91	102	93	102	96	94

Abbreviations: UA = umbilical artery; UV = umbilical vein.
From Koch G, Wendel H: Adjustment of arterial blood gases and acid base balance in the normal newborn infant during the first week of life. Biol Neonate 12:136–161, 1968. By permission of S. Karger AG, Basel.

B, CARBON DIOXIDE TENSION

	UV	UA	5–10 min	20 min	30 min	60 min	5 h	24 h	2 d	3 d	4 d	5 d	6 d	7 d
Pco$_2$ (mm Hg)	49.1	37.8	46.1	40.1	37.7	36.1	35.2	33.4	33.1	33.1	34.3	34.8	34.8	35.9
SD	5.8	5.6	7.0	6.0	5.7	4.2	3.6	3.1	3.3	3.4	3.8	3.5	3.6	3.1
Range	35	26	35	31	28	28	29	27	26	26	27	28	28	30
	60	52	65	58	54	45	45	40	43	40	43	41	42	42

From Koch G, Wendel H: Adjustment of arterial blood gases and acid base balance in the normal newborn infant during the first week of life. Biol Neonate 12:136–161, 1968. By permission of S, Karger AG, Basel.

C, pH

	UV	UA	5–10 min	20 min	30 min	60 min	5 h	24 h	2 d	3 d	4 d	5 d	6 d	7 d
pH $\bar{x}$	7.320	7.242	7.207	7.263	7.297	7.332	7.339	7.369	7.365	7.364	7.370	7.371	7.369	7.37
SD	0.055	0.059	0.051	0.040	0.044	0.031	0.028	0.032	0.028	0.027	0.027	0.031	0.032	0.02
Range	7.178	7.111	7.091	7.180	7.206	7.261	7.256	7.290	7.314	7.304	7.320	7.296	7.321	7.32
	7.414	7.375	7.302	7.330	7.380	7.394	7.389	7.448	7.438	7.419	7.440	7.430	7.423	7.43

From Koch G, Wendel H: Adjustment of arterial blood gases and acid base balance in the normal newborn infant during the first week of life. Biol Neonate 12:136–161, 1968. By permission of S. Karger AG, Basel.

D, BASE EXCESS

	UV	UA	5–10 min	20 min	30 min	60 min	5 h	24 h	2 d	3 d	4 d	5 d	6 d	7 d
BE $\bar{x}$	−5.5	−7.2	−9.8	−8.8	−7.8	−6.5	−6.3	−5.2	−5.8	−5.9	−5.0	−4.7	−4.7	−3.2
SD	1.2	1.7	2.3	1.9	1.7	1.3	1.3	1.1	1.2	1.2	1.1	1.1	1.1	0.6

Calculated from data in Koch G, Wendel H: Adjustment of arterial blood gases and acid base balance in the normal newborn infant during the first week of life. Biol Neonate 12:136–161, 1968. By permission of S. Karger AG, Basel.

APPENDIX 10
HEMOGLOBIN-OXYGEN DISSOCIATION CURVES

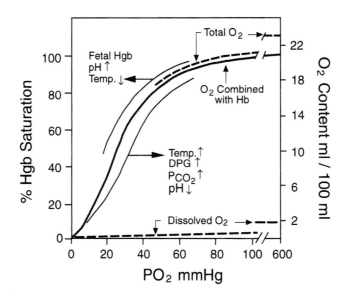

Nonlinear or S-shaped oxyhemoglibin curve and the linear or straight-line dissolved oxygen (O_2) relationships between the O_2 saturation (Sa_{O_2}) and the O_2 tension P_{O_2}). Total blood O_2 content is shown with division into a portion combined with hemoglobin and a portion physically dissolved at various levels of P_{O_2}. Also shown are the major factors that change the O_2 affinity for hemoglobin and, thus, shift the oxyhemoglobin dissociation curve either to the left or to the right (see also Appendix 11). Modified from West JB: Respiratory Physiology—the Essentials. 2nd ed. Baltimore, Williams & Wilkins, 1979, pp 71, 73.

APPENDIX 11
SIGGAARD-ANDERSEN ALIGNMENT NOMOGRAM

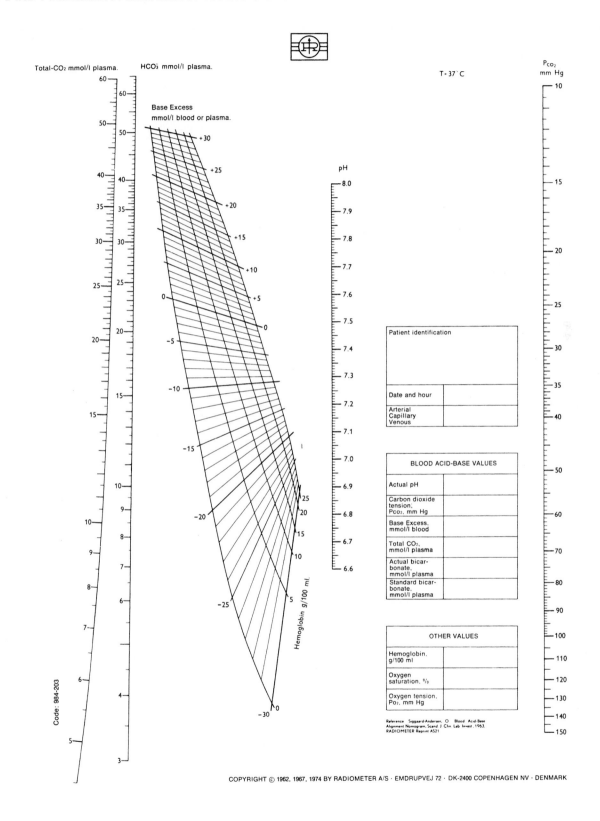

APPENDIX 12
NEUTRAL THERMAL ENVIRONMENTAL TEMPERATURES*

Age and Weight	Range of Temperature (°C)	Age and Weight	Range of Temperature (°C)
0–6 h		72–96 h	
<1200 g	34.0–35.4	<1200 g	34.0–35.0
1200–1500 g	33.9–34.4	1200–1500 g	33.0–34.0
1501–2500 g	32.8–33.8	1501–2500 g	31.1–33.2
>2500 g (and >36 wk)	32.0–33.8	>2500 g (and >36 wk)	29.8–32.8
6–12 h		4–12 d	
<1200 g	34.0–35.4	<1500 g	33.0–34.0
1200–1500 g	33.5–34.4	1501–2500 g	31.0–33.2
1501–2500 g	32.2–33.8	>2500 g (and >36 wk)	
>2500 g (and >36 wk)	31.4–33.8	4–5 d	29.5–32.6
12–24 h		5–6 d	29.4–32.3
<1200 g	34.0–35.4	6–8 d	29.0–32.2
1200–1500 g	33.3–34.3	8–10 d	29.0–31.8
1501–2500 g	31.8–33.8	10–12 d	29.0–31.4
>2500 g (and >36 wk)	31.0–33.7	12–14 d	
24–36 h		<1500 g	32.6–34.0
<1200 g	34.0–35.0	1501–2500 g	31.0–32.2
1200–1500 g	33.1–34.2	>2500 g (and >36 wk)	29.0–30.8
1501–2500 g	31.6–33.6	2–3 wk	
>2500 g (and >36 wk)	30.7–33.5	<1500 g	32.0–34.0
36–48 h		1501–2500 g	30.5–33.0
<1200 g	34.0–35.0	3–4 wk	
1200–1500 g	33.0–34.1	<1500 g	31.6–33.6
1501–2500 g	31.4–33.5	1501–2500 g	30.0–32.7
>2500 g (and >36 wk)	30.5–33.3	4–5 wk	
48–72 h		<1500 g	31.2–33.0
<1200 g	34.0–35.0	1501–2500 g	29.5–32.2
1200–1500 g	33.0–34.0	5–6 wk	
1501–2500 g	31.2–33.4	<1500 g	30.6–32.3
>2500 g (and >36 wk)	30.1–33.2	1501–2500 g	29.0–31.8

* Generally, the smaller infants in each weight group require a temperature in the higher portion of the temperature range. Within each time range, the younger the infant, the higher the temperature required.
Adapted from Scopes J, Ahmed I: Minimal rates of oxygen consumption in sick and premature newborn infants. Arch Dis Child 41:417, 1966. For their table, Scopes and Ahmed maintained the walls of the incubator at a temperature 1°C to 2°C warmer than that of the ambient air temperatures.

APPENDIX 13A

CLASSIFICATION OF NEWBORNS (BOTH SEXES)
BY INTRAUTERINE GROWTH AND GESTATIONAL AGE [1,2]

NAME_____ DATE OF EXAM_____ LENGTH_____

HOSPITAL NO._____ SEX_____ HEAD CIRC._____

RACE_____ BIRTH WEIGHT_____ GESTATIONAL AGE_____

DATE OF BIRTH_____

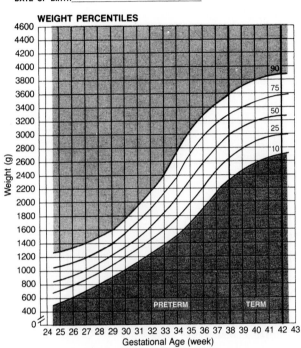

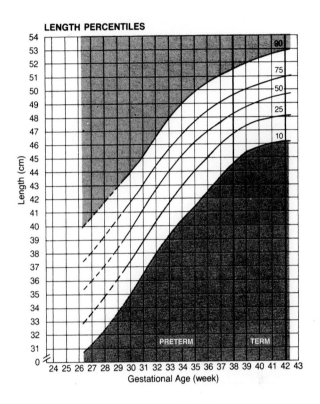

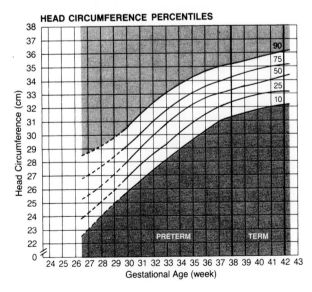

CLASSIFICATION OF INFANT*	Weight	Length	Head Circ.
Large for Gestational Age (LGA) (>90th percentile)			
Appropriate for Gestational Age (AGA) (10th to 90th percentile)			
Small for Gestational Age (SGA) (<10th percentile)			

*Place an "X" in the appropriate box (LGA, AGA or SGA) for weight, for length and for head circumference.

References
1. Battaglia FC, Lubchenco LO: A practical classification of newborn infants by weight and gestational age. J Pediatr 1967; 71:159-163.
2. Lubchenco LO, Hansman C, Boyd E: Intrauterine growth in length and head circumference as estimated from live births at gestational ages from 26 to 42 weeks. Pediatrics 1966; 37:403-408.

Reprinted by permission from Dr Battaglia, Dr Lubchenco, Journal of Pediatrics and Pediatrics.

A service of **SIMILAC® WITH IRON** Infant Formula

The Ross Hospital Formula System

A5860(0.05)/JULY 1993

ROSS PRODUCTS DIVISION
ABBOTT LABORATORIES
COLUMBUS, OHIO 43215-1724

LITHO IN USA

APPENDIX 13B

MATURATIONAL ASSESSMENT OF GESTATIONAL AGE (New Ballard Score)

NAME _____   SEX _____

HOSPITAL NO. _____   BIRTH WEIGHT _____

RACE _____   LENGTH _____

DATE/TIME OF BIRTH _____   HEAD CIRC. _____

DATE/TIME OF EXAM _____   EXAMINER _____

AGE WHEN EXAMINED _____

APGAR SCORE: 1 MINUTE _____ 5 MINUTES _____ 10 MINUTES _____

NEUROMUSCULAR MATURITY

NEUROMUSCULAR MATURITY SIGN	SCORE							RECORD SCORE HERE
	-1	0	1	2	3	4	5	
POSTURE								
SQUARE WINDOW (Wrist)	>90°	90°	60°	45°	30°	0°		
ARM RECOIL		180°	140°-180°	110°-140°	90°-110°	<90°		
POPLITEAL ANGLE	180°	160°	140°	120°	100°	90°	<90°	
SCARF SIGN								
HEEL TO EAR								

TOTAL NEUROMUSCULAR MATURITY SCORE

PHYSICAL MATURITY

PHYSICAL MATURITY SIGN	SCORE							RECORD SCORE HERE
	-1	0	1	2	3	4	5	
SKIN	sticky friable transparent	gelatinous red translucent	smooth pink visible veins	superficial peeling &/or rash, few veins	cracking pale areas rare veins	parchment deep cracking no vessels	leathery cracked wrinkled	
LANUGO	none	sparse	abundant	thinning	bald areas	mostly bald		
PLANTAR SURFACE	heel-toe 40-50 mm:-1 <40 mm:-2	>50 mm no crease	faint red marks	anterior transverse crease only	creases ant. 2/3	creases over entire sole		
BREAST	imperceptible	barely perceptible	flat areola no bud	stippled areola 1-2 mm bud	raised areola 3-4 mm bud	full areola 5-10 mm bud		
EYE/EAR	lids fused loosely: -1 tightly: -2	lids open pinna flat stays folded	sl. curved pinna; soft; slow recoil	well-curved pinna; soft but ready recoil	formed & firm instant recoil	thick cartilage ear stiff		
GENITALS (Male)	scrotum flat, smooth	scrotum empty faint rugae	testes in upper canal rare rugae	testes descending few rugae	testes down good rugae	testes pendulous deep rugae		
GENITALS (Female)	clitoris prominent & labia flat	prominent clitoris & small labia minora	prominent clitoris & enlarging minora	majora & minora equally prominent	majora large minora small	majora cover clitoris & minora		

TOTAL PHYSICAL MATURITY SCORE

SCORE

Neuromuscular _____

Physical _____

Total _____

MATURITY RATING

score	weeks
-10	20
-5	22
0	24
5	26
10	28
15	30
20	32
25	34
30	36
35	38
40	40
45	42
50	44

GESTATIONAL AGE (weeks)

By dates _____

By ultrasound _____

By exam _____

Reference
Ballard JL, Khoury JC, Wedig K, et al: New Ballard Score, expanded to include extremely premature infants. *J Pediatr* 1991; 119:417-423. Reprinted by permission of Dr Ballard and Mosby - Year Book, Inc.

APPENDIX 14
HEART RATES IN PREMATURE AND FULL-TERM NEONATES

	1–7 D			1–4 WK		
	Minimum	Mean	Maximum	Minimum	Mean	Maximum
Prematures (<1500 g)	125	145	168	110	161	192
Prematures (1500–2500 g)	100	147	195	123	157	190
Term	100	133	175	115	163	190

APPENDIX 15
SYSTOLIC AND DIASTOLIC BLOOD PRESSURE IN NEWBORN INFANTS

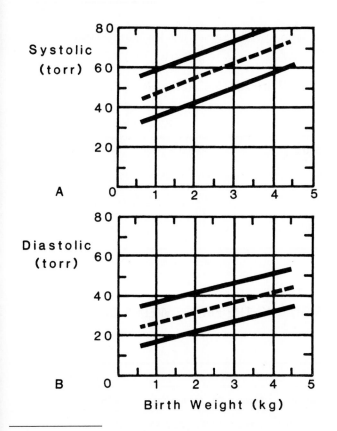

Systolic blood pressure (A) and diastolic blood pressure (B) in the first 12 hours of life as a function of birthweight. From Versmold HT, Kitterman JA, Phibbs RH, et al: Aortic blood pressure during the first 12 hours of life in infants with birth weight 610 to 4,220 grams. Pediatrics 67:607–613, 1981. Reproduced by permission of *Pediatrics*, Copyright 1981.

APPENDIX 16
MEAN BLOOD PRESSURE AND PULSE PRESSURE IN NEWBORN INFANTS

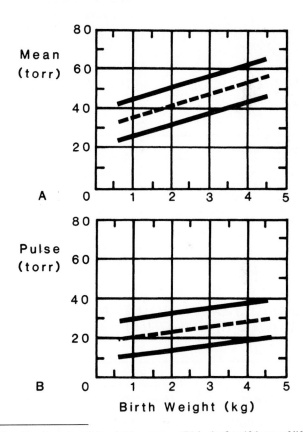

Mean blood pressure (A) and pulse pressure (B) in the first 12 hours of life as a function of birthweight. From Versmold HT, Kitterman JA, Phibbs RH, et al: Aortic blood pressure during the first 12 hours of life in infants with birth weight 610 to 4,220 grams. Pediatrics 67:607–613, 1981. Reproduced by permission of *Pediatrics*, Copyright 1981.

APPENDIX 17
BLOOD CHEMISTRIES

A, NORMAL BLOOD CHEMISTRY VALUES, TERM INFANTS

Determination	Sample Source	Cord*	1–12 h	12–24 h	24–48 h	48–72 h
Sodium (mEq/L)[†]	Capillary	147 (126–166)	143 (124–156)	145 (132–159)	148 (134–160)	149 (139–162)
Potassium (mEq/L)		7.8 (5.6–12)	6.4 (5.3–7.3)	6.3 (5.3–8.9)	6.0 (5.2–7.3)	5.9 (5.0–7.7)
Chloride (mEq/L)		103 (98–110)	100.7 (90–111)	103 (87–114)	102 (92–114)	103 (93–112)
Calcium (mg/100 mL)		9.3 (8.2–11.1)	8.4 (7.3–9.2)	7.8 (6.9–9.4)	8.0 (6.1–9.9)	7.9 (5.9–9.7)
Phosphorus (mg/100 mL)		5.6 (3.7–8.1)	6.1 (3.5–8.6)	5.7 (2.9–8.1)	5.9 (3.0–8.7)	5.8 (2.8–7.6)
Blood urea (mg/100 mL)		29 (21–40)	27 (8–34)	33 (9–63)	32 (13–77)	31 (13–68)
Total protein (g/100 mL)		6.1 (4.8–7.3)	6.6 (5.6–8.5)	6.6 (5.8–8.2)	6.9 (5.9–8.2)	7.2 (6.0–8.5)
Blood sugar (mg/100 mL)		73 (45–96)	63 (40–97)	63 (42–104)	56 (30–91)	59 (40–90)
Lactic acid (mg/100 mL)		19.5 (11–30)	14.6 (11–24)	14.0 (10–23)	14.3 (9–22)	13.5 (7–21)
Lactate (mm/L)[‡]		2.0–3.0	2.0			

* First number refers to the mean; second set of numbers refers to the range.
[†] Acharya PT, Payne WW: Blood chemistry of normal full-term infants in the first 48 hours of life. Arch Dis Child 40:430, 1965.
[‡] Daniel 55, Adamsons K Jr, James LS: Lactate and pyruvate as an index of prenatal oxygen deprivation. Pediatrics 37:942, 1966. Reprinted by permission of *Pediatrics*, Copyright 1966.

B, NORMAL BLOOD CHEMISTRY VALUES, LOW-BIRTHWEIGHT INFANTS, CAPILLARY BLOOD, FIRST DAY

Determination	<1000 g	1001–1500 g	1501–2000 g	2001–2500 g
Sodium (mEq/L)	138	133	135	134
Potassium (mEq/L)	6.4	6.0	5.4	5.6
Chloride (mEq/L)	100	101	105	104
Total CO_2 (mEq/L)	19	20	20	20
Urea (mg/100 mL)	22	21	16	16
Total serum protein (g/100 mL)	4.8	4.8	5.2	5.3

From Pincus JB, Gittleman IF, Saito M, et al: Study of plasma values of sodium, potassium, chloride, carbon dioxide, carbon dioxide tension, sugar, urea and protein base-binding power, pH, and hematocrit in prematures on the first day of life. Pediatrics 18:39, 1956. Reprinted by permission of *Pediatrics*, Copyright 1956.

C, BLOOD CHEMISTRY VALUES IN PREMATURE INFANTS DURING THE FIRST 7 WEEKS OF LIFE (BIRTHWEIGHT, 1500–1750 g)

Constituent	AGE 1 wk Mean	SD	Range	AGE 3 wk Mean	SD	Range	AGE 5 wk Mean	SD	Range	AGE 7 wk Mean	SD	Range
Sodium (mEq/L)	139.6	±3.2	133–146	136.3	±2.9	129–142	136.8	±2.5	133–148	137.2	±1.8	133–142
Potassium (mEq/L)	5.6	±0.5	4.6–6.7	5.8	±0.6	4.5–7.1	5.5	±0.6	4.5–6.6	5.7	±0.5	4.6–7.1
Chloride (mEq/L)	108.2	±3.7	100–117	108.3	±3.9	102–116	107.0	±3.5	100–115	107.0	±3.3	101–115
Carbon dioxide (mmol/L)	20.3	±2.8	13.8–27.1	18.4	±3.5	12.4–26.2	20.4	±3.4	12.5–26.1	20.6	±3.1	13.7–26.9
Calcium (mg/100 mL)	9.2	±1.1	6.1–11.6	9.6	±0.5	8.1–11.0	9.4	±0.5	8.6–10.5	9.5	±0.7	8.6–10.8
Phosphorus (mg/100 mL)	7.6	±1.1	5.4–10.9	7.5	±0.7	6.2–8.7	7.0	±0.6	5.6–7.9	6.8	±0.8	4.2–8.2
Blood urea nitrogen (mg/100 mL)	9.3	±5.2	3.1–25.5	13.3	±7.8	2.1–31.4	13.3	±7.1	2.0–26.5	13.4	±6.7	2.5–30.5
Total protein (gm/100 mL)	5.49	±0.42	4.40–6.26	5.38	±0.48	4.28–6.70	4.98	±0.50	4.14–6.90	4.93	±0.61	4.02–5.86
Albumin (g/100 mL)	3.85	±0.30	3.28–4.50	3.92	±0.42	3.16–5.26	3.73	±0.34	3.20–4.34	3.89	±0.53	3.40–4.60
Globulin (g/100 mL)	1.58	±0.33	0.88–2.20	1.44	±0.63	0.62–2.90	1.17	±0.49	0.48–1.48	1.12	±0.33	0.5–2.60
Hemoglobin (g/100 mL)	17.8	±2.7	11.4–24.8	14.7	±2.1	9.0–19.4	11.5	±2.0	7.2–18.6	10.0	±1.3	7.5–13.9

Adapted from Thomas J, Reichelderfer T: Premature infants: analysis of serum during the first seven weeks. Clin Chem 14:272, 1968.

APPENDIX 18
HEMATOLOGIC VALUES IN NEWBORN INFANTS

A, NORMAL HEMATOLOGIC VALUES DURING THE FIRST 14 DAYS OF LIFE

Value	GESTATIONAL AGE (wk)						
	28	**34**	**Full-term Cord Blood**	**Day 1**	**Day 3**	**Day 7**	**Day 14**
Hemoglobin (g/dL)	14.5	15.0	16.8	18.4	17.8	17.0	16.8
Hematocrit (%)	45	47	53	58	55	54	52
Red blood cells (mm³)	4.0	4.4	5.25	5.8	5.6	5.2	5.1
MCV (μm³)	120	118	107	108	99	98	96
MCH (pg)	40	38	34	35	33	32.5	31.5
MCHC (%)	31	32	31.7	32.5	33	33	33
Reticulocytes (%)	5–10	3–10	3–7	3–7	1–3	0–1	0–1
Platelets (1000s/mm³)			290	192	213	248	252

Abbreviations: MCV = mean corpuscular volume; MCH = mean corpuscular hemoglobin; MCHC = mean corpuscular hemoglobin concentration. From Klaus MH, Fanaroff AA: Care of the High Risk Neonate. 4th ed., Philadelphia, W.B. Saunders Co., 1993, p 486.

B, CHANGES IN HEMOGLOBIN AND RETICULOCYTE COUNT IN TERM AND PRETERM INFANTS

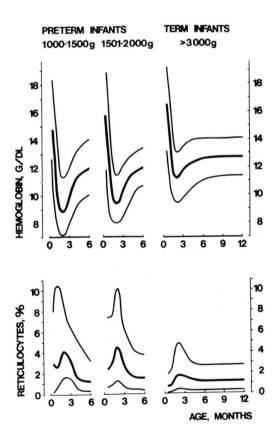

Changes in hemoglobin and reticulocyte count in two groups of preterm infants and a group of term infants (Reproduced, with permission, from Dallman PR: Anemia of prematurity. Annu Rev Med 32:143, 1981. © 1981, by Annual Reviews, Inc.)

APPENDIX 19
LEUKOCYTE VALUES AND NEUTROPHIL COUNTS IN TERM AND PREMATURE INFANTS

A, LEUKOCYTE VALUES IN TERM AND PREMATURE INFANTS (10^3 CELLS/μL)

Age (h)	Total White Cell Count	Neutrophils	Bands/Metas	Lymphocytes	Monocytes	Eosinophils
Term Infants						
0	10.0–26.0	5.0–13.0	0.4–1.8	3.5–8.5	0.7–1.5	0.2–2.0
12	13.5–31.0	9.0–18.0	0.4–2.0	3.0–7.0	1.0–2.0	0.2–2.0
72	5.0–14.5	2.0–7.0	0.2–0.4	2.0–5.0	0.5–1.0	0.2–1.0
144	6.0–14.5	2.0–6.0	0.2–0.5	3.0–6.0	0.7–1.2	0.2–0.8
Premature infants						
0	5.0–19.0	2.0–9.0	0.2–2.4	2.5–6.0	0.3–1.0	0.1–0.7
12	5.0–21.0	3.0–11.0	0.2–2.4	1.5–5.0	0.3–1.3	0.1–1.1
72	5.0–14.0	3.0–7.0	0.2–0.6	1.5–4.0	0.3–1.2	0.2–1.1
144	5.5–17.5	2.0–7.0	0.2–0.5	2.5–7.5	0.5–1.5	0.3–1.2

From Oski F, Naiman J: Hematologic Problems in the Newborn, Philadelphia, W. B. Saunders Co., 1982.

B, TOTAL NEUTROPHIL COUNT REFERENCE RANGE IN THE FIRST 60 HOURS OF LIFE

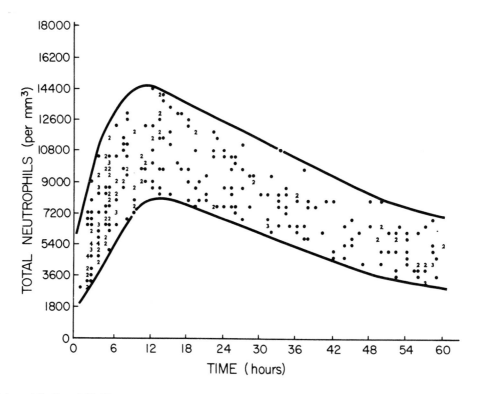

From Monroe BL, Weinberg AG, Rosenfeld CR, et al: The neonatal blood count in health and disease: I. Reference values for neutrophilic cells. J Pediatr 95:91, 1979.

APPENDIX 20
PLATELETS

A, VENOUS PLATELET COUNTS IN NORMAL LOW-BIRTHWEIGHT INFANTS

Day	No. of Infants	Mean (mm³)	Range (1000's)
0	60	203,000	80–356
3	47	207,000	61–335
5	14	233,000	100–502
7	52	319,000	124–678
10	40	399,000	172–680
14	50	386,000	147–670
21	47	388,000	201–720
28	40	384,000	212–625

From Appleyard WJ, Brinton A: Venous platelet counts in low birth weight infants. Biol Neonate 17:30, 1971.

B, PLATELET COUNTS IN FULL-TERM INFANTS

Day	Mean	Range
Cord	200,000	100,000–280,000
1	192,000	100,000–260,000
3	213,000	80,000–320,000
7	248,000	100,000–300,000
14	252,000	

From Fanaroff AA, Martin RJ (eds): Behman's Neonatal-Perinatal Medicine, 3rd ed. St. Louis, C.V. Mosby, 1983.

APPENDIX 21
COAGULATION FACTORS AND TEST VALUES IN TERM AND PREMATURE INFANTS

	Normal	Term Infant (Cord Blood)	Premature Infant (Cord Blood)
Fibrinogen (mg %)	200–400	200–250	200–250
Factor II (%)	50–150	40	25
Factor V (%)	75–125	90	60–75
Factor VII (%)	75–125	50	35
Factor VIII (%)	50–150	100	80–100
Factor IX (%)	50–150	25–40	25–40
Factor X (%)	50–150	50–60	25–40
Factor XI (%)	75–125	30–40	—
Factor XII (%)	75–125	50–100	50–100
Factor XIII (titer)	1:16	1:8	1:8
Partial thromboplastin time (s)	30–50	70	80–90
Prothrombin time (s)	10–12	12–18	14–20
Thrombin time (s)	10–12	12–16	13–20

From Avery GB: Neonatology. 2nd ed. Philadelphia, J.B. Lippincott Co., 1981, p 570.

APPENDIX 22
CEREBROSPINAL FLUID VALUES IN TERM AND PREMATURE INFANTS

	Term	Pre-term
WBC count (cells/mm³)		
No. of Infants	87	30
Mean	8.2	9.0
Median	5	6
SD	7.1	8.2
Range	0–32	0–29
±2 SD	0–22.4	0–25.4
Percentage PMN	61.3%	57.2%
Protein (mg/dL)		
No. of infants	35	17
Mean	90	115
Range	20–170	65–150
Glucose (mg/dL)		
No. of infants	51	23
Mean	52	50
Range	34–119	24–63
CSF/blood glucose (%)		
No. of infants	51	23
Mean	81	74
Range	44–248	55–105

Abbreviations: WBC = white blood cell; PMN = polymorphonuclear cells; CSF = cerebrospinal fluid.
From Sarff L, Platt L, McCracken G: Cerebrospinal fluid evaluation in neonates: comparison of high risk infants without meningitis. J Pediatr 88:473, 1976.

APPENDIX 23
DAILY MAINTENANCE, FLUID, MINERAL, AND GLUCOSE REQUIREMENTS FOR TERM NEONATES

Component	Amount
Water	100 mL/kg for each kg <10
	50 mL/kg for each kg 11–20
	20 mL/kg for each kg >20
Sodium	2–3 mEq/kg
Potassium	2–3 mEq/kg
Chloride	3–5 mEq/kg Calcium chloride is 27% Ca^{2+}
Calcium	20–40 mg/kg Calcium gluconate is 9% Ca^{2+}
Magnesium	15–25 mg/kg
Phosphorus	20–40 mg/kg
Glucose	2.4–4.8 g/kg

APPENDIX 24A
PERINATAL TRANSPORT RECORD: HISTORICAL DATA

CHILDREN'S HOSPITAL OF THE KING'S DAUGHTERS, INC.
601 Children's Lane
Norfolk, Virginia 23507-1910

NEONATAL TRANSPORT LOG/ADMISSION SCREEN

Date_____ Page 1

ADDRESSOGRAPH

1st call _____   2nd call _____   Van # _____
Time Personnel called _____   Charge_____

PERSONNEL		IN	OUT	TIME		HOSPITAL
				Departure		
				Arrival		
				Departure		
				Arrival		
				Adm. Unit		

Patient Name: BB   BG   _____   Diagnosis: _____

Membranes Ruptured: SROM / AROM   Date _____   Time _____   Obstetrician _____

Delivery: Date _____   Time _____   Apgar Scores _____ 1 & _____ 5   EGA_____
Route: Vaginal _____   C - section _____   Why?_____
Birthweight_____   Vit K_____   Erythromycin ointment_____

Prenatal History: Mother's Age _____   G _____ PARA _____ Ab _____ EDC _____ Blood Type _____
Parent's Race _____   Prenatal Care _____
Problems during this pregnancy & medications taken _____
_____
Problems with previous pregnancy/delivery_____
_____
Was the mother started on antibiotics/why? _____
Maternal substance abuse? Cigarettes: _____   ETOH: _____   Other: _____

Social Assessment: Siblings? (age & sex)_____
Are siblings in good health? _____ Does the mother work? _____ Place/Telephone # _____
Primary caretaker of the infant_____   Language spoken by the parents _____
Household composition_____   Support network_____
Did the mother see the baby?_____   Touch the baby? _____   Receive a CHKD map? _____
Receive CHKD / NICU information? _____   Receive patient's photograph? _____

Referring Physician:_____   **Primary Physician:** _____
History of infant since delivery: _____
_____
_____
_____
_____
_____
_____
_____

Hepatitis B Vaccine: _____   T4/PKU_____   Antibiotics: _____

Mileage (one way) _____   Fixed Wing / Helicopter Nautical Miles _____

_____
Transport Nurse's Signature

_____
Standard hospital transfer sheets. *Above:* Historical data to be completed by referring hospital. *Next page:* Transport data form to be completed by transport team.
(Courtesy of the Children's Hospital of the King's Daughter, Inc., Norfolk, Virginia)

A P P E N D I X   2 4 B
PERINATAL TRANSPORT RECORD: TRANSPORT DATA

Children's Hospital Of The King's Daughters, Inc.
601 Children's Lane
Norfolk, Virginia 23507-1910

TRANSPORT LOG

Date_____ Page 3

ADDRESSOGRAPH

TIME	PROCEDURES	ISOLATION CODES
	Isolation:	A = AFB
	Oximeter Placement: Alarm Limits: Hi _____ Lo_____	C = CONTACT
	IV Fluid to CHKD Pump:	D = DRAINAGE/SECRETION
	Patient placed on CHKD cardiac monitor: Alarm Limits: Hi _____ Lo_____	E = ENTERIC
	Patient placed on CHKD ventilator: Humidifier Temp._____	S = STRICT
	Xrays:	R = RESPIRATORY
		V = REVERSE
	Patient secured to stretcher/isolette: Temperature: _____	
	Physician consulted:	
	Report called to:	
	To Mom's room/room #: Family/Patient oriented to CHKD/Transport _____	
	Depart Mom's room	
	Patient secured in Mobile ICU	
	ETA called to security and admitting unit	
	Check-off List: ID Band _____ Xrays _____ Consent _____ Chart(s) _____	

TIME	PROCEDURE	PATIENT RESPONSE

TIME	MEDICATIONS	WASTE/INITIALS	TIME	PATIENT RESPONSE

_____
Transport Nurse's Signature

CHKD-0115-PT3-MR   REV. 1/99

APPENDIX 25
NEONATAL ICU FLOW SHEET

Children's Hospital Of The King's Daughters, Inc.

601 Children's Lane • Norfolk, Virginia 23507-1910

ADDRESSOGRAPH

DATE:	DAY OF ADMISSION

NEONATAL ICU FLOWSHEET

PAGE 1 OF 8

		TEMPERATURE						CARDIOVASCULAR											APNEA/BRADYCARDIA							
										BP						VENOUS										
TIME	init	PATIENT	SKIN	ENVIRONMENT	HEATER OUTPUT	% HUMIDITY	BODY HUMIDITY TEMP/REL. HUM.	HR	RR	SYSTOLIC	DIASTOLIC	MEAN	SITE	WAVE FORM	CAL	CVP	WAVE FORM	CAL	TIME / init	HR	APNEA DUR. (sec.)	APNEA	FEEDING?	COLOR CHANGE?	O_2 SAT %	STIM

Y or √ = Yes
N or Ø = No
N/A = Not Applicable

WAVE FORM
N = Normal
D = Dampened
F = Flat

BP/OXIMETER SITES:
L = Line C = Cuff
RA = R arm RL = R Leg
LA = L arm LL = L leg

STIM (STIMULATION)
G = Gentle Stimulation
M = Moderate Stimulation
V = Vigorous Stimulation
B = Manually Ventilated

CHKD #1997 REV. 12/95

APPENDIX 25
NEONATAL ICU FLOW SHEET—CONT'D

Date:	RESPIRATORY PROCEDURES	TIME
Ventilator: Mode:		
ETT: Size:		
Position:		
Suction catheter length:		
Anesthesia bag at bedside:		
Self-inflating bag/mask at bedside:		
Trach at bedside:		
HHN #1		
HHN #2		

ADDRESSOGRAPH

PAGE 2 OF 8

NEONATAL ICU FLOWSHEET

TIME	init		ASSISTED VENTILATION										BLOOD GASES							MONITORS				BREATH SOUNDS				SPUTUM				
		FIO₂/VIA	PIP OR AMPLITUDE (SET/MEASURED)	PEEP OR CPAP	TIDAL VOLUME	MEAN AIRWAY PRESSURE	RATE OR HERTZ	FLOW	I:E RATIO	INSPIRATORY TIME	TEMP/REL. HUM.	A/V/C	pH	pCO₂	pO₂	HCO₃	BE	SAT	TcCO₂	TcO₂	O₂ SAT %	OXIMETER SITE	BEFORE R/L	AFTER SXN R/L	AERATION	MECHANICS	COLOR	AMOUNT	VISCOSITY	ODOR	CPT/HHN

FIO₂ DELIVERY:
M   = Mask
H   = Oxyhood
B   = Baby Log 8000
IS = Infant Star
O   = HFOV
NC = Nasal Cannula

TC = Trach Collar
J   = HFJV
BC = Bear Cub
S   = Star 200
VB = VIP Bird

BREATH SOUNDS:
Cl = Clear   R   = Rales
C   = Coarse   D   = Diminished
W   = Wheeze   Cr = Crackles

MECHANICS:
G   = Grunting
F   = Flaring
R₁ = Sl. Retraction
R₂ = Mod. Retraction
R₃ = Severe Retraction

AERATION:
P   = Poor
Mo = Moderate
G   = Good

SPUTUM COLOR:
W   = White   Y   = Yellow
G   = Green   R   = Red
C   = Colorless   B   = Brown

AMOUNT:
N   = None
Sc = Scant
Mo = Moderate
Co = Copious

VISCOSITY:
Th = Thin
Te = Tenacious

ODOR:
P   = Present
A   = Absent

OXIMETER SITE:
*Refer to patient care note
✔ Indicates change in Probe Site

APPENDIX 25
NEONATAL ICU FLOW SHEET—CONT'D

DATE:

NEONATAL ICU FLOWSHEET

TIME	IV STARTS/LINE INSERTIONS/SITE

ADDRESSOGRAPH

PAGE 3 OF 8

	IV SOLUTIONS/ PARENTERAL NUTRITION	TUBING CHANGE	SITE	LUMEN	LINE TYPE	SITE DAY	LINE DAY
1							
2							
3							
4							
5							
6							
7							
8							

		PARENTERAL INTAKE										ENTERAL INTAKE					
TIME	init	SITE √	1	2	3	4	5	6	7	8	FLUSH	TIME	TUBE PLCMNT √	NGT LENGTH	ABD GIRTH	ROUTE*	RESIDUAL RETURNED	AMT.	FDG TYPE
			CUM	CUM	CUM	CUM	CUM	CUM	CUM	CUM									
0700																			
0800																			
0900																			
1000																			
1100																			
1200																			
1300																			
1400																			
1500																			
1600																			
1700																			
1800																			
12 HR																			
1900																			
2000																			
2100																			
2200																			
2300																			
2400																			
0100																			
0200																			
0300																			
0400																			
0500																			
0600																			
12 HR																			
24 HR																			

CUM = CUMULATIVE   *ROUTE CODES: G = GASTROSTOMY; D = DUODENAL; NG = NASO GASTRIC; OG = ORAL GASTRIC; PO - BY MOUTH

APPENDIX 25
NEONATAL ICU FLOW SHEET—CONT'D

DATE:

NEONATAL ICU FLOWSHEET

ADDRESSOGRAPH

INTAKE TOTALS

SHIFT	PARENTERAL			ENTERAL
	CRYSTALLOID	LIPIDS	COLLOID	
07-1900				
19-0600				
24 HOUR TOTAL				

OUTPUT TOTALS

SHIFT	URINE	cc/kg/HOUR	STOOL	GASTRIC	Chest Tubes		
					1	2	3
07-1900							
19-0600							
24 HOUR TOTAL							

GROWTH PARAMETER

DATE	TIME	PARAMETER	VALUE
		Admission Weight	Gms
		Current Weight	Gms
		Previous Weight	Gms
N/A	N/A	Difference	Gms ↑↓
		FOC	Cm
		Length	Cm

OUTPUT

TIME	init	URINE	GASTRIC						STOOL		BLOOD	CHEST TUBES		
			EMESIS	TUBE	IN	OUT	DIFF.	ASSESS	AMOUNT	ASSESS	PREVIOUS TOTAL:	1	2	3
		AMT	AMT	AMT	AMT	AMT	AMT				AMT	AMT	AMT	AMT
0700														
0800														
0900														
1000														
1100														
1200														
1300														
1400														
1500														
1600														
1700														
1800														
12 HR														
1900														
2000														
2100														
2200														
2300														
2400														
0100														
0200														
0300														
0400														
0500														
0600														
12 HR														

ASSESS CODES: BR = Brown, Y = Yellow, M = Meconium, S = Seedy, Blk = Black, Bld = Bloody, W = Watery, H = Hard, F = Formed, GN = Green, CG = Coffee Ground

STOOL CODES: Sm = Small, Mo = Moderate, Lg = Large

Y or √ = Yes, N or Ø = No, N/A = Not Applicable

↑ = Up, ↓ = Down

ISOLATION CODES: R = Respiratory, S = Strict, D/S = Drainage/Secretion, C = Contact, E = Enteric

APPENDIX 25
NEONATAL ICU FLOW SHEET—CONT'D

DATE:

NEONATAL ICU FLOWSHEET

ADDRESSOGRAPH

TIME						
init						
HEMATOLOGY						
WBC						
RBC						
HGB						
HCT						
Platelets						
Retic						
DIFFERENTIAL						
Polys						
Bands						
Eos						
Baso						
Lymphs						
Mono						
Meta						
Nucleated RBC						
TPN LABS						
Ca						
Phos.						
TRIG						
Mg++						
AST						
ALT						
Alk. Phos.						
GGT						

CULTURES		
Specimen Collection Date		
Source		
Results		

DIAGNOSTICS

TIME																
init																
BLOOD CHEMISTRY																
Glu																
BUN																
Na+																
K+																
Cl																
CO2																
Cr																
Dextrostix																
T. Bili																
D. Bili																
TIME																
MISCELLANEOUS																

APPENDIX 25
NEONATAL ICU FLOW SHEET—CONT'D

DATE:

ADDRESSOGRAPH

NEONATAL ICU FLOWSHEET

PUPIL SIZE (mm)

2　3　4　5　6　7　8　9

PAGE 6 OF 8

DAILY ROUTINE	A	B	DAILY ROUTINE	A	B	DAILY ROUTINE	A	B	DAILY ROUTINE	A	B
Bath			Review Plan of Care			Specialty Bed			Restraints		
Mouth Care			Side Rails			Position Change			Monitor Alarms		
Catheter Care			Code Med Sheet			Isolation Type:			MD Rounds		
Phototherapy Flux									Specialty Rounds:		

ASSESSMENT

√ = Meets all normal parameters　　* = Exception to normal parameters　　→ = Same as previous assessment

TIME													
Neuro													
Resp													
CV													
GI													
GU													
Skin													
Musc/Skel													
Lines													
Pain Score													
Initials													

FAMILY INTERACTION

TIME	init	PERSON	CALLED	VISIT	HELD	FED	BATHED	FAMILY EDUCATION	FAMILY CONSULTS

M　=　Mother
F　=　Father
GM　=　Grandmother
GF　=　Grandfather
MD　=　Physician
SW　=　Social Work
CH　-　Chaplain

01 = Other _____　PT: _____　Hospital School Teacher: _____

02 = Other _____　OT: _____　Speech: _____

Psych/Soc. Data _____

_____

_____

_____

APPENDIX 25
NEONATAL ICU FLOW SHEET—CONT'D

DATE:

NEONATAL ICU FLOWSHEET

Nursing Diagnoses from Plan of Care

1. _____

2. _____

3. _____

4. _____

ADDRESSOGRAPH

PAGE 7 OF 8

TIME	FOCUS	PATIENT CARE NOTE

APPENDIX 25
NEONATAL ICU FLOW SHEET—CONT'D

DATE:

NEONATAL ICU FLOWSHEET

ADDRESSOGRAPH

PAGE 8 OF 8

TIME	FOCUS	PATIENT CARE NOTE

SIGNATURE	INITIALS	SHIFT	SIGNATURE	INITIALS	SHIFT

(Courtesy of Children's Hospital of the King's Daugther, Inc., Norfolk, Virginia)

APPENDIX 26A
NEONATAL RESUSCITATION RECORD

OCHSNER FOUNDATION HOSPITAL
NEONATAL RESUSCITATION RECORD

Patient Name _____   Date _____

Est. Wt. _____ grams   Sex _____   Est. Gest. Age _____

Time of Birth _____ AM/PM

	Min	Heart Rate	Muscle Tone	Reflex Irritabillty	Color	Resp. Effort	Total
Time Resuscitation Procedures Initiated:	A 1						
Time Resuscitation Procedures Completed:	P 5						
Perinatal History:	G 10						
	A 15						
	R 20						
	S 25						

Amniotic Fluid: ☐ Clear   ☐ Meconium Stained

PROCEDURES	START	END	BY WHOM	
UVC or UAC				UA/UV size: 3.5 5 8
Intubation				ETT Size: 2.5 3.0 3.5 4.0
Intubation w/Ventilation				
Intubation/Suctioning Only				
Cardiac Compressions				
Positive Pressure Ventilation				
Free Flow Oxygen @ _____ L/min				
Suction				
O/G Tube In: ☐ Yes ☐ No				

DRUGS	TIME/AMT	TIME/AMT	ROUTE	FLUSH SOLUTIONS	
Epinephrine 1:10000 0.1 - 0.3 mL/kg				_____ Normal saline + 1 unit heparin/cc	
Volume Expander: 5% Albumin 10 mL/kg Normal saline Ringer's Lactate				_____ 1/2 Normal saline + 1 unit heparin/cc	
				_____ Other	
Sodium Bicarbonate 0.5 mEq/mL 2 mEq/kg (4.2% solution)				BASE I.V. SOLUTION	LABS
Naloxone Hydrochloride 0.4 mg/mL or 0.1 mg/kg 1.0 mg/mL				_____ D_5W	_____ Glucose
Blood Products				_____ $D_{10}W$	
Others					

Condition at Completion of Resuscitation: ☐ Good   ☐ Fair   ☐ Guarded   ☐ Expired

Transferred to: ☐ Newborn Nursery   ☐ NICU

Resuscitation Personnel Signatures:

M.D. _____

NNP _____

R.N. _____

Comments: _____

Recording R.N. _____

R.T. _____

APPENDIX 26B
EVALUATION OF CODE PERFORMANCE QUALITY ASSURANCE DOCUMENT

EVALUATION OF CODE PERFORMANCE
Quality Assurance Document

✦◇DO NOT COPY◇✦

MR #

Location of Code: _____   Date: _____/_____/_____

Occurrence Time: _____

Announcement Time: _____

Admitting Diagnosis/Chief Complaint: _____

Events Leading to Arrest: _____

_____

Was palpable pulse present at onset of medical emergency?   ○ Yes   ○ No

Attending Physician: _____   Attending Physician Present?   ○ Yes   ○ No

Type of Emergency

○ Respiratory Compromise
○ Cardiac Compromise
○ Other medical emergency Specify: _____

Patient Outcome

○ Remained in Department
○ Expired
○ Transferred to _____

Code Team Members/Emergency Medical Response Participants			
☆ All no answers require a comment throughout the remainder of the form			
	YES	No ☆	
Did Code Team/Emergency Medical Response Team Members Arrive?			
Did the appropriate team members fill roles?			

Emergency Medical Response Duties	Appropriate Action Taken			Comments
	YES	No☆	N/A	
Operator/Announced Overhead/Activated Pagers Correctly/Department Announcement				
Team Directed and Organized				
Defibrillated/Cardioverted *Please check:* ○ CV Tech ○ Attending MD ○ Resident ○ PICU/RN ○ Sync. Cardioverted ○ Defibrillated ○ Called "All Clear" ○ Paddles ○ Delivered energy lubricated/proper placement				
CPR not interrupted >5 seconds				
Pulse transmitted with chest compressions				
Proper chest rise and fall with ventilations				
Notifies attending physician				

APPENDIX 26B
EVALUATION OF CODE PERFORMANCE QUALITY ASSURANCE DOCUMENT—CONT'D

Emergency Medical Response Duties	Appropriate Action Taken			Comments
	YES	No☆	N/A	
Family Notified				
Needed Supplies available				
Equipment functioning properly				
Beepers/overhead speaker system/stairwell doors functioned appropriately				
Standard precautions followed				
Overall Team Effort				
All members participated in code evaluation				
Members transported patient as necessary				

Ensure the following documentation is completed:

- Complete QCC and forward to manager for signature
- Attach pink copy of Cardiac Arrest Record, if applicable, to completed evaluation form and forward to CPES for Resuscitation

Any other comments from team members to enhance response:

_____

_____

_____

_____

_____

_____   _____
Evaluation completed by   Date

_____   _____
Evaluation form reviewed by   Date

APPENDIX 26B
EVALUATION OF CODE PERFORMANCE QUALITY ASSURANCE DOCUMENT—CONT'D

Date _____ Time event recognized _____ Age _____ Weight (kg) _____

Signatures:

Was Code Team activated? ❑ Yes ❑ No

Physician in Charge: _____

Type of event: ❑ Respiratory ❑ Respiratory leading to cardiac ❑ Cardiac

Monitors on patient at onset of event: ❑ ECG ❑ Pulse oximeter ❑ Apnea ❑ None

Recording Nurse: _____

Patient conscious at onset? ❑ Yes ❑ No Pulse present at onset? ❑ Yes ❑ No

Airway/Ventilation
Breathing: ❑Spontaneous ❑Apnea ❑Agonal ❑Assisted
Type of ventilation: ❑ Mouth/Mouth ❑Mouth/Mask ❑BVM
                     ❑ETT ❑Trach ❑Other_____
Time of first assisted ventilation _____
Intubation: Time _____ Size _____
By whom: _____
Number of visualizations/attempts: _____
Confirmation:❑Auscultation ❑ETCO₂ ❑Other

Circulation
Initial Rhythm _____
Rhythm when compressions started _____
Patient Defibrillated? ❑Yes ❑No
Number of IV attempts _____
Type of Isolation _____

Outcome
Event Ended @ _____
Status: ❑Alive ❑Expired
Reason Resuscitation Ended:
❑Restored circulation ❑Restored ventilation
❑Unresponsive to ALS ❑Medical Futility
❑Restriction by family ❑Advance Directive

TIME	HR	RR	BP	O₂ Sat	INTERVENTION (CPR, Medications – Dose & Route, Defib/Cardiovert, Intubation, Vasoactive Drips)	PATIENT ASSESSMENT/RESPONSE

Addressograph

CHKD Form#0668 MR 5/02   FDB: Code Committee

Children's Hospital of The King's Daughters, Inc.
601 Children's Lane, Norfolk, VA 23507-1910

Medical Emergency Response Documentation Form
Page _____ of _____

White-Medical Record   Yellow-Pharmacy   Pink-Reviewer

APPENDIX 26B
EVALUATION OF CODE PERFORMANCE QUALITY ASSURANCE DOCUMENT—CONT'D

Date _____ Physician in Charge Signature: _____ Recording Nurse Signature: _____

Time	HR	RR	BP	O$_2$ Sat	INTERVENTION (CPR, Medications – Dose & Route, Defib/Cardiovert, Intubation, Vasoactive Drips)	Patient Assessment/Response

CHKD Form # 0669 MR 5/02   FDB: Code Committee

Children's Hospital of The King's Daughters, Inc.
601 Children's Lane, Norfolk, VA 23507-1910

Medical Emergency Response Documentation- SUPPLEMENTAL FORM
Page _____ of _____

White-Medical Record   Yellow-Pharmacy   Pink-Reviewer

Addressograph

APPENDIX 26B
EVALUATION OF CODE PERFORMANCE QUALITY ASSURANCE DOCUMENT—CONT'D

Signature _____
Print Name _____
☐ Performed artificial ventilation – Type _____
☐ Performed chest compressions
☐ Performed venipuncture - _____ attempts   ☐ Performed intraosseous
☐ Medication administration   ☐ Performed cardioversion/defibrillation
☐ Performed intubation   ☐ Other procedure –Type _____

Signature _____
Print Name _____
☐ Performed artificial ventilation – Type _____
☐ Performed chest compressions
☐ Performed venipuncture - _____ attempts   ☐ Performed intraosseous
☐ Medication administration   ☐ Performed cardioversion/defibrillation
☐ Performed intubation   ☐ Other procedure –Type _____

Signature _____
Print Name _____
☐ Performed artificial ventilation – Type _____
☐ Performed chest compressions
☐ Performed venipuncture - _____ attempts   ☐ Performed intraosseous
☐ Medication administration   ☐ Performed cardioversion/defibrillation
☐ Performed intubation   ☐ Other procedure –Type _____

Signature _____
Print Name _____
☐ Performed artificial ventilation – Type _____
☐ Performed chest compressions
☐ Performed venipuncture - _____ attempts   ☐ Performed intraosseous
☐ Medication administration   ☐ Performed cardioversion/defibrillation
☐ Performed intubation   ☐ Other procedure –Type _____

Signature _____
Print Name _____
☐ Performed artificial ventilation – Type _____
☐ Performed chest compressions
☐ Performed venipuncture - _____ attempts   ☐ Performed intraosseous
☐ Medication administration   ☐ Performed cardioversion/defibrillation
☐ Performed intubation   ☐ Other procedure –Type _____

Signature _____
Print Name _____
☐ Performed artificial ventilation – Type _____
☐ Performed chest compressions
☐ Performed venipuncture - _____ attempts   ☐ Performed intraosseous
☐ Medication administration   ☐ Performed cardioversion/defibrillation
☐ Performed intubation   ☐ Other procedure –Type _____

Signature _____
Print Name _____
☐ Performed artificial ventilation – Type _____
☐ Performed chest compressions
☐ Performed venipuncture - _____ attempts   ☐ Performed intraosseous
☐ Medication administration   ☐ Performed cardioversion/defibrillation
☐ Performed intubation   ☐ Other procedure –Type _____

Signature _____
Print Name _____
☐ Performed artificial ventilation – Type _____
☐ Performed chest compressions
☐ Performed venipuncture - _____ attempts   ☐ Performed intraosseous
☐ Medication administration   ☐ Performed cardioversion/defibrillation
☐ Performed intubation   ☐ Other procedure –Type _____

Signature _____
Print Name _____
☐ Performed artificial ventilation – Type _____
☐ Performed chest compressions
☐ Performed venipuncture - _____ attempts   ☐ Performed intraosseous
☐ Medication administration   ☐ Performed cardioversion/defibrillation
☐ Performed intubation   ☐ Other procedure –Type _____

Signature _____
Print Name _____
☐ Performed artificial ventilation – Type _____
☐ Performed chest compressions
☐ Performed venipuncture - _____ attempts   ☐ Performed intraosseous
☐ Medication administration   ☐ Performed cardioversion/defibrillation
☐ Performed intubation   ☐ Other procedure –Type _____

Addressograph

CHKD Form # 0670 MR 5./02   FDB: Code Committee

Children's Hospital of The King's Daughters, Inc.
601 Children's Lane, Norfolk, VA 23507-1910

Medical Emergency Response Documentation Form-SIGNATURES

White- Medical Record   Yellow- Reviewer

APPENDIX 26B
EVALUATION OF CODE PERFORMANCE QUALITY ASSURANCE DOCUMENT—CONT'D

Children's Hospital Of The King's Daughters, Inc.
601 Children's Lane
Norfolk, VA 23507-1911

QUALITY CARE CONTROL REPORT

(2) LOCATION	(3) STATUS	(4) SEX	(6) VARIANCE TIME
	☐ OTHER DEPART.	☐ MALE	_____ A.M.
	☐ INPATIENT	☐ FEMALE	_____ P.M.
	☐ OUTPATIENT	**(5) AGE**	**(7) VARIANCE DATE**
	☐ VISITOR		
	☐ _____ OTHER		__/__/__ (ADDRESSOGRAPH)

(8) EVENT THAT OCCURRED
- ☐ Diagnosis/Diagnostic Test
- ☐ TX/Monitoring
- ☐ Medication Event
- ☐ Product/Equipment Related
- ☐ Fall/Found on Floor
- ☐ Communication Events/ Issues
- ☐ Injury Related
- ☐ Property Related
- ☐ Other Specific Risk Issues
- ☐ Administrative Events
- ☐ Other _____

* Refer to back of form.

(9) ADMITTING DIAGNOSIS

(10) OUTCOME/SEVERITY (USE BEST JUDGEMENT ✓ ONE)
- ☐ No injury or inconsequential injury or effect
- ☐ Consequential (possible temporary injury or effect)
- ☐ Serious (possible minor permanent injury or effect)
- ☐ Severe (possible major permanent injury or effect)
- ☐ Death
- ☐ Not Applicable (e.g.; property loss; AMA/walkout)

_____ Equipment Number

(11) PHYSICIAN NOTIFIED?
- ☐ NO
- ☐ YES _____ NAME __/__/__ DATE

DID M.D. SEE PATIENT?
- ☐ NO
- ☐ YES _____ NAME __/__/__ DATE

X-RAYS TAKEN?
- ☐ NO
- ☐ YES

DOES PHYSICIAN WANT TO BE NOTIFIED OF FOLLOW-UP?
☐ NO ☐ YES

(12) BRIEFLY DESCRIBE VARIANCE (GIVE FACTS; BE BRIEF) INCLUDE INJURY/DAMAGE/LOSS, IF ANY.

(13) STATUS BEFORE FALL (MED VARIANCE)

CALL BELL ☐ Yes ☐ No   SIDE RAILS ☐ Yes ☐ No

PATIENT STATUS _____

MEDICATION
VARIANCE CATEGORY _____

(14) WAS PATIENT/SUBJECT AWARE OF VARIANCE? ☐ YES ☐ NO   GIVE PATIENT/SUBJECT RESPONSE/REACTION TO VARIANCE –

(15) COMPLETED BY (USE FOR BOXES 1 THRU 14)

X _____ SIGNATURE __/__/__ DATE

(16) OUTCOME SCREENS - TO BE COMPLETED BY HEAD NURSE / SUPERVISOR AND INCLUDE ALL MAROON BOXES ABOVE.

INPATIENT & OUTPATIENT
- ☐ DOA OR ED Death following inpatient, ED, or OPD visit - this facility past 7 days
- ☐ Return visit for **complications** following inpatient, ED, or OPD visit
- ☐ Unscheduled return visit following inpatient, ED, or OPD visit **(no complications)**
- ☐ Fracture/Burn (2° or 3°) /Tissue Necrosis with ulceration, not present on admission
- ☐ Cardiac/respiratory arrest (Exclude "No Code" patients)
- ☐ Unplanned transfer, general care to Intensive Care or to another hospital
- ☐ Admission for possible adverse result of ED/OPD management
- ☐ Readmission within 7 days of discharge
- ☐ Neurological deficit not present on admission

INFECTION CONTROL PRACTITIONER
- ☐ Severe Post-Op or other nosocomial infection
- ☐ Consent policy and procedure variance
- ☐ Foreign Body, possibly retained
- ☐ Unscheduled return to OR, same admission
- ☐ Procedure injury: removal or repair of organ or body part injured during therapeutic or diagnostic procedure
- ☐ Surgery injury: removal or repair of organ or body part injured during surgery
- ☐ Cancellation of surgery after induction of anesthesia

(17) COMPLETED BY (USE FOR OUTCOME SCREENS/ONGOING MONITORS)

X _____ SIGNATURE __/__/__ DATE

CHARTING OCCURRENCES
THIS REPORT DOES NOT REPLACE ADEQUATE CHARTING. IT IS A PERFORMANCE IMPROVEMENT TOOL, NOT A PATIENT RECORD. CHART VARIANCES CONSISTENTLY WITH HOSPITAL POLICIES.

(18) QUALITY ASSURANCE (MARK BOX 12 IF BOXES 18 OR 19 ARE COMPLETED)

_____ CONTROL NUMBER

CONCERN
☐ YES ☐ NO

HOSPITAL/FACILITY – RETAINED INFORMATION

X _____ PI SIGNATURE __/__/__ DATE

FOLLOW UP _____

RUSH
THIS REPORT TO
PERFORMANCE IMPROVEMENT
IN **24 HOURS**

(19)
SUPERVISOR X _____ SIGNATURE __/__/__ DATE   QUALITY REVIEW COORDINATOR X _____ SIGNATURE __/__/__ DATE

APPENDIX 26B
EVALUATION OF CODE PERFORMANCE QUALITY ASSURANCE DOCUMENT—CONT'D

REPORTABLE EVENT
(QUALITY/MANAGEMENT TOOL/FOR INTERNAL PURPOSES ONLY)

DIAGNOSIS/DIAGNOSTIC TEST	PRODUCT/EQUIPMENT RELATED	PROPERTY RELATED
Test Performance Related Test Selection Related Test Interpretation Related Omitted Test/Assessment Tested Incorrect Patient Test Results Related Performance of Unordered Test Other Diagnostic Event:	Equipment Selection Event Product/Equipment Failure Product/Equipment Malfunction Unavailable Product/Equipment User Related Product/Equipment Equipment Design Issue Other Product/Equipment Event: Medical Equip. Related Respiratory Equip. Related	Property Damaged/Lost (9026.02/9026.01)

TX/MONITORING	FALL/FOUND ON FLOOR	OTHER RISK ISSUES
Foreign Body Related Treatment of Incorrect Body Part Treated Incorrect Patient Treatment Order Related Performance of Unordered Treatment Infection/Contamination/Exposure Body Part Injury: Adjacent to Treatment Site Intubation/Extubation Related Omitted Treatment Treatment Performance Related Patient Monitoring Related Invasive Line Site Event (including epidurals) Intravenous Line Event (peripheral) Discharge Instruction Event (exclude Meds) Readiness for Discharge/Release (event) Unplanned Return to the ED within 72 hours for Related Symptoms UTI Post Admission w/Indwelling Urinary Cath. Treatment Refused Other Treatment Event:	CATEGORY OF FALL (CIRCLE TYPE OF FALL ALSO) Witnessed Fall Unwitnessed Fall/Found on Floor TYPE OF FALL (CIRCLE CATEGORY OF FALL ALSO) Ambulation Related Fall/Fall on Treadmill Bathroom Related Fall Bed Related Fall Chair/Commode Related Fall Transfer Related Fall Table/Stretcher Related Fall Tripped with Fall Occurring Slipped on Slick Surface/Fell Other Fall Event:	Complaint: (9024.01) Behavioral Event: (9025.01) Other Risk Issue Event: (9028.01)

OTHER SPECIFIC EVENTS

DOA w/In 7 Days of Previous Care Given
Same Facility
ED Death w/In 7 Days of Previous Care Given
  Same Facility
Unscheduled Return Visit After Previous Care
  Given Same Facility (no complications)
Fracture
Burn
Necrosis
Skin Tear
Decubitus (newly acquired)
Unplanned Transfer to ICU
Unplanned Transfer to Another Facility
Admission Related to OPD Complication
Readmission w/In 30 Days for Same/Related
  Diagnosis
Unscheduled Return to OR, Same Admission
Cancellation of surgery Post Anesthesia induction

MEDICATION EVENT	COMMUNICATION EVENTS/ISSUES
TYPE OF EVENT (CIRCLE ROUTE OF MED ALSO) Time of Administration Related Dispensing Event Dose/Rate Related MD Order Related Incorrect Patient Unordered (not ordered) Incorrect Medication Given Route of Administration Related Omitted Transcription Event Other Medication Event:	Abandonment/MD Non-attendance Allegation AMA (left after being told needed to stay) Informed Consent Issue Confidentiality Related Security Related Patient Rights Issue WALKOUTS Left After Being Seen But Before Being Told of the Need to Stay Walkout (left prior to being seen) Elopement Other Communication Event/Issue: NOC

ADVERSE REACTION (CIRCLE ROUTE ALSO)

Adverse Drug Reaction
Adverse Blood Reaction
Other Adverse Reactions:

ROUTE OF MED (CIRCLE TYPE OF EVENT ALSO)

PO
Injectable
IV/IV Med/IV Admixture
Topical
Inhalant
Transdermal
Transfusion
Other Route:

MED INSTRUCTION

Discharge Instruction - Medication(s) Related

INJURY RELATED	ADMINISTRATIVE EVENTS
Struck/Injured Against An Object Struck/Injured Against Another Person Struck/Injured by Another Person Struck/Injured by A Moving Object Self-Inflicted Injury with Survival (exclude patients w/ ICD9 codes of 436,331.0, or 294.1) Suicide Food Related Injury: Caught Between Assault: Sexual Assault: Other Medical Immobilization Patient Positioning Related Injury Occurred While Moving Patient Seclusion Related Child/Vulnerable Issue Other Injury Event:	Timeliness of Diagnosis Related Determination of Diagnosis Related Timeliness of Treatment or Admission Related EMTALA/COBRA Related Credentialing: Staff Privileges Credentialing: Peer Review Ostensible Agency/Vicarious Liability Libel/Slander/Defamation Billing Issue Contract Issue Other Regulatory Issue Deposition Request Medical Record Request

APPENDIX 26B
EVALUATION OF CODE PERFORMANCE QUALITY ASSURANCE DOCUMENT—CONT'D

FOLLOW-UP OF QCC/MEDICATION ERROR   Name _____

MR # _____

Dept. _____

Departments involved _____   _____

_____   _____

Describe occurrence _____

_____

Did you have sufficient knowledge/information to administer the medication/IV solution/treatment as prescribed?   NA ___   Yes ___   No ___   (if no comment)   medication/IV error employee # _____

_____

_____

Did anything contribute to the error? _____

_____

Treatment required: ___ No treatment required   ___ Medical &/or Diagnostic Intervention
                    ___ Nursing/Physician intervention   ___ Nursing intervention only
                    ___ Surgical Intervention   ___ Transferred to higher level of care   ___ N/A

How could this incident have been prevented? _____

_____

Outcome/significance of this occurrence:

___ Minor temporary   ___ Major temporary   ___ Unknown   ___ None
___ Major permanent   ___ Death   ___ Minor permanent

Patient's/visitor's current status: ___ Good   ___ Fair   ___ Serious
___ Discharged   ___ Transferred to: _____

Are there residual effects from occurrence? Yes ___   No ___

If yes, describe _____

_____

_____   _____
Signature   Employee number

- -

Actions: As **Department Manager**, what actions have you taken/will take to prevent a recurrence?

___ Discuss with employee   ___ Inservice   ___ Review at Staff Meeting
___ Employee counseling   ___ Discuss with Medical Director ___ Other

Additional information: _____

_____

Manager's Signature _____

APPENDIX 26B
EVALUATION OF CODE PERFORMANCE QUALITY ASSURANCE DOCUMENT—CONT'D

Children's Hospital Of The King's Daughters, Inc.
601 Children's Lane
Norfolk, VA 23507-1911

QUALITY CARE CONTROL REPORT

(2) LOCATION	(3) STATUS	(4) SEX	(6) VARIANCE TIME
	☐ OTHER DEPART. ☐ INPATIENT ☐ OUTPATIENT ☐ VISITOR ☐ _____ OTHER	☐ MALE ☐ FEMALE	_____ A.M. _____ P.M.

(5) AGE _____   **(7) VARIANCE DATE** __/__/__   (ADDRESSOGRAPH)

(8) EVENT THAT OCCURRED
- ☐ Diagnosis/Diagnostic Test
- ☐ TX/Monitoring
- ☐ Medication Event
- ☐ Product/Equipment Related
- ☐ Fall/Found on Floor
- ☐ Communication Events/ Issues
- ☐ Injury Related
- ☐ Property Related
- ☐ Other Specific Risk Issues
- ☐ Administrative Events
- ☐ Other _____

* Refer to back of form.

(9) ADMITTING DIAGNOSIS

(10) OUTCOME/SEVERITY (USE BEST JUDGEMENT ✓ ONE)
- ☐ No injury or inconsequential injury or effect
- ☐ Consequential (possible temporary injury or effect)
- ☐ Serious (possible minor permanent injury or effect)
- ☐ Severe (possible major permanent injury or effect)
- ☐ Death
- ☐ Not Applicable (e.g.; property loss; AMA/walkout)

_____ Equipment Number

(11) PHYSICIAN NOTIFIED?
- ☐ NO
- ☐ YES _____ NAME _____ /__/__ DATE

DID M.D. SEE PATIENT?
- ☐ NO
- ☐ YES _____ NAME _____ /__/__ DATE

X-RAYS TAKEN?
- ☐ NO
- ☐ YES

DOES PHYSICIAN WANT TO BE NOTIFIED OF FOLLOW-UP?
- ☐ NO ☐ YES

(12) BRIEFLY DESCRIBE VARIANCE (GIVE FACTS; BE BRIEF) INCLUDE INJURY/DAMAGE/LOSS, IF ANY.

(13) STATUS BEFORE FALL (MED VARIANCE)

CALL BELL ☐ Yes ☐ No   SIDE RAILS ☐ Yes ☐ No

PATIENT STATUS _____

MEDICATION
VARIANCE CATEGORY _____

(14) WAS PATIENT/SUBJECT AWARE OF VARIANCE? ☐ YES ☐ NO GIVE PATIENT/SUBJECT RESPONSE/REACTION TO VARIANCE –

(15) COMPLETED BY (USE FOR BOXES 1 THRU 14)

X _____ SIGNATURE   /__/__ DATE

(16) OUTCOME SCREENS - TO BE COMPLETED BY HEAD NURSE / SUPERVISOR AND INCLUDE ALL MAROON BOXES ABOVE.

INPATIENT & OUTPATIENT

- ☐ DOA OR ED Death following inpatient, ED, or OPD visit - this facility past 7 days
- ☐ Return visit for **complications** following inpatient, ED, or OPD visit
- ☐ Unscheduled return visit following inpatient, ED, or OPD visit **(no complications)**
- ☐ Fracture/Burn (2˚ or 3˚) /Tissue Necrosis with ulceration, not present on admission
- ☐ Cardiac/respiratory arrest (Exclude "No Code" patients)
- ☐ Unplanned transfer, general care to Intensive Care or to another hospital
- ☐ Admission for possible adverse result of ED/OPD management
- ☐ Readmission within 7 days of discharge
- ☐ Neurological deficit not present on admission

INFECTION CONTROL PRACTITIONER

- ☐ Severe Post-Op or other nosocomial infection
- ☐ Consent policy and procedure variance
- ☐ Foreign Body, possibly retained
- ☐ Unscheduled return to OR, same admission
- ☐ Procedure injury: removal or repair of organ or body part injured during therapeutic or diagnostic procedure
- ☐ Surgery injury: removal or repair of organ or body part injured during surgery
- ☐ Cancellation of surgery after induction of anesthesia

(17) COMPLETED BY (USE FOR OUTCOME SCREENS/ONGOING MONITORS)

X _____ SIGNATURE   /__/__ DATE

(18) QUALITY ASSURANCE (MARK BOX 12 IF BOXES 18 OR 19 ARE COMPLETED)

_____ CONTROL NUMBER

CONCERN
☐ YES ☐ NO

HOSPITAL/FACILITY –
RETAINED INFORMATION

X _____ PI SIGNATURE   /__/__ DATE

CHARTING OCCURRENCES
THIS REPORT DOES NOT REPLACE ADEQUATE CHARTING. IT IS A PERFORMANCE IMPROVEMENT TOOL, NOT A PATIENT RECORD. CHART VARIANCES CONSISTENTLY WITH HOSPITAL POLICIES.

RUSH
THIS REPORT TO
PERFORMANCE IMPROVEMENT
IN **24 HOURS**

FOLLOW UP _____

(Courtesy of Children's Hospital of the King's Daugther, Inc., Norfolk, Virginia)

APPENDIX 27
DELIVERY ROOM CARE OF THE NEONATE: NEONATAL RESUSCITATION

Both routine assessment and care of the neonate at the delivery and the possible provision of extensive resuscitation should be provided in accordance with the American Heart Association (AHA) and the American Academy of Pediatrics (AAP) Neonatal Resuscitation Program. Although the guidelines for neonatal resuscitation focus on newborns, most of the principles are applicable throughout the neonatal period and early infancy. Hospital medical staff concerned with the care and resuscitation of the newborn, including obstetricians, anesthetists, and pediatricians, should determine the qualifications needed to perform neonatal resuscitation, including completion of the AHA and AAP Neonatal Resuscitation Program. At every delivery, there should be at least one person whose primary responsibility is the neonate and who is capable of initiating resuscitation. Either that person or someone else who is capable and immediately available should have the skills required to perform a complete resuscitation, including ventilation with bag and mask, endotracheal intubation, chest compressions, and the use of medications. It is not sufficient to have someone "on call" (either at home or in another area of the hospital) for newborn resuscitations in the delivery room.

Recognition and immediate resuscitation of a distressed neonate requires an organized plan of action and the immediate availability of qualified personnel and equipment as described in the AAP and the AHA *Textbook of Neonatal Resuscitation.* Responsibility for identification and resuscitation of a distressed neonate should be assigned to a qualified individual, who may be a physician, a certified nurse-midwife, an advanced practice neonatal nurse, a labor and delivery nurse, a nurse-anesthetist, a nursery nurse, or a respiratory therapist. The provision of services and equipment for resuscitation should be planned jointly by the directors of the departments of obstetrics, anesthesia, and pediatrics, with the approval of the medical staff. A physician, usually a pediatrician, should be designated to assume primary responsibility for initiating, supervising, and reviewing the plan for management of depressed neonates in the delivery room. The following issues should be considered in this plan:

- Development of a list of maternal and fetal complications that require the presence in the delivery room of someone specifically qualified in all aspects of newborn resuscitation.
- Individuals qualified to perform neonatal resuscitation should demonstrate the following capabilities:

  - Rapid and accurate evaluation of the newborn condition, including Apgar scoring
  - Knowledge of the pathogenesis and causes of a low Apgar score (e.g., hypoxia, drugs, hypovolemia, trauma, anomalies, infections, and preterm birth), as well as specific indications for resuscitation
  - Skills in airway management (e.g., laryngoscopy, endotracheal intubation, suctioning of the airway), artificial ventilation, cardiac massage, emergency administration of drugs and fluids, and maintenance of thermal stability. Recognition and decompression of a tension pneumothorax by needle aspiration also is a desirable skill.

- Development of procedures to ensure the readiness of equipment and personnel and to provide for periodic review and evaluation of the effectiveness of the system.
- Contingency plans for multiple births and other unusual circumstances.
- The resuscitation steps should be documented in the medical record along with accurate times.
- Development of procedures for transfer of responsibility for care.

From the American Academy of Pediatrics and the American College of Obstetricians and Gynecologists: *Guidelines for Perinatal Care,* Fifth Edition, Washington, DC, 2002, pp 187–188.

APPENDIX 28
CLINICAL CONSIDERATIONS IN THE USE OF OXYGEN

The hazards associated with the nonindicated administration of supplemental oxygen to preterm neonates have been recognized for many years. Studies conducted in the 1950s indicated that prolonged oxygen therapy without clinical indication was associated with increased rates of retinopathy of prematurity, formerly called retrolental fibroplasia. The ensuing blanket restriction of ambient oxygen therapy resulted in a marked decrease in retinopathy of prematurity at the cost of a marked increase in morbidity and mortality. Current practice includes the prudent use of supplemental oxygen as needed, based on an objective determination of oxygen requirements.

When supplemental oxygen therapy is considered, the potential risks, in terms of both hypoxia and hyperoxia, should be weighed. Clinical judgment of physical signs alone as a guide to the amount of supplemental oxygen needed is acceptable for short periods, emergencies, or abrupt clinical changes. However, the ease of noninvasive determinations of oxygen saturation should preclude the continued use of supplemental oxygen without an objective assessment.

Administration and Montoring

In an emergency, high concentrations of supplemental oxygen may be administered by a face mask or endotracheal tube. When a neonate requires oxygen therapy beyond the emergency period, the oxygen should be warmed and humidified, and the concentration or flow should be carefully regulated and monitored. Oxygen can be delivered via an endotracheal tube, oxygen hood, nasal prong, or incubator. Oxygen analyzers should be calibrated in accordance with manufacturers' recommendations. Orders for oxygen therapy should be written in terms of desired ambient concentration or flow and should indicate the intervals at which the concentration (or flow rate, when nasal prongs are used) should be routinely checked. Alternatively, order should be written to adjust FIO_2 or flow within a stated range to maintain oxygen saturation within specific limits. There should be an institutional policy for ordering, delivering, and documenting oxygen therapy and monitoring.

An important development in the care of neonates who require oxygen therapy has been the ability to monitor oxygenation continuously with noninvasive techniques. The transcutaneous oxygen analyzer provides an indirect measurement of Pao_2, and the pulse oximeter measures oxyhemoglobin saturation. Because neither technique measures Pao_2 directly, they should be used as adjuncts to, rather than substitutes for, arterial blood gas sampling, especially in neonates with moderate to severe respiratory distress.

Periodic measurement of Pao_2 in samples from an umbilical or peripheral artery catheter is the most reliable method of assessing the effectiveness of oxygen therapy. If an indwelling arterial catheter is not in place, peripheral artery puncture can be used, but repeated sampling from these sites is not always possible. When arterial blood sampling is not possible, arterialized capillary sampling is an acceptable alternative. This measurement produces fairly reliable estimates of arterial pH and arterial carbon dioxide ($Paco_2$) but usually underestimates true Pao_2.

In neonates whose condition is unstable, noninvasive measurements should be correlated with Pao_2 at least every 8–12 hours. More frequent analyses of arterial blood gas may be indicated for the assessment of pH and Pao_2. In neonates whose condition is stable, correlation with arterial blood gas samples may be performed less frequently.

The use of either transcutaneous oxygen measurement or pulse oximetry may shorten the time required to determine optimum inspired oxygen concentration and ventilator settings in the acute care setting. Both measurements are particularly useful in monitoring oxygen therapy in neonates who are recovering from respiratory distress or who require long-term supplemental oxygen. Because transcutaneous oxygen measurements underestimate oxygenation in older neonates with bronchopulmonary dysplasia (BPD), pulse oximetry may be a more suitable method for monitoring oxygen therapy in these neonates.

In consideration of the current, but incomplete, understanding of the effects of oxygen administration, the following recommendations are offered:

- Supplemental oxygen should not be used without a specific indication, such as cyanosis, low Pao_2, or low oxygen saturation.
- The use of supplemental oxygen other than for resuscitation should be monitored by regular assessments of Pao_2 and oxygen saturation.
- The duration of time that oxygen therapy may be administered in nurseries lacking the capability of appropriate Pao_2 or oxygen saturation monitoring before consideration of transfer to a higher level unit is contingent on the gestational age of the neonate and the severity of the oxygenation deficit. In general, neonates delivered at less than 36 weeks of gestation or those requiring more than 40% ambient oxygen should be stabilized and transferred promptly.
- For neonates who require oxygen therapy for acute care, measurements of blood pressure levels, blood pH, and Pao_2 should accompany measurements of Pao_2. In addition, a record of blood gas measurements, details of the oxygen delivery system (e.g., ventilator, settings, continuous positive airway pressure), and ambient oxygen concentrations (or liter of flow per minute, if nasal prongs are used) should be maintained.
- When supplemental oxygen is administered to a preterm neonate, attempts should be made to maintain Pao_2 at

50–80 mm Hg. Oxygen tensions in this range should be adequate for tissue needs, given normal hemoglobin concentrations and blood flow. Even with careful monitoring, however, $Paco_2$ may fluctuate outside this range, particularly in neonates with cardiopulmonary disease.
- It is prudent when oxygen therapy is needed for a preterm neonate to discuss the reasons for using supplemental oxygen and the associated risks and benefits with parents.
- Hourly measurement and recording of the concentration of oxygen delivered to the neonate is recommended.
- Except for an emergency situation, air-oxygen mixtures should be warmed and humidified before being administered to newborns.

From the American Academy of Pediatrics and the American College of Obstetricians and Gynecologists: *Guidelines for Perinatal Care*, Fifth Edition, Washington, DC, 2002, pp 244–246.

APPENDIX 29
EXECUTIVE SUMMARY: FINAL COBRA REGULATIONS

On June 22, 1994, the Health Care Financing Administration (HCFA) published final regulations to implement the Emergency Treatment and Labor Act, commonly referred to as COBRA, a law designed to prevent patient dumping.

Since 1985, COBRA has required that all persons presenting for treatment to a hospital emergency department receive a medical screening examination by qualified personnel to determine if an emergency medical condition exists. A patient with an emergent medical condition may not be discharged or transferred to another medical facility from *anywhere* in the hospital unless any emergent condition has been stabilized to the extent possible and the physician has certified that the medical benefits of the transfer outweigh any risks. An informed consent to the transfer or discharge must also be obtained.

In large part, the final regulations merely clarify the initial legislation. However, there are a few significant additions, which are summarized below.

1. Hospitals will be required to report suspected COBRA violations to HCFA.
2. A patient who arrives on hospital property has presented to the emergency department, thus an ambulance cannot be diverted once on campus. If the ambulance is owned by the hospital, the patient is on hospital property regardless of the ambulance's location.
3. The definition of *emergency condition* is expanded to include psychiatric disturbances and symptoms of substance abuse. It has always included potential for loss of life, limb, organ or bodily function, active labor, and severe pain.
4. A hospital is required to maintain a list of physicians on-call to provide stabilizing treatment. If an on-call physician fails to respond and this prompts transfer to another facility for stabilization and treatment of an emergent medical condition, the transferring doctor *must* write the on-call physician's name and number in the medical chart, essentially documenting this as a violation of COBRA.

5. The emergency department must maintain a log of all patients showing ultimate disposition (e.g., patient refused treatment, admission, transfer, or discharge).

6. A tertiary care facility and its associated physicians may not refuse to accept an *appropriate* transfer if capacity and capability exists.

APPENDIX 30
OSHA GUIDELINES FOR OCCUPATIONAL EXPOSURE

A, UNIVERSAL PRECAUTIONS FOR USE WITH ALL PATIENTS (ADAPTED FROM THE CDC)

1. Wash hands after contact with body substances (e.g., urine, sputum, blood, etc.) before invasive procedures, and before eating or preparing food.

2. Wear gloves for direct hand contact with patient body substances (blood, urine, sputum, etc.), mucous membranes, non-intact skin, and when performing dressing changes.

3. Wear a paper isolation gown or plastic apron if soiling with any body substance is likely.

4. When performing procedures that may result in splashing of patient body fluids (e.g., tracheal suctioning, wound irrigation, endoscopy), wear a paper isolation gown or plastic apron, mask, and clear plastic goggles for eye and mouth protection.

5. Used needles shall not be bent, broken, recapped, or otherwise manipulated by hand. ONE-HANDED RECAPPING by the blood gas technician is, however, acceptable.

6. Dispose of needles and sharps in plastic needle/sharps containers provided for that purpose.

7. If exposure to blood or body fluids occurs, remove the body substance by washing hands, face, arms, or other body area affected. IMMEDIATELY report the exposure to your supervisor.

8. Treat all patient specimens as potentially infective.

9. Clean up spills of blood/body fluids with a hospital-grade disinfectant, used at manufacturer's recommended dilution. For large spills, notify environmental services immediately. They have the special equipment and information needed to handle such spills.

10. Although saliva HAS NOT been implicated in the transmission of HIV, minimize the need for mouth-to-mouth resuscitation by using one-way valve mouthpieces, resuscitation bags, or other ventilation devices in CPR situations.

Clinical Notes

- The collection of arterial blood gases has been singled out by the CDC as a procedure wherein recapping of needles is often a medical necessity. However, never recap by holding the cap in one hand and pushing the needle into the cap. When you must recap, lay the cap down on a flat surface and insert the needle into the cap, picking it up off the surface without touching the cap with your other hand. Once you have done this, you can point the needle to the ceiling and secure the cap onto the hub, touching only the base of the cap.

- As an alternative to the above, you can place the cap into the plastic shroud that the 3 mL syringes come in. The shroud can be held or left standing on a flat surface, providing a holder for the cap and allowing the needle to be recapped safely.

- Always wear the equipment that is needed to avoid contact of any kind with blood or other body fluids (e.g., gloves when handling contaminated circuits).

- Wash hands between patients even if using gloves. Never reuse gloves from patient to patient. Always wash hands even after removal of gloves.

- Use the faceshields (masks with plastic eye protection built in) when faced with any possibility of splashing or splattering body fluid into your face in other circumstances. The regular surgical masks offer less protection from penetration by fluids.

- Be sure to use the special white masks (3M PN #1814 Healthware Particulate Respirator) when giving pentamidine or working with active TB patients. Use eye protection in addition when there is any threat of splashing into your face.

- Normal prescription eyewear serves as protective equipment only if fitted with side shields.

- Procedures should always be performed in such a manner as to minimize the splashing or spraying of blood and body fluids.

From Oakes DF (ed): Neonatal/Pediatric Respiratory Care: A Critical Care Pocket Guide. Old Town, ME, Health Educator Publications, 1996, pp 9–7, 9–8, and 9–9.

APPENDIX 30
OSHA GUIDELINES FOR OCCUPATIONAL EXPOSURE—CONT'D

B, SPECIFIC GUIDELINES

(Check hospital policy for variations)

	Entry into ICU	Between Patient Contact	After Touching Hair, Face, Clothing, or Equipment	Handling Infected Patients or Equipment	After Touching Contaminated Patients or Equipment	Aseptic Techniques (Minor Proc.; ABG Sticks, IV or A-Lines, etc.)	Sterile Techniques (Major Proc., Surgery, Deliveries)	Procedures with Chance of Exposure to Body Fluids (SX, etc.)
Hands								
Wash hands vigorously for 10 s with soap and water, dry with paper towels.		×	×					
Scrub hands and arms to elbow with antiseptic for 2–5 min., clean nails, scrub again, rinse with hands up, dry with paper towels.	×				×	×		
Scrub hands and arms to elbow with antiseptic for 4–5 min., clean nails, scrub again, rinse with hands up, dry with two sterile towels (hands first).							×	
Gloves								
Wear nonsterile gloves		×		×		×		
Wear sterile gloves							×	×
Clothing								
Clean scrubs/uniforms (daily) or clean cover gown over street clothes (e.g., parents)	×							×
Cover gown over scrubs/uniform				×		×		
Sterile gown							×	
Mask—eyeshield							×	×

From Oakes DF (ed): Neonatal/Pediatric Respiratory Care: A Critical Care Pocket Guide. Old Town, ME, Health Education Publications, 1994, pp 9–7, 9–8, and 9–9.

APPENDIX 31
FDA SAFETY ALERT: HAZARDS OF HEATED-WIRE BREATHING CIRCUITS

The U.S. Food and Drug Administration has learned of instances in which improperly used heated-wire breathing circuits have overheated, softened, or melted, causing diminished gas delivery, fires, and burns to patients and caregivers.

To prevent such occurrences, it is important to take the following precautions:

1. Use only those heated-wire breathing circuits labeled for use with the specific humidifier being used. When in doubt about whether the breathing circuit is electrically compatible with the humidifier, *don't use it* without first consulting your biomedical engineering support group or the breathing circuit manufacturer.
2. Make sure the heated-wire breathing circuit has a recommended minute volume compatible with the ventilator settings.
3. Don't cover heated-wire breathing circuits with sheets, blankets, towels, clothing, or other materials.
4. Don't rest the circuits on other surfaces, such as the patient's body, bed rails, blankets, or medical equipment. Instead, use a boom arm or tube-tree to support the breathing circuit.

APPENDIX 32
EFFECTIVE FIO_2 CONVERSION TABLES FOR INFANTS ON NASAL CANNULA

1. The tables are based on those used in the STOP-ROP trials.* The data were derived from equations #3 and #4 in the paper by Benaron and Benitz, "Maximizing the stability of oxygen delivered by nasal cannula," (Arch Pediatr Adoles Med 1994; 148:294–300).
2. These tables include assumptions made by Benaron and Benitz (constant nasal flow over the inspiratory cycle and that the upper airway does not act as a reservoir) plus the follow-

ing assumptions made by the STOP-ROP investigators: Inspiration time = 0.3 seconds; tidal volume = 5 mL/kg; and that either inspiration is entirely nasal or that cannula flow is sufficiently low that on each inspiration the infant exhales all output from the cannula.

3. Example: *What is the effective FIO_2 in a 2.0–kg infant on 100% cannula at a flow of 0.15 L/min?*
Answer: Use 2.0 and 0.15 L/min in Table 1 to get a factor of 8. Then use Table 2, and the factor of 8 and 100% oxygen to yield an effective FIO_2 of 27%. Thus the effective oxygen concentration is less than 30% and the infant is eligible for the physiologic evaluation.

* The STOP-ROP Multicenter Study Group: Supplemental therapeutic oxygen for prethreshold retinopathy of prematurity (STOP-ROP): A randomized, controlled trial. I: Primary outcomes. Pediatrics 2000; 105:295–310.

TABLE 1. Factor as a Function of Flow and Weight

Flow (L/min)	Flow (L/min)	Weight (kg)								
		0.7	1.0	1.25	1.5	2	2.5	3	3.5	4
0.01		1	1	1	1	1	0	0	0	0
0.03	1/32	4	3	2	2	2	1	1	1	1
0.06	1/16	9	6	5	4	3	2	2	2	2
0.125	1/8	18	12	10	8	6	4	4	4	4
0.15		21	15	12	10	8	6	5	4	4
0.25	1/4	36	52	20	17	13	10	8	7	6
0.5	1/2	71	50	40	33	25	20	17	14	13
0.75	3/4	100	75	60	50	38	30	25	21	19
1.0	1.0	100	100	80	67	50	40	33	29	25
1.25		100	100	100	83	63	50	42	36	31
1.5		100	100	100	100	75	60	50	43	38
2.0		100	100	100	100	100	80	67	57	50

Factor = 100 • min (1 L/min/kg) (See Table 2).
Note: If your patient's exact values are not included in the table, round up or down to find the value closest to that of your patient. If the value is exactly halfway between the two values, round up.

APPENDIX 32
EFFECTIVE FIO$_2$ CONVERSION TABLES FOR INFANTS ON NASAL CANNULA—CONT'D

TABLE 2. Effective FIO$_2$ (×100) as a Function of Factor and Concentration*

Factor	Concentration (%)						
	21	22	25	30	40	50	100
0	21	21	21	21	21	21	21
1	21	21	21	21	21	21	22
2	21	21	21	21	21	22	23
3	21	21	21	21	22	22	23
4	21	21	21	21	22	22	24
5	21	21	21	21	22	22	25
6	21	21	21	22	22	23	26
7	21	21	21	22	22	23	27
8	21	21	21	22	23	23	27
9	21	21	21	22	23	24	28
10	21	21	21	22	23	24	29
11	21	21	21	22	23	24	30
12	21	21	21	22	23	24	30
13	21	21	22	22	23	25	31
14	21	21	22	22	24	25	32
15	21	21	22	22	23	25	33
17	21	21	22	23	24	26	34
18	21	21	22	23	24	26	35
19	21	21	22	23	25	27	36
20	21	21	22	23	25	27	37
21	21	21	22	23	25	27	38
22	21	21	22	23	25	27	36
23	21	21	22	23	25	28	39
25	21	21	22	23	25	28	41
27	21	21	22	23	25	29	42
28	21	21	22	24	26	29	43
29	21	21	22	24	27	29	44
30	21	21	22	24	27	30	45
31	21	21	22	24	27	31	47
33	21	21	22	24	27	31	47
36	21	21	22	24	28	31	49
38	21	21	23	24	28	32	51
40	21	21	23	25	29	33	53
42	21	21	23	25	29	33	54
43	21	21	23	25	29	33	55
44	21	21	23	25	29	34	56
50	21	21	23	25	30	35	60
55	21	22	23	26	31	37	64
57	21	22	23	26	32	38	66
60	21	22	23	26	32	38	68
63	21	22	24	27	33	39	71
67	21	22	24	27	34	40	74
71	21	22	24	27	34	42	77
75	21	22	24	28	35	43	80
80	21	22	24	28	36	44	84
83	21	22	24	28	37	45	87
86	21	22	24	29	37	46	89
100	21	22	25	30	40	50	100

* Shaded area signifies FIO$_2$ > 3.0 (i.e., O$_2$ concentration >30%).

APPENDIX 33
NEONATAL INDICATIONS AND DOSES FOR ADMINISTRATION OF SELECTED DRUGS
(SEE TABLES IN TEXT AS INDICATED FOR FURTHER COMMENTS)

Drug	Indications/Action	Dose/Route(s)
N-Acetylcysteine	Mucolytic	0.1–0.2 mL via ET tube
Adenosine (Adenocard)	Treat paroxysmal supraventricular tachycardia	37.5–100 μg/kg by rapid IV push
Albumin (human serum)	Shock, hypovolemia	1 g/kg diluted 1:1 IV (see Tables 3–7 and 3–9)
Amrinone	Inotropic agent	0.75 mg/kg IV over 10 min; then, and 5–10 mg/kg per min (see Table 15–11)
Atropine	Bradycardia Blocks muscarinic effects of neostigmine	0.01–0.03 mg/kg IV, SC, IT
Caffeine	Apneic spells	See Table 14–4
Calcium chloride, 10%	Resuscitation Hypocalcemia	Dilute 1:1 with normal saline IV (over 10 min) 0.15–0.3 mL/kg up to 1 mL/kg
Calcium gluconate	Resuscitation Hypocalcemia	100–200 mg/kg IV slowly or PO every 6 h (see Table 3–7)
Captopril	Antihypertensive	0.1–0.4 mg/kg per dose PO every 6–24 h (see Tables 15–12 and 15–17)
Diazepam	Seizures	0.1–0.3 mg/kg per dose IV, IM (see Table 3–7)
Diazoxide	Antihypertensive	5 mg/kg IV rapid bolus (see Table 15–17)
Digoxin	Heart failure	See Tables 3–7 and 15–5
Dobutamine	Inotropic agent Acute myocardial insufficiency	5–20 μg/kg per min (see Tables 14–6, 14–8, and 15–11)
Dopamine	Inotropic agent Hypotension, cardiac output	5–20 μg/kg per min (see Tables 3–7, 3–9, 14–7, 14–8, and 15–11)
Epinephrine	Resuscitation Flat-line electrocardiogram	1:10,000 aqueous solution, 0.1–0.5 mL IV, IC, IT, SC (see Tables 3–7, 3–9, 14–6, and 15–11)
Epinephrine (racemic)	Bronchoconstriction	1:100 aqueous solution, 0.5 mL in 3 mL H_2O IT via nebulizer every 4 h
Ethacrynic acid	Diuretic, fluid overload	0.5–1 mg/kg every 8–12 h, IV (see Table 15–10)
Fentanyl (Sublimaze)	Analgesia	IM or IV 2–3 μg/kg continued analgesia 1–3 μg/kg per h
Furosemide	Diuretic Increased lung water	1–5 mg/kg every 6 h IV, IM, PO (see Table 15–10)
Hydralazine	Hypertension	0.15–0.2 mg/kg IV, IM every 6 h; PO 0.5–7 mg/kg per d every 6–8 h (see Tables 15–12 and 15–17)
Hydrochlorothiazide	Diuretic	2–5 mg/kg per d every 12–24 h PO (see Table 15–10)
Indomethacin	Symptomatic patent ductus arteriosus	0.1–0.3 mg/kg every 8 h × 3 IV, PO (see Table 15–6)
Isoproterenol	Bradycardia, bronchoconstriction, pulmonary vasoconstriction	0.1–0.4 μg/min IV slowly of diluted solution 1–5 μg/mL (see Tables 3–7, 14–6, 14–8, and 15–11)
Lidocaine	Ventricular tachycardia	1 mg/kg IV bolus; maintenance 5–50 μg/kg per min IV (see Table 15–13)
Lorazepam (Ativan)	Sedation of mechanically ventilated infant	IV 0.05–0.1 mg/kg per dose
Midazolam (Versed)	Sedation	0.5 mg/kg PO 0.1–0.2 mg/kg IV
Morphine sulfate	Pain, agitation	0.05 mg/kg IM, IV, SC (see Tables 3–7 and 3–9)
Naloxone (Narcan)	Resuscitation/reverse narcotics administered to mother	IV, IM, SQ 0.1 mg/kg per dose
Neostigmine (Prostigmin)	Reverse neuromuscular blockade	0.04 mg/kg IM 0.025 mg/kg IV after atropine 0.02 mg/kg
Nitroglycerin	Acute hypertension	0.5–20 μg/kg per min (see Table 15–12)
Nitroprusside	Antihypertensive, pulmonary hypertension	0.5–8 μg/kg per min IV (see Table 15–17)
Norepinephrine	Inotropic agent	0.05–1 μg/kg per min IV (see Tables 14–6 and 15–11)
Pancuronium bromide	Paralysis Inadequate mechanical ventilation	0.03–0.1 mg/kg IV (see Table 14–3)

APPENDIX 33
NEONATAL INDICATIONS AND DOSES FOR ADMINISTRATION OF SELECTED DRUGS (SEE TABLES IN TEXT AS INDICATED FOR FURTHER COMMENTS)—CONT'D

Drug	Indications/Action	Dose/Route(s)
Phenobarbital	Seizures, sedation	Loading dose 10–20 mg/kg IV; maintenance 3–8 mg/kg per d IM, IV PO (see Table 3–7)
Phenytoin	Digoxin-related dysrhythmias	15 mg/kg IV in divided doses every 5 min over 1 h (see Table 15–13)
Procainamide	Antiarrhythmic agent, ventricular tachycardia	15 mg/kg IV slowly (see Table 15–13)
Propranolol	Supraventricular tachycardia Ventricular tachycardia Hypertension	0.05–0.2 mg/kg IV over 10 min 0.5–12 mg/kg per d PO in 4 divided doses (see Tables 15–13 and 15–17)
Prostaglandin E (Prostin VR Pediatric, alprostadil)	Keep ductus arteriosus open	IV at 0.1 μg/kg per min; increase as needed to 0.4 μg/kg per min; taper dose after desired affect achieved
Sodium bicarbonate	Resuscitation Acidosis	3 mEq/kg IV diluted 1:1 slowly (or base deficit calculation) (see Tables 3–7 and 3–9)
Spironolactone	Diuretic	1.1–3.3 mg/kg per d IV, PO in 1–2 doses (see Table 15–10)
Theophylline	Apneic spells Bronchoconstriction	See Table 14–4
Tolazoline	Pulmonary hypertension	Test dose 1–2 mg/kg IV over 5–10 min; maintenance 2–6 mg/kg per h IV (see Table 14–2)
D-Tubocurarine chloride	Paralysis, inadequate mechanical ventilation, pulmonary vasoconstriction	0.25–0.50 mg/kg IV
Verapamil	Supraventricular tachycardia	0.15–0.4 mg/kg IV slowly 10–20 mg/d PO
Vercuronium bromide (Norcuron)	Facilitate intubation and muscle relaxation	IV 0.08–0.1 mg/kg per dose Maintenance 0.01–0.1 mg/kg every hour, as needed

Abbreviations: ET = endotracheal; IV = Intravenous; SC = subcutaneous; IT = intratracheal; PO = perorally; IM = intramuscular; IC = intracardiac.

APPENDIX 34
FREQUENTLY USED ABBREVIATIONS

(A-a)DO$_2$	Alveolar-arterial oxygen gradient	g	Gram
A/C	Assist/Control	Hct	Hematocrit
ABG	Arterial blood gas	HFO	High-frequency oscillation
ADH	Antidiuretic hormone	HFV	High-frequency ventilation
ALCA	Anomalous left coronary artery	HFJV	High-frequency jet ventilation
Ao	Aorta	HFPPV	High-frequency positive-pressure ventilation
BUN	Blood urea nitrogen	Hg, Hgb	Hemoglobin
BE	Base excess	HMD	Hyaline membrane disease
BP	Blood pressure	IC	Inspiratory capacity
BPD	Bronchopulmonary dysplasia	ICP	Intracranial pressure
BPH	Bronchopulmonary hygiene	ICW	Intracellular water
bpm	Breaths per minute	ID	Internal diameter
BTPS	Body temperature and pressure saturated	I/E	Inspiratory expiratory (also I:E)
CA	Compressed air	IFR	Inspiratory flow rate
CBC	Complete blood count	IMV	Intermittent mandatory ventilation
CBF	Cerebral blood flow	IPPV	Intermittent positive-pressure ventilation
CBG	Capillary blood gas	IT	Inspiratory time
CC	Closing capacity	IVH	Intraventricular hemorrhage
CDH	Congenital diaphragmatic hernia	IWL	Insensible water loss
CDP	Continuous distending pressure	kcal	Kilocalorie
CHD	Congenital heart disease	kg	Kilogram
CHF	Congestive heart failure	LA	Left atrial
C$_{in}$	Insulin clearance	LA/Ao	Left atrium/aortic root
C$_L$	Lung compliance	LBW	Low birthweight (<2500 g)
Cm	Machine compliance	LPEP	Left ventricular pre-ejection period
CMV	Conventional mechanical ventilation	LRTI	Lower respiratory tract infection
CNAP	Continuous negative airway pressure	LVET	Left ventricular ejection time
CNEP	Continuous negative external pressure	MAC	Minimum anesthetic concentration
CNS	Central nervous system	MAP	Mean airway pressure
Cp	Patient compliance	MAS	Meconium aspiration syndrome
C$_{PAH}$	p-Aminohippurate clearance	MCT	Medium-chain triglycerides
CPAP	Continuous positive airway pressure	MPA	Main pulmonary artery
CPT	Chest physiotherapy	NICU	Neonatal intensive care unit
Cr	Creatinine	NO	Nitric oxide
CSF	Cerebrospinal fluid	NPII	Neonatal pulmonary insufficiency index
CT	Computed tomography	NRP	Neonatal Resuscitation Program
Cv	Ventilator compliance	OD	Outer diameter
CV	Closing volume	OI	Oxygen index
CVP	Central venous pressure	PAL	Pulmonary air leaks
D$_5$W	5% dextrose in water	PaCO$_2$	Partial pressure of carbon dioxide in arterial blood
D$_{10}$W	10% dextrose in water	PaO$_2$	Partial pressure of oxygen in arterial blood
ECG	Electrocardiogram	PAO$_2$ – PaO$_2$	Alveolar-arterial oxygen gradient
ECLS	Extracorporeal life support	PAP	Pulmonary arterial pressure
ECMO	Extracorporeal membrane oxygenation	PAT	Paroxysmal atrial tachycardia
ECW	Extracellular water	Paw	Mean airway pressure
EDRF	Endothelial derived relaxing factor	PDA	Patent ductus arteriosus
EEP	End-expiratory pressure	PEEP	Positive end-expiratory pressure
EFE	Endocardial fibroelastosis	PEP	Preinjection period
ERV	Expiratory reserve volume	PFC	Perfluorocarbon
ET	Endotracheal; Ethylene oxide	PFCCP	Persistence of fetal cardiopulmonary circulation pathway
ETT	Endotracheal tube		
f	Frequency (ventilator)	PG	Prostaglandin
FFP	Fresh-frozen plasma	PIE	Pulmonary interstitial emphysema
FHR	Fetal heart rate	PIP	Peak inspiratory pressure or peak inflating pressure
F$_{IO_2}$	Fraction of inspired oxygen		
FRC	Functional residual capacity	PMI	Point of maximum impulse
GFR	Glomerular filtration rate	PPHN	Persistent pulmonary hypertension of the newborn

APPENDIX 34
FREQUENTLY USED ABBREVIATIONS—CONT'D

PTV	Patient-triggered ventilation	SVT	Supraventricular tachycardia
PVR	Pulmonary vascular resistance	TAPVR	Total anomalous pulmonary venous return
R	Resistance	TBW	Total body water
RA	Right arterial	TcP_{CO_2}	Transcutaneous carbon dioxide tension
RAP	Right arterial pressure	TcP_{O_2}	Transcutaneous oxygen tension
RDS	Respiratory distress syndrome	TDD	Total digitalizing dose
REM	Rapid eye movement	TGV	Thoracic gas volume
R_L	Lung resistance	TLC	Total lung capacity
RLF	Retrolental fibroplasia	TNE	Thermal neutral environment
ROP	Retinopathy of prematurity	TPN	Total parenteral nutrition
RPEP	Right ventricular preinjection period	TTN	Transient tachypnea of the newborn
RPF	Renal plasma flow	TV or V_T	Tidal volume
RQ	Respiratory quotient	UAC	Umbilical arterial catheter
RV	Residual volume or right ventricle	UVC	Umbilical venous catheter
RVET	Right ventricular ejection time	$\dot{V}$	Ventilation per minute
Sao_2	Arterial oxygen saturation	$\dot{V}A$	Alveolar ventilation
SEH	Subependymal (germinal matrix) hemorrhage	VA	Venoarterial
SIDS	Sudden infant death syndrome	VC	Vital capacity
ST	Surface tension		